OKU 9

Orthopaedic Knowledge Update

AAOS

AMERICAN ACADEMY OF
ORTHOPAEDIC SURGEONS

OKU
9

Orthopaedic
Knowledge
Update

EDITOR:

Jeffrey S. Fischgrund, MD
Spine Fellowship Director
Department of Orthopaedic Surgery
William Beaumont Hospital
Royal Oak, Michigan

AAOS
AMERICAN ACADEMY OF
ORTHOPAEDIC SURGEONS

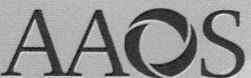

AAOS

AMERICAN ACADEMY OF ORTHOPAEDIC SURGEONS

Published 2008 by the
American Academy of Orthopaedic Surgeons
6300 North River Road
Rosemont, IL 60018

Copyright 2008
by the American Academy of Orthopaedic Surgeons

ISBN 10: 0-89203-471-8
ISBN 13: 978-0-89203-471-0

Printed in the USA
Library of Congress Cataloging-in-Publication Data

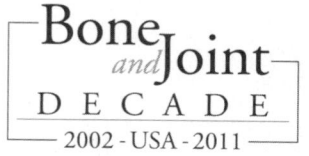

Bone *and* Joint
DECADE
— 2002 - USA - 2011 —

Acknowledgments

Editorial Board, OKU 9

JEFFREY S. FISCHGRUND, MD
Spine Fellowship Director
Department of Orthopaedic Surgery
William Beaumont Hospital
Royal Oak, Michigan

MICHAEL J. ARCHIBECK, MD
Orthopaedic Surgeon
New Mexico Center for Joint Replacement
Surgery
New Mexico Orthopaedics
Albuquerque, New Mexico

JOHN M. FLYNN, MD
Associate Chief of Orthopaedic Surgery
The Children's Hospital of Philadelphia
Associate Professor of Orthopaedic Surgery
University of Pennsylvania
Philadelphia, Pennsylvania

ALAN S. HILIBRAND, MD
Associate Professor of Orthopaedic Surgery
and Neurosurgery
Jefferson Medical College
The Rothman Institute
Philadelphia, Pennsylvania

JOSHUA J. JACOBS, MD
Crown Family Professor of Orthopaedic Surgery
Rush University Medical Center
Chicago, Illinois

MARY ANN E. KEENAN, MD
Professor and Vice Chair
Department of Orthopaedic Surgery
University of Pennsylvania
Philadelphia, Pennsylvania

THOMAS J. MOORE, MD
Associate Professor
Department of Orthopaedics
Emory School of Medicine
Atlanta, Georgia

TUSHAR PATEL, MD
Spine Surgeon
Commonwealth Orthopaedics
Herndon, Virginia

ANDREW H. SCHMIDT, MD
Associate Professor
University of Minnesota
Faculty, Hennepin County Medical Center
Minneapolis, Minnesota

SUKEN A. SHAH, MD
Attending Pediatric Orthopaedic Surgeon
Associate Professor of Orthopaedic Surgery
Department of Orthopaedics
Alfred I. DuPont Hospital for Children
Nemours Children's Clinic
Wilmington, Delaware

SCOTT P. STEINMANN, MD
Associate Professor
Shoulder, Elbow, and Hand Surgery
Mayo Clinic
Rochester, Minnesota

S. TIM YOON, MD, PHD
Assistant Professor
Department of Orthopaedic Surgery
Emory University
Atlanta, Georgia

JIM A. YOUSSEF, MD
Attending Surgeon
Durango Orthopedic Associates, P.C./Spine
Colorado
Durango, Colorado

Contributors

JULIE E. ADAMS, MD
Department of Orthopedic Surgery
Mayo Clinic
Rochester, Minnesota

CHRISTOPHER S. AHMAD, MD
Associate Professor of Orthopaedic Surgery
Columbia Orthopaedics
New York, New York

MICHAEL C. AIN, MD
Assistant Professor
Department of Orthopaedic Surgery
Johns Hopkins University
Baltimore, Maryland

HOWARD S. AN, MD
The Morton International Professor
Director of Spine Surgery and Spine Fellowship
Department of Orthopaedic Surgery
Rush University Medical Center
Chicago, Illinois

JASON ANDERSEN, AB
Research Associate
Department of Orthopaedic Surgery
Children's Hospital Boston
Boston, Massachusetts

D. GREG ANDERSON, MD
Associate Professor
Department of Orthopaedic Surgery
Thomas Jefferson University
The Rothman Institute
Philadelphia, Pennsylvania

MEGAN E. ANDERSON, MD
Attending, Orthopaedic Surgery
Harvard Medical School
Beth Israel Deaconess Medical Center and
*   Children's Hospital Boston*
Boston, Massachusetts

THOMAS P. ANDRIACCHI, PhD
Professor
Department of Mechanical Engineering and
*   Orthopedics*
Stanford University
Stanford, California

JEFFREY O. ANGLEN, MD
Director, American Board of Orthopaedic
*   Surgery*
Department of Orthopaedics
Indiana University
Indianapolis, Indiana

GEORGE S. ATHWAL, MD, FRCSC
Assistant Professor of Surgery
Hand and Upper Limb Centre
University of Western Ontario
London, Ontario, Canada

DONALD S. BAE, MD
Instructor in Orthopaedic Surgery
Department of Orthopaedic Surgery
Children's Hospital, Boston
Boston, Massachusetts

HYUN BAE, MD
Research Director
Spine Institute
St John's Hospital
Santa Monica, California

DAVID P. BAREI, MD
Assistant Professor
Department of Orthopaedics
Harborview Medical Center
Seattle, Washington

TIMOTHY C. BEALS, MD
Associate Professor of Orthopaedics
Department of Orthopaedics
University of Utah School of Medicine
Salt Lake City, Utah

DAVID P. BEASON, MS
Research Engineer
McKay Orthopaedic Research Laboratory
University of Pennsylvania
Philadelphia, Pennsylvania

R. SHAY BESS, MD
Assistant Professor
Department of Orthopaedic Surgery
University of Utah School of Medicine
Salt Lake City, Utah

NITIN N. BHATIA, MD
Assistant Professor, Orthopaedic Surgery
Chief, Spine Service
Department of Orthopaedic Surgery
University of California, Irvine
Irvine, California

R. DALE BLASIER, MD, FRCS(C)
Professor of Orthopaedic Surgery
University of Arkansas for Medical Surgery
Arkansas Children's Hospital
Little Rock, Arkansas

SCOTT D. BODEN, MD
Director, The Emory Spine Center
Professor of Orthopaedic Surgery
Emory University School of Medicine
Atlanta, Georgia

DAVID BORENSTEIN, MD
Clinical Professor of Medicine
Division of Rheumatology
Department of Medicine
The George Washington University
* Medical Center*
Washington, DC

MATHIAS P.G. BOSTROM, MD
Associate Professor
Department of Orthopaedics
Hospital for Special Surgery
New York, New York

DARREL S. BRODKE, MD
Associate Professor and Vice Chairman
Department of Orthopaedics
University of Utah
Salt Lake City, Utah

CHRISTOPHER R. BROWN, MD
Assistant Professor, Orthopaedics
Division of Orthopaedic Surgery
Duke University Medical Center
Durham, North Carolina

SUSAN V. BUKATA, MD
Assistant Professor of Orthopaedics
University of Rochester
Rochester, New York

JOSEPH P. BURNS, MD
The Southern California Orthopaedic Institute
Van Nuys, California

PATRICK J. CAHILL, MD
Spine Fellow
Department of Orthopedic Surgery
Rush University Medical Center
Chicago, Illinois

PATRICIA CAMPBELL, PhD
Associate Professor
Orthopaedic Hospital – UCLA
Department of Orthopaedic Surgery
The J. Vernon Luck Orthopaedic
* Research Center*
Los Angeles, California

LISA K. CANNADA, MD
Assistant Professor
Department of Orthopaedic Surgery
University of Texas Southwestern
* Medical Center*
Dallas, Texas

ROBERT V. CANTU, MD
Assistant Professor of Orthopaedic Surgery
Department of Orthopaedic Surgery
Dartmouth Hitchcock Medical Center
Lebanon, New Hampshire

HANS L. CARLSON, MD
Assistant Professor
Physical Medicine and Rehabilitation
Department of Orthopaedics and Rehabilitation
Oregon Health and Science University
Portland, Oregon

KENNETH O. CAYCE IV, MD
Clinical Assistant Professor
Family Medicine/Sports Medicine
Ohio State University
Columbus, Ohio

MICHAEL THOMAS CHARLTON, MD
Orthopaedic Trauma Fellow
Department of Orthopaedic Surgery
University of Texas-Southwestern
* Medical Center*
Dallas, Texas

AJIT M.W. CHAUDHARI, PhD
Assistant Professor
Department of Orthopaedics
Ohio State University
Columbus, Ohio

ROBERT H. COFIELD, MD
Professor of Orthopaedics
Department of Orthopaedic Surgery
Mayo Clinic
Rochester, Minnesota

WILLIAM P. COONEY, MD
Consultant and Emeritus Professor
Department of Orthopaedic Surgery
Mayo Clinic
Rochester, Minnesota

DENNIS CRAWFORD, MD, PhD
Assistant Professor
Surgical Director, Sports Medicine and Cartilage
    Reconstruction
Department of Orthopaedics and Rehabilitation
Oregon Health Sciences University
Portland, Oregon

CARMEN D. CROFOOT, MD
Clinical Instructor
University of Utah
Department of Orthopaedics
Salt Lake City, Utah

CRAIG J. DELLA VALLE, MD
Assistant Professor
Department of Orthopaedic Surgery
Rush University Medical Center
Chicago, Illinois

SHARI DIAMOND, MD
Fellow
Department of Rheumatology
George Washington University Hospital
Washington, DC

SETH D. DODDS, MD
Assistant Professor, Hand and Upper Extremity
    Surgery
Department of Orthopaedics and Rehabilitation
Yale University School of Medicine
New Haven, Connecticut

NEAL S. ELATTRACHE, MD
Associate and Sports Medicine Fellowship
    Director
Kerlan-Jobe Orthopaedic Clinic
Los Angeles, California

THOMAS J. ELLIS, MD
Associate Professor
Department of Orthopaedic Surgery
Ohio State University Medical Center
Columbus, Ohio

KENNETH J. FABER, MD, MHPE, FRCSC
Associate Professor of Surgery
University of Western Ontario
Hand and Upper Limb Centre
London, Ontario, Canada

LAMAR L. FLEMING, MD
Professor of Orthopaedics
Department of Orthopaedics
Emory University
Atlanta, Georgia

MARC T. GALLOWAY, MD
Cincinnati Sports Medicine and Orthopaedic
    Center
Cincinnati, Ohio

MARK C. GEBHARDT, MD
Frederick W. and Jane M. Ilfeld Professor of
    Orthopaedic Surgery
Harvard Medical School
Orthopaedic Surgeon-in-Chief
Department of Orthopaedic Surgery
Beth Israel Deaconess Medical Center
Boston, Massachusetts

JOHN T. GORCZYCA, MD
Associate Professor
Chief, Division of Orthopaedic Trauma
Department of Orthopaedics
University of Rochester Medical Center
Rochester, New York

JONATHAN N. GRAUER, MD
Associate Professor
Department of Orthopaedics and Rehabilitation
Yale University School of Medicine
New Haven, Connecticut

James T. Guille, MD
Staff Surgeon
Shriners Hospital for Children
Philadelphia, Pennsylvania

Ranjan Gupta, MD
Associate Professor and Chair
Department of Orthopaedic Surgery
University of California, Irvine
Irvine, California

E. Mark Hammerberg, MD
Assistant Professor
Department of Orthopaedic Surgery
Emory University School of Medicine
Atlanta, Georgia

John P. Heiner, MD
Professor of Orthopedics
Department of Orthopedics
University of Wisconsin
Madison, Wisconsin

Clyde A. Helms, MD
Professor of Radiology and Surgery
Director, Division of Musculoskeletal Radiology
Department of Radiology
Duke University Medical Center
Durham, North Carolina

Johnny Huard, PhD
Henry S. Mankin Professor
Vice Chair of Orthopaedic Research
Department of Orthopaedic Research
University of Pittsburgh
Pittsburgh, Pennsylvania

G. Russell Huffman, MD, MPH
Assistant Professor
Department of Orthopaedic Surgery
University of Pennsylvania
Sports Medicine Center
Philadelphia, Pennsylvania

Richard Lynn Illgen II, MD
Co-Director of the University of Wisconsin
*   Arthritis and Joint Replacement Program*
Department of Orthopedics and Rehabilitation
University of Wisconsin Hospital
Madison, Wisconsin

Claudius Jarrett, MD
Department of Orthopaedics
Emory University School of Medicine
Atlanta, Georgia

Tharun Karthikeyan, MD
Department of Orthopaedic Surgery
University of Pittsburgh
Pittsburgh, Pennsylvania

Jay D. Keener, MD
Assistant Professor
Shoulder and Elbow Service
Department of Orthopaedic Surgery
Washington University
St. Louis, Missouri

Michael W. Keith, MD
Professor, Orthopaedics and Biomedical
*   Engineering*
Case Western Reserve University
Cleveland, Ohio

Hubert T. Kim, MD, PhD
Associate Professor
Department of Orthopaedic Surgery
University of California, San Francisco
San Francisco, California

Young-Jo Kim, MD, PhD
Assistant Professor of Orthopaedic Surgery
Department of Orthopaedic Surgery
Children's Hospital
Boston, Massachusetts

Graham J.W. King, MD, MSc, FRCSC
Professor of Surgery
University of Western Ontario
Hand and Upper Limb Centre
St. Joseph's Health Care
London, Ontario, Canada

Mininder S. Kocher, MPH, MD
Associate Director, Division of Sports Medicine
Associate Professor of Orthopaedic Surgery
Children's Hospital, Boston
Harvard Medical School
Boston, Massachusetts

KENNETH J. KOVAL, MD
Professor
Department of Orthopaedics
Dartmouth Hitchcock Medical Center
Lebanon, New Hampshire

SUMANT G. KRISHNAN, MD
Attending Orthopaedic Surgeon
Shoulder and Elbow Service
W.B. Carrell Memorial Clinic
Dallas, Texas

ROBERT N. KURTZKE, MD
Neurologist, Electromyographer
Neurology Center of Fairfax
Fairfax, Virginia

ANTHONY J. LAUDER, MD
Assistant Professor
Department of Orthopaedic Surgery
University of Nebraska Medical Center
Omaha, Nebraska

CONSTANCE M. LEBRUN, MDCM, MPE, CCFP,
   FACSM, DIP. SPORTMED
Director, Primary Care Sports Medicine
Fowler Kennedy Sports Medicine Clinc
University of Western Ontario
London, Ontario, Canada

JOON Y. LEE, MD
Assistant Professor
Department of Orthopaedic and Neurological
   Surgery
University of Pittsburgh Medical Center
Pittsburgh, Pennsylvania

MICHAEL J. LEE, MD
Assistant Professor
Department of Sports Medicine and
   Orthopaedic Surgery
University of Washington
Seattle, Washington

JAY R. LIEBERMAN, MD
Director, The New England Musculoskeletal
   Institute
Professor and Chairman
Department of Orthopaedic Surgery
University of Connecticut Health Center
Farmington, Connecticut

MOE R. LIM, MD
Assistant Professor
Department of Orthopaedics
University of North Carolina
Chapel Hill, North Carolina

KENNETH C. LIN, MD
Shoulder Service
W.B. Carrell Memorial Clinic
Dallas, Texas

SUZANNE A. MAHER, PHD
Assistant Scientist
Hospital for Special Surgery
New York, New York

KAMRAN MAJID, MD
Spine Fellow
Department of Orthopaedic Surgery
William Beaumont Hospital
Royal Oak, Michigan

PETER J. MANDELL, MD
Assistant Clinical Professor
Department of Orthopaedic Surgery
University of California, San Francisco
San Francisco, California

REX MARCO, MD
Associate Professor
Departments of Orthopaedics and Neurosurgery
Chief of Spine Surgery and Musculoskeletal
   Oncology
University of Texas Medical School
Houston, Texas

TRAVIS H. MATHENEY, MD
Instructor in Orthopaedic Surgery
Harvard Medical School
Department of Orthopaedic Surgery
Children's Hospital, Boston
Boston, Massachusetts

WARREN R. MAYS, BS, CPO
Certified Prosthetist Orthotist
President, Artisan Orthotic-Prosthetic
   Technologies, Inc.
Tualatin, Oregon

JAMES J. MCCARTHY, MD
Assistant Chief of Staff
Shriners Hospital for Children
Associate Professor
Temple University
Philadelphia, Pennsylvania

HARRY A. MCKELLOP, PhD
Professor In-Residence
Department of Orthopaedic Surgery
The J. Vernon Luck Orthopaedic
  Research Center
University of California, Los Angeles
Los Angeles, California

CHARLES T. MEHLMAN, DO, MPH
Associate Professor, Pediatric Orthopaedic
  Surgery
Director, Musculoskeletal Outcomes Research
Division of Pediatric Orthopaedic Surgery
Cincinnati Children's Hospital Medical Center
University of Cincinnati College of Medicine
Cincinnati, Ohio

JAMES F. MOONEY III, MD
Chief, Pediatric Orthopaedic Surgery
Department of Orthopaedic Surgery
Medical University of South Carolina
Charleston, South Carolina

THOMAS J. MOORE, MD
Associate Professor
Department of Orthopaedics
Emory School of Medicine
Atlanta, Georgia

DANIEL B. MURREY, MD, MPP
Orthopedic Spine Surgeon
OrthoCarolina Spine Center
Charlotte, North Carolina

PETER O. NEWTON, MD
Associate Clinical Professor
Department of Orthopaedic Surgery
University of California, San Diego
San Diego, California

KENNETH J. NOONAN, MD
Associate Professor
Department of Orthopaedics
University of Wisconsin
Madison, Wisconsin

SEAN E. NORK, MD
Associate Professor
Harborview Medical Center
University of Washington
Seattle, Washington

REGIS J. O'KEEFE, MD, PhD
Chairman, Department of Orthopaedics
  and Rehabilitation
Director, Center for Musculoskeletal Research
Orthopaedics Department
University of Rochester
Rochester, New York

ALPESH A. PATEL, MD
Department of Orthopaedic Surgery
University of Utah
Salt Lake City, Utah

CHRISTOPHER L. PETERS, MD
Associate Professor
Department of Orthopedics
University of Utah
Salt Lake City, Utah

RAVI K. PONNAPPAN, MD
Spine Surgery Fellow
Department of Orthopaedics
University of Pittsburgh Medical Center
Pittsburgh, Pennsylvania

ANTHONY RINELLA, MD
Director, Spinal Deformity
Assistant Professor
Department of Orthopaedic Surgery
  and Rehabilitation
Loyola University Medical Center
Maywood, Illinois

MARCO RIZZO, MD
Assistant Professor
Department of Orthopedic Surgery
Mayo Clinic
Rochester, Minnesota

THOMAS N. SCIOSCIA, MD
West End Orthopaedic Clinic
Richmond, Virginia

ARYA NICK SHAMIE, MD
Associate Clinical Professor of Orthopaedic
    Surgery and Neurosurgery
UCLA Comprehensive Spine Center
David Geffen School of Medicine at UCLA
Los Angeles, California

ERIC D. SHIRLEY, MD, LCDR, MC, USNR
Attending, Pediatric Orthopaedics
Department of Orhtopaedics
Naval Medical Center Portsmouth
Portsmouth, Virginia

BIKRAMJIT SINGH, MD
Department of Orthopaedics
University of North Carolina – Chapel Hill
Chapel Hill, North Carolina

KERN SINGH, MD
Assistant Professor
Department of Orthopaedic Surgery
Rush University Medical Center
Chicago, Illinois

KUSH SINGH, MD
Musculoskeletal Radiology Fellow
Department of Radiology
Duke University Medical Center
Durham, North Carolina

STEPHEN J. SNYDER, MD
The Southern California Orthopedic Institute
Van Nuys, California

LOUIS J. SOSLOWSKY, PhD
Professor of Orthopaedic Surgery and
    Bioengineering
Vice Chair for Research
Director of Penn Center for Musculoskeletal
    Disorders
University of Pennsylvania
Philadelphia, Pennsylvania

SAMANTHA A. SPENCER, MD
Instructor in Orthopaedic Surgery at Harvard
    Medical School
Department of Orthopaedic Surgery
Children's Hospital, Boston
Boston, Massachusetts

JOHN W. SPERLING, MD
Associate Professor
Department of Orthopaedic Surgery
Mayo Clinic
Rochester, Minnesota

DAVID A. SPIEGEL, MD
Assistant Professor – University of Pennsylvania
Department of Orthopaedics
Children's Hospital of Philadelphia
Philadelphia, Pennsylvania

PAUL D. SPONSELLER, MD
Riley Professor and Head, Pediatric
    Orthopaedics
Johns Hopkins Medical Institution
Baltimore, Maryland

MATTHEW SQUIRE, MD, MS
Assistant Professor of Orthopedic Surgery
Department of Orthopedics and Rehabilitation
University of Wisconsin
Madison, Wisconsin

SCOTT P. STEINMANN, MD
Associate Professor
Shoulder, Elbow, and Hand Surgery
Mayo Clinic
Rochester, Minnesota

CHADI TANNOURY, MD
Thomas Jefferson University Hospital
Department of Orthopaedic Surgery
Philadelphia, Pennsylvania

DAVID TEMPLEMAN, MD
Associate Professor, Orthopedic Surgery
Hennepin County Medical Center and
    University of Minnesota
Minneapolis, Minnesota

MIHIR M. THACKER, MD
Assistant Professor, Orthopedic Surgery and
    Pediatrics
Thomas Jefferson University
Department of Orthopedic Surgery
Alfred I. DuPont Hospital for Children
Wilmington, Delaware

PAUL TORNETTA III, MD
Professor
Director of Orthopaedic Trauma
Department of Orthopaedic Surgery
Boston University Medical Center
Boston, Massachusetts

CLIFFORD TRIBUS, MD
Associate Professor
Department of Orthopedics and Rehabilitative
*   Medicine*
University of Wisconsin, Madison
Madison, Wisconsin

THOMAS E. TRUMBLE, MD
Professor and Chief
Hand and Microvascular Surgery
Department of Orthopaedics
University of Washington
Seattle, Washington

VIDYADHAR V. UPASANI, MD
Postdoctoral Research Fellow
Department of Orthopedic Surgery
University of California, San Diego
San Diego, California

JEFFREY C. WANG, MD
Chief, Spine Service
UCLA Comprehensive Spine Center
UCLA Department of Orthopaedic Surgery
UCLA School of Medicine
Los Angeles, California

PETER G. WHANG, MD
Assistant Professor
Department of Orthopaedics and Rehabilitation
Yale University School of Medicine
New Haven, Connecticut

TIMOTHY M. WRIGHT, PhD
F.M. Kirby Chair, Orthopaedic Biomechanics
Hospital for Special Surgery
New York, New York

KEN YAMAGUCHI, MD
Sam and Marilyn Fox Distinguished Professor
*   of Orthopaedic Surgery*
Chief, Shoulder and Elbow Service
Department of Orthopaedic Surgery
Washington University School of Medicine
St. Louis, Missouri

S. TIM YOON, MD, PhD
Assistant Professor
Department of Orthopaedic Surgery
Emory University
Atlanta, Georgia

MATTHEW G. ZMURKO, MD
Vermont Orthopaedic Clinic
Rutland Regional Medical Center
Rutland, Vermont

Preface

As an orthopaedic surgeon and editor, it is with great pride and pleasure that I present the latest edition of the Orthopaedic Knowledge Update Series, OKU 9. This textbook is the result of years of planning, writing, and editorial review by a large team of dedicated educators.

The goal of this publication is not only to review basic knowledge in the field of orthopaedic surgery, but to highlight the recent advances in musculoskeletal care. Therefore, this volume is not only an "update," but relies for its foundation on the knowledge accumulated over the past half century and continuously advanced by our peers. By reading and understanding this text, the orthopaedic surgeon in training and those established in practice can quickly reference the vast orthopaedic knowledge base and identify new treatment trends in patient management.

The foundation of orthopaedic knowledge must be grounded in basic science. The textbook begins with the principles of orthopaedics, including basic science, biomechanics, and principles of research. New in this edition are sections on professionalism, ethics, and the American Board of Orthopaedic Surgery. These additions are a result of the American Academy of Orthopaedic Surgeons' emphasis on standards of professionalism and outline the evolving process of the American Board of Orthopaedic Surgery's procedure for board certification and maintenance of certification.

The remainder of the textbook continues to be divided into specialty sections consistent with the subspecialty orientations of most orthopaedic surgeons. The purpose of this textbook is not to educate the subspecialists on the latest trends and techniques in their particular field. Rather, every orthopaedic surgeon should be able to understand the current trends and practices in all fields of orthopaedic surgery. To assist in this effort, and unlike in previous editions, the annotated references are cited numerically in the text to aid the clinician's efforts at more detailed study.

The effort to produce this text is enormous. I am deeply grateful to the 12 section editors and more than 100 authors who contributed to this text. The editorial process has been extensive, with multiple reviews by the section editors and me prior to the final copyedited revision by the Academy staff. As a practicing spine surgeon I have relied heavily on my section editors to ensure that the material presented is accurate, fair, unbiased, and up-to-date.

Since the completion of my training in 1992, I owe a large debt of gratitude to my mentors. Dr. Alan Levine has been instrumental in guiding me through my academic career as I advanced from chapter author to section editor and ultimately to editor of OKU 9. Dr. Harry Herkowitz has been the true guiding force behind my professional career. His continued close friendship and direction are deeply appreciated and have allowed me to reach professional and academic levels that I never thought possible.

I would also like to thank members of the Academy staff, particularly Lisa Claxton Moore and Kathleen Anderson. Their tireless efforts and continuous vigilance have allowed me and the section editors to produce this comprehensive text.

Finally, I certainly need to acknowledge the support of my wife, Laurie, and my children, Michelle, Marcy, Mark, Andrew and Melanie. The many months of editorial work on this publication were made easier by having my best friend, Laurie, at my side.

Jeffrey S. Fischgrund, MD
Editor

Table of Contents

Section 1

Principles of Orthopaedics

SECTION EDITORS:

Joshua J. Jacobs, MD
Mary Ann E. Keenan, MD
Thomas J. Moore, MD
S. Tim Yoon, MD, PhD

Chapter 1

Professionalism and Ethics

*Jeffrey O. Anglen, MD   Peter J. Mandell, MD   Thomas J. Moore, MD

1: Principles of Orthopaedics

Board Certification

Board certification is an important professional standard for physicians in the United States. Board certification influences many aspects of practice, including hospital privileges, insurance program participation, professional organization membership, partnership or employability by some groups or organizations, and the ability to market oneself successfully. Nonetheless, many young physicians sometimes do not clearly understand the purpose and process of board certification. This section will attempt to explain how and why an orthopaedic surgeon becomes board certified, and what needs to be done to maintain that certification.

Board certification is a voluntary process that is different and distinct from licensure to practice medicine, a function regulated by state government. A valid medical license is required to be board certified, but certification is not necessary for licensure. A board-certified physician has met certain standards and passed tests that are developed to ensure the public that he or she has been adequately trained in a given specialty. By 2003, more than 85% of licensed physicians in the United States were certified by at least one board.

The American Board of Medical Specialties

Advancements in medical science and treatments in the late 1800s and early 1900s led to the development of distinct medical specialties. With this development came the need to ensure the public that a physician claiming to be a specialist was indeed qualified. Medical societies and schools encouraged and assisted in the development of specialty certifying boards to define qualifying criteria and issue credentials to provide this assurance. The American Board of Medical Specialties (ABMS) was formed in 1933 to coordinate the activities of the first specialty certifying boards. ABMS is currently composed of representatives of 24 recognized specialties. This umbrella organization sets common policies and standards, helps member boards, and approves new specialty boards. More information is available at http://www.abms.org.

Jeffrey Anglen, MD serves as a Director for the American Board of Orthopaedic Surgery.

The American Board of Orthopaedic Surgery

The American Board of Orthopaedic Surgery (ABOS) was founded in 1934. It is a private nonprofit corporation that exists to serve the public interest by examining orthopaedic surgeons and certifying that they have met certain standards of education, training, and practice. ABOS is a separate organization from the American Academy of Orthopaedic Surgeons (AAOS) and other orthopaedic subspecialty organizations, with different goals, purposes, and leaders. Although many surgeons have held leadership positions in ABOS and AAOS, they are not allowed to serve both simultaneously. ABOS and AAOS communicate on many issues, but they do not routinely share information about specific individuals. A physician must be board certified to become a fellow of AAOS, but AAOS membership is not a requirement to become board certified.

The ABOS consists of 12 directors, 6 senior directors, 2 directors-elect, and 1 public member who is not an orthopaedic surgeon. Two new directors-elect are selected by ABOS each year from lists of practicing orthopaedic surgeon nominees submitted by the three founding organizations: AAOS, the American Orthopaedic Association (AOA), and the American Medical Association (AMA). ABOS derives its legitimacy from the founding organizations and from membership in the ABMS. Directors serve without pay. Hundreds of other orthopaedic surgeon volunteers serve ABOS as question writers, test task force members, case selectors, oral examiners, and site visitors. More information about ABOS is available at http://www.abos.org.

The Process of Board Certification

Board certification in orthopaedic surgery requires a multistage process involving completion of an accredited residency, a written examination (Part I), a period of 22 months in practice, peer review, and an oral examination based on the candidate's own practice (Part II). A surgeon who has passed the Part I written examination and is practicing while awaiting admission to Part II is deemed "board-eligible." This term is not appropriate for surgeons who have not passed Part I, or who have been refused admission to Part II.

Orthopaedic surgeons who have completed an accredited residency, as attested by the program director to ABOS's credentials committee, may apply and be admitted to take the written examination. This examination, which currently is a timed, secure, paper and pencil examination, consists of approximately 320 multiple choice questions covering all aspects of orthopaedics and is given on a single day in 7 hours of testing divided into two sessions. In the near future, this test will be computer-based. The examination subtest content from 2005 consisted of: basic science and tumors, 30%; adult trauma, 18%; adult orthopaedic disease, 21%; pediatric trauma, 6%; pediatric orthopaedic disease, 16%; and rehabilitation, 9% (individual items can be part of multiple subtest categories). The questions are produced through the work of more than 70 volunteer, practicing orthopaedic surgeons, with the help and professional guidance of the National Board of Medical Examiners (NBME). Each question submitted must be supported by at least two peer-reviewed references, and before a question appears on a test it is subject to review by at least three different groups of surgeons: the Question Writing Task Force, the Field Test Task Force, and the written examination committee of ABOS. Extensive statistics are kept by NBME on the performance of each question; poorly performing questions (too hard, too easy, nondiscriminating) are discarded. The passing score is set each year by the written examination committee based on an item-by-item analysis and the work of yet another group of volunteer orthopaedic surgeons, the standard setting task force. The overall pass rate in recent years has varied from 79% to 88%. The pass rate for US/Canadian medical school graduates taking the test for the first time is substantially higher.

After passing Part I, candidates have a period of 5 years to apply for and pass Part II, the oral examination. If they do not pass the test within the 5-year period, they must retake Part I to be admitted to the oral examination. It is each candidate's responsibility to know deadlines and make a correct, complete application if they wish to be board certified. To be admitted to the oral examination, a candidate must maintain a valid, unrestricted medical license, and have been in practice for 22 months (at least 12 months in a single location). ABOS will ask for peer review of the candidate from certified orthopaedic surgeons who are familiar with their work, and obtain evaluations from the hospital chief of staff, chiefs of orthopaedics, surgery, and anesthesia, and nursing staff in the operating room and orthopaedic wards. This information is reviewed by the ABOS credentials committee, which decides which applicants are admitted to sit for the Part II examination.

Once admitted to take the oral examination, a candidate must submit a list of all surgical cases performed during a defined 6-month period. Those case lists are reviewed by volunteer certified orthopaedic surgeons, and 12 cases are selected. The candidate can choose 10 of those cases to present. The examination is administered in Chicago in July of each year. The candidate must bring three copies of all pertinent medical records and one copy of imaging studies for each case presented. There are three 35-minute examination sessions conducted by two examiners each. The examiners independently grade each case presentation on six skills:

data gathering and interpretation, diagnosis, treatment plan, technical skill, outcomes, and applied knowledge. In addition, the case list is evaluated on surgical indications, handling of complications, ethics, and professionalism. The oral board examiners are all volunteer orthopaedic surgeons who have been recertified at least once. The panels are organized into subspecialty groups for general orthopaedics, trauma, spine, pediatrics, foot and ankle, sports medicine, and upper extremity.

Candidates who pass the examination are notified in the fall. After passing Part II, a surgeon receives a certificate and becomes a diplomate of ABOS for 10 years.

Recertification

During its first 50 years, ABOS issued certificates that never expired. When ABMS was first organized, there was discussion of the need for periodic recertification, based on the idea that medical knowledge and practice change over time. By 1972, the principle of recertification was adopted by all ABMS member boards. The first 10-year (time-limited) certificates were issued by the ABOS in 1986. To be recertified, a surgeon must apply and undergo a peer review process similar to that required for Part II, obtain 120 category I continuing medical education (CME) credits in the 3 years before application, and pass a secure examination. The process of recertification is based on the certification model, with CME credits taking the place of the residency education. A computer-administered examination is offered for general orthopaedics in addition to three practice profile examinations consisting of 80 core questions and 120 questions specific to either sports medicine, adult reconstruction, or spine surgery. Individuals who have a primary hand specialty certificate of added qualification (CAQ) may recertify by taking the hand specialty CAQ examination. Diplomates may recertify both the primary and hand certificates by taking an examination that has 80 core orthopaedic questions and 120 hand questions. The new CAQ in sports medicine will likely function in a manner similar to the CAQ in hand.

In early 2000, the member boards of ABMS agreed to evolve their recertification programs into a new concept called "maintenance of certification" or MOC. This path was taken in response to public and state legislative pressure to evaluate physician competence on a more frequent schedule. All ABMS member boards have adopted the MOC program and its implementation will be mandatory by 2016.

Maintenance of Certification

Beginning with certificates that expire in 2010, all ABOS diplomates with time-limited certificates who wish to remain board certified will be allowed to do so by complying with requirements of the MOC program established by ABOS. The four components of the MOC program are listed in Table 1.

The requirements for MOC will be phased in. Diplomates with certificates expiring in 2010 will have to meet the CME and self assessment examination (SAE) standards mentioned in Table 1 and submit case lists. The peer review component and secure examination will continue to be performed as part of the current, established recertification examination. The final form of MOC, Evidence of Performance in Practice, is currently under development. Web-based tools are being developed by ABOS to assist each diplomate in managing their own progress toward MOC. AAOS and some orthopaedic specialty societies are producing programs to help diplomates obtain and document CME and SAE.

More information about MOC, including a list of frequently asked questions, is available at www.abos.org. It is the responsibility of each diplomate to learn the requirements for MOC if they wish to maintain their certification.

Standards of Professionalism

Physicians around the world base their work on similar values and principles, despite differences in cultures and traditions. It is not surprising that physicians' shared humanity and common experiences, as well as the importance placed on enduring human relationships, have led to similar conclusions about values in medicine and physician virtues.[1]

For thousands of years, society and physicians have honored a tacit contract that grants extraordinary privileges to doctors in return for their behaving and performing in seemingly extraordinary ways. People have always needed medical care, and physicians have been willing and progressively able to provide that care. The Hippocratic Oath was developed to formalize concepts of compassionate care and guide physicians in their duties. With the advent of science, the idea developed that elite learned groups have particular obligations to society. In the mid 1800s, governments around the world began creating medical licensing boards to codify the tradition of self-regulation and thereby helped create the modern medical system. Licensing boards, composed of physicians, were believed to best understand whether physicians were living up to medicine's standards and society's expectations.

Prior to the 1950s, both the role of physicians in people's lives and the community and the responsibilities that accompanied professional standing were well understood. Since that time, major changes in culture, improved treatment of illness, and the progress of the information age are factors that have altered the attitudes and expectations of both the public and physicians.[2] In addition, other external factors, such as the high rate of monetary inflation during the 1970s, the changing relationship of medicine and government, and the rise of corporate medicine; and internal factors, such as increasing specialization and subspecialization, have required continuing renegotiation of society's expectations of the medical professional.[3]

Table 1
Maintenance of Certification Program Requirements*
Evidence of Professional Standing Assessed with periodic peer review, confirmation of full and unrestricted licensure in all jurisdictions where a license is held, and confirmation of hospital credentials.
Evidence of Lifelong Learning and Self-Assessment Addressed through two 3-year cycles of 120 credits of category 1 CME that include a minimum of 20 CME credits of SAE.
Evidence of Cognitive Expertise Occurs through the same secure recertification examination currently in place and required at 10-year intervals. Candidates will have the option of a practice-based oral examination to satisfy both cognitive expertise and performance in practice.
Evidence of Performance in Practice Will focus on a quality improvement model that will involve submission of case lists and patient survey information.
*CME = continuing medical education. SAE = self-assessment examination.

Defining "Profession" and "Professionalism"

Although the concept of medical professionalism has a long tradition in all human societies, there is no consensus on precise definitions of "profession" and "professionalism," nor is there an agreed-upon definition of the medical profession in the extensive literature on the subject.[4] Professionalism encompasses the actions and attitudes of physicians to fulfill society's sometimes lofty and idealized expectations of medicine. What is at stake is a set of special privileges that physicians can sometimes take for granted, including the ability to regulate themselves, set criteria for medical school accreditation and admission, define medical license requirements, accredit residency programs and CME providers, determine board certification, and set standards for hospital accreditation and physician privileges.[5]

The term "profession" as defined in the *Oxford English Dictionary* was recently modified for use by medical educators.[4] The Royal College of Physicians of London takes a somewhat different approach, pointing out that a physician's primary goal is to treat patients well[6] (Table 2). The patient's experiences, feelings, and interpretations, often in moments of fear, anxiety, or doubt, should be taken into consideration during treatment. In this position of extreme vulnerability, the patient trusts the physician based on a belief in the physician's underlying professionalism.

The medical profession has a degree of autonomy that is almost unheard of in any other sector of society. Physicians have a level of public respect surpassing that of many other occupations and an enviable measure of job security, as evidenced by almost unparalleled opportunities for well-compensated employment. If physi-

1: Principles of Orthopaedics

Table 2

Alternate Definitions of "Profession" and "Professionalism"

Source	Definition
Oxford English Dictionary	An occupation whose core element is work based upon the mastery of a complex body of knowledge and skills. It is a vocation in which knowledge of some department of science or learning or the practice of an art founded upon it is used in the service of others. Its members are governed by codes of ethics and profess a commitment to competence, integrity and morality, altruism, and the promotion of the public good within their domain. These commitments form the basis of a social contract between a profession and society, which in turn grants the profession a monopoly over the use of its knowledge base, the right to considerable autonomy in practice, and the privilege of self-regulation. Professions and their members are accountable to those served and to society.
Royal College of Physicians of London	Medical Professionalism signifies a set of values, behaviors, and relationships that underpin the trust the public has in doctors. Medicine is a vocation in which a doctor's knowledge, clinical skills, and judgment are put in the service of protecting and restoring human well being. This purpose is realized through a partnership between patient and doctor, one based on mutual respect, individual responsibility, and appropriate accountability. To be professional, doctors commit to integrity, compassion, altruism, continuous improvement, excellence, and working in partnership with members of the wider healthcare team.

cians fall short in executing their professional responsibilities and thereby fail to fulfill society's expectations, society will reassess how doctors are allowed to function in society.[5]

Medical ethics is the philosophical and aspirational set of ideal practices that form part of the medical profession's foundation. AAOS has provided this definition of medical ethics and set forth its ethical aspirations in its *Code of Medical Ethics and Professionalism for Orthopaedic Surgeons*[7] and *Medical Professionalism in the New Millennium: A Physician Charter*.[8] Many of the principles in these documents have been used to develop AAOS's *Standards of Professionalism*,[9] which are intended to guide the behavior of orthopaedic surgeons in real-life situations.

It's All About Trust

Trust is the cornerstone of professionalism. Members of the public expect a physician to be trustworthy.[6] To do a good job, physicians need to ask questions about private matters and perform invasive procedures. The prerequisite for these activities is a trusting relationship grounded in the patient's certainty that the physician will always put the patient's interests first.[2] Laws, regulations, a patient's bill of rights, watchdog government agencies, and insurance contracts are no substitute for a trustworthy physician's ability to safeguard a patient's interests.[5]

It has been suggested that self-reflection and mindfulness are indispensable qualities of the successful professional and essential to the expression of core values such as empathy, compassion, and altruism.[10] Mindfulness is basically an ongoing personal peer review. It is a constant internal check on one's personal trustworthiness. Courtesy, kindness, understanding, humility, honesty, and confidentiality strengthen patient trust and are behaviors that are recognizable to everyone.[6] Patient trust is enhanced when physicians exhibit the qualities of morality, integrity, and honesty. The public often holds professionals in general and medical professionals in particular to a higher standard than members of other occupations.

Many argue that altruism is the cornerstone of trust. The self-protective instinct to achieve survival and comfort is a strong aspect of human nature. Physicians, who are forced daily to deal with conflicts of interest, must particularly guard against temptation to promote their own self-interests.[5] Within the past two decades, physicians have had to contend with an onslaught of medical commercialism. Society has been strongly influenced by the marketplace in controlling health care costs, and some policy makers regard medicine primarily as a business. In the business model, health care focuses on achieving broad targets rather than fulfilling individual patient needs. Although businesslike procedures have made the practice of medicine less wasteful and more efficient, the business model tempts physicians to adopt the marketplace's core ideology of self-interest. Self-interest is the antithesis of the altruistic responsiveness to patients' and society's needs that underlies trust in the medical profession. Professionalism keeps physicians' recurring conflicts of interest from corrupting the patient-physician relationship and destroying trust.[5]

Altruism should not require personal sacrifice to the point of exploitation. It should not be used to justify being taken advantage of by business interests or bureaucracy, and it should not require acquiescence to poor working conditions or prolonged work hours that can lead to medical errors or damage the physician's own health. Altruism should not be achieved at the expense of a severely diminished or destroyed family life.[6] Altruism is about doing the right things for patients and thereby earning their trust.

AAOS Standards of Professionalism

AAOS bases its *Standards of Professionalism* on the public's expectations that orthopaedic surgeons will behave as competent, honest, and trustworthy professionals. Each *Standard* incorporates professional ideals and goals into a set of minimum standards related to a particular topic. The currently available topics include "Orthopaedic Expert Witness Testimony," "Professional Relationships," "Providing Musculoskeletal Services to Patients," and "Research and Academic Responsibilities."[9]

With regard to expert testimony, the public should be able to expect medical professionalism not only in the consultation room or the operating room but also in the courtroom. Society relies on expert witness testimony from a physician in resolving many legal conflicts. In a medical liability lawsuit involving orthopaedics, the jury needs expert orthopaedic guidance and opinion to distinguish orthopaedic malpractice (negligent care leading to a bad outcome) from maloccurrence (bad luck leading to a bad outcome). The orthopaedic expert witness has a serious responsibility and, therefore, a professional duty to give reputable testimony.

The perspective of doctors and scientists may be different from that of lawyers and other laypeople.[11] The development of different worldviews starts early in the educational process. Individuals with an aptitude for mathematics and science choose or are steered toward careers in related fields, including medicine. Those with other aptitudes may avoid more challenging math and science courses. Some of them may eventually become lawyers, and many more may become jurors. The differences between science and law are fundamental: science examines what is; the law determines what ought to be. Science constantly expands and improves on experience; the law rests on it. Science welcomes innovation, creativity, and challenges to the status quo; the law cherishes the status quo.[11]

The job of the orthopaedic expert witness is to bridge the divide between what science knows, what the law allows, and what actually occurs in day-to-day medical practice. He or she interprets science for jurors and judges who have not extensively studied it or do not understand it. The orthopaedic expert describes the applicable science and standard of care and gives an opinion as to whether the actual care was substandard and caused the patient's injury.

It is human nature to act as an advocate for one's own beliefs and try to win acceptance of these beliefs, but professionals resist this temptation. Jurors need to be able to clearly distinguish between an expert witness's description of facts and personal opinions. The AAOS *Standards of Professionalism* require orthopaedic surgeons to provide opinions or factual testimony in a fair and impartial manner and to state how and why their opinions vary from generally accepted standards. Acceptance of difficult-to-believe claims without corroboration may lead to unfair and biased testimony that would violate the *Standards of Profes-*

sionalism if this testimony confuses the judge and jury. This behavior is an example of unprofessional advocacy. Likewise, an expert witness must not suggest that a defendant physician should be punished by loss of medical licensure or imprisonment, unless the malpractice allegation involves a crime.

Jurors have a difficult job, especially if they do not fully understand the relevant medical science. Understandably, they may focus on an expert witness's use of absolutes, such as "always," "virtually 100%," "never," "virtually 0%," and "there is no such thing as," even though an absolutely certain diagnosis, test result, medication response, or treatment choice is rare in medicine. Thus, absolute statements can violate the requirement of the *Standards of Professionalism* that testimony be fair and impartial.

Selected Ethical Issues

Informed Consent

The concept of a patient's informed consent before either surgical procedures or involvement in clinical trials is relatively new in the history of medicine. Early documented human trials in medicine often involved the researcher or his or her family as subjects. The 20th century produced several episodes of unethical medical research and resulted in a succession of documents to formally regulate medical research. From October 1946 to August 1947, American judges presided over the Doctors Trial, part of the Nuremberg Trials, in which 23 Nazi defendants, all either scientists or physicians, were accused of medical crimes against helpless populations.[12] As a result of this trial, the Nuremberg Code was enacted to regulate human medical research. The Nuremberg Code provided for informed consent, animal trials before human trials, acceptable risks, and avoidance of research in which death or disabling injury were likely to occur. In 1964, the World Medical Association developed a further code of research ethics known as the Declaration of Helsinki.[13]

In 1966, a series of 22 unethical medical research protocols were published, including one study in which chronically ill patients were injected with cancer cells without informed consent.[14] This study, along with publication of the Tuskegee Study, in which black men with syphilis were left untreated for research purposes from 1932 to 1972, produced an outcry about unethical research.[15] The National Commission for the Protection of Human Subjects of Biomedical and Behavioral Research (Belmont Report) was enacted, which became the basis for the current Institutional Review Board (IRB) for the regulation of medical research.

IRB-Sanctioned Research

Orthopaedics, perhaps more than any other specialty, depends on the development and subsequent release of surgical procedures and implants to the general orthopaedic population. The process of development of new surgical procedures and implants, from conception and evaluation and ultimately to the release of the procedure or implant to the general orthopaedic community, has received increased scrutiny over the past several years. The formal process of regulating the development of orthopaedic implants began in 1976, when the Food and Drug Administration amended the Federal Drug and Cosmetic Act to include medical devices, in addition to pharmaceutical products. This act has various requirements for the marketing of medical devices, depending primarily on whether the proposed implant is similar to an implant in clinical use before 1976. For those implants for which there is not a demonstrated similar implant in clinical usage before 1976, the process of Food and Drug Administration approval is complex, costly and time-consuming, including a clinical trial requiring a substantial number of patients with a minimum follow-up period of 2 years.[16]

The process of obtaining informed consent for patients to be included in a clinical trial is mandated by the institution's IRB. Informed consent should include an explanation of the diagnosis or medical condition requiring treatment, a complete explanation of the proposed procedure, including its purpose and duration, and its likelihood of success. In addition, any significant risk of the procedure, reasonable alternative treatment, and the risk of nontreatment should be part of informed consent. Truly ethical informed consent should also ensure the patient's understanding of the disclosed information. There is evidence that certain groups, such as the mentally ill, the poorly educated, and the geriatric population, often do not understand informed consent. The use of multimedia has had mixed results in enhancing understanding of the information.[17]

When obtaining consent for emergency surgery or limb-salvage surgery in a patient who does not have the capacity to comprehend informed consent, a legal guardian has the authority to provide informed consent. In the absence of a designated legal guardian, most states recognize the legality of family members to provide informed consent, provided that the proposed procedure does not involve the patient's reproductive capacity, and no family member objects to the proposed procedure. In emergency situations with no legal guardian or family members present, it is appropriate to have another physician, with similar expertise and knowledge as the proposed surgeon, confirm the necessity of the procedure.[18]

Recently, a clinical trial of a hemoglobin-based oxygen-carrying blood substitute (PolyHeme Pivotal phase 3 trial) has raised significant ethical issues.[19] This trial has been conducted under an exemption from federal informed consent requirements (Code of Federal Regulations, Title 21, Section 50.24). This provision is granted in specific situations in which patients are in life-threatening situations requiring medical intervention, available medical treatments are unsatisfactory, previous studies done on the proposed treatment have shown a direct benefit (in this case, increased patient survival), and the risks are reasonable in relation to what is known about the patient's medical condition. Treatment begins at the scene of injury. Patients are randomized either to a standard treatment of traumatic hypovolemia (saline and blood transfusion) or PolyHeme (Northfield Laboratories, Evanston, IL) treatment of up to 12 hours after injury or up to six units of PolyHeme transfusion. These patients are unable to give informed consent because of their injuries. Despite the fact that this trial was conducted under appropriate exemptions from normal informed consent regulations, significant debate occurred concerning the ethical aspects of this study, both in the lay press and the scientific world. This episode has been the most visible current example of the debate between the obvious benefits of appropriately designed medical studies and the requirements to provide informed consent.

Non-IRB Sanctioned Informed Consent
According to the Regulatory Ethics Paradigm, any new drug, new medical device, or new surgical procedure should be introduced under the auspices of the IRB.[20] However, surgical techniques based on a variation of a previous surgical procedure (for example, mini-incision total joint arthroplasty) or an implant with only minor modifications from previous implants generally are not IRB-sanctioned. Off-label applications of implants (such as methylmethacrylate antibiotic beads) are by definition not IRB-sanctioned. In these instances of non-IRB sanctioned new procedures, informed consent should include a statement explaining the procedure or implant, a brief discussion of the theoretic reasons for the new procedure/implant, and alternative treatment. For procedures or implants without long-term follow-up or valid scientific studies, it has been suggested that the term "nonvalidated" be used in the informed consent discussion.[20]

In the field of orthopaedic surgery, new procedures and implants are being developed to treat a diverse array of musculoskeletal conditions. Each orthopaedic surgeon by definition will be at some time on the upward learning curve of a new procedure. Several factors can diminish medicolegal liability for obtaining informed consent. Instead of a complete list of potential complications for each procedure, it is better to document one extreme complication (such as amputation). Instead of relying solely on the preprinted informed consent form, it is desirable to have a dictated or handwritten note describing the informed consent and potential complications. It is better to obtain the informed consent in an office or clinic setting, rather than in the preoperative area.[21]

Orthopaedic Emergency Department Coverage

There has been an increasing reluctance of orthopaedic surgeons to take emergency department call. In general, hospital by-laws mandate emergency department coverage as a provision for hospital privileges. However, about two thirds of hospitals report significant uncovered periods for subspecialty coverage in the emergency department. There are several factors involved in the reluctance and avoidance of orthopaedic surgeons to take emergency department call.

On-call emergency department physicians have certain legal obligations in addition to the standard physician-patient relationship. The Emergency Medical Treatment and Active Labor Act (EMTALA) requires patients admitted to an emergency department to be evaluated by a responsible health care provider. The patient cannot be discharged from the emergency department until the patient's condition is stabilized or the patient is transferred to another hospital. To transfer the patient to another hospital, the transferring physician must document that the benefits of the transfer outweigh the risks, the outside hospital accepts the patient, and appropriate radiographs and charts are sent with the patient. A modification of EMTALA in 2003 requires hospitals to keep a current list of qualified staff physicians to provide emergency department coverage, and to have a written plan for unexpected absence of subspecialty emergency department coverage.[22]

A major reason for the reluctance of some orthopaedic surgeons to assume emergency department coverage is financial. There has been a marked increase in emergency department visits during the past 10 years, especially in large metropolitan areas. There has been a significant closure of emergency departments across the country in the past decade, resulting in overcrowding of remaining emergency departments. Ninety-one percent of all emergency departments report significant periods of overcrowding resulting in diversion, placing additional stress on the emergency departments in the United States.[23] A disproportionate number of uninsured or underinsured patients come to emergency departments for treatment. From 1995 to 2003, the number of nonelderly uninsured patients increased by more than 7 million to 45 million in the US, from 16.1% to 17.7% of the general population.[24] Uncompensated care is unevenly distributed, with a disproportionate percentage occurring in urban teaching centers (disproportionate share hospitals). In a recent, retrospective, case-controlled national database study of 97,000 patients with low injury severity scores (< 9), 27% were transferred to level 1 trauma centers. Nonmedical factors for transfer were analyzed. Patients with Medicaid insurance were transferred more often than patients with commercial insurance. There was no statistical difference in the transfer rate of self-insured patients and patients with commercial insurance.[25] In addition, there is no financial incentive for treating unscheduled emergency orthopaedic trauma patients. The Resource-Based Relative Value Scale system does not differentiate between the treatment of scheduled office patients versus the treatment of emergency hospital trauma patients. Despite the development of common procedural terminology (CPT) modifier codes to "reward" hospital on-call surgical care, Medicare, Medicaid, and most commercial insurance carriers do not recognize these codes.[26]

The American College of Surgeons has suggested a partial solution to the unwillingness of some specialists to provide emergency care. An additional period of training past general surgery residency training would designate an "acute surgeon," with the ability to deliver simple to intermediate subspecialty care. To date, the orthopaedic surgeons and neurosurgeons have managed to avoid inclusion of orthopaedic and neurosurgical procedures in the curriculum. A recent survey of AOS and OTA members was decidedly against the orthopaedic community abandoning acute orthopaedic trauma care.[26]

Another reasonable objection to orthopaedic surgeons participating in emergency department coverage is the perceived increased liability for medical malpractice in treating trauma patients. The physician-patient relationship inherent in elective surgery is usually not present in trauma surgery patients. In addition, sequelae from traumatic injuries can result in either long-term disability or death, theoretically resulting in costly malpractice suits. However, a recent retrospective study showed no increased incidence of malpractice cases in trauma surgery, excluding orthopaedic surgery, versus elective surgery.[22]

The solution for declining orthopaedic emergency department coverage is multifactorial. Obviously, more funding should be considered for uncompensated emergency care, especially increasing federal funding to disproportionate share hospitals (large urban academic centers). According to the American Hospital Association, US hospitals spent approximately $25 billion on uncompensated medical care in 2004.[24] A recent position statement by the AAOS states that it is the responsibility of government policy makers to help " the medical profession meet society's expectation for everyone's emergency care needs to be met regardless of ability to pay."[27] AAOS suggests consideration of linking federal revenue for highway construction and maintenance to establishment of a complete system of support for emergency care of trauma patients.[27] Importantly, AAOS recognizes the obligation for hospitals to fairly compensate orthopaedic surgeons who participate in emergency department call. In addition, operating room time for elective treatment of orthopaedic trauma should be made available at a reasonable time. Another reasonable objection of community orthopaedic surgeons to taking emergency department call is a perceived lack of training or expertise to treat complex musculoskeletal trauma. If adequate financial arrangements can be made, provisional emergent trauma care can be provided at the community hospital setting, and subsequent transfer can be accomplished to a trauma center where complex surgery can be done. The EMTALA Technical Advisory Group has been established by the lobbying efforts of the AAOS and other specialty groups to clarify and modify existing regulations mandated by the Centers for Medicare and Medicaid Services for the treatment of trauma patients. Further clarifications concerning obligations of receiving and transferring hospitals of trauma patients are being discussed, including geographic limitations, defining the resources of receiving hospitals to treat trauma patients, and providing the resources for follow-up of trauma patients after discharge from the emergency department.[28]

Industry-Physician Relationships

The interactions of academic research scientists and industry has become more regulated in the past several years. In the first relatively underregulated initial decade of the biotechnology era, there were few, or at least undocumented, issues with the relationship between industry and research physicians. In the late 1980s, allegations of misconduct between academic physicians and industry resulted in significant restrictions in the relationship between physicians and industry. Recently, the National Institutes of Health (NIH) abolished all corporate consulting activities of NIH researchers.[29] The potential conflicts of industry-physician collaborations are research misbehavior or bias. Research misbehavior occurs extremely rarely and consists of falsification of research results or plagiarism. Bias is the potential conflict of interest in interpreting results of research, or underreporting adverse outcomes, because of financial issues.

Another issue regarding industry-physician relationships concerns the arrangement of individual orthopaedic surgeons serving as consultants to orthopaedic implant companies. In March 2005, articles in major newspapers announced the US Justice Department's investigation into several orthopaedic companies' financial arrangements with orthopaedic surgeons.[30] It is obviously appropriate for orthopaedists-scientists to be paid for legitimate time involved in developing implants or procedures. Industry-physician interactions have been classified as type 1: intellectual property, type 2: a consulting agreement in which the orthopaedic surgeon addresses a specific issue, type 3: the orthopaedic surgeon is used as a marketing tool, and type 4: the orthopaedic surgeon is paid for using the implant.[30] Financial relationships between industry and orthopaedic surgeons should be based on a reasonable correlation of reimbursement and the actual time of involvement of the physician in the project.[31]

The mandate of disclosure of industry relationships in publications has at least allowed individuals to consider any potential bias in reporting results. The recently enacted restrictions on industry-sponsored meetings has curtailed extravagant meetings in resort-type areas paid for by industry. However, a recent survey of medical students showed that most did not consider industry gifts as unethical.[32] There was a recent proposal to develop a National Clinical Trials Consortium to eliminate direct physician-industry relationships to avoid research misconduct and bias.[33] However, it may not be feasible or even desirable to eliminate direct physician-industry relationships. It is, however, the responsibility of the orthopaedic surgeon to maintain professionalism and ethical conduct in the field of orthopaedics.

Annotated References

1. Hu P, Murray TH, Schwartz, MR: A global profession: Medical values in China and the United States. Closing Reflections. *Hastings Cent Rep* 2000;30(suppl 4):S45-S47.

2. Cruess SR: Professionalism and medicine's social contract with society. *Clin Orthop Relat Res* 2006;449: 170-176.

   The author discusses the social contract concept of professionalism and enumerates society's expectations of medicine (competence, altruism, integrity, accountability) and medicine's expectation of society (trust, autonomy, monopoly, financial and other rewards) under the terms of this tacit agreement.

3. Hafferty FW: Definitions of professionalism: A search for meaning and identity. *Clin Orthop Relat Res* 2006; 449:193-204.

   The author explores definitions of professionalism from the viewpoints of sociology, education, and medicine, highlighting the three stages in the evolution of medical professionalism and pointing out differences in the US and United Kingdom concepts of professionalism.

4. Cruess SR, Johnston S, Cruess RL: 'Profession': A working definition for medical educators. *Teach Learn Med* 2004;16:74-76.

   The authors argue that concise, inclusive definitions of professionalism are lacking. A definition is needed to teach the subject effectively, evaluate what students have learned, and form the basis of the contract between the public and medicine.

5. Cohen J: Foreword, in Stern DT (ed): *Measuring Medical Professionalism.* New York, NY, Oxford University Press, 2006, pp v-viii.

   The public, business, and government demand that physicians be accountable for their professional behavior. This book offers a theory-to-practice approach to documenting and evaluating professionalism and discusses tools for assessing a doctor's professional actions.

6. Royal College of Physicians of London: Doctors in society: Medical professionalism in a changing world. 2005, p 45. Available at: http://www.rcplondon.ac.uk/pubs/books/docinsoc/. Accessed March 9, 2007.

   This detailed report by a distinguished work group addresses events that have undermined public trust in medicine and led to questions about the traditional values and behaviors once seen as the hallmarks of professionalism.

7. American Academy of Orthopaedic Surgeons: Code of Ethics and Professionalism for Orthopaedic Surgeons. 2004. Available at: http://www.aaos.org/about/papers/ethics/code.asp. Accessed March 9, 2007.

8. Medical Professionalism Project: Medical professionalism in the new millennium: A physician charter. 2002.

Available at: http://www.aaos.org/about/papers/ethics/profess.asp. Accessed March 9, 2007.

9. American Academy of Orthopaedic Surgeons: Professional compliance program. 2005. Available at: http://www3.aaos.org/member/profcomp/profcomp.cfm. Accessed March 9, 2007.

10. Epstein RM: Mindful practice. *JAMA* 1999;282:833-839.

11. Faigman DL: *Legal Alchemy: The Use and Misuse of Science in the Law.* New York, NY, WH Freeman, 1999, pp ix-xiv.

12. Clarkfield AM: Nazi medicine and the Nuremberg trials: From medical war crimes to informed consent. *N Engl J Med* 2006;295:2668-2669.

    This article reviews a book about the Nuremberg trials.

13. Naarden AL: Informed consent. *Am J Med* 2006;119:194-197.

    The potential difficulties of informed consent are discussed in this review article.

14. Lerner BH: Sins of omission-cancer research without consent. *N Engl J Med* 2004;351:628-630.

    This historical article discusses the development of formal informed consent.

15. Baker SM, Brawley OW, Marks LS: Effects of untreated syphilis in the negro male, 1932-1972: A closure comes to the Tuskegee study, 2004. *Urology* 2005;65:1259-1262.

    This article discusses the Tuskegee study.

16. Callaghan JJ, Crowninshield RD, Greenwald AS, Lieberman JR, Rosenberg AG, Lewallen DG: Symposium: Introducing Technology into Orthopaedic Practice. *J Bone Joint Surg Am* 2005;87:1146-1158.

    A comprehensive review of the entire field of the legalities and regulation of new technology is presented.

17. Flory BA, Emanuel E: Interventions to improve participants' understanding of informed consent for research. *JAMA* 2002;292:1593-1601.

18. Suk M, Udale A, Helfet D: Orthopaedics and the law. *J Am Acad Orthop Surg* 2005;13:397-406.

    This article presents discussion of the relationship of various components of the law and surgeons, including malpractice and informed consent.

19. Moore EE, Johnson JL, Cheng AM, Masuno T, Banerjee A: Insights from studies of blood substitutes in trauma. *Shock* 2005;24:197-205.

    In a multicenter prehospital trial, severely injured patients with major blood loss (systemic blood pressure < 90 mm Hg) were randomized to initial field resuscitation with crystalloid versus hemoglobin-based oxygen carriers. Results from this study indicate that hemoglobin solutions may ultimately prove superior in delivering oxygen to ischemic or injured tissue.

20. Lieberman JR, Wenger N: New technology and the orthopaedic surgeon. *Clin Orthop Relat Res* 2004;429:338-341.

    A discussion of the responsibilities of the surgeon in introducing new technology into practice is presented.

21. Bhattacharyya T, Yeon H, Harris MB: The medical-legal aspects of informed consent in orthopaedic surgery. *J Bone Joint Surg Am* 2005;87:2395-2400.

    The risk of a malpractice claim may be decreased by obtaining informed consent in the physician's office rather than in the preoperative waiting area and by documentation of the informed consent discussion.

22. Stewart RM, Johnston J, Geoghegan K, et al: Trauma surgery malpractice risk: Perception versus reality. *Ann Surg* 2005;241:969-977.

    Data from this study indicate that the risk of lawsuit is not increased when caring for trauma patients, and the actual risk of a malpractice lawsuit is low.

23. Olshaker JS, Rathlev NK: Emergency department overcrowding and ambulance diversion: The impact and potential solutions. *J Emerg Med* 2006;30:351-356.

    This article discusses overcrowding with a focus on the significance and potential remedies of extended boarding of patients admitted to the emergency department.

24. Weissman JS: The trouble with uncompensated hospital care. *N Engl J Med* 2005;352:1171-1173.

    A discussion of the increasing problem of uncompensated health care costs and the concentration of indigent patients in large, urban academic medical centers is presented.

25. Koval KJ, Tinge C, Spratt K: Are patients being transferred to level 1 trauma centers for reasons other than medical necessity? *J Bone Joint Surg Am* 2006;88:2124-2132.

    The authors of this study evaluated possible risk factors for hospital transfer in a population of patients unlikely to require transfer to a level 1 center for medical reasons.

26. Bosse MJ, Henley MB, Bray T, Vrahas MS: An AOA critical issue: Access to emergent musculoskeletal care: Resuscitating orthopaedic emergency department coverage. *J Bone Joint Surg Am* 2006;88:1385-1394.

    A thorough discussion of the crisis in orthopaedic coverage in US emergency departments is presented.

27. Beaty J: Meeting the challenge: Orthopaedists on-call. *AAOS Bulletin* 2006;54:28-36.

    Orthopaedic on-call issues and their impact on the quality of patient care are discussed.

1: Principles of Orthopaedics

28. Pontzer K: Addressing emergency care at the federal level. *AAOS Bulletin* 2006;54:35-36.

    The goals of the Emergency Medical Treatment and Active Labor Act Technical Advisory Group are discussed.

29. Stossel TP: Regulating academic-industrial research relationships-solving or stifling progress? *N Engl J Med* 2005;353:1060-1065.

    This article discusses regulation of academic-industrial research relationships.

30. Jacobs JJ, Galante JO, Mirza SK, Zdeblick T: Relationships with industry: Critical for new technology or an unecessary evil? *J Bone Joint Surg Am* 2006;88:1650-1663.

    Legal and ethical issues related to relationships with industry are discussed.

31. Light TR: President's message. *AOA News* 2006;38:1.

    A discussion of the financial relationship between industry and the orthopaedic surgeon is presented.

32. Sierles FS, Brodkey AC, Cleary LM, et al: Medical students' exposure to and attitudes about drug company interactions: A national survey. *JAMA* 2005;294:1034-1042.

    Because little is known about relationships between drug companies and medical students, third-year medical students' exposure to and attitudes about drug company interactions were studied.

33. Weinstein JN: An altruistic approach to clinical trials: The National Clinical Trials Consortium. *Clin Orthop Rel Res* 2006;450:246-248.

    The author discusses the National Clinical Trials Consortium.

Chapter 2

Fracture Repair and Bone Grafting

Christopher R. Brown, MD   *Scott D. Boden, MD

Introduction

An understanding of bone healing and graft incorporation is fundamental to the practice of orthopaedics. Regardless of their particular specialty within orthopaedics, surgeons must have a firm grasp of the biology of bone healing and grafting. It is a necessary part of the armamentarium when treating acute fractures, nonunions, bone defects, angular deformity, limb-length inequality, and arthrodeses of the spine and extremities. The number of spinal fusion surgeries has steadily increased over the past decade. Currently there are more than 250,000 spine fusion surgeries performed in the United States each year. Since the 1990s, spinal arthrodesis has become the most common reason for autologous bone grafting. To ensure a good outcome for these patients, the surgeon must have knowledge of a broad range of treatment methods and strategies.

Bone healing and graft incorporation is a complex process that involves molecular, cellular, local, and mechanical factors. All of these processes must be effectively managed for bone healing to be successful. The surgeon must identify deficiencies in the process and intervene in an appropriate manner. Advances have been made recently in the field of bone tissue engineering, giving the surgeon practical clinical benefits in treating patients.

Bone Fracture Healing

The overall fracture incidence is 11.3 in 1,000 patients per year—11.67 in 1,000 per year in males, and 10.65 in 1,000 per year in females.[1] Acute fractures of bone result from forces to the skeleton that exceed the strength of the tissue. The severity of the injury is directly related to the intensity and duration of the force. A bone fracture initiates a cascade of events that can restore the injured bone to its original state. The first stage, inflammation, begins at the time of the impact

*Scott D. Boden, MD or the department with which he is affiliated has received research or institutional support from Medtronic, DePuy, Synthes, and Abbott, miscellaneous nonincome support, commercially derived honoraria, or other nonresearch related funding from Osteotech, royalties from Medtronic and Osteotech, and is a consultant or employee for Medtronic.

that causes the fracture. The fracture causes a disruption of both the periosteal and endosteal blood supply, leading to local necrosis. The surrounding soft tissue is usually damaged, leading to even more extensive disruption of the blood supply. Local cells release vasoactive mediators that cause increased vasodilatation and permeability. This leads to a steady increase in blood flow that peaks approximately 2 weeks after fracture. A hematoma forms that is invaded by inflammatory cells. Fibroblasts appear and produce collagen and eventually replace the hematoma with granulation tissue.

For long bone fractures, the repair phase begins with the formation of a soft callus usually between day 5 and day 21 (**Figure 1**). There is a dramatic invasion of new blood vessels formed by endothelial progenitor cells, resulting in a revascularization phase. Progenitor cells invade the environment and differentiate according to the local conditions at the site. The differentiation is mostly influenced by the oxygen tension, mechanical environment, and signals from local growth factors. High strain environments promote differentiation of cells that produce fibrous tissue. Osteoprogenitor cells proliferate in areas of increased oxygen tension and decreased strain. Areas of high oxygen tension and

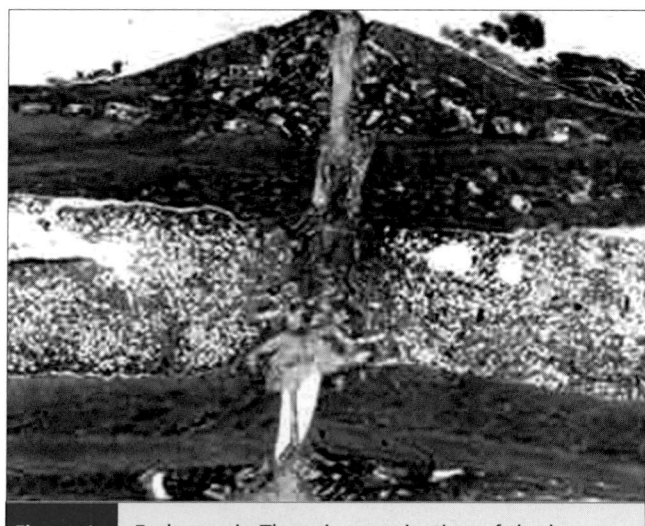

Figure 1   Early repair. There is organization of the hematoma, early primary new bone formation in subperiosteal regions, and cartilage formation in other areas.

Table 1

Local and Systemic Factors Influencing Bone Healing

Positive Factors	Negative Factors
Good vascular supply at the graft site	Radiation
Large surface area	Tumor
Mechanical stability	Mechanical instability
Mechanical loading	Infection
Growth factors	Corticosteroids
	Chemotherapy
	Smoking
	Diabetes
	Malnutrition
	Metabolic bone disease

low strain tend to promote formation of woven bone directly; this is referred to as intramembranous bone formation. Regions of intermediate strain and low oxygen tension will have chondrocyte differentiation and cartilage formation. A fibrocartilaginous callus then bridges the fracture site. The cartilage can reduce the local strain and lead to bone formation. The chondrocytes and cartilage matrix calcify, and progenitor cells develop into osteoblast and deposit new bone, replacing the calcified cartilage in a process known as endochondral bone formation.

The final stage in fracture repair, remodeling, involves conversion of immature woven bone into lamellar bone. It occurs in response to the local loading environment. Osteoclast resorption of woven bone is coupled with osteoblast deposition of mature lamellar bone. It ends when the bone has resumed its normal appearance, and the medullary canal is reconstituted. The mechanical properties of the bone return to that of the preinjured bone.

Some but not all of the basic biologic process and mechanisms involved in fracture healing apply to bone graft sites. Much has been learned about the biology of bone grafting by studying spine fusion models. This environment is very different from that of a healing long bone fracture. The biology and maturation of a spine fusion differs among the various types of fusion locations.

The interbody spine environment is rich in decorticated bone surface area, which can increase the access to bone marrow that contains osteoprogenitor cells required to form new bone. It is also subject to compressive forces that seem to stimulate remodeling and loading of bone. This biologic environment can result in generally higher fusion rates if there is adequate access to bone marrow, rigid internal fixation to avoid shearing of new blood vessels, and adequate end plate strength to prevent subsidence of the structural component of the interbody graft or spacer.[2]

An intertransverse process spine fusion is a very different environment. There is less access to bone marrow and more abundant muscle tissue, and it is subject to tensile loads. Compressive loads are less significant until the graft has consolidated. The intertransverse fusion healing process in rabbits using iliac crest bone graft has been described.[3] Analysis of histologic sections revealed three distinct and temporal phases of spine fusion healing: inflammatory, reparative, and remodeling. These phases occur throughout the fusion mass but at different times. Maturation of the fusion mass was most advanced in the regions near the decorticated transverse processes, which represent the major blood and progenitor cell supply to the fusion mass. In these transverse process zones, intramembranous formation was the major means of bone formation. In the central zone, a similar process occurred but it was delayed in time and included a period of endochondral bone formation in which cartilage was replaced by bone. This lag effect may explain why nonunions most often occur at this central zone.[3] Molecular biology studies have shown a predictable sequence of gene expression during the maturation of the fusion mass. Various proteins including collagen, osteocalcin, and bone morphogenetic proteins (BMPs) have a temporal and spatial pattern of expression. Consistent with the histologic analysis, peak expression of the genes was seen 1 to 2 weeks earlier in the areas closest to the decorticated transverse processes than in the central zones, which are farther from the decorticated host bone.[4]

Factors Affecting Bone Healing

Many factors affecting bone healing and grafting must be considered when formulating a treatment plan for a patient with a fracture or nonunion or when considering an elective arthrodesis procedure (Table 1). Some of these factors are beyond the control of the surgeon, whereas others can be manipulated to achieve a successful outcome.

Patient factors directly affect bone formation. The nutritional status of the patient must be considered and maximized before elective procedures. Medications the patient may be taking can adversely affect the biologic process needed for healing. Nonsteroidal anti-inflammatory drugs have been linked to delayed bone healing. However, it is unclear whether cyclooxygenase-2-selective nonsteroidal anti-inflammatory drugs will have less effect on healing than nonselective drugs.[5,6] Patients taking fluoroquinolones may experience decreased healing during the early stages of fracture healing.[7,8]

Nicotine, steroids, and some chemotherapeutic agents have proved to have a deleterious effect on bone healing and graft incorporation. In the rabbit spine fusion model, the administration of nicotine inhibits the gene expression of a wide range of cytokines, including those associated with neovascularization and osteoblast differentiation.[9] Using the same model, a single dose of doxorubicin at the time of surgery appears to play a significant inhibitory role in the process of spinal fusion.[10]

Patient comorbidities impact the biologic response to a fracture. Diabetes is known to cause impaired bone healing. In a 2005 study, diabetic patients with ankle fractures were retrospectively reviewed.[11] Patients with one or more comorbidities from diabetes were at an increased risk of developing complications from an ankle fracture that included nonunion, malunion, and the need for prolonged bracing.[11] The presence of human immunodeficiency virus (HIV) may increase the risk of nonunion and infection.[12]

The soft tissue surrounding the fracture can have an impact on the biology of bone healing. Surgeons are aware of the importance of limiting iatrogenic soft-tissue trauma during surgical intervention. The advent of intramedullary nails and sliding plates with percutaneous fixation allows a surgeon to avoid the injury zone, minimizing further compromise to the soft tissue and blood supply. The value of early soft-tissue coverage for open tibia fractures demonstrates the importance of the soft-tissue envelope.

Mechanical factors play a role in fracture healing and bone graft maturation. The rigidity of the fixation can affect the type of healing that occurs. Callus-free primary bone healing requires direct bone apposition and absolute stability. Rigid internal fixation using either a lag screw or a compression plate provides the mechanical stability needed for direct bone healing. Unlocked intramedullary nails and external fixators are examples of load-sharing devices that create a different biologic environment. The micromotion in the fracture leads to indirect bone healing, evidenced by the presence of a cartilaginous callus. There has been a recent shift toward the use of less rigid fixation to allow load sharing, which results in callus formation.

Classification of Graft Material

A bone grafting material may possess several properties. An osteoconductive material needs to provide the scaffolding to support new bone formation. The proper three-dimensional structure of the graft permits the ingrowth of sprouting capillaries, perivascular tissue, and osteoprogenitor cells, facilitating the process of graft incorporation known as creeping substitution. An osteoinductive substance will stimulate the recruitment and differentiation of mesenchymal stem cells (MSCs) into bone-forming cells. Specific BMPs are the primary known osteoinductive proteins BMP-2, -4, -6, -7, and -9. An osteogenic graft contains viable osteoblastic cells that are capable of direct bone formation. This potential to provide bone-forming cells is characteristic of only fresh autogenous bone graft. Other grafts rely on recruitment of host progenitor cells to differentiate into bone-forming cells.[13]

Bone graft materials can be classified into three functional biologic roles. All three roles are measured with reference to autogenous bone graft, the historic gold standard. A bone graft extender allows the use of less autogenous graft or the coverage of a larger grafting volume with similar healing success rates. A graft enhancer, when added to autogenous graft, should result in higher fusion success rates. A graft substitute can be used in place of autogenous bone graft with the requirement that it results in similar or better fusion success rates.

The specific biologic roles required of a graft will depend on the specific healing environment. For example, a tibial metaphyseal fracture is one of the least challenging healing environments after external fixation because of the high prevalence of bone marrow access, vascular supply, and protection from soft-tissue interposition. Purely osteoconductive materials usually perform well in these situations, but an osteoinductive component may be helpful in healing-impaired hosts (smokers, diabetics, steroid users). At the other extreme, posterolateral lumbar spine fusion is one of the most biologically challenging healing environments. In this case, purely conductive materials are not effective substitutes and are only variably effective as extenders. In this situation a graft enhancer or substitute with some osteoinductive properties is likely required. One exception is pediatric patients, in whom purely conductive materials function better than in adults undergoing spine fusion.

Current Graft Options
Autogenous Bone Grafts
Autogenous iliac crest bone graft is the most well-documented bone graft and has been the "gold standard" for grafting material in patients undergoing spinal fusion. It has osteogenic properties (numerous differentiated and undetermined stromal cells within the marrow cavity lining) and osteoconductive properties (ideal scaffold). Cancellous bone contains only minute amounts of BMPs, which are not active; therefore, according to strict definitions autologous bone graft material is not osteoinductive. A commonly used site for harvesting bone graft is the posterior iliac crest, because it provides a large quantity of both cancellous and corticocancellous bone. With cancellous bone grafts, approximately 15% of the osteoblasts and osteocytes of the graft survive and are capable of producing early bone.[14] The porous nature of cancellous bone permits more rapid ingrowth of new blood vessels, which allow for the influx of osteoblast precursors. Bone formation and resorption usually occur concomitantly, with osteoclasts resorbing the dead trabecular bone followed by osteoblasts depositing new bone (creeping substitution). Eventually, all grafted cancellous tissue is remodeled with new host bone and marrow.

One disadvantage of autograft is the limited amount of graft material available for use. The quantity and quality of iliac donor bone can be diminished substantially in older patients with osteoporosis or fatty marrow infiltration. Significant donor-site morbidity has been reported in as many as 25% to 40% of patients. Complications include chronic donor-site pain, infection, fracture, and hematoma.[15]

Biologic Enhancers of Bone Healing

Platelets/Autologous Growth Factor

Platelet concentrate preparation systems have gained some measure of use in spinal fusion augmentation. Platelets are rich in growth factors such as platelet-derived growth factor and transforming growth factor-β, and it has been argued that platelet concentrates therefore are helpful in bone formation. Much of the data are derived from oral and maxillofacial surgery, where membranous bone formation is much easier than spinal bone formation. Many spine surgeons believe that growth factors are good and that platelet concentrates may help and cannot hurt. Unfortunately, the evidence for efficacy in spinal surgery has not been established as clearly as the other biologics discussed above. In fact, some clinical data suggest either no efficacy or a detrimental effect. A retrospective cohort study of patients treated by a single surgeon who performed consecutive single-level posterolateral lumbar fusion showed that those with iliac crest bone alone (n = 27) had a 91% rate of fusion and those with iliac crest augmented with autologous growth factor (AGF) (n = 32) had a 62% rate of fusion.[16] In a retrospective cohort study of posterolateral lumbar fusions with autograft iliac crest mixed with a platelet concentrate (AGF) (n = 76 consecutive patients), the nonunion rate was 25%, compared with a case control cohort (n = 76 patients) in which the nonunion rate was 17%.[17] The authors noted the increase in cost and risk to the patient with use of AGF and recommended against using AGF for instrumented posterolateral lumbar fusion.

Growth and Differentiation Factor-5

Growth and differentiation factor-5 (GDF-5) is known by many different names including MP-52, LAP-4, CDMP-1, BMP-14, and radotermin. GDF-5 has been shown to promote tissue regeneration in bone, cartilage, soft tissue, and tendon in vivo. The rabbit intertransverse process fusion experiments with GDF-5 indicate that 100% fusion rates can be achieved; however, the lowest concentration used (0.5 mg/mL) resulted in the highest bone volume formation when compared with higher doses (1.0 mg/mL and 1.5 mg/mL).[18] This and other studies indicate that increasing the dose too much with this molecule may be counterproductive to bone formation. Currently, two multicenter investigational device exemption clinical trials are ongoing, one for spinal fusion and another for long bone repair.

Ultrasound

Ultrasound is acoustic radiation at frequencies beyond the limit of human hearing. It has been used as a physical signal in the detection or alteration of biologic effects for many years. Very low ultrasonic intensities (milliwatts per cm²) are applied for diagnostic purposes to avoid excessive heating of the tissues, and ultrasonic intensities of 1 to 3 W/cm² are commonly used in the treatment of joint stiffness, pain, and muscle spasm and to improve muscular mobility. Ultrasound also has some beneficial effects on wound and tendon healing. A broad spectrum of experiments performed at the basic science and clinical levels have provided substantial evidence that low-intensity ultrasound can accelerate osteogenesis and augment the fracture healing process.

Allograft

Allograft bone products are the most common substitutes for autogenous bone grafts. Some advantages of allograft include its availability in greater quantities and precut sizes/shapes than autograft and avoidance of the donor-site morbidity associated with autograft. The sterilization process kills the cells in the allograft and may damage other components including proteins. Therefore, these materials are highly osteoconductive but not osteogenic because the cells do not survive transplantation. As with mineralized autograft, mineralized allograft is not inherently osteoinductive.

In treating nonunions, bone void defects, and posterolateral spine fusions, allograft typically is used as a bone graft extender. Cancellous chips are added to local or iliac bone to increase the volume of the graft. Allograft cancellous chips function poorly when used alone for posterior lumbar fusions in adults.[19] The most suitable patient for nonstructural (morcellized) allografts in spine surgery appears to be the adolescent undergoing posterior fusion for scoliosis. Allograft chips are successful in these patients because bone heals easily in adolescents and the posterior thoracic spine is very stable with fixation and has a larger surface area for decortication.[20] Impaction bone grafting uses morcellized femoral head allograft to restore femoral and acetabular bone stock in the setting of revision joint arthroplasty. It has been shown to provide initial stability and restore long-term bone stock in the distal femur. This technique is associated with an excellent long-term prosthetic survival rate in both acetabular and femoral reconstruction.[21,22]

Allograft can also be used for its structural, weight-bearing properties. These grafts can be used in reconstructive surgery when large bony defects necessitate structural supports, such as a femoral or acetabular deficiency. Structural allograft also can be used for interbody spine fusion alone or in combination with a graft enhancer or osteoinductive material.[23]

More than 200,000 bone allografts are used in musculoskeletal procedures annually in the United States.[24] Tissue banks have been established to ensure a supply of high-quality allogenic tissue for reconstructive orthopaedic surgery. More than 50 tissue banks in the United States are accredited by the American Association of Tissue Banks (AATB). The US Food and Drug Administration (FDA) and the AATB help ensure adequate screening of tissue donors and that the allograft provided by the various tissue banks is properly processed, labeled, and distributed.

A recent event raised questions about the safety of allograft. In September 2005, the FDA received a report that a tissue recovery firm had inaccuracies in their donor records. The FDA investigation determined that human donors were not properly screened for certain infectious diseases and that some of the donors may not have met eligibility requirements. In October 2005, tissues from this tissue recovery firm were recalled and the company was ordered to cease manufacturing and to retain all cellular and tissue-based products.[25]

Screening of cadaveric donors begins with a detailed questionnaire completed by the life partner or next of kin. Donors are excluded if there is a history of the following factors or conditions: exposure to specific communicable diseases, unprotected sexual contact, drug use, neurologic diseases, autoimmune diseases, collagen disorders, or metabolic diseases. Viral disease transmission, including hepatitis C, hepatitis B, and HIV, is of utmost concern. Since 1980, two cases of HIV transmission as a result of musculoskeletal allograft have been reported.[26] However, since the AATB adopted strict screening programs and mandatory blood tests for all donors, the incidence of disease transmission has been halted.

Allograft bone can be processed many different ways, including low-dose (< 20 kGy) irradiation, physical débridement, ultrasonic or pulsatile water washes, ethanol treatment, and antibiotic soaking (4° C for at least 1 hour).[27] The goal of processing is to ensure sterility while retaining certain biologic and biomechanical properties. Terminal sterilization by gamma irradiation, electron beam irradiation, or ethylene oxide treatment may be used if there is contamination, but there is a dose-dependent effect on the mechanical strength of the graft.[28]

Osteoconductive Bone Graft Substitutes

Ceramics
Ceramics containing calcium phosphate are formed by heating and pressurizing these nonmetallic materials. The calcium phosphates are the most commonly used ceramics in orthopaedics.[29] As osteoconductive materials, they are mostly used as bone graft extenders. Ceramics have the advantage of inducing little inflammatory response and pose little or no risk of disease transmission. They are also available in unlimited quantities and have no donor-site complication. The disadvantages include low fracture resistance and tensile strength. Several animal studies using ceramics as adjuncts to posterolateral fusions have yielded conflicting results. There are clinical data showing comparable results for posterolateral lumbar fusions in patients with idiopathic scoliosis using ceramics and local bone versus local bone and autograft.[30] The best clinical experience with the ceramics has been in the setting of anterior interbody fusion in the cervical spine.[31]

Hydroxyapatite, another ceramic, has been available as a coating on joint arthroplasty implants for some time. Animal studies showed that such coatings increase fixation strength by preferential deposition of new bone at the interface, but no clear clinical advantage has been shown.[32]

Collagen
The structure of collagen is conductive to mineral deposition, vascular ingrowth, and growth factor binding; however, it provides little or no structural support. Its use as a stand-alone bone graft substitute has been unsuccessful. It does potentiate the effects of other osteoconductive and osteoinductive substances, including bone marrow and composites of hydroxyapatite and tricalcium phosphate. Its future role will most likely be as an ingredient in bone graft substitute composites.

Coralline Substitutes
The exoskeleton of certain naturally occurring marine corals has many similarities with bone. A number of animal studies have shown the biocompatibility and bioactivity of coralline implants.[33] Vascular tissue readily migrates into its matrix. Either of two general processes is used to prepare marine corals for implantation. The first is a process that uses the calcium carbonate exoskeleton directly after it has undergone a detergent-based process to remove the organic phase of the coral organism. The second general process converts calcium carbonate to hydroxyapatite by a hydrothermal reaction. Both processes result in a coralline product with an osteoconductive matrix that can be used as a bone graft extender.

Beta-Tricalcium Phosphate
Beta-tricalcium phosphate (β-TCP) bone void filler has been developed to mimic the trabecular structure of natural cancellous bone (Vitoss, Orthovita, Malvern, PA). The pores in β-TCP encourage vascularization and bone ingrowth. There has been a shift in bone void fillers from very slowly degradable ceramics (hydroxyapatite) to more rapidly resorbed materials (such as the tricalcium phosphates). A few retrospective studies have evaluated the efficacy of β-TCP in spinal surgery, and controlled clinical studies are being conducted. However, it will most likely play a role in the future as a bone graft extender in arthrodesis surgery.[34]

Osteoinductive Bone Graft Substitutes

Demineralized Bone Matrix
Demineralized bone matrix (DBM) is produced by the decalcification of cortical bone. In 1965, the osteoinductive capability of DBM was first reported.[13,35] The ideal demineralization process removes the calcium and phosphate but leaves the extracellular matrix, which consists predominantly of type I collagen and nonstructural proteins. Included in these proteins are growth factors, the most important of which is BMP. DBM provides no structural strength but it may function as an osteoinductive and conductive material if properly processed and assembled into a final formulation. The degree of osteoinductivity is highly variable between

different manufacturers of DBM and the various final formulations.[36] DBM has variable efficacy based on details of the preparation, carrier material, terminal sterilization, and the environment being tested.[37] Because DBM was regulated as a minimally manipulated tissue (until 2005), extensive studies were not required by the FDA. Therefore, most types of DBM do not have prospective clinical trials demonstrating their efficacy. A prospective randomized clinical study has shown that Grafton DBM (Osteotech, Eatontown, NJ) can be used to extend autograft iliac crest in a 2:1 ratio (Grafton to autograft) and achieve equivalent bone formation in posterolateral instrumented fusion (n = 81).[38]

Bone Morphogenetic Proteins

The BMPs comprise a family of at least 15 structurally related, low-molecular-weight noncollagenous glycoproteins that belong to the transforming growth factor-β superfamily.[39] The BMPs play an important role in embryonic organ development including endochondral and intramembranous bone formation and are believed to promote the normal healing process after fractures. BMPs are known to bind to specific receptors on a variety of different cell types, including MSCs, osteoblasts, and osteoclasts. With lower concentrations, BMPs promote the differentiation of MSCs into chondrocytes, which lay down a cartilaginous matrix. This matrix then calcifies, is invaded by blood vessels, and remodels into mature bone, a process termed endochondral bone formation. At higher concentrations, BMPs can induce direct bone formation, recapitulating normal intramembranous bone formation.[40] The proportion of intramembranous versus endochondral bone formation depends on numerous factors, including the concentration of BMP, the carrier, and the site of implantation.

BMP-2

A large body of work supports the efficacy of BMP-2 as a bone graft substitute. The efficacy of BMP-2 in the treatment of tibia fractures with cortical defects has demonstrated its ability to function as a substitute for iliac crest bone grafting.[41] Most of the work on the BMPs has been done in evaluating their efficacy as a bone graft substitute for use in patients with spinal arthrodesis. Sufficient preclinical studies were performed to determine the appropriate dose and carrier for preclinical models and resulted in 100% spinal fusion rates in most studies. This preparatory work was followed by level 1 prospective clinical trials that then resulted in FDA approval for recombinant human BMP-2 (rhBMP-2) (INFUSE, Medtronic Sofamor Danek, Minneapolis, MN) within a titanium lumbar interbody cage (LT-CAGE, Medtronic Sofamor Danek) for anterior lumbar interbody fusion. As measured by CT scans, anterior lumbar interbody fusion rates were 99.8% for rhBMP-2 (n = 143) and 95.6% for iliac crest (n = 136) at 2-year follow-up.[42] On the strength of these excellent results, INFUSE was approved by the FDA in 2002.

However, this dose and carrier of rhBMP-2 was not consistently effective in the posterolateral application, and changes were made. Using a ceramic carrier (instead of a collagen sponge) and a concentration of 2.0 mg/mL and total dose of 20 mg per side in a human posterolateral fusion pilot experiment, a fusion rate of 100% (20 of 20) for BMP-2 and 40% (2 of 5) for iliac crest was achieved.[43] In a more recent study of 74 patients with a minimum 1-year follow-up, the rhBMP-2 group had statistically higher fusion grades at both 6 months and 12 months of follow-up in comparison with the iliac crest group.[44] The concentration of rhBMP-2 used was 2.0 mg/mL in 10 mL of a ceramic matrix called compression-resistant matrix; this preparation of rhBMP-2 was placed on both sides of the spine, resulting in a total dose of 40 mg of rhBMP-2. FDA approval for posterolateral fusion application of rhBMP-2 is likely in the near future.

BMP-2 has been investigated in a prospective, randomized clinical trial of open tibia fractures. The group that received BMP-2 at the time of definitive closure had fewer bone grafting procedures, fewer patients requiring secondary invasive surgeries, and a lower rate of infection compared with the control group. These clinical trials established the clinical efficacy of BMP-2 combined with an absorbable collagen sponge in the treatment of open tibial fractures.[45]

BMP-7

BMP-7 (osteogenic protein-1 [OP-1]) is another osteoinductive molecule that has undergone extensive study. Preclinical studies have met with success, and clinical studies have been ongoing for some time. The first clinical study for OP-1 involved treatment of nonunion of open tibia fractures.[46] The authors found that 75% of those in the OP-1-treated group and 84% of the autograft-treated patients had radiographic union.[46] An uninstrumented posterolateral fusion pilot study was conducted with 3.5 mg of OP-1 in 1 g of carboxymethylcellulose resulting in 0.875 mg/mL of OP-1 concentration.[47,48] The 1-year follow-up of this study resulted in fusion rates of 74% (14 of 19) in the OP-1 patients and 60% (6 of 10) in the iliac crest bone group, but a subsequent 2-year follow-up resulted in fusion rates of 55% (11 of 20) for OP-1 and 40% (4 of 10) for iliac crest patients. The pivotal FDA study for OP-1 used in posterolateral fusion has not yet been published. However, OP-1 is now available on the basis of an FDA humanitarian device exemption for long bone fractures and spine posterolateral nonunions.

Future Directions

The future will likely provide alternative strategies for delivery of osteoinductive proteins such as BMPs. The delivery of the gene for a BMP so that the protein can be synthesized on site is one alternative that is being investigated. In a rodent study, the gene for BMP was successfully delivered by an injection of a modified adenovirus resulting in a percutaneous posterolateral spine fusion.[49] However, the challenges related to safety of gene therapy will need to be overcome.

As an alternative to delivering the gene for a single BMP, some investigators have identified a gene that seems to coordinate expression of multiple BMPs. This intracellular signaling protein is named LIM mineralization protein-1. This gene has been tranfected into bone marrow cells of rats and reimplanted into posterolateral fusion beds. It proved effective for promoting a solid fusion.[50]

The future will also bring a need for strategies to approach regional and systemic bone formation as a means of preventing fractures before they occur and treating a variety of metabolic bone disorders. A continued improved understanding of the biology of bone healing should help this effort.

Annotated References

1. Court-Brown C, Koval K: The epidemiology of fractures, in Bucholz RW, Heckman JD, Court-Brown C, et al (eds): *Rockwood and Green's Fractures in Adults*, ed 6. Philadelphia, PA, Lippincott Williams & Wilkins, 2005, pp 96-143.

   A general discussion of fracture epidemiology is presented.

2. Boden SD, Schimandle JH: Biologic enhancement of spinal fusion. *Spine* 1995;20:113S-123S.

3. Boden SD, Schimandle JH, Hutton WC, Chen MI: The use of an osteoinductive growth factor for lumbar spinal fusion: Part I. The biology of spinal fusion. *Spine* 1995;20:2626-2632.8747240

4. Morone MA, Boden SD, Martin G, et al: Gene expression during autograft lumbar spine fusion and the effect of bone morphogenetic protein-2. *Clin Orthop Relat Res* 1998;351:252-265.

5. Brown KM, Saunders MM, Kirsch T, Donahue HJ, Reid JS: Effect of COX-2-specific inhibition on fracture-healing in the rat femur. *J Bone Joint Surg Am* 2004;86-A:116-123.

   A nondisplaced unilateral fracture was created in the right femur of 57 adult male rats. Rats were given either no drug, indomethacin (1 mg/kg/d), or celecoxib (3 mg/kg/d) daily, starting on postoperative day 1. At 4 weeks, only the indomethacin group showed biomechanical and radiographic evidence of delayed healing.

6. Gerstenfeld LC, Thiede M, Seibert K, et al: Differential inhibition of fracture healing by non-selective and cyclooxygenase-2 selective non-steroidal anti-inflammatory drugs. *J Orthop Res* 2003;21:670-675.

7. Perry AC, Prpa B, Rouse MS, et al: Levofloxacin and trovafloxacin inhibition of experimental fracture-healing. *Clin Orthop Relat Res* 2003;414:95-100.

8. Huddleston PM, Steckelberg JM, Hanssen AD, Rouse MS, Bolander ME, Patel R: Ciprofloxacin inhibition of experimental fracture healing. *J Bone Joint Surg Am* 2000;82:161-173.

9. Theiss SM, Boden SD, Hair G, Titus L, Morone MA, Ugbo J: The effect of nicotine on gene expression during spine fusion. *Spine* 2000;25:2588-2594.

10. Tortolani PJ, Park AE, Louis-Ugbo J, et al: The effects of doxorubicin (adriamycin) on spinal fusion: An experimental model of posterolateral lumbar spinal arthrodesis. *Spine J* 2004;4:669-674.

    Results indicate that there were no significant differences in wound complications with doxorubicin administration in the animal model studied. A single dose of doxorubicin administered intravenously at the time of surgery appears to play a significant inhibitory role in the process of spinal fusion. If similar effects occur in humans, these data suggest that doxorubicin would be detrimental to bone healing in a spine fusion if administered during the perioperative period.

11. Jones KB, Maiers-Yelden KA, Marsh JL, Zimmerman MB, Estin M, Saltzman CL: Ankle fractures in patients with diabetes mellitus. *J Bone Joint Surg Br* 2005;87:489-495.

    In this retrospective review, 42 patients with diabetes mellitus and a closed rotational ankle fracture were compared with matched controls without diabetes mellitus. Patient's without comorbidities from diabetes mellitus had complication rates equal to controls. Those diabetics with comorbidities had a higher complication rate in regard to infection; below-knee amputation; and nonunion, malunion, or Charcot neuroarthropathy (47% versus 14%).

12. Harrison WJ, Lewis CP, Lavy CB: Open fractures of the tibia in HIV positive patients: A prospective controlled single-blind study. *Injury* 2004;35:852-856.

    The authors prospectively studied 27 patients with severe open fractures and analyzed infection and union as outcome measures. Seven patients were HIV positive, and 20 patients HIV negative. Wound infection and delayed union were more common in HIV positive patients.

13. Urist MR: Bone: Formation by autoinduction. *Science* 1965;150:893-899.

14. Ebraheim NA, Elgafy H, Xu R: Bone-graft harvesting from iliac and fibular donor sites: Techniques and complications. *J Am Acad Orthop Surg* 2001;9:210-218.

15. Arrington ED, Smith WJ, Chambers HG, Bucknell AL, Davino NA: Complications of iliac crest bone graft harvesting. *Clin Orthop Relat Res* 1996;329:300-309.

16. Weiner BK, Walker M: Efficacy of autologous growth

1: Principles of Orthopaedics

factors in lumbar intertransverse fusions. *Spine* 2003; 28:1968-1970.

17. Carreon LY, Glassman SD, Anekstein Y, et al: Platelet gel (AGF) fails to increase fusion rates in instrumented posterolateral fusions. *Spine* 2005;30:E243-E246.

    Results from this study showed that platelet gel failed to enhance the fusion rate when added to autograft in patients undergoing instrumented posterolateral spinal fusion, and is therefore not recommended to supplement autologous bone graft during instrumented posterolateral spinal fusion.

18. Magit DP, Maak T, Trioano N, et al: Healos/rhGDF-5 induces posterolateral lumbar fusion in a New Zealand white rabbit model. *Spine* 2006;31:2180-2188.

    Healos/rhGDF-5 induced fusion in 100% of the rabbits studied, compared with a 38% fusion rate induced by autograft. Overall, these results support continued research of Healos/rhGDF-5 as a potential bone graft alternative.

19. Jorgenson SS, Lowe TG, France J, Sabin J: A prospective analysis of autograft versus allograft in posterolateral lumbar fusion in the same patient: A minimum of 1-year follow-up in 144 patients. *Spine* 1994;19:2048-2053.

20. Dodd CA, Ferguson CM, Freedman L: Allograft versus autograft bone in scoliosis surgery. *J Bone Joint Surg Br* 1988;70:431-434.

21. Schreurs BW, Arts JJ, Verdonschot N, Buma P, Slooff TJ, Gardeniers JW: Femoral component revision with use of impaction bone-grafting and a cemented polished stem: Surgical technique. *J Bone Joint Surg Am* 2006; 88:259-274.

    Thirty-three consecutive femoral reconstructions that were performed between March 1991 and February 1996 with use of the X-change femoral revision system, fresh-frozen morcellized allograft, and a cemented polished Exeter stem were followed prospectively. No femoral reconstruction had been rerevised at a mean of 10.4 years postoperatively. Femoral revision with use of an impaction bone grafting technique and a cemented polished stem resulted in an excellent prosthetic survival rate at 8 to 13 years postoperatively. The major complication that occurred was a femoral fracture in four patients.

22. Schreurs BW, Busch VJ, Welten ML, Verdonschot N, Slooff TJ, Gardeniers JW: Acetabular reconstruction with impaction bone-grafting and a cemented cup in patients younger than fifty years old. *J Bone Joint Surg Am* 2004;86-A:2385-2392.

    Impaction bone grafting technique was used for 23 primary and 19 revision acetabular reconstructions. Twenty-eight patients (31 hips) were available for review after a minimum duration of follow-up of 15 years. All 28 hips (in 25 patients) had retention of the acetabular component for a minimum of 15 years.

23. Zdeblick TA, Ducker TB: The use of freeze-dried allograft bone for anterior cervical fusions. *Spine* 1991; 16:726-729.

24. Tomford WW, Mankin HJ: Bone banking: Update on methods and materials. *Orthop Clin North Am* 1999; 30:565-570.

25. Centers for Disease Control and Prevention: Brief report: Investigation into recalled human tissue for transplantation—United States, 2005-2006. *MMWR Morb Mortal Wkly Rep* 2006;55:564-566.

    This article discusses details of the FDA investigation into a human tissue processing company's violations of the Current Good Tissue Practice Rules of 2005.

26. Transmission of HIV through bone transplantation: Case report and public health recommendations. *MMWR Morb Mortal Wkly Rep* 1988;37:597-599.

27. Chase SW, Herndon CH: The fate of autogenous and homogenous bone grafts. *J Bone Joint Surg Am* 1955; 37:809-814.

28. Jinno T, Miric A, Feighan J, Kirk SK, Davy DT, Stevenson S: The effects of processing and low dose irradiation on cortical bone grafts. *Clin Orthop Relat Res* 2000; 375:275-285.

29. Muschler GF, Negami S, Hyodo A, Gaisser D, Easley K, Kambic H: Evaluation of collagen ceramic composite graft materials in a spinal fusion model. *Clin Orthop Relat Res* 1996;328:250-260.

30. Delecrin J, Takahashi S, Gouin F, Passuti N: A synthetic porous ceramic as a bone graft substitute in the surgical management of scoliosis: A prospective, randomized study. *Spine* 2000;25:563-569.

31. McConnell JR, Freeman BJ, Debnath UK, et al: A prospective randomized comparison of coralline hydroxyapatite with autograft in cervical interbody fusion. *Spine* 2003;28:317-323.

32. McPherson EJ, Dorr LK, Gruen TD, Saberi MT: Hydroxyapatite coated proximal ingrowth femoral stems: A matched pair control study. *Clin Orthop Relat Res* 1995;315:223-230.

33. Khan SN, Fraser JF, Sandhu HS, Cammisa F, Girardi FP, Lane JM: Use of osteopromotive growth factor demineralized bone matrix and ceramics to enhance spine fusions. *J Am Acad Orthop Surg* 2005;13:129-137.

    Autogenous growth factor concentrate, bovine bone-derived osteoinductive protein, and recombinant human MP52 may be used to enhance fusion rates; however, there are few studies that have assessed their efficacy.

34. Epstein NE: A preliminary study of the efficacy of beta tricalcium phosphate as a bone expander for instrumented posterolateral lumbar fusions. *J Spinal Disord Tech* 2006;19:424-429.

    The efficacy of Vitoss β-TCP, an artificial bone substitute, combined with lamina autograft (50:50 mix) in 40 prospective posterolateral fusions using pedicle/screw instrumentation was analyzed. By the sixth postoperative month, fusion was neuroradiologically confirmed on both dynamic radiographs and CT studies for 26 of 27 single level fusions (1 pseudarthrosis) and 11 of 13 two-level fusions (L4-S1).

35. Urist MR, Silverman BF, Buring K, Dubuc FL, Rosenberg JM: The bone induction principle. *Clin Orthop Relat Res* 1967;53:243-283.

36. Bae HW, Zhao L, Kanim LE, Wong P, Delamarter RB, Dawson EG: Intervariability and intravariability of bone morphogenetic proteins in commercially available demineralized bone matrix products. *Spine* 2006;31: 1299-1306.

    Enzyme-linked immunosorbent assay was used to detect BMP-2, -4, and -7 in nine commercially available ("off the shelf") DBM product formulations using three different manufacturer's production lots of each DBM formulation. There is higher variability in concentration of BMPs among three different lots of the same DBM formulation than among different DBM formulations.

37. Peterson B, Whang PG, Iglesias R, Wang JC, Lieberman JR: Osteoinductivity of commercially available demineralized bone matrix: Preparations in a spine fusion model. *J Bone Joint Surg Am* 2004;86-A:2243-2250.

    The efficacy of three different commercially available DBM products for inducing spinal fusion was compared using an athymic rat model.

38. Cammisa FP Jr, Lowery G, Garfin SR, et al: Two-year fusion rate equivalency between Grafton DBM gel and autograft in posterolateral spine fusion: A prospective controlled trial employing a side-by-side comparison in the same patient. *Spine* 2004;29:660-666.

    A total of 120 patients underwent posterolateral spine fusion with pedicle screw fixation and bone grafting. Iliac crest autograft was implanted on one side of the spine and a Grafton DBM/autograft composite was implanted on the contralateral side in the same patient.

39. Wozney JM, Rosen V: Bone morphogenetic protein and bone morphogenetic protein gene family in bone formation and repair. *Clin Orthop Relat Res* 1998;346:26-37.

40. Morone MA, Boden SD, Martin G, et al: Gene expression during autograft lumbar spine fusion and the effect of bone morphogenetic protein-2. *Clin Orthop Relat Res* 1998;351:252-265.

41. Jones AL, Bucholz RW, Bosse MJ, et al: BMP-2 Evaluation in Surgery for Tibial Trauma-Allgraft (BESTT-ALL) study group: Recombinant human BMP-2 and allograft compared with autogenous bone graft for reconstruction of diaphyseal tibial fractures with cortical defects: A randomized, controlled trial. *J Bone Joint Surg Am* 2006;88:1431-1441.

    Adult patients (15 in each study arm) with a tibial diaphyseal fracture and a residual cortical defect were randomly assigned to receive either autogenous bone graft or allograft (cancellous bone chips) for staged reconstruction of the tibial defect. Patients in the allograft group also received an onlay application of rhBMP-2 on an absorbable collagen sponge. Ten patients in the autograft group and 13 patients in the rhBMP-2/allograft group had healing without further intervention.

42. McKay B, Sandhu HS: Use of recombinant human bone morphogenetic protein-2 in spinal fusion applications. *Spine* 2002;27:S66-S85.

43. Boden SD, Kang J, Sandhu H, et al: Use of recombinant human bone morphogenetic protein-2 to achieve posterolateral lumbar spine fusion in humans: A prospective, randomized clinical pilot trial. *Spine* 2002;27:2662-2673.

44. Glassman SD, Dimar JR, Carreon LY, et al: Initial fusion rates with recombinant human bone morphogenetic protein-2/compression resistant matrix and a hydroxyapatite and tricalcium phosphate/collagen carrier in posterolateral spinal fusion. *Spine* 2005;30:1694-1698.

    This article reports a prospective, randomized, unblinded study of iliac crest bone graft versus rhBMP-2/compression-resistant matrix in a posterolateral instrumented fusion procedure. At 1 year after surgery, the mean fusion grade was 4.62 in the rhBMP-2/compression-resistant matrix group versus 3.77 in the iliac crest bone graft group ($P < 0.0023$).

45. Swiontkowski MF, Aro HT, Donell S, et al: Recombinant human bone morphogenetic protein-2 in open tibial fractures: A subgroup analysis of data combined from two prospective randomized studies. *J Bone Joint Surg Am* 2006;88:1258-1265.

    Two prospective, randomized clinical studies were conducted. A total of 510 patients with open tibial fractures were randomized to receive the control treatment (intramedullary nail fixation and routine soft-tissue management) or the control treatment and an absorbable collagen sponge impregnated with one of two concentrations of rhBMP-2. The rhBMP-2 implant was placed over the fracture at the time of definitive wound closure. Two subgroups were analyzed: (1) the 131 patients with a Gustilo-Anderson type-IIIA or IIIB open tibial fracture and (2) the 113 patients treated with reamed intramedullary nailing. The first subgroup demonstrated significant improvements in the rhBMP-2 group, with fewer bone grafting procedures ($P = 0.0005$), fewer patients requiring invasive secondary interventions ($P = 0.0065$), and a lower rate of infection ($P = 0.0234$), compared with the control group.

46. Friedlaender GE, Perry CR, Cole JD, et al: Osteogenic protein-1 (bone morphogenetic protein-7) in the treatment of tibial nonunions. *J Bone Joint Surg Am* 2001; 83(suppl 1):S151-S158.

47. Vaccaro AR, Patel T, Fischgrund J, et al: A pilot study evaluating the safety and efficacy of OP-1 Putty (rhBMP-7) as a replacement for iliac crest autograft in posterolateral lumbar arthrodesis for degenerative spondylolisthesis. *Spine* 2004;29:1885-1892.

    Thirty-six patients with degenerative lumbar spondylolisthesis and symptoms of neurogenic claudication were randomized (2:1) to either OP-1 Putty (Stryker, Kalamazoo, MI) (3.5 mg of OP-1 per side) or autogenous iliac crest bone graft for single-level uninstrumented posterolateral fusion following a decompressive laminectomy. Fourteen of 19 (74%) OP-1 Putty patients and 6 of 10 (60%) autograft patients achieved a successful posterolateral fusion, fulfilling all fusion criteria.

48. Vaccaro AR, Anderson DG, Patel T, et al: Comparison of OP-1 Putty (rhBMP-7) to iliac crest autograft for posterolateral lumbar arthrodesis: A minimum 2-year follow-up pilot study. *Spine* 2005;30:2709-2716.

Efficacy data were tabulated for 27 patients at the 24-month time point and an additional 4 patients (without evaluatable 24-month results) at the 36-month time point. A successful posterolateral fusion was achieved in 11 of 20 (55%) OP-1 Putty patients and 4 of 10 (40%) autograft patients.

49. Alden TD, Pittman DD, Beres EJ, et al: Percutaneous spinal fusion using bone morphogenetic protein-2 gene therapy. *J Neurosurg*;1999:109-114.

50. Boden SD, Titus L, Hair G, et al: Lumbar spine fusion by local gene therapy with a cDNA encoding a novel osteoinductive protein (LMP-1). *Spine* 1998;23:2486-2492.

Chapter 3

Articular Cartilage and Intervertebral Disk

Hubert T. Kim, MD, PhD   S. Tim Yoon, MD, PhD   Claudius Jarrett, MD

Articular Cartilage

Articular cartilage is a highly specialized tissue ideally suited to its function as a bearing surface for mobile joints. Biomechanically, articular cartilage acts as a fiber-reinforced composite matrix able to withstand and distribute physiologic loads without mechanical failure. For many people, articular cartilage provides a lifetime of excellent joint function. However, cartilage injury and degeneration remain major health care problems with tremendous societal costs. Recent advances in the understanding of cartilage biology and emerging technologies for the treatment of cartilage injuries may help reduce this burden.

Composition and Organization

Articular cartilage is a relatively acellular tissue; more than 90% of its volume is composed of extracellular matrix. The major components of this matrix are collagen, proteoglycans, and water.[1] Collagens account for approximately 60% of articular cartilage dry weight. Ninety percent is type II, but cartilage also contains small amounts of collagen types VI, IX, X, and XI. Collagen fibers within articular cartilage form a complex framework with a distinctive cross-sectional architecture (**Figure 1**). The superficial zone is characterized by collagen fibers oriented parallel to the joint surface; these fibers provide tensile strength and resistance to shear across the articular surface. The transitional zone contains larger diameter collagen fibers oriented in a more random manner, gradually transitioning from the horizontal arrangement in the superficial zone to the vertical columnar arrangement of the deep zone. The deep zone has the largest diameter collagen fibers. These collagen fibers insert into the tidemark that marks the transition between the deep zone and the zone of calcified cartilage.

Proteoglycans comprise 25% to 35% of cartilage dry weight. Proteoglycan content varies among the different zones, with a relatively low concentration in the superficial zone and the highest concentration in the deep zone. Large aggregating proteoglycans, or aggrecans, are the predominant proteoglycans in articular cartilage. Aggrecans consist of large numbers of extended glycosaminoglycan (GAG) chains attached to a protein core. Most aggrecans in articular cartilage are bound tightly to hyaluronic acid, forming extremely large proteoglycan aggregates of up to several hundred million daltons in size. Aggrecan molecules trapped within the collagen framework provide elastic strength to the matrix. Their strong negative charge acts as an attractant for water molecules that constitute 60% to 80% of articular cartilage wet weight. These water molecules provide fluid pressurization of the matrix, which is the primary load-support mechanism for articular cartilage.

Maintenance of this complex extracellular matrix is the responsibility of chondrocytes that reside within the matrix. Although cells in all layers of articular cartilage are termed chondrocytes, it is clear that not all chondrocytes are the same. In fact, significant differences have been shown based on location within the extracellular matrix.[2] Chondrocytes in the superficial zone are small and flattened, with small lacunae (**Figure 1**). They are aligned with their long axes parallel to the joint surface, following the orientation of the collagen network. These cells express little proteoglycan and relatively large amounts of collagen. Superficial zone cells also express lubricin and superficial zone protein, two key joint lubrication proteins. Chondrocytes in the transitional and deep zones are rounded in appearance and reside in larger lacunae. The metabolic activity of deep

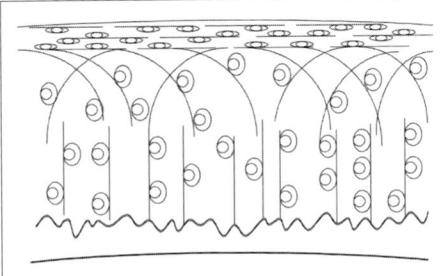

Superficial zone

Transitional zone

Deep zone

Tidemark
Calcified cartilage

Bone

Figure 1   Articular cartilage cross-sectional architecture. The chondrocytes in the superficial zone are small and flattened; in the transitional and deep zones, they are rounded and reside in larger lacunae.

zone chondrocytes may be as much as 10 times that of superficial zone cells. Studies have also shown substantial zonal differences in chondrocyte responsiveness to cytokines and other diffusible signaling molecules.[3]

Recent studies have identified a small number of cells within articular cartilage that may represent a chondrocyte stem cell population.[4] These cells, localized primarily in the superficial zone, express stem cell markers and exhibit multilineage differentiation potential. In vitro experiments have shown that these potential stem cells are responsive to growth factor stimulation and can migrate to the articular surface. However, the precise function(s) of these cells and their contribution to cartilage maintenance and/or repair are not known.

Degeneration in Osteoarthritis, Rheumatoid Arthritis, and After Mechanical Injury

One paradigm for cartilage degeneration in osteoarthritis is based on the concept of three overlapping stages: (1) matrix damage/alteration, (2) chondrocyte repair response, and (3) progressive tissue loss caused by a decline in repair effectiveness.[5] The first stage may be initiated by mechanical overload, inflammation, and/or metabolic perturbations that affect normal matrix maintenance. This stage is characterized by decreased organization of the collagen framework with altered relationships between minor collagens and the type II collagen fibrils. Matrix proteoglycan content is decreased, with less proteoglycan aggregation and shorter GAG chains. These changes negatively affect the mechanical properties of the cartilage matrix, reducing its ability to function in a normal manner and making it more susceptible to further damage. The second stage is marked by chondrocyte responses directed toward repair of the damaged matrix. These responses include chondrocyte proliferation (cloning), as well as enhanced chondrocyte anabolic activity with markedly increased synthesis of matrix components. At the same time, catabolic activity is increased, presumably to remove damaged matrix components and to facilitate matrix remodeling. Paradoxically, this upregulation of matrix-degrading enzymes likely contributes to the progression of cartilage degeneration. The extent to which these repair responses can halt or slow cartilage degeneration is quite variable. Eventually, chondrocyte repair responses decline with aging, leading to progressive cartilage tissue loss that marks the third phase of cartilage degeneration. This decline in biosynthetic capacity is caused by a combination of chondrocyte death, limited proliferative capacity, and decreased responsiveness to anabolic signals.

Cartilage degeneration in rheumatoid arthritis is driven by an autoimmune inflammatory response that is likely initiated by activation of antigen-specific T cells. This activation initiates a cascade of events including endothelial and synovial cell proliferation, and production of proinflammatory cytokines including tumor necrosis factor-alpha (TNF-α) and interleukin (IL)-1. The development of an invasive synovial tissue (pannus) composed of synoviocytes, lymphocytes, and macrophages results in erosive destruction of articular cartilage and adjacent bone. Proinflammatory cytokines induce chondrocytes to secrete matrix-degrading enzymes and osteoclasts to resorb bone. Thus, cartilage and bone, as well as supporting soft-tissue structures, are degraded by both intrinsic and extrinsic mechanisms, eventually leading to a characteristic clinical picture of cartilage loss, bony erosion, joint instability, and deformity.

Cartilage degeneration after mechanical injury shares many of the same processes seen in osteoarthritis, but often progresses at a more rapid pace. Factors contributing to this accelerated time course include catastrophic disruption of cartilage matrix integrity and structure; extensive chondrocyte death in the area of cartilage injury; expansion of this "zone of injury" facilitated by diffusible mediators; and persistent mechanical overload caused by associated joint incongruity, instability, and/or limb malalignment.[6] In vitro data show that the extent of cartilage damage is related to both the peak strain and strain rate. Injurious compression disrupts the collagen framework, resulting in decreased load-carrying capacity. Mechanical injury is also associated with proteoglycan loss, both from alterations to the chondrocyte biosynthetic activity and from chondrocyte death. Mechanical overload causes chondrocytes to upregulate their expression of matrix-degrading enzymes including ADAMTS-5 and several matrix metalloproteinases (MMPs), which may play a major role in subsequent cartilage degeneration.

Apoptosis

Apoptosis (programmed cell death) is a highly regulated process that plays a critical role in normal skeletal growth and development. Apoptosis in normal adult articular cartilage is a rare event. However, abnormally increased chondrocyte apoptosis is associated with cartilage damage and degeneration. Several studies have shown elevated levels of chondrocyte apoptosis in samples of cartilage obtained from patients with arthritis.[7,8] Very high levels of chondrocyte apoptosis are associated with intra-articular fractures and acute cartilage injury. The specific factors that promote chondrocyte apoptosis are not fully understood. However, it is likely that matrix disruption plays a major role through the loss of integrin-mediated survival signals. Other contributing factors that are likely to promote apoptosis include the release of proapoptotic cytokines and reactive oxygen species by infiltrating inflammatory cells, as well as exposure of the chondrocytes to blood.

Perhaps the most intriguing aspect of chondrocyte apoptosis is the possibility that blockade of the pathways responsible for the initiation and/or execution of apoptosis may prevent chondrocyte loss associated with cartilage injury. A series of recent studies have shown that growth factors and inhibitors of key apoptotic mediators can block chondrocyte apoptosis both in vitro and in vivo. For example, Z-VAD-fmk, a broad-spectrum caspase inhibitor, was shown to block chondrocyte apoptosis and subsequent cartilage loss in vivo in animal models of cartilage injury and osteoarthritis.[9] Collectively, this area of research suggests apoptosis inhibition may be a useful therapeutic approach for both acute and chronic forms of cartilage injury and degeneration.

Biomarkers

Articular cartilage degeneration is associated with increased synthesis and degradation of matrix molecules. These degradation products can be detected in joint fluid, blood, and urine. The development of analytical techniques to measure these biomarkers has advanced rapidly and may soon represent a useful set of tools for the analysis of articular cartilage degeneration. Theoretically, biomarkers could provide a way to identify patients with very early arthritis before radiographic changes are apparent, or patients at high risk for rapid disease progression. Biomarkers also could be used as a sensitive tool to monitor the effects of emerging treatments of cartilage degeneration.[10] For example, elevated urinary levels of specific type II collagen cleavage products (Helix-II and CTX-II) were shown to be associated with rapidly destructive hip osteoarthritis. Similarly, in a 3-year study of 333 patients with hip osteoarthritis, urinary CTX-II and serum hyaluronan levels were identified as positive predictors of disease progression. Markedly elevated concentrations of CTX-II, as well as proteoglycan fragments, were found in joint fluid obtained after anterior cruciate ligament and meniscus surgeries. These findings demonstrate the potential utility of matrix degradation products as useful markers. However, a recent study of 120 women with knee arthritis failed to show a correlation between CTX-II and disease progression, indicating that interpretation and application of these new tools remains a work in progress.[11]

Cartilage breakdown products are not the only biomarkers that may prove useful. In a recent study, microarray and reverse transcription-polymerase chain reaction analyses of blood from patients with early osteoarthritis identified a set of genes that were consistently downregulated.[12] Using a linear combination of nine marker genes, the investigators were able to distinguish patients with mild arthritis from normal control patients with a sensitivity of 86% and a specificity of 83%. However, blinded application of this tool to a second set of patients yielded a decrease in sensitivity and specificity to 72% and 66%, respectively. Nevertheless, this study provided proof of the concept of "gene profiling" as a potentially useful biomarker, and it is certain that this technology will advance rapidly.

Genetic Factors

It is commonly believed that the pathophysiology of osteoarthritis involves both genetic and physical factors. Recently, experiments using knockout mice have identified some of the genes that may contribute to the development of arthritis. A pair of studies identified ADAMTS-5, an aggrecanase, as a critical mediator of cartilage degradation. In these studies, deletion of the ADAMTS-5 gene protected mice from cartilage degeneration in models of osteoarthritis and inflammatory arthritis.[13] Other studies demonstrated that deletion of the collagen IX gene in mice also produces early arthritis. Genetic defects in ADAMTS-5 have not, so far, been directly associated with osteoarthritis in humans. However, a recent genetic analysis of 481 families with arthritis found strong linkage of the type IX collagen gene to female patients with osteoarthritis.[14] Together, these and other studies strongly suggest that genes involved in matrix production and degradation contribute to the development and progression of cartilage degeneration.

Treatment and Repair

Disease-Modifying Drugs

Although disease-modifying antirheumatic drugs are extremely effective treatments of patients with inflammatory joint diseases, no drugs have been proven definitively to prevent or delay the progression of cartilage degeneration in patients with osteoarthritis. Drugs most commonly used for the management of osteoarthritis include acetaminophen, nonsteroidal anti-inflammatory drugs, and narcotics. All are effective analgesics, but none have a significant effect on cartilage degeneration. Similarly, intra-articular injection of steroids or hyaluronic acid can provide short-term symptomatic relief, but neither appears to slow disease progression. Therefore, the search for effective disease-modifying osteoarthritis drugs continues.

Nutritional supplements, most commonly glucosamine and chondroitin sulfate, are widely promoted as effective treatments of cartilage degeneration. Several European prospective randomized clinical studies have reported radiographic evidence of cartilage preservation in patients with knee osteoarthritis. In a study of 202 patients, glucosamine (1,500 mg daily) maintained joint space over a 3-year period compared with placebo (treated = + 0.04 mm, 95% confidence interval [CI] − 0.06 to + 0.14; control = − 0.19 mm, 95% CI − 0.29 to − 0.09; $P = 0.001$), suggesting disease-modifying activity. Similarly, in a 2-year study of 300 patients, chondroitin sulfate (800 mg daily) prevented progression of joint-space narrowing (treated = 0.00 ± 0.61 mm; control = 0.14 loss ± 0.61 mm; $P = 0.04$), but yielded no symptomatic benefit.[15,16] However, data from other similar studies have provided conflicting results, rendering assertions about disease modification somewhat weaker. The National Institutes of Health Glucosamine/Chondroitin Arthritis Intervention Trial, involving over 1,500 patients, did not find clear evidence for symptomatic benefit for the group as a whole; however, a subgroup analysis of patients with moderate to severe pain did show some benefit from oral glucosamine/chondroitin in regard to pain relief.[17] Analyses of the effects on disease progression have not yet been released.

Other candidate disease-modifying osteoarthritis drugs have shown some potential benefit in clinical tri-

1: Principles of Orthopaedics

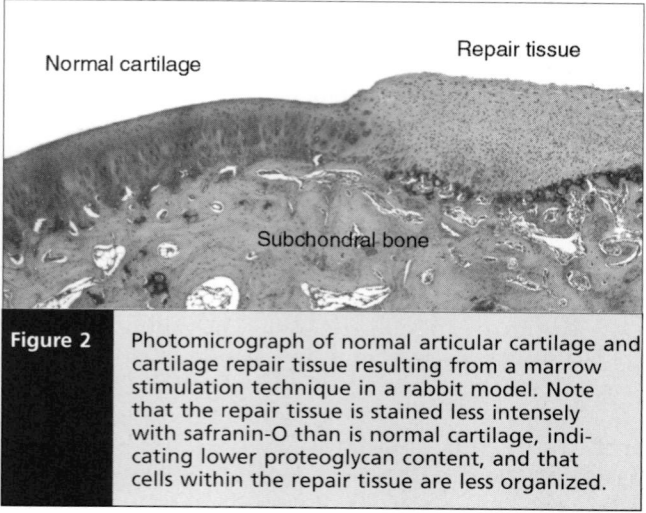

Figure 2 Photomicrograph of normal articular cartilage and cartilage repair tissue resulting from a marrow stimulation technique in a rabbit model. Note that the repair tissue is stained less intensely with safranin-O than is normal cartilage, indicating lower proteoglycan content, and that cells within the repair tissue are less organized.

als. Diacetylrhein (diacerein) has been shown to block the catabolic mediator IL-1 and decrease production of cartilage matrix-degrading enzymes. Modest pain relief appears to be a consistent finding for hip and knee osteoarthritis patients receiving diacerein.[18] In a large 3-year randomized controlled clinical trial of patients with hip osteoarthritis, progressive joint-space narrowing was decreased in patients receiving diacerein (100 mg/d). However, the difference was relatively small (treated = 0.18 ± 0.25 mm/y; placebo = 0.23 ± 0.23 mm/y; $P = 0.042$), and similar trials conducted on patients with knee osteoarthritis have yielded conflicting results. Tetracycline-class antibiotics such as doxycycline and minocycline also block cytokine-mediated catabolic pathways. In a large clinical trial of obese women with knee osteoarthritis, patients receiving doxycycline (200 mg/d) had 40% less joint-space loss compared with control patients over the 16-month treatment period, and 33% less after 30 months.[19]

At the present time, potential disease-modifying osteoarthritis drugs such as recombinant growth factors, specific MMP inhibitors, and cytokine antagonists have not been proven to be safe and effective enough for general clinical use. However, preclinical and clinical data from ongoing trials of related drugs are encouraging and may yield effective therapeutic options in the near future.

Repair Procedures
Cartilage repair technology has advanced rapidly over the past decade. The three most commonly performed cartilage repair procedures are microfracture, mosaicplasty, and autologous chondrocyte implantation (ACI). Microfracture and related marrow-stimulation techniques are based on mechanical débridement of damaged and/or unstable cartilage followed by penetration of the subchondral bone in the area of cartilage damage to allow the egress of marrow elements. These marrow elements, which include cells capable of differentiating into cartilage, fill the defect and mature over time into cartilage repair tissue (**Figure 2**). The repair

tissue is composed primarily of fibrocartilage, although some of the repair tissue may have a hyaline-like appearance. Animal studies have demonstrated that the formation of hyaline cartilage is enhanced by continuous passive motion, which is typically part of the postoperative therapy. Clinical studies on the use of continuous passive motion for cartilage repair are limited, and the results are mixed. For small (< 4 cm²) focal articular cartilage defects, microfracture appears to be effective. A recent short-term prospective cohort study reported good or excellent knee function in 32 of 48 patients (67%) at 2 years. Improvement correlated with good defect filling on MRI, low body mass index, and a short duration of symptoms.[20] Long-term data are sparse, but one study of 72 patients (75 knees) reported 80% patients "improved" based on self-administered questionnaires.[21] However, normal cartilage composition and structure are never restored, and it is commonly accepted that the eventual fate of this repair tissue is progressive degeneration.

Mosaicplasty involves the transfer of cylindrical osteochondral plugs from an area of normal cartilage to size-matched recipient sites. An advantage of this technique is that the area of damaged or missing cartilage is replaced by mature, normal cartilage tissue and underlying bone. However, factors that are of concern include donor-site morbidity, inability to completely fill defects, and difficulty restoring the contour of the articular surface. The developers of the technique have reported encouraging short- and intermediate-term results. Of their 831 patients, good to excellent clinical results were achieved in 92% of the patients treated for femoral condyle lesions, 87% of those treated for tibial lesions, 79% of those treated for patellar and/or trochlear lesions, and in 94% of the patients treated for talar lesions.[22] A similar procedure using osteochondral allograft tissue in place of autologous tissue may be particularly useful for very large chondral lesions and for osteochondral lesions with significant bone loss or necrosis. However, rigorous clinical outcomes data for this procedure are limited.

ACI represents the first use of a tissue engineering approach to address orthopaedic pathology. In this procedure, cartilage biopsies are obtained in the first of two surgical procedures. Chondrocytes are released from the tissue by enzymatic digestion and expanded in tissue culture. The cells are then injected as a cell suspension under a periosteal patch sewn over the cartilage defect site. These cells produce repair tissue that is a mixture of hyaline-like cartilage and fibrocartilage. Interestingly, there is some evidence that the repair tissue matures over time and becomes more hyaline-like. Short- and intermediate-term clinical results have been encouraging, with favorable clinical results reported by multiple groups. The developers of the ACI technique reported their 2- to 9-year outcomes on 94 patients.[23] Good or excellent clinical results were seen in 92% of those with an isolated femoral condylar lesion. Results were not as good for those with multiple lesions (67% good or excellent) or patellar lesions (65% good or excellent). "Second generation" techniques incorporate a synthetic matrix to retain the cultured chondrocytes and eliminate the need for periosteum, thus simplifying the procedure and reducing morbidity. Matrices synthesized from porcine collagen and hyaluronic acid both have been shown to be clinically effective, with short-term results comparable to those obtained with traditional ACI.

Despite several clinical series reporting better results from ACI, randomized clinical trials have not demonstrated clear superiority of ACI over microfracture or mosaicplasty.[24] All three techniques appear to be reasonably effective, at least in the short- or intermediate-term, given the right clinical situation. However, each has significant limitations, and none of them can completely restore an area of damaged cartilage to a normal state. However, as understanding of these techniques is increased, it is likely that their use can be optimized by manipulating the biologic processes that impact their success.

Intervertebral Disk

Intervertebral disks are essential components of the axial skeleton that allow for a combination of stability and mobility of the spine. Disks are articulating cartilaginous units between adjacent vertebrae that bind the vertebrae together while permitting physiologic motion. The superior and inferior boundaries of the disk are composed of the disk end plates, which provide the bulk of the nutritional pathway for the intradiskal cells. Between the end plates, the disk is composed of a firm fibrosus ring, the anulus fibrosus, and a softer gelatinous interior structure, the nucleus pulposus. Each element has its own unique structure and mechanical properties. Analogous to other connective tissues, the extracellular matrix found within intervertebral disk allows for its mechanical characteristics. The cellular population is more abundant during juvenile life and becomes relatively sparse in the adult, comprising only 1% of the total volume in the adult disk. The intradiskal cells manufacture and maintain the disk matrix.[25]

Gross Morphologic Structure
The anulus fibrosus is made of an outer and an inner segment. The outer layers are filled with tightly packed, highly organized type I collagen arranged in sheets. The inner portion is larger and less organized, and has an increasing concentration of proteoglycans toward the center of the disk. Early in life, the lamellae in the anulus fibrosus is composed of distinct individual bundles. By adulthood, they transform into intricate interdigitating, branching layers with increasing thickness. The cells in the anulus fibrosus are fibroblast-like, appear elongated, generally align with the collagen fibers, and produce varying amounts of collagen types I and II. The anulus fibrosus is connected to the adjacent vertebrae by collagen fibers that pierce the vertebral end plates. This anatomic relationship between the anulus

fibrosus and end plate connects and stabilizes the anterior portion of the spinal column.[25]

The nucleus pulposus is positioned centrally within the disk and takes up approximately one half of the volume of a normal disk. Water comprises approximately 70% of the nucleus pulposus of a normal disk by adulthood. The nucleus pulposus has a paucity of cells when compared with the anulus fibrosus. Unlike those found in the anulus fibrosus, cells in the nucleus pulposus are spherical or oval in shape and are referred to as being chondrocyte-like. The nucleus pulposus cells typically generate a higher proportion of type II collagen than those found in the anulus fibrosus. The nucleus pulposus cells also produce a disk matrix composed of a diverse population of proteoglycans and collagen molecules. Morphologically, the nucleus pulposus appears gel-like and translucent in younger adults and gradually becomes more fibrous and opaque with age.

The vertebral end plates form the superior and inferior boundaries of the intervertebral disk. The end plates are composed of bony and cartilaginous components. The bony end plate consists of a condensation of cancellous bone that is much denser than cancellous bone and more like cortical bone. Subadjacent to the dense bone is a heavily vascularized bed of cancellous bone, which forms the major route for nutrients to cross into the disk by diffusion. The cartilaginous component of the end plate is adjacent to the bony end plate and within the disk. The cartilaginous tissue is high in collagen type II and proteoglycans.[25,26]

Composition and Organization
The two major constituents of the extracellular matrix in intervertebral disks are proteoglycans and collagens. The concentration of collagen and proteoglycan molecules varies depending on the location within the disk. Collagen comprises a far larger percentage of the dry weight of the anulus fibrosus (as much as 70%) than of the nucleus pulposus (15% to 20%). In comparison, proteoglycans form a greater portion, as much as 60%, of the nucleus pulposus compared with the anulus fibrosus. In the aging disk, the proteoglycan content progressively decreases.[27]

The proteoglycans in the disks can be grouped into the large aggregating proteoglycans and the small leucine-rich proteoglycans (SLRPs). Aggrecan is the prototypical large aggregating proteoglycan found in the extracellular matrix of the disk. Large numbers of aggregan molecules are grouped together by a long chain of hyaluronic acid molecules. Aggrecan itself is composed of a core protein that forms the chain to which hundreds of sulfated GAGs are attached. Chondroitin sulfate and keratan sulfate are the most common GAGs associated with aggrecans. Keratan sulfate is less abundant in a normal disk, but increases in concentration as the disk degenerates. The fixed negative charges found on aggrecan are mainly attributed to the sulfated GAGs. This large net negative charge attracts and retains water molecules, thus creating a swelling pressure within the disk. This provides the characteris-

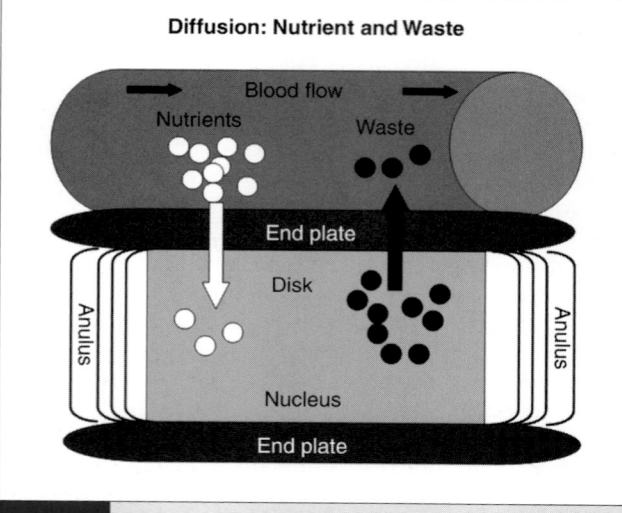

Diffusion: Nutrient and Waste

Blood flow

Nutrients

Waste

End plate

Disk

Anulus

Anulus

Nucleus

End plate

Figure 3	Illustration of intervertebral disk nutritional flow. Vertebral body blood flow brings nutrients to the end plate. Then the nutrients diffuse across the end plate to reach disk cells. The metabolic waste products leave the disk tissue across the end plate by diffusion, to be carried away by blood flow.

tic compressive strength of normal intervertebral disks.[27]

Versican is another aggregating large molecular weight proteoglycan found in the disk. It is organized in much the same way as aggrecan, with a core protein and associated GAG molecules. Versican, however, has fewer GAG binding sites than aggrecan and therefore is potentially less effective at attracting water as compared with aggrecan. Versican also has messenger RNA splice variants that result in slightly different compositions, but the significance of these variants is not yet known.

Several different SLRPs are found in the disk (fibromodulin, decorin, lumican, and biglycan). These molecules are small in comparison with aggrecan and versican. SLRPs do not contain the large negative charges necessary to be efficient at attracting water. Rather, SLRPs have different functions including binding to collagens, growth factors, and other matrix components. SLRPs are believed to play important roles in the regulation of extracellular matrix assembly and cell-matrix interaction.

Multiple collagen types are found in the disk. Fibrillar collagens form well-ordered sheets in the anulus fibrosus and a network of collagen fibers within the nucleus pulposus. To maximize their stability and ability to handle high mechanical loads, collagen fibers are heavily cross-linked with various molecules coupled to their surfaces such as collagen types V and XI. Type V is often bound directly to the surface of type I collagen (anulus fibrosus) and thus has a higher concentration in the regions of the disks where type I predominates. Type XI is covalently cross-linked to type II collagen and is present at higher levels where type II prevails

(nucleus pulposus).[27] The concentration of type II collagen is higher in the nucleus pulposus and rises progressively toward the center of the disk. Approximately 80% of the total collagen content in the nucleus pulposus is type II. Collagen types III, V, and XI are present but in low concentrations in the intervertebral disk. Short collagen fibers that do not form fibrils, such as collagen type VI, also are present in the disks. An assortment of noncollagenous proteins such as elastin and cartilage intermediate-layer protein also are present and account for 20% to 45% of the dry weight of the nucleus pulposus.

Disk Nutrition

The intervertebral disk in a normal adult is largely avascular. There are only meager capillary endings along the superficial perimeter of the anulus fibrosus, and the rest of the disk acquires its nutritional supply through diffusion. Most of the diffusion into the disk occurs through the disk end plates via a rich network of capillaries that terminate on the vertebral body side of the end plate. The highest concentration of capillaries is found within the center of the end plates, and there are lower concentrations of capillaries toward the periphery of the disk. A diffusion gradient exists such that glucose, amino acids, and other nutrients diffuse into the disk, and waste products diffuse out of the disk into the capillary bed[28,29] (Figure 3). The diffusion gradient is such that at the center of the disk there are lower concentrations of glucose and oxygen compared with the regions closer to the end plate. Thus, cells further away from the end plates and superficial anulus fibrosus are in a more hypoxic and nutritionally challenging environment. Nucleus pulposus cells have adapted to these conditions and actually synthesize more proteoglycans in hypoxic environments. Insufficient nutrient transport to the disk can theoretically occur with end-plate pathology, and such pathology would be expected to cause degenerative changes in the center of the disk first. Studies have shown that critical imbalance between disk cell nutrition and cell density can lead to cell death.[28]

Disk Changes With Age and Degeneration

The morphology of the intervertebral disk in the juvenile is different from that of the mature adult. In the newborn, the nucleus pulposus occupies nearly one half of the total disk volume, a larger percentage than that at maturity. The gross appearance of the nucleus pulposus is a clear, watery gelatinous matrix in the very young disk, but with age the nucleus pulposus becomes more opaque, less hydrated, and firm. In the young disk, there is a clear boundary between the anulus fibrosus and nucleus pulposus, but with age the boundary becomes less well delineated. The degree of disorganization between the anulus fibrosus and the nucleus pulposus has been used as a measure of disk degeneration. With age, the disks increase significantly in size, thus increasing the distance of the central cells from the surrounding blood supply. Furthermore, many of the blood vessels found in the outer anulus fibrosus in children disappear with age. This change in size and vascularity leads to greater challenges in supplying nutrients to the central portion of the disk.

The cellular composition of the young disk consists of many notochordal cells, but after 10 years of age notochordal cells are not seen in the disk. Rather, in the more mature disk, the nucleus pulposus cells are more chondrocyte-like. Recent animal experiments suggest that end-plate chondrocytes invade into the nucleus during the degenerative process. During adolescence, the notochordal cells, found in ample supply in the newborn nucleus pulposus, are gradually replaced by more adult chondrocyte-like cells. With age, there is a significant decrease in the total number of viable cells in the disk. By adulthood, the disk is the most sparsely populated tissue throughout the entire body.[30]

The nucleus pulposus has its highest proteoglycan and water content during the juvenile years and it gradually diminishes with age. By adolescence, there is a notable increase in the number of collagen fibers and a decrease in the concentration of proteoglycans in the nucleus pulposus compared with that of early childhood. It seems that the production of newly synthesized aggrecan diminishes with age in the nucleus pulposus. In the adult, the inner anulus fibrosus increases in thickness and replaces the region previously occupied by the outer nucleus pulposus. As the amount of proteoglycans and thus water decreases while the concentration of fibrous tissue increases, the nucleus pulposus transforms into a firmer, less spongy, and less translucent substance. In the adult, the collagen layers of the outer anulus fibrosus start to degenerate. More variability in the diameter and the space between collagen fibrils develop. The development of noncollagenous granular material in the extracellular matrix also disrupts the neatly organized layering found in the newborn and adolescent anulus fibrosus. By late adulthood, the nucleus pulposus has continued to increase in its fibrous tissue content and becomes a very rigid fibrocartilaginous structure. In elderly people, it is difficult to distinguish the nucleus pulposus from its surrounding inner anulus fibrosus. The disk continues to lose its height and structure, allowing it to bulge at the periphery.[30]

Causes of Disk Degeneration

Genetic causes seem to be the largest known factor that contributes to disk degeneration. A Scandinavian study of identical twins was performed and various factors that might be important in disk degeneration were analyzed.[31] Factors that were considered included age, smoking, mechanical loads, and genetics. The factor that had the most impact on disk degeneration was genetics, accounting for approximately 30% to 50% of the variability in disk degeneration in the lumbar spine. However, genetic factors were not perfect predictors of disk degeneration. In the low lumbar region (L4 to S1), more than 50% of the disk degeneration could not be attributed to any known factor. Thus, genetic factors seem to indicate a predilection for disk degeneration

but are not directly predictive. Furthermore, a genetic predilection does not indicate that biologic interventions cannot be effective in preventing or reversing disk degeneration, much like individuals with a genetic predisposition to cardiac disease may modify their risk profile with diet and exercise.

Individual genes have been implicated in disk degeneration. This includes aggrecan, vitamin D receptor, aspirin, and cartilage intermediate-layer protein. Gene disruption experiments also have indicated that mutation in structural genes such as collagens and SLRPs can lead to accelerated disk degeneration. However, it is unclear how important any of these genes are in contributing to disk degeneration in most humans under normal conditions.

Mechanical loading can be another cause of disk degeneration. There are clear instances in which abnormal loading of the disk leads to disk degeneration. A well-recognized example is adjacent disk disease after spinal fusion. Long fusions that end at the L5 vertebra can often lead to L5-S1 disk degeneration. This clinical finding has been reinforced by animal experiments in which abnormal loading was created. One example involved rabbits that had simulated lumbar fusions. Degeneration at the disk adjacent to the fusion developed much like in the human example. In another animal model, rats that have been forced to become bipedal by forelimb amputation showed accelerated disk degeneration. Excessive vibration has been proposed as a cause for disk degeneration; however, the data on this cause are inconclusive.

Disk degeneration is associated with age. Imaging studies indicate that 90% of individuals older than 60 years have disk degeneration.[32] However, the correlation between age and disk degeneration is not entirely predictive, and there is a significant amount of variability in disk degeneration status even among equal-aged individuals. Age-related disk degeneration should not be considered a disease, because individuals may have disk degeneration without any clinical ill effects. In fact, most individuals with significant disk degeneration are asymptomatic.[32]

In the adult intervertebral disk, most of the disk volume consists of the extracellular matrix; only a small percentage of the overall volume is occupied by disk cells. Thus, the mechanical properties of the disk are essentially determined by the matrix. The role of the disk cells are to maintain the disk matrix, breaking down and rebuilding the extracellular matrix by removing old molecules and synthesizing new ones. Disk matrix metabolism is a slow process; the turnover of the proteoglycan component of the disk matrix has been estimated to occur over a period of many years and the turnover of collagen fibers is even slower. It is the imbalance in this disk matrix metabolism that results in matrix degradation and loss.

Inadequate nutritional supply to the disks may be a critical factor in disk degeneration. As disks become larger during skeletal maturation, the diffusion distance to supply the disk center become longer. This may explain why in human disks, the most proteoglycan syn-

1: Principles of Orthopaedics

thesis occurs in the outer nucleus pulposus and inner anulus fibrosus zones. The diffusion limitation may also place a limit on cell density as this parameter seems to be inversely proportional to the volumetric size of the disk as found in cross-species comparison.[30]

Inflammatory mediators have also been implicated in the degeneration of the extracellular matrix of the disk. TNF-α, IL-1, IL-6, and MMPs, for example, have been shown to be major players in the breakdown of proteoglycans. TNF-α, once activated, can induce multiple cellular responses, including decreased production of both aggrecan and type II collagen as well as increased expression of enzymes that promote proteoglycan destruction.

Association of Disk Degeneration With Pain

Although the disk is believed to be a source of pain in some patients, disk degeneration by itself does not constitute a painful or disease process. In fact, most disks that are classified as degenerated do not cause pain. However, there is a statistical correlation between lumbar disk degeneration and low back pain. Imaging modalities such as radiography, CT, and MRI can indicate morphologic evidence of disk degeneration; however, imaging studies cannot accurately identify painful disks, as many asymptomatic individuals have degenerated disks and some individuals with apparently normal disks have pain. Diskography has been developed to assist in identifying painful disks. However, recent studies indicate that diskography can have high false-positive results in patients with chronic pain or somatization disorders.[33]

Degenerative disks may produce pain via at least four different mechanisms. One method is from disk mechanical hypermobility leading to abnormal mechanical forces applied to the disk. Another mechanism is the local production of one or more inflammatory molecules (such as TNF-α, IL-1, IL-6, or IL-8). When disk herniation occurs, the inflammatory response is even more dramatic and includes a cellular response with macrophages. This inflammatory response may be painful. Another mechanism is from the production of mediators that sensitize surrounding nociceptors in the outer anulus fibrosus and the neighboring end plates. Disks are innervated along its periphery by myelinated A delta fibers and unmyelinated C fibers that travel to the dorsal root ganglion. These pain receptors can be stimulated chemically or mechanically to induce pain signals that propagate to the somatosensory cortex. Finally, new nerve endings have been found to grow into degenerative disks. Studies have found that anulus fibrosus cells can produce nerve growth factors, especially during disk degeneration. Despite the new insights on pain generation in the disk, it is still unknown why some degenerating intervertebral disks cause pain while others do not.[34,35]

Molecular Therapy for Disk Degeneration

Molecules that can have therapeutic effects on the disk matrix can be classified as anticatabolic molecules or anabolic molecules. Within each of these two categories, there are many different subgroups. Some of these molecules are classic growth factors or cytokines, but many do not fit into that nomenclature. Therefore, the more general term molecular therapy is used to describe the totality of different molecules that can be used for potential disk therapy.

Anticatabolic agents act by reducing the activity of the catabolic enzymes found in the degenerating disk. MMPs are important catabolic enzymes found in the normal and degenerating disk. MMPs such as stromelysin, collagenase, and gelatinase are dispersed throughout the disk and act by degrading collagen, aggrecans, and link proteins. Tissue inhibitors of MMPs are normal physiologic molecules that inhibit the activity of MMPs. In a proof-of-concept experiment, researchers have been able to successfully introduce the *TIMP-1* gene into disk cells using viral vectors and cause higher levels of proteoglycans in tissue culture.[36] Other potential anticatabolic enzymes include inhibitors of specific inflammatory molecules such as TNF-α and IL-1. A theoretic benefit of using anticatabolic therapy is the avoidance of increasing the metabolic demands on disk cells.

Anabolic molecules constitute the other group of potentially therapeutic molecules. This group can be subgrouped into mitogenic molecules, morphogenic molecules, or intracellular regulators. Mitogenic molecules work by increasing cell proliferation and thereby increasing cell number and disk matrix synthesis. Examples are insulin-like growth factor, epidermal growth factor, and fibroblast growth factor. Morphogenic molecules are distinct from mitogens because morphogens function primarily by changing the phenotype of the target cells without necessarily increasing the cell number. Thus morphogens have the potential to restore the chondrogenic phenotype of nucleus pulposus cells and increase the production of a superior quantity and quality of disk matrix. Examples of morphogenic molecules include bone morphogenetic protein (BMP)-2, BMP-7, growth and development factor-5, and transforming growth factor-beta. Each of these has been shown to increase the chondrogenic phenotype of disk cells and increase disk matrix synthesis either in culture or in small animal models.[37,38] Intracellular molecules constitute a distinct subgroup because these molecules have to be present in the intracellular compartment to have activity. Classic growth factors work by binding a receptor found on the cell membrane; however, intracellular regulators such as SOX9, Smads, and latent membrane protein-1 cannot be merely injected into the disk and expected to have activity. With these molecules, the delivery mechanism is more complex and can involve gene therapy approaches to produce the molecule inside the cell or involve the use of protein transduction domains to translocate the molecule into the intracellular domain. Anabolic molecules address a fundamental cause of disk degeneration—the poor synthetic activity of cells in the degenerated disk. Therefore, anabolic molecules will most likely be a critical part of any molecular therapy strategy.

Summary

Articular cartilage and intervertebral disk constitute important cartilaginous structures that have separate mechanical and biologic functions. Articular cartilage provides the joint with a bearing surface that has a combination of extremely low friction and excellent wear characteristics, far superior to any man-made substitute. The intervertebral disk provides the axial skeleton multiaxial mobility while preserving structural stability. Both articular cartilage and intervertebral disk have a cellular population that actively maintains the extracellular matrix through a homeostatic balance between synthesis and degradation. When the cells are unable to sustain the normal composition of the extracellular matrix, tissue structure and performance becomes degraded. Several promising avenues aimed at preventing this downward spiral, including anticatabolics, mitogens, morphogens, intracellular regulators, and antiapoptotic agents, are actively being investigated.

Annotated References

1. Ulrich-Vinther M, Maloney MD, Schwarz EM, Rosier R, O'Keefe RJ: Articular cartilage biology. *J Am Acad Orthop Surg* 2003;11:421-430.

2. Darling EM, Hu JC, Athanasiou KA: Zonal and topographical differences in articular cartilage gene expression. *J Orthop Res* 2004;22:1182-1187.

   The authors present data on the differences in zonal expression of type II collagen, superficial zone protein, and aggrecan in goat articular cartilage.

3. Eleswarapu SV, Leipzig ND, Athanasiou KA: Gene expression of single articular chondrocytes. *Cell Tissue Res* 2007;327:43-54.

   The authors review the composition, structure, and biomechanics of articular cartilage. They also review mechanisms of cartilage degeneration and provide an extensive reference list.

4. Dowthwaite GP, Bishop JC, Redman SN, et al: The surface of articular cartilage contains a progenitor cell population. *J Cell Sci* 2004;117:889-897.

   The authors identify and characterize a progenitor cell population from the superficial zone of articular cartilage. Labeled progenitor cells injected into chick embryos homed to relevant tissues including articular fibrocartilage and bone.

5. Buckwalter JA, Mankin HJ, Grodzinsky AJ: Articular cartilage and osteoarthritis. *Instr Course Lect* 2005;54: 465-480.

   The authors review the composition, structure, and biomechanics of articular cartilage. They also review mechanisms of cartilage degeneration and provide an extensive reference list.

6. Kurz B, Lemke AK, Fay J, Pufe T, Grodzinsky AJ, Schunke M: Pathomechanisms of cartilage destruction by mechanical injury. *Ann Anat* 2005;187:473-485.

   The authors review models and mechanisms of cartilage degeneration after mechanical injury, focusing primarily on in vitro studies.

7. Blanco F, Guitian R, Vazquez-Martul E, de Toro FJ, Galdo F: Osteoarthritis chondrocytes die by apoptosis: A possible pathway for osteoarthritis pathology. *Arthritis Rheum* 1998;41:284-289.

   The pancaspase inhibitor Z-VAD-fmk is shown to block chondrocyte apoptosis, decrease cartilage degeneration, and enhance cartilage repair after osteochondral injury in a rabbit model.

8. Hashimoto S, Ochs RL, Komiya S, Lotz M: Linkage of chondrocyte apoptosis and cartilage degradation in human osteoarthritis. *Arthritis Rheum* 1998;41:1632-1638.

9. Dang AC, Warren AP, Kim HT: Beneficial effects of intra-articular caspase inhibition therapy following osteochondral injury. *Osteoarthritis Cartilage* 2006;14: 526-532.

   The pan-caspase inhibitor Z-VAD-fmk is shown to block chondrocyte apoptosis, decrease cartilage degeneration, and enhance cartilage repair after osteochondral injury in a rabbit model.

10. Kraus VB: Biomarkers in osteoarthritis. *Curr Opin Rheumatol* 2005;17:641-646.

    The author discusses current approaches to the use of biochemical markers for osteoarthritis and reviews several recent studies that include the use of biomarkers to measure the effects of therapeutic interventions.

11. Mazzuca SA, Brandt SA, Eyre DR, Katz BP, Askew J, Lane KA: Urinary levels of type II collagen C-telopeptide crosslink are unrelated to joint space narrowing in patients with knee osteoarthritis. *Ann Rheum Dis* 2006;65:1055-1059.

    In a study of women with knee osteoarthritis, serial CTx-II levels did not distinguish subjects with progressive radiographic or symptomatic knee osteoarthritis from those with stable disease.

12. Marshall KW, Zhang H, Yager TD, et al: Blood-based biomarkers for detecting mild osteoarthritis in the human knee. *Osteoarthritis Cartilage* 2005;13:861-871.

    Microarray technology and real-time RT-PCR were used to identify differentially expressed genes in RNA isolated from peripheral blood obtained from normal patients and those with OA. This study provides proof of concept for gene expression profiling as a biomarker for early OA.

13. Glasson SS, Askew R, Sheppard B, et al: Deletion of active ADAMTS5 prevents cartilage degradation in a murine model of osteoarthritis. *Nature* 2005;434:644-648.

    Deletion of the gene encoding the aggrecanase ADAMTS-5 is shown to protect mice from developing

1: Principles of Orthopaedics

osteoarthritis-like cartilage degeneration after knee ligament transection.

14. Mustafa Z, Chapman K, Irven C, et al: Linkage analysis of candidate genes as susceptibility loci for osteoarthritis-suggestive linkage of COL9A1 to female hip osteoarthritis. *Rheumatology* 2000;39:299-306.

15. Pavelka K, Gatterova J, Olejarova M, et al: Glucosamine sulfate use and delay of progression of knee osteoarthritis: A 3-year, randomized, placebo-controlled, double-blind study. *Arch Intern Med* 2002; 162:2113-2123.

16. Michel BA, Stucki G, Frey D, et al: Chondroitins 4 and 6 sulfate in osteoarthritis of the knee: A randomized, controlled trial. *Arthritis Rheum* 2005;52:779-786.

    The authors report the results of a randomized, double-blind, placebo-controlled trial of chondroitin sulfate in 300 patients with knee OA. Level of evidence: I.

17. Clegg DO, Reda DJ, Harris CL, et al: Glucosamine, chondroitin sulfate, and the two in combination for painful knee osteoarthritis. *N Engl J Med* 2006;354: 795-808.

    The authors report results from the GAIT (Glucosamine/ Chondroitin Arthritis Intervention Trial) study funded by the National Institutes of Health. Level of evidence: I.

18. Fidelix TS, Soares BG, Trevisani VF: Diacerein for osteoarthritis. *Cochrane Database Syst Rev* 2006;1: CD005117.

    The authors report the results of a comprehensive meta-analysis of clinical trials of diacerein for osteoarthritis.

19. Brandt KD, Mazzuca SA, Katz BP, et al: Effects of doxy-cycline on progression of osteoarthritis: Results of a randomized, placebo-controlled, double-blind trial. *Arthritis Rheum* 2005;52:2015-2025.

    The authors report the results of a large clinical trial involving 431 obese women with knee OA. Doxycycline was shown to be effective as a disease-modifying osteoarthritis drug in this population. Level of evidence: I.

20. Mithoefer K, Williams RJ III, Warren RF, et al: The microfracture technique for the treatment of articular cartilage lesions in the knee: A prospective cohort study. *J Bone Joint Surg Am* 2005;87:1911-1920.

    The authors present short-term (2-year) data on the results of microfracture using subjective and objective (MRI) outcome measures. Level of evidence: IV.

21. Steadman JR, Briggs KK, Rodrigo JJ, et al: Outcomes of microfracture for traumatic chondral defects of the knee: Average 11-year follow-up. *Arthroscopy* 2003;19: 477-484.

22. Szerb I, Hangody L, Duska Z, Kaposi NP: Mosaicplasty: Long-term follow-up. *Bull Hosp Jt Dis* 2005;63:54-62.

    The developers of the mosaicplasty technique report their results from over 800 cases performed since 1992.

23. Peterson L, Minas T, Brittberg M, Nilsson A, Sjogren-Jansson E, Lindahl A: Two- to 9-year outcome after autologous chondrocyte transplantation of the knee. *Clin Orthop Relat Res* 2000;374:212-234.

    This paper also provides a description of the technique and rehabilitation protocol. Level of evidence: IV.

24. Wasiak J, Clar C, Villanueva E: Autologous cartilage implantation for full thickness articular cartilage defects of the knee. *Cochrane Database Syst Rev* 2006;3: CD003323.

    The authors report the results of a meta-analysis of clinical trials of ACI compared with alternative cartilage repair techniques. Each of the relevant clinical trials is reviewed.

25. Buckwalter JA, Mow VC, Boden SD, Eyre DR, Weidenbaum M: Intervertebral disk structure, composition, and mechanical function, in Buckwalter JA, Einhorn TA, Simon SR (eds): *Orthopaedic Basic Science: Biology and Biomechanics of the Musculoskeletal System*, ed 2. Rosemont, IL, American Academy of Orthopaedic Surgeons, 2000, pp 548-555.

26. Gruber HE, Ashraf N, Kilburn J, et al: Vertebral endplate architecture and vascularization: Application of micro-computerized tomography, a vascular tracer, and immunocytochemistry in analyses of disc degeneration in the aging sand rat. *Spine* 2005;30:2593-2600.

    The authors used a micro CT architectural model, vascular tracer, and immunocytochemical identification to investigate the porosity and vascularization of lumbar vertebral end plates from young and old sand rats. Their results included the inability to find vascular connections between the end plate and disk.

27. Feng H, Danfelter M, Stromqvist B, Heinegard D: Extracellular matrix in disc degeneration. *J Bone Joint Surg Am* 2006;88(suppl 2):25-29.

    The authors present a review of the molecular components of the extracellular matrix in the intervertebral disk as well as the interactions that maintain and lead to its early degradation.

28. Boos N, Weissbach S, Rohrbach H, Weiler C, Spratt KF, Nerlich AG: Classification of age-related changes in lumbar intervertebral discs. *Spine* 2002;27:2631-2644.

29. Grunhagen T, Wilde G, Soukane DM, Shirazi-Adl SA, Urban JP: Nutrient supply and intervertebral disc metabolism. *J Bone Joint Surg Am* 2006;88(Suppl 2):30-35.

    The authors discuss key concepts of intervertebral disk metabolism, including the method of nutrient delivery and waste removal.

30. Kim KW, Lim TH, Kim JG, Jeong ST, Masuda K, An HS: The origin of chondrocytes in the nucleus pulposus and histologic findings associated with the transition of a notochordal nucleus pulposus to a fibrocartilaginous nucleus pulposus in intact rabbit intervertebral discs. *Spine* 2003;28:982-990.

31. Battie MC, Videman T, Gibbons LE, Fisher LD, Man-ninen H, Gill K: Determinants of lumbar disc degenera-tion: A study relating lifetime exposures and magnetic resonance imaging findings in identical twins. *Spine* 1995;20:2601-2612.

32. Boden SD, McCowin PR, Davis DO, Dina TS, Mark AS, Wiesel S: Abnormal magnetic-resonance scans of the cervical spine in asymptomatic subjects: A prospec-tive investigation. *J Bone Joint Surg Am* 1990;72:1178-1184.

33. Carragee EJ, Alamin TF, Carragee JM: Low-pressure positive discography in subjects asymptomatic of signif-icant low back pain illness. *Spine* 2006;31:505-509.

The authors investigated the hypothesis that low-pressure diskography may eliminate false-positive injec-tions. Their analysis found a false-positive rate of 25% in patients without chronic low back pain symptoms.

34. Lotz JC, Ulrich JA: Innervation, inflammation, and hy-permobility may characterize pathologic disc degenera-tion: Review of animal model data. *J Bone Joint Surg Am* 2006;88(suppl 2):76-82.

The authors provide an up-to-date review of the patho-logic mechanisms of disk degeneration via animal model-based evidence.

35. Brisby H: Pathology and possible mechanisms of ner-vous system response to disc degeneration. *J Bone Joint Surg Am* 2006;88(suppl 2):68-71.

The author discusses the interplay of the nervous system with disk degeneration and how it may influence our subjective perception of disk degeneration.

36. Wallach CJ, Sobajima S, Watanabe Y, et al: Gene trans-fer of the catabolic inhibitor TIMP-1 increases mea-sured proteoglycans in cells from degenerated human intervertebral discs. *Spine* 2003;28:2331-2337.

37. Yoon S, Kim K, Li J, et al: The effect of bone morpho-genetic protein-2 on rat intervertebral disc cells in vitro. *Spine* 2003;28:1773-1780.

38. Masuda K, Imai Y, Okuma M, et al: Osteogenic protein-1 injection into a degenerated disc induces the restoration of disc height and structural changes in the rabbit annular puncture model. *Spine* 2006;31:742-754.

The authors evaluated the changes observed following the injection of osteogenic protein-1 into a needle punc-ture disk degeneration model. The authors found a res-toration of disk height as well as a high proteoglycan content and a lower degeneration grade when compared with their control group.

Chapter 4

Muscle, Tendon, and Ligament

David P. Beason, MS   Louis J. Soslowsky, PhD   Tharun Karthikeyan, MD   *Johnny Huard, PhD

Skeletal Muscle

Structure and Function

Skeletal muscle represents the largest tissue mass in the human body, comprising 40% to 50% of total body weight.[1] Components of muscle include muscle cells, a complex network of blood vessels and nerves, and the extracellular connective tissue matrix. The most fundamental structural unit is the myofiber, which is actually a syncytium formed by the fusion of several individual myoblasts (muscle precursor cells). Newly formed myofibers possess multiple nuclei, which are centrally located initially, but eventually move to the periphery of the fiber as it matures (central nucleation is an indicator of newly regenerating myofibers following muscle injury). Mature myofibers are among the longest cells in the body, with lengths that can reach more than 10 cm in some individuals.[2] A hierarchy of connective tissue layers exists, beginning with the endomysium or basement membrane, which surrounds individual myofibers. The perimysium surrounds each fascicle or bundle of myofibers, and the epimysium surrounds the entire muscle (which is composed of several fascicles) (Figure 1).

The intracellular organelles of the myofiber are highly specialized for the function of muscle contraction, which is reflected in their structure as well as their nomenclature. The cell membrane of myofibers is called the sarcolemma; it possesses channels called transverse tubules that permit the passage of action potentials from the membrane surface to the sarcoplasmic reticulum (SR). The SR is the repository of calcium ions within the myofiber, and the action potential triggers release of these ions into the sarcoplasma, which in turn stimulates muscular contraction.

The contractile elements within a myofiber are the myofibrils, which are made up of an organized network of actin and myosin filaments, along with other structural proteins. The myofibril contains regularly repeating units, or sarcomeres, which can be generally defined as the region between two adjacent Z-lines within a myofibril.

Nerves exert the primary control over muscle contraction. Each myofiber is contacted by a separate axon branch at its motor end plate. The total of all myofibers contacted by branches from a single axon are known as a motor unit. Muscles requiring fine motor control may contain as few as 10 myofibers per motor unit, whereas larger muscles may have as many as 1,000. The neuromuscular junction contains three major structures: the presynaptic axon, the synaptic cleft, and the postsynaptic area of the muscle fiber.

As an action potential reaches the axon terminal, acetylcholine is released and diffuses across the synaptic cleft, binding to postsynaptic receptors on the myofiber. This process then causes sodium influx and another action potential in the myofiber, which is transmitted to the SR via the transverse tubules, resulting in calcium efflux into the cell. The calcium interacts with the myofilaments via its binding to troponin, inducing a conformational change that allows the actin and myosin filaments to slide along each other in a process that uses adenosine triphosphate and generates a muscular contraction. Contraction stops when acetylcholine at the postsynaptic receptor is degraded, and the calcium within the cell is resequestered in the SR.

Not all muscle contraction results in muscle shortening. Although the cellular and molecular events are similar, there are three different types of contractions. In a concentric contraction, the force generated by the muscle exceeds that of the resistive force, and the muscle shortens. Conversely, the force generated by an eccentric contraction is less than the resistive force, and the muscle lengthens despite contraction of the individual sarcomeres. In isometric contractions, the force generated by the muscle is equal to the resistive force, and the muscle length is therefore unchanged.

There are three main types of myofibers, each of which is suited to different functions (Table 1). Type I (slow-twitch fibers) are resistant to fatigue but have a relatively slow contraction velocity and time to maximum force output. Type IIB (fast-twitch fibers) are capable of sudden forceful contraction, but fatigue easily. Type IIA fibers also are capable of fast contractions, but are more resistant to fatigue than are type IIB fibers. It is important to note that these fiber types do not differ significantly in the total amount of force produced but differ in the rate of force production.

Most muscles are made up of a combination of different fiber types, but some are composed of a preponderance of one type of fiber because that fiber type re-

---

Johnny Huard, PhD or the department with which he is affiliated has received research or institutional support from Cook MyoSite and is a consultant or employee for Cook MyoSite.

1: Principles of Orthopaedics

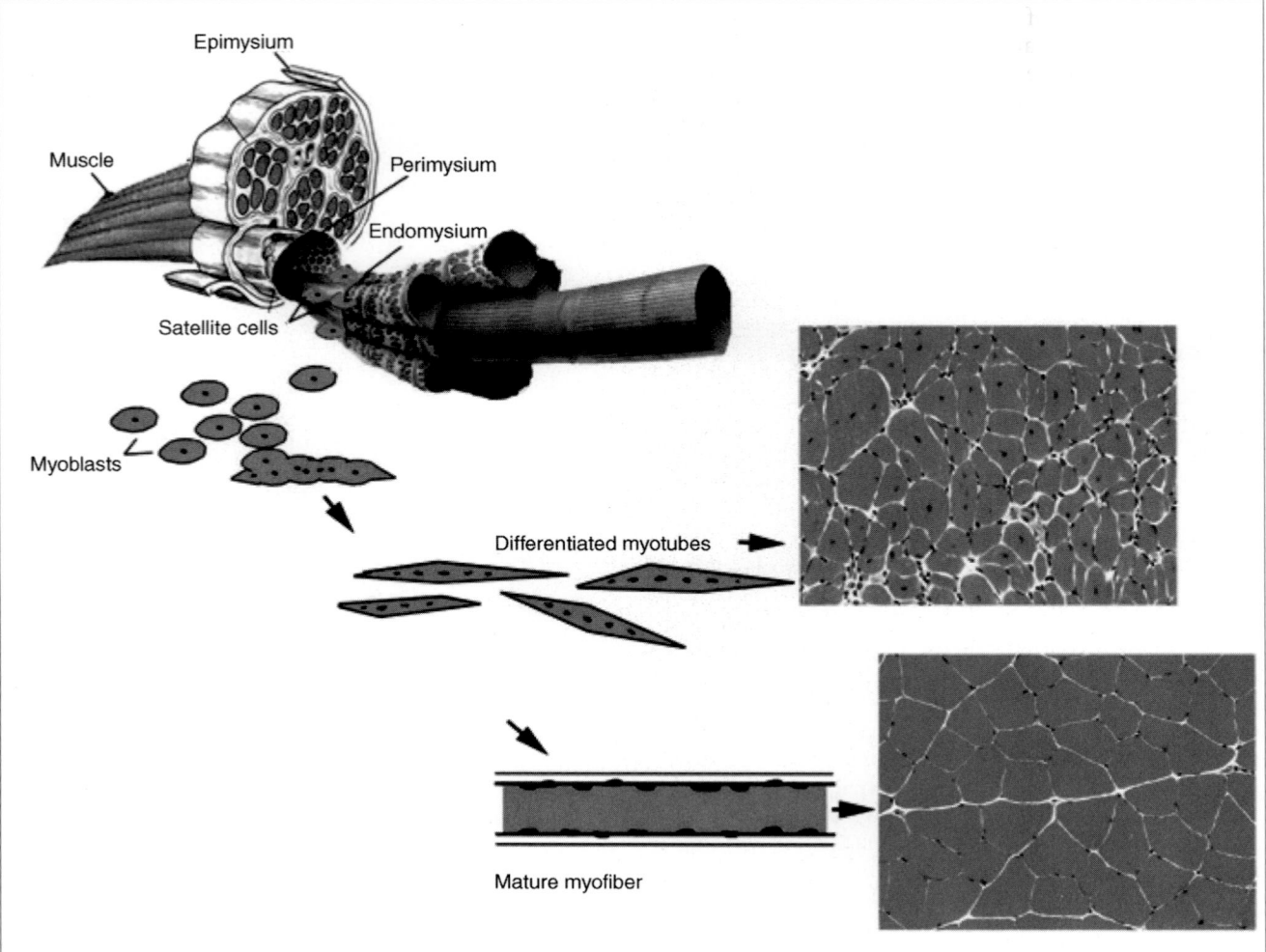

Figure 1 Schematic drawing of the structural design of skeletal muscle. The endomysium or basement membrane is the connective tissue layer that surrounds individual myofibers, the perimysium surrounds fascicles of myofibers, and the epimysium is the outermost connective tissue layer that surrounds the entire muscle. When a muscle is injured, satellite cells are released and activated to become myoblasts, which differentiate into immature myotubes, and eventually mature into muscle fibers. The histologic panels show that nuclei are centrally located within immature or regenerating myotubes, but migrate to the periphery of the myofiber as it matures.

Table 1

The Three Main Types of Myofibers and Their Characteristics

Fiber Type	Contraction Velocity	Fatigue Resistance
Type I	Slow	Greatest
Type II-A	Fast	Intermediate
Type II-B	Fast	Least

lates to the primary function of that muscle. For example, the soleus muscle is primarily involved in balance, and thus contains mostly type I fibers, whereas the quadriceps muscle contains fewer type I and a greater proportion of type IIB fibers.

Conditions Affecting Muscle Function

It is a well-known fact that proper training can enhance the function of specific muscles or muscle groups. Muscle training can generally be categorized as either resistance or endurance training, although some training modalities have considerable overlap of these categories.

The maximum force generated by a muscle is proportional to its cross-sectional area. However, the initial strength gains observed with resistance training (for example, weight lifting) are caused primarily by an increase in the number of motor units recruited to execute a particular movement, as well as other "neural modifications."[3] After approximately 4 to 6 weeks, individual myofibers begin to exhibit hypertrophy, primarily by synthesis of additional myofibrils within each fiber.[4] Formation of additional myofibers (hyperplasia) appears to contribute little to overall muscle hypertrophy. Other changes that occur with muscular resistance training include an increase in the number of type IIA fibers with a concomitant decrease in type IIB fibers.[4]

Endurance training primarily involves aerobic activities and results in different muscular adaptations compared with resistance training. Perhaps the most important adaptation is a significant increase in the capillary density of active muscles.[5] The respiratory capacity of mitochondria in recruited muscle fibers is increased, resulting in greater maximal oxygen consumption; however, there are no significant changes in the activity of glycolytic enzymes.[5] Conversion of fiber type from type IIB to type IIA also occurs; however, there is not a significant increase in the proportion of type I fibers.[6]

Important changes in muscle structure and function also occur with age. Age-related loss of muscle mass is known as sarcopenia. This condition results in a subsequent loss of function, which leads to an increase in the incidence of osteoporosis, falls, and certain fractures.[5] Loss of muscle mass in sarcopenia is caused by a reduction in both the size and number of muscle fibers. The reduction in the number of muscle fibers appears to be related to a denervation of muscle fibers (primarily type II fibers), which leads to denervation atrophy. In addition, aging results in a decrease in capillary density, aerobic energy production, and muscle relaxation velocity.[7,8] The capacity of satellite cells to participate in normal muscle turnover also appears to diminish with age and is likely caused by a decrease in notch signaling.

Muscular Dystrophies

Derangements of the structure of skeletal muscle inevitably lead to suboptimal function. The most common of these disorders are the muscular dystrophies, of which Duchenne muscular dystrophy (DMD) is perhaps the best characterized.

DMD is an X-linked genetic disorder affecting approximately 1 in 3,500 male births. The affected gene codes for dystrophin, a structural protein found in skeletal and cardiac muscle, which links the intracellular actin framework of muscle cells to the extracellular matrix (ECM).[9,10] Absence of this link makes the sarcolemma extremely fragile and subject to degradation and subsequent fibrosis following even routine activity. Clinical symptoms begin to manifest between 3 and 5 years of age, and may include leg weakness, progressive scoliosis, dilated cardiomyopathy, and a characteristic "pseudohypertrophy" of the calf muscles. Diagnosis is usually suspected based on the presence of these symptoms and a positive family history of the disease, and is confirmed by muscle biopsy, which shows a lack of dystrophin with immunohistochemical staining. Genetic detection is difficult because of the large variety of point mutations that can cause the disease. The prognosis of DMD is dire—patients are usually confined to a wheelchair by age 10 years, and succumb to respiratory or cardiac complications by the second or third decade of life.

Becker muscular dystrophy (BMD) is a related disorder that results from a deficiency in dystrophin rather than the total absence of the protein. It is phenotypically more variable than DMD but generally follows a milder course; however, cardiac involvement can be severe. Patients with BMD are ambulatory into their teen years and usually survive into the fourth decade of life.

Corticosteroids have been the mainstay of treatment for these and other muscular dystrophies. Although steroids are effective in slowing the progression of DMD, they do not alter the underlying pathology; the adverse effects of these drugs hamper their widespread use. Much research in recent years has focused on molecular and cell-based therapies for DMD; several strategies have been used in an effort to restore the absent or deficient dystrophin protein. The most basic strategy attempted is to directly inject naked plasmid DNA engineered to contain a "minidystrophin" gene (a full-length dystrophin at 2.3 million base pairs is too large to be incorporated into a plasmid) into dystrophic muscle.[11] However, gene delivery in this manner is extremely inefficient, and stimulates a vigorous antibody response to the newly synthesized dystrophin. Viral vectors such as adeno-associated virus have also been used as a means of introducing the dystrophin gene into DMD muscle fibers, but have met similar challenges in terms of efficiency of transduction and immune responses.[12] Perhaps the most promising therapies involve ex vivo gene transfer. In this technique, muscle cells from dystrophic muscle are harvested and expanded in tissue culture, and are then genetically modified to express dystrophin (usually through adeno-associated virus mediated transduction). These cells are then reimplanted, either systemically or directly into dystrophic muscle. A parallel approach involves implantation of normal myoblasts or other myogenic precursor cells (including muscle-derived stem cells) in an effort to restore dystrophin expression.[13] Although preliminary results using some of these therapies are encouraging, more research is needed before they can be translated into effective clinical treatments for DMD and BMD.

Phases of Skeletal Muscle Healing Following Injury

Muscle injuries can occur in a variety of circumstances. Participation in sports is an especially likely scenario, and by some estimates, muscle injuries comprise as much as 55% of all sports-related injuries.[2] Muscle injury can consist of contusion, strain, or laceration. Although the mechanism and forces involved with each of these injury types may differ significantly, the biologic processes of repair are basically similar. In general, there are three phases of healing following a muscle injury, all of which are interrelated and time dependent (Figure 2).

Immediately following injury, the muscle undergoes an initial period of degeneration and inflammation.

1: Principles of Orthopaedics

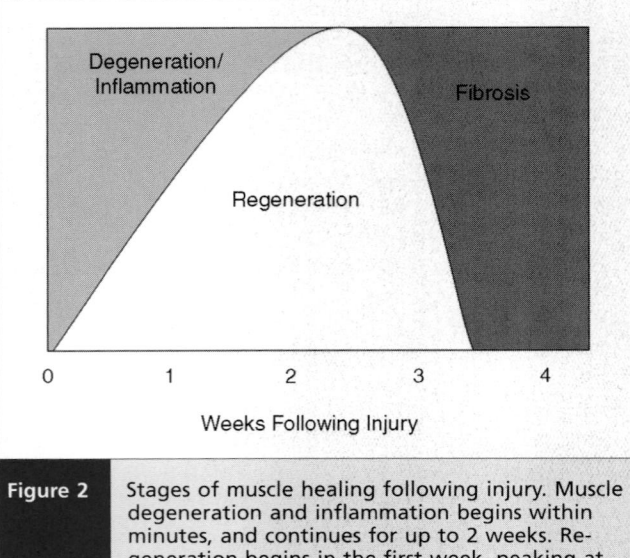

Figure 2 Stages of muscle healing following injury. Muscle degeneration and inflammation begins within minutes, and continues for up to 2 weeks. Regeneration begins in the first week, peaking at approximately 2 weeks after injury. Fibrosis usually begins approximately 2 weeks after injury and continues until approximately 4 weeks after the initial injury.

The muscle fibers are torn, as is the surrounding basement membrane or endomysium. This injury initiates necrosis of the myofibers, mediated primarily by intrinsic proteases. Although the myofiber can be quite long, the area of necrosis is contained through the formation of contraction bands that "wall off" the damaged myofiber and allow repair of the sarcolemma.[2] Injury to the muscle is also accompanied by injury to the local capillary bed and vasculature, which stimulates an influx of inflammatory cells (as does the localized necrosis). For the first day or so following injury, neutrophils are the most abundant cells, but are replaced by monocytes within approximately 24 hours. These monocytes eventually mature into activated macrophages under the influence of local cytokines, and are responsible for the phagocytosis of necrotic material. The invading mononuclear cells, activated macrophages, and T-lymphocytes secrete a variety of cytokines (for example, interleukin [IL]-8,-6, and-1 and tumor necrosis factor-alpha) and adhesion molecules (P-selectin, L-selectin), which further stimulate the inflammatory process.[1]

The second phase of healing is the regeneration phase, which usually begins 7 to 10 days following injury. The release of growth factors (insulin-like growth factor [IGF]-1, transforming growth factor-beta [TGF-β], and platelet-derived growth factor [PDGF]) by inflammatory cells at the injury site triggers the activation of satellite cells, which are normally quiescent muscle progenitor cells that reside within the basal lamina. These growth factors stimulate the satellite cells to proliferate, differentiate, and eventually fuse with the residually injured myofibers, helping to reconstitute them. As noted above, these newly formed fibers can be easily identified by their central nuclei. Recent studies also have shown the existence of a pool of stem cells lo-

cated within the muscle (muscle-derived stem cells) that also contribute to regeneration.[9] The process of regeneration peaks at 2 weeks following injury, then begins to slow significantly by 3 to 4 weeks.

The final phase of muscle healing is fibrosis, or the formation of a connective tissue scar. The first steps in this phase actually occur immediately following the injury, when fibrin and fibronectin from the initial hematoma form an early granulation tissue at the site of injury.[2] Fibroblasts accompany the influx of inflammatory cells and initially secrete more fibronectin, which adds strength and elasticity to the granulation tissue. However, within 2 to 3 weeks following injury, secretion of various growth factors (especially TGF-β) causes the fibroblasts to begin producing type I collagen, which is the primary constituent of the ensuing fibrotic scar. Type I collagen greatly increases the strength of the injured area; soon after it is laid down, the scar itself is no longer the weakest point in the injured muscle. Most instances of rerupture after 10 days usually occur at the junction of the scar and adjacent regenerated myofibers.[2]

Biologic Approaches to Improve Muscle Healing After Injury

Current treatments immediately following injury are generally limited to rest, ice, compression, and elevation. These measures attempt to decrease bleeding into the zone of injury, although there is sparse evidence of their efficacy. Immobilization is of some benefit in the early phases of muscle regeneration because it prevents further retraction of the muscle stumps and minimizes hematoma and the size of the ensuing fibrotic scar;[14] however, in a mouse laceration model, immobilization for 5 days appeared to hamper histologic and functional healing.[15] It is clear, however, that prolonged immobilization leads to atrophy, excessive connective tissue deposition, and a slower recovery of muscle strength.[14]

These traditional treatments do not alter the natural course of muscle healing. As previously described, injured muscle undergoes a sequential cycle of healing phases, including muscle degeneration/inflammation, regeneration, and fibrosis. In many instances, the development of excessive fibrosis inhibits complete muscle recovery. The development of biologic approaches to modulate these different phases of muscle healing as a means of improving muscle healing after injury is an area of intense study (**Figure 3**).

Nonsteroidal anti-inflammatory drugs (NSAIDs) are often prescribed to relieve pain after muscle injury. However, the effect of this group of drugs on the muscle-healing process remains controversial. Studies performed in vitro to determine the role of cyclooxygenase-2 (COX-2) in muscle healing have shown that NS-398 (a COX-2 specific inhibitor) hinders the proliferation and maturation of differentiated muscle precursor cells, suggesting that NS-398 may have a detrimental effect on skeletal muscle healing.[16] In vivo studies using a laceration model in mouse skel-

1: Principles of Orthopaedics

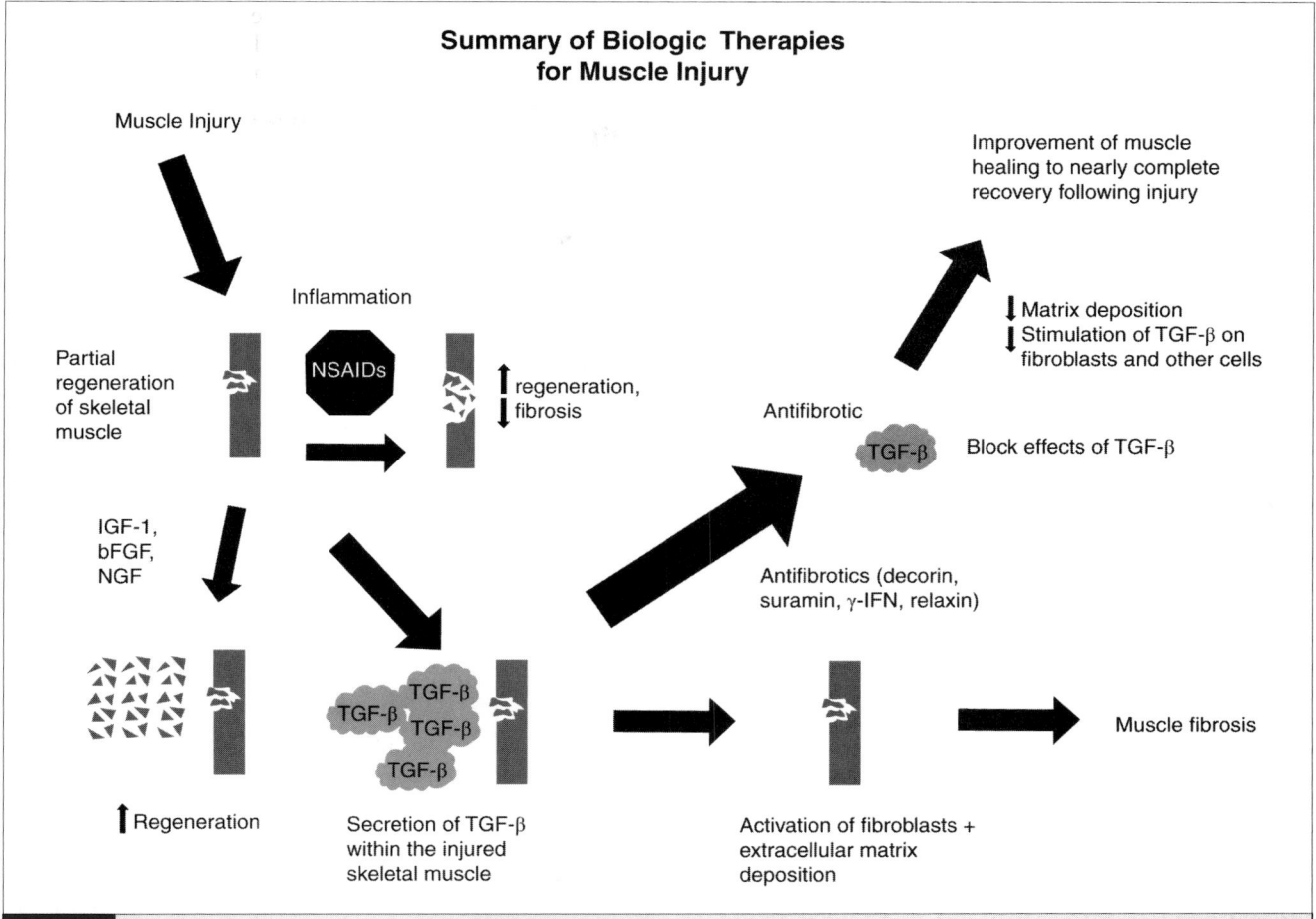

Summary of Biologic Therapies for Muscle Injury

Figure 3	Summary of biologic approaches to affect muscle healing. Following the initial injury, inflammation occurs, which may be crucial in the initial regenerative process because NSAIDs appear to inhibit healing. Gene therapy with IGF-1, bFGF and nerve growth factor (NGF) appear to enhance regeneration. Following the period of inflammation and regeneration, the injured muscle begins to secrete TGF-β, which can lead to fibrosis and incomplete recovery. Gene therapy with antifibrotic factors such as decorin, relaxin, suramin, and γ-interferon (γ-IFN) may inhibit TGF-β, which can decrease deposition of ECM and ultimately improve muscle healing.

etal muscles also showed delayed muscle regeneration at early time points after injury in mice treated with NS-398.[16] The lacerated muscles treated with NS-398 expressed higher levels of TGF-β1 than did control muscles, which corresponded with increased fibrosis. Less neutrophil and macrophage infiltration occurred in the treated muscles, which indicates that the delayed skeletal muscle healing observed after injection of NS-398 could be caused by the inhibitory effect of NS-398 on inflammatory responses.[16] Histologic and functional assessments of lacerated tibialis anterior muscles in COX-2 knockout mice also showed decreased regeneration relative to that observed in the wild-type mice. These findings show that the COX-2 pathway plays an important role in muscle healing and suggest that the use of NSAIDs to treat muscle injuries warrants critical evaluation because NSAIDs may actually impair muscle healing.

Many studies have shown that growth factors play a variety of roles during muscle regeneration.[17] In a mouse model, direct injections of IGF-1, basic fibroblast growth factor (bFGF), and, to a lesser extent, nerve growth factor, have enhanced muscle healing in lacerated, contused, and strain-injured muscle.[17,18] One potential advantage of using human recombinant growth factors to treat muscle injuries is the ease and safety of the injection. However, the efficacy of direct injection of recombinant proteins (growth factors) is limited by the high concentration of the factor typically required to elicit a measurable effect. Whereas growth factors have a dose-dependent effect on myoblast proliferation and differentiation in vitro, several consecutive injections of relatively high concentrations of nerve growth factor, IGF-1, or bFGF (100 ng/growth factor) are usually necessary to achieve detectable enhancement of skeletal muscle healing in mice.[19] The ability of the bloodstream to rapidly clear these molecules and their relatively short biologic half-lives are the main reasons that such large concentrations of growth factors are typically required. Gene therapy may prove to

1: Principles of Orthopaedics

be an effective method for delivering high, maintainable concentrations of growth factor to injured muscle. Myoblast-mediated ex vivo gene transfer (myoblasts harvested, transduced with the engineered adenovirus, then reintroduced into the animal) of an adenovirus carrying the gene encoding for IGF-1 improved healing of lacerated muscle in immunocompetent mice.[19] However, histology of the injected muscle showed muscle fibrosis within the lacerated site, despite the production of a high level of IGF-1.[19] Taken together, these results suggest that, although the high level of IGF-1 secretion mediated by adenoviral-based gene therapy can improve muscle healing, the functional recovery of the injured muscle remains incomplete. Some research suggests that the stimulatory action of IGF-1 on myofibroblast proliferation and the deposition of scar tissue may interfere with the ability of this growth factor (even at high concentrations) to improve muscle healing after injury. Prevention of muscle fibrosis may be a better approach to improve muscle healing.

Research results strongly indicate that scar tissue formation precludes complete regeneration of muscle tissue. Although various studies have implicated the role of TGF-β1 in the onset of fibrosis in various tissues, very few studies have examined the role of this cytokine in skeletal muscle fibrosis.[20] Research has shown that TGF-β1 is expressed at high levels and is associated with fibrosis in the skeletal muscle of patients with DMD.[21,22] Studies also have shown excess TGF-β1 in muscle biopsy specimens of patients with dermatomyositis.[23,24] This excess TGF-β1 leads to chronic inflammation, fibrosis, and the accumulation of ECM.[23,24] Strong expression of TGF-β1 also has been observed in injured skeletal muscle.[25] These results support the hypothesis that the expression of TGF-β1 in skeletal muscle plays an important role in the fibrotic cascade that occurs after the onset of muscle disease or trauma. Therefore, it is feasible that neutralization of TGF-β1 expression in injured muscle could inhibit the formation of scar tissue. The use of antifibrotic agents that inactivate TGF-β1 appear to reduce muscle fibrosis and, consequently, improve muscle healing, leading to nearly complete recovery of lacerated muscle.[25,26]

Various approaches to block the effect of TGF-β1 include treatment with a neutralizing TGF-β1 antibody, with the antisense and ribozyme to TGF-β1, with suramin, with relaxin, and with interferon-γ.[27-30] However, the unique ability of decorin (a small proteoglycan present in the ECM of muscle tissue) to both neutralize the fibrotic effect of TGF-β1 and enhance muscle regeneration makes this molecule particularly well suited for use in applications intended to improve muscle healing after injury.[25,26] Further evaluation of the beneficial effect of decorin on muscle regeneration and its mechanism(s) of action is extremely important because an improved understanding of these mechanisms could lead to the identification of novel therapies to promote muscle growth and regeneration.

Tendon and Ligament

Composition, Structure, and Function

Tendons and ligaments are soft connective tissues that serve to stabilize joints, aid in providing gliding motion, and carry loads between the respective structures that they join. Functionally, tendons join muscle and bone, whereas ligaments connect bone to bone. Both are composed primarily of water, type I collagen (roughly 70% to 90% of dry weight), and to a lesser extent, type III collagen. In general, the structure of these tissues can be described as building in structural complexity from the ECM. At this level, groups of collagen molecules form fibrils, which are embedded in the ECM. Also within the ECM are numerous proteoglycans, which consist of a core protein with chains of negatively charged glycosaminoglycans (GAGs). As a result of this large accumulated negative charge, proteoglycans have an affinity for binding water molecules, which gives the ECM its gel-like composition and also affects its rate-dependent response to mechanical loading. This combination of collagen fibrils and proteoglycans is mainly responsible for the tensile strength of the tissue. The crimped bundles of fibrils packed together comprise fascicles, which combine to complete the structure up to the tissue level. These bundles are typically parallel and longitudinally oriented; however, orientation can be affected by native loading conditions. It has been suggested that tendon and ligament properties are also dependent on their location and function.[31] Collagen organization and tissue structure have a profound effect on biomechanical function.

Biomechanics of Tendon and Ligament

Because one of the primary functions of tendon and ligament is load transmission, discussion of the mechanical integrity of these tissues is important. Understanding tendon and ligament biomechanics is vital to developing strategies for surgical repair and for potential tissue-engineered replacement or regeneration.

Experimentally, the shape and function of tendons and ligaments lend themselves to quasistatic tensile testing. Testing can focus on obtaining either structural properties of the entire complex (muscle-tendon-bone or bone-ligament-bone), or material properties of the tissue itself. Structural properties are discerned from the load-deformation curve, whereas material properties are determined from a similar analysis of stress and strain. Like other biologic soft tissues, tendons and ligaments exhibit both nonlinear and viscoelastic behavior. The nonlinear behavior is characterized initially by a relatively large increase in deformation/strain with respect to load/stress (**Figure 4**). During tensile tests, this region represents the longitudinal aligning and uncrimping of relaxed collagen fibers. This period is referred to as the toe region and is followed by a linear phase of constant load-elongation behavior. Structural and material properties such as stiffness and modulus can be obtained from the slope of this region. The en-

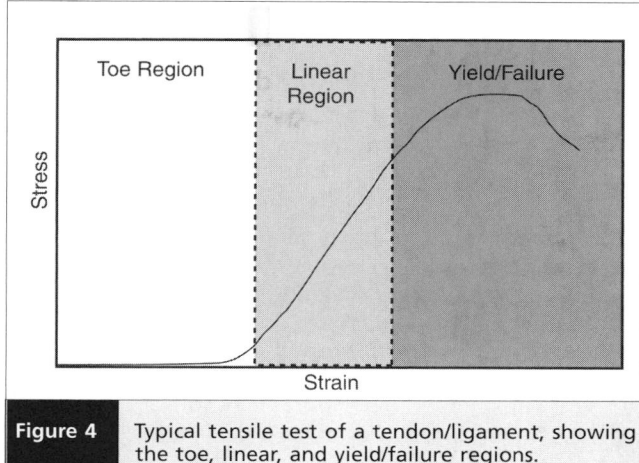

Figure 4 Typical tensile test of a tendon/ligament, showing the toe, linear, and yield/failure regions.

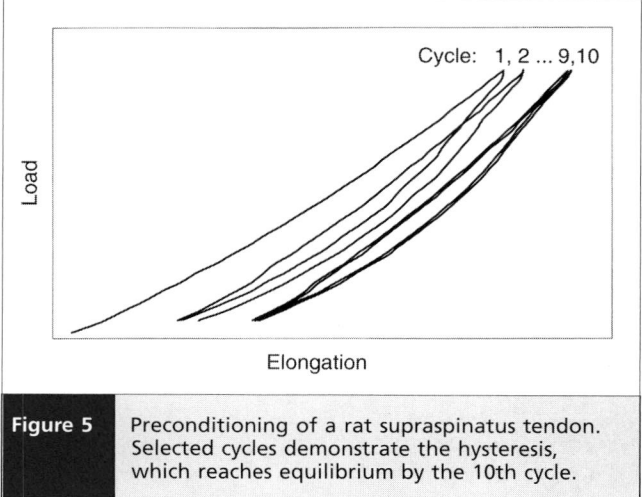

Figure 5 Preconditioning of a rat supraspinatus tendon. Selected cycles demonstrate the hysteresis, which reaches equilibrium by the 10th cycle.

suing region of nonlinear yield culminates with the ultimate failure of the specimen.

In addition to showing nonlinear behavior, tendons and ligaments are also viscoelastic in that their tensile properties are rate dependent. This characteristic is a product of the amount of water brought into the tissue because of the presence of proteoglycans and their GAGs. As a result, the water acts as a dashpot, in that rapid loading tends to cause the tissue to be stiffer than when loaded more gradually. When viscoelastic materials are cyclically loaded, there is a hysteresis characterized by a shift in the load-deformation response until equilibrium is reached (**Figure 5**). This potential variability can be experimentally eliminated by preconditioning specimens to 10 to 20 cycles at loads well within their normal physiologic range.

Although studies quantifying human cadaver ligament and tendon tensile properties have proven to be immensely beneficial, only limited information can be obtained. The use of animal models in the basic science setting has allowed a more detailed approach to studying how different constituents affect the overall properties of the tissue. Results from some recent studies using transgenic knockout mice have shown that estrogen and growth/differentiation factor-7 (GDF-7) have no significant effect on knee ligament and Achilles tendon biomechanics, respectively.[32,33] Another study has shown increased modulus in patellar tendons from mice deficient in proinflammatory cytokine, IL-6.[34] Another study has elucidated the role of TGF-β inducible early gene-1 using knockout mice. This study showed decreased viscoelastic peak and equilibrium stresses for mice deficient in TGF-β inducible early gene-1 at 3 months of age, and increased fibril diameters at 1 and 3 months of age.[35] Yet another study examined different tendons from mice that were deficient in small leucine-rich proteoglycans (biglycan and decorin), and showed that the biglycan deletion lowered maximum stress and elastic modulus of flexor tendons, whereas patellar tendons from decorin-null mice exhibited higher modulus and percent of stress relaxation. These differences, combined with the fact that tail tendon fas-

cicles showed no differences, led to the conclusion that tendon properties are tissue- and location-specific.[31]

One limitation to these types of studies is the potential during the animal's development for compensation in response to the missing gene. One study used multiple regression statistical models to evaluate the relative contributions of several different parameters.[36] This method also can be used to eliminate the possibility of genetic compensatory mechanisms. It has been recently reported that biomechanical properties differ between inbred mouse strains; this finding should be considered when comparing transgenic mice bred on different strains.[37]

Injury and Repair of Tendon and Ligament

When tendon or ligament injury occurs, a natural healing process ensues, which can be divided into three overlapping phases: inflammation, regeneration, and remodeling. During the initial phase, there is an influx of inflammatory cells such as neutrophils into the wound area. The type of collagen synthesis following injury is progressive in nature, with the synthesis of type III collagen (initiated during inflammation) peaking during the regeneration phase, replaced after a few weeks by the initiation of type I collagen production. The tissue during this phase is also characterized by a high content of water, proteoglycan, and GAGs, which helps to increase the organization of the matrix of granulation tissue that is present. During remodeling, the final stage, there is a notable decrease in cellularity, an increase in fibrosis, and a characteristic longitudinal orientation to the collagen fibers. As the remodeling phase concludes, the wound matures, and slowly changes in nature and appearance from fibrotic to scarred over the course of 1 year or longer. It is believed that these healing processes can occur either extrinsically through infiltration of external cells, or intrinsically via proliferation of cells contained within the tissue.

Recent experiments using human cadaver tissue have yielded useful data on the potential viability of certain

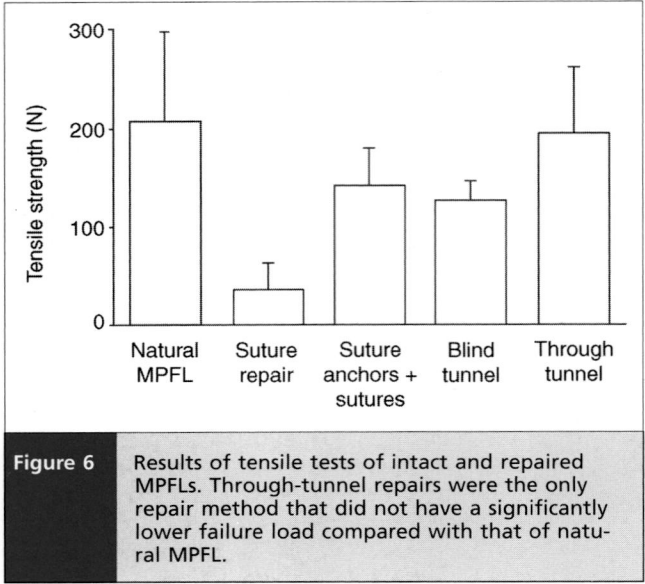

Figure 6 Results of tensile tests of intact and repaired MPFLs. Through-tunnel repairs were the only repair method that did not have a significantly lower failure load compared with that of natural MPFL.

surgical repair techniques for tendon and ligament injury. In medial patellofemoral ligaments (MPFLs) that had been tensile tested to failure, evaluation of four different surgical techniques showed that a through-tunnel tendon graft technique using bovine extensor tendon resulted in comparable failure load levels when compared with intact MPFLs, whereas corkscrew suture anchors, blind-tunnel tendon grafts, and Kessler suture techniques produced more fragile repair and failure-load levels significantly different than those of the intact ligament[38] (**Figure 6**). Suture anchor repairs also result in reduced failure loads in failed and repaired ulnar collateral ligaments of the thumb when compared with intact values.[39] Flexor digitorum profundus tendon-to-bone properties were improved immediately following repair when using a tunnel method with a peripheral suture compared with tunnel-only and volar cortical surface techniques.[40] For anterior cruciate ligament (ACL) avulsion fractures, three different fixation techniques were compared under cyclic loading conditions. Although all techniques were deemed effective through measures of anterior tibial translation, antegrade screw fixation performed significantly better than pullout suture fixation and marginally better than retrograde screw fixation.[41]

Experimental animal models can be especially useful when studying injury and repair because reproducible injuries can be created and the subsequent repair process evaluated. Models of tendon and ligament injury are available for many animals including dogs, mice, pigs, rabbits, rats, and sheep.[42-66] Rat rotator cuff injury models have been used to show inferior healing at 2 weeks postinjury of detached supraspinatus tendons with either no repair or 3-week delayed repair; however, properties are shown to rebound in the absence of repair beginning at 4 weeks, and eventually surpass normal control values.[56,57] Canine flexor tendons have also been shown to increase in size and resistance to su-

ture pullout within the first 3 weeks following detachment from the bony insertion without repair.[42]

A recent study has shown reduced mechanics and collagen organization in injured patellar tendons of mice deficient in IL-6, indicating the importance of this inflammatory cytokine in tendon healing.[46] Additional studies to isolate the specific constituents involved in tendon and ligament healing will provide valuable insight into the mechanisms behind this process.

Growth factors are known to play a role in the wound healing process of tendons and ligaments. Recent studies of growth factors involved measuring the levels of several different growth factors and their effect on the production of cells and collagen in healing dissected canine flexor tendons.[43,44] Immunohistochemistry has shown expression of TGF-β, epidermal growth factor, PDGF-AA, PDGF-BB, IGF, bFGF, and vascular endothelial growth factor within the first 10 days following laceration, but at different sites in the tendon.[44] PDGF-BB and bFGF have been shown to increase fibroblast proliferation and collagen production, with the effect on cell proliferation being magnified when the two growth factors are combined.[45]

Several studies have investigated the use of pulsed ultrasound as a potential treatment for improving and accelerating tendon and ligament healing. This treatment has improved healing time of the rat Achilles tendon and medial collateral ligament (MCL) compared with groups who did not receive active pulsed ultrasound.[60,61] One study also showed that administering a NSAID to treat a ruptured ligament actually delays ligament healing.[60] Rat rotator cuff tendon-to-bone healing has also been shown to be significantly hindered by postoperative treatment with traditional and COX-2–inhibiting NSAIDs.[59] Another study using a rat model showed improved knee ligament healing with one selected NSAID, but reported no overall effect for nonselective NSAIDs and COX-2 inhibitors.[58]

Following surgical repair, a fine balance exists between providing sufficient exercise to foster tissue remodeling and sufficiently restricting motion to prevent failure of the repair. Stress deprivation leads to inferior tensile strength and modulus in normal rat tail tendons.[62] The level of in vitro static tensile loading in rat tail tendons is inversely proportional to the level of expression of interstitial collagenase (matrix metalloproteinase-1).[63] Two other recent studies examined the effects of immobilization following rabbit patellar tendon and MCL collagen shrinkage techniques; however, conclusions on the effect of immobilization were conflicting.[50,52] It is believed that immobilization and stress deprivation can be detrimental to the quality of the healing tissue; however, some level of immobilization seems to be necessary to prevent a level of motion that may damage newly repaired tissue.

Tendons and ligaments heal by forming a fibrous scar, which tends to reduce mechanical function. Recent studies have investigated the use of collagen-platelet-rich plasma hydrogel scaffolds to enhance ACL healing.[45,47] Canine central defects[45] and porcine complete transections[47] treated with such a scaffold have shown improved primary repair healing when compared with untreated controls as late as 6 weeks after injury. Some studies have focused on regenerative rather than reparative healing through the use of fetal tissue. Lateral extensor tendons of fetal sheep receiving 50% tenotomies have been shown, histologically, to heal without scar.[64] It appears that this regenerative response is inherent to the fetal tissue itself, because transplantation into an adult mouse environment does not result in differences in histology or tensile properties between injured fetal sheep tendons and uninjured controls.[65] In contrast, adult tendons show significantly compromised healing compared with controls.

In general, tendon and ligament properties tend to reduce as a function of age. Two recent studies have shown interesting results regarding the capacity for healing in aged tendon. In a patellar tendon injury model, mesenchymal stem cells (MSCs) were harvested from young adult rabbits and were cryogenically preserved. Three years later, MSCs were again harvested from the same (now geriatric) rabbits and both sets of harvested MSCs were implanted into patellar tendon defects. Mechanical testing showed that, surprisingly, the elderly MSCs were no less effective than their younger counterparts.[53] Using the same injury model (without MSCs), tendon healing at various postinjury time points was again observed to be no worse in older age groups.[54]

Functional Tissue Engineering for Tendon and Ligament

In recent years, the field of tissue engineering has been receiving increased attention. At its core, tissue engineering attempts to combine the concepts of biology and engineering for the purposes of repair and even replacement of injured tissue. A novel, bioartificial tendon construct made from tendon fibroblasts has been developed that mimics the composition of native tendon, but is drastically inferior biomechanically.[67] Treatment with IL-1β reduces strength and elastic modulus of bioartificial tendon constructs and modulus of tenocytes, whereas cyclic loading of the constructs increases these properties to levels that remain nearly an order of magnitude below native values.[67-69] To ensure the practical quality of functional tissue engineering, engineered tissues must be capable of performing the mechanical function of the original tissues, particularly those that serve primarily biomechanical purposes.[70]

Tissue-engineered constructs such as porcine small intestine submucosa have been used in current experimental research to evaluate their potential as scaffolds in tendon and ligament repair. At 12 weeks after injury, tissues treated with small intestine submucosa have shown significant increases in stiffness ranging from 39% to 56%, and improvements in failure load from 27% (not significant) to 77% compared with surgical controls (with untreated constructs) in sheep tendon and rabbit ligament injury models.[49,66] Ligaments also have been reported to be 50% stronger than those of untreated controls at 26 weeks after injury.[55] In all cases, however, properties remained significantly inferior to sham controls.

One of the predominant principles governing functional tissue engineering is the idea that in vivo experimental measurements are important in providing valuable thresholds for tissue-engineered constructs. Since this concept was adopted, many studies have focused on in vivo measurement of tendon and ligament for this purpose. In vivo measurements in the rabbit patellar and Achilles tendons during locomotion have shown that peak loads and loading rates within the tendon increase significantly with increased activity level (such as inclination).[48,51] Other in vivo techniques suitable for use in human patients, such as ultrasonography, also have been used. Measurements of the elastic moduli of human patellar and Achilles tendon using this technique under various conditions have been reported to be on the order of 1 GPa.[71-73] In vivo data of this nature could provide valuable information to both clinicians and engineers regarding the functional properties of tendons and ligaments during normal usage.

Summary

Collectively, muscles, tendons, and ligaments are soft, connective tissues that make skeletal motion possible. Skeletal muscle is a large and complex organ with microscopic and macroscopic structure that reflects its specialized functions. Following injury, skeletal muscle undergoes a predictable pattern of healing, including inflammation, regeneration, and fibrosis. Recovery of skeletal muscle following injury may be hampered by incomplete muscle regeneration and by the production of fibrosis. Along with stabilization and gliding, tendons and ligaments are responsible for transmitting muscle loads. Considering the vital nature of their function, research involving biomechanics, injury, repair, and tissue-engineered repair and replacement strategies is crucial to achieving strides in clinical practice and patient care for tendon and ligament injuries.

Annotated References

1. Huard J, Li Y, Fu FH: Muscle injuries and repair: Current trends in research. *J Bone Joint Surg Am* 2002;84: 822-832.

2. Jarvinen TA, Jarvinen TL, Kaariainen M, Kalimo H, Jarvinen M: Muscle injuries: Biology and treatment. *Am J Sports Med* 2005;33:745-764.

   The authors present a summary of the prevailing understanding of the biology of muscle injury and regeneration and a review of the existing data on various treatment modalities.

3. Moritani T, deVries HA: Neural factors versus hypertrophy in the time course of muscle strength gain. *Am J Phys Med* 1979;58:115-130.

4. Deschenes MR, Kraemer WJ: Performance and physiologic adaptations to resistance training. *Am J Phys Med Rehabil* 2002;81(suppl 11):S3-16.

5. Kirkendall DT, Garrett WE: The effects of aging and training on skeletal muscle. *Am J Sports Med* 1998;26: 598-602.

6. Pollock ML, Foster C, Knapp D, et al: Effect of age and training on aerobic capacity and body composition of master athletes. *J Appl Physiol* 1987;62:725-731.

7. Proctor DN, Sinning WE, Walro JM, Sieck GC, Lemon PW: Oxidative capacity of human muscle fiber types: Effects of aging and training status. *J Appl Physiol* 1995;78:2033-2038.

8. Coggan AR, Spina RJ, King DS, et al: Skeletal muscle adaptations to endurance training in 60- to 70-yr-old men and women. *J Appl Physiol* 1992;72:1780-1786.

9. Hoffman EP, Brown RH Jr, Kunkel LM: Dystrophin: The protein product of the Duchenne muscular dystrophy locus. *Cell* 1987;51:919-928.

10. Zubrzycka-Gaarn EE, Bulman DE, Karpati G, et al: The Duchenne muscular dystrophy gene product is localized in sarcolemma of human skeletal muscle. *Nature* 1988; 333:466-469.

11. Acsadi G, Dickson G, Love DR, et al: Human dystrophin expression in mdx mice after intramuscular injection of DNA constructs. *Nature* 1991;352:815-818.

12. Gregorevic P, Blankinship MJ, Allen JM, et al: Systemic delivery of genes to striated muscles using adeno-associated viral vectors. *Nat Med* 2004;10:828-834.

    Systemic gene transfer to striated muscles resulted in widespread transduction of the muscles.

13. Qu-Petersen Z, Deasy B, Jankowski RJ, et al: Identification of a novel population of muscle stem cells in mice: Potential for muscle regeneration. *J Cell Biol* 2002;157: 851-864.

14. Jarvinen MJ, Lehto MUK: The effect of early mobilization and immobilization on the healing process following muscle injuries. *Sports Med* 1993;15:78-79.

15. Menetrey J, Kasemkijwattana C, Fu FH, Moreland MS, Huard J: Suturing versus immobilization of a muscle laceration: A morphological and functional study in a mouse model. *Am J Sports Med* 1999;27:222-229.

16. Shen W, Li Y, Tang Y, Cummins J, Huard J: NS-398, a cyclooxygenase-2-specific inhibitor, delays skeletal muscle healing by decreasing regeneration and promoting fibrosis. *Am J Pathol* 2005;167:1105-1117.

    The use of a COX-2 inhibitor in a mouse model of muscle injury was associated with decreased proliferation and maturation of myogenic precursor cells, delayed muscle regeneration, increased levels of TGF-β1 and fibrosis, and decreased neutrophil and macrophage infiltration.

17. Barton-Davis ER, Shoturma DI, Musaro A, Rosenthal N, Sweeney HL: Viral mediated expression of insulin-like growth factor I blocks the aging-related loss of skeletal muscle function. *Proc Natl Acad Sci USA* 1998;95: 15603-15607.

18. Menetrey J, Kasemkijwattana C, Day CS, et al: Growth factors improve muscle healing in vivo. *J Bone Joint Surg Br* 2000;82:131-137.

19. Lee CW, Fukushima K, Usas A, et al: Biological intervention based on cell and gene therapy to improve muscle healing following laceration. *Musculoskeletal Res* 2000;4:265-277.

20. Czaja MJ, Weiner FR, Flanders KC, et al: In vitro and in vivo association of transforming growth factor-beta 1 with hepatic fibrosis. *J Cell Biol* 1989;108:2477-2482.

21. Bernasconi P, Torchiana E, Confalonieri P, et al: Expression of transforming growth factor-beta 1 in dystrophic patient muscles correlates with fibrosis: Pathogenetic role of a fibrogenic cytokine. *J Clin Invest* 1995; 96:1137-1144.

22. Zanotti S, Negri T, Cappelletti C, et al: Decorin and biglycan expression is differentially altered in several muscular dystrophies. *Brain* 2005;128:2546-2555.

    The evaluation of muscle biopsies of several patients with eight different types of muscular dystrophy showed (among other findings) an elevated level of TGF-β1 and decreased levels of decorin messenger RNA in patients with DMD, suggesting that the two may be related.

23. Amemiya K, Semino-Mora C, Granger R, Dalakas M: Downregulation of TGF-beta1 mRNA and protein in the muscles of patients with inflammatory myopathies after treatment with high-dose intravenous immunoglobulin. *Clin Immunol* 2000;94:99-104.

24. Confalonieri P, Bernasconi P, Cornelio F, Mantegazza R: Transforming growth factor-beta 1 in polymyositis and dermatomyositis correlates with fibrosis but not with mononuclear cell infiltrate. *J Neuropathol Exp Neurol* 1997;56:479-484.

25. Li Y, Foster W, Deasy BM, et al: Transforming growth factor-beta1 induces the differentiation of myogenic cells into fibrotic cells in injured skeletal muscle: A key event in muscle fibrogenesis. *Am J Pathol* 2004;164: 1007-1019.

    Injection of recombinant human TGF-β1 into mouse muscle resulted in autocrine secretion of endogenous TGF-β1, increased fibrosis, and differentiation of myoblasts into myofibroblasts. The addition of decorin appeared to block this differentiation by blocking TGF-β1.

26. Fukushima K, Badlani N, Usas A, Riano F, Fu FH, Huard J: The use of an antifibrosis agent to improve

1: Principles of Orthopaedics

muscle recovery after laceration. *Am J Sports Med* 2001;29:394-402.

27. Shah M, Foreman DM, Ferguson MW: Control of scarring in adult wounds by neutralizing antibody to transforming growth factor beta. *Lancet* 1992;339:213-214.

28. Chan YS, Li Y, Foster W, Fu FH, Huard J: The use of suramin, an antifibrotic agent, to improve muscle recovery after strain injury. *Am J Sports Med* 2005;33:43-51.

    Suramin decreased the stimulating effect of TGF-β1 on the growth of muscle-derived fibroblasts in vitro. Significantly less fibrous scar formation was observed in suramin-treated muscles than in sham-injected muscles. The fast-twitch and tetanus strength of suramin-treated muscles was also significantly greater relative to that of control muscles.

29. Negishi S, Li Y, Kuroda R, Foster W, Fu FH, Huard J: The effect of relaxin treatment on skeletal muscle injuries. *Am J Sports Med* 2005;33:1816-1824.

    Relaxin treatment resulted in a dose-dependent decrease in myofibroblast proliferation, downregulated expression of the fibrotic protein α-smooth muscle actin, and promoted the proliferation and differentiation of myoblasts in vitro. Relaxin therapy enhanced muscle regeneration, reduced fibrosis, and improved injured muscle strength in vivo.

30. Foster W, Li Y, Usas A, Somogyi G, Huard J: Gamma interferon as an antifibrosis agent in skeletal muscle. *J Orthop Res* 2003;21:798-804.

31. Robinson PS, Huang TF, Kazam E, Iozzo RV, Birk DE, Soslowsky LJ: Influence of decorin and biglycan on mechanical properties of multiple tendons in knockout mice. *J Biomech Eng* 2005;127:181-185.

    This study evaluates mechanical behavior of multiple types of tendons from wild-type, decorin knockout, and biglycan knockout mice. Results show significant differences in mechanical properties between wild-type controls and knockout mice; however, differences are dependent on tendon location and function.

32. Warden SJ, Saxon LK, Castillo AB, Turner CH: Knee ligament mechanical properties are not influenced by estrogen or its receptors. *Am J Physiol Endocrinol Metab* 2006;290:E1034-E1040.

    The role of estrogen and its receptors on knee ligament properties was investigated using knockout mice. The authors concluded that estrogen is not a significant factor in determining normal ligament tensile properties.

33. Mikic B, Bierwert L, Tsou D: Achilles tendon characterization in GDF-7 deficient mice. *J Orthop Res* 2006;24:831-841.

    The role of GDF-7 on Achilles tendon properties was investigated using knockout mice and built on previous research with GDF-5. No reported differences in tendon mechanical properties resulted from the GDF-7 deficiency.

34. Lin TW, Cardenas L, Soslowsky LJ: Tendon properties in interleukin-4 and interleukin-6 knockout mice. *J Biomech* 2005;38:99-105.

    Organizational, geometric, and tensile properties in patellar tendons of mice deficient in pro- and anti-inflammatory cytokines IL-6 and IL-4 were compared with those of wild-type controls. Results showed differences that supported the use of transgenic mice and provided support for a subsequent study on healing.

35. Bensamoun SF, Tsubone T, Subramaniam M, et al: Age-dependent changes in the mechanical properties of tail tendons in TGF-beta inducible early gene-1 knockout mice. *J Appl Physiol* 2006;101:1419-1424.

    Tail tendons from mice deficient in TGF-β inducible early gene 1 were studied at 1, 3, and 9 months of age. Viscoelastic properties peak and equilibrium stress were reduced at 3 months, and fibril size was increased at 3 and 9 months.

36. Robinson PS, Lin TW, Jawad AF, Iozzo RV, Soslowsky LJ: Investigating tendon fascicle structure-function relationships in a transgenic-age mouse model using multiple regression models. *Ann Biomed Eng* 2004;32:924-931.

    A multiple regression statistical model was used to simultaneously evaluate seven different transgenic mouse tail tendon fascicle properties. Overall, GAG properties are the strongest predictors of mechanics.

37. Wang VM, Banack TM, Tsai CW, Flatow EL, Jepsen KJ: Variability in tendon and knee joint biomechanics among inbred mouse strains. *J Orthop Res* 2006;24:1200-1207.

    Biomechanical data were collected and analyzed from three different strains of inbred mice. The authors found that properties differed across the groups, indicating that genetic factors have an important impact on mechanics.

38. Mountney J, Senavongse W, Amis AA, Thomas NP: Tensile strength of the medial patellofemoral ligament before and after repair or reconstruction. *J Bone Joint Surg Br* 2005;87:36-40.

    Human cadaver specimens of MPFL were tested to failure and subsequently repaired using four techniques: Kessler suture, corkscrew suture anchor, blind-tunnel tendon graft, and through-tunnel tendon graft. Failure load in the through-tunnel technique was shown to be no different than that in the intact ligament.

39. Harley BJ, Werner FW, Green JK: A biomechanical modeling of injury, repair, and rehabilitation of ulnar collateral ligament injuries of the thumb. *J Hand Surg Am* 2004;29:915-920.

    Thumb ulnar collateral ligaments were tested to failure and subsequently repaired using suture anchors. Failure loads were shown to be significantly reduced in the repaired group compared with those of intact ligaments.

40. Dovan TT, Gelberman RH, Kusano N, Calcaterra M, Silva MJ, Zone I: Flexor digitorum profundus repair: An ex vivo biomechanical analysis of tendon to bone repair in cadavera. *J Hand Surg Am* 2005;30:258-266.

1: Principles of Orthopaedics

Three repair techniques for flexor tendon repair were compared in cadaver hands. Results showed that the use of a tunnel method with a peripheral suture performs better than tunnel-only and volar cortical surface methods.

41. Tsukada H, Ishibashi Y, Tsuda E, Hiraga Y, Toh S: A biomechanical comparison of repair techniques for anterior cruciate ligament tibial avulsion fracture under cyclic loading. *Arthroscopy* 2005;21:1197-1201.

    ACL avulsion fractures were created in human cadaver knees. Three fixation repair techniques were evaluated, based largely on measurements of anterior tibial translation. Antegrade screw fixation was shown to be the most effective repair method when compared with methods using retrograde screws and pullout sutures.

42. Silva MJ, Ritty TM, Ditsios K, Burns ME, Boyer MI, Gelberman RH: Tendon injury response: Assessment of biomechanical properties, tissue morphology and viability following flexor digitorum profundus tendon transection. *J Orthop Res* 2004;22:990-997.

    This study used a canine injury model in which the flexor digitorum profundus tendon was detached from its bony insertion, with no reattachment. Due in part to a measured increase in resistance to suture pullout and maintenance of cell viability, the authors concluded that the practice of reattachment within 3 weeks is supported.

43. Tsubone T, Moran SL, Amadio PC, Zhao C, An KN: Expression of growth factors in canine flexor tendon after laceration in vivo. *Ann Plast Surg* 2004;53:393-397.

    An in vivo canine flexor tendon injury model showed expression of seven growth factors in this immunohistochemical study. Growth factors are expressed by different cell types and at different locations.

44. Thomopoulos S, Harwood FL, Silva MJ, Amiel D, Gelberman RH: Effect of several growth factors on canine flexor tendon fibroblast proliferation and collagen synthesis in vitro. *J Hand Surg Am* 2005;30:441-447.

    Canine flexor tendon cell proliferation and collagen production were measured in this study. PDGF-BB and bFGF increased both properties, whereas bone morphogenetic protein-2 and vascular endothelial growth factor did not. The combination of PDGF-BB and bFGF further increased fibroblast proliferation.

45. Murray MM, Spindler KP, Devin C, et al: Use of a collagen-platelet rich plasma scaffold to stimulate healing of a central defect in the canine ACL. *J Orthop Res* 2006;24:820-830.

    ACL healing was studied by implanting a collagen-platelet rich plasma hydrogel scaffold into central defects in a canine injury model. Results indicated improved healing in the treated group.

46. Lin TW, Cardenas L, Glaser DL, Soslowsky LJ: Tendon healing in interleukin-4 and interleukin-6 knockout mice. *J Biomech* 2006;39:61-69.

    This study was a follow-up to a previous study by the authors who examined tendon properties in the same mouse patellar tendon model. Evaluation of injury showed that IL-6 plays an important role in healing as measured through biomechanics and collagen organization.

47. Murray MM, Spindler KP, Abreu E, et al: Collagen-platelet rich plasma hydrogel enhances primary repair of the porcine anterior cruciate ligament. *J Orthop Res* 2007;25:81-91.

    ACL healing was studied by implanting a collagen-platelet rich plasma hydrogel scaffold into sutured, complete transections of porcine ACL. Results indicated improved healing in treated ligaments.

48. Juncosa N, West JR, Galloway MT, Boivin GP, Butler DL: In vivo forces used to develop design parameters for tissue engineered implants for rabbit patellar tendon repair. *J Biomech* 2003;36:483-488.

49. Musahl V, Abramowitch SD, Gilbert TW, et al: The use of porcine small intestine submucosa to enhance the healing of the medial collateral ligament: A functional tissue engineering study. *J Orthop Res* 2004;22:214-220.

    The ability of porcine small intestine submucosa to improve healing in a rabbit MCL-injury model was evaluated at 12 weeks after injury. Stiffness, failure load, and tangent modulus in the group treated with small intestine submucosa were superior compared with results in the untreated controls.

50. Pötzl W, Heusner T, Kümpers P, Marquardt B, Steinbeck J: Does immobilization after radiofrequency-induced shrinkage influence the biomechanical properties of collagenous tissue? An in vivo rabbit study. *Am J Sports Med* 2004;32:681-687.

    Rabbit patellar tendons were subjected to radiofrequency-induced shrinkage. Immobilized tendons showed faster recovery of immediate postoperative properties than did nonimmobilized tendons; however, neither group recovered completely at any time point.

51. West JR, Juncosa N, Galloway MT, Biovin GP, Butler DL: Characterization of in vivo Achilles tendon forces in rabbits during treadmill locomotion at varying speeds and inclinations. *J Biomech* 2004;37:1647-1653.

    Implantable force transducers were used to record in vivo forces during rabbit hopping. Peak loads and rates of rise and fall in loads were correlated with an increasing level of incline, but not with speed. Safety factors were developed for standing, level hopping, and hopping on an inclined surface.

52. Demirhan M, Uysal M, Kilicoglu O, et al: Tensile strength of ligaments after thermal shrinkage depending on time and immobilization: In vivo study in the rabbit. *J Shoulder Elbow Surg* 2005;14:193-200.

    In this study, rabbit knee ligaments were treated with thermal shrinkage. Immobilized ligaments showed reduced failure loads compared with nonimmobilized ligaments, with a significant difference at 9 weeks after treatment.

53. Dressler MR, Butler DL, Boivin GP: Effects of age on

the repair ability of mesenchymal stem cells in rabbit tendon. *J Orthop Res* 2005;23:287-293.

Young adult and aged rabbit patellar tendon MSCs were harvested and implanted in patellar tendon defects of aged rabbits. Specimens treated with aged MSCs did not show a reduction in properties.

54. Dressler MR, Butler DL, Boivin GP: Age-related changes in the biomechanics of healing patellar tendon. *J Biomech* 2006;39:2205-2212.

Young adult and aged rabbits were subjected to a patellar tendon defect. Healing was assessed through biomechanical testing. Aged specimens did not show a reduced healing response.

55. Liang R, Woo SL-Y, Takakura Y, Moon DK, Jia F, Abramowitch SD: Long-term effects of porcine small intestine submucosa on the healing of medial collateral ligament: A functional tissue engineering study. *J Orthop Res* 2006;24:811-819.

This study extended a previous study that evaluated the ability of porcine small intestine submucosa to improve healing in a rabbit MCL injury model at 26 weeks after injury. Maximum stress and tangent modulus were superior in the group treated with small intestine submucosa compared with the untreated control group. These findings provide additional support for the use of small intestine submucosa as a bioscaffold.

56. Gimbel JA, Van Kleunen JP, Mehta S, Perry SM, Williams GR, Soslowsky LJ: Supraspinatus tendon organizational and mechanical properties in a chronic rotator cuff tear animal model. *J Biomech* 2004;37:739-749.

A rat rotator cuff injury model was used to investigate supraspinatus tendon healing over time following humeral detachment and in the absence of repair. Tendon mechanics and organization decreased substantially immediately following injury, but began to increase at 4 weeks after detachment.

57. Galatz LM, Rothermich SY, Zaegel M, Silva MJ, Havlioglu N, Thomopolous S: Delayed repair of tendon to bone injuries leads to decreased biomechanical properties and bone loss. *J Orthop Res* 2005;23:1441-1447.

In a study of tendon-to-bone healing in a rat rotator cuff model, it was shown that reduced mechanical properties and bone mineral density resulted from a 3-week delay in repair of a supraspinatus transection from the humerus when compared with immediate repair.

58. Hanson CA, Weinhold PS, Afshari HM, Dahners LE: The effect of analgesic agents on the healing rat medial collateral ligament. *Am J Sports Med* 2005;33:674-679.

Ligament healing was investigated using a rat injury model with seven analgesic treatment groups. Although piroxicam increased failure loads, the authors concluded that nonselective NSAIDs and COX-2 inhibitors have little positive or negative effect on ligament healing.

59. Cohen DB, Kawamura S, Ehteshami JR, Rodeo SA: Indomethacin and celecoxib impair rotator cuff tendon-to-bone healing. *Am J Sports Med* 2006;34:362-369.

The authors of this study reported on the effect of both traditional NSAIDs and COX-2 inhibitors on tendon-to-bone healing in a rat rotator cuff injury model. Both drug groups significantly reduced healing as assessed through failure loads and collagen organization.

60. Warden SJ, Avin KG, Beck EM, DeWolf ME, Hagemeier MA, Martin KM: Low-intensity pulsed ultrasound accelerates and a nonsteroidal anti-inflammatory drug delays knee ligament healing. *Am J Sports Med* 2006;34: 1094-1102.

This study examined the effect of both low-intensity pulsed ultrasound and a NSAID on MCL healing in rats. The authors found that pulsed ultrasound accelerates (but does not improve) ligament healing and the use of a NSAID delays (but does not diminish) healing.

61. Yeung CK, Guo X, Ng YF: Pulsed ultrasound treatment accelerates the repair of Achilles tendon rupture in rats. *J Orthop Res* 2006;24:193-201.

Rat Achilles tendons were partially transected to evaluate the effect of pulsed ultrasound on the healing of the injured tendons. Histologic and mechanical evaluation showed significant improvements in healing in the group treated with pulsed ultrasound compared with the untreated group at each time point.

62. Lavagnino M, Arnoczky SP, Frank K, Tian T: Collagen fibril diameter distribution does not reflect changes in the mechanical properties of in vitro stress-deprived tendons. *J Biomech* 2005;38:69-75.

Rat tail tendons were tested to determine if an association exists between collagen fibril diameter distribution and tensile properties. Stress-deprived tendon tensile properties were significantly lower than those in the control group; however, this decrease in properties was not solely governed by collagen fibril diameter distribution.

63. Arnoczky SP, Tian T, Lavagnino M, Gardner K: Ex vivo static tensile loading inhibits MMP-1 expression in rat tail tendons through a cytoskeletally based mechanotransduction mechanism. *J Orthop Res* 2004;22: 328-333.

Rat tail tendons were treated with stress deprivation in addition to various static tensile loads. Matrix metalloproteinase-1 expression was increased with stress deprivation and proportionally inhibited with increasing static loads.

64. Beredjiklian PK, Favata M, Cartmell JS, Flanagan CL, Crombleholme TM, Soslowsky LJ: Regenerative versus reparative healing in tendon: A study of biomechanical and histological properties in fetal sheep. *Ann Biomed Eng* 2003;31:1143-1152.

65. Favata M, Beredjiklian PK, Zgonis MH, et al: Regenerative properties of fetal sheep tendon are not adversely affected by transplantation into an adult environment. *J Orthop Res* 2006;24:2124-2132.

Fetal and adult sheep extensor tendons were treated with a partial tenotomy and were subcutaneously transplanted into adult severe combined immune deficiency mice. Organizational and mechanical properties were

1: Principles of Orthopaedics

decreased in adult tendons compared with uninjured controls, whereas fetal tendons showed no differences.

66. Schlegel TF, Hawkins RJ, Lewis CW, Motta T, Turner AS: The effects of augmentation with swine small intestine submucosa on tendon healing under tension: Histologic and mechanical evaluations in sheep. *Am J Sports Med* 2006;34:275-280.

    The ability of porcine small intestine submucosa to improve healing in a sheep infraspinatus tendon injury model was evaluated at 12 weeks after injury. Stiffness was superior in the group treated with small intestine submucosa compared with untreated controls.

67. Garvin J, Qie J, Maloney M, Banes AJ: Novel system for engineering bioartificial tendons and application of mechanical load. *Tissue Eng* 2003;9:967-979.

68. Qi J, Chi L, Maloney M, Yang X, Bynum D, Banes AJ: Interleukin-1β increases elasticity of human bioartificial tendons. *Tissue Eng* 2006;12:2913-2925.

    Human bioartificial tendons were treated with IL-1β. Strength and modulus were reduced as a result of the treatment; however, it is proposed that the increase in elasticity actually protects the tendons from failure.

69. Qi J, Fox AM, Alexopoulos LG, et al: IL-1β decreases the elastic modulus of human tenocytes. *J Appl Physiol* 2006;101:189-195.

    Human tenocytes were incubated with IL-1β, which reduced elastic modulus. The authors concluded that reduced elastic modulus may actually contribute to increased cell survival.

70. Butler DL, Goldstein SA, Guilak F: Functional tissue engineering: The role of biomechanics. *J Biomech Eng* 2000;122:570-575.

71. Muraoka T, Muramatsu T, Fukunaga T, Kanehisa H: Geometric and elastic properties of in vivo human Achilles tendon in young adults. *Cells Tissues Organs* 2004;178:197-203.

    In vivo measurements were made in Achilles tendons of young adult humans. It was shown that the tendon's extendibility was not caused by its geometry.

72. Lichtwark GA, Wilson AM: In vivo mechanical properties of the human Achilles tendon during one-legged hopping. *J Exp Biol* 2005;208:4715-4725.

    The dynamic in vivo mechanical properties of human Achilles tendon were measured. The relative contribution of the Achilles tendon to the total energy required to produce one-legged hopping was appreciable.

73. Hansen P, Bojsen-Moller J, Aagaard P, Kjaer M, Magnusson SP: Mechanical properties of the human patellar tendon, in vivo. *Clin Biomech (Bristol, Avon)* 2006;21:54-58.

    The in vivo mechanical properties of human patellar tendon were measured using ultrasonography and the accuracy and precision of the method were assessed. It was determined that the technique was a repeatable method for measuring patellar tendon properties in vivo.

Chapter 5

Spinal Cord Injury and Peripheral Nerve Injury

Nitin N. Bhatia, MD   Hyun Bae, MD   *Ranjan Gupta, MD

Spinal Cord Injury

Spinal cord injury (SCI), first described as early as 1700 BC, is a significant cause of morbidity, mortality, and financial hardship.[1] The annual incidence of SCI in the United States is approximately 11,000 cases.[2,3] Although approximately one third of these patients die during or before hospitalization,[4] the care of SCI patients has improved tremendously over the past several decades due in part to the advent of centralized SCI treatment centers. In 1974, the average length of the hospital stay for patients entering an SCI center was 26 days, but that length had decreased to 16 days by 1999. The average length of rehabilitation also decreased from 115 days to 44 days over the same period.[3,5] The life expectancy of SCI patients remains lower than that of the general population, a discrepancy mainly caused by pulmonary complications.[3]

SCI continues to exact an enormous financial toll on patients and the US economy as a whole. The average age of the patient with SCI is 32 years, and approximately 81% of patients are male. The postinjury rate of employment for these patients is only 25%. This combination of young patient age and low likelihood of postinjury employment results in an annual cost of $4 billion in the United States.[6] The lifetime costs of care are dependent on the severity and level of injury, ranging from almost $500,000 for the patient with incomplete spinal injuries to over $2 million for the patient with cervical quadriplegia.

The nature of the trauma causing SCI has changed recently; violence has become a more important cause of SCI, whereas motor vehicle and sporting accidents have steadily decreased in number as causes of annual SCI cases. Over the past 15 years, motor vehicle crashes have been the most common cause of SCI (38.5%). Violent acts (24.5%), falls (21.8%), and sports accidents (7.2%) are the next three most common causes of SCI. Incomplete quadriplegia (29.6%) is the most common SCI pattern seen at presentation, followed by complete

paraplegia (27.3%), incomplete paraplegia (20.6%), and complete quadriplegia (18.6%), although the latter is decreasing in annual incidence.[3]

The severity of the SCI is frequently dependent on the level of the injury and the anatomy of the spine and cord at that particular level. Hence, different patterns of injury are seen at the different anatomic levels of the spine.

Anatomy

The spinal cord exits at the base of the skull and travels through the cervical and thoracic spine. Injuries at these levels can cause one of several SCI patterns. In the cervical spine, patients with smaller sagittal diameters have a higher risk of neurologic deficit following injury.[7] The thoracic spine is more rigid than the cervical or lumbar regions because of its rib articulations and coronal facet orientation. The lower two ribs do not articulate with the sternum, which causes decreased stability at the thoracolumbar junction. This area is further susceptible to injury because of the increased forces caused by the long rigid lever arm of the thoracic spine.

The spinal cord anatomy also changes at the thoracolumbar junction. The spinal cord terminates as the conus medullaris, which exists at the lower portion of L1 in women and the pedicle of L1 in men. The sacral nuclei are contained within the conus medullaris, and their nerve rootlets continue distally with the lumbar rootlets as the cauda equina. Injuries at the level of the conus medullaris can cause upper motor neuron injuries to the sacral nuclei, lower motor neuron injuries to the rootlets, or a combination of both. Injuries below the conus medullaris will cause a lower motor neuron injury to the cauda equina and possibly include either the lumbar or sacral levels.

Classification

The clinical manifestation of SCI is dependent on a variety of factors including the location, mechanism, and severity of the injury. Additionally, the cross-sectional location of the ascending and descending axonal tracts influences the syndromes seen after SCI (Table 1). A variety of different neurologic syndromes may occur, and orthopaedic surgeons must be familiar with these to make an accurate diagnosis and ensure appropriate treatment.

*Ranjan Gupta, MD or the department with which he is affiliated has received research or institutional support from NIH-NINDS.

1: Principles of Orthopaedics

Table 1

Axonal Tracts Within the Spinal Cord

Axonial Tracts	Function	Ascending or Descending
Dorsal column	Proprioception, vibratory sense, discriminative touch	Ascending
Spinothalamic	Pain, crude temperature, light touch	Ascending
Spinocerebellar	Subconscious regulation of muscle position and tone	Ascending
Corticospinal	Voluntary motor function	Descending
Rubrospinal	Flexor muscle tone control	Descending
Vestibulospinal	Spinal cord reflexes and muscle tone regulation	Descending
Reticulospinal	Influence voluntary movements, head position, muscle tone	Descending
Autonomic pathway	Autonomic control	Descending

Table 2

Clinical Deficit and Functional Outcome After SCI

Level of Injury	Motor Function	Mobility
C1-C3	Ventilator-dependent with limited talking	Electric wheelchair with head or chin control
C3-C4	Initially ventilator-dependent, but can become independent	Electric wheelchair with head or chin control
C5	Ventilator-independent, biceps and deltoid function, independent activities of daily living	Electric wheelchair with hand control, minimal manual wheelchair function
C6	Wrist flexion and extension, independent living	Improved manual wheelchair function, can drive a car with manual controls
C7	Improved triceps strength	Daily use of manual wheelchair
C8-T1	Improved hand and finger strength and dexterity	Fully independent transfers
T2-T6	Normal upper extremity function, improved trunk control	Wheelchair-dependent
T7-T12	Increased abdominal muscle control, able to perform unsupported seated activities	With extensive bracing, walking may be possible
L1-L5	Variable lower extremity and bowel/bladder function	Assistive devices and bracing may be needed
S1-S5	Various return of bowel, bladder, and sexual function	Walking with minimal or no assistance

SCIs can be classified as complete or incomplete. Complete SCI involves complete loss of all motor and sensory function below the level of injury and carries a poor prognosis. The exact clinical syndrome depends on the level of the injury (**Table 2**). An upper motor neuron picture will ultimately develop, including spastic paraplegia and hyperreflexia. Spinal shock can occur during the first 24 to 48 hours following any SCI and can mimic a complete injury in this setting. During spinal shock, the reliability of the neurologic examination may be limited. The absence of the bulbocavernosus reflex indicates that a patient is in spinal shock, and its return signifies that the patient is no longer in a state of spinal shock and that a reliable examination can be obtained.

Incomplete SCI is defined as partial motor or sensory loss below the level of the injury. This category is further subdivided into the central cord, anterior cord, Brown-Séquard, and posterior cord syndromes. The clinical findings and prognosis are dependent on the specific subcategory of incomplete injury; as a group, incomplete injuries have a better prognosis for neurologic improvement than do the complete lesions.

Central cord syndrome is the most common incomplete SCI syndrome. Older patients with underlying spinal stenosis are susceptible to central cord injuries following hyperextension injuries. The central spinal tracts are more affected by the compressive lesions that involve anterior osteophytes and buckling posterior ligamentum flavum. Greater weakness develops in the upper extremity versus the lower extremity, and the overall prognosis is favorable for both motor improvement and bowel and bladder function.

Anterior cord syndrome occurs following injuries to

the anterior spinal cord from vascular insults, disk herniations, and vertebral body fracture displacement. Motor function is significantly impaired, as is light touch and pain sensation. The deep pressure, proprioception, and vibratory senses of the dorsal spinal columns are relatively spared, however. Of the incomplete lesions, anterior cord syndrome carries the worst prognosis for functional recovery.

Brown-Séquard syndrome is a functional hemisection injury to the spinal cord. Motor function and proprioception are impaired ipsilateral to the side of injury, whereas pain and temperature sensation are decreased on the contralateral side. A classic scenario for Brown-Séquard syndrome is the penetrating knife wound to the spinal cord. More than 90% of these patients will regain the ability to walk and control their bowel and bladder function, giving Brown-Séquard syndrome the best prognosis for recovery of all of the SCI syndromes.

Posterior cord syndrome is extremely rare and results in loss of proprioception, deep pressure, and vibratory sense. Because only the dorsal columns are affected, motor function is retained.

Pathophysiology of SCI

The neurologic deficits related to SCI develop as a result of both primary and secondary injury processes. The primary mechanisms are those caused by the initial injury, including energy transfer to the spinal cord, spinal cord deformation, and persistent postinjury cord compression. These primary injury mechanisms cause immediate cell death, axonal disruption, and ongoing vascular changes that lead to further cellular disruptions.

The secondary mechanisms of SCI are a complex set of biochemical interactions that lead to ongoing and prolonged cellular derangements, instability, and ultimately cell death over several hours or days following the initial injury. The various causes of secondary injury include free radical formation, calcium homeostasis disruption, opiate receptor abnormalities, lipid peroxidation, and excitatory neurotransmitter accumulation. Each of these possible causes likely plays some role in the secondary mechanisms of SCI, and as a group they have become a focal point for SCI-related research.

Excitotoxic neurotransmitters, such as glutamate, accumulate in the extracellular environment in patients with SCI because of presynaptic and postsynaptic dysfunction. Excessive glutamate receptor activation leads to an abnormal influx of calcium into the cell. Once the cell's buffering mechanisms are overwhelmed, the intracellular free calcium activates enzymes, changes gene expression, causes cell membrane failure, and ultimately leads to cell death.

Oxygen radicals are known to form following SCI. These radicals cause lipid peroxidation, cell membrane dysfunction, and cell death. Furthermore, this process is enhanced by a positive feedback loop that occurs when more free radicals are created by cell membrane lysis.[5,8]

The cellular mechanisms of SCI are caused by immediate anatomic and vascular injury as well as complex ongoing biochemical insults. The specific causes and possible treatments of these mechanisms remain elusive and are the focus of substantial ongoing basic science and clinical research.

Evaluation and Diagnosis

The evaluation of the SCI patient begins with a thorough examination, including a mandatory complete neurologic examination. Close attention should be paid to whether the patient is in spinal shock as well as the level of injury and any distal sparing. These elements are critical to the correct diagnosis of SCI, evaluation of the prognosis for recovery, and development of an appropriate treatment plan. For patients with injury at the thoracolumbar junction, bowel and bladder function must be evaluated in detail to rule out an otherwise subclinical conus medullaris or cauda equina injury. Serial examinations should be performed in high-risk patients, and all SCI patients should be reexamined after therapeutic and diagnostic interventions because neurologic deterioration is most likely to occur following these interventions.[9]

The American Spinal Injury Association impairment scale is a commonly used, reproducible grading system for characterizing the severity of SCI[10] (**Figure 1**). Standardized grading is critical to ensure the accurate and understandable assessment of a patient's disability and rapid recognition of any deterioration in function.

Imaging studies are pivotal in the workup of the SCI patient. Multiple noncontiguous spine fractures occur in 7% to 34% of patients, and imaging of the entire spine is needed to evaluate these injuries.[11,12] Advanced studies including MRI scans, CT scans, and bone scans can be used to better delineate vertebral involvement, canal compromise, and spinal cord edema. Imaging studies are also used to evaluate damage to other organs such as the intestinal, pulmonary, and vascular systems that commonly occurs in conjunction with SCI.

Medical Management

Optimal medical management of the patient with acute SCI remains the subject of much debate and controversy. The lack of high-quality human studies in this field has led to an absence of definitive treatment algorithms. Hence, there is no uniformly accepted recommendation regarding the medical treatment of acute SCI including the possible use or nonuse of systemic steroids. A few of the studies in this field are summarized in the following paragraphs, but this should not be construed to be a recommendation of any particular treatment.

The initial steps of management for the SCI patient include immobilization, evaluation, and medical stabilization. Further management is focused on preventing neurologic deterioration and can be based on both surgical and medical therapies. Medical therapy aims to minimize damage caused by the primary and secondary mediators of SCI. One of the important primary causes

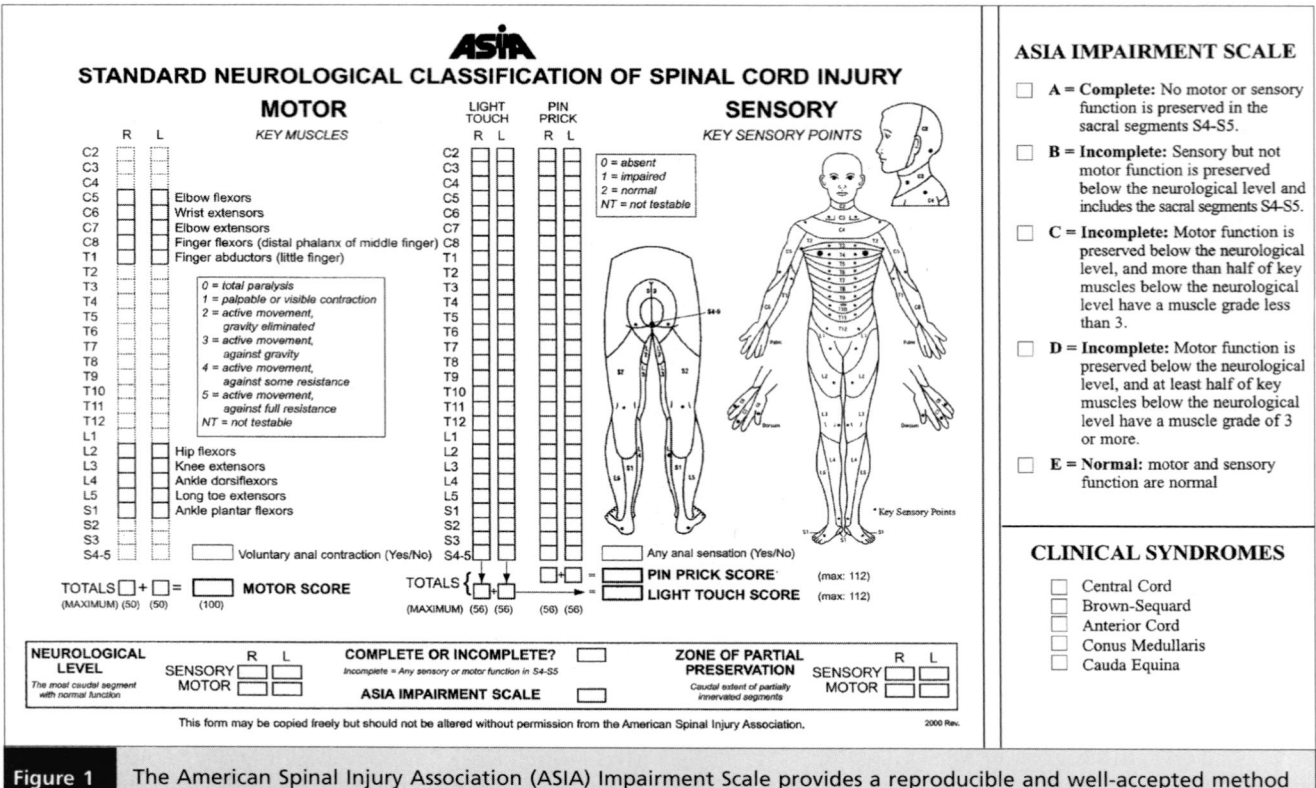

Figure 1 The American Spinal Injury Association (ASIA) Impairment Scale provides a reproducible and well-accepted method for grading SCI. (*Reproduced from the American Spinal Injury Association.*)

of SCI is local hypoxemia, which can be caused by a combination of impaired systemic oxygenation and hypotension. Oxygen supplementation should be used to maintain appropriate saturation levels, and ventilatory support may be required for patients with cervical-level SCI or other pulmonary injuries. Systemic hypotension can exacerbate local blood vessel dysfunction and should be treated. Vasopressors may be required to improve the impaired sympathetic tone seen in SCI-associated neurogenic shock. Neurogenic shock is characterized by hypotension with relative bradycardia, in contrast to hypovolemic shock, which presents with hypotension and tachycardia.

Ongoing nerve damage may occur following the initial insult because of the secondary mechanisms of SCI. These secondary mechanisms begin hours and days following the injury, and this delay may provide a therapeutic opportunity for stabilization or improvement of a patient's condition. Some agents that have been studied include corticosteroids, opiate antagonists, calcium-channel blockers, and glutamate receptor antagonists. Only one medical treatment, methylprednisolone, has been shown to possibly improve recovery following SCI, although its effectiveness has been recently questioned.[13-20]

The success of glucocorticoids in the treatment of closed head injuries and in animal studies for SCI led to the development of the National Acute Spinal Cord Injury Study (NASCIS). The results of this prospective,

randomized, double-blind, multicenter study evaluating high- and low-dose methylprednisolone treatment of SCI were published in 1984. No improvement was seen in either patient group, although there was concern that the steroid dose was lower than that required to see efficacy in humans.

A second study, NASCIS II, was designed to evaluate a higher dose of methylprednisolone (30 mg/kg intravenous bolus followed by 5.4 mg/kg for 23 hours), naloxone, or placebo.[15] As with the first NASCIS study, a prospective, randomized, double-blind, multicenter study was performed. Initial data analysis showed no difference in recovery for any of the groups at either a 6-month or 12-month follow-up. Upon further stratification, the patients who received steroids within 8 hours of injury did show improved neurologic improvement versus other patients. This steroid patient subgroup also had twice the wound infection and pulmonary embolism rates, although these differences were not found to be statistically significant. Patients treated with steroids outside of the 8-hour postinjury window had impaired recovery versus those who were administered a placebo.

Because of the clinical improvement seen in the steroid group of the NASCIS II trial, a third study, NASCIS III, was developed.[17,18] This investigation was a prospective, multicenter, randomized, double-blind study that evaluated steroid use for 24 hours, steroid use for 48 hours, and tirilazad for 48 hours. All pa-

1: Principles of Orthopaedics

tients received a 30 mg/kg bolus of steroids on initiation of treatment because of the findings of the NASCIS II trial. Patients were stratified based on time after injury for initiation of the treatment protocols. For the patients treated within 3 hours of injury, no difference was seen between the treatment groups. For patients treated from 3 to 8 hours postinjury, the 48-hour steroid group had a statistically significant improvement over the 24-hour steroid group. The 48-hour group, however, also had increased rates of pneumonia and sepsis, although these increases were not statistically significant.

The authors of the NASCIS trial reports have recommended that patients treated within 3 hours of SCI should receive 24 hours of methylprednisolone treatment in addition to the bolus dose, whereas patients seen 3 to 8 hours postinjury should be treated with 48 hours of steroids as well as the bolus dose. Patients seen outside of this 8-hour time period should not be given steroids for SCI because of their lack of improvement and significant complications associated with the treatment.

The NASCIS trials suggested that methylprednisolone treatment may be beneficial for a selected group of SCI patients with nonpenetrating trauma. However, significant controversy regarding these results exists. The stratification into subgroups based on postinjury timing in the NASCIS II trial was performed following completion of the study[20] and was not performed prospectively during the trial. Furthermore, no patients with penetrating trauma or life-threatening comorbidities were included in the trials. The neurologic improvement seen in the steroid patients did not result in any clinically relevant functional improvements. Finally, multiple other studies have evaluated steroid treatment of SCI, and most of these have not shown any improvement of neurologic function with steroid treatment.[21-27] Given the increased complication rate with steroid treatment and lack of evidence corroborating the results of the NASCIS trials, a growing controversy over steroid treatment of SCI has developed.[28-32] Further well-designed investigations will likely be necessary to fully define the role of steroids and other medications in the medical treatment of SCI. Currently, the lack of evidence-based criteria regarding steroids does not support either their use or nonuse for the treatment of SCI.

Surgical Management
A full discussion regarding the appropriate surgical management of patients with SCI is beyond the scope of this chapter. Many aspects regarding surgical treatment of these patients remain controversial. Each case needs to be evaluated individually for a variety of factors including: spinal stability or lack thereof; ongoing canal compromise with neural compression; neurologic deficit and deterioration; and patient-related factors including comorbidities, age, osteoporosis, and related injuries. Most physicians would agree that patients with persistent neural compression and neurologic deterioration should undergo surgical decompression.

Outside of this scenario, however, a variety of options are likely available.

Patients with posttraumatic spinal instability will likely benefit from surgical treatment including fracture reduction, instrumentation, and fusion. Surgical stabilization helps to prevent further injury and allows rapid and safe mobilization and rehabilitation. Canal compromise alone may not be an indication for surgical intervention. If a patient has canal compromise with a neurologic deficit, however, surgical decompression may be beneficial although the timing of the surgical decompression remains controversial.[33-35] Patients should be medically optimized before surgery to avoid potential postoperative complications.

Developing Technologies
The potential for successful treatment of SCI, either to preserve or restore function, exists because most traumatic injuries do not involve transection of the cord but stretching, contusion, or compression of the cord as the primary mechanism of injury. The initial trauma is followed by a complex pathogenic cascade including hemorrhage, vasospasm, ischemia, all of which, on a cellular level, lead to the invasion of inflammatory cells, the production of cytokines, apoptotic degeneration, free radical generation, and ultimately, cell destruction. This secondary injury cascade increases the devastation and damage to the spinal cord well after the initial insult has occurred. If the secondary injury cascade could somehow be minimized or attenuated, cell destruction could be halted and the chances of functional recovery after SCI could be improved. This premise of using a neuroprotective pharmacologic agent to limit destruction and/or improve neurologic function is the focus of most of the clinical research currently performed. The results, however, reveal only modest improvement at best. Thus, at present there is no consensus for acute treatment or rehabilitative therapy.[15-18,36-44]

Neuroprotection
Neuroprotection as a concept has been proven many times over in preclinical animal studies. A variety of pharmacologic agents have shown great potential in their ability to improve neurologic function in SCI models in animals. However, these agents have been disappointing once translated into human clinical trials. Naloxone, nimodipine, thyrotropin-releasing hormone, and GM-1 ganglioside are examples of such agents that have demonstrated encouraging results in animal models yet have failed to achieve significant functional improvement in human trials. However, additional pharmacologic agents, especially those with an established safety profile in humans, are a target of ongoing research.[45,46] Of these agents, minocycline and erythropoietin have been cited in a recent review as clinically promising.[47]

Minocycline is a synthetic tetracycline derivative used clinically as an antimicrobial agent for the treatment of conditions such as acne. In recent years it has been shown to have many neuroprotective properties, such as the inhibition of apoptosis or programmed cell death, inhibition of microglia or the neuronal equivalent of scar, and inhibition of metalloproteinases or inflammatory activators. Most importantly, many different laboratories have corroborated improvement in functional recovery after SCI in different animal models when minocycline was administered. It has also shown promise in other disease models including Parkinson's disease, Huntington's disease, amyotrophic lateral sclerosis, and ischemic stroke in animals. Currently, a pilot study using minocycline to treat acute SCI in patients has been initiated in Canada.[44,48]

Erythropoietin is known for its ability to stimulate erythropoiesis. Its use is widespread in the treatment of anemia and anemia related to chronic renal failure and chemotherapy. It has also been used preoperatively in orthopaedics, mostly in arthroplasty to decrease perioperative transfusions. Erythropoietin also seems to have tissue preservation and protective effects. It has been shown to be beneficial in animal models of Parkinson's disease, multiple sclerosis, diabetic neuropathy, and stroke. In animal models of SCI, it has demonstrated the ability to decrease neuronal apoptosis and promote neuroregeneration resulting in improved functional recovery.[49,50-52] It has also been directly compared to bolus dosing of methylprednisolone, with superior histologic appearance and control of lipid peroxidation, the proposed primary mechanism of methylprednisolone-associated functional improvement in the NASCIS II clinical trial.[53] Although the difficulty of translating promising animal results to human results has already been discussed, a small human trial using erythropoietin in patients with acute strokes has demonstrated improved neurologic recovery at an early stage.[54] There is an ongoing phase II trial of erythropoietin in patients with malignant spinal cord compression who are paraparetic or paraplegic. A clinical trial using erythropoietin for treatment of acute SCI has not been initiated.

Neurorestoration

The injured spinal cord presents an inhibiting environment for axonal regeneration or growth. A common idea for stimulating axonal growth or regeneration is to deliver a neurotrophic growth factor to the injury site. Neurotrophic growth factors have been implicated in the processes of neuronal homeostasis and survival, axonal growth and development, synaptic plasticity, and neurotransmission. The most vigorously studied is brain-derived neurotrophic factor (BDNF). Significant axonal regeneration has been shown when this growth factor is delivered acutely after injury in an animal model.[55] Also, cell-mediated gene therapy using fibroblasts genetically modified to produce BDNF and neurotrophin-3 (NT-3) have been transplanted into a thoracic cord transection model in rats.[56] The animals transplanted with the fibroblasts producing BDNF and NT-3, with daily cycling exercise and serotonin agonists, displayed the greatest gains in functional recovery

compared with those transplanted with fibroblasts or any other treatment alone. Limitations are noted when BDNF is administered at a later time point 6 to 8 weeks after injury, when no beneficial effect was demonstrated on axonal regeneration.[57,58] This emphasizes that affecting cell restoration at later stages of SCI may be more difficult. In chronic SCI, the intrinsic damage presents a hostile environment for neuronal growth and regeneration.[59,60] First, the area of injury is colonized with astrocytes causing gliosis, the central nervous system (CNS) equivalent of scar, which surrounds a cystic zone devoid of cells or tissue. This glial scar not only serves as a mechanical barrier but also secretes a complement of inhibitory proteins that prevent axonal regeneration.[61-64] Second, there is a reduction in viable cells available to regenerate. If more cells could be recruited they still would have to find a way to cross the impermissive glial border and resynapse with other neurons. In the face of these problems, cell transplantation may be an attractive solution. Yet cell survival after allogeneic transplantation may require host immune suppression or appropriate encapsulation.[62,63]

Currently, cell-based strategies for transplantation in SCI patients include stem cells, bone marrow stromal cells, fetal tissue, Schwann cells, and olfactory ensheathing cells (OECs). The cellular substrate with the greatest human experience is the OEC. Human trials have been performed in four countries—China, Portugal, Australia, and Russia. The primary olfactory system is an unusual tissue and an attractive site for transplantation because it supports neurogenesis throughout life. In addition, newly generated olfactory neurons are able to grow into the inhibitory CNS environment of the olfactory bulb tissue and reform synapses. It is believed that this unique regenerative property depends in part on the presence of OECs. OECs are distinct glial cells that ensheathe the olfactory neuron and direct axonal regeneration from the nasal mucosa located across the cribriform plate, and synapse with second-order neurons in the CNS. The ability of the OECs to cross from the peripheral nervous system (PNS) through the cribriform plate into the CNS is unique. This ability to bridge the PNS-CNS interface has stimulated the concept that OECs could also serve as a conduit of axonal regeneration across the inhibitory glial scar that is inherent in SCI. Researchers have demonstrated that OECs have the ability to survive, migrate, remyelinate axons like Schwann cells, and even regenerate axons across the injury site in SCI animal models.[64] In humans, the most controversial study obtains OECs from aborted fetuses for transplantation into the spinal cord of the patient via injection. This technique has been performed in more than 300 patients in China; however, the technique has been criticized because of a lack of standardized protocol for treatment, poor follow-up of patients, and the lack of monitored outcomes, systematic reporting of adverse events or safety, and peer-reviewed evaluation of results.[47]

In brief, advanced techniques of molecular and cell biology may enable a combination therapy that combines the limitation of secondary injury with treatments that promote remyelination of damaged axons, axonal regeneration, and restoration of the spinal cord. These techniques, although complex, will hopefully provide novel therapeutic strategies that will restore function in what is currently considered a devastating injury.

Peripheral Nerve Injury

Peripheral nerves are heterogeneous composite structures composed of multiple cell types including neurons, Schwann cells, macrophages, and fibroblasts. The primary function of peripheral nerves is the propagation of action potentials. To improve the speed of action potential propagation (such as nerve conduction velocity) without increasing the diameter of the axon, the Schwann cell—the primary glial cell of the PNS—forms a myelin sheath around the axon to insulate the axon and reduce dissipation of the action potential. Between each myelinated segment are periodic interruptions in the myelin sheath, or nodes of Ranvier. These nodes and the regions of membrane that surround the nodes, the paranode and juxtaparanode, are critical to the rapid, efficient conduction of the action potential. Although the central dogma of neuroscience for the past century has been that the PNS regenerates while the CNS does not, functional reinnervation after a peripheral nerve injury in adults remains quite limited.[65,66] As such, this arena of orthopaedic surgery warrants continued, vigorous exploration and research so as to improve patient outcomes.

Adult Brachial Plexus Injury
Mechanism of Injury
The brachial plexus is the critical link between the spinal cord and the upper extremity. Although the brachial plexus is a portion of the PNS, regeneration after injury is quite limited secondary to numerous issues including the distance that the regenerating axon must travel to reach the terminal end organ. These devastating injuries have a lasting impact on patients because these injuries most often occur as closed trauma in young adults secondary to motor vehicle crashes including motorcycles and bicycles. The nerve injury is most often secondary to traction forces that may induce a root avulsion, nerve rupture, or significant nerve stretch. The nerve may be injured at the root, anterior branch of the spinal nerve, the trunk, the cord, or at the peripheral nerve itself.

When the brachial plexus injury is at the level of the root, it must be classified relative to the dorsal root ganglion, for example, either preganglionic (supraganglionic) or postganglionic (infraganglionic). With both types of injury, there are distinct motor/muscle changes. With postganglionic lesions, there is also loss of sensory function; these injuries may be treated with surgical repair and grafting. In contrast, sensory nerve action potentials are retained with preganglionic lesions as the cell body and peripheral neurites/axons remain in continuity. The efferent or central neurite is no longer in continuity with the spinal cord and currently is only amenable to neurotization procedures. Root avulsions tend to be primarily supraclavicular injuries and may occur secondary to either central or peripheral loading. With a central mechanism of injury, direct cervical trauma may cause the spinal cord to move either longitudinally or transversely. With this mechanism, the root remains with the neural foramen as the epidural sleeve is preserved. In contrast, traction forces avulse the rootlets with the peripheral mechanism. Here, the epidural sleeve may be altered as the epidural cone tends to move into the neural foramina. The C7-T1 nerve roots have relatively weaker fascial attachments at the spine and thus are more likely to be injured than the C5 and C6 nerve roots.[67]

Although the brachial plexus may be injured anywhere along its course, it is more likely to be injured supraclavicularly within the root and trunk regions (approximately 75% of all brachial plexus injuries). Moreover, if the head rapidly moves away from the shoulder, then the injury tends more often to be an upper trunk or C5 and C6 lesion. In contrast, if the arm is violently abducted, then the traction injury tends to be localized to the lower trunk or C8-T1 nerve roots. Injuries to the shoulder girdle such as an anterior dislocation tend to create the less common infraclavicular lesions. For a nerve rupture to occur, the nerve must be fixed at two distinct locations. Because the suprascapular, axillary, and musculocutaneous nerves may be fixed within either the scapular notch or coracobrachialis, these nerves are most susceptible to rupture.

Electrodiagnostic and Imaging Modalities
After most musculoskeletal injuries, radiographs are obtained to provide objective evidence of bony pathology. After a brachial plexus injury, cervical spine, shoulder, and chest radiographs should be obtained to evaluate for possible associated fractures. A CT myelogram may be obtained 3 to 4 weeks after injury as the presence of a pseudomeningocele is highly suggestive of a root avulsion. MRI and magnetic resonance neurography studies are continuing to evolve as potential diagnostic tests. Yet, the objective testing that must be performed after a brachial plexus injury is electrodiagnostic testing. A combination of electromyography (EMG) and nerve conduction velocity studies (NCS) will help to determine which nerves are injured, the location of injury, the extent of the damage, and if there is ongoing reinnervation. With NCS, the nerve is stimulated both proximally and distally with recordings from the nerve to assess sensory function and from the muscle to assess motor function. The amplitude, latency, and velocity all must be measured to help assess the severity of damage. The compound action potential is lost immediately after nerve injury with the response proportional to the remaining active axons distal to the site of injury. It is important to remember that axonal disruption may be distinguished from a conduction block 5 days after injury. Yet a conduction block, which manifests as a focal amplitude change, may last for months if there is axonal

distortion with preserved architecture after injury. If there is axonal disruption, the accompanying low-amplitude response and fibrillation potentials may last for years. Fibrillation potentials are spontaneous discharges within the muscle fibers after neural injury and are always a sign of pathology. The number of fibrillation potentials is usually proportional to the amount of axonal loss. The EMG changes after nerve trauma change from reduced recruitment and fibrillation potentials secondary to the axonal loss to signs of collateral sprouting at a later point. By 1 month after injury, the collateral sprouting and signs of recovery include an increasing number of motor unit potentials, nascent motor unit potentials, increasing compound action potentials, and decreasing number of fibrillation potentials. As an adjunct to standard electrodiagnostic testing, there is increasing use of somatosensory-evoked potentials to evaluate nerve trauma.

Fibrillations and positive sharp waves occur on average about 3 weeks following injury. Electrodiagnostic studies should initially be performed at this time point to establish a baseline. If a root avulsion is expected, careful examination of the posterior cervical musculature is required because these muscles are innervated by the posterior primary rami that provide the anterior primary rami. If there is evidence for denervation, then a root avulsion should be strongly considered. Additionally, sensory conduction will remain intact unless there is an additional infraganglionic or distal rupture. At 7 days following injury, abnormal spontaneous activity begins in the paraspinal muscles and then progresses to the limb muscles after a few weeks. Fibrillation potentials decrease with time; at 6 months, they are approximately one half of the initial amplitude. Abnormal spontaneous activity will not occur if there is concurrent demyelination. Assessment for the possibility of a root avulsion type of injury is critical at the early juncture because this impacts treatment management.

If there is a clinical deficit after a brachial plexus injury, then NCS must be performed for motor function in the median, ulnar, radial, and musculocutaneous nerves as well as sensory function in the median, ulnar, radial, and lateral antebrachial cutaneous nerves. EMG evaluation of the cervical paraspinal, biceps, triceps, and first dorsal interosseous muscles should also be performed to help localize the site of injury. After these initial studies, additional evaluation may be performed based on the suspected level of injury. For upper trunk lesions, the rhomboids, deltoid, infraspinatus, and brachioradialis should be evaluated to assess C5 and C6 integrity. The pronator teres and extensor carpi radialis localize the lesion to the middle trunk or C7 level. To assess the lower trunk, the C8 muscles (extensor carpi ulnaris, flexor carpi ulnaris, and flexor pollicis longus) should be evaluated.

Priorities for Reconstruction

Based on the level and extent of injury, a complete recovery may not be a reasonable expectation.[68] As such, a hierarchy of reconstruction must be established to optimize function. Most surgeons would prioritize in the following manner: elbow flexion, shoulder stability, protective hand sensation, stable wrist extension, dynamic finger flexion, and finally intrinsic muscle function. To achieve scapulohumeral stability, the trapezius, rhomboids, and serratus anterior need to be functional. Because shoulder abduction requires both the deltoid and supraspinatus, ideally they both should be reinnervated. Shoulder external rotation occurs via the infraspinatus whereas the pectoralis and subscapularis provide internal rotation. Although most patients prefer a dynamic, active shoulder, a shoulder arthrodesis in a position of function (30° of abduction, internal rotation, and flexion) needs to be an option that is discussed with all patients, especially if they lack the critical function of elbow flexion. To regain the ability of bringing the hand to the mouth, active elbow flexion is considered the highest priority. As such, the biceps and brachialis must be reinnervated or functionally replaced with either a free muscle transfer or a tendon transfer procedure.[69] For reinnervation of these muscles, the techniques include a plexus repair and neurotization procedures based on the level of injury. If these techniques fail, then tendon transfers and free muscle transfers may be considered as either primary or salvage procedures.

Methods of Repair

There are two primary anterior exposures that can be used to approach the brachial plexus, the supraclavicular and the infraclavicular. The C5-T1 nerve roots travel beneath and between the scalene muscles. Immediately lateral to the scalene muscles, the plexus divides into the trunks with the divisions beneath the clavicle. A supraclavicular approach may be used to treat injury to these regions; the platysma is divided and the sternocleidomastoid is retracted away from the zone of dissection. The phrenic nerve (C3-C5) is identified and used to identify the C5 nerve root. The infraclavicular approach is often used for injuries to the divisions or cords of the brachial plexus. This area is posterior to the clavicle and is particularly difficult with revision surgery (that is, after a vascular repair). The relationships of the neurovascular structures to the pectoralis minor are important to help guide the dissection. Once the site of injury is identified, a nerve repair may be performed using standard microsurgical techniques. These repairs are being increasingly augmented with the use of a fibrin sealant.[70] This sealant requires the mixing of two self-activating components—fibrinogen with aprotinin and thrombin with calcium chloride. These agents form a solid coagulum within minutes and can be used to create a stable, watertight seal. Currently in the United States, this remains an off-label use of this product. If a direct repair is not possible, nerve grafting from the sural nerves has been the traditional donor source.[71] Vascularized nerve grafts are alternative sources. The rationale remains that the vascularized nerve inherently has greater blood supply, may prevent neural fibrosis, and may be used in scarred beds. Graft sources include the anterior tibial, superficial peroneal, saphenous, superficial radial, and ulnar nerves. These vascularized grafts create donor-site morbidity and are extremely surgically challenging; furthermore, improvements in functional outcomes have not been clearly demonstrated and remain controversial.

Nerve Transfers

One of the most exciting new areas of peripheral nerve surgery is the increasing use of nerve transfers or neurotization procedures. Nerve transfers are procedures in which a functional donor nerve is directly coapted close to the target end organ of the injured nerve to theoretically encourage faster recovery while limiting secondary muscle atrophy and neuromuscular junction degeneration. There must be a motor nerve with a significant number of axons in relative proximity to the denervated muscle to act as a donor nerve. If this donor nerve innervates muscles synergistic to the denervated muscles, then postoperative motor reeducation is more effective. The donor nerve may be either extraplexal (outside the brachial plexus) or intraplexal (inside the brachial plexus). The extraplexal donor nerves that are primarily used are the spinal accessory nerve or cranial nerve XI, the phrenic nerve, intercostal nerves, and the C7 nerve root from the contralateral extremity.[72] The primary intraplexal donor nerves are the ulnar and radial nerves. These surgical procedures should be performed within the first 6 months after the brachial plexus injury. To achieve functional reinnervation, significant postoperative rehabilitation is required for both sensory and motor reeducation.

A variety of nerve transfers are currently being used by different surgical teams. One of the most popular and straightforward procedures is the Oberlin procedure because of its predictable, favorable results.[73] This intraplexal neurotization procedure is used to achieve active biceps function after either a C5-C6 palsy or a C5-C6-C7 palsy by transferring ulnar nerve fascicles in the upper arm to the motor branch of the musculocutaneous nerve. For upper plexus lesions, several transfers may be performed, including (1) the spinal accessory to the suprascapular nerve, (2) triceps branch of the radial nerve to the axillary nerve, and (3) a double fascicular transfer for elbow flexion (flexor carpi radialis fascicle of the median nerve to the biceps branch of the musculocutaneous nerve and flexor carpi ulnaris fascicle of the ulnar nerve to the brachialis branch). Other procedures include the use of intercostal nerves as donors for transfer to the musculocutaneous nerve or to innervate a free functioning muscle transfer such as the gracilis. Nerve transfers offer a possibility for function after preganglionic lesions that otherwise are considered irreparable. For postganglionic lesions, where large nerve gaps exist or there is a tremendous distance for axonal regeneration to occur, they provide an alternative to nerve grafting and serve to power free muscle transfers. As surgeons continue to champion these innovative techniques, these patients are offered hope that they may regain function of their injured extremities.

Traumatic/Acute Peripheral Nerve Injury
Mechanisms of Injury

Most orthopaedic surgeons treat acute nerve injuries whether they are nerve transection or crush injuries. After the axon is injured, the distal stump undergoes a process known as wallerian degeneration to clear axonal and myelin debris while creating an environment hospitable for regeneration.[74] The breakdown of axoplasm and cytoskeleton is triggered by increased production of axoplasmic calcium with the granular disintegration of the axonal cytoskeleton considered as the hallmark of the initiation of wallerian degeneration. Whereas normal Schwann cells do not divide, Schwann cells within the distal segment divide within 24 hours of injury with peak response by 72 hours. They form Büngner's bands, which are cytoplasmic processes that interdigitate and line up in rows under the original basal lamina of the nerve fiber. Regenerating axons travel within these channels to reach their target end organ. The macrophage is the primary phagocyte of myelin and accumulates by 72 hours. Early on, the macrophages express major histocompatibility complex class II antigen 1a and are not phagocytic. Later, the hematogenously derived macrophages penetrate the basal lamina, lose 1a expression and become phagocytic, produce interleukin-1, and stimulate Schwann cells to produce nerve growth factor to enhance regeneration.

There is also a profound nerve cell body response with a significant alteration of metabolic priority. There is a decrease of neurotransmitter production with an ensuing increase in protein production such as tubulin, actin, and growth-associated proteins. The proximal nerve segment response will degenerate if the cell body dies, but will regenerate if the cell body survives. There is an early decrease in myelin thickness relative to the axon diameter after injury that gradually increases but remains smaller than the original thickness. It is important to recognize that collateral sprouts occur from nodes of Ranvier whereas terminal sprouts arise from tips of remaining axons. Axonal regeneration across the zone of injury is limited by scar tissue between stumps that may be obstructive to axonal advancement. Within the distal segment, there is a variable rate of axonal regeneration based on type/location of injury. On average, axonal growth occurs at a rate of 1 to 2 mm/day with a decreased rate in distal regions.

Techniques for Surgical Repair

After a nerve transection, the objectives of surgical repair are to maximize the number of axons regenerating across the injury site and to maximize the accuracy of reinnervation. Younger patients usually have better functional outcome for still unknown reasons. A primary nerve repair is defined as an immediate repair or a repair performed within several hours of injury.[75] It is the treatment of choice if conditions permit, including a clean wound, healthy tissue bed, appropriate surgical equipment/surgeon/staff, and a physically and emotionally stable patient. Although immediate primary repair may be appropriate for a sharp nerve transection injury, crushed nerve segments must be excised before repair. If there is an open fracture, then the nerve may be explored (radial nerve exploration with open humerus fracture). A delayed primary repair is defined as a repair that is performed within 5 to 7 days and is best with avulsive and crush-type injuries in which the zone of injury is not initially defined. A secondary repair is performed more than 7 days from the time of injury.

Microsurgical technique includes the use of microscopes/loupes, microsurgical instruments, and appropriate sutures. Because the nerve repair should be tension-free, interpositional nerve grafting is required if a tension-free repair is not possible. An epineurial repair should be performed if the nerve includes mixed sensory and motor fibers without well-defined fascicular groups. It may be possible to attempt a grouped fascicular repair if a particular fascicle is recognized that mediates a specific function. For an epineurial repair, the surgeon must identify the proximal and distal nerve ends in a bloodless field. Fascicular or vascular landmarks are identified with coapted epineurial sleeves. The repair is performed with the first suture farthest from the surgeon and the second suture 180° from the first suture. Uniform tension is desired, with additional sutures placed sparingly. For a group fascicular repair, higher magnification is needed as nerve ends are inspected to determine alignment of fascicles so that the fascicular groups may be matched, trimmed, and repaired. It is quite rare to perform individual fascicular repair except for digital nerve repairs. To date, no study has demonstrated the superiority of one single technique. The potential benefits of fascicular repair may be lost because of increased surgical manipulation; the repair of inappropriate fascicles leads to poor results.

Fascicle matching techniques may be attempted with intraoperative nerve stimulation. This technique may identify the proximal sensory and distal motor fascicles but does require patient cooperation. Alternatively, immunohistochemical identification may be used up to 9 days after injury. Acetylcholinesterase is present in axoplasm of myelinated motor axons and many unmyelinated axons, but is not present within the sensory axons. In contrast, carbonic anhydrase is present in myelin and axoplasm of sensory axons. To attempt this technique, nerve tissue from proximal and distal stumps must be sacrificed. Although the technique does require 1 to 2 hours of processing time, patient cooperation is not necessary. Although both of these techniques have not convincingly demonstrated superior results, they may have a role in late nerve reconstruction.

At the time of surgical reconstruction, the surgeon must determine if a nerve gap or defect is present. If an end-to-end repair cannot be performed without undue tension, then a nerve graft should be considered.[76] The ideal graft should have large fascicles, little connective tissue, separate parallel fascicles, accessible location, little variability, and little branching. The functional outcome of the graft decreases as the length of the graft increases. Donor nerves include sural, anterior branch of the medial antebrachial cutaneous, lateral antebrachial, and terminal branch of posterior interosseous nerves.

The role of vascularized nerve grafts has not been clearly established, but potential indications include large nerve gaps, very proximal injuries, compromised tissue beds (radiated tissue), and large-caliber donor nerve grafts. An alternative to nerve grafting is the use of nerve tubes or axonal guidance channels.[77,78] These may be either vascular channels from the patient such as redundant arteries and veins or may be commercially available composite structures, collagen, silicone, and/or components of the extracellular matrix (laminin and fibronectin). Although there are reports of increased rates of axonal regeneration across a gap when a nerve guide tube is used to bridge the gap, these axonal guidance channels are currently primarily used for gaps with digital nerve repairs.

Chronic Nerve Compression

Compression neuropathies are some of the most common conditions that orthopaedic surgeons routinely treat, from carpal tunnel syndrome to spinal nerve root stenosis. Because these conditions most often develop over the course of weeks to months, they are by their nature chronic nerve injuries. Until recently, they were simply considered variants of acute nerve injuries that simply developed over time and had a similar pathogenesis.

Pathogenesis

Much of the earlier literature described compression neuropathies as the by-product of mild wallerian degeneration that occurred at the site of injury. Recent research using both in vivo and in vitro modeling systems has called that notion into question.[79] The hallmark of compression neuropathies is a progressive decrease in the nerve conduction velocity at the site of injury that occurs over time. Yet, there are numerous changes at the site of injury that actually occur before the nerve conduction velocity changes. Among them, one of the primary features is a dramatic Schwann cell turnover that induces both Schwann cell proliferation and apoptosis in the absence of any evidence of axonal pathology. This finding was quite remarkable because glial cells such as Schwann cells most often respond secondarily to the cues from neurons, as with acute nerve injuries and wallerian degeneration. Moreover, there is a progressive change in the Schwann cell phenotype as these cells become less promyelinogenic, with a decrease in myelin-specific proteins such as myelin basic protein and myelin-associated glycoprotein (MAG). In turn, they upregulate proregenerative molecules such as vascular endothelial growth factor. These changes alter their primary function of myelination, with changes in internodal length and myelin thickness. Of interest, there is also a change in the occurrence of Schmidt-Lanterman incisures after compressive neuropathies. The Schmidt-Lanterman incisures are channels within the myelin that allow communication between the Schwann cell nucleus and the axon and have been hypothesized to be actively involved in the metabolic function within the myelin sheath. The thinner myelin produced by the new Schwann cells may be the result of increased energy requirements.

In addition to the Schwann cell changes that occur after the induction of compression neuropathies, there is a slow, gradual recruitment of macrophages to the site of injury over weeks and months. This is in contrast to acute nerve injuries, which induce a rapid recruitment of macrophages over 48 to 72 hours that then declines. These macrophages upregulate the enzyme-inducible nitric oxide synthase and are responsible for the altered blood-nerve barrier that develops with compression neuropathies. As macrophages may produce Schwann cell mitogens, macrophage depletion experiments have demonstrated that macrophages play an integral role with the altered vascular permeability, but not the altered Schwann cell function with compression neuropathies.

Although there is a profound early glial cell response by the Schwann cells and macrophages with compression neuropathies, axonal architecture and integrity is maintained. Although rigorous evaluation fails to find any morphometric changes to the axonal cytoskeleton, the neuron does respond. Recent work has demonstrated that the Schwann cells locally downregulate the production of MAG at the site of injury. As MAG helps to maintain normal axonal architecture, the downregulation of MAG creates an environment that permits axonal sprouting at the nodes of Ranvier. As the MAG levels eventually return to baseline levels, this sprouting response is abrogated.[80] Behavioral and immunohistochemical data support the idea that this sprouting is responsible for the pain that occurs early with compression neuropathies. Clinically, this pain eventually diminishes while the patient is left with profound sensory and motor deficits. A continued understanding of the pathogenesis of compression neuropathies will help improve management of these conditions with the potential of developing effective treatment regimens to reverse this pathology.

Objective Testing

Electrodiagnostic testing including NCS and EMG are considered the gold standard to objectively evaluate patients with compression neuropathies. Traditional NCS studies routinely evaluate the health and function of the largest, myelinated fibers. As early data seem to indicate that smaller fibers may preferentially be affected early in the disease course, additional electrodiagnostic testing such as near-nerve studies and motor unit nerve number estimation studies may prove to be beneficial with early diagnosis. There are also an increasing number of reports in the literature detailing the use of magnetic resonance neurography to make the diagnosis. With continued improvements in the development of magnetic resonance sequences, changes in nerve size and water content may be appreciated to help localize the site of pathology. Gray-scale and color Doppler ultrasonography are also being reported as viable techniques to objectively diagnose compression neuropathies of the upper extremity such as cubital syndrome.

As with most ultrasonography techniques, these techniques are heavily operator-dependent and require significant experience and practice to establish proficiency.

Outcomes of Surgical Management

There have been several recent reports in the literature advocating the use of decompression of symptomatic diabetic neuropathies. The rationale for this treatment is that as diabetes induces metabolic changes to the peripheral nerve, these nerves are more susceptible to compression neuropathies. Retrospective studies have reported successful management of neuropathies involving the common peroneal, deep peroneal, and tarsal tunnel nerves.[81] Although the promise of reduced pain, improved sensation, and reduced rates of amputation is quite alluring, a systematic review of the literature detailed that only class IV studies exist to support such bold claims.[82] Furthermore, these techniques do create incisions and potential nonhealing wounds in patients with little reserve and significant medical problems. Further exploration with prospective, randomized studies needs to be conducted before widespread acceptance of these techniques.

With the increased rates of surgical decompression for entrapment neuropathies, there has been increased interest in determining if there is a genetic component to these conditions. One such neurologic disorder that seems likely to reduce the threshold for inducing pathology is hereditary neuropathy with liability to pressure palsies (HNPP).[83] This disorder is an autosomal-dominant peripheral neuropathy that results from deletion of a 1.5-megabase pair segment of the short arm of chromosome 17. A recent study analyzed the genomic DNA from blood obtained from patients that had more than one surgical release for compression neuropathy. Polymerase chain reaction amplification and polyacrylamide gel electrophoresis failed to detect the chromosomal anomaly associated with HNPP that was detected in positive control subjects. As such, although it seems unlikely that HNPP is the genetic predisposition for orthopaedic patients who undergo several releases for compression neuropathies, it is still a distinct possibility that a currently undetected genetic predisposition for compression neuropathies does exist.

With the increasing age of the US population, an increased awareness of medical conditions afflicting older patients is required by all health care providers. Although carpal tunnel syndrome is not a condition that is age-specific, it does manifest differently in elderly patients with increased thenar atrophy and weakness and decreased subjective reports of pain. Furthermore, the surgical outcomes after carpal tunnel release may not be equivalent to outcomes after similar treatment in younger patients.[84,85] Whereas patients in several studies did detect an improvement after surgical release of the carpal canal, symptoms of persistent numbness and loss of manual dexterity and grip strength persisted. Fundamentally, a carpal tunnel release changes the size of the carpal canal and decreases the sustained mechan-

1: Principles of Orthopaedics

ical forces on the median nerve. The nerve itself must then regenerate and hopefully return to its native, pre-injured condition. As neural plasticity is increasingly limited with advanced age, it is not surprising that similar surgical management would yield different results across the age distribution. These data simply provide further support that while surgical management of older patients with carpal tunnel syndrome should be undertaken when appropriate indications are met, surgical management alone is not sufficient to address this pathology and pharmacologic adjuvant may be warranted in the future to maximize functional recovery.

Summary

Nerve injuries, whether in the spinal cord or peripherally, can be devastating and life-changing events. Current treatment modalities are focused on improving function and preventing further injury. Ongoing research in both medical and surgical therapies may improve the ability to treat these injuries in the near future.

Annotated References

1. Breasted JH: *The Edwin Smith Surgical Papyrus*. Chicago, IL, University of Chicago Press, 1930.

2. Ergas Z: Spinal cord injury in the United States: A statistical update. *Cent Nerv Syst Trauma* 1985;2:19-32.

3. *Spinal Cord Injury: Facts and Figures at a Glance*. Birmingham, AL, National Spinal Cord Injury Statistical Center, 2001.

4. Albin MS, White RJ: Epidemiology, physiopathology, and experimental therapeutics of acute spinal cord injury. *Crit Care Clin* 1987;3:441-452.

5. Sekhon LH, Fehlings MG: Epidemiology, demographics, and pathophysiology of acute spinal cord injury. *Spine* 2001;26:S2-S12.

6. Stripling TE: The cost of economic consequences of traumatic spinal cord injury. *Paraplegia News* 1990; 8:50-54.

7. Eismont FJ, Clifford S, Goldberg M, Green B: Cervical sagittal spinal canal size in spine injury. *Spine* 1984; 9:663-666.

8. Hall ED, Braughler JM: Free radicals in CNS injury. *Res Publ Assoc Res Nerv Ment Dis* 1993;71:81-105.

9. Marshall LF, Knowlton S, Garfin SR, et al: Deterioration following spinal cord injury: A multicenter study. *J Neurosurg* 1987;66:400-404.

10. American College of Surgeons: *Advanced Trauma Life Support*, ed 5. Chicago, IL, American College of Surgeons, 1995.

11. Keenen TL, Antony J, Benson DR: Non-contiguous spinal fractures. *J Trauma* 1990;30:489-491.

12. Green RA, Saifuddin A: Whole spine MRI in the assessment of acute vertebral body trauma. *Skeletal Radiol* 2004;33:129-135.

   The authors present whole-spine MRI as a tool for assessing occult vertebral body fracture and show that it may detect more injuries than plain radiographic evaluation.

13. Bracken MB, Collins WF, Freeman DF, et al: Efficacy of methylprednisolone in acute spinal cord injury. *JAMA* 1984;251:45-52.

14. Bracken MB, Shepard MJ, Hellenbrand KG, et al: Methylprednisolone and neurological function 1 year after spinal cord injury: Results of the National Acute Spinal Cord Injury Study. *J Neurosurg* 1985;63:704-713.

15. Bracken MB, Shepard MJ, Collins WF, et al: A randomized, controlled trial of methylprednisolone or naloxone in the treatment of acute spinal-cord injury: Results of the Second National Acute Spinal Cord Injury Study. *N Engl J Med* 1990;322:1405-1411.

16. Bracken MB, Shepard MJ, Collins WF Jr , et al: Methylprednisolone or naloxone treatment after acute spinal cord injury: 1-year follow-up data: Results of the second National Acute Spinal Cord Injury Study. *J Neurosurg* 1992;76:23-31.

17. Bracken MB, Shepard MJ, Holford TR, et al: Administration of methylprednisolone for 24 or 48 hours or tirilazad mesylate for 48 hours in the treatment of acute spinal cord injury: Results of the Third National Acute Spinal Cord Injury Randomized Controlled Trial. National Acute Spinal Cord Injury Study. *JAMA* 1997;277: 1597-1604.

18. Bracken MB, Shepard MJ, Holford TR, et al: Methylprednisolone or tirilazad mesylate administration after acute spinal cord injury: 1-year follow up. Results of the third National Acute Spinal Cord Injury randomized controlled trial. *J Neurosurg* 1998;89:699-706.

19. Hurlbert RJ: The role of steroids in acute spinal cord injury: An evidence-based analysis. *Spine* 2001;26: S39-S46.

20. Hurlbert RJ: Methylprednisolone for acute spinal cord injury: An inappropriate standard of care. *J Neurosurg* 2000;93:1-7.

21. Kiwerski JE: Application of dexamethasone in the treatment of acute spinal cord injury. *Injury* 1993;24: 457-460.

22. George ER, Scholten DJ, Buechler CM, Jordan-Tibbs J,

Mattice C, Albrecht RM: Failure of methylprednisolone to improve the outcome of spinal cord injuries. *Am Surg* 1995;61:659-664.

23. Prendergast MR, Saxe JM, Ledgerwood AM, Lucas CE, Lucas WF: Massive steroids do not reduce the zone of injury after penetrating spinal cord injury. *J Trauma* 1994;37:576-579.

24. Poynton AR, O'Farrell DA, Shannon F, Murray P, McManus F, Walsh MG: An evaluation of the factors affecting neurological recovery following spinal cord injury. *Injury* 1997;28:545-548.

25. Pointillart V, Petitjean ME, Wiart L, et al: Pharmacological therapy of spinal cord injury during the acute phase. *Spinal Cord* 2000;38:71-76.

26. Pollard ME, Apple DF: Factors associated with improved neurologic outcomes in patients with incomplete tetraplegia. *Spine* 2003;28:33-39.

27. Matsumoto T, Tamaki T, Kawakami M, Yoshida M, Ando M, Yamada H: Early complications of high-dose methylprednisolone sodium succinate treatment in the follow-up of acute cervical spinal cord injury. *Spine* 2001;26:426-430.

28. Molano Mdel R, Broton JG, Bean JA, Calancie B: Complications associated with the prophylactic use of methylprednisolone during surgical stabilization after spinal cord injury. *J Neurosurg* 2002;96:267-272.

29. Short DJ, El Masry WS, Jones PW: High dose methylprednisolone in the management of acute spinal cord injury: A systematic review from a clinical perspective. *Spinal Cord* 2000;38:273-286.

30. Hugenholtz H, Cass DE, Dvorak MF, et al: High-dose methylprednisolone for acute closed spinal cord injury: Only a treatment option. *Can J Neurol Sci* 2002;29:227-235.

31. O'Connor PA, McCormack O, Gavin C, et al: Methylprednisolone in acute spinal cord injuries. *Ir J Med Sci* 2003;172:24-26.

32. Molloy S, Middleton F, Casey AT: Failure to administer methylprednisolone for acute traumatic spinal cord injury: A prospective audit of 100 patients from a regional spinal injuries unit. *Injury* 2002;33:575-578.

33. Delamarter RB, Sherman J, Carr JB: Pathophysiology of spinal cord injury: Recovery after immediate and delayed compression. *J Bone Joint Surg Am* 1995;77:1042-1049.

34. Fehlings MG, Sekhon LH, Tator C: The role and timing of decompression in acute spinal cord injury: What do we know? What should we do? *Spine* 2001;26:S101-S110.

35. Tator CH, Fehlings MG, Thorpe K, Taylor W: Current use and timing of spinal surgery for management of acute spinal surgery for management of acute spinal cord injury in North America: Results of a retrospective multicenter study. *J Neurosurg* 1999;91(suppl 1):12-18.

36. Hurlbert RJ: Strategies of medical intervention in the management of acute spinal cord injury. *Spine* 2006;31 (suppl 11):S16-S21.

This review is a literature search from 1996 to 2006 of specialized pharmacologic agents that may prevent secondary injury and promote repair or regeneration. Steroids continue to be administered clinically for acute spinal cord injury. Modulation of posttraumatic inflammation may provide the best opportunity to arrest secondary injury. Protein kinase and metalloproteinase inhibition are promising treatment strategies. Regeneration techniques are concentrating on cell transplantation and manipulating glial receptors and protein production. There are clinical trials on few of these agents.

37. Sayer FT, Kronvall E, Nilsson OG: Methylprednisolone treatment in acute spinal cord injury: The myth challenged through a structured analysis of published literature. *Spine J* 2006;6:335-343.

In this systematic review of literature accumulated on the use of methylprednisolone with subgroup analyses, the authors conclude that there is insufficient evidence to support methylprednisolone as a standard treatment in acute spinal cord injury.

38. Eck JC, Nachtigall D, Humphreys SC, Hodges SD: Questionnaire survey of spine surgeons on the use of methylprednisolone for acute spinal cord injury. *Spine* 2006;31:E250-E253.

The authors present the results of a survey of 305 surgeons on the use of methylprednisolone in patients with acute spinal cord injury. Fourteen surgeons (4.6%) used steroids only if initiated before their consultation, 262 (85.9%) would initiate if within 8 hours of injury, 20 (6.6%) did not use steroids, and 9 (3.0%) used alternative protocols. Only 24% of surgeons followed strict steroid protocol; decisions were made on a case-by-case basis.

39. Sipski ML, Pearse DD: Methylprednisolone and other confounders to spinal cord injury clinical trials. *Nat Clin Pract Neurol* 2006;2:402-403.

The authors comment that current studies are inconsistent in controlling or accounting for methylprednisolone use, and medical and rehabilitative management. They recommend that design of future clinical trials include sensitive outcome measures and control variables such as level/degree of injury, and inconsistent acute surgical, medical, and rehabilitation management. They suggest that trials should target patients with incomplete SCI because they are likely to benefit from neuroprotective therapies.

40. Coleman WP, Benzel D, Cahill DW, et al: A critical appraisal of the reporting of the National Acute Spinal Cord Injury Studies (II and III) of methylprednisolone in acute spinal cord injury. *J Spinal Disord* 2000;13:185-199.

1: Principles of Orthopaedics

41. Bracken MB: Methylprednisolone and acute spinal cord injury: An update of the randomized evidence. *Spine* 2001;26(suppl 24):S47-S54.

42. Bracken MB, Holford TR: Neurological and functional status 1 year after acute spinal cord injury: Estimates of functional recovery in National Acute Spinal Cord Injury Study II from results modeled in National Acute Spinal Cord Injury Study III. *J Neurosurg* 2002;96 (suppl 3):259-266.

43. Bracken MB: Methylprednisolone and spinal cord injury. *J Neurosurg* 2002;96(suppl 1):140-141.

44. Fehlings MG, Baptiste DC: Current status of clinical trials for acute spinal cord injury. *Injury* 2005;36(suppl 2): B113-B122.

   Research has identified pharmacologic compounds that specifically antagonize primary and secondary mechanisms contributing to the etiology of acute SCI. Methylprednisolone and GM-1 ganglioside have shown evidence of modest benefits on all test subjects. Trials on promising neuroprotectives (riluzole, minocycline, erythropoietin, and the fusogen polyethylene glycol), and mild hypothermia are recommended.

45. Hall ED, Springer JE: Neuroprotection and acute spinal cord injury: A reappraisal. *NeuroRx* 2004;1:80-100.

   The authors present a review of the methylprednisolone-SCI controversy, and of agents for neuroprotection after SCI.

46. Anderson DK, Beattie M, Blesch A, et al: Recommended guidelines for studies of human subjects with spinal cord injury. *Spinal Cord* 2005;43:453-458.

   The authors discuss issues to consider in planning and initiation of human clinical trials in SCI.

47. Kwon BK, Fisher CG, Dvorak MF, Tetzlaff W: Strategies to promote neural repair and regeneration after spinal cord injury. *Spine* 2005;30(suppl 17):S3-S13.

   In this excellent review of current literature on neuroprotection and axonal regeneration, the authors urge rigorous design and execution of clinical trials with an emphasis on agents with long-established safety, such as as minocycline, erythropoietin, or those proposed for regeneration as OECs.

48. Baptiste DC, Fehlings MG: Pharmacological approaches to repair the injured spinal cord. *J Neurotrauma* 2006; 23:318-334.

   This is a review of promising neuroprotective pharmacologic treatments in animal models of SCI: sodium (Na$^+$) channel blocker riluzole, the tetracycline derivative minocycline, the fusogen copolymer polyethylene glycol, and the tissue-protective hormone erythropoietin. Neuroprotective and neuroregenerative properties ascribed to the rho pathway antagonist Cethrin (BioAxone Therapeutic, Montreal, Canada) and implantation of activated autologous macrophages (ProCord, Proneuron Biotechnologies, Israel) were recently tested in patients with thoracic and cervical SCI.

49. Arishima Y, Setoguchi T, Yamaura I, Yone K, Komiya S: Preventive effect of erythropoietin on spinal cord cell apoptosis following acute traumatic injury in rats. *Spine* 2006;31:2432-2438.

   An antiapoptotic effect of erythropoietin was found after SCI in rats. Erythropoietin treatment significantly decreased TUNEL-positive apoptotic neurons and oligodendrocytes as early as 6 hours and as long as 7 days after SCI in rats. Erythropoietin treatment significantly decreased the number of active caspase-3 immunoreactive cells within the SCI.

50. Coleman T, Brines M: Science review: Recombinant human erythropoietin in critical illness: A role beyond anemia? *Crit Care* 2004;8:337-341.

   The authors discuss erythropoietin, which rescues cells from apoptosis, reduces inflammatory responses, restores vascular autoregulation, and promotes healing. Erythropoietin has been studied in a phase II clinical trial of ischemic stroke; recombinant human Erythropoietin protects the brain, spinal cord, retina, heart, and kidney from ischemic injury.

51. Celik M, Gokmen N, Erbayraktar S, et al: Erythropoietin prevents motor neuron apoptosis and neurologic disability in experimental spinal cord ischemic injury. *Proc Natl Acad Sci USA* 2002;99:2258-2263.

52. Gorio A, Gokmen N, Erbayraktar S, et al: Recombinant human erythropoietin counteracts secondary injury and markedly enhances neurological recovery from experimental spinal cord trauma. *Proc Natl Acad Sci USA* 2002;99:9450-9455.

53. Gorio A, Madaschi L, Di Stefano B, et al: Methylprednisolone neutralizes the beneficial effects of erythropoietin in experimental spinal cord injury. *Proc Natl Acad Sci USA* 2005;102:16379-16384.

   High-dose erythropoietin and methylprednisolone suppressed proinflammatory cytokines. Only erythropoietin reduced microglial infiltration and scar formation, and improved neurologic function after contusive SCI in rats. Coadministration of methylprednisolone antagonized effects of erythropoietin. Suppression of proinflammatory cytokines alone does not prevent secondary injury. Glucocorticoids should not be coadministered with erythropoietin for treatment of SCI.

54. Ehrenreich H, Aust C, Krampe H, et al: Erythropoietin: Novel approaches to neuroprotection in human brain disease. *Metab Brain Dis* 2004;19:195-206.

   This review presents a neuroprotective approach using erythropoietin in brain disease. The "Gottingen erythropoietin-stroke trial" represents the first effective use of a neuroprotective therapy in an acute brain disease.

55. Vavrek R, Girgis J, Tetzlaff W, Hiebert GW, Fouad K: BDNF promotes connections of corticospinal neurons onto spared descending interneurons in spinal cord injured rats. *Brain* 2006;129:1534-1545.

   BDNF promotes connections of corticospinal neurons onto spared descending interneurons in rats after a dorsal overhemisection of the thoracic spinal cord sparing only the left ventrolateral quadrant. Rats receiving BDNF at the cell bodies of lesioned corticospinal neurons showed a significant increase in collateral sprouting and in the number of contacts with propriospinal interneurons. Increase in collateral sprouting and number of contacts correlated with functional recovery.

56. Nothias JM, Mitsui T, Shumsky JS, Fischer I, Antonacci MD, Murray M: Combined effects of neurotrophin secreting transplants, exercise, and serotonergic drug challenge improve function in spinal rats. *Neurorehabil Neural Repair* 2005;19:296-312.

Spinalized rats received transplants of fibroblasts genetically modified to express BDNF and NT-3, with daily cycling exercise, and with serotonin agonists. Combined treatments of fibroblasts expressing BDNF and NT-3, exercise, and serotonergic agonists produced the greatest improvements in motor function versus individual treatments.

57. Shumsky JS, Tobias CA, Tumolo M, Long WD, Giszter SF, Murray M: Delayed transplantation of fibroblasts genetically modified to secrete BDNF and NT-3 into a spinal cord injury site is associated with limited recovery of function. *Exp Neurol* 2003;184:114-130.

58. Kwon BK, Liu J, Oschipok L, Teh J, Liu ZW, Tetzlaff W: Rubrospinal neurons fail to respond to brain-derived neurotrophic factor applied to the spinal cord injury site 2 months after cervical axotomy. *Exp Neurol* 2004;189:45-57.

BDNF applied at the injury site 2 months after cervical axotomy in rats did not reverse rubrospinal neuronal atrophy nor promote GAP-43, Talpha1 tubulin messenger RNA expression, or axonal regeneration into peripheral nerve transplants. TrkB receptor immunohistochemistry demonstrated immunoreactivity on the neuronal cells, but not on anterograde-labeled rubrospinal axons at the injury site. This finding was due to loss of trkB receptors on the injured axons over time in chronic injury.

59. Kwon BK, Liu J, Messerer C, et al: Survival and regeneration of rubrospinal neurons 1 year after spinal cord injury. *Proc Natl Acad Sci USA* 2002;99:3246-3251.

60. Hermanns S, Klapka N, Gasis M, Muller HW: The collagenous wound healing scar in the injured central nervous system inhibits axonal regeneration. *Adv Exp Med Biol* 2006;557:177-190.

The prevention of collagen scar formation after traumatic CNS injury is important to allow severed axons to regenerate fibers to their former targets, develop chemical synapses, become remyelinated by resident oligodendrocytes, elongate into the uninjured CNS, and conduct action potentials in the brain and spinal cord.

61. Tan AM, Zhang W, Levine JM: NG2: A component of the glial scar that inhibits axon growth. *J Anat* 2005; 207:717-725.

This article is a review of high-molecular-weight chondroitin sulphate proteoglycan (NG2), found on oligodendrocyte precursor cells in the glial scar forming after injury to the brain or spinal cord. The glial scar is considered a biochemical and physical barrier to successful axon regeneration. NG2 and other macromolecules represent an important target for therapies designed to promote axon regrowth.

62. Swanger SA, Neuhuber B, Himes BT, Bakshi A, Fischer I: Analysis of allogeneic and syngeneic bone marrow stromal cell graft survival in the spinal cord. *Cell Transplant* 2005;14:775-786.

The authors present an analysis of allogeneic and syngeneic bone marrow stromal cell graft survival. Allogeneic transplantation with appropriate immune suppression permits long-term survival of bone marrow stromal cells; thus, both allogeneic and syngeneic strategies could be used in devising cell-based therapies for CNS injury.

63. Tobias CA, Han SS, Shumsky JS, et al: Alginate encapsulated BDNF-producing fibroblast grafts permit recovery of function after spinal cord injury in the absence of immune suppression. *J Neurotrauma* 2005;22:138-156.

Alginate-encapsulated fibroblasts expressing BDNF (Fb/BDNF) were grafted into cervical hemisection. Rats treated with encapsulated Fb/BDNF had partial recovery of forelimb usage and hindlimb function that was greater than those with unencapsulated Fb/BDNF without immune suppression, but similar to immune-suppressed rats with unencapsulated Fb/BDNF. Alginate encapsulation has the potential to provide a protective barrier against host immune cell interactions.

64. Fouad K, Schnell L, Bunge MB, Schwab ME, Liebscher T, Pearse DD: Combining Schwann cell bridges and olfactory-ensheathing glia grafts with chondroitinase promotes locomotor recovery after complete transection of the spinal cord. *J Neurosci* 2005;25:1169-1178.

The authors used a combination intervention to reduce scar (chondroitinase ABC) and provide a supportive substrate bridge of Schwann cells for axonal regeneration of olfactory-ensheathing glia grafts after complete transection of the spinal cord at T8. A significant improvement in locomotion was observed with treatment of olfactory-ensheathing glia plus chondroitinase ABC compared to untreated and merely grafted rats.

65. Lundborg G: The intrinsic vascularization of human peripheral nerves: Structural and functional aspects. *J Hand Surg Am* 1979;4:34-41.

66. Sunderland S: The intraneural topography of the radial, ulnar, and median nerves. *Brain* 1945;68:243.

67. Shin AY, Spinner RJ, Steinmann SP, Bishop AT: Adult traumatic brachial plexus injuries. *J Am Acad Orthop Surg* 2005;13:382-396.

This article provides a comprehensive review of the evaluation and management of adult traumatic brachial plexus injuries.

68. Hentz VR, Narakas A: The results of microneurosurgical reconstruction in complete brachial plexus palsy: Assessing outcome and predicting results. *Orthop Clin North Am* 1988;19:107-114.

1: Principles of Orthopaedics

69. Mackinnon SE, Novak CB, Myckatyn TM, Tung TH: Results of reinnervation of the biceps and brachialis muscles with a double fascicular transfer for elbow flexion. *J Hand Surg Am* 2005;30:978-985.

This article describes how the successful transfer of expendable motor fascicles from the ulnar and median nerves can reinnervate the biceps and brachialis muscles for strong elbow flexion. The authors report that direct coaptation of the nerve fascicles may be performed without the need for nerve grafts. There was no subsequent functional or sensory donor morbidity.

70. Jubran M, Widenfalk J: Repair of peripheral nerve transections with fibrin sealant containing neurotrophic factors. *Exp Neurol* 2003;181:204-212.

71. Seddon HJ: Nerve grafting. *J Bone Joint Surg Br* 1963; 45:447-461.

72. Songcharoen P, Wongtrakul S, Mahaisavariya B, Spinner RJ: Hemi-contralateral C7 transfer to median nerve in the treatment of root avulsion brachial plexus injury. *J Hand Surg Am* 2001;26:1058-1064.

73. Oberlin C, Beal D, Leechavengvongs S, Salon A, Dauge MC, Sarcy JJ: Nerve transfer to biceps muscle using a part of ulnar nerve for C5-C6 avulsion of the brachial plexus: Anatomical study and report of four cases. *J Hand Surg Am* 1994;19:232-237.

74. Lee SK, Wolfe SW: Peripheral nerve injury and repair. *J Am Acad Orthop Surg* 2000;8:243-252.

75. Rowshan K, Jones NF, Gupta R: Current surgical techniques of peripheral nerve repair. *Op Tech Orthopedics* 2004;14:163-170.

This review provides a clinically relevant discussion of the widely accepted surgical approaches to the repair of peripheral nerves and the issues to consider when selecting the appropriate surgical technique.

76. Hentz VR, Rosen JM, Xiao SJ, et al: The nerve gap dilemma: A comparison of nerves repaired end to end under tension with nerve grafts in a primate model. *J Hand Surg Am* 1993;18:417-425.

77. Raimondo S, Nicolino S, Tos P, et al: Schwann cell behavior after nerve repair by means of tissue-engineered muscle-vein combined guides. *J Comp Neurol* 2005; 489:249-259.

The authors detail the behavior of migratory glial/Schwann cells along a particular type of autologous tissue-engineered conduit made of a vein filled with fresh skeletal muscle. Their data help to explain the effectiveness of these fresh muscle-vein combined nerve guides in improving neural regeneration.

78. Midha R, Munro CA, Dalton PD, Tator CH, Shoichet MS: Growth factor enhancement of peripheral nerve regeneration through a novel synthetic hydrogel tube. *J Neurosurg* 2003;99:555-565.

79. Gupta R, Rummler LS, Steward O: Understanding the biology of compressive neuropathies. *Clin Orthop Relat Res* 2005;436:251-260.

This article is a review of data that expand our understanding of the pathogenesis of compression neuropathies. These studies suggest that while the reciprocal relationship between neurons and glial cells is maintained, chronic nerve compression injury is a Schwann cell-mediated disease.

80. Gupta R, Rummler LS, Palispis W, et al: Local downregulation of myelin-associated glycoprotein permits axonal sprouting with chronic nerve compression injury. *Exp Neurol* 2006;200:418-429.

Chronic nerve compression injuries induce a robust Schwann cell proliferation in a distinct spatial and temporal pattern, which is accompanied by an increase in the number of small unmyelinated axons in the area of the injury. These data show that a local downregulation of myelin-associated glycoprotein within the peripheral nerve secondary to chronic nerve compression injury is the critical signal for the sprouting response.

81. Dellon AL: Diabetic neuropathy: Review of a surgical approach to restore sensation, relieve pain, and prevent ulceration and amputation. *Foot Ankle Int* 2004;25: 749-755.

This review article provides a synopsis of rationale and treatment results of surgical decompression for diabetic neuropathy.

82. Therapeutics and Technology Assessment Subcommittee of the American Academy of Neurology, Chaudhry V, Stevens JC, Kincaid J, So YT: Practice advisory: Utility of surgical decompression for treatment of diabetic neuropathy: Report of the Therapeutics and Technology Assessment Subcommittee of the American Academy of Neurology. *Neurology* 2006;66:1805-1808.

This systematic review of the literature indicates that there is limited hard evidence to support widespread use of surgical management of diabetic neuropathy without further rigorous studies.

83. Sander MD, Abbasi D, Ferguson AL, Steyers CM, Wang K, Morcuende JA: The prevalence of hereditary neuropathy with liability to pressure palsies in patients with multiple surgically treated entrapment neuropathies. *J Hand Surg Am* 2005;30:1236-1241.

HNPP increases susceptibility of peripheral nerves to pressure and trauma and can be associated with symptoms at multiple anatomic entrapment sites. This study evaluated the genomic DNA from patients with a history of more than one carpal tunnel release and/or ulnar nerve transposition. They did not find any evidence for an association between HNPP and patients who have multiple surgical releases for upper extremity entrapment neuropathies.

84. Hobby JL, Venkatesh R, Motkur P: The effect of age and gender upon symptoms and surgical outcomes in carpal tunnel syndrome. *J Hand Surg Br* 2005;30:599-604.

The outcome of carpal tunnel release in terms of improvement in the symptom and functional scores is sufficient to justify surgery in elderly patients, but surgical outcomes are less predictable than in younger patients, with continued loss of manual dexterity and thenar atrophy. The authors recommend that this discrepancy be explained to patients preoperatively.

85. Weber RA, Rude MJ: Clinical outcomes of carpal tunnel release in patients 65 and older. *J Hand Surg Am* 2005; 30:75-80.

Patients 65 years of age or older objectively benefit and have improved clinical outcomes after carpal tunnel release. As such, age alone should not be a contraindication to carpal tunnel release.

1: Principles of Orthopaedics

Chapter 6
Musculoskeletal Biomechanics

Timothy M. Wright, PhD   Suzanne A. Maher, PhD

Introduction

Musculoskeletal biomechanics is the study of the effect of forces on the skeletal system. Forces can be generated from muscle contraction or from external sources such as gravity. Forces act externally to cause accelerations and, therefore, movements of the extremities. They also act internally, placing a mechanical burden on the tissues that comprise the musculoskeletal system and the biomaterials that are used in implants that reinforce or replace skeletal parts. The principles governing musculoskeletal biomechanics have been outlined in the literature.[1-3] One key concept is that external effects can be understood by applying Newton's laws of motion, which allow calculation of muscle and joint loads required to resist functional loads such as gravity. A similar approach can be used to determine the ability of materials to withstand the mechanical burdens imposed by the external loads. This approach is guided by defining the state of stress and strain in the material.

Forces, Moments, and Static Equilibrium

Forces and moments affect the way in which all body segments move. A force is the quantity that changes the velocity and/or direction of an object. Its magnitude is equal to the mass of the object multiplied by the acceleration of the object. The unit of force is kg·m/s², which is a newton (N).

A moment is the quantity that changes the angular velocity of an object. For example, when a power reamer is used in the operating room, the angular velocity at which the reamer turns can be increased only by applying a moment to the reamer. The magnitude of moment is equal to the mass moment of inertia of the object (a term that combines the object's mass and the distribution of the mass) and its angular acceleration. The unit of the moment is the newton-meter (N·m).

When an external force is applied to a limb, such as a weight being held by the upper extremity, the magnitude of the moment created about the elbow can be calculated as the product of the force acting on the hand and the perpendicular distance between the line of action of the force and the center of rotation of the joint (often called the moment arm of the force). Thus, the force applied to the outstretched hand in **Figure 1** is the 10-N gravitational force from the weight multiplied by the 0.2-m moment arm, creating a moment of 2 N·m.

To resist the external load and maintain the elbow in its flexed position, internal forces must be generated by contraction of the biceps muscle.

The concept of static equilibrium can be used to calculate the required biceps force. Static equilibrium is the situation in which no accelerations are occurring in the system (that is, the system is at rest or moving at a constant velocity). With no acceleration, the forces and the moments acting on the system must both sum to 0. If the weight in the hand and the biceps force are considered to be the only forces generating moments about the elbow, then the extension moment caused by the weight (2 N·m) must be offset by the flexion moment created in the biceps. Because the moment arm of the biceps muscle about the elbow is an order of magnitude smaller than the moment arm of the weight (2 cm compared to 20 cm), the muscle must generate 10 times the

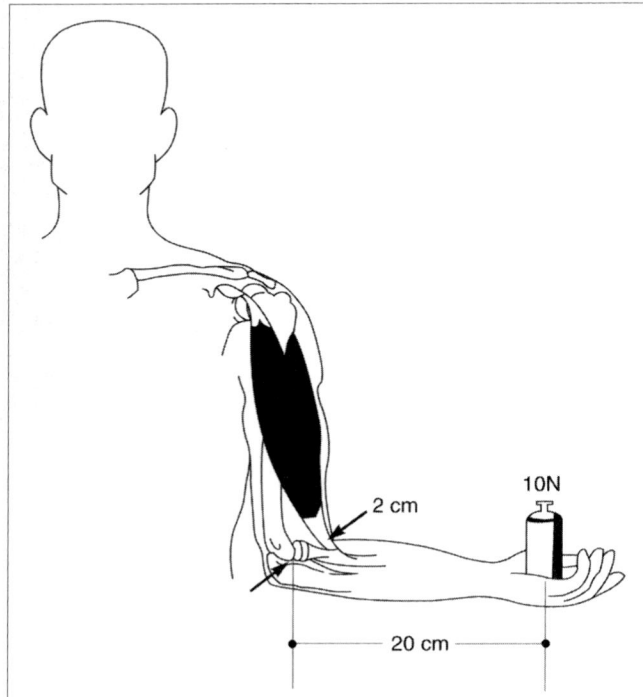

Figure 1   A 10-N weight in the hand creates a 2-N·m moment about the elbow. *(Reproduced with permission from Burstein AH, Wright TM: Fundamentals of Orthopaedic Biomechanics. Philadelphia, PA, Lippincott Williams & Wilkins, 1994, p 7.)*

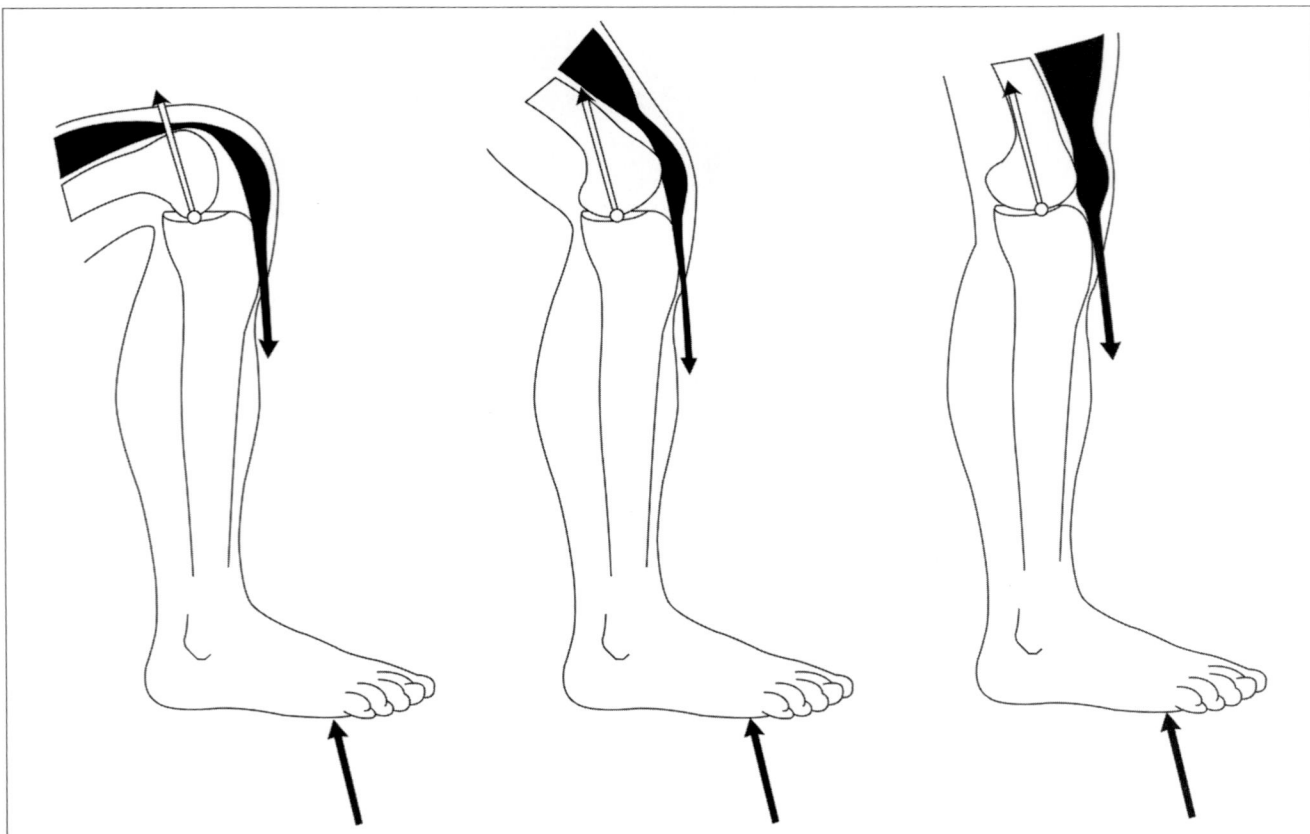

Figure 2   Regardless of the position of the knee joint, if the functional load remains constant, the orientation of the joint compressive force does not move substantially because the line of application of the muscle force does not change dramatically. *(Reproduced with permission from Burstein AH, Wright TM:* Fundamentals of Orthopaedic Biomechanics. *Philadelphia, PA, Lippincott Williams & Wilkins, 1994, p 67.)*

force (100 N) to create the same magnitude moment about the elbow as was created by the weight.

Functional loads, including the ground reaction force during gait, generally have a mechanical advantage around joints because their line of action passes far away from the joint. Muscles, therefore, must generate large loads to resist the moments caused by the functional loads. Because muscles pass close to the joint centers, the muscle force also acts to compress the joint surfaces together, creating large joint contact forces. Joint forces in the lower extremities often reach multiples of body weight for routine daily activities.[4-6]

Joint Stability

A joint is stable if, when moving through a normal range of motion, it can carry the required functional loads without pain and produce joint contact forces of normal intensity on its articular cartilage surfaces. In stable joints, peripheral or edge loading does not occur. Furthermore, small changes in the direction of the functional load do not produce large, sudden changes in joint contact position. Thus, if a knee joint is supporting a flexion moment, a small torque applied to the tibia should not produce a sudden, large angular displacement.

The most passive mechanism of joint stability is the control of the location of the joint contact force by the curvature of the articular surfaces. The joint involuntarily seeks a contact position consistent with the production of an appropriately directed joint reaction force. The stability provided by surface curvature varies greatly among joints. The hip joint, for example, can provide compression forces throughout the large range of orientation of required joint reaction forces because of the large included angle of the acetabulum. Although the shoulder joint is analogous to the hip joint with respect to its range of motion, the range of orientation of the compressive joint contact forces is much more limited because of the rather small included angle of the glenoid.

When the knee is in its fully flexed, partially flexed, and fully extended positions, the same external load (the ground reaction force) is applied to the foot in all three positions, and the orientation of the patellar ligament with respect to the tibial plateau is maintained; thus, the direction of the ligament force varies little between the three positions (**Figure 2**). The contacting surface of the tibial plateau has a much smaller variation in surface curvature than the femoral condyles.

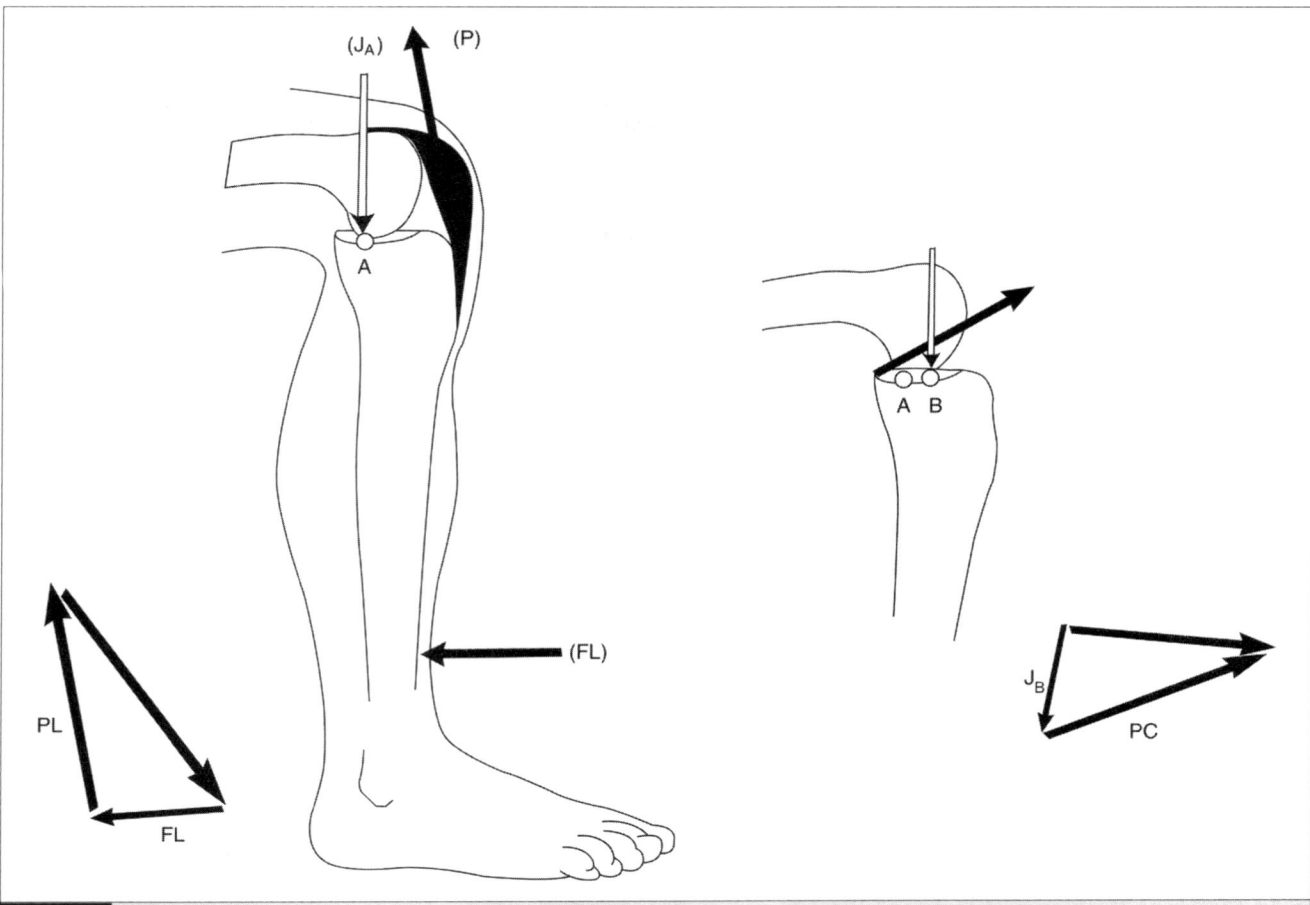

Figure 3 At the contact position shown (point A), the joint contact force (J_A) cannot provide the required joint reaction to offset the functional load (FL) and the patellar ligament load (PL). The femur moves to contact at point B, and the posterior cruciate ligament stretches, pulling anteriorly and proximally on the tibia with a force (PC). The sum of the two forces (J_B and PC) produces the required joint reaction force. *(Reproduced with permission from Burstein AH, Wright TM: Fundamentals of Orthopaedic Biomechanics. Philadelphia, PA, Lippincott Williams & Wilkins, 1994, p 70.)*

These characteristics combine to ensure that the joint reaction force on the plateau required for equilibrium varies little relative to the plateau in all three orientations.

In addition to surface geometry and muscle forces, passive ligament forces also provide for joint stability.[7] When an external functional load creates a joint reaction force in the knee that does not lie perpendicular to the tibial plateau, the femur slides anteriorly on the tibia, stretching the posterior cruciate ligament and thereby creating tension in the ligament (**Figure 3**). This tensile force provides the missing component of the joint reaction force. The joint remains stable, because it has undergone only 2 to 3 mm of displacement while maintaining contact on the articular regions of its surfaces.

In a laboratory simulation of an anterior drawer test, under the anterior load, the tibia translates anteriorly with respect to the femur. The amount of translation depends on the original neutral position and the final position of the tibia under load. A small region exists in the center of the load versus the displacement curve for the knee that is relatively flat, called the dead zone (**Figure 4**). In this region, the position of the knee is extremely sensitive to the imposed load; very little force can produce a big change in displacement. If the anterior cruciate ligament (ACL) is then cut and the test repeated, the curve corresponding to anterior translation is altered. Therefore, sectioning the ACL allows increased anterior translation, creating an unstable situation because of the broad region of translation without additional load.

The dead zone is an important property affecting joint stability. In the dead zone, the joint finds a stable position based only on the curvature of its surfaces and the direction of the joint reaction force. If there is no equilibrium position within this zone, increased joint excursion must induce ligament tension to contribute directly to joint stability. The stabilizing ligament forces should be oriented as close as possible to the direction of the joint excursion. For the ACL to prevent anteroposterior motion without also creating moments that would disturb joint equilibrium, its line of action must also pass close to the center of rotation of the joint.

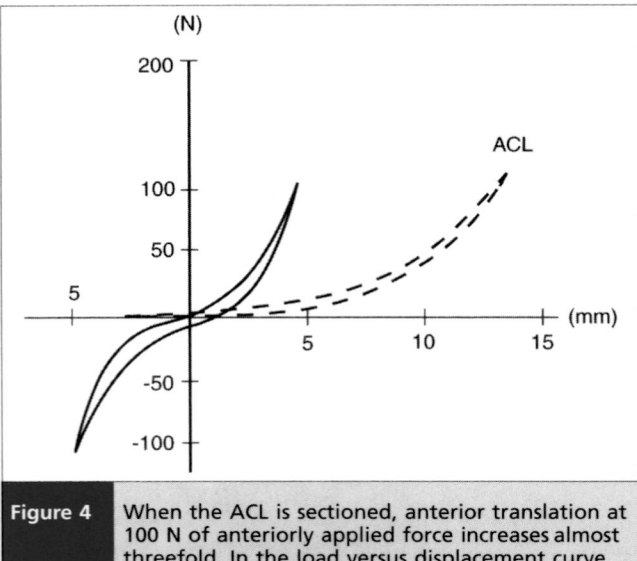

Figure 4 When the ACL is sectioned, anterior translation at 100 N of anteriorly applied force increases almost threefold. In the load versus displacement curve for intact and sectioned ACL, a small, relatively flat region exists in the center of the curve, denoting that very little force produces a big change in displacement. *(Reproduced with permission from Burstein AH, Wright TM: Fundamentals of Orthopaedic Biomechanics. Philadelphia, PA, Lippincott Williams & Wilkins, 1994, p 88.)*

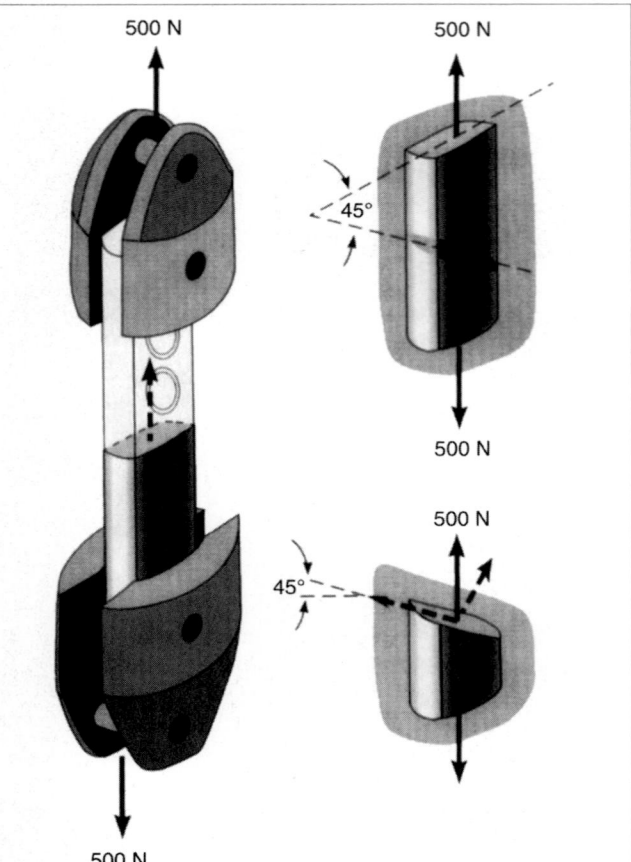

Figure 5 A bone plate is gripped at its ends and loaded in tension by a 500-N load. On the plane perpendicular to the load, the stress is normal tensile stress (magnitude = 500 N divided by the plate's cross-sectional area). On a plane at 45°, the 500-N load has components both perpendicular and parallel to the plane, creating normal and shear stresses, respectively. *Reproduced with permission from Burstein AH, Wright TM: Fundamentals of Orthopaedic Biomechanics. Philadelphia, PA, Lippincott Williams & Wilkins, 1994, p 105.)*

Knee arthrometers were developed to provide objective measurements of anteroposterior motion of the tibia relative to the femur in a clinical setting (often called an anterior drawer test). Unlike measurements made in a controlled laboratory test, many variables can affect results, such as patient muscle activity, knee flexion angle, magnitude of force applied, and tibial rotation. Nonetheless, differences of 2 to 3 mm of anterior tibial displacement between injured and noninjured knees are considered indicative of ACL injury. Arthrometers have been used to identify abnormal joint laxity related to ligament injury, to assess restoration of constraint in the operating room, and to assess functional outcome following surgical intervention.[8-10]

In the spine, intervertebral stability is provided by the disk and the facet joints. With total disk arthroplasty, the constraint afforded by the implant can have a profound effect on the joint kinematics, the loads transferred to the facet joints, and the likelihood of developing facet arthritis. In the immediate postoperative period, for example, total disk replacements with less constraint can result in increased facet forces relative to an intact spine, particularly during lateral bending. Although designs with higher levels of constraint appear to protect the facet joints from adverse kinematics, joint kinematics can be significantly altered.[11]

Mechanical Behavior of Materials

Predicting performance limits for skeletal structures (bones or implants) depends on knowing the forces to which the structure is subjected, the burdens placed on the materials that comprise the structure, and the extent to which the materials can sustain those burdens.

Stress

When a bone plate is tested in the laboratory, the external load applied to the plate is an axial tensile load. Using the concept of static equilibrium, this external axial load must be resisted internally in some continuous manner over the surface of the plate's cross section (**Figure 5**). The stress on every small piece of the cross section is defined as the internal force divided by the surface area over which it acts: stress = force/area. The units of stress are newtons/meter^2; 1 N/m^2 is called a pascal (Pa).

For the bone plate, the force was perpendicular to the cross section. This condition is called normal stress.

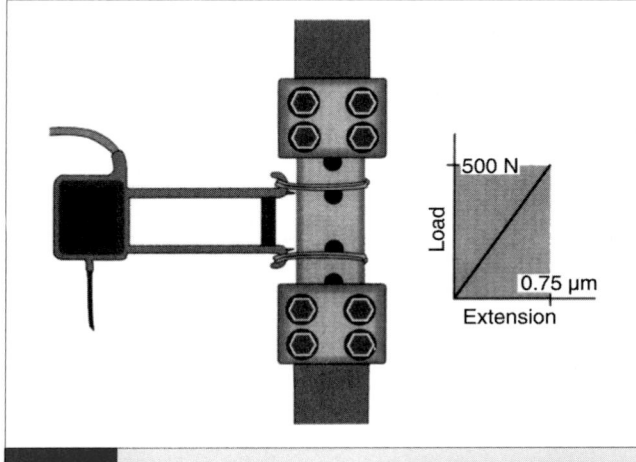

Figure 6 An extensometer measures the change in length between the two knife edges contacting the surface of the bone plate. The accompanying graph shows the applied load (up to 500 N) plotted against the extension measured by the extensometer. *(Reproduced with permission from Burstein AH, Wright TM: Fundamentals of Orthopaedic Biomechanics. Philadelphia, PA, Lippincott Williams & Wilkins, 1994, p 107.)*

On cross sections that are not perpendicular to the applied load, the force acting on the plate has a component acting parallel to the surface of the cross section (**Figure 5**). The condition produced by this component is called shear stress.

Strain

Stress in the bone plate could be easily calculated. However, in most musculoskeletal situations, shapes are more complex and structures are composed of several materials; consequently, such a simple calculation is impossible. Thus, a measurement tool is necessary that provides for direct observations of physical phenomena that can be correlated with stresses. In the bone plate example, an instrument called an extensometer is attached; it measures the change in distance between its two attachment points on the plate (**Figure 6**). As load is applied, the curve produced on the graph is a straight line. When the load reaches 500 N, the extension of the extensometer is 0.00075 mm. At this point, the load is released, and the curve is retraced back to the origin. Repeating the loading process up to 500 N reproduces the original straight line.

Corresponding to the 500-N load, 750 microns (750×10^{-6} m) of elongation were observed in the plate. This elongation took place between measuring points on the extensometer that were spaced 15 mm apart (**Figure 6**). Therefore, each millimeter of plate length experienced an elongation of 5×10^{-5} mm. This ratio of elongation to unit length (7.5×10^{-4} mm/15 mm = 0.00005) is defined as normal strain. Accordingly, normal strain = change in length/unit length, and can be positive (tensile) or negative (compressive).

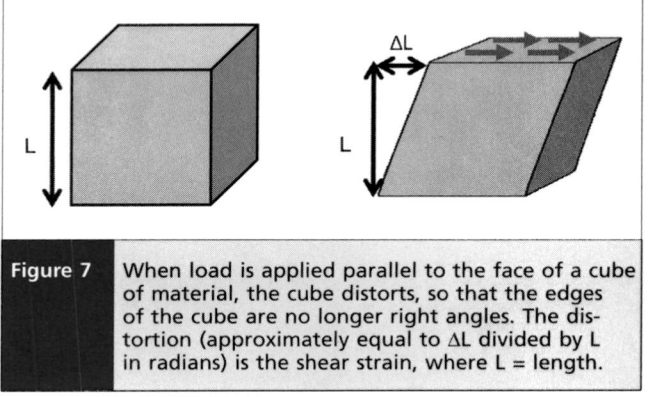

Figure 7 When load is applied parallel to the face of a cube of material, the cube distorts, so that the edges of the cube are no longer right angles. The distortion (approximately equal to ΔL divided by L in radians) is the shear strain, where L = length.

Strain is a ratio with no units, and because strains are often very small quantities, strain is often presented as a percentage or as microstrain. In the example, the elongation created a tensile strain of 50 microstrain.

Another type of strain occurs when the foot is externally rotated under a torsional load of 10 N·m; the distal tibia is externally rotated with respect to the proximal tibia. A small piece of bone tissue within the tibial cortex undergoes a similar distortion, but on a smaller scale. What were once longitudinal edges become oriented in an oblique direction. The change in angle between two adjacent faces of the piece that were formerly perpendicular to one another is defined as shear strain (**Figure 7**). In this instance, the change in angle between the faces is 0.05°. By convention, shear strain is always expressed in units of radians ($360° = 2\pi$ radians). The change in angle of 0.05° corresponds to a shear strain of 0.00094 radians.

Modulus of Elasticity

As noted above, loading and unloading the bone plate demonstrates a constant linear relationship between load and extension (**Figure 6**). Because the load versus elongation curve is fully reversible, the material is said to behave elastically; when the load is released, there is no permanent change in the shape. If the stress in the plate is plotted versus the strain, the relationship between the calculated stress and the measured strain is linear, so the ratio of stress to strain (the slope of the line) is constant. For the example of the stainless steel bone plate, the stress was 500 N/Area$_{plate}$ = 500 N/50 mm² = 10 MPa when the strain was 50 microstrain, so the ratio is: stress/strain = 10 MPa/50 microstrain = 10×10^{6} Pa/50×10^{-6} = 200×10^{9} Pa = 200 GPa, where the unit GPa (gigapascal) is equal to one billion (10^{9}) pascals.

Many such tension or compression experiments are conducted on different sizes and shapes of stainless steel specimens, and this ratio does not change. The ratio of stress to strain depends, therefore, on the material being tested and not on the shape of the structure being tested. This ratio is termed the modulus of elasticity, and is usually denoted by the letter E.

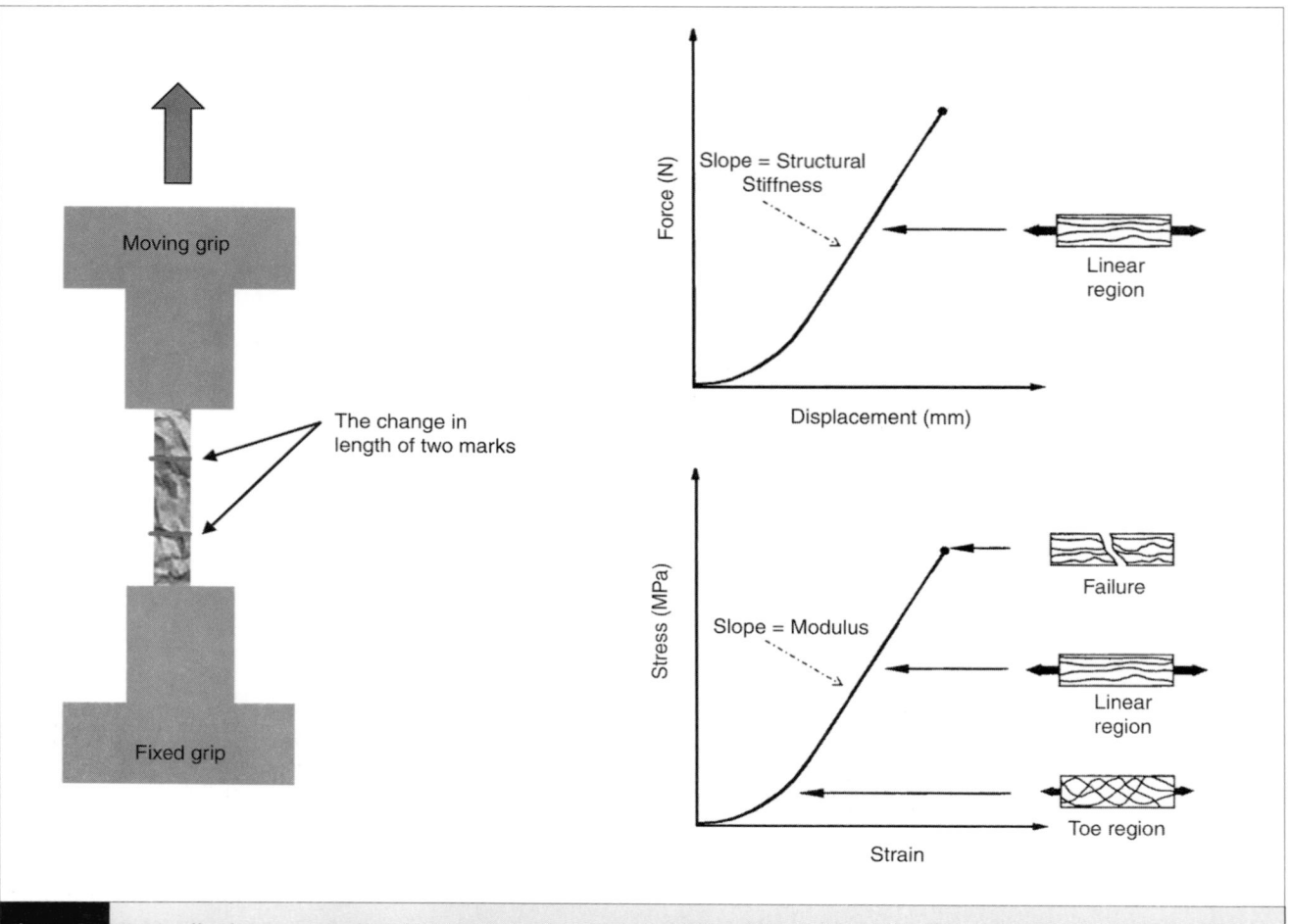

Figure 8	A patellar ligament is subjected to a uniaxial tensile test. The stiffness is the slope of the linear portion of the resulting force-versus-displacement graph. If load is converted to stress and displacement to strain, the slope of the stress-versus-strain graph is the elastic modulus of the ligament tissue. The strength is the maximum stress that the ligament can withstand before rupture.

Mechanical Behavior of Skeletal Structures

Structures can best be categorized mechanically according to the types of loads to which they are subjected. Skeletal structures are subjected to combinations of axial, bending, and torsional loads.

Axial Load

Axial load is the simplest loading situation that a structure can experience. Ligamentous structures, for example, only support loads that pull the tissue fibers in the direction of their axis. This situation is termed tensile axial loading. The ligament elongates because the tissue elastically deforms. When a ligament is subjected to a tensile test (**Figure 8**), elongation is measured as the change in length of two marks placed on the tissue while the tensile force is applied.

The resulting force versus displacement graph helps define the stiffness of the structure. Structural stiffness is the ratio of the applied load (in this case the tensile force) to the resulting distortion (in this case the displacement). The stiffness is the slope of the linear portion of the graph (structural stiffness = load/displacement). Structural stiffness reflects the ability of a structure to maintain its shape while under load. It depends on the geometry of the structure (length and cross-sectional area for the case of axial loading) and the material properties of the ligament tissue (modulus of elasticity for the case of axial loading). These two factors are independent, and therefore structural stiffness can be altered either by changes in geometry or elastic modulus.

The strength of a structure is usually defined as the maximum load that the structure can withstand without causing material failure. As with structural stiffness, strength is also dependent on a geometric property (the cross-sectional area for the case of axial loading) and a material property (the ultimate stress that the ligament tissue can withstand).

Bending Loads

Understanding the stresses placed on a structure in bending, hence the ability of musculoskeletal tissues

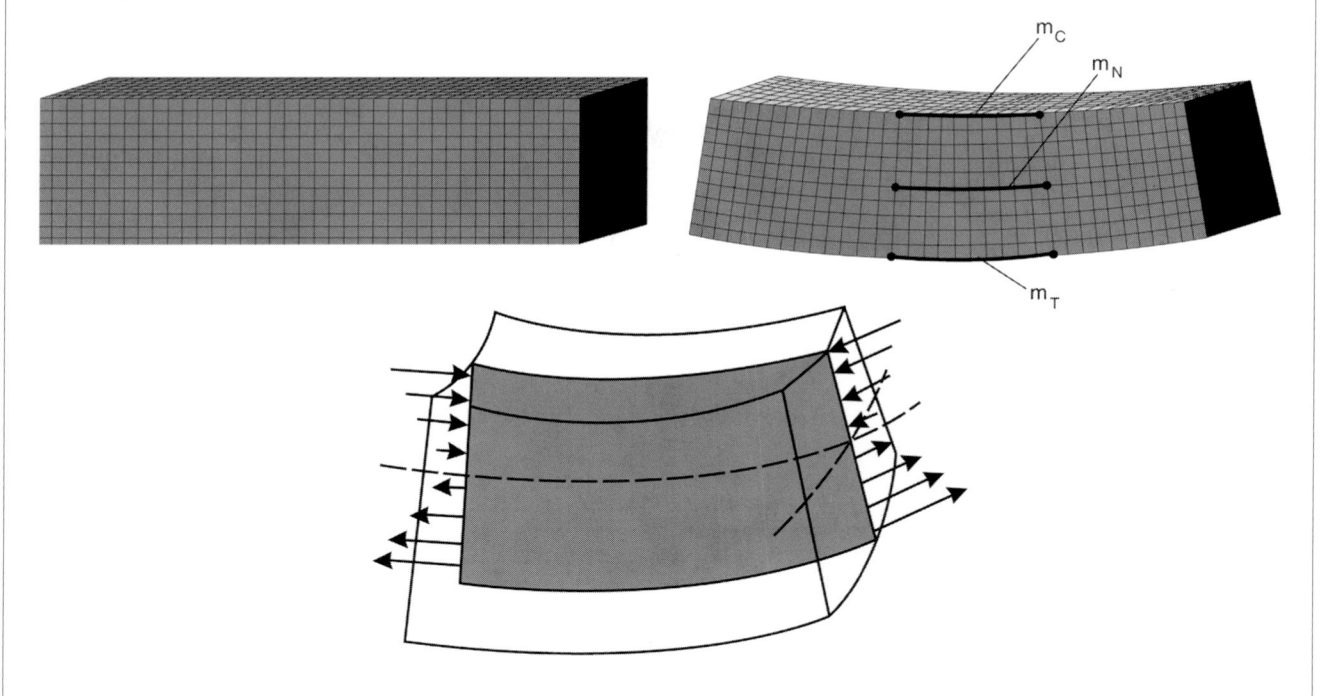

Figure 9	Under the influence of bending loads, the longitudinal lines curve and the transverse lines are no longer parallel. The line segment m_T lengthens, m_C shortens, and m_N does not change in length. The pattern of stress is therefore a linear distribution. Material further away from the midline, or neutral axis, experiences higher stress than material at the midline, which experiences no stress. *(Reproduced with permission from Burstein AH, Wright TM:* Fundamentals of Orthopaedic Biomechanics. *Philadelphia, PA, Lippincott Williams & Wilkins, 1994, pp 143-146.)*

(such as bone) to support bending loads, requires an understanding of how loads are distributed through a structure in bending. When a bending load is applied to a long, rectangular piece of rubber with longitudinal and transverse lines inscribed on its surface (**Figure 9**), the lines no longer form a rectangular grid. Rather, the longitudinal lines become curved, whereas the transverse lines, although still essentially straight, are no longer parallel.

The line segment m_T lengthens when the load is applied, corresponding to a tensile strain. This occurrence implies that a tensile stress is present on the transverse surfaces on this side of the beam. Similarly, line segment m_C shortens under load, corresponding to a compressive strain (an implication of compressive stress). At the midline of the beam, line segment m_N has no length change, so it has no tensile or compressive strain. Thus, the midline of the beam (often called the neutral axis) experiences neither tensile nor compressive stress.

Because transverse lines have remained as straight lines under load, the amount of shortening or elongation of any particular longitudinal line segment is proportional to its location between the midline axis and the outer surface of the beam. The pattern of stresses implied by this observed deformation pattern is a linear distribution. Material in the beam farther away from the midline experiences higher stresses than material at the midline (which experiences no stress at all). If ma-

terial in the beam were reconfigured so that more of it were placed nearer the outer surface, the stresses would be lower (because more material would be present to resist the applied load). The distribution of mass about the midline can be described by the area moment of inertia, derived from adding together each increment of cross-sectional area in the beam multiplied by the square of the distance from the increment of cross section to the neutral axis.

The strength of a beam is the largest bending moment that the beam can carry without causing the stress within the material to exceed a critical limit. For skeletal structures and implants that experience cyclic bending loads, this critical limit is the fatigue strength of the material. The strength of the beam is controlled by two factors—the maximum tolerable stress in the material and the area moment of inertia divided by the distance from the neutral axis to the outer beam surface (half the height of the beam). Therefore, in a situation analogous to axial loading, the bending strength depends on a material property and a geometric property.

When bending loads are applied to the long bones of the limbs, the intensities of the induced compressive and tensile stresses are approximately equal because of the relative symmetry of the bones. Because bone tissue is weaker under tensile loading than under compressive loading, failure will be initiated in the region of highest tensile stress.

1: Principles of Orthopaedics

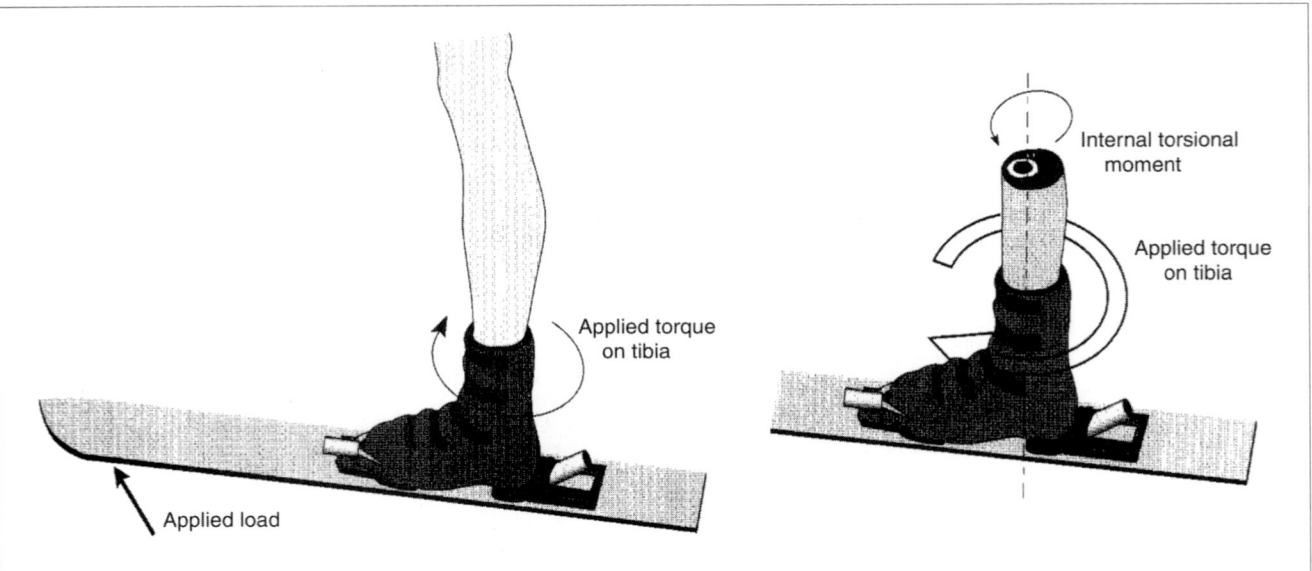

Figure 10   A large externally applied torque is created by the force applied at the ski tip. A free body of the distal tibia shows that equilibrium is satisfied if an internal torque of equal magnitude but opposite direction is applied at the upper boundary. *(Reproduced with permission from Burstein AH, Wright TM:* Fundamentals of Orthopaedic Biomechanics. *Philadelphia, PA, Lippincott Williams & Wilkins, 1994, pp 160-161.)*

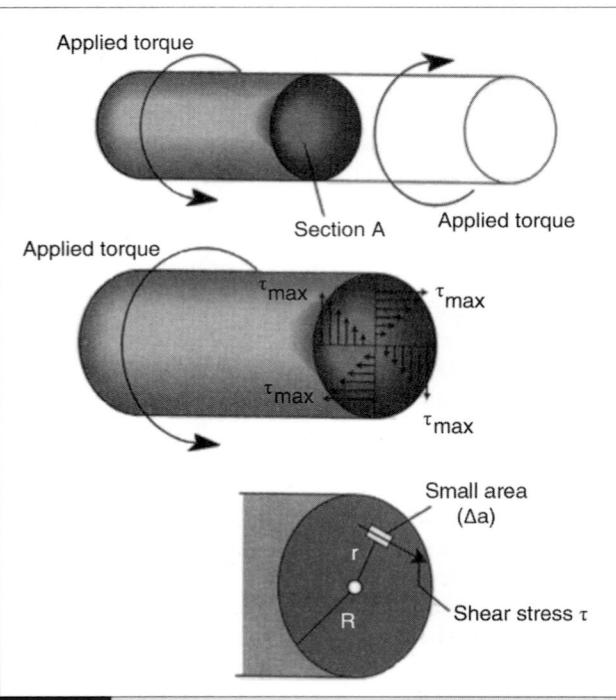

Figure 11   A circular bar of radius R is loaded with a torsional moment. The shear stress at any point on section A is proportional to the distance from the center of the bar. The shear stresses generate an internal torque equal in magnitude, but opposite in direction, to the applied torque. *(Reproduced with permission from Burstein AH, Wright TM:* Fundamentals of Orthopaedic Biomechanics. *Philadelphia, PA, Lippincott Williams & Wilkins, 1994, p 162.)*

Torsional Loads

The third common mode of loading is torsional load. Torsional loads produce moments that tend to twist the structure. A typical example of torsional loading occurs while skiing. If a load is applied perpendicular to the ski tip, a torsional moment is produced that causes external rotation of the tibia. For static equilibrium, the moment applied to the internal cross section of the tibia at the proximal end must be equal in magnitude to the applied moment, but in the opposite direction (**Figure 10**). This internal torque is constant along the length of the tibia in direct contrast to the bending moments produced by transverse loads, which vary along the length of the bone.

When a circular bar is subjected to torsional loading (**Figure 11**), the stress distribution on the internal cross section (A) consists of a set of shear stresses that are greatest in magnitude at the periphery and diminish linearly to 0 at the center. In a manner analogous to bending, the shear stress (τ) at any point (r) will be influenced by its distance from the central axis. Similar to the area moment of inertia, the polar moment of inertia is represented by the sum of each segment of area multiplied by the square of its distance from the center.

When torsional load is applied to the cylinder, one end rotates with respect to the other. A straight longitudinal line on the surface of the cylinder will twist into a helix (**Figure 12**). The helix angle (α) increases proportionally with the torque. The total deformation (θ) is proportional to both the applied torque (T) and the length of the rod (L): $\theta \propto T \times L$. As with beams in bending, the proportionality constant between the torque and the angle of deformation (the torsional stiffness) depends on a material property and a geometric property of the structure. The material property is the shear modulus. For materials such as metallic alloys, the shear modulus is related to the elastic modulus; for example, because the elastic modulus of 316L-type stainless steel is approximately twice that of titanium alloy, its shear modulus is also twice as great.

Torsional strength also depends on a material property and a cross-sectional property. The material property is the ultimate shear stress and the cross-sectional property is the ratio of the polar moment of inertia to the radius.

Unlike bending of long bones, where the moments vary along the length, torsional loading of bones produces a constant moment. Therefore, fracture initiates at the weakest section, that is, the section that produces the highest stress in response to the applied torque. Because the strength of the cross section depends on the radius, torsional fractures initiate at the surface of the cross section that is closest to the centroid of the section (the section with the smallest radius).

Effects of Altered Geometry

An important biomechanical question relates to the weakening effect of surgically induced defects in bone. Virtually all open reduction and internal fixation result in holes filled with screws. What happens to the strength of the bone in the presence of these defects? In general, larger holes create greater weakening effects. The amount of weakening depends on the size of the hole and its location. For example, a hole in the proximal tibial will not reduce the strength of the tibia subjected to torsional loading because of the large strength (large polar moment and large radius) compared with that of the distal/middle third junction. For a bending load applied at the midsection of a tibia, the strains created in the region of the hole in the proximal tibia are a small fraction of those seen in the region of the midshaft where the fracture will originate. Thus, even doubling the strains in the proximal tibia will not induce failure at that site and, of course, if a failure is not induced at the hole, then the hole will not adversely affect the strength of the bone. A more serious situation is one in which a hole is located at the bending loading site or near the weakest section under torsion. In such a situation, the weakening effect is profound. For example, a hole with a diameter approximately 30% that of the bone will create a 40% reduction in torsional strength.

Load Transfer and Load-Sharing Characteristics of Orthopaedic Implants

Orthopaedic implants must interface with the skeletal system to transmit loads between biologic structures. The interfaces are either with cortical bone, such as is required by a bone plate on the midshaft of a long bone, or cancellous bone, such as with the tibia component of a total knee replacement. In each situation, load is transmitted either at discrete points, usually by

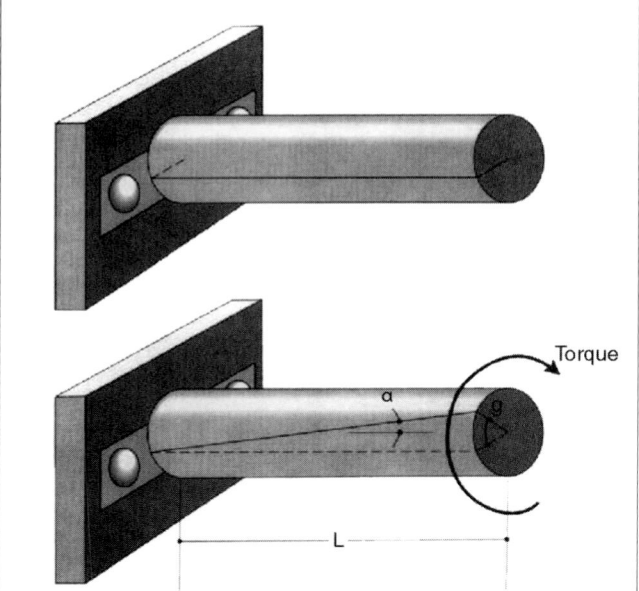

Figure 12 A cylinder is fixed at one end and has a torque applied to the other end. The torque causes an angular twist to the rod. *(Reproduced with permission from Burstein AH, Wright TM: Fundamentals of Orthopaedic Biomechanics. Philadelphia, PA, Lippincott Williams & Wilkins, 1994, p 167.)*

screws or pins, or over broad surfaces, usually by press-fitting, cementing, or porous ingrowth. To have a stable interface with adjacent tissue, the implant structure must be designed so that the tissue is not subjected to loads high enough to cause local fracture or low enough to induce osteopenia.

Orthopaedic devices can be categorized by their load transmission mechanism: load sharing and load transfer. The concept of load sharing is important for understanding the performance of plates, rods, and stems. The implant-bone interface of a plate, for example, is load sharing. At the fracture site, all load is carried within the plate. Beyond the last attachment point (the most distal screw), all load is carried by the bone. Between these two points, some fraction of load is carried by the plate, while the remainder is carried by the bone. In another example, that of a cemented stem, if the stem and bone are subject to a bending moment, much of the moment is carried by the rod throughout the rod's length. However, closer to the tip of the rod, a more rapid transition occurs, with a large fraction of the moment transmitted to the bone over a short distance.

In the extreme, load sharing raises two deleterious outcomes. Wolff's law suggests that in situations where bone loads are reduced, bone mass is resorbed. If bone is resorbed, the bone stiffness will decrease. Decreasing the stiffness in the presence of an implant will result in even less of the shared load being carried by the bone, which should lead to further reduction in bone mass. Although clinical evidence for this cycle exists (for ex-

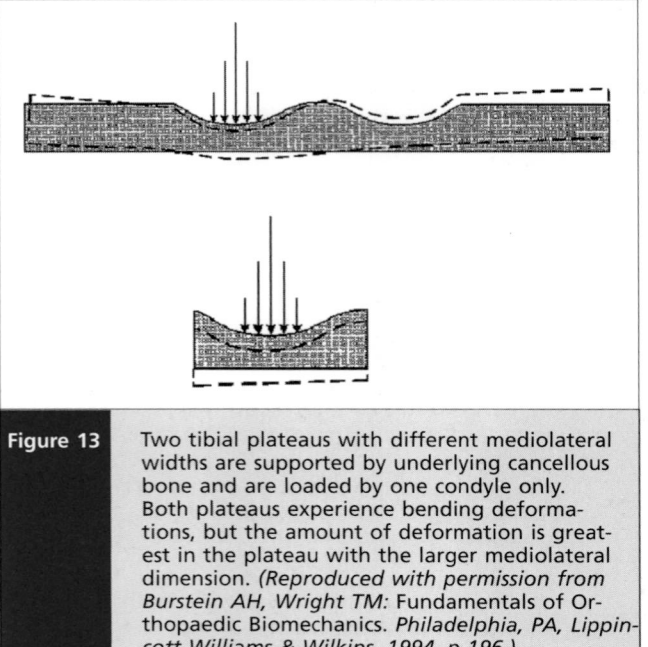

Figure 13 Two tibial plateaus with different mediolateral widths are supported by underlying cancellous bone and are loaded by one condyle only. Both plateaus experience bending deformations, but the amount of deformation is greatest in the plateau with the larger mediolateral dimension. *(Reproduced with permission from Burstein AH, Wright TM:* Fundamentals of Orthopaedic Biomechanics. *Philadelphia, PA, Lippincott Williams & Wilkins, 1994, p 196.)*

ample, in fully porous-coated femoral stems for hip replacement), fortunately the biologic control system does not rapidly push the process to the extreme. The second deleterious outcome deals with the implant; as the load shared by the implant increases, so too does the probability for mechanical failure.

Load transfer devices transfer load directly between the implant and the bone across a contact surface. The distribution of contact pressure is often complex and depends on the shape and rigidity of both the biologic and mechanical structures. Surface replacements for hemiarthroplasty and total joint prostheses have broad areas of contact with epiphyseal cancellous bone. In essence, the entire load imposed on the device is carried within the device until the load transfers to the supporting cancellous bone.

The load transfer process depends on three factors: how the load is distributed onto the implant's surface, how the load distribution results in distortion of the implant, and how the combination of load distribution and implant distortion affects load distribution to the bone. In the load transfer pathway, regardless of fixation technique (cement or porous bone ingrowth), cancellous bone is the weak link.

Load distribution and hence contact stresses on the bearing surface depend on the shape of the contacting surfaces and the elastic moduli of the contacting materials.[12] For thin implants made from low modulus materials or implants whose contacting surfaces have greatly differing elastic moduli, component thickness also influences load distribution. If the modulus of a modern total knee tibial component made from conventional polyethylene (modulus of 1 GPa) with a minimum thickness of 8 mm is doubled (such as might happen with oxidative degradation of the polyethylene),

the peak contact stress increases by 40%, because the load imposed by the femoral component is distributed over a smaller contact area than with the conventional material. Similarly, if the conformity between the surfaces is decreased by making the tibial component flatter (a larger radius of curvature), the peak contact stress increases markedly, again because the contact area is smaller with the flatter component. Finally, if the curvature and material properties of the component example were maintained but the polyethylene thickness were decreased from 8 to 5 mm, the peak contact stress again increases substantially.

If the load distribution is concentrated on the component surface, implant distortion will be a problem. In the case of a tibial plateau with the entire load applied on one condyle, if load transfer to the bone is to be uniform, then the shape of the prosthesis should not change appreciably under load. A tibial plateau with an exaggerated mediolateral width serves to depict the mechanics of the situation (**Figure 13**). When the load is applied to the joint surface, a bending moment distribution in the implant creates concave upward deformation. The deformed implant is no longer contiguous with the bony surface. Depending on the attachment mode with the bone, no load transfer would occur in the separated regions; such a case would exist with a cementless implant that failed to achieve bone ingrowth. The fixation mode must allow tensile forces to develop at the interface to limit the distortion. Therefore, total joint components that are relatively thin can have complex load transfer patterns that depend on the thickness-to-width ratio of the component, as well as on the conditions of surface attachment.

For a tibial component with a narrow mediolateral width (for example, a unicondylar implant), the bending effect is minimized. The implant transfers load to the cancellous bone in a uniform manner. Unfortunately, whenever a region of sudden change in load distribution occurs on a contact surface, such as at the outer edges of the component, high shear stresses are induced in the bone. Therefore, the length-to-thickness ratio for a load transfer component should be sufficient to allow reasonably uniform load transfer intensities and avoid large regions of separation, yet cover enough of the surface to avoid abrupt loading changes at the edge of contact. A compound structure, such as a metallic tray to support the polyethylene bearing insert, will increase the effective thickness (by increasing the actual thickness, but more importantly by adding material with a much higher elastic modulus), thus stiffening the component.

Summary

An understanding of the biomechanical response of musculoskeletal tissues is crucial to establishing their function, whether a tissue is required to carry loads transmitted to it via an orthopaedic device or to confer stability to an articular joint. The magnitude and direction of external forces and moments acting on the tissue and its inherent material properties can be combined to facilitate a true interpretation of the response to loading. The same mechanical principles apply to the implant systems that impact so much of orthopaedic surgical treatment. Material properties and geometry control the mechanical behavior of implants and provide the designer and the surgeon with choices that can significantly impact implant performance.

Annotated References

1. Nigg BM, Herzog W: *Biomechanics of the Musculoskeletal System*. West Sussex, United Kingdom, John Wiley & Sons, 1999.

2. Hall SJ: *Basic Biomechanics*. St Louis, MO, Mosby-Year Book, 1995.

3. Nordin M, Frankel VH: *Basic Biomechanics of the Musculoskeletal System*. Hagerstown, MD, Lippincott Williams & Wilkins, 2001.

4. D'Lima DD, Patil S, Steklov N, Slamin JE, Colwell CW Jr: The Chitranjan Ranawat Award: In vivo knee forces after total knee arthroplasty. *Clin Orthop Relat Res* 2005;440:45-49.

   Tibial forces were measured in vivo using a telemetrized knee replacement and found to reach values of 2.6 times body weight when rising from a chair and 3.3 times body weight during stair descent.

5. Bergmann G, Deuretzbacher G, Heller M, et al: Hip contact forces and gait patterns from routine activities. *J Biomech* 2001;34:859-871.

6. Davy DT, Kotzar GM, Brown RH, et al: Telemetric force measurements across the hip after total arthroplasty. *J Bone Joint Surg Am* 1988;70:45-50.

7. Fukubayashi T, Torzilli PA, Sherman MF, Warren RF: An in vitro biomechanical evaluation of anterior-posterior motion of the knee: Tibial displacement, rotation, and torque. *J Bone Joint Surg Am* 1982;64:258-264.

8. Daniel DM, Malcom LL, Losse G, Stone ML, Sachs R, Burks R: Instrumented measurement of anterior laxity of the knee. *J Bone Joint Surg Am* 1985;67:720-726.

9. Malcom LL, Daniel DM, Stone ML, Sachs R: The measurement of anterior knee laxity after ACL reconstructive surgery. *Clin Orthop Relat Res* 1985;196:35-41.

10. Maletis GB, Cameron SL, Tengan JJ, Burchette RJ: A prospective randomized study of anterior cruciate ligament reconstruction: A comparison of patellar tendon and quadruple-strand semitendinosus/gracilis tendons fixed with bioabsorbable interference screws. *Am J Sports Med* 2007;35:384-394.

    A randomized controlled clinical trial found significant improvement in outcomes after ACL reconstruction with bone-patellar tendon-bone versus that with quadruple-strand semitendinosus/gracilis. Outcome measures included KT-1000 arthrometer measurements.

11. Rousseau MA, Bradford DS, Bertagnoli R, Hu SS, Lotz JC: Disc arthroplasty design influences intervertebral kinematics and facet forces. *Spine J* 2006;6:258-266.

    Facet forces and instant axes of rotation secondary to disk replacement were characterized in a biomechanical test. The degree of constraint afforded by disk replacement designs was found to affect postimplantation kinematics and load transfer.

12. Bartel DL, Bicknell VL, Wright TM: The effect of conformity, thickness, and material on stresses in ultra-high molecular weight components for total joint replacement. *J Bone Joint Surg Am* 1986;68:1041-1051.

1: Principles of Orthopaedics

Chapter 7

Bearing Materials for Hip, Knee, and Spinal Disk Replacement

*Harry A. McKellop, PhD   *Patricia Campbell, PhD

Introduction

Over the past three decades, total joint arthroplasty, particularly for the hip and knee, has proved to be one of the most effective surgical procedures in orthopaedics. Nevertheless, during this period, it became increasingly apparent that even a well-performing prosthetic joint releases billions of microscopic wear particles (debris) into the joint space. When an excessive amount of debris is generated, it may stimulate a severe foreign body reaction in the capsular tissues and bone, leading to inflammation and osteolysis. The resulting loss of supporting bone may lead to loosening of the implant and require difficult and dangerous revision surgery.[1] Consequently, there has been an explosion of research over the past 10 years, with the goal of developing more wear-resistant bearing materials for prosthetic joints. This chapter summarizes recent improvements in bearing technology, midterm clinical results, and the prospects for future improvements.

Metal-on-Metal Bearings in Total Hip Replacements

The modern generation of metal-on-metal bearings began in Europe in the late 1980s, with the introduction of total hip replacements (THRs) using a metal-on-metal bearing couple.[2] As with other new bearing materials, modern metal-on-metal bearings were devel-

*Harry A. McKellop, PhD or the department with which he is affiliated has received research or institutional support from Wright Medical, Encore Medical, Exactech, and DePuy, miscellaneous nonincome support, commercially-derived honoraria, or other nonresearch-related funding from DePuy, royalties from DePuy, and is a consultant or employee for DePuy. Patricia Campbell, PhD or the department with which she is affiliated has received research or institutional support from Wright Medical and Zimmer and miscellaneous nonincome support, commercially-derived honoraria, or other nonresearch-related funding from Wright Medical, Stryker, and Smith & Nephew.

oped as one approach to avoiding osteolysis caused by the billions of submicron polyethylene wear particles that were generated in hips using even the best polyethylene available at that time. Presently, almost all implant manufacturers offer a metal-on-metal couple as one of their bearing options.

In laboratory wear tests using hip joint simulators, metal-on-metal bearings consistently have demonstrated a "wear in" phase, during which the rate of wear typically is tens of microns per million cycles, followed by a "steady state" phase, with wear of a few microns per million cycles or less.[3] For comparison, a typical patient walks about one to two million cycles per year. The preponderance of hip simulator testing has indicated that metal-on-metal bearings undergo less wear when at least one of the surfaces is high carbon (0.2%) rather than low carbon (0.07%). Metal-on-metal bearings are produced either by forging or casting. Cast components may be used in the as-cast condition, or they may be solution-annealed to improve their ultimate strength and ductility, or they may be hot isostatic pressed to reduce porosity. Some investigators maintain that the as-cast material has superior wear properties,[4] but others have found no effect on the wear resistance.[5,6]

In hip simulator tests, the amount of wear and its distribution over the bearing surface can be determined with a coordinate measuring machine (CMM). These machines use a computer-controlled robot arm to record the x-y-z coordinates on a grid of hundreds of points on the surface of the implant. The dimensional data then can be analyzed to identify the nominal spherical shape of the ball or cup and the location and depth of wear. Although the accuracy of a specific point is approximately 2 μm, the overall surface can be identified with high precision because of the large number of data points.

Although there is no comparably accurate way to measure the amount of wear of a metal-on-metal hip prosthesis while it is in the patient, CMM analysis also can be used to determine the amount of wear present on retrieved implants. The retrieval studies have tended to confirm the predictions of the hip simulator testing, that is, an initial wear-in phase lasting about 1 year, followed by a steady state, with a much lower wear rate of a few microns per year or less.[7]

In view of these very low steady-state wear rates, it

is not likely that a modern, properly manufactured metal-on-metal hip will fail because of excessive wear during the patient's lifetime. However, there is concern regarding the long-term biologic effects of the metal ions (chiefly cobalt and chromium) that are released directly from the metal bearing surfaces and from the wear debris. The concentration of these ions in the blood and urine of patients with metal-on-metal hips, as measured by atomic absorption analysis, has been reported as 5 to 10 times normal with well-functioning implants, but can be several hundred times higher if the wear rate is abnormally high, for example, as a result of surface damage caused by impingement or a malpositioned implant.[8] The concentration of metal ions in the tissues directly adjacent to the prosthesis could be many times higher than in the blood and urine.[9]

The relationship between activity level and ion concentration is a controversial subject. One study reported that blood ion concentration increased only after 1 hour of walking on a treadmill.[10] In contrast, another study reported only a small, transient increase in ion levels in a triathlete after 11 hours of intense exercise, whereas a third study reported that neither 1 hour of treadmill walking nor 1 week of increased activity caused a systematic increase in ion concentrations in the blood or urine.[11]

Because metal ions are eliminated from the body by the kidneys, it may be that the increased body burden of metal ions does not have a substantial negative impact on the patient's health. For example, in one study with a follow-up of 28 years, the incidence of cancers in patients with metal-on-metal hips was closely comparable to the incidence of cancers for patients without a hip prosthesis.[12] Nevertheless, it is possible that an elevated concentration of metal ions could have other, more subtle, negative effects, including changes to the DNA.[13] Consequently, many surgeons recommend against the use of metal-on-metal bearings in female patients who could become pregnant, in patients with kidney disorders, and in those with known sensitivity to metals.

Although there are no firm data to show that dermal sensitivity is related to a poor clinical outcome, on rare occasions, metal-on-metal hips have failed because of metal sensitivity.[14] It is not clear whether the presence of a metal-on-metal hip can induce metal sensitivity, and it has occurred in patients whose metal-on-metal hips had both normal and high rates of wear. Furthermore, it often is difficult to diagnose metal sensitivity with certainty, because the symptoms vary from chronic groin pain to rapid and extensive osteolysis.[14]

If left untreated, soft-tissue involvement from wear or sensitivity reactions can lead to the expansion of soft-tissue bursas, with subsequent vascular occlusion and necrosis of the muscle and bone. Radiologically and clinically, the bursae may resemble pseudo-tumors.[15] Histologically, the tissues from hips with metal sensitivity exhibit extensive infiltration of perivascular lymphocytes, plasma cells and, often, tissue necrosis and deposition of fibrin, characteristics that are collectively referred to as aseptic lymphocytic

vasculitis-associated lesions.[14] If other causes such as infection or loosening have been eliminated, the only effective treatment is to replace the cobalt-chromium components with more inert materials (typically, ceramic, titanium alloy, and polyethylene).

Hip Resurfacing Arthroplasty

The first generation of hip resurfacing arthroplasties that were developed in the 1970s featured a metal femoral head bearing against a polyethylene socket.[4,16] During that period, the polyethylene components typically were packaged in air during sterilization with gamma radiation and during subsequent storage, which often led to oxidative degradation of the polyethylene. Consequently, these hip resurfacing arthroplasties generated large volumes of polyethylene wear debris and were highly susceptible to osteolytic destruction of the adjacent bone, particularly bone underlying the femoral head.[17] Because of this, metal-polyethylene hip surface replacement was largely abandoned as an alternative to THR.

The clinical success of modern metal-on-metal bearing in THRs has encouraged their use in hip resurfacing arthroplasty. One manufacturer recently received Food and Drug Administration (FDA) approval, a second has received conditional approval, and clinical trials are underway with several others. As with conventional THRs, in hip simulator testing, hip resurfacing arthroplasty bearings typically exhibit a higher wear-in period, followed by lower steady-state wear. In comparison with metal-on-metal THR, the total volume of wear during the wear-in period tends to be slightly greater with the larger diameter hip resurfacing arthroplasties, but the steady-state wear rate can be as low or lower.[18]

The explanation for this difference is somewhat complex. Historically, the rate of wear of polyethylene increased approximately in proportion to the bearing diameter, simply because of the longer sliding distance per walking cycle. Because of this finding, the diameters of the femoral components used with historical polyethylene cups were 32 mm or less. In contrast, with metal-on-metal bearings, the steady-state wear rate does not appear to increase with increasing diameter. One possible reason for this difference is that the initial wear-in of the metal-on-metal bearing reduces the clearance between the ball and socket in the bearing zone, favoring fluid-film separation and, with a larger diameter bearing, the film tends to be thicker because of the greater surface sliding speed. These two factors apparently offset the longer sliding distance that occurs with a larger diameter.

Thus, with total amount of wear being a nonissue (provided that the implants are correctly positioned, as with all hip prostheses), the chief advantage of a hip resurfacing arthroplasty over a THR is the preservation of the bone of the proximal femur, which may be an advantage if revision to THR is necessary. The chief disadvantages of a hip resurfacing arthroplasty are the greater technical difficulty of the surgery and the small but substantial risk of femoral neck fracture that, of course, is not a complication with a conventional THR.

Ceramic Bearings for Hip Replacements

Alumina Ceramic

Alumina was the first ceramic to be widely used in THR, either as a femoral ball articulating against a polyethylene socket or in a ceramic-ceramic configuration. In hip simulator testing and clinical studies, the wear rate of polyethylene against alumina has been comparable to or lower than the wear rate against metal, with the wear advantage being increased in the presence of third-body abrasive particles because of the superior scratch resistance of alumina.[19] The chief disadvantage has been brittle fracture of alumina components, a rare but devastating complication.[20] Fortunately, during the past two decades, several modifications have substantially increased the strength of alumina, including increased purity and decreased grain size, with a corresponding reduction in the incidence of fracture. For example, there were no component fractures at 7 years in a recent clinical trial of 316 patients with ceramic-ceramic hips.[21]

Clinically, alumina-alumina bearings have exhibited wear properties consistent with the results of hip simulator testing, with long-term wear rates on the order of a few microns per year or less. The bearing surfaces of retrieved alumina-alumina hips may exhibit several distinct textures, including the highly polished original surface, a mildly damaged main contact zone, and a more roughened wear "stripe" that apparently is caused by contact between the surface of the ball and the rim of the cup during partial subluxation.[22,23] Although the overall wear rate of alumina-alumina remains low, the potential for stripe wear emphasizes the importance of proper positioning of the acetabular cup to minimize the chance of subluxation, which can be more damaging in ceramic-ceramic or metal-metal bearings than with a polyethylene acetabular cup.

Squeaking, ranging from barely audible to severely annoying, has been reported to occur in 1% to 3% of hips with alumina-alumina bearings.[24] Although the cause of squeaking has not yet been determined, one hypothesis is that it is initiated by microseparation of the bearing surfaces that, particularly in a malpositioned implant, can lead to rim impingement and stripe wear. In some patients, the squeaking has resolved spontaneously over time.

Zirconia Ceramic

Yttrium-stabilized zirconia (Y-zirconia) ceramic was introduced as an alternative to alumina primarily because of its superior toughness, which allowed Y-zirconia ceramic to be used in smaller diameter femoral heads with less risk of fracture while minimizing the wear of the opposing polyethylene cup. Hip simulator tests also indicated slower wear of the polyethylene with Y-zirconia ceramic, even for the same diameter, essentially providing a double advantage. However, the wear advantage exhibited in the laboratory tests has not been realized clinically, and the incidence of osteolysis has been greater than for comparable hips using metal-polyethylene bearings.[25] A close examination of retrieved Y-zirconia femoral components has indicated that they sometimes exhibit a gradual phase transformation during use in vivo, which can weaken the component and roughen the surface, increasing the rate of wear.[26] In addition, several Y-zirconia components from one production run from one manufacturer apparently were improperly fabricated and exhibited an unusually high incidence of fracture in clinical use, necessitating their recall. Because of these developments, and in view of the availability of zirconia-toughened alumina, the use of Y-zirconia is being questioned.[26]

Zirconia also may be stabilized using magnesium.[27] To date, magnesium-zirconia components have not exhibited the susceptibility to phase transformation that has been problematic with Y-zirconia ceramic.

Alumina-Zirconia Composite

Clinical trials are underway with a mixed ceramic that contains 75% alumina and 24% zirconia, a combination that is tougher than pure alumina but not susceptible to the phase transformation that occurs with Y-zirconia. In hip simulator testing of the mixed ceramic femoral balls and cups, the rate of wear has been more than tenfold lower than with alumina-alumina.[28]

Oxidized Zirconium

One manufacturer has combined the fracture resistance of a metal with the abrasion resistance of a ceramic by generating a layer of zirconia on the surface of a substrate of zirconium metal alloy. In hip simulator testing under clean conditions, the wear of polyethylene against this "oxidized zirconium" was comparable to that against conventional cobalt chromium. In contrast, when the femoral heads were tumbled in an abrasive slurry, the harder ceramic experienced less scratching and, therefore, generated less wear of the polyethylene.[29] However, the oxidized zirconia surface can be severely damaged by contact with the rim of the metal acetabular shell during dislocation.[30] Again, the need for accurate placement of the prosthetic components, regardless of the materials used for the bearings, is emphasized.

Ceramic on Metal

In recent hip simulator testing, the wear rate of an alumina ball against a cobalt-chromium alloy cup has been well below the range with a metal-on-metal bearing and comparable to that with an alumina-alumina bearing.[31] Clinical trials of hips with these "hybrid" bearings are in progress. The advantage of an alumina-metal bearing over metal-on-metal would be the reduction in the volume of wear particles and a lower concentration of metal ions in the body. The advantage over an alumina-alumina bearing would be the elimina-

1: Principles of Orthopaedics

tion of the potential for fracture of the alumina acetabular component.

Diamond Coatings

In industrial applications, such as bits for drilling oil wells, artificial diamond coatings on a metal substrate have demonstrated remarkably low friction and extremely high resistance to scratching and wear, two properties that make them attractive for use in joint arthroplasties. However, the process for applying a diamond coating is technically complex and expensive. It remains to be seen whether this technology will prove practical as an alternative bearing surface for joint arthroplasty.

Most THRs in clinical use currently use either a metal-on-polyethylene, ceramic-on-polyethylene, metal-on-metal, or ceramic-on-ceramic bearing combination, and each of these can provide overall excellent performance. Surgeons should take their relative advantages and disadvantages (Table 1) into account when deciding on the optimum bearing for a given patient.

Cross-Linked Polyethylenes in Hip Replacement

The polyethylenes with elevated cross-linking that were introduced clinically during the past decade have come to be referred to as the "first generation" materials. Unfortunately, this designation ignores several types of cross-linked polyethylenes (gamma sterilized in acetylene, 100 Mrad gamma cross-linked, and silane cross-linked) that were introduced as early as the 1970s and have shown excellent clinical performance to date.[32] Nevertheless, because it is established in the literature, "first generation" will be used here to refer to the cross-linked polyethylenes that were developed and introduced clinically in the 1990s.

There are strong similarities among the first generation cross-linked polyethylene (Table 2). Each uses high-energy radiation to cross-link the polyethylene, followed by a thermal treatment intended to reduce the free radicals that are generated during radiation that otherwise would predispose the cross-linked polyethylene to long-term oxidative degradation. At the same radiation dose, the type of radiation used (electron-beam or gamma) does not appear to markedly affect the wear resistance or other physical properties.

The postirradiation thermal treatments include either melting or annealing. Most of the free radicals that are generated by the radiation remain trapped within the crystalline regions of the polyethylene. When the polyethylene is heated above its melt temperature, the crystal regions break up (become amorphous), releasing the free radicals, which are then neutralized. In con-

Table 1

Tradeoffs Among State-of-the-Art Hip Bearings

Bearing	Advantages	Concerns
Cross-linked Polyethylene	Lowest cost Surgically "forgiving" Low wear High oxidation resistance	Clinical use less than 8 years Long-term potential for fatigue fracture?
Metal-Metal	Lower wear Self-polishing	Cost Biologic effects of metal ions?
Ceramic-Ceramic	Least wear High biocompatibility	Cost Surgical technique sensitive Squeaking Fracture

Title 2

Comparisons Among Cross-Linked Thermally Stabilized Polyethylenes Introduced in the 1990s*

Name and Manufacturer	Radiation Type and Dose	Thermal Stabilization	Final Sterilization
Marathon (DePuy Orthopaedics, Warsaw, IN)	Gamma radiation to 5 Mrads at room temperature	Remelted at 155°C for 24 hours	Gas plasma
XLPE (Smith & Nephew, Memphis, TN)	Gamma radiation to 10 Mrads at room temperature	Remelted at 150°C for 2 hours	Ethylene oxide
Longevity (Zimmer, Warsaw, IN)	Electron beam radiation to 10 Mrads at warm temperature	Remelted at 150°C for about 6 hours	Gas plasma
Durasul (Zimmer, Warsaw, IN)	Electron beam radiation to 9.5 Mrads at 125°C	Remelted at 150°C for about 2 hours	Ethylene oxide
Crossfire (Stryker-Howmedica-Osteonics, Mahway, NJ)	Gamma radiation to 7.5 Mrads at room temperature	Annealed at about 120°C for a proprietary duration	Gamma at 2.5 to 3.5 Mrads while packaged in nitrogen

*The processing parameters shown in this table were compiled from various publications, and information provided by the manufacturers, and are subject to ongoing modification.

trast, when the cross-linked polyethylene is annealed (by definition, heated below the melt temperature) the crystals do not break up and many of the free radicals are not neutralized. After only a few years of clinical use, substantial oxidation has been measured in cross-linked polyethylene cups that had been annealed after cross-linking.[33] Although it is not yet clear that this oxidation will have a detrimental effect on the clinical performance of the cups, it has motivated the development of a second-generation annealing method that is more effective in neutralizing the residual free radicals.

Remelting is highly effective in neutralizing free radicals, so there should be negligible oxidation of these components during clinical use. However, remelting causes a partial reduction in crystallinity that, in turn, can reduce the resistance to crack propagation.[34] This tradeoff also has motivated the development of second generation methods that remove free radicals by other means.

Clinical Performance to Date of Cross-Linked Polyethylene Acetabular Components
In clinical use, the amount of wear that has occurred on a polyethylene cup typically is measured radiographically. A template or computer-based image analysis system is used to measure the distance between the centers of the cup and ball. The change in this distance over time indicates the "penetration" of the ball into the cup. It is important to note that the total penetration includes the change in thickness of the cup caused by creep (plastic flow) and actual wear (loss of material in the form of wear debris). Particularly with the highly wear-resistant cross-linked polyethylenes, most of the penetration during the first 2 years is caused by creep, and the amount of this creep is comparable to that for historical polyethylenes. Fortunately, the rate of creep decreases exponentially, becoming negligible after approximately 2 years, and investigators typically ignore the penetration during this "bedding-in" period to obtain a more accurate comparison between the steady-state rates of wear of two types of polyethylene.

In contrast, in laboratory testing in a hip simulator, the amount of wear is typically determined by periodically weighing the polyethylene cup, and plotting the cumulative weight loss as a function of cycles, thereby avoiding any error resulting from creep deformation. In several independent hip simulator studies,[32,35,36] the greatest reduction in polyethylene wear occurred for the first few Mrads of cross-linking, with progressively less reduction per Mrad thereafter, and wear became too small to measure for doses of 15 to 20 Mrads (**Figure 1**). In most instances the percent reductions in wear rate of the cross-linked polyethylene that have been reported in clinical studies to date have equaled or exceeded those predicted by the preclinical hip simulator testing.[37-41]

Osteolysis With Cross-Linked Polyethylene
Reviews of the literature found a strong positive correlation between the rate of wear of historical polyethy-

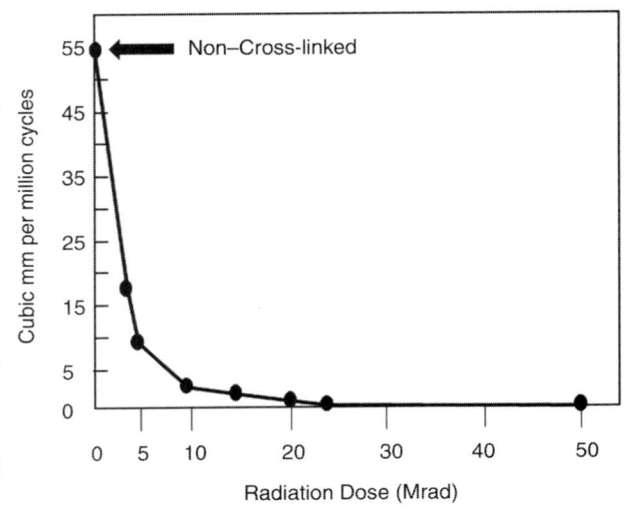

Figure 1   Wear rate of ultra high molecular weight polyethylene versus cross-linking dose. In hip simulator testing, the greatest decrease in the rate of wear occurred for a cross-linking dose ranging from 5 to 10 Mrads, induced using gamma radiation, with less decrease per Mrad thereafter. Above approximately 20 Mrads, the wear rate was negligible, but brittleness also increases with higher cross-linking. *(Reproduced with permission from McKellop H, Shen F-W, Lu B, Campbell P, Salovey R: Development of an extremely wear-resistant ultra high molecular weight polyethylene for total hip replacements. J Orthop Res 1999;17:157-167.)*

lene and the incidence and severity of osteolysis.[42,43] As a general rule, lysis was either absent or negligible in hips for which the rate of polyethylene wear was 0.1 mm or less, but was observed with increasing frequency and severity when the wear rate was substantially greater than this "threshold" level. Fortunately, the steady-state wear rates (at 2 years and beyond) that have been reported for the cross-linked polyethylenes all are well below 0.1 mm per year, and clinically significant lysis has not yet been observed.[37-41] If these promising midterm results continue through the next decade of use, osteolysis in response to polyethylene wear may cease to be a factor in limiting the lifespan of a THR.

Fracture of Cross-Linked Polyethylene Components
Oxidation breaks the molecular chains in the polyethylene, causing increased brittleness and reduced resistance to crack propagation. With historical gamma-air sterilized polyethylene, there was a strong association between severe oxidation and fracture of the polyethylene components during clinical use (including hip and knee prostheses).[44] During the development of the first-generation cross-linked polyethylenes, it was well recognized that, as the level of cross-linking was increased, there was a progressive reduction in some mechanical

1: Principles of Orthopaedics

Table 3

Alternatives to Remelting for Neutralizing Free Radicals

Antioxidant polyethylene: An antioxidant, such as vitamin E (α tocopherol), can be mixed with the polyethylene powder before fusing it into a solid by extrusion or molding. When the polyethylene is subsequently cross-linked using radiation, the antioxidant neutralizes the free radicals, eliminating the need for subsequent melting or annealing.

Vitamin E doping: After irradiation cross-linking, the components are soaked in vitamin E, which diffuses into the polyethylene and neutralizes the free radicals.

Mechanical deformation: After irradiation cross-linking, the polyethylene is stretched, which mechanically quenches the free radicals. It is then annealed to eliminate the residual stresses caused by the stretching, machined into a component, and sterilized without irradiation.

Multistage annealing: Cross-linking is generated by three separate exposures to gamma radiation (at one third of the total dose each time), with annealing after each dose. Based on laboratory testing, the developers have reported that this process removes free radicals as effectively as melting, but without causing a degradation of crack resistance.

properties, including crack resistance. However, the justification for the clinical use of the cross-linked polyethylenes was that, even at the highest level of cross-linking (approximately 10 Mrads), the fracture toughness remained well above that of the badly oxidized polyethylene that had been a problem historically[44,45] (Table 2).

The clinical results thus far with the first-generation cross-linked polyethylenes are consistent with this premise. For example, it has been estimated that nearly three million cross-linked polyethylene acetabular cups have been implanted, with the longest follow-up period exceeding 7 years. As of June 2006, the FDA's Center for Devices and Radiological Health MAUDE Website contained reports of 75 failed and/or revised THRs that were implanted with cross-linked polyethylene acetabular cups. Sixty-one of these reports included the reason for the revision. Of these, only 10 cups had been revised because of a fracture of the liner, primarily in highly cross-linked cups (10 Mrads).

A recent case report on the fracture of a cross-linked polyethylene cup has been published in the peer-reviewed literature.[46] This fracture occurred in a cup fabricated from 10 Mrad–remelted polyethylene, and the crack apparently was initiated by impingement of the neck of the femoral component on the rim of the cup. Although it is not possible to determine whether this incidence of fracture with the cross-linked polyethylene components is greater or worse than with the historical polyethylenes, in view of the markedly reduced wear rates and corresponding reductions in the incidence and severity of osteolysis it would appear that the rate of fracture of the cross-linked polyethylene components to date is acceptably low. Nevertheless, because fatigue fracture is a time-dependent process, close monitoring of the clinical performance of all of the first-generation cross-linked polyethylenes should continue.

Newer Cross-Linked Polyethylenes

One manufacturer has recently introduced a cross-linked polyethylene based on GUR 1020 resin (molecular weight of 2 to 4 million) in place of GUR 1050 (molecular weight of 4 to 6 million). Because, in laboratory testing, 1020 polyethylene that is cross-linked at 7.5 Mrads has mechanical properties comparable to those of 1050 polyethylene cross-linked at 5 Mrads,[47] acetabular cups fabricated from the 7.5 Mrad–1020 polyethylene may provide about 50% less wear, with no further reduction in toughness.

Several manufacturers have developed alternatives to remelting for neutralizing free radicals, thereby avoiding the reduction in crystallinity and fracture toughness.[48] These processes and methods are presented in Table 3. As with the first-generation cross-linked polyethylenes, the clinical performance of these "second-generation" materials should be closely monitored to detect any unsuspected complications as early as possible.

Bearing Surfaces in Total Knee Replacement

Compared with hip replacements, there are fewer choices for bearing materials for total knee replacements (TKRs). Most TKRs use a cobalt-chromium femoral component articulating against a tibial plateau of ultra-high molecular weight polyethylene. As with THRs, wear of the polyethylene components of TKRs can generate billions of submicron polyethylene particles that, in turn, may stimulate a substantial osteolytic reaction.[49] Although osteolysis historically has been less frequent and less severe with TKRs than with THRs, failure as a result of gross fracture of the polyethylene components has been more of a clinical complication associated with TKRs. The higher incidence of fracture is undoubtedly caused by the stresses that are generated in a polyethylene tibial plateau being greater than in a typical polyethylene acetabular component.

Retrieval analysis has shown that, in modular TKRs, unintentional micromotion between the polyethylene tibial insert and the underlying metal tray can be a substantial source of wear debris.[49] Although manufacturers have attempted to minimize this "backside wear" by improving the fixation between the polyethylene and metal components, it may be impossible to completely eliminate the micromotion and, therefore, the wear at this interface. Another approach is the use of mobile-bearing designs, which intentionally allow motion between the polyethylene and a highly polished tibial plate. In some designs, the interface motion is nearly linear or circular, rather than cross-path motion, which helps to reduce the rate of wear of the polyethylene.

The improved resistance to wear also has made cross-linked polyethylene attractive for use in TKRs. However, there has been greater initial concern regarding the corresponding reduction in fracture toughness. The manufacturers have addressed these concerns through several approaches. For example, one manufacturer uses GUR 1020 polyethylene as the base resin, instead of the GUR 1050, which provides superior mechanical properties (and equal wear resistance) at an equal level of cross-linking.[47] Other manufacturers have used a lower cross-linking dose for TKR components than for THRs to better preserve the mechanical properties of the polyethylene. The second-generation crosslinked polyethylenes that are being introduced in THRs also may be attractive for use in TKRs because of their superior mechanical properties. As with THRs, the suitability of the cross-linked polyethylene components for TKR will be determined through close monitoring of their clinical performance in the coming years.

Bearing Surfaces in Spinal Disk Arthroplasty

During the past 10 years, interest in replacing degenerated spinal disks with an arthroplasty has increased dramatically.[50] The underlying assumption is that, by preserving motion, a disk arthroplasty will reduce the tendency for degeneration to spread to the adjacent disks, as often occurs with disk fusion. Three implants have received FDA approval, two for the lumbar spine featuring a polyethylene component between two cobalt-chromium end plates, and one for the cervical spine using stainless steel versus stainless steel. Several other designs in various stages of development use a cobalt-chromium versus cobalt-chromium bearing. However, because of substantial differences in loading, motion, and possibly lubrication, bearing combinations that have functioned well in a hip or knee prosthesis may have uncertain long-term performance in a particular type of disk arthroplasty,[51] and some combinations are being considered that have not been used in hips or knees, such as titanium versus polyurethane, polyurethane, polyetheretherketone versus itself, and titanium-metal matrix composites. Furthermore, because of their placement directly adjacent to the spinal cord, the consequences of excessive wear and/or gross mechanical failure of spinal disk arthroplasties may be substantially more serious than for hip or knee joints, and revision surgery in the lumbar spine can be much more problematic. Because of these possible consequences, it is imperative that prototype disk arthroplasties undergo extensive and realistic preclinical laboratory testing, and that the clinical trials be closely monitored for early detection of excessive wear, mechanical failure, or loosening.

Annotated References

1. Schmalzried TP, Jasty M, Harris WH: Periprosthetic bone loss in total hip arthroplasty: Polyethylene wear debris and the concept of the effective joint space. *J Bone Joint Surg Am* 1992;74:849-863.

2. Weber BG: Experience with the Metasul total hip bearing system. *Clin Orthop Relat Res* 1996;329:S69-S77.

3. Rieker C, Konrad R, Schon R: In vitro comparison of the two hard-hard articulations for total hip replacements. *Proc Inst Mech Eng [H]* 2001;215:153-160.

4. McMinn D, Daniel J: History and modern concepts in surface replacement. *Proc Inst Mech Eng [H]* 2006;220: 239-251.
   This review article documents the evolution of one particular design for metal-on-metal hip resurfacing by the surgeon designer.

5. Dowson D, Hardaker C, Flett M, Isaac G: A hip joint simulator study of the performance of metal on metal joints: Part 1. Materials. *J Arthroplasty* 2004;19:118-123.
   This article describes a hip simulator study of various combinations of 36 mm high- and low-carbon wrought and cast femoral heads and acetabular components. Low carbon showed the highest wear; volumetric wear decreased as diametral clearance decreased.

6. Bowsher JG, Nevelos J, Williams PA, Shelton JC: 'Severe' wear challenge to 'as-cast' and 'double heat-treated' large-diameter metal-on-metal hip bearings. *Proc Inst Mech Eng [H]* 2006;220:135-143.
   This article presents a hip simulator wear study incorporating features to exacerbate wear in metal-on-metal bearings.

7. Sieber HP, Rieker CB, Kottig P: Analysis of 118 second-generation metal-on-metal retrieved hip implants. *J Bone Joint Surg Br* 1999;81:46-50.

8. Witzleb WC, Ziegler J, Krummenauer F, Neumeister V, Guenther KP: Exposure to chromium, cobalt and molybdenum from metal-on-metal total hip replacement and hip resurfacing arthroplasty. *Acta Orthop* 2006;77: 697-705.
   In this clinical study of ion levels in 74 total hip arthroplasty patients and 111 resurfacing arthroplasties there was a higher rise in ion levels in the first 2 years for the resurfacing group.

9. Betts F, Wright T, Salvati EA, Boskey A, Bansal M: Cobalt-alloy metal debris in periarticular tissues from total hip revision arthroplasties: Metal contents and associated histologic findings. *Clin Orthop Relat Res* 1992;276:75-82.

10. Khan M, Takahashi T, Kuiper JH, Sieniawska CE, Takagi K, Richardson JB: Current in vivo wear of metal-on-metal bearings assessed by exercise-related rise in

1: Principles of Orthopaedics

plasma cobalt level. *J Orthop Res* 2006;24:2029-2035.

This study of patients with a metal-on-metal hip resurfacing found a significant rise of serum ion levels after a short period of exercise and suggest that this is a method to monitor the in vivo performance of a metal-on-metal bearing.

11. Heisel C, Silva M, Skipor AK, Jacobs JJ, Schmalzried TP: The relationship between activity and ions in patients with metal-on-metal bearing hip prostheses. *J Bone Joint Surg Am* 2005;87:781-787.

Patients with metal-on-metal hip joints provided blood samples during low and high activity periods. Serum cobalt and chromium ion levels were not acutely affected by patient activity.

12. Visuri TI, Pukkala E, Pulkkinen P, Paavolainen P: Cancer incidence and causes of death among total hip replacement patients: A review based on Nordic cohorts with a special emphasis on metal-on-metal bearings. *Proc Inst Mech Eng [H]* 2006;220:399-407.

Data from Nordic registries was used to estimate adverse effects on a large population of mostly metal-on-polyethylene bearings, but including McKee-Farrar metal-on-metal hips. Temporary increases in hematopoietic cancers at different follow-up periods were seen in some cohorts but cancer incidence overall was in line with that of the general population.

13. Ladon D, Doherty A, Newson R, Turner J, Bhamra M, Case CP: Changes in metal levels and chromosome aberrations in the peripheral blood of patients after metal-on-metal hip arthroplasty. *J Arthroplasty* 2004;19:78-83.

Using blood from patients with metal-on-metal implants, these researchers found evidence of DNA damage that they attribute to metal, although no direct correlation to cobalt or chromium levels was found.

14. Willert HG, Buchhorn GH, Fayyazi A, et al: Metal-on-metal bearings and hypersensitivity in patients with artificial hip joints: A clinical and histomorphological study. *J Bone Joint Surg Am* 2005;87:28-36.

This article presents a histopathologic and clinical study of a group of patients who had a failed metal-on-metal THR in association with apparent metal sensitivity reactions, including pain, osteolysis, and tissues showing extensive lymphocytic infiltrates.

15. Boardman DR, Middleton FR, Kavanagh TG: A benign psoas mass following metal-on-metal resurfacing of the hip. *J Bone Joint Surg Br* 2006;88:402-404.

This case report describes a benign psoas mass secondary to the tissue reaction to a metal-on-metal hip resurfacing arthroplasty.

16. Amstutz HC: Hip resurfacing arthroplasty. *J Am Acad Orthop Surg* 2006;14:452-453.

This article presents an overview of metal-on-metal hip resurfacing and discusses the underlying technology, patient selection, surgical technique, and 1- to 5-year clinical results.

17. Howie DW, Cornish BL, Vernon-Roberts B: Resurfacing hip arthroplasty: Classification of loosening and the role of prosthetic wear particles. *Clin Orthop Relat Res* 1990;255:144-159.

18. Rieker CB, Schon R, Konrad R, et al: Influence of the clearance on in-vitro tribology of large diameter metal-on-metal articulations pertaining to resurfacing hip implants. *Orthop Clin North Am* 2005;36:135-142.

An experimental study of the influence of diameter and clearance on the lubrication and wear of large diameter metal-on-metal hip resurfacing prostheses is presented.

19. Nizard R, Sedel L, Hannouche D, Hamadouche M, Bizot P: Alumina pairing in total hip replacement. *J Bone Joint Surg Br* 2005;87:755-758.

A summary of the technology and clinical performance of alumina bearing in hip arthroplasty from 1971 to 2005 is presented.

20. Hannouche D, Nich C, Bizot P, Meunier A, Nizard R, Sedel L: Fractures of ceramic bearings: History and present status. *Clin Orthop Relat Res* 2003;417:19-26.

21. D'Antonio J, Capello W, Manley M, Naughton M, Sutton K: Alumina ceramic bearings for total hip arthroplasty: Five-year results of a prospective randomized study. *Clin Orthop Relat Res* 2005;436:164-171.

A summary of the clinical performance up to 7 years of 328 hips with alumina ceramic bearings compared with hips with conventional metal-on-polyethylene bearings is presented.

22. Manaka M, Clarke IC, Yamamoto K, Shishido T, Gustafson A, Imakiire A: Stripe wear rates in alumina THR: Comparison of microseparation simulator study with retrieved implants. *J Biomed Mater Res B Appl Biomater* 2004;69:149-157.

This article describes a hip simulator study of wear of alumina-alumina hip bearings under normal conditions and with edge contact caused by microseparation causing stripe wear.

23. Walter WL, Insley GM, Walter WK, Tuke MA: Edge loading in third generation alumina ceramic-on-ceramic bearings: Stripe wear. *J Arthroplasty* 2004;19:402-413.

An analysis of 16 bearings retrieved from a series of 1,588 cementless hip arthroplasties with third-generation alumina ceramic-on-ceramic bearings was performed to characterize the mechanism of formation of stripe wear.

24. Walter WL, O'Toole GC, Walter WK, Ellis A, Zicat BA: Squeaking in ceramic-on-ceramic hips: The importance of acetabular component orientation. *J Arthroplasty* 2007;22:496-503.

Acetabular component orientation for 17 alumina-alumina hips with squeaking and 17 matched controls was compared.

25. Hernigou P, Bahrami T: Zirconia and alumina ceramics in comparison with stainless-steel heads: Polyethylene

wear after a minimum ten-year followup. *J Bone Joint Surg Br* 2003;85:504-509.

26. Clarke IC, Manaka M, Green DD, et al: Current status of zirconia used in total hip implants. *J Bone Joint Surg Am* 2003;85:73-84.

27. Willmann G: The evolution of ceramics in total hip replacement. *Hip International* 2000;10:193-203.

28. Stewart TD, Tipper JL, Insley G, Streicher RM, Ingham E, Fisher J: Long-term wear of ceramic matrix composite materials for hip prostheses under severe swing phase microseparation. *J Biomed Mater Res B Appl Biomater* 2003;66:567-573.

29. Good V, Ries M, Barrack RL, Widding K, Hunter G, Heuer D: Reduced wear with oxidized zirconium femoral heads. *J Bone Joint Surg Am* 2003;85:105-110.

30. Evangelista GT, Fulkerson E, Kummer F, Di Cesare PE: Surface damage to an Oxinium femoral head prosthesis after dislocation. *J Bone Joint Surg Br* 2007;89:535-537.

   This article describes a case report of severe damage to a femoral ball made of oxidized zirconium that occurred during open reduction of a dislocation.

31. Brockett C, Williams S, Jin Z, Isaac G, Fisher J: Friction of total hip replacements with different bearings and loading conditions. *J Biomed Mater Res B Appl Biomater* 2007;81:508-515.

   The friction of 28-mm diameter hip bearings, including conventional material combinations such as metal-on-ultra-high molecular weight polyethylene, ceramic-on-ceramic, and metal-on-metal, as well as novel ceramic-on-metal pairings, was compared in a laboratory study.

32. Kurtz SM, Muratoglu OK, Evans M, Edidin AA: Advances in the processing, sterilization, and crosslinking of ultra-high molecular weight polyethylene for total joint arthroplasty. *Biomaterials* 1999;20:1659-1688.

33. Wannomae KK, Bhattacharyya S, Freiberg A, Estok D, Harris WH, Muratoglu O: In vivo oxidation of retrieved cross-linked ultra-high-molecular-weight polyethylene acetabular components with residual free radicals. *J Arthroplasty* 2006;21:1005-1011.

   A study of the level of oxidation in retrieved acetabular liners, comparing cross-linked–annealed to cross-linked–remelted polyethylenes, is presented.

34. Gencur SJ, Rimnac CM, Kurtz SM: Fatigue crack propagation resistance of virgin and highly crosslinked, thermally treated ultra-high molecular weight polyethylene. *Biomaterials* 2006;27:1550-1557.

   This article describes a study of the effects of gamma radiation-induced cross-linking combined with annealing or melting on the resistance to crack propagation of two highly cross-linked polyethylenes compared with non–cross-linked polyethylene.

35. Wang A, Essner A, Polineni VK, Stark C, Dumbleton JH: Lubrication and wear of ultra-high molecular weight polyethylene in total joint replacements. *Tribology International* 1998;31:17-33.

36. McKellop H, Shen FW, Lu B, Campbell P, Salovey R: Development of an extremely wear-resistant ultra high molecular weight polyethylene for total hip replacements. *J Orthop Res* 1999;17:157-167.

37. Heisel C, Silva M, Dela Rosa MA, Schmalzried TP: Short-term in vivo wear of cross-linked polyethylene. *J Bone Joint Surg Am* 2004;86:748-751.

   This article presents a comparison of the wear rates in vivo of acetabular liners of conventional polyethylene (moderately cross-linked during gamma sterilization) and cross-linked poly (5 Mrads, remelted), with 24 patients in each group and with the wear rates normalized to the activity levels of the individual patients. Level of evidence: II-1.

38. Engh CA Jr , Stepniewski AS, Ginn SD, et al: A randomized prospective evaluation of outcomes after total hip arthroplasty using cross-linked marathon and non-cross-linked Enduron polyethylene liners. *J Arthroplasty* 2006;21:17-25.

   The wear rates in vivo of acetabular liners of noncross-linked polyethylene (gas plasma sterilized) and cross-linked polyethylene (5 Mrads, remelted) were compared at a mean follow-up of 5.7 years.

39. Dorr LD, Wan Z, Shahrdar C, Sirianni L, Boutary M, Yun A: Clinical performance of a Durasul highly cross-linked polyethylene acetabular liner for total hip arthroplasty at five years. *J Bone Joint Surg Am* 2005;87:1816-1821.

   This article presents a comparison of the wear rates in vivo of 35 hips with conventional polyethylene liners to 31 hips with highly cross-linked remelted liners, with a minimum 5 year follow-up. Level of evidence: III.

40. D'Antonio JA, Manley MT, Capello WN, et al: Five-year experience with crossfire(r) highly cross-linked polyethylene. *Clin Orthop Relat Res* 2005;441:143-150.

   This article compares the wear rates in vivo of 53 hips with conventional polyethylene (moderately cross-linked during gamma sterilization) and 56 hips of highly cross-linked–annealed polyethylene at 5 years average follow-up.

41. Digas G, Karrholm J, Thanner J, Malchau H, Herberts P: Highly cross-linked polyethylene in total hip arthroplasty: Randomized evaluation of penetration rate in cemented and uncemented sockets using radiostereometric analysis. *Clin Orthop Relat Res* 2004;429:6-16.

   This article discusses a comparison of the wear rates in vivo of 32 patients with one hip having a highly cross-linked polyethylene liner and the opposite hip having conventional polyethylene. Twenty-seven patients were evaluated at more than 2-year follow-up. A second study of 60 patients randomized to receive either highly

1: Principles of Orthopaedics

cross-linked or conventional polyethylene is also presented.

42. Oparaugo PC, Clarke IC, Malchau H, Herberts P: Correlation of wear debris-induced osteolysis and revision with volumetric wear-rates of polyethylene: A survey of 8 reports in the literature. *Acta Orthop Scand* 2001;72: 22-28.

43. Dumbleton JH, Manley MT, Edidin AA: A literature review of the association between wear rate and osteolysis in total hip arthroplasty. *J Arthroplasty* 2002;17:649-661.

44. Birman MV, Noble PC, Conditt MA, Li S, Mathis KB: Cracking and impingement in ultra-high-molecular-weight polyethylene acetabular liners. *J Arthroplasty* 2005;20:87-92.

    The authors assessed the prevalence of crack formation in conventional polyethylene cups and its association with rim impingement, oxidation, and time in situ in 120 retrieved acetabular cups.

45. Collier JP, Currier BH, Kennedy FE, et al: Comparison of cross-linked polyethylene materials for orthopaedic applications. *Clin Orthop Relat Res* 2003;414: 289-304.

46. Halley D, Glassman A, Crowninshield RD: Recurrent dislocation after revision total hip replacement with a large prosthetic femoral head: A case report. *J Bone Joint Surg Am* 2004;86:827-830.

    A case report of rim damage and fracture of a highly cross-linked acetabular liner that occurred in conjunction with multiple dislocations and closed reductions of a hip prosthesis is presented.

47. Greer KW, King RS, Chan FW: The effects of raw material, irradiation dose, and irradiation source on crosslinking of UHMWPE, in Kurtz RG, Martell J (eds): *Crosslinked and Thermally Treated Ultra-High Molecular Weight Polyethylene for Joint Replacements*. West Conshohocken, PA, ASTM, 1996, pp 209-220.

48. Oral E, Rowell SL, Muratoglu OK: The effect of alpha-tocopherol on the oxidation and free radical decay in irradiated UHMWPE. *Biomaterials* 2006;27:5580-5587.

    This article compared the resistance to oxidation of ultra-high molecular weight polyethylene with and without soaking in vitamin E after radiation cross-linking.

49. Collier MB, Engh CA Jr, McAuley JP, Ginn SD, Engh GA: Osteolysis after total knee arthroplasty: Influence of tibial baseplate surface finish and sterilization of polyethylene insert. Findings at five to ten years postoperatively. *J Bone Joint Surg Am* 2005;87:2702-2708.

    This article describes radiographic study of the incidence and severity of osteolysis in 242 knees with a polyethylene insert that had been gamma-irradiated in air and affixed to a rough baseplate surface, compared with 98 knees with a polyethylene insert that had been gamma-irradiated in an inert gas, or had not been irradiated, and joined to a polished surface.

50. Vaccaro AR, Papadopoulos S, Traynelis VC, Haid RW, Sasso RC: *Spinal Arthroplasty: The Preservation of Motion*. Philadelphia, PA, Saunders Elsevier, 2007.

    The state of the art of spinal disk replacement, in comparison with other treatments including fusion, is presented.

51. van Ooij A, Kurtz SM, Stessels F, Noten H, van Rhijn L: Polyethylene wear debris and long-term clinical failure of the Charite disc prosthesis: A study of 4 patients. *Spine* 2007;32:223-229.

    The clinical significance of polyethylene wear debris in salvage surgery after initial total disk replacement, the pattern and the mechanisms of polyethylene wear in the retrieved cores, and the extent of polyethylene debris in the periprosthetic tissues obtained from four patients were assessed.

Chapter 8

Musculoskeletal Imaging

Kern Singh, MD   Kush Singh, MD   Clyde A. Helms, MD   Howard S. An, MD

Introduction

The field of musculoskeletal radiology continues to expand at an ever-increasing rate. The introduction of new imaging modalities as well as the increasing sophistication of current technology have allowed the radiologist to play an invaluable complementary role in the field of orthopaedic surgery.

Imaging Modalities

Selected imaging studies should aid in determining the clinical diagnosis, use available resources, and minimize the radiation dose to the patient. The most commonly ordered studies in the field of musculoskeletal radiology include plain films, CT, and MRI. Recent advances in nuclear medicine, MRI, and ultrasonography now provide the orthopaedic surgeon with an increased number of diagnostic modalities.

Plain Film Radiography

With the rapid growth in the field of musculoskeletal radiology, both the orthopaedic surgeon and the musculoskeletal radiologist have many choices to aid in diagnosis. Many of these new techniques, although commonly used, are expensive, provide unnecessary radiation to the patient, and have contributed to the dramatic increase in the cost of medical care.

From the emergency department to the clinic, the plain film is perhaps the most versatile imaging modality. Indications for plain films are wide-ranging and their use is extremely cost-effective. Almost every orthopaedic imaging evaluation should begin with a plain radiograph, allowing the clinician to choose a subsequent imaging study that will aid in the correct diagnosis and evaluation of a given disorder.

Several key issues are raised when using conventional radiography. At least two views of the area should be obtained, ideally with views that are at 90° angles to each other, with each view including two adjacent joints. This decreases the risk of missing an associated fracture, subluxation, and/or dislocation at a site remote from the apparent injury. Comparison views are occasionally helpful, particularly in the pediatric population.

The standard radiographic series comprises the AP and lateral views. A weight-bearing view should be used and may be of value for a dynamic evaluation of the joint space under the weight of the body.

Occasionally, oblique and special views are necessary, particularly in evaluation of complex structures such as the elbow, wrist, ankle, and pelvis. Extensive discussion of each of these views is beyond the scope of this chapter, and the reader is directed to a more comprehensive text on radiography or a text on musculoskeletal imaging.[1] However, several of the more common special views are discussed in this chapter.

Shoulder

The Grashey view is an AP view that demonstrates the glenoid in profile, allowing for an unobstructed view of the glenoid and glenohumeral joint space without overlap of the humeral head. This view is particularly useful in posterior shoulder dislocations. The patient can be erect or supine and rotated approximately 40° toward the side of the suspected injury.

The axillary view, a superoinferior view of the shoulder, is helpful in determining the exact relationship of the humeral head and the glenoid fossa. The axillary view is useful for the detection of anterior or posterior shoulder dislocations. With the patient seated at the side of the radiographic table and the arm abducted so that the axilla is positioned over the cassette, the radiographic tube is angled approximately 5° to 10° toward the elbow, and the central beam is directed through the shoulder joint. The axillary view is important in traumatic situations where a glenohumeral dislocation may be missed with an AP radiograph.

Although similar to the axillary view, the West Point view also demonstrates the anteroinferior rim of the glenoid. With the patient prone, a pillow is placed under the shoulder, raising it approximately 8 cm. The film cassette is positioned against the superior aspect of the shoulder. The radiographic tube is angled toward the axilla at 25° to the patient's midline and 25° to the table's surface.

Elbow

The radial head-capitellum view allows an unobstructed view of the radial head; this view is often limited on the lateral film by the coronoid process. The capitellum, coronoid process, and humeroradial and humeroulnar articulations are also well demonstrated. To obtain this view, the patient is seated at the side of the radiographic table, with the forearm resting on its ulnar side, the elbow joint flexed 90°, and the thumb

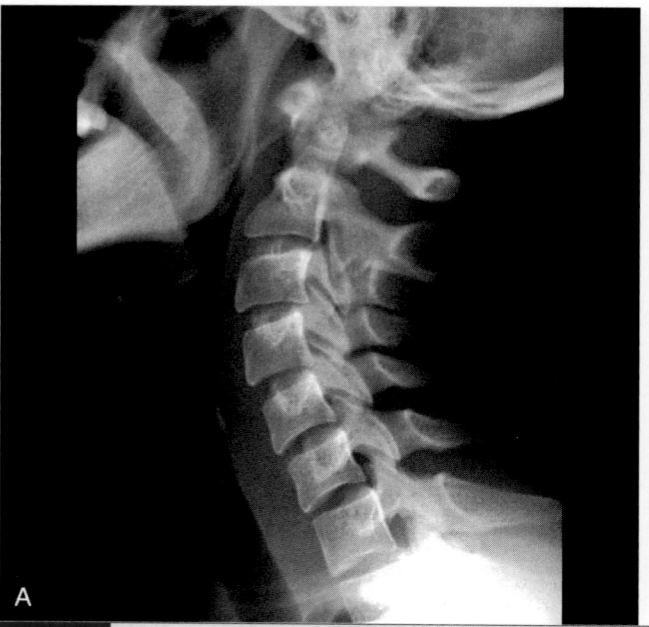
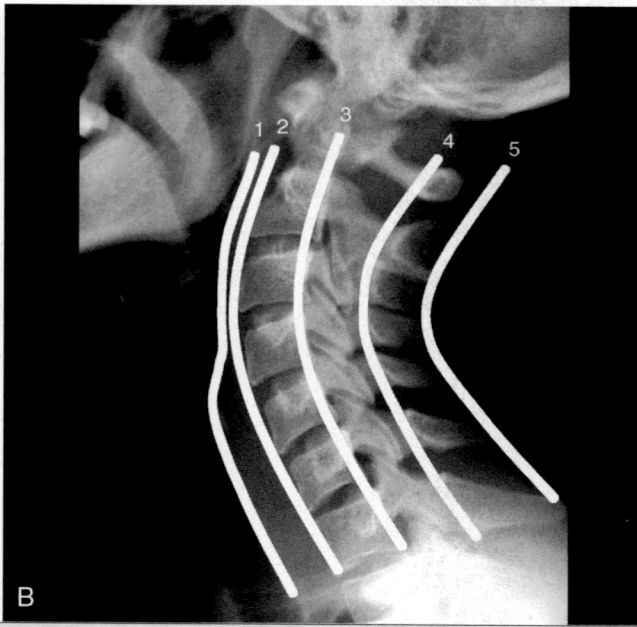

Figure 1 **A,** Normal lateral plain film of the cervical spine. **B,** Normal lateral plain film of the cervical spine labeled with the standard five lines used to evaluate the cervical spine. Line 1, prevertebral soft tissues; line 2, anterior vertebral line; line 3, posterior vertebral line; line 4, spinolaminar line; line 5, posterior spinous line.

pointing upward. The central beam is directed toward the radial head at a 45° angle to the forearm.

Pelvis

The Ferguson view provides a tangential view of the sacroiliac joints and the sacral bone. The pubic and ischial rami are also well demonstrated. With the patient supine and the radiographic tube angled approximately 30° to 35° cephalad, the central beam is directed toward the midportion of the pelvis.

Also known as oblique projections of the pelvis, Judet views are used in the evaluation of the acetabulum as well as for evaluating heterotopic ossification and ankylosis of the hip joint. For the anterior oblique view of the pelvis, the patient is supine and anteriorly rotated, with the affected hip elevated 45°. The central beam is directed vertically toward the affected hip. This allows visualization of the iliopubic (anterior) column and posterior lip of the acetabulum. The posterior Judet views evaluate the ilioischial (posterior) column, the posterior acetabular lip, and the anterior acetabular rim. Inlet and outlet views are also helpful for evaluating the competency of the pelvic ring in traumatic conditions.

Knee

The sunrise view provides a tangential (axial) view of the patella and demonstrates the femoropatellar joint compartment. The view is obtained with the patient prone and the knee flexed 115°. The central beam is directed toward the patella with approximately 15° of cephalad angulation.

The articular facets of the patella and femur are well demonstrated on the Merchant view. With the patient supine and the knee flexed approximately 45° at the table's edge, a device is used to hold the film cassette and the knee in position. The central beam is directed caudally through the patella at a 60° angle from the vertical. Weight-bearing PA views help to best assess potential articular cartilage narrowing between the femoral condyles and the tibial plateau.

The tunnel view demonstrates the posterior aspect of the femoral condyles, the intercondylar notch, and the intercondylar eminence of the tibia. With the patient prone and the knee flexed approximately 40°, and the foot supported by a cylindrical sponge, the central beam is directed caudally toward the knee joint at a 40° angle from the vertical.

Foot

The Harris-Beath view shows the body of the calcaneus, as well as the middle and posterior facets of the subtalar joints. With the patient erect and the sole of the foot flat on the film cassette, the central beam is aligned 45° toward the midline of the heel.

Axial Skeleton

Trauma

Radiographic examination of a patient with cervical spine trauma may be difficult, particularly if the patient is unconscious, because there are often undiagnosed injuries. Views are usually limited to one or two projections because unnecessary movement risks damage to the cervical cord. The single most valuable projection in these instances is the lateral cervical view, which may be obtained in the standard fashion or with the patient supine (**Figure 1**). This projection shows the most trau-

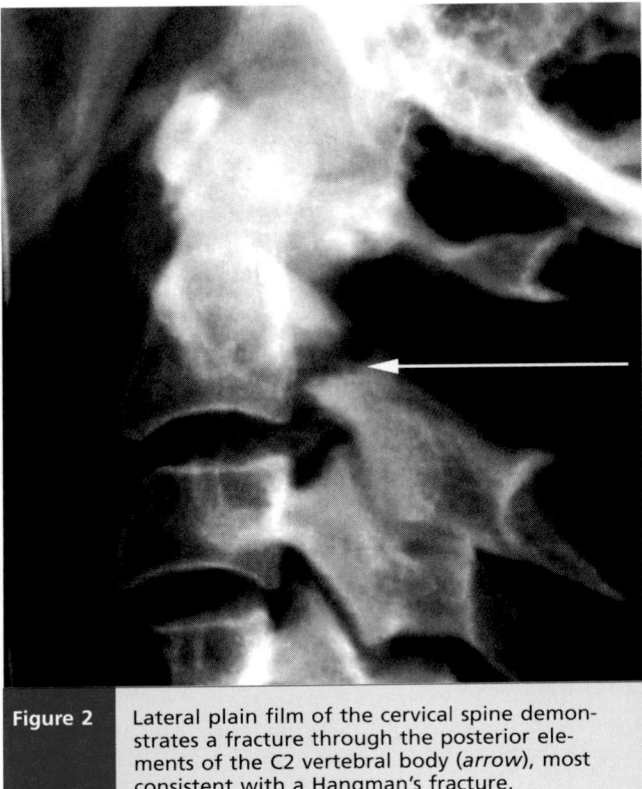

Figure 2 Lateral plain film of the cervical spine demonstrates a fracture through the posterior elements of the C2 vertebral body (*arrow*), most consistent with a Hangman's fracture.

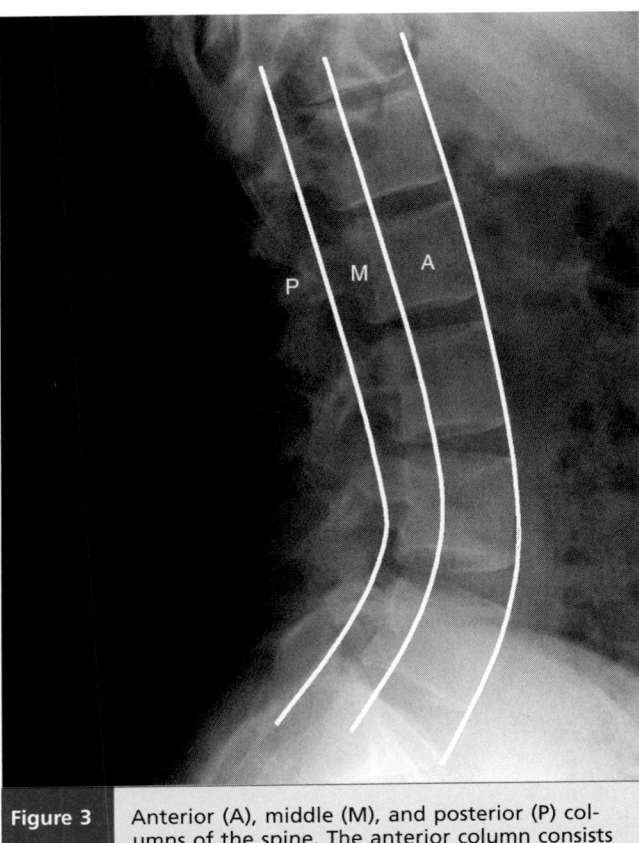

Figure 3 Anterior (A), middle (M), and posterior (P) columns of the spine. The anterior column consists of the anterior two thirds of the anulus fibrosus and vertebral body, and the anterior longitudinal ligament. The middle column consists of the posterior longitudinal ligament, the posterior one third of the vertebral body, and, the anulus fibrosus. The posterior column consists of the posterior ligament complex, which includes the supraspinous and infraspinous ligaments, the capsule of the intervertebral joints, the ligamentum flavum, and the posterior elements of the bony spine.

matic conditions of the cervical cord, including injuries involving the anterior and posterior arches of C1, the odontoid process that is seen in profile, and the anterior atlantodental interval (**Figure 2**). It is essential to visualize the complete cervical spine to exclude traumatic injury at the cervicothoracic junction.

Standard radiographic projections for evaluating injury to the thoracic and lumbar spine include AP and lateral projections with additional coned-down views of the lumbosacral (L5-S1) junction. In the setting of trauma, these views are often supplemented by CT and MRI as dictated by the clinical scenario.

Fractures of the thoracolumbar segment of the spine may involve the vertebral body and arch, as well as the transverse, spinous, and articular processes. They can generally be grouped by mechanism of injury as compression fractures, burst fractures, distraction fractures (Chance fractures and other seat-belt injuries), and fracture-dislocations.

In 1983, Denis introduced the concept of the three-column spine classification of acute injuries to the thoracic and lumbar segments[2] (**Figure 3**). This system determines the stability of the various fractures based on the site of injury of one or more of the spinal columns or elements.

Nontrauma
Plain radiographs of the spine are commonly used in the evaluation of nontraumatic disorders such as in degenerative and arthritic conditions. The initial workup of neck and low back pain may begin with a cervical or lumbar series, respectively, to exclude degenerative disk disease or occult fracture as the cause. Plain films are often limited in their evaluation in these settings and are often supplemented with CT and MRI.

Appendicular Skeleton
Trauma
Fracture of the extremities is a common indication for plain films, particularly in the acute setting. Fractures are characterized on plain films and radiopaque foreign bodies can be identified. Prereduction and postreduction films are usually obtained to ensure proper alignment after reduction. CT is usually not indicated in the setting of trauma to the extremities other than for preoperative planning. Orthogonal views of the fracture, as well as the two adjacent joints, should be obtained to exclude a remote fracture or dislocation.

1: Principles of Orthopaedics

Neoplasms

Plain films are very helpful in the diagnosis of osseous neoplasms. A lesion can be characterized on plain films as lytic or sclerotic; this information, along with the patient's age, can subsequently narrow the differential diagnosis of the lesion. Other important plain film findings include the presence or absence of calcification, as well as the presence or absence of a pathologic fracture. Although it is often easy to separate a lesion into benign or malignant categories and to provide a succinct differential diagnosis, pathologic specimens are required in many instances to establish the correct diagnosis.

When evaluating a plain film in the setting of an osseous neoplasm, three criteria should be used to differentiate a benign versus a malignant bone process. First, the presence or absence of cortical destruction is important to note because malignant processes will often show cortical destruction (**Figure 4**). Second, the presence or absence of periostitis should not only be addressed, it should also be characterized as benign or aggressive. Benign periostitis usually is thick, wavy, uniform, or dense because it is a low-grade, chronic irritation that gives the periosteum time to lay down thick new bone and remodel into more normal cortex. A malignant tumor causes a periosteal reaction that is high-grade and more acute; as a result, the periosteum does not have time to consolidate. Consequently, the periosteum may appear lamellated (onion-skinned), amorphous, or even sunburst (**Figure 5**). Third, the zone of transition should be evaluated. This is the most reliable indicator in determining benign versus malignant lesions. The zone of transition is the border between the normal bone and the lesion. A general rule is that if the margins of a lesion can be traced with a pencil, the zone of transition is narrow. If the margin is imperceptible and cannot be easily drawn, it is said to be wide (**Figure 6**). Lesions that demonstrate a permeative appearance, or the appearance of multiple small holes, do not fit into either of these two categories and include processes such as multiple myeloma, primary lymphoma of bone, and Ewing's sarcoma (**Figure 7**).

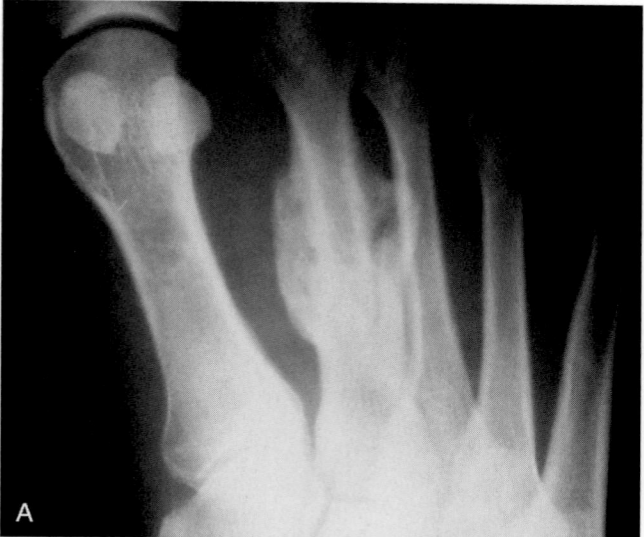

| Figure 4 | Plain film of the humerus of a patient with Ewing's sarcoma shows malignant, amorphous periostitis, a wide zone of transition, and cortical destruction. |

A   B

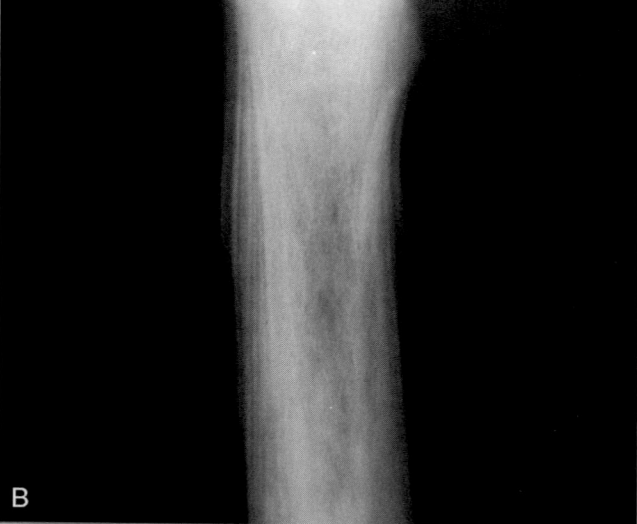

| Figure 5 | **A,** Plain film of the right foot of a patient with foot pain shows thick benign periostitis of the second metatarsal associated with a stress fracture of the middiaphysis. **B,** Aggressive, lamellated (onion-skinned) periostitis. |

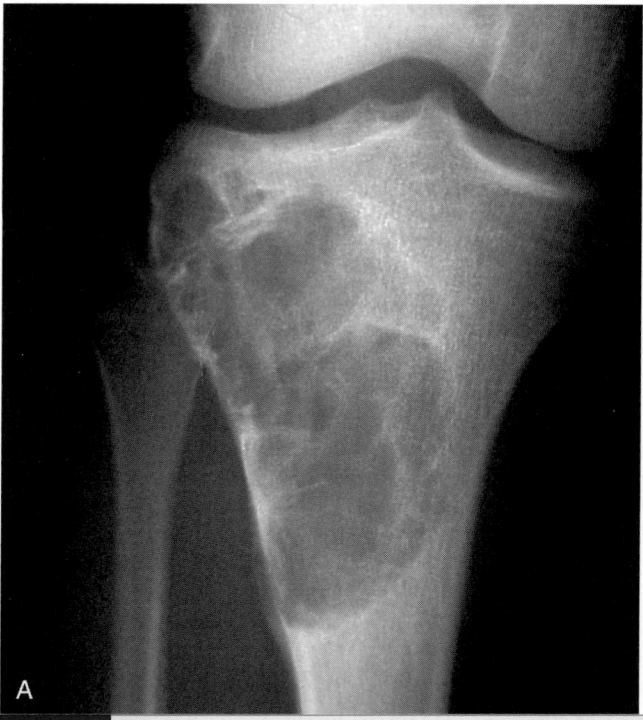
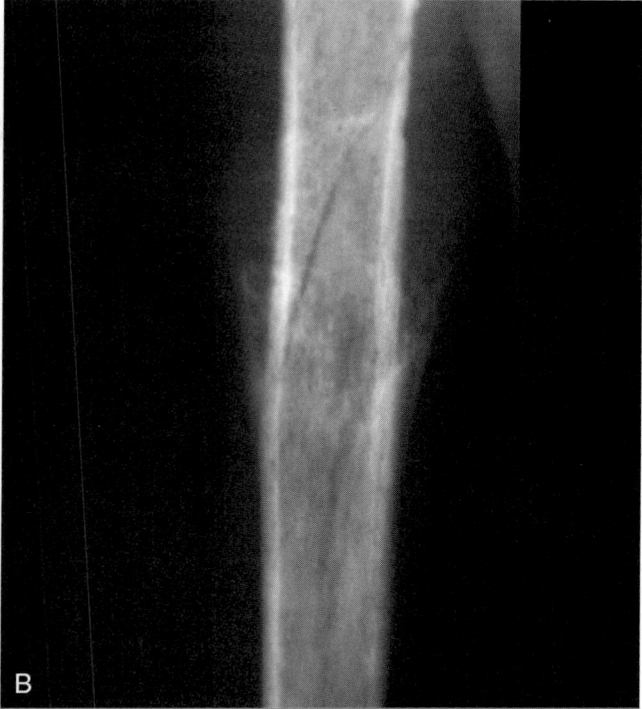

| Figure 6 | **A,** Plain film of the proximal right tibia shows the classic appearance of a cortically based nonossifying fibroma arising from the tibial metadiaphysis with a sclerotic, narrow zone of transition. **B,** Plain film of the right humerus in a patient with Ewing's sarcoma shows typical aggressive appearance, with a wide zone of transition and malignant periostitis. Also note the oblique fracture through the midhumeral diaphysis. |

Arthritis

The radiologic modalities used to evaluate arthritis are very similar to those used in traumatic conditions involving the bones and joints, although there are some modifications. The most important modality for the evaluation of arthritis is conventional radiography. Weight-bearing views may be of value, particularly for a dynamic evaluation of the joint space.

Pertinent radiographic findings in the setting of arthritis include bone mineralization, distribution of disease, alignment, presence or absence of erosive change, and any soft-tissue findings. Each of the arthritides can often be characterized by using these radiographic findings. However, classification is often very difficult; clinical as well as laboratory analysis may be necessary.

Osteoarthritis, or degenerative joint disease (DJD), is the most common arthritide. DJD, most commonly caused by trauma, is also known as secondary osteoarthritis, although a less common hereditary form also exists (primary osteoarthritis) that occurs primarily in middle-aged women. The hallmarks of DJD are joint space narrowing, sclerosis, and osteophytosis. Another diagnosis should be considered if all three of these findings are not present on a radiograph.

Unless severe osteoporosis is present, sclerosis should be present in varying amounts in all patients with DJD. Osteoporosis will cause the sclerosis to be diminished. Osteophytosis also will be diminished in

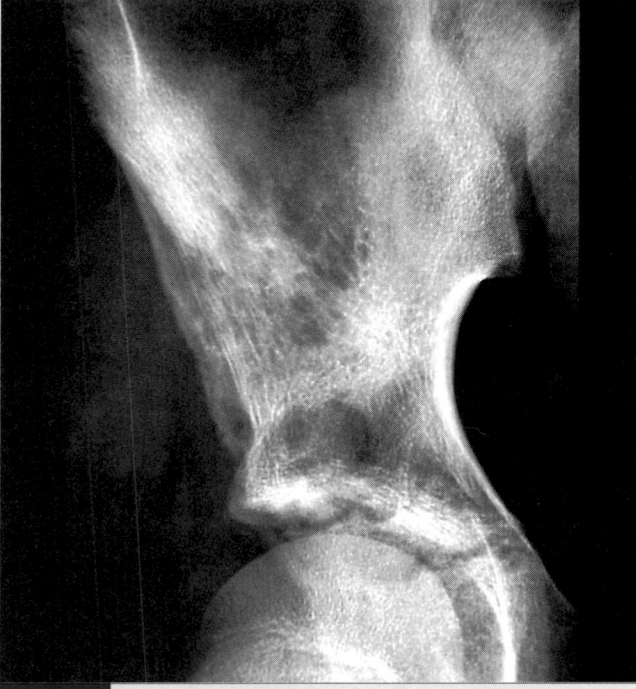

| Figure 7 | Coned-down plain film of the right pelvis in a patient with multiple myeloma shows permeative appearance of the right iliac wing and supra-acetabular region. |

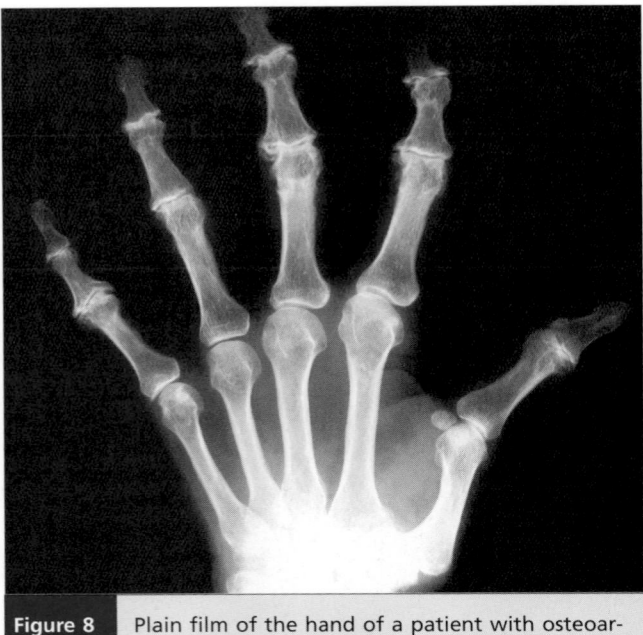

Figure 8 Plain film of the hand of a patient with osteoarthritis. Notice the distal distribution predominantly involving the DIP and PIP joints with joint space narrowing, subchondral sclerosis, and osteophyte formation.

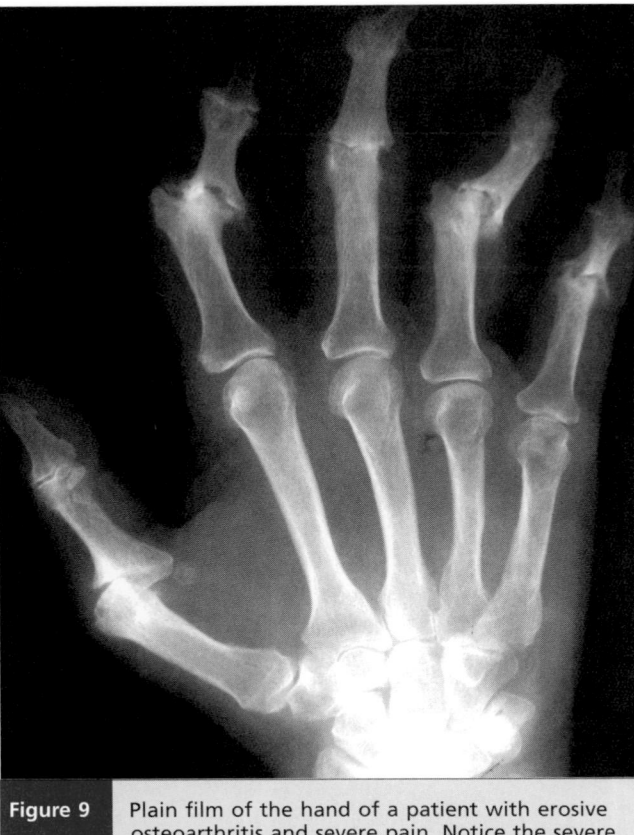

Figure 9 Plain film of the hand of a patient with erosive osteoarthritis and severe pain. Notice the severe osteoporosis with distal predominance (PIP and DIP joints) of joint involvement with joint space narrowing, subchondral sclerosis, and osteophyte formation. Also, erosions are present within these joints. The base of the thumb is not affected in this patient.

the setting of osteoporosis. Otherwise, sclerosis and osteophytosis should be prominent in DJD.

Secondary osteoarthritis can occur in any joint in the body but is most common in the hands, knees, hips, and spine. Within the hands, the distribution is distal and typically involves the distal interphalangeal (DIP) and proximal interphalangeal (PIP) joints (**Figure 8**).

Primary osteoarthritis is a familial arthritis that affects middle-aged women almost exclusively and is only seen in the hands. It affects the DIP joints, PIP joints, and the base of the thumb in a bilaterally symmetric fashion. Erosive osteoarthritis is a subset of primary osteoarthritis that is uncommon but can be very painful and debilitating. It has the identical distribution mentioned for primary osteoarthritis but is associated with severe osteoporosis of the hands as well as erosions (**Figure 9**).

There are a few exceptions to the classic triad of findings seen in DJD (sclerosis, joint space narrowing, and osteophytes). Several joints also exhibit erosions as a manifestation of DJD: the temporomandibular joint, the acromioclavicular joint, the sacroiliac joints, and the symphysis pubis. When erosions are seen in one of these joints, DJD must be considered.

A subchondral cyst, or geode, is often found in joints affected with DJD. Geodes are cystic formations that occur around joints in a variety of disorders, including DJD, rheumatoid arthritis, osteonecrosis, and crystalline pyrophosphate dihydrate crystal deposition disease.

Rheumatoid arthritis is a connective tissue disorder of unknown etiology that can affect any synovial joint in the body. The radiographic hallmarks are soft-tissue swelling, osteoporosis, joint space narrowing, and mar-

ginal erosions. In the hands, it is classically a proximal process that is bilaterally symmetric. However, rheumatoid arthritis has a variety of appearances; from its radiographic appearance alone, it can be very difficult to diagnose (**Figure 10**).

Rheumatoid arthritis causes fairly characteristic findings in large joints, including marked joint space narrowing and associated osteoporosis. Erosions may occur and tend to be marginal (away from the weight-bearing portion of the joint). In the hip, the femoral head tends to migrate axially or superomedially, whereas the hip tends to migrate more superolaterally in osteoarthritis. In the shoulder, the humeral head tends to be high-riding, which can also be seen in the setting of rotator cuff tears as well as crystalline pyrophosphate dehydrate crystal deposition disease (**Figure 11**). In long-standing cases of rheumatoid arthritis, it is not uncommon for secondary DJD to superimpose itself on the findings one would expect with rheumatoid arthritis.

Psoriatic arthritis is classified as an HLA-B27 spondyloarthropathy and has many findings that are similar to osteoarthritis in the hands. Psoriatic arthritis causes a distinctive arthropathy that is characterized by

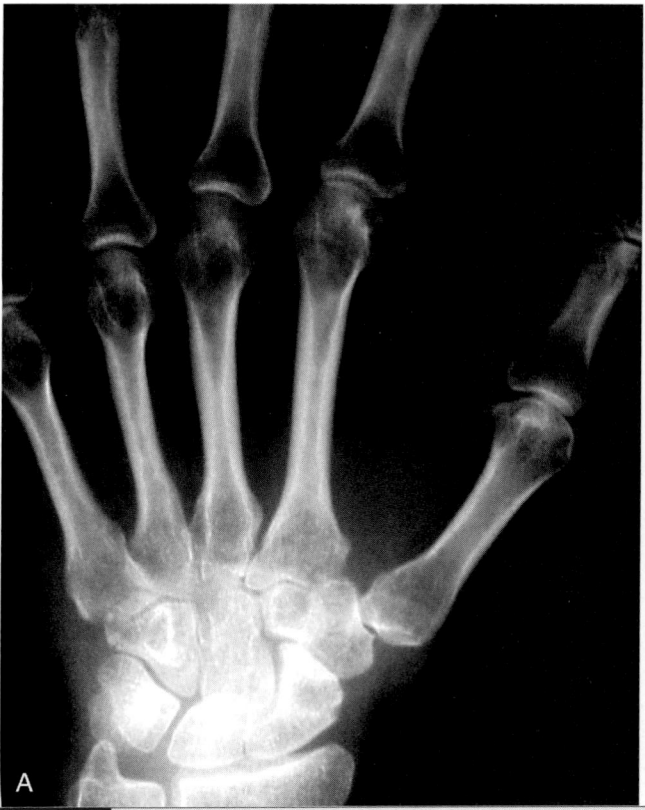
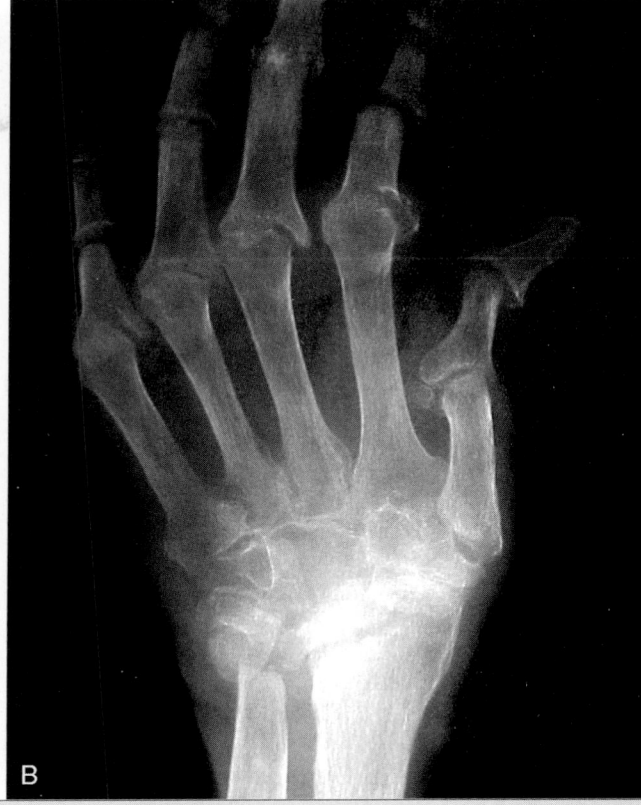

Figure 10 **A,** Plain film of the hand of a patient with positive rheumatoid factor. Subtle periarticular osteopenia is the only apparent finding. **B,** Plain film of the hand of the same patient several years later. Findings of late-stage rheumatoid arthritis are now very apparent, including diffuse osteopenia, carpal crowding, and erosive changes of the metacarpophalangeal and PIP joints with relative sparing of the DIP joints. Subtle soft-tissue nodule is present along the radial aspect of the wrist.

its distal predominance, proliferative erosions, soft-tissue swelling, and periostitis (**Figure 12**). Proliferative erosions are different from the clean-cut, sharply marginated erosions seen in all other erosive arthritides in that they have fuzzy margins with wisps of periostitis emanating from them. Severe forms are often associated with bony ankylosis across joints and arthritis mutilans deformities. Reiter syndrome causes identical changes in every respect to psoriatic arthritis, with the exception that the hands are not as commonly involved as the feet.

Computed Tomography

Accessibility, rapid image acquisition, excellent contrast resolution, and multiplanar capability make CT indispensable in the setting of trauma as well as in the evaluation of bone and soft-tissue tumors. CT can be used to define intra-articular abnormalities such as articular cartilage damage, aid in the evaluation of foreign bodies (both calcified and noncalcified), and localize fracture fragments. CT is of particular importance in the detection of small bone fragments displaced into the joints; detection of small, displaced fragments of the fractured vertebral body; and in the assessment of concomitant injury to the cord or thecal sac.

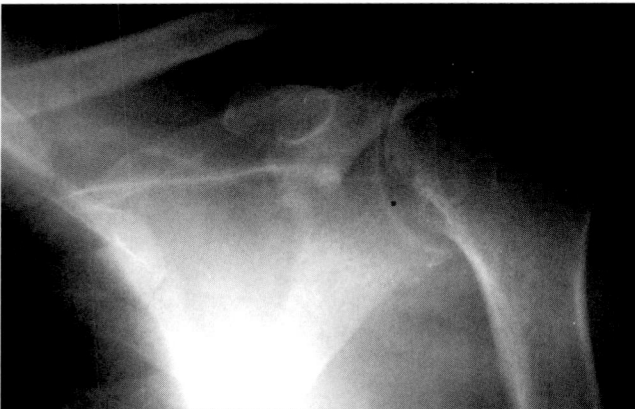

Figure 11 Plain film of the shoulder of a patient with rheumatoid arthritis. Notice the high-riding humeral head, which almost abuts the under-surface of the acromion. This may also be seen in chronic rotator cuff tears and crystalline pyrophosphate dehydrate crystal deposition.

CT myelography provides sensitive information regarding the status of neural compression and is of particular importance when MRI may be contraindicated

1: Principles of Orthopaedics

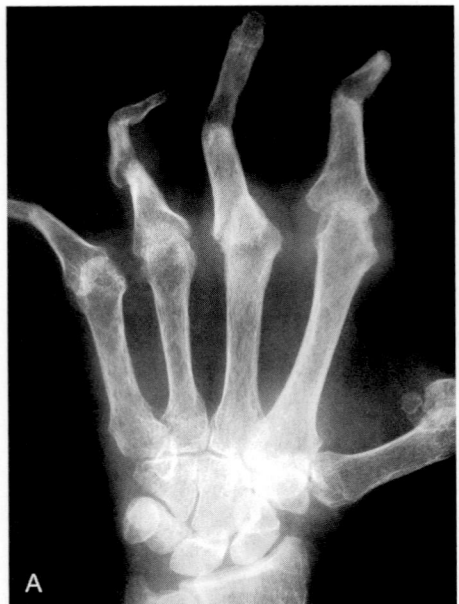 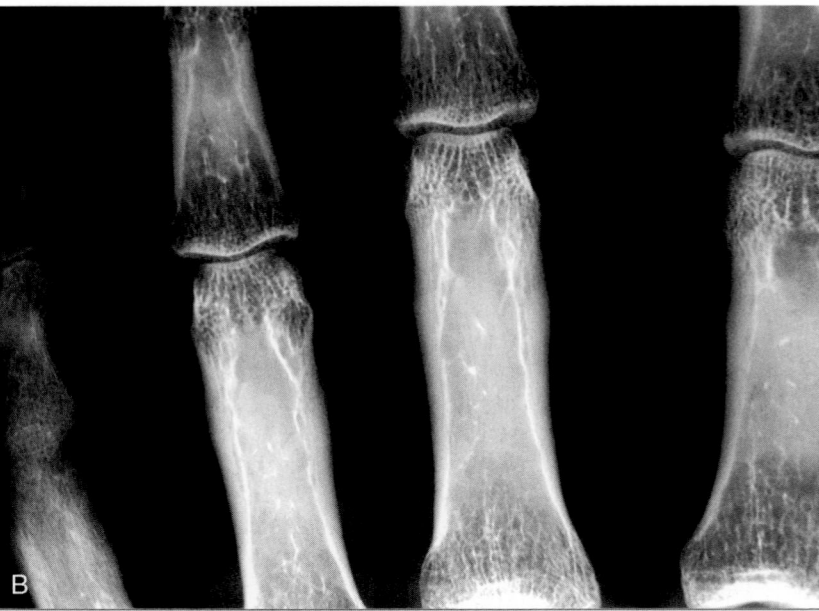

Figure 12 **A,** Radiograph of the hand in a patient with late, severe psoriatic arthritis. Note the distal predominance of the arthropathy with bony ankylosis of several of the joints. **B,** Coned-down view of the fingers of a different patient with psoriatic arthritis demonstrates mild soft-tissue swelling of the digits with associated periostitis of the phalanges. Cortical and periosteal thickening is present as a result of chronic periostitis, particularly within the shaft of the third metacarpal (second from right).

(ocular implants, vascular clips, cardiac pacemakers, claustrophobia). CT myelography is often used in the setting of neurologic compression (tumor or metastatic disease, stenosis, herniated disk, degenerative changes of the spine), and symptoms of radiculopathy characterized by weakness or pain that is not responsive to conservative therapy. In most clinical scenarios, CT myelography has fallen out of favor compared with MRI because of the significantly increased radiation exposure and risks associated with the procedure, including seizures, contrast reaction, and trauma related to cervical or lumbar puncture.[3]

CT arteriography allows for a precise interpretation of the circulatory system without the cumbersome filming methods previously used in standard angiograms. Additional software capabilities now allow a three-dimensional evaluation of the vascular system. This study is particularly useful in the setting of oncology in which tumor vascularity can be shown as well as extent of disease. Additionally, it is also useful to locate vessels suitable for preoperative intra-arterial chemotherapy.

Recent Advances
Recent advances have been made in the imaging of bone and soft-tissue masses. Although most workups consist of plain film and MRI, results from a recent study indicated that multidetector CT (MDCT) following intravenous enhancement is helpful in the preoperative assessment of musculoskeletal masses when compared with MRI and plain radiographs.[4] In a prospective study of 68 patients, MDCT provided more detailed information than MRI and plain radiographs

with regard to calcification/ossification (Figure 13) and cortical/marrow involvement. This information is of particular importance in the estimation of cortical destruction and bone marrow extension during the preoperative evaluation. Limitations of MDCT were noted when detecting the histologic properties (benign versus malignant) and the vascularity of musculoskeletal masses.

Advances in Interventional CT
Depending on the comfort level of the musculoskeletal radiologist, CT-guided intervention can be used in both the diagnosis and treatment of several musculoskeletal conditions.

Open biopsy usually serves as the final procedure in the diagnosis of musculoskeletal lesions with reported accuracy rates as high as 98%. However, open biopsy has potential for significant complications. As a result, percutaneous needle biopsy and fine needle aspiration biopsy, usually CT-guided, have supplanted open biopsy because of increased safety, lower costs, and reduced pain. The diagnostic accuracy rate for these procedures is as high as 96% in some reports, with complication rates ranging from 0% to 7.4%. CT-guided core biopsy is often performed initially for diagnosis and repeat needle biopsy, or open biopsy is subsequently performed if the diagnosis is still in question or if the results vary from what is suspected clinically.

CT-guided percutaneous biopsies are generally performed using local anesthesia, although conscious sedation is usually used for children. Potential complications are minimal and include bleeding, infection, and

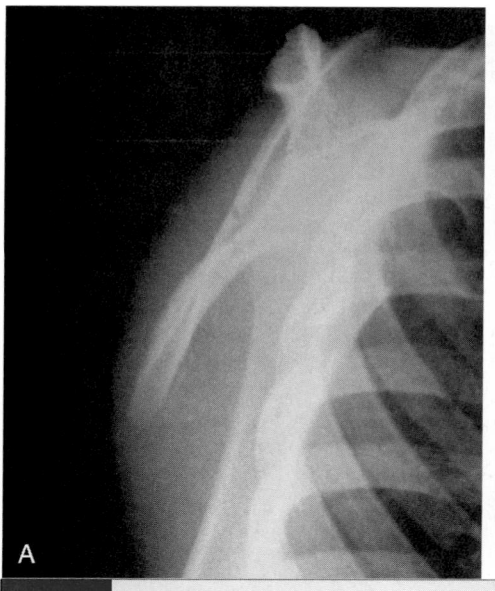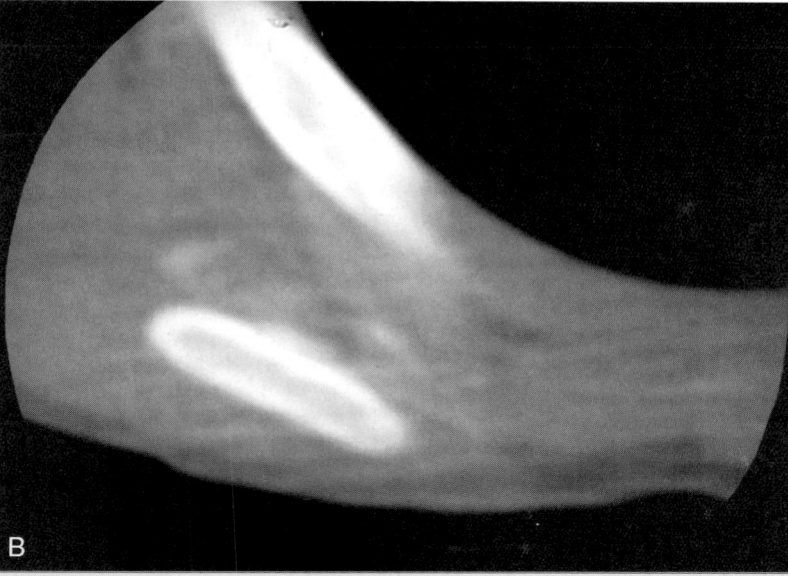

Figure 13	A, Plain film of the right scapula of a patient with a history of recent trauma. Subtle calcifications are present just deep to the body of the scapula, but are very difficult to visualize on this radiograph. B, Coned-down axial CT image of the right hemithorax provides much better visualization of subtle calcification just deep to the scapula. Findings were most consistent with myositis ossificans.

contamination of the needle tract. The benefit is more obvious when the lesion is deep seated, located in the pelvis or spine, or very closely related to neurovascular structures.

A 2002 study found that anatomic site has a significant influence on the accuracy of the biopsy.[5] Pelvic biopsy has the highest accuracy rate (81%), whereas spine biopsy has the lowest diagnostic accuracy (61%). The discrepancy of accuracy was postulated to be a result of pelvic lesions being larger on presentation than those in other more cloistered anatomic sites. Biopsy of nonpelvic and nonspinal lesions has an accuracy rate of approximately 73%.

An additional benefit of CT guidance is facilitation of definitive therapy, avoiding the need for an open surgical procedure for diagnosis. In a recent prospective study, the efficacy and safety of CT-guided percutaneous biopsies for the evaluation of deep-seated musculoskeletal lesions was demonstrated.[6] The overall diagnostic yield and accuracy rate for bony lesions were 81.03% and 95.74%, respectively; for soft-tissue lesions, 70% and 92.85%, respectively.

Limitations to the procedure vary, the most significant being ionizing radiation. As a result, CT-guided percutaneous biopsy is often limited to spinal, paraspinal, and pelvic lesions. These lesions are difficult to target and benefit from CT guidance to improve the accuracy of the biopsy. Biopsy of large lesions of the limbs can easily be done without image guidance.

CT-guided radiofrequency coagulation of osteoid osteomas has become a common procedure. CT-guided radiofrequency ablation has been shown to successfully treat osteoid osteomas while reducing surrounding bone loss during its removal.[7] CT is extremely effective

at locating the tumor nidus and guiding accurate needle placement (**Figure 14**). The authors describe three preprocedural requirements: (1) high probability of diagnosis based on clinical and imaging evidence; (2) safe access for a 16-gauge needle, permitting placement such that no part of the tumor is more than 5 mm from the needle; and (3) no vital structures within 1 cm of the tip of the electrode.

Magnetic Resonance Imaging
Sequences
Ideally suited for the evaluation of the musculoskeletal system, MRI distinguishes tissues by displaying different signal intensities on T1- and T2-weighted images.[8] Proton density represents a mixture of T1 and T2 weighting, with contrast being primarily a function of the number of protons within each tissue.

Fast spin-echo (FSE) sequences allow for a more rapid acquisition of images than the conventional spin-echo method. However, as a result, the signal intensity of fat remains bright on both FSE T1- and T2-weighted images. Consequently, pathology in subcutaneous fat or marrow may be obscured because of the similar signal intensity of fat and fluid. This limitation can be overcome by the use of fat saturation. Two different techniques are use to accomplish this: frequency-selective (chemical) fat saturation and short tau inversion recovery (STIR) imaging.

Frequency-selective (chemical) fat saturation is based on differences in resonant frequencies between fat and water. A pulse is applied at the frequency of fat to nullify the signal from fat without affecting the signal from water. This sequence is compatible with the use of gadolinium, either intra-articular or intravenous. Limitations in-

1: Principles of Orthopaedics

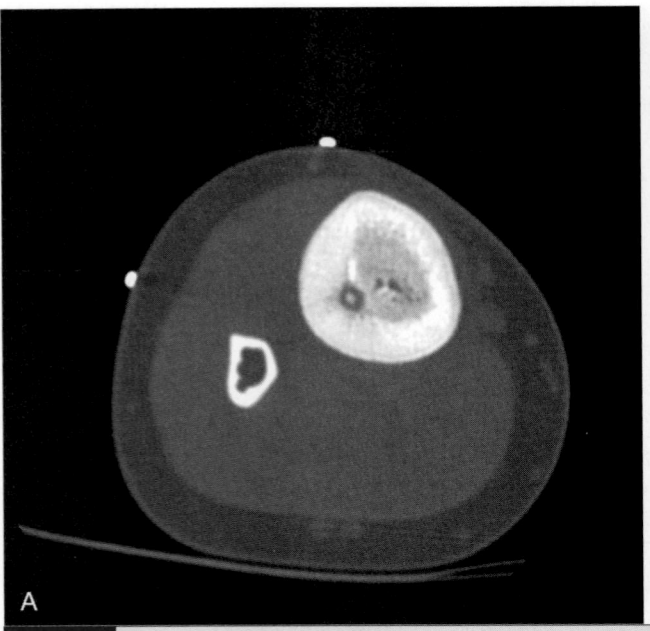 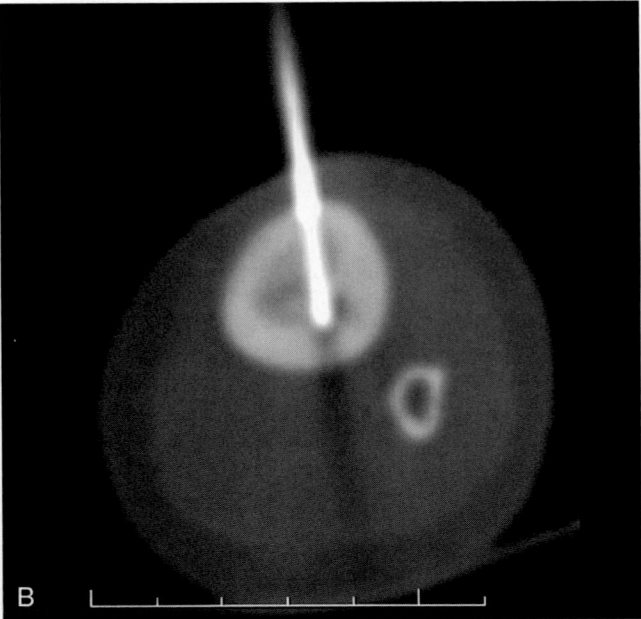

Figure 14 **A,** Axial CT image of the lower extremity shows classic appearance of an osteoid osteoma with a calcified nidus within the tibia. **B,** Axial CT image demonstrates radiofrequency ablation needle placed directly into the calcified nidus under CT guidance. The lesion was successfully treated and the patient's symptoms subsequently resolved.

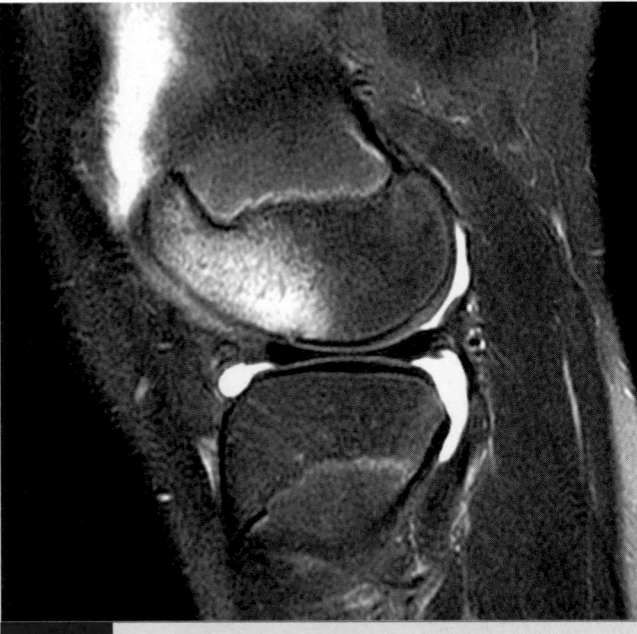

Figure 15 Sagittal FSE T2-weighted image with fat saturation of the knee demonstrates amorphous increased T2 signal within the lateral femoral condyle anteriorly in the setting of lateral patellar dislocation, most consistent with a bone contusion.

that mimics pathology. This often can be identified by noticing the lack of suppression of the overlying subcutaneous fat signal in these regions, but it can be difficult to recognize and may result in diagnostic errors.

A STIR sequence is a fat saturation technique that results in markedly decreased signal intensity from fat and strikingly increased signal from fluid and edema. This technique is based on the relaxation properties of fat protons rather than their resonant frequency, as is the case with frequency selective fat saturation. A FSE T2-weighted sequence is often used with fat saturation rather than STIR imaging; although these appear very similar in terms of image contrast, differences are related to varying mechanisms. STIR images are generally more homogeneous in fat suppression because they are not as sensitive to field heterogeneity as the frequency-selective technique. Additionally, STIR sequences should not be used with intravenous or intra-articular gadolinium because the contrast agent has similar relaxation properties to fat protons and its signal intensity will be saturated along with fat.

Indications

Traumatic musculoskeletal injures are effectively evaluated by MRI. Certain abnormalities, such as bone contusions or trabecular microfractures not typically seen on radiography and CT, are particularly well demonstrated on MRI (**Figure 15**). Occult fractures, which can be missed on conventional radiographs, are often much more apparent on MRI.

Gadolinium (Gd-gadopentetic acid) is a contrast agent that demonstrates increased signal intensity on

clude potential for heterogeneous fat suppression, particularly along curved surfaces such as the shoulder and ankle. This may result in spurious signal intensity

T1-weighted images. This MRI contrast agent can be used intravenously in the evaluation of soft-tissue masses, which demonstrate diffuse enhancement. Conversely, fluid collections such as abscesses typically demonstrate peripheral enhancement.

It was noted in a recent study that the use of MRI of the extremities has markedly increased from the early 1990s.[9] During the same time period, the use of diagnostic arthroscopy has decreased and that of therapeutic arthroscopy has increased. These findings support the hypothesis that there is an increased reliance of clinical practitioners on the diagnostic information provided by MRI in preoperative clinical decision making.

Recent Advances

Many technological advances have been made in the field of MRI; in particular, there has been a growing interest in increasing field strength using a 3-Tesla (T) magnet. Many theoretic advantages to 3-T MRI exist, although clinical application remains limited. The increased field strength provides a higher signal-to-noise ratio (SNR), improving image quality and potentially increasing diagnostic accuracy. The higher field strength also provides images with higher spatial resolution, decreases time to produce images, and enhances contrast mechanisms (T2-weighted gradient echo).

For musculoskeletal applications, higher SNR is used primarily to increase imaging speed or spatial resolution. However, it is not clear that improved image quality leads to improved diagnostic accuracy. For example, previous studies have found no difference between low-field scanners (< 0.5 T) and 1.5-T instruments in the diagnosis of anterior cruciate ligament and meniscal tears, although high-field strength images may improve diagnostic confidence. Diagnostic accuracy is high for these common indications and does not seem to be limited by SNR efficiency. The relative advantage of 3-T MRI for these studies is related to faster imaging time with an equivalent level of contrast resolution.

Indications in which accurate diagnosis is limited by available SNR include shoulder labral pathology, evaluation of early cartilage lesions, preoperative spine assessment, or small ligaments.[10] In other situations, such as unilateral hip evaluations or peripheral nerve lesions, current MRI studies at 1.5 T are technically challenging because of the simultaneous need for large field-of-view coverage as well as high spatial resolution to resolve small structures (such as the acetabular labrum). For these applications, a higher SNR afforded by 3-T magnets allows acquisition of high-image matrices while effectively using techniques that maintain reasonable image acquisition times. Finally, the higher SNR that is available at 3 T may lead to new musculoskeletal applications of MRI that are not feasible at lower field strength, such as new forms of image contrast, nonproton MRI, and functional MRI.[11,12]

Low-field MRI magnets are defined by a field strength less than 0.5 T. They consist of open-configured whole-body MRI systems or dedicated extremity scanners. Initial studies performed with low-field strength have reported unsatisfactory results in the assessment of the musculoskeletal system. Limitations of the low-field MRI primarily result from a lower SNR, which has to be compensated for by increasing the section thickness and subsequently reducing in-plane resolution, increasing the number of acquisitions, and decreasing the bandwidth. Furthermore, low-field scanners lack the capability of using sophisticated image analysis techniques that require a strong and homogeneous magnetic field.

Recent improvements in low-field-strength MRI such as better magnet homogeneity and improved receiving coil technology, however, have generated a renewed interest in low-field-strength MRI.[13] Advantages of low-field systems include decreased purchase, installation, and maintenance costs.[14] Additional advantages include higher comfort for claustrophobic patients and children, the possibility of MRI-guided interventions and kinematic studies, increased tissue contrast (T1-weighted sequences), less metallic artifacts in postoperative patients,[15] and the absence of phase artifacts from pulsatile blood flow (especially at the knee). Stray fields of several dedicated low-field scanners may be so small that cardiac pacemakers and implantable cardioverter defibrillators may not be affected during imaging of the extremity.

Multiparametric and flexible image contrast provides not only characterization of diseased tissue but also definition of related anatomy and functionally relevant tissue parameters (flow, perfusion, diffusion, tissue temperature). These advantages have allowed for a variety of MRI-guided therapeutic procedures including tumor ablation.[16]

Additional advantages such as the lack of ionizing radiation, interactive multiplanar imaging, volumetric imaging, and the ability to perform real-time imaging updates make MRI a superb modality for integration with therapy. The result is a remarkable tool that allows for minimally invasive surgical and percutaneous procedures.[17,18]

Because many of the advances in MRI technology are relatively recent, costs continue to be a prohibitive barrier. Research is still needed to determine whether MRI-guided therapy definitively improves clinical outcomes and reduces complication rates, or whether the effects of electromagnetic field exposure will ultimately limit the use of interventional MRI.[19,20]

Significant progress has been made in the field of intraoperative MRI. Much of the recent published literature has discussed the use of intraoperative MRI in the neurosurgical patient. However, many of the same concepts apply to the field of orthopaedics.

Initially, the closed-bore design and the strong fringe magnetic fields of the first MRI devices prevented their use in the operating room. In the mid 1990s, the development of open MRI systems made intraoperative MRI possible for the first time.

The image quality generated by various intraoperative low-field-strength MRI systems did not compare well with the diagnostic image quality obtained with

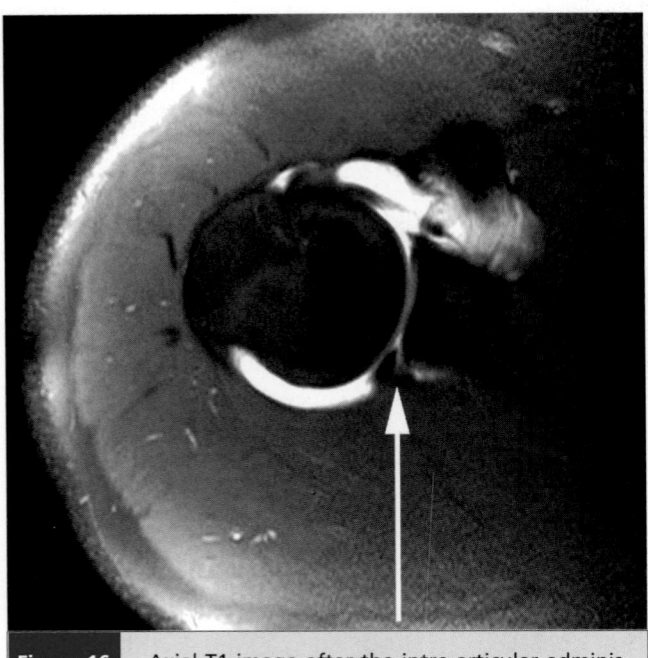

Figure 16 Axial T1 image after the intra-articular administration of gadolinium shows a labral tear (*arrow*) to much better advantage.

high-field-strength imagers. Intraoperative high-field strength MRI magnets were relatively uncommon until recently. A standard 1.5-T imager was adapted for the surgical environment. In addition, a 1.5-T imager was designed specifically for the requirements of the operating room, including a mobile ceiling-mounted magnet that can be moved into the appropriate imaging position intraoperatively. Since the initial introduction of high-field intraoperative MRI, many improvements have been made on the concept, currently making its use more common.

The benefits of intraoperative MRI are numerous. In the oncologic setting, intraoperative imaging allows the surgeon to determine whether or not the entire tumor has been removed. If the resection is incomplete, the surgeon's efforts can subsequently be directed to the site of residual tumor. Moreover, higher field strength allows for more complex imaging techniques such as diffusion weighted imaging and angiography both of which have applications in the field of neurosurgery.

Direct magnetic resonance arthrography extends the capabilities of conventional MRI by using the natural advantage gained from joint effusions.[21] This technique can be used in several different joints, including the hip, elbow, knee, wrist, and ankle. Either saline or diluted gadolinium may be injected as the arthrographic contrast material that serves to distend the joint capsule and outline intra-articular structures (**Figure 16**). Saline magnetic resonance arthrography may not differentiate partial-thickness from full-thickness rotator cuff tears because native fluid in the subacromial-subdeltoid space resulting from bursitis may have the same magnetic resonance appearance.

Magnetic resonance neurography is a relatively new technique used in the evaluation of the peripheral nervous system. Multiple advances in the field of MRI have allowed for more accurate detail of the peripheral nervous system. Higher field-strength magnets allow for increased SNR, faster imaging times, and whole-body techniques. Nerve courses may be mapped and presented in such a way that clinicians are afforded a "virtual" look at the peripheral nervous system. Two different types of studies have been described, diffusion neurography and T2-based neurography. Diffusion neurography was the first to be reported and has extremely high selectivity for nerves, allowing for identification of a variety of types of pathology. However, technical demands have delayed its clinical application. T2-based neurography is more commonly used and is based on the suppression of signals from fat as well as the signals from flowing blood, allowing for increased conspicuity of endoneurial fluid.

Tissue-specific imaging of nerves is useful in many clinical scenarios because it is capable of demonstrating detailed information about pathology, particularly in the setting of small nerve tumors that are difficult to localize precisely using electromyography. In the past, low-field-strength MRI was inaccurate in diagnosing small nerve tumors.

Now, for example, tumors of the sciatic nerve are readily distinguished from other nonneurologic causes of sciatica. Magnetic resonance neurography can distinguish between tumor types, including distinguishing perineuriomas from schwannomas. Magnetic resonance neurography also can be extremely helpful in surgical planning for the treatment of these lesions, allowing for evaluation of the specific elements of a nerve involved by tumor and identifying the relationship of the main nerve trunk to the mass of the tumor so that an appropriate surgical approach can be determined.

In the setting of acute trauma, imaging can provide information about the continuity of a nerve. Magnetic resonance neurography can establish the existence of significant nerve injury[22] and any neural discontinuities, although hemorrhage in the acute setting does limit evaluation somewhat. In the evaluation of nerve compression syndromes, magnetic resonance neurography demonstrates sensitivity and specificity similar to needle electromyography. For instance, magnetic resonance neurography was useful in predicting positive outcomes for surgical intervention in those patients with carpal tunnel and ulnar release surgeries.[23]

Ultrasound

Indications

Although not as commonly used in musculoskeletal radiology, ultrasound possesses potential advantages over MRI. Ultrasound machines are portable, usually more accessible, and less expensive than MRI equipment. Additional benefits include the absence of radiation exposure, multiplanar imaging capability, and dynamic real-time image acquisition. Ultrasound imaging is extremely operator-dependent, however. A secondary limitation is the lack of familiarity of many musculo-skeletal radiologists with ultrasound musculoskeletal images. Like MRI, ultrasound is limited by artifact secondary to metallic hardware. Common indications for musculoskeletal ultrasound include evaluation of hip dysplasia in newborns and evaluation of rotator cuff pathology in adults.[24]

Recent Advances
Musculoskeletal ultrasound has become an established imaging method for the diagnosis and follow-up of patients with rheumatic diseases. Although MRI may be the standard, high cost limits its widespread use, especially in countries where the availability of modern MRI systems is limited. Some researchers have found ultrasound as sensitive as MRI in the detection of synovitis and tenosynovitis. In addition, power Doppler ultrasonography has proved to be a valuable tool for the assessment of synovial and entheseal inflammation.[25] High-resolution ultrasound has proven useful in the detection of median nerve enlargement at the distal wrist crease in symptomatic patients with carpal tunnel syndrome.[26]

Additional advances in musculoskeletal ultrasound have been made in the setting of trauma.[27] Ultrasound provides valuable diagnostic information serving as an adjunct to CT and MRI. For example, ultrasound may be useful in the evaluation of bony union. Plain films have traditionally been used to evaluate bone healing. However, metallic hardware can sometimes obscure evidence of healing. Although ultrasound cannot penetrate hardware, the ultrasonographer can effectively position the probe to image the region of interest while avoiding artifact. Fracture callus appears more echogenic as the callus ossifies, a finding that may be identified earlier than on plain radiographs.

Ultrasound is useful in the evaluation of soft tissues and joints for evidence of infection. Fluid collections may develop and can be well localized by ultrasound for aspiration. Joints may be examined to determine whether fluid is present and when there are specific fluid collections, such as bursitis or soft-tissue abscesses outside the joint, ultrasound can differentiate a bursa or soft-tissue abscesses from intra-articular effusions. This technique is particularly useful in patients with cellulitis, soft-tissue edema, or a body habitus that limits physical examination.

Additionally, ultrasound is useful in the evaluation of the interosseous ligament complex of the ankle. The continuity of these ligaments is accurately assessed with ultrasound. Ultrasound is useful for evaluating the integrity of the interosseous ligament in "high" ankle sprains as well as suspected or known syndesmotic injuries associated with ankle fracture. Disruption of the anterior talofibular ligament and calcaneofibular ligament is also well documented on ultrasound. Ultrasound has also been shown to identify ligamentous pathology in the posterolateral corner of the knee.[28] The ability to assess ligamentous injury via ultrasound has proved to be a useful adjunct to MRI in evaluating

multiligamentous knee injuries. A significant limitation exists in the evaluation of the cruciate ligaments, particularly the posterior cruciate ligament, which are seen to much better advantage with MRI.

Nuclear Medicine
A myriad of radiopharmaceutical agents are available to facilitate diagnosis in different clinical settings. In the setting of trauma, plain radiographs are the mainstay of diagnosis, but may be normal early in the course of a fracture. Although fractures are radiologically obvious in 95% of patients younger than 65 years of age within 24 hours of injury, in older patients it may be up to 72 hours before fractures are apparent on plain radiographs. Bone scans will demonstrate uptake on both the early blood pool and on the late images.

In the setting of spinal infections, gallium-67 is still the radiopharmaceutical agent of choice. Indium-111 (In-111) oxine-labeled leukocytes and technetium-Tc 99m hexamethylpropylenamine oxine-(Tc 99m HMPAO) labeled leukocytes are the preferred agent for the diagnosis of infection in the appendicular spine. In-111 and Tc 99m HMPAO require handling of blood products. Additionally, In-111 requires 24 hours to prepare before imaging and delivers a large dose to the spleen, limiting its use in the pediatric population. The drawbacks to each of these agents have led to the increased use of several newer radiopharmaceutical agents.

Recent Advances
Fluorine-18 deoxyglucose positron emission tomography (FDG-PET) has been used in the localization of infections within bone. Clinical studies have shown diagnostic accuracy of up to 96% to 100% in the skeleton. The use of FDG-PET has the potential advantages of being a single-step procedure with imaging 1 hour after the injection, rapid loss of radioactivity from the patient, and a radiation dose comparable with that of leukocyte-imaging techniques.

Bone scintigraphy is inadequate for the detection of myeloma secondary to minimal osteoblastic activity and hypovascularity of the lesion.[29] Radiographs are usually obtained for staging, but are of limited value in the evaluation of early disease (stages I and II) (Figure 17). Several studies have shown that multifocal disease may be present despite normal radiographs.

In a recent study, it was shown that FDG-PET was able to detect medullary involvement in 13 patients with multiple myeloma.[30] FDG-PET resulted in upstaging of disease in four patients, influencing subsequent treatments. The sensitivity of FDG-PET in detecting myelomatous involvement was 85% and the specificity was 92%. One false-positive result was identified in a patient who had undergone radiation therapy 3 weeks before FDG-PET. Two false-negative studies were identified, one in which the radiographic skeletal survey showed subcentimeter lytic lesions within the ribs that were not detected on FDG-PET and in another study, a lytic lesion detected on radiography showed only

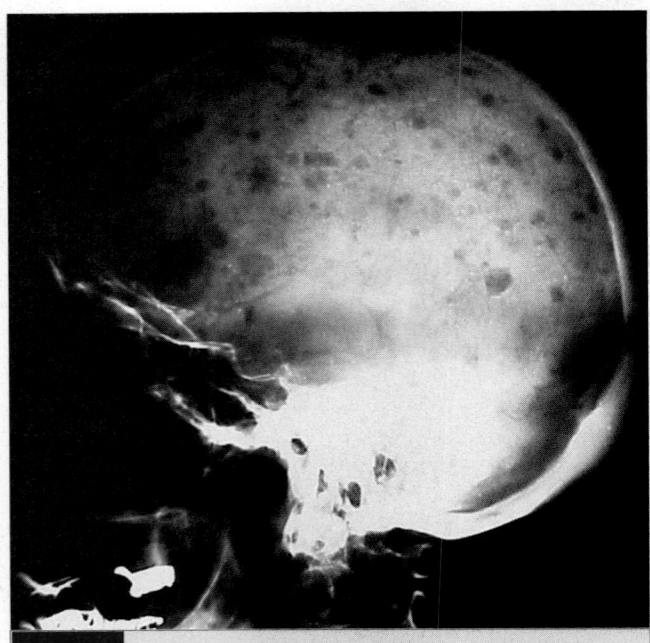

Figure 17 Lateral plain film of the skull demonstrates innumerable lytic lesions in the skull in a patient with known diagnosis of multiple myeloma. Plain films of the skull 1 year earlier were normal.

mildly increased FDG uptake and was not identified prospectively.

Summary

The field of musculoskeletal radiology is rapidly advancing. The evolution of diagnostic imaging modalities has altered the physician's approach to patients with musculoskeletal conditions. Earlier diagnosis of pathologic, traumatic, and degenerative musculoskeletal conditions can have a profound effect on the management of orthopaedic patients. As musculoskeletal imaging advances continue to accelerate, it becomes more imperative that the musculoskeletal radiologist and orthopaedic surgeon work in tandem to ensure a higher quality of patient care.

Annotated References

1. Greenspan A: *Orthopedic Imaging: A Practical Approach*, ed 4. Philadelphia, PA, Lippincott Williams & Wilkins, 2004, p 982.

   This textbook discusses musculoskeletal imaging for radiologists and orthopaedic surgeons.

2. Denis F: The three column spine and its significance in the classification of acute thoracolumbar spinal injuries. *Spine* 1983;8:817-831.

3. Sandow BA, Donnal JF: Myelography complications and current practice patterns. *AJR Am J Roentgenol* 2005;185:768-771.

   A survey of practicing radiologists and procedural-related complications associated with myelography are presented. Level of evidence: IV.

4. Mori T, Fujii M, Akisue T, Yamamoto T, Kurosaka M, Sugimura K: Three-dimensional images of contrast-enhanced MDCT for preoperative assessment of musculoskeletal masses: Comparison with MRI and plain radiographs. *Radiat Med* 2005;23:398-406.

   An evaluation of MDCT versus MRI in 68 patients is presented. Level of evidence: III.

5. Hau A, Kim I, Kattapuram S, et al: Accuracy of CT-guided biopsies in 359 patients with musculoskeletal lesions. *Skeletal Radiol* 2002;31:349-353.

6. Puri A, Shingade VU, Agarwal MG, et al: CT-guided percutaneous core needle biopsy in deep seated musculoskeletal lesions: A prospective study of 128 cases. *Skeletal Radiol* 2006;35:138-143.

   According to this study, CT-guided percutaneous core needle biopsy had a high rate of diagnostic yield and accuracy.

7. Torriani M, Rosenthal DI: Percutaneous radiofrequency treatment of osteoid osteoma. *Pediatr Radiol* 2002;32:615-618.

8. Westbrook C, Kaut-Roth C, Talbot J: *MRI in Practice*, ed 3. Malden, MA, Blackwell Publishing, 2005, p 410.

   This textbook discusses MRI indications in clinical practice.

9. Glynn N, Morrison WB, Parker L, Schweitzer ME, Carrino JA: Trends in utilization: Has extremity MR imaging replaced diagnostic arthroscopy? *Skeletal Radiol* 2004;33:272-276.

   This study demonstrates increasing reliance on preoperative MRI versus diagnostic arthroscopy. Level of evidence: III.

10. Magee T, Shapiro M, Williams D: Comparison of high-field-strength versus low-field-strength MRI of the shoulder. *AJR Am J Roentgenol* 2003;181:1211-1215.

11. Berg A, Singer T, Moser E: High-resolution diffusivity imaging at 3.0 T for the detection of degenerative changes: A trypsin-based arthritis model. *Invest Radiol* 2003;38:460-466.

12. Mosher TJ, Smith HE, Collins C, et al: Change in knee cartilage T2 at MR imaging after running: A feasibility study. *Radiology* 2005;234:245-249.

    This study demonstrates that cartilage compression results in greater anisotropy of superficial collagen fibers. Level of evidence: II.

13. Ma QY, Chan KC, Kacher DF, et al: Superconducting

RF coils for clinical MR imaging at low field. *Acad Radiol* 2003;10:978-987.

14. Tavernier T , Cotten A : High- versus low-field MR imaging. *Radiol Clin North Am* 2005;43:673-681.

    This article presents a review of the literature on high versus low field MRI. Level of evidence: V.

15. Sugimoto H, Hirose I, Miyaoka E, et al: Low-field-strength MR imaging of failed hip arthroplasty: Association of femoral periprosthetic signal intensity with radiographic, surgical, and pathologic findings. *Radiology* 2003;229:718-723.

16. Nour SG: MRI-guided and monitored radiofrequency tumor ablation. *Acad Radiol* 2005;12:1110-1120.

    A review of current radiofrequency ablation techniques used in oncologic settings is presented. Level of evidence: V.

17. Elgort DR, Duerk JL: A review of technical advances in interventional magnetic resonance imaging. *Acad Radiol* 2005;12:1089-1099.

    Current developments and new applications for interventional MRI are described. Level of evidence: V.

18. Schulz T, Trobs RB, Schneider JP, Hirsch W, Schmidt F, Kahn T: MR imaging-guided percutaneous procedures in children. *Acad Radiol* 2005;12:1128-1134.

    Available MRI procedures are presented and clinical examples and indications are discussed. Level of evidence: V.

19. Hill DL, McLeish K, Keevil SF: Impact of electromagnetic field exposure limits in Europe: Is the future of interventional MRI safe? *Acad Radiol* 2005;12:1135-1142.

    An evaluation of occupational exposure hazards to electromagnetic fields is presented. Level of evidence: V.

20. Atalar E: Radiofrequency safety for interventional MRI procedures. *Acad Radiol* 2005;12:1149-1157.

    The radiofrequency safety aspects of interventional MRI are discussed. Level of evidence: V.

21. Elentuck D, Palmer WE: Direct magnetic resonance arthrography. *Eur Radiol* 2004;14:1956-1967.

    The current role, technique, and applications of direct magnetic resonance arthrography are discussed.

22. Cornwall R, Radomisli TE: Nerve injury in traumatic dislocation of the hip. *Clin Orthop Relat Res* 2000;377:84-91.

23. Cudlip SA, Howe FA, Clifton A, Schwartz MS, Bell BA: Magnetic resonance neurography studies of the median nerve before and after carpal tunnel decompression. *J Neurosurg* 2002;96:1046-1051.

24. Churchill RS, Fehringer EV, Dubinsky TJ, Matsen FA III: Rotator cuff ultrasonography: Diagnostic capabilities. *J Am Acad Orthop Surg* 2004;12:6-11.

    Ultrasonography is an accurate, noninvasive, inexpensive imaging method for assessing the rotator cuff. Level of evidence: V.

25. D'Agostino MA, Said-Nahal R, Hacquard-Bouder C, Brasseur JL, Dougados M, Breban M: Assessment of peripheral enthesitis in the spondylarthropathies by ultrasonography combined with power Doppler: A cross-sectional study. *Arthritis Rheum* 2003;48:523-533.

26. Wiesler ER, Chloros GD, Cartwright MS, Smith BP, Rushing J, Walker FO: The use of diagnostic ultrasound in carpal tunnel syndrome. *J Hand Surg [Am]* 2006;31:726-732.

    High-resolution ultrasound provides diagnostic information in patients with carpal tunnel syndrome. Level of evidence: III.

27. Weiss DB, Jacobson JA, Karunakar MA: The use of ultrasound in evaluating orthopaedic trauma patients. *J Am Acad Orthop Surg* 2005;13:525-533.

    The authors found that ultrasound is helpful in identifying pathology in orthopaedic trauma patients. Level of evidence: V.

28. Sekiya JK, Jacobson JA, Wojtys EM: Sonographic imaging of the posterolateral structures of the knee: Findings in human cadavers. *Arthroscopy* 2002;18:872-881.

29. Angtuaco EJ, Fassas AB, Walker R, Sethi R, Barlogie B: Multiple myeloma: Clinical review and diagnostic imaging. *Radiology* 2004;231:11-23.

    MRI studies of marrow have improved detection of the extent and location of multiple myeloma. Level of evidence: V.

30. Bredella MA, Steinbach L, Caputo G, Segall G, Hawkins R: Value of FDG PET in the assessment of patients with multiple myeloma. *AJR Am J Roentgenol* 2005;184:1199-1204.

    FDG-PET is able to detect bone marrow involvement in patients with multiple myeloma and may help assess the extent of disease and staging. Level of evidence: III.

1: Principles of Orthopaedics

Chapter 9

Perioperative Medical Management

Thomas J. Moore, MD

Introduction

Perioperative mortality is approximately 3% after emergency surgery, and is less than 0.5% for elective surgery.[1] It has been estimated that anesthesia-related mortality accounts for approximately 10% of all perioperative mortality.[1] Despite these relatively low figures, there has been a significant effort recently to develop indices to assess preoperative medical risk for surgery. The obvious goal is to determine clinical situations that, if corrected, will decrease mortality and morbidity in elective surgery. In emergency surgery, the use of preoperative testing can allow the determination of potential morbidity and mortality versus the potential benefit of the surgery. Preoperative tests, as a component of preoperative clinical evaluation, may be indicated for discovery of a preexisting medical condition that may affect perioperative outcome; assessment of an already known medical condition that may affect perioperative management; and formation of specific plans and alternatives for anesthetic care based on preoperative medical assessment.

According to the American Society of Anesthesiologists (ASA) in 2003, routine preoperative tests (performance of tests in the absence of specific clinical indications in an individual patient) are not specifically recommended. Individual anesthesiology departments or health care facilities should develop appropriate guidelines for preanesthetic screening tests in selected patient populations. Appropriate indications for preoperative tests relate to specific clinical risk factors such as age, preexisting disease such as a recent myocardial infarction, or the magnitude of the proposed surgical procedure. General guidelines for preoperative testing have been developed (Table 1). ASA provides a classification of physical status (Table 2).

A recent ASA task force on preoperative evaluation attempted to use evidence-based medical data to determine the correlation of specific preoperative tests and eventual postoperative outcomes. In a meta-analysis of more than 1,000 studies, only 30 met sufficient criteria for evaluation. Therefore, current ASA recommendations on preoperative testing are based on consensus opinion rather than evidence-based criteria.[2]

More than 30 million surgical procedures are performed yearly in the United States, and approximately 60% are outpatient procedures, with an additional 10% to 15% performed on a same-day admission basis.[2] There have been some conflicting studies concerning the need, as well as the timing, of preoperative medical "clearance" before elective surgery. Some studies have suggested that preoperative evaluation performed days before elective surgery can decrease the number of cancellations and surgical delays, whereas other studies have shown that same-day medical "clearance" of elective surgical patients can be done without negative sequelae.[2]

Cardiac Assessment

Assessment of preoperative cardiac risk has been studied extensively. The incidence of perioperative cardiac arrest has decreased over the past 25 years. The incidence of anesthesia-related cardiac arrest is reportedly 0.12-1.4 per 10,000 patients.[1] In general, preoperative cardiac assessment should determine any acutely correctable conditions in patients undergoing emergent surgery. In patients with known cardiac risk factors who are undergoing elective surgery, preoperative cardiac assessment should determine any potential preoperative cardiac intervention that would lessen perioperative cardiac morbidity or mortality.

The generally accepted cardiac assessment methods are available in most hospitals. A 12-lead electrocardiogram (EKG) is a screening test for arrhythmias, remote myocardial infarction, or acute cardiac ischemia. In addition, in asymptomatic postmenopausal women, even minor EKG abnormalities (such as first- and second-degree atrioventricular block, left ventricular hypertrophy without ST-T abnormalities, or frequent atrial or ventricular premature beats) are independently associated with increased risk of cardiac events and mortality.[3] The risk of elective surgery in patients with minor EKG abnormalities has not been determined, but in truly elective surgery, further evaluation may be indicated. Resting two-dimensional echocardiography determines left ventricular ejection fraction (a left ventricular ejection fraction of less than 35% increases cardiac complications in the perioperative period in patients

1: Principles of Orthopaedics

Table 1

Suggested Preoperative Testing Guidelines

Preoperative Condition	HGB (M)	HGB (F)	WBC	PT/PPT	PLT	Electrolytes	Creat/ BUN	Blood Glucose	SGOT/ Alk/ PTAse	Radiographs PA/LAT	EKG	Pregnancy	Type and Screen
Procedure with blood loss	X	X		X									X
Neonates	X	X											
Age < 45	X	X								If symptomatic	If symptomatic		
Age 45-49	X	X								If symptomatic	X		
Age 50-64	X	X					X			X	X		
Age 65-74	X	X					X	X		X	X		
Age 75 and >	X	X					X	X		X	X		
Cardiovascular disease							X			X	X		
Pulmonary disease										X	X		
Malignancy	X	X	****	****						X	X		
Radiation therapy			X							X	X		
Hepatic disease				X					X		X		
Exposure to hepatitis									X				
Renal disease	X	X		X		X	X				X		
Bleeding disorders and/or hemoglobinopathy (these patients will require an appropriate hematology workup)					X								
Diabetes						X	X	X					
Possible pregnancy — All women of childbearing age except those who have had a hysterectomy												X	
Steroids						X		X					
Anticoagulants	X	X		X							X		
CNS disease	X	X	X			X	X	X					

HGB = hemoglobin; WBC = white blood cells; PT/PPT = prothrombin time/partial prothrombin time; PLT = platelet count; Creat/BUN = creatinine/blood urea nitrogen; SGOT/Alk/PTAse = serum glutamate oxaloacetate transaminase/alkaline phosphatase; PA/LAT = posteroanterior/lateral; EKG = electrocardiogram; CNS = central nervous system.

undergoing noncardiac surgery).[4] Preoperative stress cardiac testing is an accurate predictor of cardiac complications following noncardiac surgery. The rapidity of onset and duration of ST segment depression during exercise testing correlates with ischemic heart disease. Vasodilation stress testing (with dipyridamole or adenosine thallium) has high sensitivity and specificity in detecting clinically significant cardiac ischemia. Dobutamine stress echocardiography evaluates cardiac ischemia, but also allows assessment of ventricular contractile function. Coronary angiography detects anatomic coronary artery stenosis amenable to surgical intervention.

The most commonly used algorithm to assess perioperative cardiac risk in patients with known cardiac ischemic disease was published by the American Heart Association.[4] In emergency surgery, the focus of cardiac assessment is perioperative medical management to decrease cardiac morbidity and mortality. If the patient has had coronary revascularization procedures within 5 years and is asymptomatic, no further workup is necessary. If the patient has undergone a cardiac workup within 2 years and is asymptomatic, no further tests are indicated. If the patient has unstable coronary artery syndrome or major clinical predictors of cardiac disease (uncompensated congestive heart failure, symptomatic arrhythmias, high-grade atrioventricular block, or significant valvular disease), cardiac catheterization is indicated before elective surgery. If the patient has intermittent predictors of cardiac risk (stable angina, prior history of myocardial infarction compensated congestive heart failure, diabetes, and possibly chronic renal failure) but has minimal functional limitations, then elective surgeries can proceed with little cardiac risk. In patients with intermittent predictive parameters of cardiac risk that also have significant functional limitations, further cardiac testing should be done before elective surgery. If a noninvasive cardiac workup suggests significant ischemic cardiac disease, then coronary angiography should be considered before elective surgery.[4]

In addition to cardiac ischemic disease, other cardiac and medical conditions can impact cardiac function in the perioperative period. Cardiac valvular disease (aortic stenosis and mitral stenosis are more clinically significant than regurgitate lesions) is associated with postoperative congestive heart failure. Cardiomyopathy is associated with congestive heart failure in the postoperative period; fluid management, including central line placement, is important to avoid fluid overload. The treatment of hypertension should continue preoperatively and postoperatively. Preoperative cessation of β-blockers and clonidine can result in significant postoperative rebound hypertension. The incidence of adverse cardiac effects postoperatively can be reduced by modulating the adrenergic surge caused by the stress of surgery by the use of β-blockers, and by decreasing platelet adherence with aspirin.

Table 2

ASA Physical Status Classification System

P1	A normal healthy patient
P2	A patient with mild systemic disease
P3	A patient with severe systemic disease
P4	A patient with severe systemic disease that is a constant threat to life
P5	A moribund patient who is not expected to survive without the operation
P6	A declared brain-dead patient whose organs are being removed for donor purposes

Modifier: Emergency operation (E): Any patient in one of the above classes who undergoes emergency surgery is considered to be in poorer physical condition
Reproduced with permission from Classification of Physical Status: Manual for Anesthesia Department Organization and Management. *Park Ridge, IL, American Society of Anesthesiologists, 2005. Acessed 10/1/07 at http://www.asahg.org/clinical/physicalstatus.htm.*

Pulmonary Assessment

Pulmonary complications in the perioperative period include pneumonia, atelectasis, and bronchial spasm. In contrast to cardiac assessment, there are fewer studies of preoperative pulmonary assessment in preoperative planning. In patients who smoke, pulmonary complications have decreased with smoking cessation at least 8 weeks before elective surgery. In patients with asthma, bronchodilators should be considered if the peak expiratory flow rate is less than 80% of normal or 80% of individual baseline levels.

Perioperative pulmonary management of obese patients calls for special considerations. The incidence of obesity (defined as body mass index greater than 30 kg/m²) has increased 110% over the past 25 years. An estimated 30.5% of the US population is obese.[5] Obesity affects almost every organ system. The pulmonary system is especially affected in patients with significant obesity (body mass index greater than 40 kg/m²). Chest wall excursion is limited, and overall pulmonary compliance is decreased. In patients with significant obesity, pulmonary compliance may be only 35% of normal, requiring special considerations for anesthesia. In addition, obese patients may have a reduced CO_2 induced respiratory drive (obesity hypoventilation syndrome) and may develop hypoxemia in the postoperative period, especially with excessive narcotic analgesia. In addition, obese patients also have an increased incidence of obstructive sleep apnea.

Renal and Hepatic Assessment

Approximately 5% of the general population has some form of chronic renal failure. The importance of preoperative evaluation of renal compromised patients is the potential effect of chronic renal failure on metabolic function (electrolyte abnormalities), hematopoietic function (chronic anemia), coagulopathy, and excretion of medications (requiring alteration of dosage of certain medications). In addition, certain anesthetic drugs and medications (aminoglycoside antibiotics) that are known to be nephrotoxic should be avoided or their dosages regulated by serum levels in renal compromised patients.

An elevated serum potassium level is the most important clinically significant electrolyte abnormality that occurs in patients with chronic renal failure; it is recommended that potassium levels remain less than 5.5 mmol/L to reduce the incidence of cardiac arrhythmias in the perioperative period. Uremia-induced platelet dysfunction can lead to prolonged bleeding time, causing increased intraoperative blood loss. The bleeding time before surgery should be 10 to 15 minutes or less. Hemodialysis should be done on the day before surgery. A hematocrit of at least 20% in patients with chronic anemia is suggested before major surgery is attempted.

Patients with hepatic disease have significant perioperative mortality and morbidity. Vitamin K-deficient coagulopathy should be corrected with vitamin K replacement and fresh frozen plasma. Perioperatively, there should be careful fluid maintenance to avoid worsening of ascites. The Child-Turcotte-Pugh scale has been used to evaluate the risk factors for elective surgery in patients with hepatic disease.

Coagulation Assessment and Transfusion Indications

The physician should be aware of preoperative coagulopathy, either a hypocoagulable or a hypercoagulable state. The diagnosis can be made by the history and/or physical examination. In patients in a hypocoagulable state, there is usually a known coagulopathy, either anticoagulation for medical reasons, a known intrinsic deficiency of coagulation factors, or a history of a bleeding diathesis, such as excessive bleeding during menstruation, excessive bruising, or unexpected blood loss during minor surgery. A hypocoagulable state should be confirmed by standard laboratory tests. Normal hemostasis involves primary hemostasis, the acute activation of platelets to form a temporary clot, and secondary hemostasis, which involves a complex cascade of activation of factors V, VII, and XI leading to production of thrombin and conversion of fibrinogen to fibrin, ultimately forming a durable clot. Laboratory tests for primary hemostasis include tests for platelet function. A manual platelet count is available at most hospitals. The minimum platelet count acceptable to proceed with elective surgery varies. The bleeding time is a test of platelet function, usually prolonged in primary hemostasis dysfunction. Specific tests for factor deficiencies can be done to further investigate primary hemostasis coagulopathy. The most common laboratory tests for secondary hemostasis are the activated partial thromboplastin time and the prothrombin time. The international normalized ratio diminishes individual laboratory variants in reporting prothrombin times and allows more accurate monitoring of coagulation status, especially with patients treated with oral anticoagulation (warfarin) therapy.

Several inherited and acquired hematologic abnormalities have been associated with venous thromboembolism. Acquired etiologies of a hypercoagulable state include pregnancy, malignancy, nephrotic syndrome, estrogen use, and trauma. Known inherited thrombophilic defects include deficiencies of protein S or protein C, antithrombin, presence of factor V Lieden, the prothrombin mutation G20210A, high levels of factors VIII, IX, or XI, hyperhomocysteinemia, and antiphospholipid antibodies. In a retrospective study, 723 first and second degree relatives of index patients with known hereditary deficiencies of protein S, protein C, or antithrombin, or the presence of factor V Leiden, were followed for thromboembolic events. It was found that thrombotic events, especially deep vein thrombosis with or without pulmonary embolism, were increased with the thrombophilic genetic risk factors. There was a predisposing risk factor for thromboembolism, such as the use of birth control pills, in approximately 50% of patients with genetic thrombophilia who developed thromboembolic disease.[6] In a preoperative patient with a history compatible with a hypercoagulable state, postoperative precautions for venous thromboembolism should include mechanical and chemotherapeutic prophylaxis and placement of inferior vena cava filters when indicated.

Although there are no specific guidelines for canceling elective surgery for a coagulopathy, the presence of abnormal laboratory values requires investigation of the etiology of the coagulopathy and possible correction before surgery. If a coagulopathy exists before elective surgery and is not correctable or is present during emergency surgery, several steps can be taken to decrease blood loss during surgery. Erythropoietin given preoperatively can decrease the need for perioperative blood transfusions. The use of a tourniquet during limb surgery, intraoperative salvage of blood (using a cell-saver machine), and preoperative self-directed autogenous blood donation may lessen the need for perioperative allogenic blood transfusions. Hypotensive anesthesia has been used to decrease blood loss during surgery. Results from a study of total hip replacements in 100 Jehovah's Witnesses treated with hypotensive anesthesia showed a 40% decrease in intraoperative blood loss in comparison with matched controls.[7] The safety of allogenic blood transfusions has been well documented. A mild allergic response (mild fever and/or chills) occurs in approximately 1% to 3% of the more than 4 million allogenic blood transfusions done yearly in the United States.[7] A more serious allergic reaction to allogenic blood occurs in patients previously sensitized to blood transfusions and who are usually deficient in immunoglobulin A. This major allergic reaction rarely occurs (in about 5% of the 4 million blood transfusions done yearly).[7] The incidence of transmission of infectious agents in allogenic blood transfusion is relatively low. The reported risk of transmission of hepatitis B is 1 in 200,000 transfusions; hepatitis C, 1 in 5,000 transfusions; and human immunodeficiency virus (HIV) transmission, 1 in 2,000 to 1 in 800,000 transfusions.[7]

The indication for preoperative allogenic blood transfusion for elective surgery has evolved throughout the decades. The concept of 30/10 (hematocrit 30%, hemoglobin 10 g) as a minimal requirement to proceed with elective surgery began in the 1940s. There was little physiologic or scientific basis for this concept. Currently hemoglobin levels much lower than 10 g have been shown to be safe for surgery, particularly in young, healthy patients. Preoperative hemoglobin levels as low as 5.5 g have been tolerated in Jehovah's Witness patients undergoing surgery. Currently, treatment of preoperative anemia should be determined by several factors, including the likelihood of significant intraoperative blood loss and the physiologic status of the patient.

The Preoperative Assessment of the Geriatric Patient

Hip fracture is the most common condition for which the elderly seek orthopaedic care. Because of the increasing age of the US population, the annual number of hip fractures will double from 250,000 in 1990 to 500,000 by 2040.[8] Despite improvements in medical management, surgical implants, and treatment techniques for patients with hip fractures, the condition is associated with significant mortality. Approximately 5% of all fracture patients die during initial hospitalization, and the mortality rate in the first year after hip fracture is between 20% to 25%. Several factors have been shown to be predictive of early mortality following a hip fracture, including age older than 85 years, lack of independence in activities of daily living before the hip fracture, poor nutrition, and preoperative ASA class 3 to 4. In addition, if significant postoperative medical complications occur, the mortality rate is increased following hip fractures.

The optimal timing of surgical intervention for hip fracture has not been well defined. Some studies have reported an increased mortality for surgical delay of greater than 48 hours. In a retrospective study of 2,660 patients with hip fractures, the overall 30-day mortality was 9%. A delay in surgery for up to 4 days in patients with no significant medical comorbidity did not increase the mortality rate. In patients with a hip fracture and an acute medical comorbidity (such as pneumonia) who had a delay in surgery longer than 4 days, the mortality rate was 22.5%, more than double the 30-day mortality rate, in comparison with hip fracture patients without medical comorbidity and a delay in surgery.[9] In general, surgical intervention for patients with hip fractures should proceed as rapidly as possible. However, in healthy patients with a hip fracture, surgery can be delayed for up to 4 days without increased mortality. In hip fracture patients with significant medical comorbidities, surgical intervention should proceed

as soon as medical optimization of acute conditions is accomplished. In a randomized, prospective study of postoperative arthroplasty patients, patients were divided into two groups: the first group was treated in the standard manner, with each patient managed during the postoperative period by the orthopaedic surgeon with internal medicine consultation only as indicated, and the second group of patients were managed hospital-based physicians specializing in internal medicine.. The second group had fewer postoperative complications, but length of stay and cost were the same in both groups.[10]

Nutritional Assessment

There is a retrospective correlation between a patient's nutritional status and postoperative morbidity. Clinically, a patient's nutritional status can be determined by a history of weight loss of 10% of body weight over 6 months or 5% of weight loss over 1 month, and physically by cachectic appearance, temporal wasting, ascites, or poor dentition.[11] Laboratory tests of several serum markers, proteins produced in the liver, can detect acute versus chronic malnutrition (albumin: half-life of 21 days, transferrin: half-life of 8 days, and prealbumin: half-life of 2 to 3 days). Serum albumin and total lymphocyte count, found on routine tests, can be used as a general parameter of nutritional status. A serum albumin of less than 2.0 and/or a total lymphocyte count of less than 1,000 is indicative of severe malnutrition, whereas a serum albumin of less than 3.5 and/or a total lymphocyte count of less than 2,000 is suggestive of mild malnutrition.[12]

There is conflicting data on whether enhancement of a patient's nutritional status preoperatively can decrease postoperative morbidity and mortality. However, before elective surgery in significantly malnourished patients or in malnourished patients with planned surgical procedures with known wound healing issues (pressure sore surgery or surgical treatment of osteomyelitis) enhancement of the patient's nutritional status is probably beneficial. Oral enhancement of nutritional status is associated with a decreased incidence of infection and metabolic complications and is less costly than parenteral enhancement (total parenteral nutrition).[12]

Immune Status Assessment

Over the past several decades, the number of surgical procedures done in immunosuppressed patients has increased. Chemotherapy for cancer, corticosteroid usage for rheumatologic diseases, immunosuppressive drugs for transplant patients, and acquired immunodeficiency syndrome (AIDS) all are factors that have led to an increase in immunosuppressed patients, with an associated increase in surgical procedures.

HIV infection results in a decrease in CD4 positive T-lymphocytes, resulting in impairment of cell-mediated immunity. The immune status of patients

1: Principles of Orthopaedics

with HIV infection, if left untreated, results in progressive deterioration, resulting in severe opportunistic infections and tumors (AIDS). However, the development of highly active antiretroviral therapy (HAART) has significantly altered the progression of HIV infection in the United States. HAART treatment, if effective, decreases viral load and increases CD4 count. The mortality in HIV-positive patients has decreased 50% from 1995 to 2000 in the United States.[13] This longer life expectancy in patients with HIV infection in the United States makes it likely that HIV-positive patients will undergo more elective and emergent surgical procedures. For example, there has been a significant increase in the diagnosis of osteonecrosis, particularly in the femoral head, in HIV-positive patients. The etiology of the increased rate of osteonecrosis is multifactorial. Known risk factors for osteonecrosis, such as alcoholism and corticosteroid usage, are often present in HIV-positive patients. HAART, which has known lipid metabolic effects, is believed to be an independent risk factor for the development of osteoporosis. However, many patients on HAART have concomitant known risk factors for osteonecrosis, and the increased life expectancy associated with HAART makes the development of osteonecrosis more likely. Despite the etiology of osteonecrosis, there is likely to be an increase in candidates for total joint arthroplasty in HIV-positive patients in the future.

There has been logical concern for potential postoperative infection after elective and emergent surgery in patients with HIV infection. Several studies done before HAART was initiated have shown a slight increase in postoperative complications in HIV-positive patients, especially wound sepsis. HIV-positive patients with a severely compromised immune system (CD4 positive lymphocyte count less than 200/mm³) are believed to be especially at risk for postoperative sepsis. However, recent evidence suggests that surgical treatment of closed tibial fractures in HIV-positive patients, even with CD4 counts below 200/mm³, can be done without any significant increased risk of surgical site infections.[14] Treatment of open fractures, especially open tibial fractures, may lead to an increased rate of infection in HIV-positive patients.[15]

Despite the lack of evidence-based data, it seems reasonable for HIV-positive patients with severely compromised immune systems to undergo HAART therapy to enhance their immune status before elective surgery. In emergency surgery in severely immune compromised patients, additional attention should be given to known risk factors for postoperative morbidity, such as malnutrition. Prophylactic antibiotics, perhaps broad spectrum, should be used in the perioperative period.

Perioperative Antibiotics

Surgical site infections occur at a rate of 500,000 per year in the United States. A patient who develops a surgical site infection is 60% more likely to spend time in an intensive care unit, and twice as likely to die during

the perioperative period than a patient without a surgical site infection.[16] In 2002, the Centers for Medicare and Medicaid Services and the Centers for Disease Control and Prevention initiated the National Surgical Infection Prevention Project to decrease morbidity and mortality in surgical site infections by promoting appropriate preoperative antibiotic prophylaxis.[16] Three performance parameters have been developed for national surveillance and quality improvement in antibiotic prophylaxis. The first is initiation of parenteral antibiotics within 1 hour of surgical incision. The entire antibiotic dose should be administered before inflation of the tourniquet. When allergies to antibiotics are suspected, test doses should be done 1 hour before surgery. Second, an appropriate antibiotic should be selected. For total joint arthroplasty, cefazolin or cefuroxime is the preferred prophylactic antibiotic. Vancomycin or clindamycin is indicated for patients with severe allergies or adverse reactions to β-lactams. In hospitals with a "high" frequency of methicillin-resistant *Staphylococcus aureus* (exact incidence not defined) vancomycin should be used for antibiotic prophylaxis. In obese patients undergoing gastroplasty, there is evidence that 1 g of cephalosporin antibiotic did not provide adequate minimal inhibitory concentration for prophylaxis for gram-positive or gram-negative organisms. Those patients who received 2 g of cephalosporins had a lower incidence of surgical site infections than the patients who received 1 g of cephalosporin antibiotics.[17] The third performance parameter is duration of prophylaxis. Prophylactic antimicrobial therapy should be discontinued within 24 hours of the end of surgery. There is no evidence that the continuation of antibiotics until removal of surgical drains provides additional protection against surgical site infection. A national surveillance performance analysis of 34,133 Medicare patients undergoing five major surgical procedures, including total joint arthroplasty, revealed appropriate antimicrobial agents were given for surgical prophylaxis 92.6% of the time, but were administered within 1 hour of the surgical incision only 55.7% of the time and discontinued within 24 hours of the end of surgery only 40.7% of the time.[16]

Preoperative Medications

It is important to assess a preoperative patient's medication usage. Certain medications can interfere with perioperative medical management. In elective surgery, drugs that affect coagulation status should be discontinued before surgery. Aspirin irreversibly inhibits platelet cyclooxygenase (COX). Aspirin and clopidogrel both interfere with platelet function and if feasible should be discontinued 1 week before elective surgery.

Nonsteroidal anti-inflammatory drugs (NSAIDs) alleviate or modify pain through two mechanisms. The first is by inhibition of COX-1 and COX-2, thereby inhibiting the production of prostaglandins, prostacyclins, and thromboxanes. The inhibition of prostaglan-

Table 3

Perioperative Concerns and Recommendations for Eight Herbal Medicines

Common Name of Herb	Perioperative Concerns	Preoperative Recommendations
Echinacea	Allergic reactions; decreased effectiveness of immunosuppressants; potential for immunosuppression with long-term use	No data
Ephedra	Risk of myocardial ischemia and stroke from tachycardia and hypertension; ventricular arrhythmias with halothane; long-term use depletes endogenous catecholamines and may cause intraoperative hemodynamic instability; life-threatening interaction with monoamine oxidase inhibitors	At lease 24 h before surgery
Garlic	Potential to increase risk of bleeding, especially when combined with other medications that inhibit platelet aggregation	At least 7 days before surgery
Ginkgo	Potential to increase risk of bleeding, especially when combined with other medications that inhibit platelet aggregation	At least 36 h before surgery
Ginseng	Hypoglycemia; potential to increase risk of bleeding; potential to decrease anticoagulation effect of warfarin	At least 36 h before surgery
Kava	Potential to increase sedative effect of anesthetics; potential to addiction, tolerance, and withdrawal after abstinence unstudied	At least 24 h before surgery
St. John's wort	Induction of cytochrome P450 enzymes, affecting cyclosporine, warfarin, steroids, protease inhibitors, and possible benzodiazepines, calcium-channel blockers, and many other drugs; decreased serum digoxin levels.	At least 5 days before surgery
Valerian	Potential to increase sedative effect of anesthetics; benzodiazepine-like acute withdrawal; potential to increase anesthetic requirements with long-term use	No data

(Reproduced with permission from Ang-Lee MK, Moss J, Yuan C-S: Herbal medicines and perioperative care. JAMA 2001;286:208-216.)

dins is responsible for the platelet function interference and resultant coagulopathy. The second mechanism of pain and inflammation modulation is inhibition of white blood cell activation and function, which usually occurs when high doses of NSAIDs are administered.

Although there is some evidence that NSAIDs do not significantly increase intraoperative blood loss, general recommendations are to discontinue NSAIDs before elective surgery.[18] NSAIDs with a short half-life (ibuprofen and indomethacin) should be discontinued 1 to 2 days before surgery. NSAIDs with longer half-lives (naproxen, piroxicam) should be discontinued 6 days before surgery.

Discontinuation of certain medications before surgery should be done with caution. Significant cardiac abnormalities have been reported with the abrupt cessation of β-blockers. In general, psychiatric medications, pulmonary medications, and cardiac medications should be continued until the time of surgery, and if possible, taken with a sip of water on the morning of surgery. In patients taking long-term corticosteroids preoperatively, perioperative corticosteroid treatment should be considered if the hypothalamus-pituitary-adrenal axis is suppressed. Common dosages of prednisone known to suppress the hypothalamus-pituitary-adrenal axis are 5 mg per day long term, 7.5 to 10 mg per day for 1 month, or more than 20 mg per day for

1 week. The time for the hypothalamus-pituitary-adrenal axis to reverse postcessation of corticosteroid treatment varies from a few days to several months. Therefore, for patients taking preoperative corticosteroids at any of the above dosages, 25 to 100 mg of hydrocortisone should be given at the time of minor surgery, with the patient resuming a preoperative regimen in the immediate postoperative period. In patients who have had major surgery, 100 mg of hydrocortisone should be given every 8 hours for a total of 24 hours in the postoperative period. The patient should resume preoperative corticosteroid treatment when oral intake is reestablished.

Chondroitin and glucosamine supplements are frequently used by orthopaedic preoperative patients, especially patients undergoing joint arthroplasty or patients with sport medicine injuries. Both supplements are components of cartilaginous matrix. Their potential adverse effect in the perioperative period derives from their similar structure to heparin (chondroitin) and plant insulin (glucosamine). In addition, chondroitin is known to inhibit glucose transport. Although the potential anticoagulative effect (chondroitin) and hypoglycemia (glucosamine) have not been formally studied, ASA recommends cessation of chondroitin and glucosamine 2 to 3 weeks prior to elective surgery.[18]

Patients with rheumatoid arthritis frequently undergo orthopaedic surgery. Medications for rheumatoid arthritis have significant potential perioperative effects. The potential benefit of stopping antirheumatoid medications in the perioperative period has to be balanced by the possible negative effect of stopping the medications in the rehabilitative period. Methotrexate has been a commonly used drug to treat rheumatoid arthritis since the 1970s, because of its efficacy (approximately 60% response rate) and relative safety.[19] Methotrexate is a folate analog that has significant anti-inflammatory properties. Older studies suggested fewer complications with cessation of methotrexate in the perioperative period. In a more recent prospective randomized study of methotrexate in the perioperative period, patients were divided into three groups. One group discontinued methotrexate 2 weeks before and after surgery, a second group continued methotrexate therapy, and the third control group had not been on methotrexate. The group that continued the therapy had fewer postoperative complications and rheumatoid flares.[20] Methotrexate can produce nephrotoxic effects; in patients with abnormal renal function in the postoperative period, methotrexate should be discontinued. In patients with poor oral intake in the postoperative period, folate supplements should be considered, as folate deficiency can potentiate methotrexate toxicity, including bone marrow suppression. In patients with certain chronic diseases, such as pulmonary disease, liver disease, alcoholism, or poorly controlled diabetes, methotrexate should be discontinued 1 week prior to and 1 week after surgery.[19]

Hydroxychloroquine is an antimalarial drug long used for treatment of rheumatoid arthritis. Hydroxychloroquine can be continued during the perioperative period. Newer antirheumatoid drugs have not been extensively studied for perioperative complications. Leflunomide is an inhibiter of pyrimidine synthesis, a component of DNA, and targets rapidly dividing cells. Several biologic agents have been developed to treat rheumatoid arthritis. Etanercept inhibits a proinflammatory cytokine causing joint destruction in rheumatoid arthritis. Adalimumab and infliximab are other biologic agents used in rheumatoid arthritis. In the absence of significant data, it is recommended that these biologic agents can be continued for minor orthopaedic procedures and probably should be discontinued temporarily for major procedures in the perioperative period.[19]

Recently, there has been an increase in use of over-the-counter herbal medications. It has been estimated that up to 70% of the general public do not report over-the-counter medications to their physicians.[18] Although considered without serious systemic side effects by the general public, over-the-counter herbal medications can have effects on various systems (**Table 3**). In general, herbal medications should be discontinued 1 week before elective surgery. rheumatoid arthritis are reviewed.

Annotated References

1. Jenkins K, Baker A: Consent and anesthetic risk. *Anesthesia* 2003;58:962-984.

   A meta-analysis of known anesthetic perioperative risk factors and complications and the experience of the Australian Anesthesia Society are discussed.

2. Pasternak R: Chapter 1: Anesthetic management of the surgical patient, in Lubin M (ed): *Medical Management of the Surgical Patient*. Cambridge, England: Cambridge University Press, 2006, pp 7-20.

   The first chapter in this book details the interaction of primary care physicians and anesthesiologists to provide perioperative care.

3. Denes P, Larson D: Major and minor ECG abnormalities in asymptomatic females and risk of cardiovascular events and mortality. *JAMA* 2007;297:978-985.

   A retrospective study of the Women's Health Initiative to correlate clinically relevant minor electrocardiogram findings and subsequent cardiovascular morbidity and mortality is presented. Level of evidence: III.

4. Kang Y, Lazarus M: Chapter 1: Perioperative medicine, in *Washington Manual of Medical Therapeutics*, ed 31. Philadelphia, PA, Lippincott Williams & Wilkins, 2004.

   This text is the definitive quick source for medical evaluation of the perioperative patient.

5. Guss D, Bhattacharyya Y: Perioperative management of the obese orthopaedic patient. *J Am Acad Orthop Surg* 2006;14:425-432.

   An analysis of the known studies documenting the perioperative care of the obese patient is presented.

6. Martinelli I, Mannucci P, DeStefano V: Different risks of thrombosis in coagulation defects associated with inherited thrombophilia: A study of 150 families. *Blood* 1998;92:2353-2358.

7. Lemos MJ, Healy WL: Current concept review: Blood transfusions in orthopaedic operations. *J Bone Joint Surg Am* 1996;78:1260-1271.

8. Lindskog DM, Baumgaertner MR: Unstable intertrochanteric hip fractures in the elderly. *J Am Acad Orthop Surg* 2004;12:179-190.

   A review of the literature is presented, discussing treatment of intertrochanteric hip fractures in elderly patients (epidemiology, preoperative and postoperative care, and analysis of the various implants used).

9. Moran CG, Wenn RT, Sikand M, Taylor AM: Early mortality after hip fracture: Is delay before surgery important? *J Bone Joint Surg Am* 2005;87:483-489.

   This is a prospective observational study of 2,660 patients who were surgically treated for hip fractures. The 30-day postoperative mortality of hip fracture patients was 9%. Patients who had medical comorbidities that delayed surgery had 2.5 times the 30-day mortality compared with patients without medical comorbidities that delayed surgery. Patients who had surgery delayed for up to 4 days for nonmedical reasons had no increase in mortality.

10. Huddleston JM, Long KH, Naessens JM, et al: Medical and surgical comanagement after elective hip and knee arthroplasty: A randomized, controlled trial. *Ann Intern Med* 2004;141:28-38.

    In this study, 526 patients were randomized into two groups: one group was treated in the standard way (orthopaedists and medical consultants as needed) and the second group was comanaged by orthopaedic surgeons and hospital-based physicians specializing in internal medicine (hospitalists). The second group experienced a reduction in minor postoperative complications but there was no statistically significant difference in length of stay or cost. Subjectively, the orthopaedic surgeons and the nurses preferred the second treatment model.

11. Weintraub S, Wang Y, Hunt J, O'Leary P: Preoperative preparation of the patient. *Sabiston Textbook of Surgery*, ed 17. Oxford, England, Elsevier Health Sciences, 2004.

    A definitive analysis of preoperative assessment of patients is presented.

12. Ansley J: Nutrition, in Lubin M (ed): *Medical Management of the Surgical Patient*, ed 4. Cambridge, England, Cambridge University Press, 2006.

    This chapter analyzes the nutritional status and metabolic response to injury as components of care of the perioperative patient.

13. Lennox J: Medical care of the HIV infected surgical patient, in Lubin M (ed): *Medical Management of the Surgical Patient*, ed 4. Cambridge, England, Cambridge University Press, 2006.

    The general assessment and treatment of HIV positive patients regarding optimal perioperative management is discussed.

14. Harrison WJ: HIV/AIDS in trauma and orthopedic surgery. *J Bone Joint Surg Br* 2005;87:1178-1182.

    The treatment of HIV-positive patients with traumatic injuries and those undergoing arthroplasty in Malawi is discussed. Level of evidence: IV.

15. Harrison WJ, Lewis CP, Lavy CB: Open fractures of the tibia in HIV positive patients: A prospective controlled single-blind study. *Injury* 2004;35:852-856.

    In a prospective study of 27 patients with open fractures of the tibia, 7 patients were HIV positive and 20 were HIV negative. The rate of infection was increased in the HIV-positive group ($P = 0.020$). Level of evidence: IV.

16. Bratzler DW, Hunt DR: The surgical infection prevention and surgical care improvement projects: National incentives to improve outcomes for patients having surgery. *Clin Infect Dis* 2006;43:322-330.

    The Centers for Medicare and Medicaid Services have implemented several initiatives to improve outcomes after surgery. This article provides an overview of the Surgical Infection Prevention Project, specifically discussing antibiotic prophylaxis.

17. Forse RA, Karem B, MacLean LD, Christou NV: Antibiotic prophylaxis for surgery in morbidly obese patients. *Surgery* 1989;106:750-756.

18. Heller J, Gabby J, Ghadjank K: Top 10 list of herbal and supplemental medicines used by cosmetic patients: What the plastic surgeon needs to know. *Plast Reconst Surg* 2006;117:436-445.

    A discussion is presented of the most common over-the-counter medications taken electively by patients who have had plastic surgery. These medications are most likely comparable to those taken by orthopaedic patients. Current recommendations for perioperative use are suggested.

19. Howe CR, Gardner GC, Kadel NJ: Perioperative management of the patient with rheumatoid arthritis. *J Am Acad Orthop Surg* 2006;14:544-551.

    Recommendations for medication use in patients with rheumatoid arthritis are reviewed.

20. Grennan D, Gray J, Loudan J, Fear S: Methotrexate and early postoperative complications in patients with rheumatoid arthritis undergoing elective orthopaedic surgery. *Ann Rheum Dis* 2001;60:214-217.

1: Principles of Orthopaedics

Chapter 10
Medical Care of Athletes

Constance M. Lebrun, MDCM, CCFP, MPE, FACSM, Dip Sport Med

Introduction

The roles and responsibilities of the team physician may call for a multidisciplinary approach, including care from specialist physicians, physiotherapists, athletic therapists, nutritionists, and/or sports psychologists. However, the team physician still needs to have at least a working knowledge of these areas to be an effective gatekeeper.[1,2] Several basic fundamentals of medical care can easily be assimilated into a busy orthopaedic practice. The ultimate goal is the physical and mental well-being of the athlete. Success of the athlete and/or team is a secondary goal, and the physician must never let the desires of administrative or coaching staff interfere with good evidence-based medical decisions. A physician who agrees to be a team physician is often held to a higher standard of care and accountability for his or her services. These services may include preparticipation physical evaluations (PPEs), injury prevention programs, plans for rehabilitation, and safe return to participation.

Liability and Ethical Issues

The athlete-physician relationship is somewhat unique.[3] The sports medicine physician often faces additional challenges, with medical decisions complicated by influences by the team or school that may be employing the physician, the athlete's desire to play at all costs, and possible economic consequences of the athlete's having to take time off. Ethical issues include scenarios such as injecting local or long-acting anesthetic agents into joints or soft tissues, or the overuse of medications (such as injectable ketorolac, a strong anti-inflammatory drug) or other oral narcotic analgesics (such as propoxyphene or codeine) to allow the athlete to continue playing with pain, as well as recommending or prescribing performance-enhancing or illicit drugs. Professional athletes and teams present special challenges to the team physician.[4] The team physician is usually under contract to the team owners, or is even an employee of the team, and there may be an initial lack of trust by the athletes. Nevertheless, the same principles apply in terms of privacy, ensuring both consent for treatment and authorization to release information, in accordance with the Health Information Portability and Accountability Act (HIPAA). The interests of the patient or athlete should remain paramount

in the practice of medicine. In the setting of a PPE, the physician is acting as an agent for the team and will decide if the athlete is a good risk in terms of future health issues. It is critical to discuss all findings with the athlete (as well as with family, coaches, and agents). It is essential to document everything, including discussions about informed consent, treatments, and phone consultations. Although legal issues differ somewhat from moral ethics, the two entities are often intertwined.[5] The physician should be fully cognizant of the specific regional and local rules in any jurisdiction in which they choose to practice. For example, the Canadian Medical Protective Association recently stopped providing malpractice insurance for physicians who work with professional teams. Therefore, unless the physician (or their team) purchases additional liability coverage, these physicians cannot treat athletes on the sidelines, on the field, or the rink, but are still allowed to see athletes in consultation in their office or clinic. Lawsuits for medical negligence and malpractice may arise when a breach of the physician's duty has occurred and medical conduct has failed to meet the standard of care, directly causing injury or death. The most common areas relate to issues such as sudden cardiac death, concussion and return to play, heat illness, knee dislocation, and cervical spine injuries. Litigation may occasionally arise when the team physician excludes an athlete from participation and the athlete demands to participate. Legal precedence has also been established whereby student-athletes must be provided with adequate emergency medical care for any institutionally organized athletic activity. This mandates the establishment and implementation of specific written policies and procedures and emergency action plans. Consensus statements and position statements prepared by sports medicine associations are guidelines consistent with reasonable objective practice, but despite disclaimers in these publications that they should not be interpreted as the standard of care, increasingly the courts are turning to them for reference. In addition to remaining current in the field of sport medicine, the physician must maintain up-to-date knowledge of new pronouncements and regulations.

Preparticipation Physical Evaluation Guidelines

The PPE is designed to assess whether or not individual athletes can participate safely in their chosen sport(s),

Supplementary Health History Questionnaire for the female athlete

1. How old were you when you had your first menstrual period?
2. How often do you have a period?
3. How long do your periods last?
4. How many periods have you had in the last year?
5. When was your last period?
6. Do you ever have trouble with heavy bleeding?
7. Do you have questions about tampon use?
8. Do you ever experience cramps during your period? If so, how do you treat them?
9. Are you currently on birth control pills or hormones? Previously? What type? For how long? Any side effects?
10. Do you have any unusual discharge from your vagina?
11. When was your last pelvic examination?
12. Have you ever had an abnormal Pap smear?
13. How many urinary tract infections (bladder or kidney) have you had?
14. Have you ever been treated for anaemia?
15. How many meals do you eat each day? How many snacks?
16. What have you eaten in the last 24 hours?
17. Are there certain food groups that you refuse to eat (meat, breads, ets.?)
18. Have you ever been on a diet?
19. What is your present weight?
20. Are you happy with this weight? If not, what would you like to weigh?
21. Have you ever tried to lost weight by vomiting? Using laxatives? Diuretics? Diet pills?
22. Have you ever been diagnosed as having an eating disorder?
23. Do you have questions about healthy ways to control your weight?
24. How often do you drink alcohol?
25. How often do you use drugs? Smoke cigarettes?
26. Do you wear your seat belt when in a car?
27. Do you wear a helmet when you bike?
28. Do you have any questions about health or personal issues?

Figure 1 Sample of supplemental health questionnaire for female athletes.(*Reproduced with permission from Lebrun CM: The female athlete triad. Women's Health Medicine 2006;3:1-5.*)

sports such as football, hockey, or rugby may mandate frequent reassessments, whereas for other sports such as rowing, tennis, or golf a review of medical questionnaires may be sufficient. It is preferable that the PPE be conducted by a physician so that a complete physical examination can be given to address other possible sports-related medical conditions (for example, amenorrhea). For many athletes, especially adolescents, the PPE represents their only contact with a health care professional if they do not have a family physician or fail to visit their physician regularly.

Many standardized health history forms exist for PPEs. A recent monograph,[6] written and approved by the Preparticipation Physical Examination Task Force (whose participating organizations include the American Academy of Family Physicians, the American Academy of Pediatrics, the American College of Sports Medicine, the American Medical Society for Sports Medicine, the American Orthopaedic Society for Sports Medicine, and the American Osteopathic Academy of Sports Medicine), has an outline for the PPE and details for subsequent physical examination. This monograph also covers medical conditions affecting sports participation and an excellent explanation of the rationale behind their recommendations. Some institutions amend this basic form for their own use, and many also add a supplemental history form to cover selected issues for the female athlete[7] (**Figure 1**). Currently there is a trend toward using computerized Internet-based medical questionnaires, which can be modified for certain sports. Computer-savvy athletes can easily complete and print out these questionnaires in advance of the examination. These questionnaires can also be linked to a database for tracking illnesses and injuries, and for research purposes. An athlete authorization form regarding disclosure of personal health information to the school and possibly the coaches is also essential (**Figure 2**).

The physical examination should include assessment of height, weight, body mass index, visual acuity, heart rate, blood pressure, examination of various organ systems (especially cardiovascular and pulmonary), and a sport-specific detailed musculoskeletal examination. Completion of the proper forms for notification of use of banned or restricted medications can also be done at this time. Workshops or lectures for the athletes at the start of a season will clear up confusion as to what medications are allowed and establish a conduit for future communication. Although the office-based PPE offers more privacy and opportunity for one-on-one communications, station-based examinations can make use of ancillary personnel such as athletic trainers. Other stations, such as a concussion station with baseline testing (either pen and paper tests, or the newer computerized neuropsychological tests) can easily be included. The yield of laboratory tests such as urinalysis, complete blood cell counts, and determination of serum ferritin level is poor in asymptomatic healthy sports participants; a possible exception is female endurance athletes in whom iron deficiency anemia is commonly found. The physician should approve the final written documents,

and to identify those at risk of significant injury or illness. It requires that the physician have a working knowledge of sport-specific demands as well as conditions that may preclude participation or require further investigation. A thorough history and focused physical examination are standard. A more sophisticated preseason PPE may also include assessment of functional fitness, detection of muscle weakness and imbalance, and an exercise prescription. Ideally, these assessments should be completed 4 to 6 weeks before the competitive season, but practically (particularly for fall sports, when the athletes are just returning after a summer away) this is sometimes difficult. Some schools require "signing off" by the team physician before an athlete's participation. It is recommended that PPEs be conducted at least at the start of school, with updates focusing on intervening illnesses or injuries. Contact

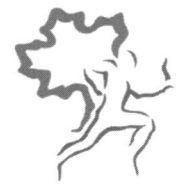

Varsity Athlete Pre-participation Physical
Medical Staff Recommendation Form

Name : _____ Date: _____ Varsity year _____

Please Print   *1 2 3 4 5*

Sport: _____ **PPE Type: Full Physical /Patient Interview** ☐

Forms Only / Review of History Forms ☐

PART 1   *Medical Clearance*

☐   Cleared to play - no Restrictions

☐   Cleared to Play - with Restrictions

☐   Disqualification: _____Temporary or _____ Season _____

☐   Clearance Deferred_____Pending, following referral/investigation : _____

| **MD to complete: Signature** |
| _____ |

PART 2   *MSK Clearance*

☐   Cleared to play - no Restrictions

☐   Cleared to Play - with Restrictions

☐   Disqualification:____Temporary or _____Season

☐   Clearance Deferred:_____ pending

following referral/investigation _____

| ***Athletic Therapist, Physiotherapist*** ***MD to complete and Sign_____*** |

Restricted or *Disqualified:*   Please indicate reasons and conditions of play

Notes:

| |
| |
| |

Confidentiality of Information & Release Form

We maintain protocols to ensure the security and confidentiality of your personal information. It is difficult to achieve absolute confidentiality in a screening such as the PPE, in training rooms or at sporting events, but every effort will be made to accomplish this.

Your pre-participation exam (PPE) clearance forms will be collected and stored in a confidential manner at the PPE. Information pertaining to clearance and/or restrictions will be shared only with those in the school administration who need to know. By signing this form, you are giving us permission to share information from the PPE and information that may arise during the next academic year that could impact sports participation with those essential to the process of evaluation and future participation. This may include your personal physician, team physicians, physiotherapist, athletic trainers, and if appropriate, coaches and /or UWO administration. Specific medical information will not be discussed with non-healthcare professionals, but final clearance or disqualification decisions may be reviewed with school officials.

We will attempt to maintain your privacy the best that we can during the PPE screening and during the upcoming sports season.

_____   _____

Athlete Signature   Date

| *Office Use :* |
| *Reviewed* _____*Date*_____ |

| **Figure 2** | Sample PPE medical staff recommendation/disclosure form. *(Courtesy of Fowler Kennedy Sport Medicine Clinic, University of Western Ontario, Canada.)* |

indicating full clearance, modified clearance, or no clearance for participation. It is critical that the coach and/or athletic director commit to making this system work effectively.

Duties of the Team Physician

Sideline Coverage of Events

The principles of sideline coverage of events are identification of and planning for medical services to promote the safety of the athletes, limiting injury, and providing appropriate medical care. Knowledge of the range of potential medical problems is essential.[8] Preseason or preevent planning benefits from access to health information on the participants, whether through means such as a pre-event medical questionnaire or information printed on the back of race numbers worn by the athletes. It is important to know participant demographics and environmental conditions as well as the demands of and inherent risks of the sport.[9] Outlines with additional information can be obtained from the Team Physician Consensus Statements, jointly produced by the same professional organizations that participate in the Preparticipation Physical Examination Task Force. These have been published, but are also available on organization Websites.

lp;&3qEmergency Preparedness

An emergency action plan is essential, with a designated chain of command and plans for evacuation. Usual information is the nature of the emergency, the location and phone number of the venue, and the nearest street address or intersection for ambulance access. A responsible person should be sent to meet and direct the ambulance; the team physician stays with the injured athlete. For larger events, it is courteous to speak with local emergency medical services personnel and hospitals well ahead of time to prepare for potential problems. In terms of sideline medical coverage, standard established guidelines for return-to-play decisions following common injuries such as concussions are helpful. The first rule of thumb is always "primum non nocere" (first do no harm).

Assessment of Environmental Conditions

Plans for inclement weather must include dealing with heat, cold, high altitude, and lightning.[10] It is necessary to involve the referees and the head organizer of the event in these deliberations well ahead of time. Some national sport organizations, such as Rowing Canada Aviron, have specific printed protocols,[11] but a document from the National Athletic Trainers' Association (NATA) outlines reasonable precautions.[12]

When traveling with a team, particularly when out of the country, it is important to note in advance the location and scope of other medical services, including imaging, medications, ambulance, hospital, access to specialists, and language considerations. After the com-

petition, a summary of injuries and assessment of policies and procedures provide recommendations for the next event or season in terms of injury prevention and management of medical care.

Equipment for the Team Physician

The Medical Bag and Associated Equipment

The contents of the team physician's medical bag and the need for associated equipment will vary with the nature of the event and proximity to more definitive and tertiary medical care. Good guidelines exist for suggested contents, with a modular approach that can be built on as necessary. **Table 1** lists the possible contents in an emergency medical bag.

Automated External Defibrillators

Automated external defibrillators (AEDs) are fast becoming a standard piece of equipment—not only in airports, shopping malls, and casinos, but also in health and fitness facilities,[13] training rooms, and on the sidelines.[14] There are many available models, but all are now relatively inexpensive, easy to use, and proven to improve patient survival after certain cardiac events. AEDs are used mainly for ventricular tachycardia or ventricular fibrillation, for which early defibrillation increases the chances of success. For each minute that elapses before defibrillation is started, the survival rate diminishes by 2% to 10%. Portable oxygen tanks and/or a pulse oximeter round out the equipment for cardiovascular emergencies.

It is helpful to hold a training session on the use of AEDs and other emergency procedures for all medical and paramedical personnel at the start of season. The athletic trainer is often the ideal person to coordinate this training session. Practical sessions on topics such as helmet removal and management of the spine-injured athlete[15] can also be included. For example, current teaching is to remove the face mask, but not the helmet or pads; this allows access to airway and minimizes movement of the cervical spine. For sports such as football, hockey, or lacrosse, it is critical to know in advance which tools are available for face mask removal and which types of face masks are likely to be encountered.

Management of Medical Conditions Encountered on the Field

The Collapsed Athlete

Management of the collapsed athlete is described by the acronym ABCDE: a primary survey with management of Airway (with cervical spine precautions), establishment and maintenance of Breathing and Circulation, a limited neurologic examination (Disability), removal of the athlete from hazardous Environment

(Exposure and Environment), and further assessment and treatment as necessary. Specific airway management involves the use of oral or nasal airways and artificial ventilation—mouth-to-mouth, facemask-to-mouth, bag-mask, endotracheal intubation, or needle cricothyrotomy, depending on the skills, training, and comfort level of the first responder. Regular recertification in Advanced Cardiac Life Support, Advanced Trauma Life Support, or equivalent courses is recommended for all team physicians.

It is critical to document the initial level of disability and neurologic status, and continue monitoring it at frequent intervals. Commonly used scales are AVPU (Alertness, response to Vocal or Painful stimuli, Unresponsive) or the Glasgow Coma Scale. In obtunded athletes, all potential causes must be considered, such as hypoxia, hypovolemia (shock), concussion and loss of consciousness, seizures, hyperthermia, hypothermia, and possible illicit drug use. During the secondary survey a more thorough head-to-toe examination is conducted and vital signs are measured (including core body temperature); decisions are then made regarding further treatment and/or transfer to another facility (**Figure 3**).

Concussion and Head Injuries

Marked progress has been made in the definition and management of concussion or mild traumatic brain injury. Loss of consciousness is not believed to be as important a prognosticator of recovery and/or long-term disability as immediate anterograde or retrograde amnesia.[16,17] The previous concussion grading scales (of which there were many different versions) have largely been discontinued because scientific evidence of their reliability and validity is lacking. In a summary and agreement statement presented at the Second International Conference on Concussion in Sport, it was recommended that concussions be characterized as either simple or complex (if the symptoms are more severe and persistent and cognitive impairment is prolonged).[18] Guidelines for return to play follow a graduated progression, provided that there are no signs or symptoms at rest. The Sport Concussion Assessment Tool (SCAT) cards for medical evaluation (**Figure 4**) and athlete information (**Figure 5**) are recent additions to the clinician's armamentarium. These handy-to-use clinical tools incorporate all of the previous sideline assessment questions, signs and symptoms of concussion, and appropriate instructions for medical follow-up and return to play. Another major advance in the field is the evolution of computerized neuropsychological testing. The four commonly used programs are Immediate Post-Concussion Assessment and Cognitive Testing (ImPACT), CogSport, Automated Neuropsychological Assessment Metric (ANAM) and HeadMinder. Most of the research to date has been performed with the first two instruments, which are the most commonly used in North America.

<table>
<tr><td>**Table 1**</td></tr>
</table>

Contents of a Basic Emergency Bag

Small bag
Fanny pack
Cell phone with important phone numbers (hospital, orthopaedic surgeon, etc)
Mouth-to-mouth cardiopulmonary resuscitation mask
Nonsterile gloves
Alcohol swabs
Sterile gauze pads
Bandage scissors, tape, and adhesive strip bandages
Minimal medications (beta-agonist inhaler for patients with asthma, a source of glucose for suspected hypoglycemia, regular strength aspirin or baby aspirin for an athlete or spectator with suspected myocardial infarction, and epinephrine for allergic reactions and anaphylaxis (a small needle and syringe with a vial of 1:1000 epinephrine or an auto-injector [EpiPen or Twinject])
Larger bag (organized into compartments)
Medication kit
Airways kit
Intravenous kit
Wound procedure kit (suture material, disposable stapler, small portable sharps container, biohazard bags)
Eye kit
Ear kit
Prepackaged dental trauma kit (tooth transport medium)
Stethoscope
Sphygmomanometer
Penlight
Reflex hammer
Tuning fork
Tongue depressor
Otoscope/ophthalmoscope
Thermometer (including a low-reading model for hypothermia)
Finger splints
Slings
Knee immobilizers
Crutches
Elastic wraps, self-adhesive wrap, and splinting materials
Preassembled fiberglass splints
Miscellaneous items
Prescription pads and business cards
Pen and notebook
Plastic bags
Forms (radiograph requisitions, a list of banned substances, injury reporting forms, copies of cards for sideline assessment of concussion)
Sunglasses and hat, raingear
Insect repellent and sunscreen
Camera

Other Medical Conditions Related to Athletic Participation

Cardiovascular Conditions

The PPE can be used to screen for some cardiovascular conditions that limit or preclude athletic participation. The American Heart Association guidelines suggest specific questions on the history portion regarding sudden death of a family member younger than 50 years of

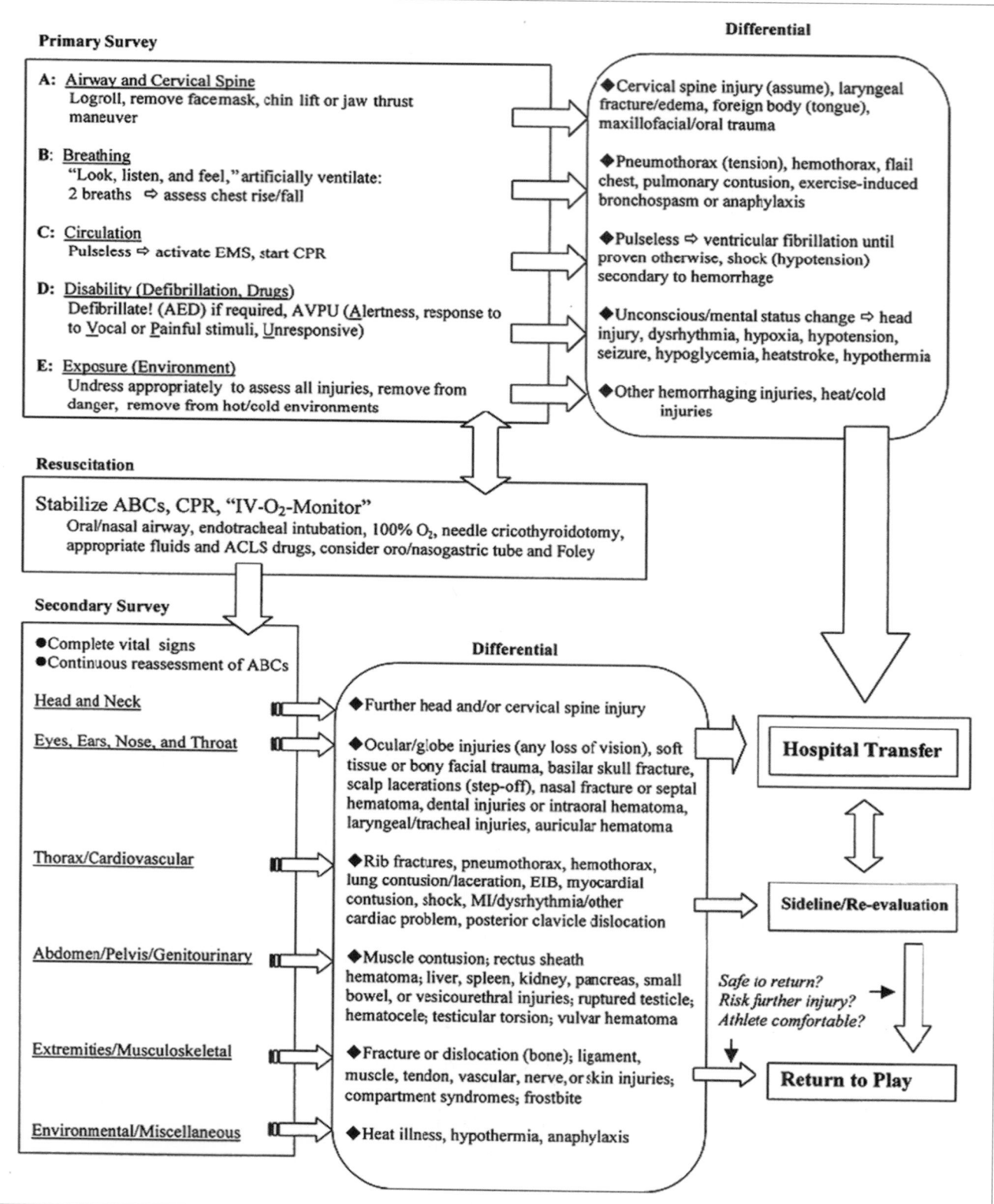

Primary Survey

A: Airway and Cervical Spine
Logroll, remove facemask, chin lift or jaw thrust
maneuver

B: Breathing
"Look, listen, and feel," artificially ventilate:
2 breaths ⇨ assess chest rise/fall

C: Circulation
Pulseless ⇨ activate EMS, start CPR

D: Disability (Defibrillation, Drugs)
Defibrillate! (AED) if required, AVPU (Alertness, response to
to Vocal or Painful stimuli, Unresponsive)

E: Exposure (Environment)
Undress appropriately to assess all injuries, remove from
danger, remove from hot/cold environments

Differential

◆ Cervical spine injury (assume), laryngeal fracture/edema, foreign body (tongue), maxillofacial/oral trauma

◆ Pneumothorax (tension), hemothorax, flail chest, pulmonary contusion, exercise-induced bronchospasm or anaphylaxis

◆ Pulseless ⇨ ventricular fibrillation until proven otherwise, shock (hypotension) secondary to hemorrhage

◆ Unconscious/mental status change ⇨ head injury, dysrhythmia, hypoxia, hypotension, seizure, hypoglycemia, heatstroke, hypothermia

◆ Other hemorrhaging injuries, heat/cold injuries

Resuscitation

Stabilize ABCs, CPR, "IV-O_2-Monitor"
Oral/nasal airway, endotracheal intubation, 100% O_2, needle cricothyroidotomy, appropriate fluids and ACLS drugs, consider oro/nasogastric tube and Foley

Secondary Survey

● Complete vital signs
● Continuous reassessment of ABCs

Differential

Head and Neck

◆ Further head and/or cervical spine injury

Eyes, Ears, Nose, and Throat

◆ Ocular/globe injuries (any loss of vision), soft tissue or bony facial trauma, basilar skull fracture, scalp lacerations (step-off), nasal fracture or septal hematoma, dental injuries or intraoral hematoma, laryngeal/tracheal injuries, auricular hematoma

Thorax/Cardiovascular

◆ Rib fractures, pneumothorax, hemothorax, lung contusion/laceration, EIB, myocardial contusion, shock, MI/dysrhythmia/other cardiac problem, posterior clavicle dislocation

Abdomen/Pelvis/Genitourinary

◆ Muscle contusion; rectus sheath hematoma; liver, spleen, kidney, pancreas, small bowel, or vesicourethral injuries; ruptured testicle; hematocele; testicular torsion; vulvar hematoma

Extremities/Musculoskeletal

◆ Fracture or dislocation (bone); ligament, muscle, tendon, vascular, nerve, or skin injuries; compartment syndromes; frostbite

Environmental/Miscellaneous

◆ Heat illness, hypothermia, anaphylaxis

Hospital Transfer

Sideline/Re-evaluation

Safe to return?
Risk further injury?
Athlete comfortable?

Return to Play

Figure 3 Treatment chart for emergency injury assessment. *(Reproduced with permission from Madden CC, Walsh WM, Mellion MB: The team physician: The prepartication examination and on-field emergencies in DeLee JC, Drez D JR, Miller MD (eds): DeLee and Drez's Orthopaedic Sports Medicine: Principles and Practice, ed 2. Philadelphia, PA, WB Saunders, 2003, vol 1, p 754.)*

Sport Concussion Assessment Tool (SCAT)

This tool represents a standardized method of evaluating people after concussion in sport. This Tool has been produced as part of the Summary and Agreement Statement of the Second International Symposium on Concussion in Sport, Prague 2004

Sports concussion is defined as a complex pathophysiological process affecting the brain, induced by traumatic biomechanical forces. Several common features that incorporate clinical, pathological and biomechanical injury constructs that may be utilized in defining the nature of a concussive head injury include:

1. Concussion may be caused either by a direct blow to the head, face, neck or elsewhere on the body with an 'impulsive' force transmitted to the head.
2. Concussion typically results in the rapid onset of short-lived impairment of neurological function that resolves spontaneously.
3. Concussion may result in neuropathological changes but the acute clinical symptoms largely reflect a functional disturbance rather than structural injury.
4. Concussion results in a graded set of clinical syndromes that may or may not involve loss of consciousness. Resolution of the clinical and cognitive symptoms typically follows a sequential course.
5. Concussion is typically associated with grossly normal structural neuroimaging studies.

Post Concussion Symptoms

Ask the athlete to score themselves based on how they feel now. It is recognized that a low score may be normal for some athletes, but clinical judgment should be exercised to determine if a change in symptoms has occurred following the suspected concussion event.

It should be recognized that the reporting of symptoms may not be entirely reliable. This may be due to the effects of a concussion or because the athlete's passionate desire to return to competition outweighs their natural inclination to give an honest response.

If possible, ask someone who knows the athlete well about changes in affect, personality, behavior, etc.

Remember, concussion should be suspected in the presence of ANY ONE or more of the following:
- Symptoms (such as headache), or
- Signs (such as loss of consciousness), or
- Memory problems

Any athlete with a suspected concussion should be monitored for deterioration (i.e., should not be left alone) and should not drive a motor vehicle.

For more information see the "Summary and Agreement Statement of the Second International Symposium on Concussion in Sport" in the April, 2005 edition of the Clinical Journal of Sport Medicine (vol 15), British Journal of Sports Medicine (vol 39), Neurosurgery (vol 59) and the Physician and Sportsmedicine (vol 33). This tool may be copied for distribution to teams, groups and organizations. ©2005 Concussion in Sport Group

The SCAT Card
(Sport Concussion Assessment Tool)
Athlete Information

What is a concussion? A concussion is a disturbance in the function of the brain caused by a direct or indirect force to the head. It results in a variety of symptoms (like those listed below) and may, or may not, involve memory problems or loss of consciousness.

How do you feel? You should score yourself on the following symptoms, based on how you feel now.

Post Concussion Symptom Scale

	None		Moderate			Severe	
Headache	0	1	2	3	4	5	6
"Pressure in head"	0	1	2	3	4	5	6
Neck Pain	0	1	2	3	4	5	6
Balance problems or dizzy	0	1	2	3	4	5	6
Nausea or vomiting	0	1	2	3	4	5	6
Vision problems	0	1	2	3	4	5	6
Hearing problems / ringing	0	1	2	3	4	5	6
"Don't feel right"	0	1	2	3	4	5	6
Feeling "dinged" or "dazed"	0	1	2	3	4	5	6
Confusion	0	1	2	3	4	5	6
Feeling slowed down	0	1	2	3	4	5	6
Feeling like "in a fog"	0	1	2	3	4	5	6
Drowsiness	0	1	2	3	4	5	6
Fatigue or low energy	0	1	2	3	4	5	6
More emotional than usual	0	1	2	3	4	5	6
Irritability	0	1	2	3	4	5	6
Difficulty concentrating	0	1	2	3	4	5	6
Difficulty remembering	0	1	2	3	4	5	6

(follow up symptoms only)

Sadness	0	1	2	3	4	5	6
Nervous or Anxious	0	1	2	3	4	5	6
Trouble falling asleep	0	1	2	3	4	5	6
Sleeping more than usual	0	1	2	3	4	5	6
Sensitivity to light	0	1	2	3	4	5	6
Sensitivity to noise	0	1	2	3	4	5	6
Other: _____	0	1	2	3	4	5	6

What should I do?
Any athlete suspected of having a concussion should be removed from play, and then seek medical evaluation.

Signs to watch for:
Problems could arise over the first 24-48 hours. You should not be left alone and must go to a hospital at once if you:
- Have a headache that gets worse
- Are very drowsy or can't be awakened (woken up)
- Can't recognize people or places
- Have repeated vomiting
- Behave unusually or seem confused; are very irritable
- Have seizures (arms and legs jerk uncontrollably)
- Have weak or numb arms or legs
- Are unsteady on your feet; have slurred speech

Remember, it is better to be safe. Consult your doctor after a suspected concussion.

What can I expect?
Concussion typically results in the rapid onset of short-lived impairment that resolves spontaneously over time. You can expect that you will be told to rest until you are fully recovered (that means resting your body and your mind). Then, your doctor will likely advise that you go through a gradual increase in exercise over several days (or longer) before returning to sport.

Figure 4 Sport Concussion Assessment Tool (SCAT) medical evaluation form. *(Reproduced with permission from McCrory P, Johnston K, Meeuwisse W, et al: Summary and agreement statement of the 2nd International Conference on Concussion in Sport, Prague 2004. Br J Sports Med 2005;39:196-204.)*

1: Principles of Orthopaedics

Sport Concussion Assessment Tool (SCAT)

The SCAT Card
(Sport Concussion Assessment Tool)
Medical Evaluation

Name: _____ Date _____

Sport/Team: _____ Mouth guard? Y N

1) SIGNS
Was there loss of consciousness or unresponsiveness? Y N
Was there seizure or convulsive activity? Y N
Was there a balance problem / unsteadiness? Y N

2) MEMORY
Modified Maddocks questions (check correct)

At what venue are we? __; Which half is it? __; Who scored last?__

What team did we play last? __; Did we win last game? __?

3) SYMPTOM SCORE
Total number of positive symptoms (from reverse side of the card) = _____

4) COGNITIVE ASSESSMENT

5 word recall

	(Examples)	Immediate	Delayed (after concentration tasks)
Word 1 _____	cat	___	___
Word 2_____	pen	___	___
Word 3 _____	shoe	___	___
Word 4 _____	book	___	___
Word 5 _____	car	___	___

Months in reverse order:
Jun-May-Apr-Mar-Feb-Jan-Dec-Nov-Oct-Sep-Aug-Jul (circle incorrect)

or

Digits backwards (check correct)
5-2-8   3-9-1   _____
6-2-9-4   4-3-7-1   _____
8-3-2-7-9   1-4-9-3-6   _____
7-3-9-1-4-2   5-1-8-4-6-8   _____

Ask delayed 5-word recall now

5) NEUROLOGIC SCREENING

	Pass	Fail
Speech	___	___
Eye Motion and Pupils	___	___
Pronator Drift	___	___
Gait Assessment	___	___

Any neurologic screening abnormality necessitates formal neurologic or hospital assessment

6) RETURN TO PLAY
Athletes should not be returned to play the same day of injury.
When returning athletes to play, they should follow a stepwise symptom-limited program, with stages of progression. For example:
1. rest until asymptomatic (physical and mental rest)
2. light aerobic exercise (e.g. stationary cycle)
3. sport-specific exercise
4. non-contact training drills (start light resistance training)
5. full contact training after medical clearance
6. return to competition (game play)

There should be approximately 24 hours (or longer) for each stage and the athlete should return to stage 1 if symptoms recur. Resistance training should only be added in the later stages. Medical clearance should be given before return to play.

Instructions:
This side of the card is for the use of medical doctors, physiotherapists or athletic therapists. In order to maximize the information gathered from the card, it is strongly suggested that all athletes participating in contact sports complete a baseline evaluation prior to the beginning of their competitive season. This card is a suggested guide only for sports concussion and is not meant to assess more severe forms of brain injury. **Please give a COPY of this card to the athlete for their information and to guide follow-up assessment.**

Signs:
Assess for each of these items and circle Y (yes) or N (no).

Memory: If needed, questions can be modified to make them specific to the sport (e.g. "period" versus "half")

Cognitive Assessment:
Select any 5 words (an example is given). Avoid choosing related words such as "dark" and "moon" which can be recalled by means of word association. Read each word at a rate of one word per second. The athlete should not be informed of the delayed testing of memory (to be done after the reverse months and/or digits). Choose a different set of words each time you perform a follow-up exam with the same candidate.
Ask the athlete to recite the months of the year in reverse order, starting with a random month. Do not start with December or January. Circle any months not recited in the correct sequence.
For digits backwards, if correct, go to the next string length. If incorrect, read trial 2. Stop after incorrect on both trials.

Neurologic Screening:
Trained medical personnel must administer this examination. These individuals might include medical doctors, physiotherapists or athletic therapists. Speech should be assessed for fluency and lack of slurring. Eye motion should reveal no diplopia in any of the 4 planes of movement (vertical, horizontal and both diagonal planes). The pronator drift is performed by asking the patient to hold both arms in front of them, palms up, with eyes closed. A positive test is pronating the forearm, dropping the arm, or drift away from midline. For gait assessment, ask the patient to walk away from you, turn and walk back.

Return to Play:
A structured, graded exertion protocol should be developed; individualized on the basis of sport, age and the concussion history of the athlete. Exercise or training should be commenced only after the athlete is clearly asymptomatic with physical and cognitive rest. Final decision for clearance to return to competition should ideally be made by a medical doctor.

For more information see the "Summary and Agreement Statement of the Second International Symposium on Concussion in Sport" in the April, 2005 Clinical Journal of Sport Medicine (vol 15), British Journal of Sports Medicine (vol 39), Neurosurgery (vol 59) and the Physician and Sportsmedicine (vol 33). ©2005 Concussion in Sport Group

Figure 5 Sport Concussion Assessment Tool (SCAT) athlete information form. *(Reproduced with permission from McCrory P, Johnston K, Meeuwisse W, et al: Summary and agreement statement of the 2nd International Conference on Concussion in Sport, Prague, 2004. Br J Sports Med 2005;38:196-204.)*

age, family history of heart disease, exertional dyspnea or chest pain, unexplained syncope, excessive fatiguability, history of heart murmur, and systemic hypertension.[19] Routine electrocardiograms (ECGs) and echocardiograms (both three-dimensional and limited two-dimensional) have not generally been used because of expense and the potential for false positive results.[20] However, ECGs have recently been recommended as practical and cost-effective strategic alternatives to routine echocardiograms for population-based PPE screening.[21]

Physical examination should include measurement of blood pressure in both arms, precordial auscultation (supine or sitting, and standing) assessment of peripheral (femoral) pulses, and examination for stigmata of Marfan syndrome.

The most common risk factors for sudden cardiac death (SCD) in athletes in general include hypertrophic cardiomyopathy, congenital coronary artery anomalies, and Marfan syndrome. Only some of these will be evident with common screening procedures, including a medical history questionnaire. Hypertrophic cardiomyopathy is an autosomal dominant condition; 60% of affected individuals have an affected first-degree relative. The ventricular septal wall is symmetrically thickened, producing a systolic murmur that decreases in supine position, and increases with standing or during the Valsalva maneuver. Up to 95% of cases can be detected on a standard ECG. It is important, however, to distinguish hypertrophic cardiomyopathy from "athlete's heart," which is a spectrum of abnormal but benign ECG changes reflecting physiologic variations that may occur in up to 40% of healthy, highly trained athletes (Table 2). For example, athletes who engage in endurance or isometric sports may develop an increase in cardiac mass and chamber size, but this increase may regress with cessation of intensive training.

Marfan syndrome, an inherited disorder of connective tissue, is also autosomal dominant, but up to 25% of cases can result from sporadic de novo gene mutation.[22] It is not uncommon in taller athletes, such as volleyball and basketball players. SCD can occur from aortic root aneurysm and dissection and rupture caused by cystic medial necrosis. Common physical findings include tall stature, arachnodactyly (long, thin spidery fingers), narrow, high-arched palate, increased joint laxity, kyphoscoliosis, anterior chest deformity (pectus excavatum [funnel chest] or pectus carinatum [pigeon breast]), arm span greater than height, murmur of mitral or aortic regurgitation or midsystolic click of mitral valve prolapse. An ophthalmologic slit lamp examination may reveal ectopic lens and myopia. Some sources recommend that all male athletes taller than 6 feet and all female athletes taller than 5 feet 10 inches be screened with an ECG, echocardiogram, and slit lamp examination. Therapy includes beta-blockers to delay or prevent aortic aneurysm and dissection, and restriction of activities such as contact or physically competitive sports and heavy isometric exercise or lifting. In some instances, aortic surgical intervention will be necessary. These athletes are best managed with a mul-

Table 2

Electrocardiographic Changes in "Athlete's Heart"

Sinus bradycardia
Sinus pauses
Sinus arrhythmia
Atrial or ventricular premature beats
  Atrioventricular (AV) blocks
  First degree block
  Second degree block, type 1 (Wenckebach)
  Advanced AV block
Voltage criteria of right/left ventricular hypertrophy
ST elevations
T wave changes

tidisciplinary team. The National Marfan Foundation (http://www.marfan.org) is a resource for patients, family members, and health care professionals.

Commotio Cordis

Commotio cordis is a unique cause of ventricular arrhythmias (primarily ventricular fibrillation), initiated by a sudden blow to the anterior chest during a vulnerable time in the cardiac cycle.[23] If witnessed, either defibrillation with an AED or immediate administration of a "precordial thump" may help to start the heart again. This condition has been documented mainly in youth baseball, but also in hockey, lacrosse, cricket, soccer, and other sport and nonsport situations. Safety measures include the use of chest protector plates and softer baseballs.

There are many other cardiovascular conditions that affect athletic participation or cause SCD that can be screened for effectively.[20] For example, in Wolff-Parkinson-White syndrome, the presence of an aberrant accessory bypass tract can cause reentry type of arrhythmias. The diagnosis can be made on ECG, with a characteristic delta wave preceding the QRS complex. Congenital long QT syndrome is a group of disorders of cardiac repolarization characterized by prolongation of the QT interval, leading to syncope and SCD as a result of ventricular tachyarrhythmias. Another condition, arrhythmogenic right ventricular dysplasia, is seen primarily in certain populations in Italy. This is also a hereditary condition, and screening programs there have been very effective. The most recent recommendations for participation in sports by athletes with various cardiovascular conditions can be found in the *36th Bethesda Guidelines*, a publication of the American College of Cardiology.[24]

Asthma, Exercise-Induced Asthma, and Exercise-Induced Bronchospasm

The prevalence of asthma in elite athletes is believed to vary from 3.7% to 22.8% in summer sports, and from 14.1% to 54.8% in winter sports. Mechanisms include prolonged airway dehydration or hypertonicity of air-

1: Principles of Orthopaedics

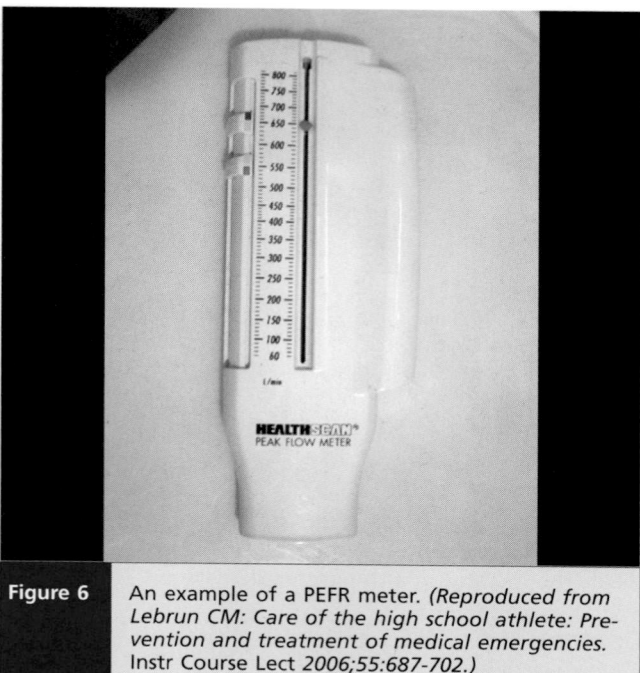

Figure 6 An example of a PEFR meter. *(Reproduced from Lebrun CM: Care of the high school athlete: Prevention and treatment of medical emergencies. Instr Course Lect 2006;55:687-702.)*

way fluid.[25] High-minute ventilation during exercise (often up to 200 L/min for short periods in speed and power athletes, and for longer periods in endurance athletes such as cross-country skiers) dries and cools the airway. The subsequent water loss triggers mast cell release and smooth muscle constriction. Type, intensity, and duration of exercise as well as external environment influence both onset and severity of exercise-induced asthma (EIA), and exercise-induced bronchospasm (EIB). The former term refers to patients with chronic asthma who experience more symptoms with exercise, whereas EIB occurs only during exercise.

Newer treatment concepts include the model of airway inflammation, in which some form of repeated thermal, mechanical, or osmotic airway trauma results in a healing or remodeling process. Inhaled irritants, pollen allergens, and cold exposure may all precipitate EIA/EIB. Swimmers may microaspirate water in the trachea and bronchi. Both chlorine gas and hypochlorite liquid are irritants. In ice arenas, pollutants such as gas and particulate exhausts from ice resurfacing machines are the culprits. For these reasons, electric machines are preferable to combustion engines.

Some individuals have underlying atopy, with immunoglobulin E-mediated allergy. These athletes typically have seasonal variation in their condition, as well as symptoms such as allergic rhinitis (hay fever), general skin itching, watery eyes, hives, and anaphylaxis. True asthmatics may have bronchospasm at other times, but always experience falls in peak expiratory flow rate (PEFR) with exercise. In patients with demonstrated sensitivity to acetylsalicylic acid, the use of other non-steroidal anti-inflammatory drugs and over-the-counter products containing acetylsalicylic acid can also worsen symptoms.

The diagnosis of asthma and EIA/EIB can be made with baseline pulmonary function tests, PEFR, and measurements of forced expiratory volume in 1 second. Screening on the PPE can be done through an addition to the medical questionnaire and/or spirometry and simple on-field exercise challenge tests.[26] Sometimes an empirical trial of therapy with inhaled bronchodilators is warranted. In such cases, a 10% to 15% increase in PEFR is good evidence of efficacy.

Both behavioral and pharmacologic measures are helpful in managing EIA and EIB.[27] A physical warmup with either continuous low-intensity exercise or a short burst of 80% to 90% of a maximum workload 15 to 20 minutes before practice or competition can induce a refractory period of up to several hours. Nasal breathing and the use of breathing filters or face masks will warm the inspired air and decrease bronchoconstriction. Viral infections increase the risk of asthma attacks, and therefore athletes with asthma or EIA/EIB should not engage in endurance sports if they have a viral respiratory infection. Athletes, trainers, and physicians on the sidelines should use a simple PEFR meter to monitor symptoms and response to treatment (Figure 6).

The mainstay of treatment of asthma and EIA/EIB is inhaled beta 2-adrenoceptor agonists, such as salbutamol. The International Olympic Committee mandates documentation of reduced forced expiratory volume in 1 second on testing in an approved laboratory using certain tests: the exercise challenge test, methacholine challenge, thermal challenge, hypertonic saline, or eucapnic voluntary hyperpnea or hyperventilation (in which the athlete voluntarily hyperventilates on dry air containing 4.9% carbon dioxide). A specific threshold on one of these tests is necessary before permission to use inhaled beta-agonists is granted. The International Association of Athletic Federations (IAAF) has decided to follow these instructions in all IAAF-sanctioned competitions through an Olympic quadrennium. For competitions at a lower level, the World Anti-Doping Agency only requires notification by the treating or prescribing physician before issuing an abbreviated therapeutic use exemption. These measures were instituted because of theoretic ergogenic effects on skeletal muscle anabolism and anaerobic and aerobic performance. This potential competitive advantage in athletes using these inhaled medications has never been scientifically documented.

Salbutamol is used 20 to 30 minutes before exercise and at intervals as needed, whereas longer-acting salmeterol can be inhaled 1 hour before exercise but should not be used for rescue situations. Other long-acting beta 2 agonists such as formoterol offer a protective effect that lasts 4 hours, which is better for endurance athletes. Inhaled corticosteroids seem to be less beneficial for EIB, but oral leukotriene antagonists (montelukast and zafirlukast) have an immediate protective effect. Montelukast reduces eosinophilic inflammation, whereas others (pranleukast, zileuton) prevent mast cell degranulation. Nedocromil or cromolyn sodium can be administered by inhalation to stabilize mast cells.

Omega-e polyunsaturated fatty acids, such as eicos-apentaenoic acid and docosahexaenoic acid in fish oils, compete with arachidonic acid as substrates for formation of inflammatory mediators, such as the leukotrienes and prostaglandins. These anti-inflammatory effects have been shown to be helpful for athletes with EIB.[28] Other measures include treatment of seasonal allergic rhinitis with nonsedating antihistamines or prophylactic intranasal corticosteroids, or the use of histamine blockers to prevent contributing gastroesophageal acid reflux disease. Immunotherapy for specific antigens can also be helpful.

More acute, severe attacks may require either oral or intravenous corticosteroids (60 to 80 mg per day for 5 to 7 days with tapering or intravenous methylprednisolone 0.5 to 2 mg/kg every 6 hours). Treatment of emergent episodes on the sidelines may include subcutaneous epinephrine (up to 0.3 mL of 1:1000 solution). Use of a spacer (Figure 7) with an albuterol (salbutamol) metered-dose inhaler (4 to 8 puffs every 20 to 30 minutes for up to 3 doses) has been shown to be as effective as a nebulizer in delivering the medication to the lower airways. Supplemental oxygen may also be necessary.[29]

The differential diagnosis has to include vocal cord dysfunction. This condition is more common in female athletes[30] and is characterized by inspiratory stridor during exercise that resolves spontaneously after activity cessation. It is frequently audible with auscultation over the laryngeal area instead of over the lung fields. Stress can precipitate vocal cord dysfunction, and management includes speech therapy, breathing exercises, and behavioral modification. Definitive diagnosis can only be made by direct laryngoscopy during exercise, and visualization of the abnormal adduction of the anterior two thirds of the vocal cords. Other conditions that can mimic asthma and EIB are central airway obstruction, cardiac disease, and other restrictive or obstructive pulmonary diseases.

Anaphylaxis

Anaphylaxis or acute allergic reactions can be idiopathic, triggered by an allergen (most commonly food, medication, or an insect sting), or may actually be induced by exercise. Latex allergy is becoming increasingly more common.[31] Bronchospasm, laryngospasm, urticaria, hives, and/or vascular collapse can occur in rapid succession; immediate treatment with intravenous access, fluids, and epinephrine is critical.[32] Epinephrine can be administered subcutaneously or intramuscularly (0.3 to 0.5 mL of 1:1000 solution) or intravenously (0.3 to 0.5 mL 1;10,000 solution); diphenhydramine (25 to 50 mg) should be given concurrently either intramuscularly or intravenously, followed by immediate transport to a hospital facility.

Hypertension

Athletes can be affected by hypertension.[33] The incidence of hypertension is increased in African Americans, the elderly, the obese, and those with diabetes, re-

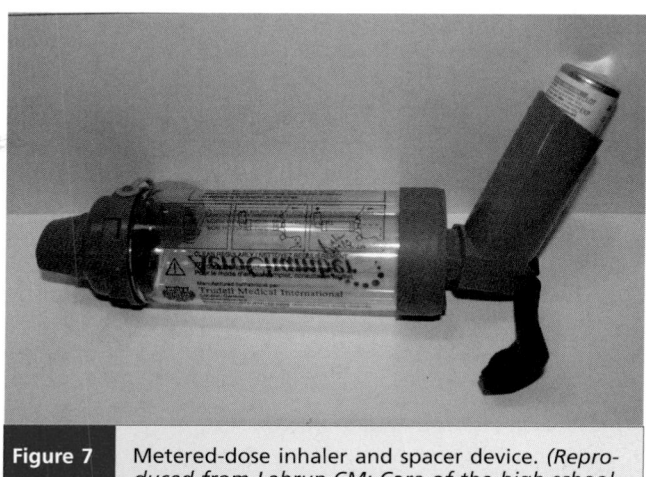

Figure 7 Metered-dose inhaler and spacer device. *(Reproduced from Lebrun CM: Care of the high school athlete: Prevention and treatment of medical emergencies. Instr Course Lect 2006;55:687-702.)*

nal disease, or a family history of hypertension. Wheelchair athletes with spinal cord injuries may also develop hypertension because of the loss of autonomic control of blood pressure. In terms of screening for hypertension on the PPE, it is important to use a larger cuff size (thigh cuff) for bigger athletes to avoid falsely elevated readings that can be generated with the smaller cuff. Hypertension can be primary (where a single reversible cause of hypertension cannot be found, which occurs in 95% of patients) or secondary (for example, resulting from the additional estrogen in oral contraceptives; approximately 5% of all women who take oral contraceptive pills develop hypertension over a 5-year period). Other risk factors include high sodium intake, excessive alcohol (binge drinking), illicit drug use (cocaine), stimulants taken before competition, tobacco, anabolic steroids, and, in certain people, the use of nonsteroidal anti-inflammatory drugs. Many over-the-counter herbs and dietary supplements contain naturally-occurring stimulants such as ma huang or ephedra.

Nonpharmacologic measures such as dietary therapy, weight loss, lifestyle changes, stress reduction, and regular aerobic exercise will decrease blood pressure. There are many pharmacologic treatments, each with their own risk-benefit ratio. Low-dose therapy with angiotensin-converting enzyme inhibitors may cause a nonproductive cough as an adverse effect. There are anecdotal reports of postural hypotension after intense exercise; therefore, an adequate cool-down period is recommended. Alpha-blockers have no major effects on energy metabolism during exercise and no effects on diabetes, but adverse effects may include mild to moderate drowsiness, dry mouth, and impotence. Calcium-channel blockers (such as verapamil) are generally good choices for the hypertensive athlete. Thiazide diuretics may not be appropriate for the endurance athlete, and will create problems for doping control. The use of oral beta-blockers in athletes is also banned, and these substances will frequently cause fatigue. It is critical to be aware of such effects of medication on exercise tolerance.

Diabetes Mellitus

Athletes may have either type 1 (insulin-dependent) or type 2 (non–insulin-dependent) diabetes mellitus. Both conditions require specific strategies for adequate control, planning for optimal training and competition, and prevention of complications.[34,35] Type 2 diabetes is more common in older, obese patients, but the disease is being diagnosed in an increasing number of adolescents. Approximately 20% of patients with type 2 diabetes will eventually develop impaired insulin secretion and will require exogenous insulin in addition to the other treatments of dietary restriction, weight loss, exercise, and administration of oral hypoglycemic agents. Athletes with type 1 diabetes usually manage their disease through regular monitoring by glucometer and a once or twice daily regimen of injected insulin. Some

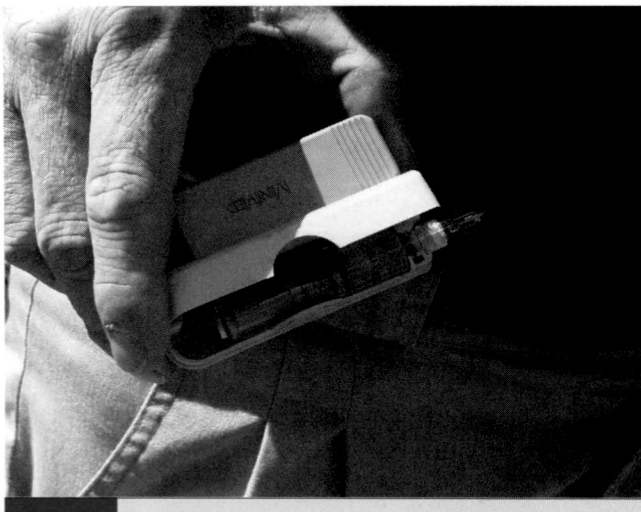

Figure 8 Insulin pump. *(Reproduced from Lebrun CM: Care of the high school athlete: Prevention and treatment of medical emergencies.* Instr Course Lect *2006;55:687-702.)*

will use an insulin pump (also known as continuous subcutaneous insulin infusion), which delivers a constant amount of insulin through a subcutaneous catheter, and has the ability to add in a bolus as needed (Figure 8). Newer therapies include insulin glargine (a longer-acting, once-daily insulin) and inhaled insulin.[36,37] Different types of insulin have variable onset of action and peak levels and are frequently given as combined therapy (Table 3).

Complications of exercise in the diabetic athlete include hypoglycemia secondary to insufficient glucose stores and/or excessive insulin dose, and hyperglycemia, in which insulin levels are insufficient. Emergency treatment of hypoglycemia is immediate administration of glucose, orally or intravenously (50 mL of 50% solution), or glucagon (1 mg intramuscularly or subcutaneously) to release hepatic stores of glucose. Diabetic ketoacidosis occurs when circulating insulin levels are too low, and blood glucoses rise to dangerous levels (> 250 mg/dL), leading to ketosis, hyperosmolar coma, and possibly death. Rapid transportation to an emergency facility is of paramount importance.

In general, athletes with diabetes, particularly those at significant risk of hypoglycemia or hyperglycemia, should not engage in sports in which they are a risk to themselves or others should they become incapacitated (for example, rock climbing or scuba diving). Good metabolic control is desirable, with blood glucose levels slightly elevated before exercise (> 100 mg/dL), and provision of a source of glucose for prolonged exercise. The athlete must take into account other factors such as travel, timing of training or competition, and concomitant illnesses such as upper respiratory infections. Keeping a food/training/insulin diary is essential, as is regular monitoring of blood glucose levels with a glucometer before, during, and after exercise. Postexercise hypoglycemia can occur in the patient with type 1 diabetes 6 to 24 hours after exercise. This late-onset hypoglycemia can therefore occur during the night, and the subsequent reactive hyperglycemia sometimes complicates interpretation of the morning blood glucose levels. Athletes who have had diabetes for some time as well as their physicians need to be cognizant of other

Table 3			
Insulin Profiles			
Type*	Onset of Action	Peak	Duration
Actrapid (human soluble insulin, Humalog (insulin lispro injection)	Rapid	45 min	Gone in 2 hours
Regular insulin	30 min	90 min	Gone in 6 to 8 hours
Lente, NPH insulin	5 to 6 hours	8 hours	Gone in 12 to 18 hours
Ultralente insulin	4 hours	10 hours	Gone in 12 to 20 hours
Lantus (glargine) and Levemir (detemir)	2 hours	No peak	Gone in 12 to 24 hours

*Actrapid and Levemir, Novo Norkisk, Denmark; Humalog, Eli Lilly and Company, Indianapolis, IN; Lantus, Sanofi Aventis, Paris, France.
NPH = neutral protamine Hagedorn insulin.

complications such as peripheral neuropathy, cardiovascular disease, autonomic neuropathy, nephropathy, and retinopathy.

Heat Illness/Dehydration

Heat illness and/or dehydration are conditions that occur during certain sports and athletic populations.[38,39] As little as 2% body weight loss or a 1% drop in total body water and intravascular volume can affect performance and hinder thermoregulatory function. There are both intrinsic and extrinsic risk factors for exertional heat illness. The wet globe bulb temperature (WGBT) is a measure that takes into account radiation, humidity, and convection to give a more accurate assessment of heat stress (**Figure** 9), and recommendations exist for assessment of risk at athletic events (**Table** 4). In the absence of a WGBT thermometer, heat stress risk temperature and humidity graphs can be used to predict dangerous temperatures; however, these may not be practical, especially in the southern United States, where both values are routinely elevated. It is necessary to educate athletes, coaches, athletic trainers, and other health professionals about hydration needs, acclimatization, work/rest ratio, signs and symptoms of heat illness, and treatment. In addition to frequent use of dietary supplements, other nutritional issues and fitness status also play a part.

Thirst is generally a late sign, but dry mouth, irritability, general discomfort, headache, apathy, weakness, dizziness, cramps, chills, vomiting, nausea, heat (particularly neck heat) sensations, excessive fatigue, and/or decreased performance may signal heat illness.

Treatment includes moving the athlete to a cool place, and rehydration with fluids such as a sports drink containing carbohydrate and electrolytes (sodium, potassium).

Exertional heat stroke involves significant central nervous system abnormalities such as altered consciousness, coma, convulsions, disorientation, irrational behavior, decreased mental acuity, irritability, confusion, and combativeness. The skin may be hot and wet or hot and dry. Other physical findings are increased heart rate, decreased blood pressure, and increased respiratory rate. Hemodynamic collapse leads to lower cardiac output and decreased blood flow to the skin, vital organs, and kidneys. The elevated body temperature has the potential to cause permanent tissue damage. Core temperature (usually 104°F [40°C] in these patients) should be measured by rectal thermometer as oral, axillary, and tympanic temperatures are

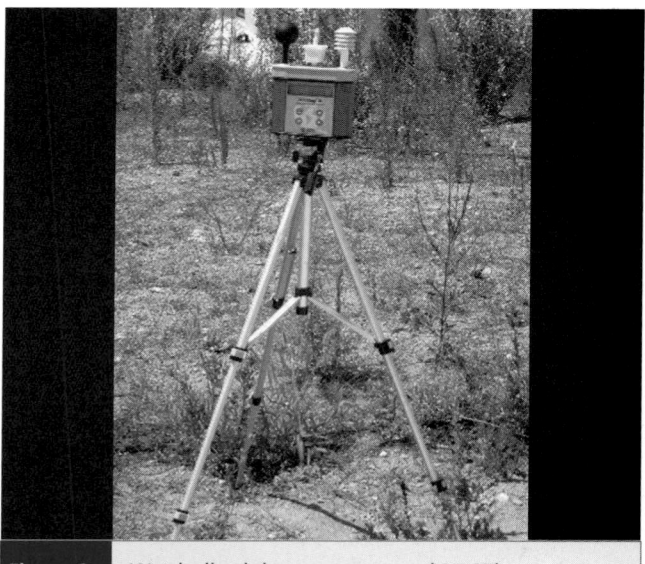

| Figure 9 | Wet bulb globe temperature (WBGT) thermometer. |

Table 4

Guidelines for Assessment of Heat Risk for Athletic Competitions

WBGT	Flag Color	Level of Risk	Comments
< 65°F (< 18°C)	Green	Low	Risk low but still exists on the basis of risk factors
65° to 73°F (18° to 23°C)	Yellow	Moderate	Risk level increases as event progresses through the day
73° to 82°F (23° to 28°C)	Red	High	Everyone should be aware of injury potential Individuals at risk should not compete
> 82°F (> 28°C)	Black	Extreme or hazardous	Consider rescheduling or delaying the event until safer conditions prevail If the event must take place, be on high alert Take steps to reduce risk factors (for example, more and longer rest breaks, reduced practice time, reduced exercise intensity, access to shade, minimal clothing and equipment, cold tubs at practice site)

WBGT = wet bulb globe temperature
The WBGT can be measured with a WBGT meter. The calculation for the determination of WBGT is WBGT = 0.7 (wet bulb temperature) + 0.2 (black globe temperature) + 0.1 (dry bulb temperature).

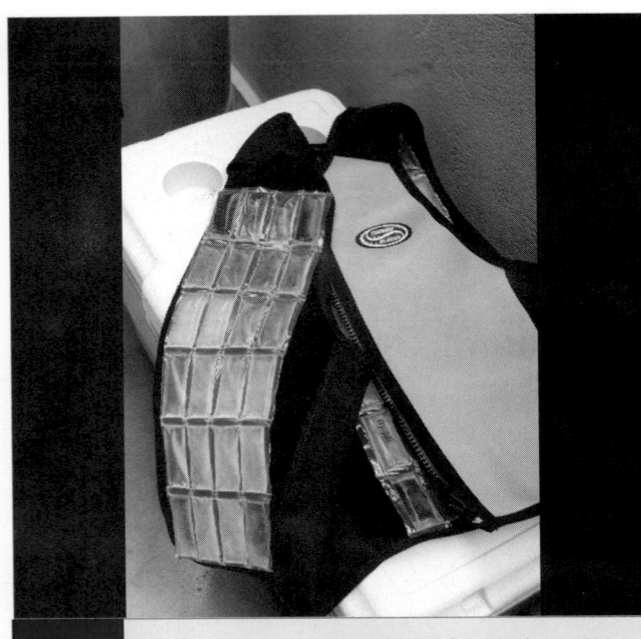

Figure 10 A cooling vest. *(Reproduced from Lebrun CM: Care of the high school athlete: Prevention and treatment of medical emergencies. Instr Course Lect 2006;55:687-702.)*

not accurate in this setting. Aggressive immediate whole-body cooling is warranted, through cold water immersion, spraying the body with cold water, using fans, and placing ice bags over areas of the large vessels in the groin, axilla, and neck. Cooling should cease when the core temperature reaches 101° to 102°F (38.3° to 38.9°C). It is essential to monitor vital signs, start an intravenous line with normal saline, and arrange for rapid transport to a nearby hospital.

Heat exhaustion is characterized by the lack of central nervous system changes and a lower core body temperature. Nevertheless, the athlete is often unable to continue sports participation, and may experience syncope, ataxia, incoordination, and profuse sweating. These symptoms may respond rapidly to postural positioning and to having the legs propped up.

Heat cramps (muscle cramps and/or intense pain) may or may not be heat-related. Common causes are believed to be dehydration, a diet poor in minerals, and large losses of sodium and other electrolytes in sweat. Some individuals are "salty sweaters," and may benefit from estimation of sweat loss during exercise to determine adequate replacement.

Prevention of heat illness can be accomplished with proper hydration and gradual acclimation to heat stress during exercise. Liberal use of sports drinks and calculation of body weight losses secondary to dehydration will also help. More recently, cooling vests (**Figure 10**) and cooling before exercise have been used to lower the core body temperature either during exercise or between episodes of repeated exercise in the heat. Return to play after heat illness or exertional heat stroke depends on the severity of the episode. General guide-

lines are to avoid strenuous exercise for a minimum of 1 week, followed by a gradual return to the previous level of physical activity.

Hyponatremia, Fluid and Electrolyte Requirements

If an athlete consumes more fluids (especially water) than necessary and/or the sodium losses in sweat are not adequately replaced, hyponatremia (serum sodium < 130 mmol/L) may occur. Some cases are iatrogenic, with too-rapid rehydration of a collapsed athlete with improper intravenous fluids. Symptoms frequently seen with this condition are headache, nausea, vomiting, swelling of the hands/feet, and cerebral and/or pulmonary edema. If unrecognized and untreated, coma and death can result. Specific guidelines exist for prevention and management.[40]

Infectious Diseases (Viral/Bacterial Infections)

Infectious diseases of the upper and lower respiratory system, as well as the gastrointestinal tract, can sideline athletes and even entire teams. Examples include upper respiratory infections, pharyngitis, sinusitis, otitis media/externa, conjunctivitis, meningitis, and gastroenteritis.[41] Proper hygienic practices will minimize transmission of disease. With upper respiratory infections, which are frequently viral in nature, a simple "neck check" can help to guide management. Symptoms such as stuffy nose and sore throat do not necessarily preclude athletic participation, but fever and generalized myalgias are usually good indications for rest.[42] Of particular concern is the possibility of myocarditis, an acute inflammatory condition of myocardium secondary to viral, bacterial, or fungal infection.[43] Coxsackie B virus accounts for more than 50% of cases. Symptoms and signs include dyspnea, orthopnea, cough, exercise intolerance, and findings of congestive heart failure. Diagnosis is made by myocardial biopsy, and return to training and competition may take 6 months or longer.

Transmission of blood-borne pathogens such as human immunodeficiency virus and hepatitis B and C are theoretic risks in sporting activities, but are more likely to occur as a result of unprotected sexual activities or intravenous drug abuse. Universal precautions and the removal of blood from skin and other surfaces such as clothing will help with prevention of these diseases. Immunization against hepatitis B and C is available as single or combined vaccines. It is also a good practice to implement annual influenza vaccinations for college-age athletes.

Infectious Mononucleosis

Infectious mononucleosis is a common medical occurrence, particularly in high school and college-age athletes. In addition to sore throat and swollen glands, which may sometimes compromise nutrition and fluid replacement, general malaise and fatigue take their toll. The biggest risk, however, is rupture of the enlarged, congested spleen. Although spontaneous ruptures have

1: Principles of Orthopaedics

been reported, this usually occurs in the setting of contact sports; therefore, participation must be restricted during the time of highest risk (the first 3 weeks), and gradual return to sport activities can commence when symptoms resolve and laboratory values return to normal (**Figure 11**). Because clinical examination can be unreliable, serial ultrasound measurements of spleen size are recommended.[44]

Dermatologic Conditions/Infections

Skin infections, whether viral (herpes simplex or herpes gladiatorum), fungal (jock itch), or bacterial (impetigo, folliculitis) are common in athletes.[45] Recently, methicillin-resistant *Staphylococcus aureus* (MRSA) has been reported in the locker room.[46] Whereas MRSA was previously found primarily in hospitals, particularly intensive care units and surgical units, there has now been an alarming increase in community-acquired soft-tissue infections in young, immunocompetent hosts such as football players. The preventive role of actions such as frequent hand washing, cleaning of equipment and surfaces, and not sharing water bottles is currently a topic of debate. MRSA causes a range of disease including boils (furuncles), folliculitis, impetigo, cellulitis, necrotizing fasciitis, endocarditis, pneumonia, empyema, septic arthritis or bursitis, and osteomyelitis. Bacteremia, septic shock, toxic shock-like symptoms, and other systemic complications have been reported. Current therapy, besides general hygienic measures, dictates the covering of draining wounds, and avoidance of contact sports, whirlpools, and saunas if a potential participant has an open lesion. Suitable antibiotic therapies include penicillinase-resistant penicillin (oral dicloxacillin, or intravenous oxacillin or nafcillin), first-generation cephalosporins (cephalexin), trimethoprim-sulfamethoxazole, doxycycline, or clindamycin. Vancomycin is discouraged for empirical treatment of furuncles and nonsevere skin and soft-tissue infections and should be reserved for more serious cases or for patients with health care-associated risk factors.[47]

Medical Care of the Female Athlete

The female athlete has some unique orthopaedic and medical issues. Most injuries are sport- rather than gender-specific, with a few notable exceptions. Women seem to be more prone to patellofemoral pain, possibly certain shoulder pathologies (because of lesser upper body strength), and anterior cruciate ligament injuries. Medical concerns revolve around the female athlete triad, an interrelationship between three entities—disordered eating, amenorrhea or other menstrual dysfunction, and altered bone mineral density (BMD). A small proportion of susceptible individuals may develop one or more of these conditions, and estimates of their incidence varies with the population under study.[48-50]

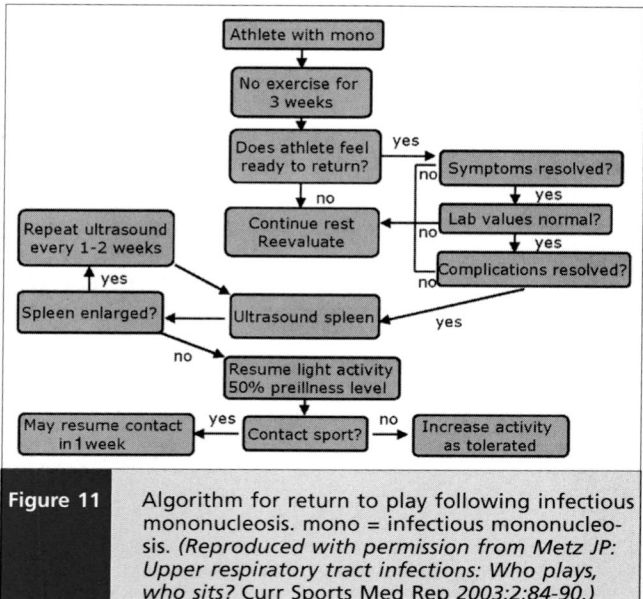

Figure 11 Algorithm for return to play following infectious mononucleosis. mono = infectious mononucleosis. (Reproduced with permission from Metz JP: Upper respiratory tract infections: Who plays, who sits? Curr Sports Med Rep 2003;2:84-90.)

Disordered Eating and Inadequate Energy Intake

Disordered eating encompasses the true eating disorders of anorexia nervosa, bulimia nervosa, and eating disorders not otherwise specified as defined in the *Diagnostic and Statistical Manual DSM IV* of the American Psychiatric Association,[51] and also includes disordered eating whether intentional or inadvertent. Some researchers have coined the term "anorexia athletica" to describe the specifics of this disorder in athletes, reflecting a slightly different psychological makeup.[52] Criteria include weight loss, gastrointestinal complaints, absence of a medical or affective disorder explaining the weight loss, excessive fear of becoming obese, and restriction of caloric intake. The athlete must also exhibit either delayed puberty, menstrual dysfunction, disturbance in body image, use of purging methods, binge eating, or compulsive exercising.

Energy intake is basically inadequate for the needs of basal body metabolism plus the additional demands of physical activity, giving rise to the concept of "energy drain."[53] This condition is even believed to be dose-specific.[54] Alteration of the pulsatile secretion of reproductive hormones (luteinizing hormone and follicle-stimulating hormone) from the hypothalamus and pituitary glands leads to menstrual dysfunction, with a subsequent relative deficiency in estrogen and/or progesterone. The lack of these important hormones creates an environment similar to the postmenopausal state, with altered BMD that may be at least partially irreversible, even with resumption of normal menstrual cycles. Therefore, efforts should be mainly focused on prevention of the triad disorders. Organizations such as the American College of Sports Medicine (ACSM) and the International Olympic Committee have published position statements.[55,56] The ACSM document has recently been rewritten and updated according to evidence-based standards.

Menstrual Dysfunction/Altered Bone Mineral Density

Menstrual dysfunction exists along a spectrum, and can vary even month to month in the same individual. It is not uncommon for female athletes to stop having menstrual cycles during times of intense training or the competitive season, and to resume them in the off-season. Amenorrhea or lack of menstrual cycles can be primary or secondary. Recently, because of the earlier age of menarche in North American women, the Practice Committee of the American Society of Reproductive Medicine has revised the definition of primary amenorrhea to having not started menstruation by 15 years of age.[57] Secondary amenorrhea can result from a variety of medical causes that must be excluded before terming it hypothalamic amenorrhea[58] (Table 5). Athletes may also develop oligomenorrhea (menstrual cycles occurring at intervals of more than 3 months), anovulatory cycles (in which regular menstrual bleeding takes place in the absence of ovulation), and shortened luteal phase (less than 10 days).[59] All have implications for the athlete's health, including infertility, altered BMD, and potentially an increased risk of cardiovascular disease because of the loss of the protective effect of estrogen.[60] However, it is the energy imbalance, not the exercise itself, that is the culprit. Frequently only a slight improvement in caloric intake or increase in weight or a decrease in training will be sufficient to restore normal menstrual function.

Although most clinicians are familiar with the World Health Organization classification of osteoporosis and osteopenia, researchers have questioned the use of these terms in describing the female athlete triad.[61] Most recently, the International Society for Clinical Densitometry issued a statement that these categories are not appropriate for premenopausal women, children, or men.[62] Instead, the term "low BMD for chronological age" is more appropriate. Especially because weight-bearing exercise should be protective for BMD, it is important to be aware of the potential for low BMD in women with menstrual dysfunction. A minimal screening procedure on the PPE includes asking about a history of recurrent stress fractures, menstrual dysfunction, and/or poor nutritional practices.

Treatment of any aspect of the female athlete triad frequently requires a multidisciplinary approach, including a primary care physician, the coach, and the athlete and her family.[63] Particularly if frank eating disorders are present, it is critical to involve a psychiatrist or clinical psychologist for immediate and ongoing care. Sometimes, education about nutrition[64] and promotion of healthy weight-control practices are sufficient.[65]

Formal measurement of BMD will depend on the clinical scenario. If regular ovulation and normal menstrual function cannot be restored with a reasonable trial (3 to 6 months) of nonpharmacologic means, then hormonal replacement therapy is indicated. For most young women, this may be in the form of combination oral contraceptives containing some form of synthetic estrogen and progestin.[66] There is some debate as to whether these medications can actually be "osteoprotective."[67] The injectable contraceptive medroxyprogesterone acetate works by inhibiting ovulation, and as a result may be detrimental for BMD. Female athletes using this method should be regularly monitored. Optimal BMD is reached in the first few decades of life by ensuring adequate estrogen levels, sufficient caloric and nutritional intake (especially calcium and vitamin D), and regular weight-bearing exercise. Thus, the female athlete will not be at a disadvantage when entering the postmenopausal years, where loss of BMD occurs much more rapidly. Men can also develop low BMD. If a male athlete presents with a stress fracture consideration should be given to assessment of BMD and other endocrinologic functions.

Pregnancy

There are several important considerations for the pregnant athlete. As scientific data accumulate on the benefits of exercise throughout pregnancy and during the postpartum period, more guidelines are available for the practicing physician. The Canadian Society for Exercise Physiology has developed the Physical Activity Readiness Medical Questionnaire (PARmed-X) for Pregnancy. This simple four-page pamphlet contains screening questions for the physician and the pregnant athlete (preexercise health checklist), relative and absolute contraindications for exercise during pregnancy (Table 6), and information on physical training and safety considerations, including possible complications.[68] Other studies and guidelines summarize the evidence regarding exercising throughout pregnancy and the postpartum period and give suggestions for exercise prescription.[69-71]

Anabolic Steroids

Performance-enhancing or ergogenic aids have been used as long as there has been human competition. These substances can be broadly classified into five categories: physiologic, physical, psychologic, nutritional, and chemical (or pharmacologic), with the latter being the most frequently abused.[72] After World War II, the use of drugs such as amphetamines was routine to improve endurance, and steroids were the muscle builder of choice. In 1994, the Dietary Supplement and Health Act made supplements available over the counter, meaning that they did not have to pass the efficacy and safety requirements of the Food and Drug Administration. These supplements included the naturally occurring (produced in the adrenals and gonads) testosterone precursors dehydroepiandrosterone (DHEAS) and androstenedione. Although banned by the National Football League, the National Collegiate Athletics Association and the International Olympic Committee,

Table 5

Possible Causes of Secondary Amenorrhea

Pregnancy
Hypothalamic defect
  Absence of GnRH
  Constitutional delay
  Psychological or physical stress
  Anorexia nervosa
  Idiopathic
  Kallmann's syndrome (olefactogenital dysplasia)
Pituitary defect
  Inability to make gonadotropins
  Tumors (prolactinomas)
  Granulomatous disease
  Sheehan's syndrome
Ovarian defect
  Turner's syndrome (45, X)
  Gonadal dysgenesis (46, XY)
  Polycystic ovary syndrome
  Autoimmune disease
  Idiopathic premature ovarian failure
Uterine defect
  Isolated absence of uterus
  Male pseudohermaphrodism syndromes (46, XY)
  Asherman's syndrome
  Granulomatous disease

GnRH = gonadotropin-releasing hormone.
(Reproduced with permission from Fagan KM: Pharmacologic management of athletic amenorrhea. Clin Sports Med 1998;17:327-341.)

Table 6

Contraindications to Exercise During Pregnancy

Absolute Contraindications

Ruptured membranes, premature labor

Persistent second or third trimester bleeding/placenta previa

Pregnancy-induced hypertension or preeclampsia

Incompetent cervix

Evidence of intrauterine growth restriction

High order pregnancy (for example, triplets)

Uncontrolled type 1 diabetes; hypertension or thyroid disease; other serious cardiovascular, respiratory, or systemic disorder

Relative Contraindications

History of spontaneous abortion or premature labor in previous pregnancies

Mild/moderate cardiovascular or respiratory disease (eg, chronic hypertension, asthma)

Anemia or iron deficiency (hemoglobin < 100 g/L)

Very low body fat, eating disorder (anorexia, bulimia)

Twin pregnancy after 28th week

Other significant medical condition

(Reproduced with permission from Physical Activity Readiness Medical Examination for Pregnancy. *Ottawa, Ontario, Canada, Canadian Society for Exercise Physiology, 2002, pp 1-4.)*

androstenedione is often used in combination with human growth hormone to enhance sports performance. The Food and Drug Administration has recently issued an edict to discontinue manufacture, marketing, and distribution of androstenedione-containing products to companies producing these dietary supplements.

More commonly abused are the higher profile androgenic anabolic steroids, variously known as roids, juice, hype, or pump. As a result of the 1990 Anabolic Steroid Control Act, these medications are Schedule III drugs and require prescription by a physician. Formulations include tablets (such as stanozolol), injections (nandrolone decanoate or nandrolone phenpropionate), patches, or gels. These agents help to build muscle tissue through increased production of messenger RNA for protein synthesis, leading to an increase in lean body mass and a positive nitrogen balance. Anticatabolic effects attenuate the effects of cortisol in the body—the steroids displace cortisol from receptors and prevent tissue degradation, allowing athletes to train harder and more frequently. Rampant use of these agents by power lifters from the Soviet Union became evident in the 1950s, and spread to Germany and the United States by 1964. Systematic testing of athletes for steroid abuse began in 1976 at the Olympic Games in Montreal, but also led to the development of new "designer steroids," meant to both minimize adverse side effects and escape detection. For example, tetrahydrogestrinone is an oral liquid recently placed on the market. A body cream has also been manufactured that contains both testosterone and epitestosterone, and was designed to mask steroid use by keeping the ratio of testosterone to epitestosterone in the normal range (under 6:1).

Estimates of use of anabolic steroids in young athletes ranges from 3% to 7%, with athletes participating in weight training, bodybuilding, football, endurance sports, track and field, cycling, or swimming being more likely to use these agents.[73] Athletes take steroids in supraphysiologic doses (10 to 40 times the prescribed levels). Frequent practices include "stacking" (mixing different kinds of steroids, and possibly other drugs), "cycling" (starting and discontinuing androgens for periods of 7 to 14 weeks), and "pyramiding" (increasing dosages over a longer period). For ethical reasons it is difficult to perform extensive research on the effects of these agents, but one study did demonstrate increased size and strength in males using higher doses of testosterone for 6 weeks, but only in the presence of weight training.[74]

Complications related to steroid abuse include increased acne, mood swings, striae, sleep disturbances, baldness, and sexual dysfunction. Testicular atrophy, infertility, and gynecomastia in males, as well as virilization in females, may be irreversible conditions. More worrisome conditions affecting long-term health are cardiac muscle hypertrophy, increase in low-density lipoprotein cholesterol, decrease in high-density lipopro-

1: Principles of Orthopaedics

tein cholesterol, and increased risk of thrombosis. Elevations in heart rate and blood pressure have been reported, as have sudden cardiac death, myocardial infarction, and atrial fibrillation. There are also many effects on the liver: abnormal liver function tests, toxic hepatitis, and liver cancers including hepatocellular carcinoma. In the musculoskeletal system, there is acceleration of maturation and early epiphyseal closure, as well as a propensity for tendon ruptures. Patients who abuse steroids often experience an increase in aggressive behavior ("roid rage") and/or depression when steroids are discontinued. Shared needles carry the concomitant risks of hepatitis B and C and human immunodeficiency virus/acquired immunodeficiency syndrome. In addition to addressing the ethical issues of maintaining a "level playing field," the efforts of government and professional organizations should be directed toward strategies to prevent abuse of steroids in athletes of all ages.

Annotated References

1. Madden CC, Walsh WM, Mellion MB: Roles and functions of the team physician, in DeLee JC, Drez D JR, Miller MD (eds): *DeLee and Drez's Orthopaedic Sport Medicine: Principles and Practice*, ed 2. Philadelphia, PA, WB Saunders, 2003, pp 738-764.

2. Team physician consensus statement. *MSSE* 2000;32:877-888.

3. Johnson R: The unique ethics of sports medicine. *Clin Sports Med* 2004;23:175-182.

   The many facets of ethics and liability for the sports medicine practitioner are presented.

4. Tucker AM: Ethics and the professional team physician. *Clin Sports Med* 2004;23:227-241.

   Major ethical issues and potential conflicts confronting the professional team physician are discussed, including controversies around advertising and marketing.

5. Pearsall AE: Kovaleski JE, Madanagopal SG: Medicolegal issues affecting sports medicine practitioners. *Clin Orthop Relat Res* 2005;433:50-57.

   This review outlines legal obligations and risks for all physicians who take care of athletes.

6. *Preparticipation Physical Evaluation*, ed 3. Minneapolis, MN, McGraw-Hill 2004.

   This is the updated version of the monograph copublished by six participating organizations—the American Academy of Family Physicians, American Academy of Pediatrics, American College of Sports Medicine, American Medical Society for Sports Medicine, the American Orthopaedic Society for Sports Medicine, and the American Osteopathic Academy of Sports Medicine. It contains the latest information on all aspects of the PPE.

7. Rumball JS, Lebrun CM: Preparticipation physical examination: Selected issues for the female athlete. *Clin J Sport Med* 2004;14:153-160.

   This article reviews the salient potential disorders that need to be screened for in the female athlete. The entire issue of this journal is a thematic issue, devoted to the PPE.

8. Lebrun CM: Care of the high school athletes: Prevention and treatment of medical emergencies. *Instr Course Lect* 2006;55:687-702.

9. Franc-Law JM: A community-based model for medical management of a large scale sporting event. *Clin J Sport Med* 2006;16:406-411.

   This article details the preparation for medical care for the World Masters Games, which were held in Edmonton, Alberta, Canada during the summer of 2005.

10. Seto CK, Way D, O'Connor N: Environmental illness in athletes. *Clin Sports Med* 2005;24:695-718.

    Environmental illnesses in athletes include hyperthermia, hypothermia, and high altitude sickness. Diagnosis and management of these conditions are covered in this article.

11. Millikin R: Rowing Canada Aviron. Weather Protocol. Available from Rowing Canada Aviron website: http://www.rowingcanada.org/safety/weather. Accessed October 16, 2006.

    Rowing Canada Aviron introduced its first weather protocol document to help regatta organizers better monitor and predict weather conditions.

12. Walsh KM, Bennett B, Cooper MA, Holle RL, Kithil R, Lopez RE: National Athletic Trainers' Association position statement: Lightning safety for athletics and recreation. *J Athl Train* 2000;35:471-477.

13. American College of Sports Medicine and American Heart Association joint position statement: Automated external defibrillators in health/fitness facilities. *MSSE* 2002;34:561-564.

14. Courson R, Drezner J: Inter-Association Task Force Recommendations on Emergency Preparedness and Management of Sudden Cardiac Arrest in High School and College Athletic Programs. National Association of Athletic Trainers website. Available at: http:/www.nata.org/statements/consensus/SCA_statement.pdg. Accessed October 16, 2006.

    Emergency preparedness and treatment of sudden cardiac arrest in high school and college-age athletes is discussed.

15. Inter-Association Task Force for Appropriate Care of the Spine-Injured Athlete: Prehospital care of the spine-injured athlete. National Association of Athletic Trainers Website. Available at: http://www.nata.org/spineinjuredathlete/main.htm. Accessed May 4, 2007.

    A task force composed of representatives from 26 associations wrote guidelines outlining appropriate management of athletic spine injuries. An updated position statement is expected to be available in May/June 2008.

16. Concussion (mild traumatic brain injury) and the team physician: A consensus statement. *MSSE* 2006;38: 22012-22016.

    This joint consensus statement, together with the following references from NATA and the Prague conference, summarize the current thinking in terms of diagnosis and management of concussion (mild traumatic brain injury).

17. Guskiewicz KM, Bruce SL, Cantu RC, et al: Recommendations on management of sport-related concussion: Summary of the National Athletic Trainers' Association position statement. *Neurosurgery* 2004;55:891-892.

18. McCrory P, Johnston K, Meeuwisse W, et al: Summary and agreement statement of the 2nd International Conference on Concussion in Sport, Prague 2004. *Br J Sports Med* 2005;39:196-204.

    At this conference, background issues, including definition of concussion, pathophysiologic basis, grading scales, and subtypes were reviewed, and a new classification proposed (simple and complex concussion). This summary document covers clinical issues, investigations, management, and prevention. The Sport Concussion Assessment Tool (SCAT) and a guide for its use are included.

19. American Heart Association: Cardiovascular preparticipation screening of competitive athletes. *Circulation* 1996;94:850-856.

20. Bader RS, Goldberg L, Sahn DJ: Risk of sudden cardiac death in young athletes: Which screening strategies are appropriate? *Pediatr Clin North Am* 2004;51:1421-1441.

    The most common causes of sudden cardiac death in young athletes are reviewed, along with appropriate screening strategies, based on current scientific evidence.

21. Bille K, Figueiras D, Schamasch P, et al: Sudden cardiac death in athletes: The Lavsanne Recommendations. *Eur J Cardiovasc Prev Rehabil* 2006;13:859-875.

    Guidelines for PPE cardiovascular screening of athletes are outlined.

22. Grimes SJ, Acheson LS, Matthews AL, Wiesner GL: Clinical consult: Marfan syndrome. *Prim Care* 2004;31: 739-742.

    In this case study of Marfan syndrome, disease characteristics and natural history, inheritance and genetics, diagnosis, differential diagnosis, and management are discussed.

23. Geddes LA, Roeder RA: Evolution of our knowledge of sudden death due to commotio cordis. *Am J Emerg Med* 2005;23:67-75.

    This article summarizes current knowledge on the mechanisms of commotio cordis (nature of blow-producing

agent and victim-related factors), beginning with the first case report in 1978.

24. Maron BJ, Zipes DP: Introduction: Eligibility recommendations for competitive athletes with cardiovascular abnormalities: General considerations. *J Am Coll Cardiol* 2005;45:1318-1321.

    This article covers eligibility recommendations for competitive athletes with cardiovascular abnormalities; other aspects of management of cardiovascular conditions in this population are also discussed in the article.

25. Helenius I, Lumme A, Haahtela T: Asthma, airway inflammation and treatment in elite athletes. *Sports Med* 2005;35:565-574.

    This review highlights some of the controversies in diagnosis and management of asthma and exercise-induced bronchospasm in elite athletes.

26. Holzer K, Brukner P: Screening of athletes for exercise-induced bronchoconstriction. *Clin J Sport Med* 2004; 14:134-138.

    Screening methods for exercise-induced bronchoconstriction are reviewed.

27. Miller MG, Weiler JM, Baker R, Collins J, D'Alonzo G: National Athletic Trainers' Association position statement: Management of asthma in athletes. *J Athl Train* 2005;40:224-245.

    Based on current research and literature, guidelines for recognition, prophylaxis, and management of asthma in an exercising population are outlined in detail.

28. Mickleborough TD: Protective effect of fish oil supplementation on exercise-induced bronchoconstriction in asthma. *Chest* 2006;129:39-49.

    In a randomized double-blind crossover study in 16 asthmatic patients with documented EIB, fish oil supplementation improved pulmonary function to below the diagnostic EIB threshold.

29. Higgins JC: The "crashing asthmatic". *Am Fam Physician* 2003;67:997-1004.

30. Parker JM, Guerrero ML: Airway function in women: Bronchial hyperresponsiveness, cough, and vocal cord dysfunction. *Clin Chest Med* 2004;25:321-330.

    The entity of vocal cord dysfunction as a differential diagnosis is explored.

31. Binkley HM, Schroyer T, Catalfano J: Latex allergies: A review of recognition, evaluation, management, prevention, education and alternative product use. *J Athl Train* 2003;38:133-140.

32. Ellis AK, Day JH: Diagnosis and management of anaphylaxis. *CMAJ* 2003;169:307-312.

33. Niedfeldt MW: Managing hypertension in athletes and physically active patients. *Am Fam Physician* 2002;66: 445-458.

34. Lisle DK, Trojian TH: Managing the athlete with type 1 diabetes. *Curr Sports Med Rep* 2006;5:93-98.

    This article provides an excellent overview of type 1 diabetes in the athlete, including strategies for PPE evaluation and management of the disease.

35. Colberg S: *The Diabetic Athlete.* Champaign, IL, Human Kinetics, 2001.

36. Rosenstock J: Basal insulin supplementation in type 2 diabetes: Refining the tactics. *Am J Med* 2004;116:10S-16S.

    This article discusses the standard of care for the treatment of type 2 diabetes, and reviews two recent randomized controlled trials supporting the clinical usefulness of once-daily insulin glargine in optimal management.

37. Borja N, Daniel K, Tourtelot JB: Insulin inhalation powder (Exubera) for diabetes mellitus. *Am Fam Phys* 2007;75:1546-1547.

    This independent review is part of the STEPS review series in this journal and covers safety, tolerability, effectiveness, price, and simplicity of new drugs.

38. Binkley HM, Bechett J, Casa DJ, Kleiner DM, Plummer PE: National Athletic Trainers' Association position statement: Exertional heat illnesses. *J Athl Train* 2002;37:329-343.

39. Inter-Association Task Force on Exertional Heat Illnesses Consensus Statement: National Association of Athletic Trainers website. Available at: http://www.nata.org/statements/consensus/heatillness.pdf. Accessed October 16, 2006.

    Representatives from 16 associations established guidelines to increase safety and performance for individuals engaged in physical activity, especially in warm and hot environments.

40. Hew-Butler T, Almond C, Ayus JC, et al: Consensus statement of the 1st International Exercise-Associated Hyponatremia Consensus Development Conference, Cape Town, South Africa 2005. *Clin J Sport Med* 2005;15:208-213.

    A panel of 12 experts from a variety of backgrounds reviewed the existing data on exercise-associated hyponatremia and summarize current knowledge on diagnosis and management.

41. Hosey RG: Training room management of medical conditions: Infectious diseases. *Clin Sports Med* 2005;24:745-506.

    This article covers diagnosis and management of the most common infectious diseases seen in this population.

42. Metz JP: Upper respiratory infections: Who plays, who sits? *Curr Sports Med Rep* 2003;2:84-90.

43. Brady WJ, Ferguson JD, Ullman EA, Perron AD: Myocarditis: Emergency department recognition and management. *Emerg Med Clin North Am* 2004;22:865-885.

    Diagnosis and management of acute myocarditis, including aggressive cardiorespiratory support, is discussed.

44. Waninger KN, Harcke HT: Determination of safe return to play for athletes recovering from infectious mononucleosis: A review of the literature. *Clin J Sport Med* 2005;15:410-416.

    Because no strong evidence-based information exists on this topic, current consensus on optimal management of athletes with infectious mononucleosis is reviewed.

45. Cordoro KM, Ganz JE: Training room management of medical conditions: Sports dermatology. *Clin Sports Med* 2005;24:565-598.

    Common skin conditions in athletes are reviewed. Diagnosis, management, and guidelines for training and competition are discussed.

46. Zetola N, Francis JS, Nuermberger, Bishai WR: Community-acquired methicillin-resistant Staphylococcus aureus: An emerging threat. *Lancet Infect Dis* 2005;5:275-286.

    The authors review the characteristics of the new strains of community-acquired MRSA, and also discusses new approaches to diagnosis and management.

47. Bamberger DM, Boyd SE: Management of Staphylococcus aureus infections. *Am Fam Physician* 2005;72:2474-2481.

    This article discusses the spectrum of disease caused by *Staphylococcus aureus* , including MRSA, and gives key recommendations for practice (SORT evidence rating C) and therapy.

48. Cobb KL, Bachrach LK, Greendale G, et al: Disordered eating, menstrual irregularity, and bone mineral density in female runners. *Med Sci Sports Exerc* 2003;35:711-719.

49. Beals KA, Hill AK: The prevalence of disordered eating, menstrual dysfunction and low bone mineral density among US collegiate athletes. *Int J Sport Nutr Exerc Metab* 2006;16:1-23.

    One hundred twelve US collegiate athletes representing seven different sports were assessed by health, weight, dieting, and menstrual history questionnaire as well as with dual energy x-ray absorptiometry for spinal bone density. Level of evidence: II.

50. Torstveit MK, Sundgot-Borgen J: The female athlete triad exists in both elite athletes and controls. *Med Sci Sports Exerc* 2005;37:1449-1459.

    Norwegian elite athletes and control patients were screened using a detailed questionnaire, measurement of BMD, and clinical interview to assess for components of the female athlete triad. Level of evidence: II.

51. American Psychiatric Association: *Diagnostic and Statistical Manual of Mental Disorders (DSM IV).* Washington, DC, American Psychiatric Association, 1994.

52. Sundgot-Borgen J: Eating disorders, in Drinkwater B (ed): *IOC Sport Medicine Encyclopedia Volume IV: Women in Sport.* London, England, Blackwell, 2000, pp 364-376.

53. Loucks AB, Thuma JR: Luteinizing hormone pulsatility is disrupted at a threshold of energy availability in regularly menstruating women. *J Clin Endocrinol Metab* 2003;88:297-311.

54. Ihle R, Loucks AB: Dose-response relationships between energy availability and bone turnover in young exercising women. *J Bone Miner Res* 2004;19:1231-1240.

    This study assessed markers of bone turnover in 29 young women after manipulating energy availability. Bone formation was impaired by less severe energy restrictions than those that increased bone resorption.

55. Otis CL, Drinkwater B, Johnson MD, Loucks A, Wilmore J: American College of Sports Medicine position stand on the female athlete triad. *Med Sci Sports Exerc* 1997;29:i-ix.

56. International Olympic Committee Medical Commission Working Group Women in Sport: Position Stand on the Female Athlete Triad 2005. Available at: http://multimedia.olympic.org/pdf/en_report_917.pdf. Accessed May 4, 2007.

    A position statement on the female athlete triad is presented.

57. Practice Committee of the American Society of Reproductive Medicine: Current evaluation of amenorrhea. *Fertil Steril* 2006;86:S148-S155.

    Current standardized diagnostic criteria and evaluation of amenorrhea are reviewed.

58. Master-Hunter T, Heiman DL: Amenorrhea: Evaluation and treatment. *Am Fam Physician* 2006;73:1374-1382.

    A clinical summary of the evaluation and treatment of primary and secondary amenorrhea is presented.

59. Redman LM, Loucks AB: Menstrual disorders in athletes. *Sports Med* 2005;35:747-755.

    Current literature on menstrual disorders in athletes discussing incidence, clinical consequences, and mechanism is reviewed.

60. O'Donnell E, DeSouza MJ: The cardiovascular effects of chronic hypoestrogenism in amenorrheic athletes: A critical review. *Sports Med* 2004;34:601-627.

    Evidence and studies on the cardiovascular effects of chronic hypoestrogenism in amenorrheic athletes is reviewed and recommendations made for future research.

61. Khan KM, Liu-Ambrose T, Sran MM, Ashe MC, Donaldson MG, Wark JD: New criteria for female athlete triad syndrome? As osteoporosis is rare, should osteopenia be among the criteria for defining the female athlete triad syndrome? *Br J Sports Med* 2002;36:10-13.

62. Writing Group for the International Society for Clinical Densitometry Position Development Conference: The diagnosis of osteoporosis in men, premenopausal women, and children. *J Clin Densitom* 2004;7:17-26.

    The previous use of WHO criteria using bone densitometry for the diagnosis of osteoporosis in men, premenopausal women, and children is questioned. New characterizations are recommended, using Z scores, not T scores, when reporting bone density results.

63. Currie A, Morse ED: Eating disorders in athletes: Managing the risks. *Clin Sports Med* 2005;24:871-883.

    This article assesses the risks and consequences of eating disorders in athletes and methods of prevention and treatment.

64. Manore MM: Dietary recommendations and athletic menstrual dysfunction. *Sports Med* 2002;32:887-901.

65. Committee on Sports Medicine and Fitness: Promotion of healthy weight-control practices in young athletes: Policy statement. *Pediatrics* 2005;116:1557-1564.

    Unhealthy weight control practices are described, along with healthy methods of weight loss and gain.

66. Leib ES: Treatment of low bone mass in premenopausal women: When may it be appropriate? *Curr Osteoporos Rep* 2005;3:13-18.

    The risks and benefits of pharmacologic treatment of premenopausal women with low bone mass are discussed.

67. Liu SL, Lebrun CM: Effect of oral contraceptives and hormone replacement therapy on bone mineral density in premenopausal and perimenopausal women: A systematic review. *Br J Sports Med* 2006;40:11-24.

    A systematic review of current literature about possible osteogenic effects of oral contraceptives and other hormonal replacement therapy is presented. Level of evidence: II.

68. Wolfe LA, Mottola MF: *PARmed-X for Pregnancy. Physical Activity Readiness Medical Examination.* Ottawa, Canada, Canadian Society for Exercise Physiology. 2002. Available at: http://www.csep.ca/communities/c574/files/hidden/pdfs/parmed-xpreg.pdf. Accessed August 2007.

    Current literature on physical activity and bone health is reviewed.

69. American College of Obstetricians and Gynecologists: Exercise during pregnancy and the postpartum period. ACOG Committee opinion 267. *Obstet Gynecol* 2002;99:171-173.

70. Pivarnik JM, Chambliss HO, Clapp FJ, et al: Roundtable consensus statement: Impact of physical activity during pregnancy and postpartum on chronic disease risk. *MSSE* 2006; 989-1006.

    This article discusses physical activity and pregnancy, along with factors such as preeclampsia, gestational diabetes, breastfeeding and weight loss, musculoskeletal

1: Principles of Orthopaedics

disorders, mental health, and offspring health and development.

71. Davies GAL, Wolfe MF, Mottola MF, MacKinnon C: Joint SOGC/CSEP clinical practice guideline: Exercise in pregnancy and the postpartum period. *Can J Appl Physiol* 2003;28:329-341.

72. Carpenter PC: Performance-enhancing drugs in sport. *Endocrinol Metab Clin N Am* 2007;36:481-495.

    The concept and history of ergogenic aides and the role of the clinician/endocrinologist in managing patient drug use is discussed.

73. Laos C, Metzl JD: Performance-enhancing drug use in young athletes. *Adolesc Med* 2006;17:719-731.

    Ergogenic aids most commonly abused by young athletes are discussed in detail, and strategies are outlined to prevent their use.

74. Bhasin S, Storer TW, Berman N, et al: The effects of supraphysiologic doses of testosterone on muscle size and strength in normal men. *N Engl J Med* 1996;335: 1-7.

Chapter 11
The Polytrauma Patient

*E. Mark Hammerberg, MD

1: Principles of Orthopaedics

Initial Management of the Multiple Trauma Patient

The American College of Surgeons has established a stepwise protocol for the evaluation and management of all trauma patients, presented in the Advanced Trauma Life Support (ATLS) manual. The so-called ABCs of trauma reflect priorities in initial trauma management: A, airway management with protection of the cervical spine; B, breathing and ventilation; C, circulation with hemorrhage control; D, disability: neurologic status; and E, exposure/environment (remove clothes to evaluate external wounds, but avoid hypothermia). Each of these areas is addressed simultaneously by the trauma team. Treatment is initiated as diagnostic workup continues. For example, if a patient requires intubation for airway management, chest tube placement for a tension pneumothorax, and transfusion for hypovolemia, different members of the trauma team can be mobilized to address these issues in a coordinated fashion.[1]

Primary Survey

During the primary survey, each of the treatment priorities outlined above is addressed by a rapid stepwise physical assessment of each system, and resuscitation is initiated as appropriate. Adjuncts to the primary survey include blood pressure monitoring, pulse oximetry, arterial blood gas monitoring, and electrocardiographs. Urinary catheters are typically placed to monitor urine output, but placement should be avoided if urethral injury is suspected (blood at the penile meatus, high-riding or nonpalpable prostate). Nasogastric tubes may be placed to decompress the stomach and reduce the risk of aspiration. Radiographs taken during the primary survey include AP chest, AP pelvis, and lateral cervical spine; these are obtained in the trauma unit and should not interfere with or delay resuscitation efforts. Once the primary survey has been completed, the patient is reevaluated to determine the response to re-

suscitation. If the patient is not responding to resuscitation, the process should be repeated and treatment modified as needed.

Early identification and treatment of shock in the trauma patient is important in successful overall treatment. The most common etiology of shock in the trauma setting is hypovolemia resulting from hemorrhage. There are also several forms of nonhemorrhagic shock. Neurogenic shock results from injury to the central nervous system and is characterized by hypotension without associated tachycardia. Cardiogenic shock may result from direct trauma to the heart, myocardial infarction, or pericardial tamponade. These conditions can be distinguished with auscultation, electrocardiogram, and ultrasound in the trauma bay. Tension pneumothorax results from the collection of intrapleural air with resultant lung collapse and shifting of the mediastinum. Cardiac output falls as a result of limited venous return. Diagnosis is made by physical examination, checking for respiratory distress, subcutaneous emphysema, absent breath sounds, and tracheal shift. Immediate thoracic decompression is accomplished with a large bore spinal needle or chest tube.[1]

Hemorrhagic shock is treated with volume replacement. Two large-caliber intravenous catheters should be established. Depending on the patient's physiologic reserve, varying degrees of total blood volume may be lost before frank hypotension is observed. The extent of blood loss is best assessed by the response to initial fluid bolus (lactated Ringer's solution or normal saline: 1 to 2 L for adults, 20 mL/kg for children). If the patient's vitals signs are weak or absent, severe blood loss (> 40%) is suspected, and additional transfusion with untyped blood is required. If a transient response is noted but vital signs begin to deteriorate again, moderate blood loss (20% to 40%) is suspected, and blood should be secured for potential transfusion requirements (type-specific or cross-matched as available). If vital signs normalize and remain stable after initial fluid bolus, blood loss is minimal and blood transfusion may be avoided. The source of bleeding should be identified and the hemorrhage controlled, with surgical intervention if necessary. If the source of hemorrhage is not obvious, additional tests such as diagnostic peritoneal lavage or ultrasound examination (FAST: Focused Assessment Sonography in Trauma) may identify the source of bleeding. Although CT may prove useful in the diagnosis of patients with blunt trauma, CT scans should be reserved for patients with normal hemody-

*E. Mark Hammerberg, MD or the department with which he is affiliated has received research or institutional support from Synthes and Osteotech, and miscellaneous nonincome support, commercially-derived honoraria, or other nonresearch-related funding from Synthes, Smith & Nephew, and DePuy.

namic function. For patients requiring emergent surgical intervention, CT scanning may cause unwarranted delays in surgical treatment.[1]

Secondary Survey

The secondary survey is meant to provide a conceptual framework for the ongoing diagnostic work-up and treatment of a trauma patient. It is a tool to organize the process of the trauma workup. The secondary survey marks no specific phase or period of stabilization. There is no specific time when the primary survey ends and the secondary survey begins. Throughout the process of resuscitation, the priorities emphasized in the primary survey must be revisited. In many ways, the primary survey never really ends. Conceptually, the secondary survey begins after the primary survey is completed, but it is often completed during the process of treating the priorities identified by the primary survey. The treatment of trauma is a fluid process that changes even during the course of the diagnostic workup. The primary and secondary surveys are intended to organize the workup according to the priorities of resuscitation. They do not mark specific boundaries in the course of treatment.

The secondary survey is essentially a detailed inventory of all anatomic regions, from head to toe, including a thorough musculoskeletal examination. If the patient is medically stable, then this detailed examination can be completed in the emergency department. If the patient fails to respond to initial resuscitation, then the secondary survey must be postponed until the treatment priorities set forth in the primary survey have been met.

At many centers, the workup of the trauma patient involves a multidisciplinary team approach, so priorities of the primary and secondary surveys can be addressed simultaneously. If a patient's life is threatened by an exsanguinating intra-abdominal hemorrhage, for example, it would be inappropriate to delay an emergency laparotomy to investigate a closed tibial fracture. However, with the same patient, there is no reason why a tibia fracture should be ignored if adequate personnel are available to treat the fracture. It may be possible to initiate treatment of the fracture with splinting, even as the patient is being transported to the operating room. In this manner, certain elements of the secondary survey can be addressed simultaneously with the primary survey. After the patient has been stabilized, the various elements of the secondary survey can be addressed in a stepwise fashion, and a formal investigation of musculoskeletal injuries can be completed.

Evaluation and Early Management of Orthopaedic Emergencies

Pelvic Ring Injuries

The role of the orthopaedic surgeon in the emergent management of unstable pelvic ring injuries continues to evolve. In many instances, the presence of a pelvic fracture serves as a marker for high-energy trauma, alerting emergency department personnel and trauma surgeons to look for associated injuries. The treatment of pelvic ring injury in hemodynamically unstable patients has received particular attention. The etiology of hypovolemic shock in such patients is multifactorial, and patients may have blood loss from associated thoracic, intra-abdominal, or extremity injuries. The extent of blood loss referable to a patient's pelvic injury and the degree to which such blood loss may be controlled by emergent pelvic stabilization is a topic of ongoing debate.

Anterior external fixation frames have been advocated as a method to provide rapid reduction and fixation of pelvic ring injuries.[2] Early fixation limits ongoing injury from unstable fracture fragments. Anteroposterior compression fractures, also called openbook injuries, with widening of the pelvic ring and increasing pelvic volume, have received particular attention. Reduction of open-book injuries decreases pelvic volume, promoting self-tamponade of retroperitoneal venous bleeding and thus reducing blood loss. Posterior pelvic clamps have been designed with the same goals of early stabilization with reduction of the pelvic volume.[3] However, both forms of early pelvic fixation have their drawbacks. In inexperienced hands, both forms of fixation may be time-consuming in their application or may be misapplied, possibly leading to further injury or hindering definitive stabilization.

More recently, authors have advocated pelvic sheets or binders in the emergency treatment of pelvic ring injuries.[4] A circumferential pelvic binder or sheet can be applied in the field or in the emergency department. Such treatment is noninvasive, and it can be applied in minutes. It does not delay transfer to the operating room, and it can be left in place during an emergency laparotomy. When compared with external fixation systems, pelvic binders are equally capable of reducing pelvic volume, and they provide comparable biomechanical stability. As a result, several authors have begun to advocate pelvic sheets or binders as part of the routine treatment of pelvic ring injuries in hemodynamically unstable patients.

The theory of self-tamponade of pelvic bleeding currently remains unproven, and some authors have begun to question whether simple reduction of pelvic volume will allow retroperitoneal pressures to increase to levels sufficient to limit blood loss.[3,5] Laparotomy with direct packing of venous bleeding may be required in some patients. Angiography may identify bleeding from an arterial source that can be controlled with selective embolization. Some studies demonstrate a relatively low yield for pelvic angiography, suggesting that other sources of bleeding should be investigated as the cause of hypovolemia. However, more recent studies indicate that the incidence of pelvic arterial bleeding may be higher than previously suggested, and the rate of arterial injury increases with respect to the severity of skeletal injury to the pelvic ring.[6,7] Many centers have adopted algorithms that include pelvic angiography early during the resuscitative process.

Cervical Spine Injuries

Appropriate management of spine injuries in patients with multiple trauma begins in the field. Initial management consists of immobilization, and the patient should be transferred and secured to a spine board using log-roll precautions. Manual in-line traction should be used during initial resuscitative efforts, and a rigid cervical collar should be placed. When patients need to be removed from a motor vehicle, a cervical collar should be placed before extrication. During transport to the hospital, the patient remains secured to the spine board, with the head taped to the board and sandbags secured on either side.

The management of spine injuries in the emergency department continues as part of the primary and secondary surveys. Usually, formal evaluation of the spine proceeds as part of the stepwise progression of the ATLS protocol, when the trauma team log-rolls the patient to remove the spine board. At this point, the spine should be examined for any deformity and palpated to detect any areas of tenderness. In many instances, a formal neurologic examination is not possible because the patient has been intubated to protect the airway. For this reason, it is important to document whether the patient had been moving his or her extremities at the scene of injury or before intubation. In patients with associated extremity trauma, formal testing is not feasible because muscle function will be limited by pain and potential skeletal deformity. In such instances, it is more appropriate to document voluntary contraction of different muscle groups than to attempt formal strength testing. Absence of spinal reflexes, including the bulbocavernosus reflex, indicates the presence of spinal shock, and the level of spinal injury cannot be determined until reflexes have returned.

Traditionally, ATLS protocols have included lateral C-spine radiographs obtained during initial trauma evaluation as part of the primary survey. With a well-coordinated trauma team, radiographs can be obtained rapidly in the trauma bay, without interruption of ongoing workup and resuscitation efforts. In patients who would otherwise require a CT scan of the head, chest, or abdomen, cervical spine CT scans can be added without significant additional cost or time. In comparison with plain radiography, CT is more sensitive for the detection of cervical spine injuries.[8] For this reason, it has been suggested that helical CT scanning should replace plain radiography as the primary screening test for cervical trauma in obtunded patients.[9] For patients who are medically unstable and unable to undergo CT scanning, lateral cervical spine imaging in the trauma bay remains useful, especially if an injury is identified.

To date, there have been several studies, including five randomized controlled trials, investigating the use of high-dose corticosteroids for the treatment of acute spinal cord injury. The evidence from the randomized trials suggests that motor function scores improve when high-dose steroid therapy is initiated within 8 hours of injury.[10] The guidelines generated from the National Acute Spinal Cord Injury Study (NASCIS) call for a 30 mg/kg loading dose of methylprednisolone.[11] When initiated within 3 hours of injury, a maintenance dose of 5.4 mg/kg/hour is continued for 24 hours. When initiated 3 to 8 hours following injury, the maintenance dose is extended to 48 hours. It is clear that these recommendations have not been universally accepted, and many surgeons question the merits of high-dose steroid therapy.[12,13] It is uncertain whether improvements in motor scores reflect meaningful improvements in functional outcome, and critics suggest that the evidence demonstrating harmful side effects is stronger than the evidence suggesting a clinical benefit.[14]

Displaced fracture-dislocations of the cervical spine should be reduced as quickly as possible to minimize injury to the cervical spinal cord. In awake, cooperative patients, closed reduction, usually with Gardner-Wells tongs and traction, can be performed safely. Serial neurologic function is performed while traction is increased incrementally, and serial radiographs are obtained to document when satisfactory reduction is obtained. Because patients may experience neurologic deterioration during closed reduction, the safety of the procedure has been questioned for obtunded patients. The presence of a posterior herniated nucleus pulposus has been implicated as a potential cause of spinal cord injury during reduction of cervical spine dislocations, so prereduction MRI has been recommended by some authors. Others have demonstrated that closed reduction can be accomplished safely without neurologic compromise despite the presence of herniated disk material, so the significance of prereduction MRI findings remains uncertain.[15] Depending on the time of presentation and location, MRI resources may not be readily available, and it is doubtful that reduction of cervical spine dislocations should be delayed for the purpose of patient transfer or to wait for available personnel.

Open Fractures

The optimal management of open fractures requires timely and thorough wound débridement, fracture fixation, and soft-tissue closure. As soon as a patient is adequately resuscitated and medically stable, wound débridement should be performed on an urgent basis in the operating room. Historically, there has been an emphasis on early débridement within 6 to 8 hours of injury, but there is little evidence to support the notion that infection rates increase when débridement is delayed beyond 8 hours.[16,17] Nevertheless, most authors continue to recommend that surgical débridement should be performed as soon as the patient is deemed medically stable.

Administration of appropriate intravenous antibiotics is perhaps the most important intervention for the prevention of infection following open fracture. Delay in antibiotic administration is known to increase the rate of infection.[18] For Gustilo-Anderson type I open fractures, a broad-spectrum, first-generation cephalosporin is appropriate. For type II and type III injuries, combination therapy using a cephalosporin and aminoglycoside has been recommended. For wounds

1: Principles of Orthopaedics

Table 1

Example Injury Severity Score Calculation

Region	Injury	AIS Score	(AIS)^2
Head and Neck	Cerebral contusion	1	1
Face	Mandible fracture	1	1
Thorax	Tension pneumothorax	5	25
Abdomen	Grade II splenic laceration	3	9
Pelvis/Extremity	Right femur fracture	3	9
	Left femur fracture	3	9
	Pelvic ring fracure	3	9
External	No injury	0	0
	ISS: 25+9+9 = 43		

AIS = Abbreviated Injury Scale;
ISS = Injury Severity Score

heavily contaminated with soil, penicillin should be added.

Recommendations regarding closure of open fracture wounds continue to change. Previously, primary closure of open fracture wounds has been discouraged, for it was believed that primary closure would result in increased rates of deep infection. As a result, formal repair of open fracture wounds was delayed until a repeat débridement could be accomplished. Recently, it has been suggested that primary closure of open fracture wounds may be safe if a thorough débridement has been achieved and a clean wound can been ensured. A recent multicenter randomized study has investigated the safety of primary closure in the setting of open tibial fractures. In this study of type II and type IIIA open tibial fractures, primary closure and delayed closure were noted to have the same rates of infection and nonunion, but delayed closure was noted to have a higher rate of local wound complications.[19] For this reason, the doctrine of delayed closure for open fracture wounds has been called into question.

Compartment Syndrome

Although compartment syndrome usually occurs after an extremity fracture, most commonly a tibia fracture, it can result from isolated muscle trauma following a direct blow or crushing type of injury.[20] Muscle contusion leads to edema, and tissue pressures begin to increase within unyielding fascial compartments. When tissue pressure approaches or exceeds perfusion pressure, tissue ischemia results. Once ischemia has developed, muscle and nerve function are compromised, and irreversible damage will occur unless compartment pressures are released and perfusion restored. This is generally accomplished by timely fasciotomy.

If a patient has tense, painful compartments, with pain upon passive stretching of the involved musculature, then the diagnosis of compartment syndrome should be considered and urgent fasciotomies planned.

Dysesthesia or paresthesia may or may not be present. Although the diagnosis is made clinically, compartment pressure measurement may prove to be a useful adjunct. In an obtunded patient, in whom clinical examination is impossible, the diagnosis may rely entirely on compartment pressure measurement. The exact tissue pressure threshold, beyond which ischemia ensues, has been a topic of debate, but a safe threshold for fasciotomy appears to be 30 mm Hg below diastolic blood pressure.[21] It should be noted that this threshold is not a static value, but it changes according to the hemodynamic status of the patient.

Trauma Scores

Trauma scoring systems have been devised to quantify and compare the total "dose" of trauma sustained by patients with multiple injuries. Valid scoring systems allow for more meaningful comparison between patients with similar injuries, and the effectiveness of various treatments can be judged accordingly. In the clinical setting, trauma scoring allows for better prediction of outcomes such as sepsis, multiple organ failure, intensive care unit admission, and mortality. To date, one of the most widely used trauma scoring systems has been the Injury Severity Score (ISS).[22] To calculate the ISS, the body is divided into six regions: head and neck, face, thorax, abdomen, pelvis/extremity, and external. Each region is assigned an Abbreviated Injury Scale (AIS) score (0 to 5), and the worst scores from the three most severely injured regions are squared and summed to provide the ISS. The popularity of the ISS relates to its relative simplicity, and the fact that it can be calculated rapidly once a patient's injuries are known (Table 1).

One of the drawbacks with the use of ISS is that it factors only one injury per region. A patient with bilateral femur factures and a pelvic fracture would have the same score as a patient with an isolated femur fracture. This issue has been addressed with the development of the New Injury Severity Score (NISS).[23] When using the NISS, the three most severe AIS scores are used whether or not they are from the same body region. Using NISS, the example patient with bilateral femur factures and a pelvic fracture would have a score of 27, whereas the patient with an isolated femur fracture would have a score of 9. The NISS is a better predictor of mortality, sepsis, multiple organ failure, and intensive care unit stay than ISS.[24]

Systemic Inflammatory Response, Adult Respiratory Distress Syndrome, and Multiple Organ Failure

In response to trauma, the body demonstrates a systemic inflammatory response that varies in intensity according to the severity of the injuries sustained. Increased production of proinflammatory cytokines serves to activate the host immune system. Immunocompetent cells are recruited to the site of primary injuries, and the complement cascade is activated. In some patients, a compensatory anti-inflammatory response may be generated, resulting in a period of post-traumatic immunosuppression. The recruitment of inflammatory cells is necessary for the initiation of the healing response to injured tissue, but an exaggerated inflammatory response may actually serve to worsen the initial injury. Furthermore, the activation of a systemic inflammatory response may lead to remote end-organ damage with neutrophil demargination and disruption of the vascular endothelium. Disturbances in microcirculation exacerbate local tissue hypoxia, and parenchymal necrosis may ensue. In this way, the systemic inflammatory response serves as the basis for the development of adult respiratory distress syndrome (ARDS) and multiple organ failure following trauma.[25]

The development of ARDS following trauma is rare but potentially fatal. The most common cause of ARDS is sepsis caused by gram-negative bacteremia, but it can result from direct injury to the lung parenchyma, or as a consequence of a prolonged systemic inflammatory response to trauma. ARDS resulting from direct lung injury is called pulmonary ARDS. When ARDS results from systemic inflammation or sepsis, it is called extra-pulmonary ARDS. In pulmonary ARDS, the locus of injury is the pulmonary epithelium, with subsequent activation of the pulmonary macrophages. Loss of epithelial integrity results in alveolar filling and subsequent fibrosis. In extrapulmonary ARDS, the primary locus of injury is the endothelium of the pulmonary capillaries. Microvascular congestion results from the recruitment of monocytes, neutrophils, and platelets, and interstitial edema results from increased capillary permeability. Given the varying pathophysiology of ARDS, specifically during its early stages, strategies for successful mechanical ventilation may be tailored accordingly.[26]

The rate of ARDS following blunt trauma has been evaluated by a recent prospective study showing an overall incidence of 0.5%. The rate of ARDS appears to be proportional to the severity of injury sustained. For example, no patient with an ISS of 9 or less developed ARDS. Also, patients with injuries to more than one anatomic region were observed to be at higher risk for ARDS than patients with injury to an isolated anatomic region. Of particular interest is the fact that higher rates of ARDS can be predicted for patients with femoral fractures as well as for patients with combined trauma to the abdomen and extremities.[27]

Multiple organ failure refers to the potential final fatal pathway for patients with severe multiple trauma. Its etiology is multifactorial, but the final common pathway is cellular hypoxia and parenchymal necrosis, with end-organ failure. Although pulmonary failure is often discussed separately, it is a component of multiple organ failure and contributes to its etiology. Ultimately, hypoxia resulting from ARDS combines with microcirculatory disturbances resulting from hemorrhagic shock and/or sustained systemic inflammation. The result is inadequate oxygenation at the tissue level. This process may be exacerbated by disseminated intravascular coagulation with intravascular fibrin clots con-

tributing to microcirculatory disturbances. End-organ failure occurs as a result of tissue hypoxia. The renal and gastrointestinal systems appear to be especially sensitive. Necrosis of the renal tubules results in renal failure and anuria. Disruption of the intestinal mucosa can result in translocation of bacteria with resultant sepsis.[25]

The "two-hit" hypothesis refers to the fact that many patients with severe injuries are subjected to two traumatic events: the initial trauma related to the injury, and a second trauma related to surgical intervention. The extent of the inflammatory response has been investigated in patients undergoing secondary procedures after trauma, and increases in inflammatory markers have been observed.[28] Furthermore, the subsequent development of ARDS and multiple-organ failure has been correlated with the severity of the inflammatory response. When early fracture fixation (within 2 days of injury) is compared with delayed fracture fixation (5 to 8 days following injury), the inflammatory response is noted to be markedly elevated for patients undergoing early fixation.[29] With this in mind, it has been recommended that surgery for definitive fracture fixation should be delayed in patients with multiple trauma to minimize the so-called second hit of surgery.

Several serologic inflammatory markers have been investigated for their potential usefulness in measuring and monitoring the inflammatory response to major trauma. These markers include interleukin (IL)-1, IL-6, IL-8, and IL-10, as well as C-reactive protein and tumor necrosis factor-α. For many of these markers, serum concentration is noted to increase following severe trauma, but the extent and duration of elevation have been too variable to allow for clinical application.[30] IL-6 has been shown to be a reliable measure of systemic inflammatory response, correlating with injury severity and outcome.[29] For this reason, some authors have recommended measurement of IL-6 concentration to trace the severity of the inflammatory response. In this way, it may be possible to clarify the risks associated with secondary procedures such as fracture fixation and to determine when these procedures should be performed.

Damage Control Orthopaedic Surgery

The concept of damage control surgery was first defined for the purposes of treating medically unstable patients with abdominal trauma. The purpose of such surgery is rapid control of hemorrhage and contamination, not definitive repair of injuries. The goal is to improve survival of those patients with the potentially lethal triad of hypothermia, acidosis, and coagulopathy. Definitive repair of injuries and abdominal closure are not performed at the time of initial laparotomy. Rather, the abdominal wound is left open, a dressing is secured, and the patient is transported to the intensive care unit for continued resuscitation. This includes optimization of hemodynamic condition, ventilatory support, warming, and correction of coagulopathy. Following successful resuscitation, when the patient is medically stable, a return to the operating room is scheduled for repair of injuries and abdominal closure.

Damage control orthopaedics represents the application of this methodology for treating musculoskeletal injuries in patients with multiple trauma. The goal is to provide rapid stabilization of orthopaedic injuries while avoiding prolonged surgical procedures, giving the surgical team the best opportunity at minimizing hypothermia, acidosis, and coagulopathy. Open wounds and mangled extremities are washed out and débrided as necessary, and fractures are reduced and stabilized provisionally. For long bone fractures, external fixation frames are applied to provide temporary fixation. Definitive treatment is postponed until the patient is successfully resuscitated and medically stable. In this way, prolonged surgical interventions and excessive blood loss are avoided, and the patient can be transferred to the intensive care unit as quickly as possible. Damage control orthopaedic surgery should minimize the systemic inflammatory response by reducing the effect of the second hit associated with prolonged orthopaedic procedures.

The consensus statement of the Eastern Association for the Surgery of Trauma relating to the timing of long bone fracture fixation in patients with multiple trauma is instructive. This group performed a systematic review of the literature regarding the timing of fracture fixation in different subsets of patients with multiple trauma. Specifically, the group concluded that there is no compelling evidence that early long bone stabilization either enhances or worsens outcome for patients with severe head injury or for patients with associated pulmonary trauma. Although it is suggested that early fracture fixation may reduce associated morbidity for certain patients with multiple trauma, the study stops short of recommending early fixation for all patients. Instead, the authors recommend that the timing of fracture fixation be individualized according to the patient's clinical condition. If a patient has severe pulmonary dysfunction, remains hemodynamically unstable, or has severely elevated intracranial pressures, then prolonged surgery for extremity fractures should be delayed.[31]

The application of temporary external fixation for femur fractures, with planned conversion to intramedullary nailing, has been advocated for patients with multiple trauma.[32,33] It is believed that external fixation allows for some of the benefits of early fracture fixation while avoiding the pitfalls associated with prolonged orthopaedic procedures. Surgical time and blood loss are minimized, and the potential pulmonary morbidity associated with intramedullary nailing is postponed until the patient has had a chance to recover from the initial traumatic insult. Compared with patients undergoing early femoral nailing, patients treated with external fixation demonstrate a blunted inflammatory response as measured by serologic inflammatory markers.[34] Furthermore, when patients undergo staged intramedullary nailing after temporary external fixation, they demonstrate a decreased inflammatory re-

sponse following the nailing procedure. For this reason, it has been suggested that a protocol including damage control orthopaedic surgery may improve the outcomes for the most severely injured patients.

However, it must be recognized that the clinical significance of a decreased inflammatory response remains uncertain. There are few prospective data to show that that damage control orthopaedics can actually reduce the rate of ARDS, multiple organ failure, or mortality. Critics argue that damage control protocols contradict decades of experience and the accumulation of data supporting the superiority of early fracture fixation in patients with multiple trauma.[35] Proponents infer the success of damage control orthopaedics based on studies showing that patients treated with damage control orthopaedics seem to have results that are better than might have been expected based on their ISS scores.[33,36,37] With this in mind, temporary external fixation makes sense for those patients too sick to undergo early definitive fixation of their orthopaedic injuries. Although damage control protocols do make theoretic sense, prospective data are lacking. Additional study may be required before damage control protocols are universally accepted.

Annotated References

1. American College of Surgeons Committee on Trauma: *Advanced Trauma Life Support for Doctors*, ed 7. Chicago, IL, American College of Surgeons, 2004.

   The treatment recommendations of the American College of Surgeons for the evaluation and treatment of trauma patients are presented in concise format. Emphasis is placed on emergent management and initial resuscitation. Any physician who participates in the care of trauma patients should be familiar with the ATLS guidelines. Level of evidence: V.

2. Riemer BL, Butterfield SL, Diamond DL, et al: Acute mortality associated with injuries to the pelvic ring: The role of early patient mobilization and external fixation. *J Trauma* 1993;35:671-675.

3. Ertel W, Keel M, Eid K, et al: Control of severe hemorrhage using C-clamp and pelvic packing in multiply injured patients with pelvic ring disruption. *J Orthop Trauma* 2001;15:468-474.

4. Krieg JC, Mohr M, Ellis TJ, et al: Emergent stabilization of pelvic ring injuries by controlled circumferential compression: A clinical trial. *J Trauma* 2005;59:659-664.

   A series of 16 patients is managed with temporary stabilization using a pelvic binder applied at the level of the greater trochanter. No complications were observed. The quality of reduction for open-book injuries in the binder was noted to be comparable the reduction obtained with definitive surgery. Level of evidence: IV.

5. Grimm MR, Vrahas M, Thomas K: Pressure-volume characteristic of the intact and disrupted pelvic retro-

peritoneum. *J Trauma* 1998;44:454-459.

6. Eastridge BJ, Starr A, Minei JP: The importance of fracture pattern in guiding therapeutic decision-making in patients with hemorrhagic shock and pelvic ring disruptions. *J Trauma* 2002;53:446-450.

7. Miller PR, Moore PS, Mansell E, et al: External fixation or arteriogram in bleeding pelvic fracture: Initial therapy guided by markers of arterial hemorrhage. *J Trauma* 2003;54:437-443.

8. Widder S, Doig C, Burrows P, Larsen G, Hurlbert RJ, Kortbeek JB: Prospective evaluation of computed tomographic scanning for the spinal clearance of obtunded trauma patients: Preliminary results. *Trauma* 2004;56: 1179-1184.

    This is a prospective cohort study of 102 severely injured patients. All patients were evaluated with three-view plain radiography and CT scans. Independent blind review by two radiologists demonstrated CT scanning to be more sensitive for the diagnosis of cervical spine trauma. Level of evidence: I.

9. Holmes JF, Akkinepalli R: Computed tomography versus plain radiography to screen for cervical spine injury: a meta-analysis. *J Trauma* 2005;58:902-905.

    Seven of 712 studies identified through a MEDLINE search met the inclusion criteria for this meta-analysis. Pooled data demonstrate that CT is superior to plain radiography for the purposes of screening patients with a high risk of cervical spine injury. Level of evidence: I.

10. Bracken MB: Methylprednisolone and acute spinal cord injury: An update of the randomized evidence. *Spine* 2001;26 (suppl 24):S47-S54.

11. Bracken MB, Shepard MJ, Holford TR, et al: Administration of methylprednisolone for 24 to 48 hours or tirilazad mesylate for 48 hours in the treatment of acute spinal cord injury: Results of the third national acute spinal cord injury randomized controlled trial. *JAMA* 1997;277:1597-1604.

12. Frampton AE, Eynon CA: High dose methylprednisolone in the immediate management of acute, blunt spinal cord injury: What is the current practice in emergency departments, spinal units, and neurosurgical units in the UK? *Emerg Med J* 2006;23:550-553.

    Use of high-dose methylprednisolone for cervical spine trauma was investigated using a questionnaire sent to different emergency departments and neurosurgical and spinal units in the United Kingdom. No consistent approach was identified for the emergency departments, and only a minority of the neurosurgical and spinal units advocated routine steroid use. Level of evidence: V.

13. Chappell ET: Pharmacological therapy after acute cervical spinal cord injury. *Neurosurgery* 2002;51:855-856.

14. Pharmacological therapy after acute cervical spinal cord injury. *Neurosurgery* 2002;50:S63-S72.

15. Darsaut TE, Ashforth R, Bhargava R, et al: A pilot study of magnetic resonance imaging-guided closed reduction of cervical spine fractures. *Spine* 2006;31:2085-2090.

    In this study, 17 patients underwent MRI-guided reduction of cervical dislocations using traction. The diameter of the spinal canal at the injured level was followed throughout reduction. No patients experienced a decrease in canal diameter during traction. Posterior disk herniations were noted to return toward the disk space. No neurologic deterioration was noted during the process of reduction. Level of evidence: IV.

16. Khatod M, Botte MJ, Hoyt DB, et al: Outcomes in open tibia fractures: Relationship between delay in treatment and infection. *J Trauma* 2003;55:949-954.

17. Harley BJ, Beaupre LA, Jones A, et al: The effect of time to definitive treatment on the rate of nonunion and infection in open fractures. *J Orthop Trauma* 2002;16: 484-490.

18. Patzakis MJ, Wilkins J: Factors influencing infection rate in open fracture wounds. *Clin Orthop Relat Res* 1989;243:36-40.

19. Russell GV, Laurent S, Sasser H, et al: Immediate versus delayed closure of grade II and IIIA tibial fractures: A prospective, randomized, multicenter study. *22nd Annual Meeting Proceedings*. Rosemont, IL, Orthopaedic Trauma Association, 2005.

    This Orthopaedic Trauma Association-sponsored study was conducted at 30 trauma centers in the United States. Four hundred fifty-one patients with type II or type IIIA open tibia fractures were treated with débridement and reamed intramedullary nails. Following débridement, patients were randomized to receive either immediate or delayed closure. There were no significant differences in the rates of infection, delayed union, or nonunion. Delayed closure was associated with a higher rate of wound problems. Level of evidence: I.

20. Hope MJ, McQueen MM: Acute compartment syndrome in the absence of fracture. *J Orthop Trauma* 2004;18:220-224.

    In a consecutive series of 164 patients treated for acute compartment syndrome, 38 patients with no fracture were identified and compared with patients with associated fracture. Patients without fracture tended to be older and to have more comorbidities. Muscle necrosis was noted more frequently in patients without fracture. This finding may relate to observed delays for fasciotomy in patients without fracture. Level of evidence: III.

21. McQueen MM, Court-Brown CM: Compartment monitoring in tibial fractures: The pressure threshold for decompression. *J Bone Joint Surg Br* 1996;78:99-104.

22. Baker SP, O'Neill B, Haddon W Jr, et al: The injury severity score: A method for describing patients with multiple injuries and evaluating emergency care. *J Trauma* 1974;14:187-196.

1: Principles of Orthopaedics

23. Osler T, Baker SP, Long W: A modification of the injury severity score that both improves accuracy and simplifies scoring. *J Trauma* 1997;43:922-925.

24. Harwood PJ, Giannoudis PV, Probst C, et al: Which AIS based scoring system is the best predictor of outcome in orthopaedic blunt trauma patient? *J Trauma* 2006;60:334-340.

    The NISS is compared with the ISS for 10,062 patients with blunt trauma. The NISS was found to be a better predictor of sepsis, multiple organ failure, length of intensive care unit admission, length of hospital stay, and mortality. Level of evidence: I.

25. Keel M, Trentz O: Pathophysiology of polytrauma. *Injury* 2005;36:691-709.

    The authors present a thorough review of the pathophysiologic response to trauma. Level of evidence: V.

26. Rocco PR, Zin WA: Pulmonary and extrapulmonary acute respiratory distress syndrome: Are they different? *Curr Opin Crit Care* 2005;11:10-17.

    The distinction between pulmonary and extrapulmonary ARDS is defined. The distinct histopathology, radiology, and pathophysiology of the two forms of ARDS are outlined, and different strategies for ventilatory management are provided.

27. White TO, Jenkins PJ, Smith RD, et al: The epidemiology of posttraumatic adult respiratory distress syndrome. *J Bone Joint Surg Am* 2004;86-A:2366-2376.

    The incidence of ARDS is evaluated in a population of 7,192 trauma patients admitted to a single hospital over an 8-year period. The relationship between ARDS and ISS is evaluated along with various injury combinations. Femoral fracture was found to be an independent risk factor for ARDS. Similarly, the combination of an extremity injury with an abdominal injury is related to an increased risk for ARDS. Level of evidence: II.

28. Waydhas C, Nast-Kolb D, Trupka A, et al: Posttraumatic inflammatory response, secondary operations, and late multiple organ failure. *J Trauma* 1996;40:624-631.

29. Pape HC, van Griensven M, Rice J, et al: Major secondary surgery in blunt trauma patients and perioperative cytokine liberation: Determination of the clinical relevance of biochemical markers. *J Trauma* 2001;50:989-1000.

30. Roberts CS, Pape HC, Jones AL, et al: Damage control orthopaedics: Evolving concepts in the treatment of patients who have sustained orthopaedic trauma. *J Bone Joint Surg Am* 2005;87:434-449.

    In this article, the argument for damage control orthopaedics is presented along with a detailed review of the systemic inflammatory response to trauma. Level of evidence: V.

31. Dunham CM, Bosse MJ, Clancy TV, et al: Practice management guidelines for the optimal timing of long-bone fracture stabilization in polytrauma patients: The EAST practice management guidelines work group. *J Trauma* 2001;50:958-967.

32. Nowotarski PJ, Turen CH, Brumback RJ, Scarboro JM: Conversion of external fixation to intramedullary nailing for fractures of the shaft of the femur in multiply injured patients. *J Bone Joint Surg Am* 2000;82:781-788.

33. Pape HC, Hildebrand F, Pertschy S, et al: Changes in the management of femoral shaft fractures in polytrauma patients: From early total care to damage control orthopaedic surgery. *J Trauma* 2002;53:452-462.

34. Pape HC, Grimme K, van Griensven M, et al: Impact of intramedullary instrumentation versus damage control for femoral fractures on immunoinflammatory parameters: Prospective randomized analysis by the EPOFF Study Group. *J Trauma* 2003;55:7-13.

35. Meek RN: The John Border Memorial Lecture: Delaying emergency fracture surgery: Fact or fad. *J Orthop Trauma* 2006;20:337-340.

    This article highlights the relative paucity of clinical data supporting delayed fixation of femur fractures. Special consideration is given to the article by Pape et al. (*J Trauma* 2002;53:452-462), and correction of the statistics shows that the benefits of damage control orthopaedics may have been overstated.

36. Harwood PJ, Giannoudis PV, van Griensven M, et al: Alterations in the systemic inflammatory response after early total care and damage control procedures for femoral shaft fracture in severely injured patients. *J Trauma* 2005;58:446-454.

    In this study, the systemic inflammatory response syndrome (SIRS) score and the Marshall multiorgan dysfunction score were calculated at different points for patients undergoing immediate femoral nailing and damage control procedures. Despite higher NISS scores, patients treated with damage control procedures demonstrated lower SIRS scores. Level of evidence: III.

37. Harwood PJ, Giannoudis PV, Probst C, et al: The risk of local infective complications after damage control procedures for femoral shaft fracture. *J Orthop Trauma* 2006;20:181-189.

    It has been suggested that planned conversion to intramedullary fixation following temporary external fixation may expose the patient to an increased risk of infection. This study evaluates the infection rate in 172 patients treated with staged external fixation before intramedullary fixation. Overall, rates of infection were not significantly different between the damage control group and the group treated with primary intramedullary nailing. However, when conversion to intramedullary nailing was delayed more than 2 weeks, an increased risk of infection was noted. The authors stress the importance of timely conversion.

Chapter 12

Coagulation, Thromboembolism, and Blood Management in Orthopaedic Surgery

*Jay R. Lieberman, MD   *Craig J. Della Valle, MD

Coagulation and Thromboembolism

Venous thromboembolic disease is associated with significant morbidity and mortality and acute pulmonary embolism (PE) is responsible for more than 150,000 deaths per year in the United States. Patients undergoing major orthopaedic surgery procedures involving the pelvis, hip, and knee, multiple trauma patients with lower extremity fractures, and spinal cord injury patients are at increased risk for developing venous thromboembolic disease.[1,2] This risk of venous thromboembolic disease is exacerbated in patients with hypercoagulable states that may be classified as either primary (inherited) or secondary (Table 1).

The Coagulation Cascade

The coagulation system is a complex cascade that involves activation of enzymes and cofactors that leads to fibrin formation, a critical component of blood clots. The coagulation cascade consists of two pathways, the intrinsic and extrinsic, which converge downstream with the activation of factor X. Both pathways lead to the eventual formation of thrombin, which activates the conversion of fibrinogen to fibrin. The intrinsic pathway is activated by components of blood such as factor XII in plasma interacting with exposed collagen fibrils in damaged vessel walls. In contrast, the extrinsic pathway is activated by tissue damage that occurs with either fracture or soft-issue injury, which leads to expo-

sure of tissue factor to activated factor VIIa. The formation of this complex in conjunction with calcium and phospholipids promotes the activation of factors IX and X. Both pathways lead to the formation of thrombin, which is essential for normal hemostasis and the conversion of fibrinogen to fibrin. The prothrombin time is used to measure the level of activation of the extrinsic pathway and the partial thromboplastin time is used to measure the intrinsic and common pathways.

The fibrinolytic system modulates the coagulation cascade to limit clot formation to the local site of a vascular injury. The fibrinolytic system consists of several groups of naturally occurring anticoagulants. The plasminogen-plasma system inhibits fibrin polymeriza-

*Jay R. Lieberman, MD or the department with which he is affiliated has received miscellaneous nonincome support, commercially derived honoraria, or other non-research-related funding from Boehringer-Ingelheim, Bayer HealthCare, and Daiichi Sankyo. Craig J. Della Valle, MD or the department with which he is affiliated has received research or institutional support from Zimmer, miscellaneous nonincome support, commercially derived honoraria, or other nonresearch-related funding from Ortho Biotech and Zimmer, and is a consultant or employee for Zimmer.

Table 1

Risk Factors for Venous Thromboembolic Disease

Primary hypercoagulable states
Antithrombin III deficiency
Protein C deficiency
Protein S deficiency
Activated protein C resistance
Secondary hypercoagulable states
Bed rest or immobility longer than 5 days
Malignancy
Congestive heart failure
Estrogen use or hormone replacement therapy
Fractures of pelvis, hip, or leg
History of myocardial infarction
History of stroke
Indwelling femoral vein catheter
Inflammatory bowel disease
Major surgery (particularly operations involving abdomen, pelvis, and lower extremities)
Multiple trauma
Obesity
Paralysis
Prior venous thromboembolic disease
Varicose veins
History of smoking

1: Principles of Orthopaedics

tion and directly breaks down fibrin, and proteins C and S inactivate cofactors Va, VIIIa, and antithrombin.[3]

Pathogenesis of Venous Thromboembolic Disease

Three essential elements are associated with thrombus formation. These elements, called Virchow's triad, are endothelial injury, venous stasis, and a hypercoagulable state. Endothelial injury alone can induce thrombosis and can occur during the course of a total hip or knee arthroplasty. For example, kinking of veins during the course of a total hip or knee arthroplasty can lead to local endothelial injury, which can ultimately lead to clot formation. Venous stasis may occur as a result of limb positioning during the course of the procedure, the use of a tourniquet, or a general decrease in mobility that occurs after surgery. It is hypothesized that stasis can lead to platelet contact with the endothelium, which can prevent the inflow of clotting factor inhibitors or limit dilution of activated clotting factors. The mechanism by which hypercoagulability leads to clot formation is poorly understood. In the normal physiologic state there is a balance between the coagulation and fibrinolytic systems. Total joint arthroplasty is a potent stimulus for thrombus formation. Studies have shown that there is an increase in a variety of markers of both thrombosis and fibrinolysis during a total joint arthroplasty, including fibrinopeptide A, prothrombin F1.2, and thrombin-antithrombin complexes.[4] During a total hip arthroplasty, activation of these factors usually occurs during manipulation of the femoral canal.

Epidemiology of Venous Thromboembolic Disease

Multiple trauma patients with lower extremity fractures, patients undergoing total hip or knee arthroplasty or spine surgery, and patients who have sustained a spinal cord injury have variable risks of the development of venous thromboembolic disease whether or not prophylaxis is used. In patients not receiving either mechanical or pharmacologic prophylaxis, asymptomatic deep venous thrombosis (DVT) will develop in approximately 40% to 60% of patients undergoing total hip or knee arthroplasty. Proximal DVT occurs in 15% to 25% of these patients and a fatal PE in 0.5% to 2%. Symptomatic and fatal PEs are less common after total knee than total hip arthroplasty. Patients undergoing hip fracture surgery and multiple trauma patients, especially those with pelvic or lower extremity fractures, are also at increased risk for thrombus formation. The incidence of DVT is approximately 20% to 60% in patients with prior pelvic trauma. Several factors pose a risk for the development of DVT, including hypercoagulable states, advanced age, prior history of thromboembolic disease, immobility, smoking, obesity, stroke and cancer (**Table 1**). The primary goal of prophylaxis is to prevent symptomatic and fatal PE.

Pharmacologic Prophylaxis

It has been shown in a variety of studies that thrombus formation actually begins intraoperatively. Therefore, in most instances thromboembolic prophylaxis is initiated either before or just after surgery. At the present time a combination of prophylaxis, early mobilization, and expeditious surgery has reduced the risk of fatal PE after total joint arthroplasty to less than 1%. Regional anesthesia may also reduce thrombus formation because it is associated with lower extremity venodilation; however, this has not been proven in a randomized trial compared it with general anesthesia.[2] The selection of a prophylactic agent is a balance between efficacy and safety. Surgeons are particularly concerned about the development of bleeding, which can lead to local hematoma formation and subsequent reoperation. DVT prophylaxis may include pharmacologic or mechanical options or a combination of the two. Pharmacologic options for DVT prophylaxis include warfarin, low molecular weight heparin (LMWH), fondaparinux, and aspirin. Mechanical approaches include pneumatic compression boots, intermittent plantar compression, and early mobilization. In general, a short-course of prophylaxis during hospitalization followed by screening is not recommended.

Warfarin

Warfarin inhibits the production of vitamin K-dependent clotting factors II, VII, IX, and X by blocking the transformation of vitamin K in the liver. Warfarin prophylaxis is usually administered either the evening before or after surgery in a dose that ranges between 5 and 10 mg. Subsequent doses are usually determined via a sliding scale method using a target international normalized ratio (INR) to determine the appropriate levels of anticoagulation. The target INR is 2.0. The incidence of local and systemic bleeding varies between 1% and 5%.[5,6]

Although warfarin has been demonstrated to be a safe and effective agent, in several randomized trials LMWH has been found to be more effective in preventing asymptomatic clot formation than warfarin after both total knee and hip arthroplasty. However, there is no significant difference in the risk of symptomatic proximal clot formation or fatal PE between LMWHs and warfarin. There are some limitations associated with the use of warfarin. Warfarin requires frequent monitoring of the INR. In addition, there are potential interactions with other medications. Simultaneous use of nonsteroidal anti-inflammatory drugs is associated with an increased risk of bleeding gastric ulcers. Other medications such as trimethoprim, cimetidine, phenytoin, and cefamandole can potentiate the anticoagulation effect of warfarin and may also increase the risk of bleeding. The delayed action of warfarin leaves the patient relatively unprotected during the early postoperative period. Therefore, the goal of warfarin prophylaxis is really not to prevent clot formation in the perioperative period but to limit the propagation of these clots.

Low Molecular Weight Heparin

LMWH is formed by the depolymerization of standard unfractionated heparin. The molecular weight of these compounds ranges between 3,000 and 10,000 daltons. LMWH has different properties than standard unfractionated heparin. LMWH has decreased ability to inactivate thrombin and is unable to simultaneously bind antithrombin and thrombin. Therefore, LMWH is associated with less bleeding than standard unfractionated heparin but has greater Xa activity. LMWH has a bioavailability of 90% and it also has a prolonged half-life, which enables it to be given in either a once-daily or twice-daily dosing regimen. LMWH does not require monitoring. At the present time, there are two different LMWHs available for use in North America. One requires twice-daily dosing beginning a minimum of 12 hours after the surgical procedure and the other is given in a once-daily dose with a half dose administered approximately 6 hours after the procedure.[2] There has been no direct comparison of the efficacy of these agents. In addition, the LMWHs are associated with increased bleeding when compared with warfarin. There are also concerns about the use of LMWH in conjunction with epidural anesthesia and analgesia, and guidelines have been established for the use of these agents when using epidural catheters. LMWHs are metabolized in the kidney and must be administered carefully in patients with renal impairment.

Potential limitations of LMWH include the cost and the need for parenteral administration. In a series of randomized trials, LMWHs were noted to be more effective than warfarin in preventing asymptomatic clots in both total hip and knee arthroplasty patients.[7,8] However, in a study of symptomatic DVT and PE after total hip arthroplasty, there was no difference in outpatient symptomatic DVT rates between LMWH and warfarin.[9]

Fondaparinux

Fondaparinux is a synthetic pentasaccharide that selectively inhibits factor Xa. The inactivation of factor Xa leads to inhibition of fibrin formation. Fondaparinux has been compared with the LMWH enoxaparin in randomized trials in both total hip and knee arthroplasty patients. In a study of total hip arthroplasty patients receiving 7 days of prophylaxis there was no significant difference in DVT rates between the fondaparinux (5.6%) and the LMWH groups (5.6% versus 8.2%). There were also no differences in PE or major bleeding episodes. In another randomized trial in total knee arthroplasty patients, the overall DVT rates were significantly less in patients who were treated with fondaparinux (12.5%) versus enoxaparin (27.8%), but there was an associated increase in major bleeding episodes in the fondaparinux group.[10]

Fondaparinux may be administered via a once-daily subcutaneous dose (2.5 mg) beginning either 8 hours after surgery or the morning after surgery. According to results from several studies, there was no increase in DVT rates in total hip arthroplasty patients who received the agent the morning after surgery.[11] Fondaparinux is metabolized in the kidney and should not be prescribed for patients with renal failure. Fondaparinux provides effective and safe prophylaxis for total hip and knee arthroplasty and hip fracture patients.

Aspirin

Aspirin works by irreversibly binding and inactivating cyclooxygenase in both immature and circulating platelets. Aspirin inhibits thrombin plug formation by inhibiting platelet aggregation. The use of aspirin for total hip and knee arthroplasty patients is favorable because of its ease of administration, and no monitoring is required. In addition, aspirin is associated with few side effects and is relatively inexpensive. Unfortunately, few randomized trials exist that assess the efficacy of aspirin prophylaxis. One trial compared aspirin prophylaxis to placebo in total hip arthroplasty patients. There was no difference in overall clot rates in patients receiving aspirin prophylaxis versus those receiving a placebo; however, there were multiple protocol violations in this study. Approximately one third of patients received either a nonsteroidal anti-inflammatory drug or a LMWH.[12] In a meta-analysis, proximal and overall DVT rates were higher in patients who had received aspirin compared with warfarin or LMWH for prophylaxis after total hip arthroplasty.[13] Randomized trials are necessary to evaluate the efficacy of aspirin in preventing symptomatic DVT or PE after total hip or knee arthroplasty.

Mechanical Prophylaxis

There is significant interest in the use of mechanical prophylaxis because no monitoring is required and there is no risk of bleeding. The mechanism of action of external pneumatic compression boots is to decrease venous stasis by accelerating venous emptying and to increase fibrinolysis. Plantar compression devices work by mimicking the hemodynamic effect of plantar arch compression observed with normal ambulation. In studies of total hip arthroplasty patients, pneumatic compression boots were found to be less effective in preventing asymptomatic proximal clot formation than warfarin. There is one study comparing the foot pump with LMWH after total hip arthroplasty and there was no difference in the asymptomatic clot formation between the groups.[14] There are several randomized trials in the literature demonstrating the efficacy of external pneumatic compression boots in preventing DVT after total knee arthroplasty. Many orthopaedic surgeons stack modalities by combining warfarin, LMWH, or aspirin with pneumatic compression boots or plantar compression devices. These regimens compared with chemoprophylaxis alone have not been studied in large multicenter randomized trials to conclusively determine that they provide increased efficacy.

Thromboembolic Disease After Hip Fracture

Hip fracture patients are also at an increased risk for thromboembolic disease. In a variety of studies, DVT rates have been reported to be between 20% and 60%.

The risk of bleeding is a major concern in patients with hip fractures because these patients have a decreased ability to tolerate more than one surgery. Fondaparinux is the only agent presently approved by the Food and Drug Administration for the management of hip fracture patients. In several randomized trials, fondaparinux was found to be more effective than LMWH in preventing asymptomatic clot formation after hip fracture surgery.[15,16] Other agents such as warfarin and LMWH have also been shown to be effective, but further studies are necessary to optimize prophylaxis in this patient population. The surgeon must carefully weigh safety and efficacy when choosing a regimen for prophylaxis in this fragile patient population.

Thromboembolic Disease After Pelvic Fractures and Major Orthopaedic Trauma

Patients with pelvic fractures and multiple trauma patients with pelvic fractures or lower extremity fractures have an increased risk of formation of DVT, particularly pelvic thrombi. These pelvic thrombi are of concern because they have a predilection to migrate proximally. LMWH has been shown to be effective in reducing the rate of proximal DVT after major orthopaedic trauma, but the overall rate of DVT may not change significantly. Pneumatic compression boots or plantar compression may be an appropriate alternative for multiple trauma patients, particularly those with increased risk of bleeding. However, the efficacy of these agents in trauma patients clearly requires further study.[17,18]

Thromboembolic Disease After Spine Surgery

DVT also develops in patients who have had spine surgery or spinal cord trauma. Because of concerns with respect to the development of epidural hematomas, pharmacologic prophylaxis is not routinely used in patients after spine surgery. Mechanical prophylaxis with compression stockings and pneumatic boots may provide adequate anticoagulation for most posterior spinal fusions. Chemoprophylaxis or vena cava filter placement should be considered for patients who are at higher risk for thrombus formation, particularly those with spinal cord injuries, or for combined anterior and posterior spinal procedures. The prophylaxis could be delayed until the risk of bleeding has diminished.

Thromboembolic Disease After Total Hip and Knee Arthroplasty

Several different agents have been shown to provide safe and effective prophylaxis after total hip and knee arthroplasty. The risk of DVT remains between 15% and 25% after total hip arthroplasty and 35% to 50% after total knee arthroplasty. However, the rate of PE is approximately 0.2%. Recently, guidelines for DVT prophylaxis have been set forth by the Surgical Care Improvement Project, sponsored by the Centers for Medicare and Medicaid Services. LMWH, warfarin, and fondaparinux were the drugs selected to provide the best prophylaxis after total hip arthroplasty.

LMWH, warfarin, fondaparinux, and pneumonic compression boots were the agents of choice for prophylaxis after total knee arthroplasty. Further studies assessing the efficacy of different regimens in preventing symptomatic DVT are necessary. Surgeons are particularly concerned about bleeding in these patients because hematoma formation is not well tolerated after knee surgery. Recently the American Academy of Orthopaedic Surgeons has developed guidelines for the prevention of symptomatic PE in patients after total hip and knee replacement. In light of concerns about both bleeding and efficacy, recommendations for prophylaxis to prevent symptomatic PE for total hip and knee arthroplasty included LMWH, warfarin, fondaparinux, and aspirin. However, the recommendation for aspirin was not based on data obtained from randomized trials and clearly, additional studies of randomized trials that assess symptomatic events are necessary to determine the efficacy and safety of aspirin.

There is no consensus regarding the appropriate duration of prophylaxis after total hip and knee arthroplasty. In general, 10 to 14 days of prophylaxis is adequate for most regimens. There are no data available to indicate that prolonged prophylaxis is beneficial after routine total knee replacement. However, there are data available that suggest prolonged prophylaxis (28 to 35 days) after total hip arthroplasty reduces asymptomatic DVT rates. Further study of this issue is necessary and risk stratification may be appropriate in the future. A short period of prophylaxis during hospitalization followed by a screening study is not recommended.[19]

PE and DVT: Diagnosis and Treatment

PE may cause a variety of symptoms or hemodynamic instability, resulting in death within 1 hour of acute onset. Patients may present with dyspnea and tachypnea, tachycardia, pleuritic chest pain, or hemoptysis. In most instances, PE will go undetected. Because of the lack of sensitivity and specificity associated with the aforementioned clinical findings, they cannot be relied on to confirm the diagnosis of PE. Arterial blood gas, chest radiography, and electrocardiography findings must be incorporated in the diagnosis and workup of PE; however, diagnostic findings are only seen in 25% of patients with an acute PE. The most frequent abnormal electrocardiographic finding is T wave inversion, especially in leads 1 through 4.

Pulmonary angiography is still the gold standard diagnostic test for PE because it allows direct visualization of acute obstructions of filling defects in pulmonary vessels. However, the test is invasive, costly, and has a 1% risk of major complications including death, renal failure, and cardiac arrhythmias. Currently, pulmonary angiography is only used for patients in whom noninvasive testing has proved inconclusive. The ventilation profusion scan (V/Q) is the modality more frequently used in the diagnosis of an acute PE. The major concern associated with V/Q scans is that there is a high percentage of indeterminate studies; 30% of all patients with an indeterminate scan will have an angiographically proven PE. Therefore, these patients require further study with either a spiral CT, pulmonary angiography, or duplex ultrasound to establish a definitive diagnosis. When PE is suspected, a V/Q scan can be obtained. The "low probability" scan usually does not warrant further investigation unless clinical suspicion remains high. A "high probability" V/Q scan means that the patient should be treated with either intravenous heparin or LMWH therapy.

Because of the high rate of such indeterminate V/Q scans, spiral CT scanning is an attractive option and is now used more frequently when evaluating a patient with a possible PE. The spiral CT scan is more accurate in diagnosing a central lobar PE than a segmental PE. Spiral CT has a sensitivity of approximately 70% and a specificity of approximately 88%, but there is concern that this technology will detect small emboli that are not clinically relevant.[20]

There is no reliable clinical test for diagnosis of a DVT. Swelling, chest pain, and a positive Homans' sign are not specific for the presence of a DVT. In addition, there is no laboratory test that can make a definitive diagnosis of DVT. Recently, there has been increased interest in using D-dimer as an adjunct to noninvasive testing because there is a high negative predictive value. Screening studies appear to be the most reliable method to determine the presence of DVT in symptomatic patients. Various screening studies have different ranges of sensitivity, specificity, and accuracy. Currently the most reliable screening method is venous ultrasonography. This test is painless and offers a two-dimensional cross section representation of tissue and direct visualization of the thrombus. Thrombi can be detected in the proximal veins of symptomatic patients especially those having total joint arthroplasty but ultrasonography has not been shown to be an effective screening tool in asymptomatic patients after total hip or knee arthroplasty.[19] The sensitivity of this test is highly technician dependent.[21,22]

Because many clinically significant thrombi probably arise from the pelvic veins there has been interest in using magnetic resonance venography for the diagnosis of thrombosis formation in patients with major orthopaedic trauma and after total joint arthroplasty. Although this technology has been shown to be effective in identifying pelvic thrombi, it has not been used routinely because of concerns about cost and the clinical relevance of asymptomatic pelvic thrombi. Further study of this technology, particularly in multiple trauma patients, is necessary for it to be used cost-effectively.

Immediate treatment is necessary once a patient has been diagnosed with PE. Intravenous heparin has been used to treat PE for many years. Heparin accelerates the activity of antithrombin III, which normally prevents the formation of additional thrombi and allows dissolution of some clot via the endogenous fibrinolytic system. Patients are given a bolus of unfractionated heparin followed by a continuous infusion and the goal is to obtain a therapeutic partial thromboplastin time between 60 and 80 seconds. To limit the bleeding it is important that the bolus dose of heparin not be administered to patients who have had major surgery (such as total hip or knee arthroplasty) within 1 week of the diagnosis of PE. It has been demonstrated in several studies that LMWH is as effective and safe as unfractionated heparin in the management of acute PE. The advantage of the LMWH is that no monitoring is required and, if the patient is stable, outpatient management is appropriate. LMWH or standard heparin therapy should be used as bridge therapy when treatment with oral warfarin is begun. In general, it is recommended that the target INR value for treatment is 3.0. The optimal duration of anticoagulation after PE has not been determined. Current guidelines state that 3 to 6 months of anticoagulable therapy is ideal for preventing recurrence of PE. Contraindications to the use of extended warfarin therapy include liver insufficiency, alcoholism, uncontrolled hypertension, and pregnancy. An inferior vena cava filter is generally reserved for those patients in whom anticoagulation is contraindicated or in the event of a reoccurring PE despite the use of adequate intravenous heparin therapy.

A diagnosis of DVT proximal to the popliteal vessels requires treatment, but whether or not a calf vein thrombosis should be treated is controversial. In general, calf vein thrombi are asymptomatic. These thrombi usually resolve without treatment and have a low risk of embolization. If it is decided to withhold heparinization and the use of warfarin therapy in the presence of a calf clot, close surveillance with serial duplex scans to identify proximal propagation is advisable.[23]

Blood Management in Orthopaedic Surgery

In an era when cost containment, length of hospital stay, and patient concerns over the transmission of disease have become increasingly important, it is critical for the orthopaedic surgeon to be aware of the issues surrounding blood management. Many orthopaedic procedures, both elective and nonelective, are associated with substantial perioperative blood loss and thus blood management is among the most important factors in optimizing the orthopaedic patient's perioperative outcome. Research over the past several years has revealed that a given patient's blood management should be individualized based on the procedure performed, preoperative hemoglobin (Hb) levels, age, and general medical status (presence of cardiac, pulmonary, or vascular disease).[24-26] The indiscriminate use of allogenic blood is discouraged because transfusions can be associated with immunocompromise and an increased risk of infection,[27] pulmonary injury, the transmission of both viral and bacterial pathogens, and transfusion reactions. Further, there is not only concern over the transmission of known pathogens but also of unknown pathogens as highlighted by the recent concern of the potential transfusion-related transmission of variant Creutzfeldt-Jakob disease.[28] Surgeons should strive to decrease the risk of allogenic transfusions because the demand for allogenic blood products is already high, is expected to increase in the future, and already exceeds supply in many areas.

Preoperative Blood Management

Preoperative Evaluation

Patients undergoing elective primary and revision total hip arthroplasty, primary and revision total knee arthroplasty, complex spinal surgery, oncologic procedures, and related long bone and pelvic procedures can be expected to be at risk for substantial perioperative blood loss and consideration should be given to how that blood loss will be managed. Several studies have indicated that the patient's preoperative Hb level is the strongest predictor of the need for perioperative transfusion; therefore, a preoperative complete blood count should be among the preoperative laboratory tests ordered when patients are scheduled for elective surgery.[24-26,29] Patients who have a preoperative Hb level of less than 10 g/dL should be evaluated by an internist and/or hematologist to determine the cause of their anemia, and consideration given to delaying elective procedures until the cause is determined and corrected. These patients may have unrecognized medical conditions such as malignancy or gastrointestinal bleeding that not only places them at high risk for allogenic transfusion but also for other perioperative medical complications.

For patients with Hb levels of more than 10 g/dL, multiple options for blood management are possible and decisions should be made, in conjunction with the patient's wishes, to prepare them for elective procedures. An important part of a blood management program is patient education on the various options available. The use of an algorithmic approach to perioperative blood management for elective orthopaedic procedures has been recommended.[30-32] In one study of 500 consecutive total hip and knee arthroplasties, the use of the algorithm was associated with a statistically and clinically relevant reduction in blood transfusions.[32] This algorithm uses a mathematical formula to identify patients at high risk for transfusion (defined as a predicted lowest Hb of less than 7.0 g/dL; preoperative Hb procedure-specific expected Hb drop plus 1 SD [5.1 for primary total hip arthroplasty and 4.8 for primary total knee arthroplasty]). For patients with a predicted lowest Hb of less than 7.0 g/dL the use of erythropoietin α was recommended and in those with a predicted lowest Hb of more than 7.0 g/dL the recommendation was for observation only. The prevalence of a transfusion (both allogenic and autologous) was 16.4% in patients who did not follow the algorithm and 2.1% in the group that did ($P = 0.0001$).

Autologous Donation

The preoperative donation of autologous blood is among the most popular methods of blood management for patients undergoing elective orthopaedic surgery and has been shown to decrease the risk of allogenic transfusion. Both patients and surgeons are comfortable with the technique given increasing concerns and awareness over the risks of transfusion-related disease transmission. Negative factors associated with this approach include a high percentage of units that are not transfused (greater than 50% in some studies)[33] and thus discarded; most blood banks do not incorporate these units into the general supply because most donors do not meet the general health requirements typically required for donation, and the shelf life of a given unit is short once no longer needed by the donor. Discarding this unused blood is expensive, and this expense is sometimes directly charged back to the patient.

Autologous blood, like any transfusion, is susceptible to clerical error when retransfused; this effect is magnified by the anemia that is often induced by the preoperative donation of blood, leading to a higher rate of transfusion overall. The risk of a clerical error for a predonated unit is estimated at 1:30,000 to 1:50,000 units transfused. Further, febrile nonhemolytic transfusion reactions can still occur even with an autologously donated unit.

Although it is intuitive that a patient's Hb level should rapidly return to predonation levels prior to the planned surgical procedure, studies suggest that this typically does not occur[34-36] and that recovery to normal Hb levels is only stimulated when more severe levels of anemia are induced. The National Heart, Lung, and Blood Institute does not recommend autologous donation for patients who are expected to have a risk of transfusion of less than 10%.[37] Autologous donation should be considered more strongly in patients with alloantibodies that make crossmatching of a unit postoperatively more difficult.

To donate autologous blood, patients must have a Hb level of more than 11 g/dL and not have a risk factor predisposing for bacteremia (such as an indwelling urinary catheter or venous access port) because bacteria collected in predonated blood can multiply during storage. For a full donation, patients must weigh more than 110 lb. Patients with a history of aortic stenosis, unstable angina, or recent myocardial infarction are discouraged from donating. Patients donating autologous blood should be given supplemental iron and should predonate at least 5 to 7 days before the surgical procedure. A cost that is often unrecognized and difficult to quantify is the time required for the patient to predonate blood. Donation itself is not without risks and in one report, the risk of a donation-related complication that required hospitalization was approximately 1:17,000.[38] The most frequently reported complication is vasovagal reactions. However, exacerbations of coronary artery disease, tetany, compartment syndrome, and vascular injury have all been reported. Stored autologous blood is generally considered usable for 35 to 42 days after collection unless frozen.

Studies that have examined risk factors for transfusion in patients undergoing primary total hip arthroplasty, primary total knee arthroplasty, and total shoulder arthroplasty have consistently found that patients with a preoperative Hb level of less than 13 g/dL are at highest risk for transfusion, whereas those with a preoperative Hb of more than 15 g/dL are at low risk for transfusion and in these cases autologous donation is discouraged[24-26,31] In one study, patients with a preoperative Hb level of 13 to 15 g/dL only required transfusion if they were older than 65 years.[29]

Donor-Directed Donations

Another approach to blood management is the donation of blood by a family member or friend that is specifically designated for a particular patient. Although viewed by patients as having the same risks as autologous donation, the two approaches should not be considered as equivalent because donor-directed blood may not be as safe.[39] A potentially unsafe donor (one with a risk factor for transmissible blood borne disease) may feel pressured to donate blood when asked by a friend or family member. Also, it may be difficult to find a suitable type-match donor, increasing costs if multiple screenings are required to find an appropriate match.

Erythropoietin

Recombinant erythropoietin is genetically engineered to replicate the naturally occurring glycoprotein hormone and stimulates erythropoiesis. It is typically dosed at 600 IU administered subcutaneously 21, 14, and 7 days before surgery, with a final dose given on the day of surgery. Erythropoietin has been shown to be effective for reducing transfusions in orthopaedic surgery with a trend toward reduced allogenic transfusion.[37] It is currently indicated for patients with a Hb level of 10 to 13 g/dL who are unwilling to donate autologous blood. Erythropoietin has been successfully used in several centers as part of a comprehensive blood management program for patients undergoing total hip arthroplasty, total knee arthroplasty, and spinal surgery. However, the dosing regimen has decreased its acceptance among many surgeons. The concomitant administration of oral iron is recommended during treatment. Recently the US Food and Drug Administration issued a "black box warning" for all erythropoiesis-stimulating medications. Specifically, concern was raised over elevating Hb to a level greater than 12 mg/dL secondary to an increased risk of thromboembolic events noted in patients undergoing spinal surgery without the use of chemoprophylaxis for thromboembolic events, those with malignancies, and patients with chronic renal failure. Although a higher rate of thromboembolic events has not been noted in prior, prospective, randomized trials of hip and knee arthroplasty where pharmacologic prophylaxis against thromboembolic events was used, present recommendations from the Food and Drug Administration include raising a given patient's Hb to the lowest level that will avoid the need for transfusion.

Intraoperative Blood Management

Effect of Anesthetic Techniques

Several studies, including a recent meta-analysis, suggest that the amount of blood lost intraoperatively (which in turn affects a given patient's risk for transfusion) can be influenced by the type of anesthetic technique used.[40] Specifically, a neuraxial anesthetic (spinal or epidural) is associated with not only decreased blood loss but also a decreased risk of transfusion, shorter surgical time, and a decreased risk of thromboembolic events.

Intraoperative Blood Salvage

Intraoperative blood salvage systems have been used extensively in orthopaedic procedures. With the use of these techniques, typically one third to one half of shed blood can be recovered and transfused back to the patient. Red blood cell viability is generally equivalent to that of autologous blood, and in orthopaedic applications the blood must be washed to prevent the transfusion of debris and hemolyzed blood products. The main disadvantage of this technique is cost and thus it is most cost effective for procedures with high expected blood loss where a tourniquet is not used such as revision total hip arthroplasty (particularly if both components are to be revised or an extensile approach such as an extended trochanteric osteotomy is performed),[40-44] pelvic fracture surgery, and complex spinal procedures. If high volumes of blood are reinfused, the patient must be monitored carefully for the development of coagulopathy, because the reinfused blood is often deficient in both platelets and coagulation factors. If there is a high quantity of hemolyzed red blood cells in the fluid that is retransfused, renal function should be monitored because renal failure can ensue, particularly in those with preoperative renal dysfunction. Intraoperative blood salvage should not be attempted in a patient who has an infection that is being treated surgically or who is undergoing surgery for the treatment of cancer.

Acute Normovolemic Hemodilution

Acute normovolemic hemodilution involves the withdrawal of whole blood in the operating room just before the surgical procedure and replacing that volume with crystalloid and/or colloid solutions so that the shed blood during the procedure has a lower red blood cell content. The whole blood is then retransfused to the patient within 8 hours of its collection. This technique has been recommended for procedures with a high anticipated perioperative blood loss where a tourniquet cannot be used. Although this technique has been shown to be effective, it is time intensive and not practiced regularly at most centers.

Antifibrinolytic Agents

Tranexamic acid and ε-aminocaproic acid (EACA) are synthetic agents that act by inhibiting the fibrinolytic system (specifically retarding plasmin-mediated fibrin clot dissolution) and thereby potentially reducing blood loss. Tranexamic acid has been most extensively tested in total knee arthroplasty where it is typically administered as a bolus before tourniquet release, with the use of a second bolus given 3 hours postoperatively in some studies (dosing ranges from 10 to 20 mg/kg). Several reports suggest a decrease in total blood loss without an increased risk of thromboembolic events; a

1: Principles of Orthopaedics

meta-analysis suggested an overall decreased risk of transfusion when tranexamic acid was used for primary total hip arthroplasty and total knee arthroplasty.[45,46] EACA has been tested in major spinal surgery and is associated with decreases in both perioperative blood loss and transfusion requirements; however, a meta-analysis did not support the use of EACA in orthopaedic surgery because such benefits were not consistently documented in the literature.

Aprotinin has a similar effect; however, its mechanism of action is unclear. It is typically administered as a bolus at the initiation of the procedure (typically 2 million kallikrein inhibitory units [KIU]) and continued as an infusion during the procedure (0.5 million KIU per hour) and in some instances in the early postoperative period. Meta-analysis has shown that it was effective in both primary and revision total hip arthroplasty and major spinal surgery with clinically relevant reductions in both blood loss and transfusion requirements without an increase in thromboembolic events.[45,46] The efficacy of aprotinin seems optimal with large expected blood loss and extended surgical times. The drug, however, is expensive and cost effectiveness has not yet been determined. Further, concern has been raised recently of an increased risk of renal toxicity, cerebrovascular events, and death when aprotinin was used in cardiothoracic surgery, dampening enthusiasm for this particular agent. An additional advantage of the antifibrinolytics is the ability to use them in situations such as infection or tumor when red cell salvage is not an option and expected blood loss is high.

Bipolar Sealing Device

A recent addition to the potential tools for reducing perioperative blood loss includes the use of a bipolar sealing device. This device uses radiofrequency energy to reduce blood loss by shrinking collagen in blood vessels. It can be used on both soft tissue and bone and is unique in that the temperature is kept at less than 100°C so that hemostasis is obtained but damage to surrounding tissues is minimized. Limited data are presently available and cost effectiveness has not been proven.

Perioperative Injection

Perioperative injections with epinephrine into the soft tissues at the time of total knee arthroplasty (typically used in combination with a local anesthetic agent and other analgesic medications) is associated with modest decreases in blood loss.[47] Given the relatively low costs of this intervention, and the benefits in terms of pain control, this approach has garnered interest and merits further study.

Topical Agents

The topical application of fibrin or a combination of fibrin and thrombin has been investigated to enhance hemostasis and decrease blood loss. In one study, the combination of thrombin, fibrin, and tranexamic acid was associated with decreased drainage from the wound, a lower mean drop in Hb levels, and a reduced

risk of transfusion in primary, cemented TKA.[48] This formulation includes virally inactivated human blood products. These agents cannot be used intravascularly; thus, the use of reinfusion drains is not recommended. The use of autologous platelet gel and fibrin sealant placed in and around the wound at the time of closure has also been studied and was found to be associated with both decreased blood loss and transfusion requirements as well as a decreased risk of wound-related complications.[49] Concerns with these agents include disease transmission (viral and prion), sensitization that can lead to an inhibition of hemostasis if reused in the same patient, and cost effectiveness; however, further study in this area is warranted.

Postoperative Blood Management

Reinfusion Drains

The use of a reinfusion drain involves the collection of blood in the immediate postoperative period (typically 4 to 6 hours after surgery) and then filtering or washing the blood before retransfusion. Various studies have examined the efficacy of this approach with mixed results in terms of reducing total blood loss and transfusion requirements.[50-53] Similar to a cell saver device, reinfusion drains are contraindicated in patients with infection or malignancy.

Allogenic Blood Transfusion

The most common complications associated with allogenic blood transfusion are nonhemolytic transfusion reactions, alloimmunization, and febrile reactions. The more feared complications of viral disease transmission are rarer and have declined precipitously since the initiation of improved donor screening programs and more sensitive screening tests for the detection of the human immunodeficiency virus and the hepatitis-C virus.

Indications for Transfusion

The indications for postoperative transfusion are both controversial and unclear. Most authors currently recommend a transfusion when the Hb level is less than 7.0 or 8.0 g/dL, when patients have symptoms that require additional oxygen-carrying capacity (and not hypovolemia), or when patients have medical comorbidities (including cardiac, pulmonary, or vascular disease) that place them at high risk for anemia-induced complications. It is even more unclear whether or not the transfusion indications for autologous blood should be different than those for allogenic blood. Although the risks of an autologous transfusion are less than an allogenic transfusion, the risks of a clerical error, for example, are still present and thus allogenic blood should not be transfused unless clinically indicated.

Annotated References

1. Geerts WH, Pineo GF, Hut JA, et al: Prevention of venous thromboembolism: The Seventh ACCP Confer-

ence on Antithrombotic and Thrombolytic Therapy. *Chest* 2004;126(suppl 3):338s-400s.

2. Lieberman JR, Hsu WK: Prevention of venous thromboembolic disease after total hip and knee arthroplasty. *J Bone Joint Surg Am* 2005;87:2097-2112.

   A comprehensive review of DVT prophylaxis after total joint arthroplasty is presented.

3. Millenson MM, Bauer KA: Pathogenesis of venous thromboembolism, in Hull R, Pineo GD (eds): *Disorders of Thrombosis.* Philadelphia, PA, WB Saunders, 1996, pp 175-190.

4. Sharrock NE, Go G, Harpel PC, Ranawat CS, Sculco TP, Salvati EA: The John Charnley Award: Thrombogenesis during total hip arthroplasty. *Clin Orthop Relat Res* 1995;319:16-27.

5. Pellegrini VD Jr, Donaldson CT, Forbes DC, Lehman EB, Evarts CM: The John Charnley Award: Prevention of readmission for venous thromboembolic disease after total hip arthroplasty. *Clin Orthop Relat Res* 2005;441:56-62.

   Warfarin prophylaxis for 6 weeks provided more effective protection against readmission for DVT after total hip arthroplasty (0.27%, 1 of 360 patients) than stopping warfarin prophylaxis at the time of discharge after a negative venogram (2.2%, 19 of 880 patients).

6. Lieberman JR, Wollaeger J, Dorey F, et al: The efficacy of prophylaxis with low-dose warfarin for prevention of pulmonary embolism following total hip arthroplasty. *J Bone Joint Surg Am* 1997;79:319-325.

7. Hull RD, Pineo GF, Francis C, et al: Low molecular weight heparin prophylaxis using dalteparin extended out-of-hospital vs in-hospital warfarin/out-of-hospital placebo in hip arthroplasty patients: A double-blind, randomized comparison: North American Fragmin Trial Investigators. *Arch Intern Med* 2000;160:2208-2215.

8. Leclerc JR, Geerts WH, Desjardins L, et al: Prevention of venous thromboembolism after knee arthroplasty: A randomized, double-blind trial comparing enoxaparin with warfarin. *Ann Intern Med* 1996;124:619-626.

9. Colwell CW Jr, Collis DK, Paulson R, et al: Comparison of enoxaparin and warfarin for the prevention of venous thromboembolic disease after total hip arthroplasty: Evaluation during hospitalization and three months after discharge. *J Bone Joint Surg Am* 1999;81:932-940.

10. Bauer KA, Eriksson BL, Lassen MR, Turpie AG: Fondaparinux compared with enoxaparin for the prevention of venous thromboembolism after elective major knee surgery. *N Engl J Med* 2001;345:1305-1310.

11. Colwell CW, Kwong LM, Turpie AG, Davidson BL: Flexibility in administration of fondaparinux for prevention of symptomatic venous thromboembolism in orthopaedic surgery. *J Arthroplasty* 2006;21:36-45.

    This study examined flexibility in the timing of the first dose of fondaparinux and found no significant difference in the incidence of symptomatic venous thromboembolism.

12. Prevention of pulmonary embolism and deep vein thrombosis with low dose aspirin: Pulmonary Embolism Prevention trial. *Lancet* 2000;355:1295-1302.

13. Freedman KB, Brookenthal KR, Fitzgerald RH Jr, Williams S, Lonner JH: A meta-analysis of thromboembolic prophylaxis following elective total hip arthroplasty. *J Bone Joint Surg Am* 2000;82:929-938.

14. Warwick D, Harrison J, Whitehouse S, Mitchelmore A, Thronton M: A randomized comparison of a foot pump with the use of low molecular weight heparin for the prevention of deep-vein thrombosis after total hip replacement: A prospective, randomized trial. *J Bone Joint Surg Am* 1998;80:1158-1166.

15. Eriksson BI, Lassen MR: Duration of prophylaxis against venous thromboembolism with fondaparinux after hip fracture surgery: A multicenter, randomized, placebo-controlled, double-blind study. *Arch Intern Med* 2003;163:1137-1142.

16. Ericksson BI, Bauer KA, Lassen MR, Turpie AG: Steering Committee of the Pentasaccharide in Hip-Fracture Surgery Study: Fondaparinux compared with enoxaparin for the prevention of venous thromboembolism after hip-fracture surgery. *N Engl J Med* 2001;345:1298-1304.

17. Geerts WH, Code KI, Jay RM, Chen E, Szalai JP: A prospective study of venous thromboembolism after major trauma. *N Engl J Med* 1994;331:1601-1606.

18. Geerts WH, Jay RM, Code KI, et al: A comparison of low-dose heparin with low molecular weight heparin as prophylaxis against venous thromboembolism after major trauma. *N Engl J Med* 1996;335:701-707.

19. Robinson KS, Anderson DR, Gross M, et al: Ultrasonographic screening before hospital discharge for deep venous thrombosis after arthroplasty: The postarthroplasty screening study. A randomized controlled trial. *Ann Intern Med* 1997;127:439-445.

20. Cross JJ, Kemp PM, Walsh CG, Flower CD, Dixon AK: A randomized trial of spiral CT and ventilation perfusion scintigraphy for the diagnosis of pulmonary embolism. *Clin Radiol* 1998;53:177-182.

21. Garino JP, Lotke PA, Kitziger KJ, Steinberg ME: Deep venous thrombosis after total joint arthroplasty: The role of compression ultrasonography and the importance of the experience of the technician. *J Bone Joint Surg* 1996;78:1359-1365.

22. Montgomery KD, Potter HG, Helfet DL: The detection and management of proximal deep venous thrombosis in patients with acute acetabular fractures: A follow-up

1: Principles of Orthopaedics

report. *J Orthop Trauma* 1997;11:330-336.

23. Conduah AH, Lieberman JR: Thromboembolism and pulmonary distress in the setting of orthopaedic surgery, in Einhorn TA, O'Keefe RJ, Buckwalter JA (eds), *Orthopaedic Basic Science*, ed 3. Rosemont, IL, American Academy of Orthopaedic Surgeons, 2007, pp 105-114.

    A comprehensive review of the factors associated with thromboembolism and fat embolism is presented.

24. Bierbaum BE, Callaghan JJ, Galante JO, Rubash HE, Tooms RE, Welch RB: An analysis of blood management in patients having a total hip or knee arthroplasty. *J Bone Joint Surg Am* 1999;81:2-10.

25. Bong MR, Patel V, Chang E, Issack PS, Hebert R, Di Cesare PE: Risks associated with blood transfusion after total knee arthroplasty. *J Arthroplasty* 2004;19:281-287.

    In this retrospective review of 1,402 patients undergoing primary total knee arthroplasty, age, Hb level, and the use of LMWH were found to be the strongest predictors of allogenic transfusion.

26. Millett PJ, Porramatikul M, Chen N, Zurakowski D, Warner JJ: Analysis of transfusion predictors in shoulder arthroplasty. *J Bone Joint Surg Am* 2006;88:1223-1230.

    In a retrospective review of 124 consecutive total should arthroplasties, the preoperative Hb level was found to be the strongest predictor of the need for a transfusion. Patients with a Hb level of more than 13 g/dL had a low risk of transfusion. Level of evidence: II.

27. Weber EW, Slappendel R, Prins MH, van der Schaaf DB, Durieux ME, Strumper D: Perioperative blood transfusions and delayed wound healing after hip replacement surgery: Effects on duration of hospitalization. *Anesth Analg* 2005;100:1416-1421.

    In this observational study of 444 patients undergoing total hip arthroplasty, there was a statistically significant increase in wound healing complications and a longer length of stay in patients requiring allogenic blood.

28. Wroe SJ, Pal S, Siddique D, et al: Clinical presentation and pre-mortem diagnosis of variant Creutzfeldt-Jakob disease associated with blood transfusion: A case report. *Lancet* 2006;368:2061-2067.

    The risk of transfusion-associated variant Creutzfeldt-Jakob infection is likely high in patients who received a transfusion from donors who subsequently developed variant Creutzfeldt-Jakob disease.

29. Hatzidakis AM, Mendlick RM, McKillip T, Reddy RL, Garvin KL: Preoperative autologous donation for total joint arthroplasty: An analysis of risk factors for allogenic transfusion. *J Bone Joint Surg Am* 2000;82:89-100.

30. Callaghan JJ, O'Rourke MR, Liu SS: Blood management: Issues and options. *J Arthroplasty* 2005;20:51-54.

    This review article outlines options for blood management in total hip arthroplasty and total knee arthroplasty and presents an algorithm for blood management.

31. Keating EM, Meding JB, Faris PM, Ritter MA: Predictors of transfusion risk in elective knee surgery. *Clin Orthop Relat Res* 1998;357:50-59.

32. Pierson JL, Hannon TJ, Earles DR: A blood-conservation algorithm to reduce blood transfusions after total hip and knee arthroplasty. *J Bone Joint Surg Am* 2004;86-A:1512-1518.

    The authors retrospectively reviewed the outcomes of 500 primary total hip arthroplasties and total knee arthroplasties where an algorithmic approach to blood management was used that emphasized the use of epoetin α based on an expected lowest Hb of less than 7.0. Level of evidence: III (therapeutic study).

33. Bess RS, Lenke LG, Bridwell KH, Steger-May K, Hensley M: Wasting of preoperatively donated autologous blood in the surgical treatment of adolescent idiopathic scoliosis. *Spine* 2006;31:2375-2380.

    This retrospective review of 123 patients treated for adolescent idiopathic scoliosis showed a high rate of wastage of autologous blood and recommended more precise guidelines for autologous donation.

34. Bezwada HP, Nazarian DG, Henry DH, Booth RE Jr: Preoperative use of recombinant human erythropoietin before total joint arthroplasty. *J Bone Joint Surg Am* 2003;85-A:1795-1800.

35. Hardwick ME, Morris BM, Colwell CW Jr: Two-dose epoetin alfa reduces blood transfusions compared with autologous donation. *Clin Orthop Relat Res* 2004;423:240-244.

    This prospecitve randomized trial of 40 patients undergoing primary total hip arthroplasty found that a two-dose regimen of epoetin alfa was a safe alternative to autologous donation.

36. Stowell CP, Chandler H, Jove M, Guilfoyle M, Wacholtz MC: An open-label, randomized study to compare the safety and efficacy of perioperative epoetin alfa with preoperative autologous blood donation in total joint arthroplasty. *Orthopedics* 1999;22:s105-s112.

37. Transfusion alert: Use of autologous blood. National Heart, Lung, and Blood Institute expert panel on the use of autologous blood. *Transfusion* 1995;35:703-711.

38. Popovsky MA, Whitaker B, Arnold NL: Severe outcomes of allogeneic and autologous blood donation: Frequency and characterization. *Transfusion* 1995;35:734-737.

39. Cordell RR, Yalon VA, Cigahn-Haskell C, McDonough BP, Perkins HA: Experience with 11,916 designated donors. *Transfusion* 1986;26:484-486.

40. Mauermann WJ, Shilling AM, Zuo Z: A comparison of neuraxial block versus general anesthesia for elective to-

tal hip replacement: A meta-analysis. *Anesth Analg* 2006;103:1018-1025.

This meta-analysis showed that neuraxial anesthesia was associated with less blood loss, a lower risk of transfusion, faster surgical times, and a lower risk of thromboembolic events compared with general anesthesia.

41. Bridgens JP, Evans CR, Dobson PM, Hamer AJ: Intraoperative red blood-cell salvage in revision hip surgery: A case-matched study. *J Bone Joint Surg Am* 2007;89: 270-275.

    This case-matched analysis of 94 patients who underwent revision total hip arthroplasty found that the use of intraoperative cell salvage was associated with a decreased volume of allogenic blood transfused. Level of evidence: III (therapeutic).

42. Garvin KL, Feschuk CA, Sekundiak TD, Lyden ER: Blood salvage and allogenic transfusion needs in revision hip arthroplasty. *Clin Orthop Relat Res* 2005;441: 205-209.

    This retrospective review of 147 patients who underwent revision total hip arthroplasty showed a decreased risk of allogenic transfusion associated with a cell saver and that transfusion risk was associated with the complexity of the revision and the preoperative Hb level. Level of evidence: IV (therapeutic study, case series).

43. Phillips SJ, Chavan R, Porter ML, et al: Does salvage and tranexamic acid reduce the need for blood transfusion in revision hip surgery? *J Bone Joint Surg Br* 2006; 88:1141-1142.

    This retrospective case control study of 80 patients who underwent revision total hip arthroplasty showed that the use of a cell saver and tranexamic acid was associated with a lower risk of transfusion and that this technique was cost effective.

44. Zarin J, Grosvenor D, Schurman D, Goodman S: Efficacy of intraoperative blood collection and reinfusion in revision total hip arthroplasty. *J Bone Joint Surg Am* 2003;85-A:2147-2151.

45. Gill JB, Rosenstein A: The use of antifibrinolytic agents in total hip arthroplasty: A meta-analysis. *J Arthroplasty* 2006;21:869-873.

    This meta-anlaysis showed that aprotinin was effective in reducing both blood loss and transfusion in patients who underwent revision total hip arthroplasty.

46. Zufferey P, Merquiol F, Laporte S, et al: Do antifibrin-olytics reduce allogeneic blood transfusion in orthopedic surgery? *Anesthesiology* 2006;105:1034-1046.

    This meta-analysis of 43 randomized trials showed that aprotinin and tranexamic acid reduced the risk of allogenic transfusion in orthopaedic procedures.

47. Lombardi AV Jr, Berend KR, Mallory TH, Dodds KL, Adams JB: Soft tissue and intra-articular injection of bupivacaine, epinephrine, and morphine has a beneficial effect after total knee arthroplasty. *Clin Orthop Relat Res* 2004;428:125-130.

    In this report, patients who received an intra-articular and soft-tissue injection of local anesthetic combined with epinephrine and morphine required less narcotic pain medication and had less blood loss.

48. Wang GJ, Hungerford DS, Savory CG, et al: Use of fibrin sealant to reduce bloody drainage and hemoglobin loss after total knee arthroplasty: A brief note on a randomized prospective trial. *J Bone Joint Surg Am* 2001; 83-A:1503-1505.

49. Everts PA, Devilee RJ, Brown Mahoney C, et al: Platelet gel and fibrin sealant reduce allogeneic blood transfusions in total knee arthroplasty. *Acta Anaesthesiol Scand* 2006;50:593-599.

    Patients treated with autologous platelet gel and fibrin sealant following primary total knee arthroplasty had higher Hb levels, a decreased risk of allogenic transfusion, and were less likely to have wound healing complications.

50. Grosvenor D, Goyal V, Goodman S: Efficacy of postoperative blood salvage following total hip arthroplasty in patients with and without deposited autologous units. *J Bone Joint Surg Am* 2000;82-A:951-954.

51. Han CD, Shin DE: Postoperative blood salvage and reinfusion after total joint arthroplasty. *J Arthroplasty* 1997;12:511-516.

52. Mauerhan DR, Nussman D, Mokris JG, Beaver WB: Effect of postoperative reinfusion systems on hemoglobin levels in primary total hip and total knee arthroplasties: A prospective randomized study. *J Arthroplasty* 1993;8: 523-527.

53. Rizzi L, Bertacchi P, Ghezzi LM, Bellavita P, Scudeller G: Postoperative blood salvage in hip and knee arthroplasty: A prospective study on cost effectiveness in 161 patients. *Acta Orthop Scand* 1998;69:31-34.

1: Principles of Orthopaedics

Chapter 13

Work-Related Illnesses, Cumulative Trauma, and Compensation

*E. Mark Hammerberg, MD   Lamar L. Fleming, MD

Introduction

A physician who undertakes the care of injured workers is required to consider and negotiate a variety of societal, psychological, and economic factors that are normally outside the scope of traditional medical intervention. In this context, a physician's recommendations have an impact that reaches beyond the successful evaluation and treatment of the injury in question. Medical recommendations may require work restrictions or time off from work. Depending on the injury, a worker may require extended therapy or reeducation. Workers with permanent injury may not return to the preinjury level of function, and a physician's input is required to determine the degree of impairment. At each step in the treatment, medical recommendations have the potential to determine the expenditure of considerable resources. For this reason, the traditional doctor-patient relationship is expanded to include employers, insurance carriers, governmental agencies, and the legal system.

In 1970, the US Congress passed the Occupational Safety and Health Act. At the time of its passage, the responsibility for defining and enforcing regulations for workplace safety was left to the individual state governments. The act established the Occupational Safety and Health Administration (OSHA) in the Department of Labor, empowering it to protect the health of workers by setting and enforcing safety standards. In addition, the act established the National Institute for Occupational Safety and Health (NIOSH) in the Department of Health and Human Services. NIOSH was charged to conduct research on matters affecting the safety of workers and thereby to develop and establish recommended health standards. Initially, the act was intended to enforce uniform federal standards. However, it was amended to allow individual states to continue their own systems. The National Commission

on State Workman's Compensation Laws was set up to evaluate and oversee these plans.[1]

Workers' compensation laws currently vary considerably, and a physician who treats occupational injuries should be familiar with the laws and regulatory agencies particular to his or her state of practice. Although the state laws are different, there are four basic concepts similar to each system. Workers are covered for any work-related injury, regardless of negligence. Employees injured at work are entitled to wages and medical care during a term of temporary disability before maximal medical improvement (MMI). After MMI, employees may be entitled to continued medical benefits if a disability persists. The employer covers the costs, usually by premiums paid to a private workers' compensation insurance plan. After MMI is reached, a level of permanent partial or total disability is established, and benefits are assigned accordingly.[2]

Cumulative Trauma Disorder

The notion that some employees may be at risk of sustaining subacute injury as the result of prolonged exposure to certain repetitive activities has received considerable attention. Repetitive strain injury, repetitive trauma injury, and cumulative trauma disorder are terms that have been used to categorize several upper extremity symptoms supposedly brought about by repetitive motions or exacerbated by extreme postures required by certain occupations. The use of these terms has been criticized because of the relative lack of evidence to support a causal link between repetitive motion and the development of any objective upper extremity disorder.[3,4] For this reason, a newer term, work-related musculoskeletal disorder, has been offered to describe the same constellation of ailments. With this newer designation, the terms injury and trauma, which imply the presence of tissue damage, are avoided, and the role of repetitive stress is excluded.

The topic of work-related musculoskeletal disorders is perplexing to physicians for several reasons. One reason is that this category of illness encompasses a variety of potential symptoms that are not necessarily representative of any specific medical condition or diagnosis. Some patients may manifest signs and symptoms refer-

*E. Mark Hammerberg, MD or the department with which he is affiliated has received research or institutional support from Synthes and Osteotech and miscellaneous nonincome support, commercially-derived honoraria, or other nonresearch-related funding from Synthes, Smith & Nephew, and DePuy.

1: Principles of Orthopaedics

able to a well-defined clinical entity such as carpal tunnel syndrome. In such instances, the diagnosis can be established by discrete clinical examination findings and abnormalities noted on electrodiagnostic studies. However, patients with work-related musculoskeletal disorders often present with a vague pattern of upper extremity pain and a relative paucity of objective clinical findings. For example, in one cross-sectional study evaluating a series of 229 patients with a diagnosis of repetitive stress injury, only 29 patients demonstrated objective findings referable to a well-defined musculoskeletal disorder. The remaining 200 patients were characterized by a variety of psychological disturbances, including anxiety, irritability, affective changes, and chronic fatigue.[5]

Some authors have classified repetition strain injury as a functional somatic syndrome.[6] Viewed in this manner, vague reports of upper extremity pain or dysfunction may not be manifestations of actual injury or tissue abnormality. Rather, when reports of pain are associated with nonspecific clinical findings, it has been suggested that such symptoms may relate more to psychosocial or psychiatric phenomena than to workplace exposures or activities.[7] Such symptoms are understood to be the result of somatization, a coping mechanism whereby unresolved or unacceptable psychological conflicts are expressed as physical symptoms.

It has been suggested that patients reporting arm pain in general demonstrate a greater somatizing tendency, increased health anxiety, and increased rates of chronic fatigue syndrome and chronic widespread pain.[8] Patients with vague complaints appear to be most at risk for this type of extremity disorder; those patients with idiopathic pain have been shown to demonstrate more anxiety, helplessness, and fear.[9] Such patients have a greater tendency toward somatic complaints, and they are more likely to rate their pain as severe.[9]

It is understandable that orthopaedic surgeons, trained in the treatment of objectively identifiable anatomic abnormalities, may be apprehensive about directing treatment of this population of patients. It is understandable, also, that this patient population includes those who are least likely to accept a medical opinion that their somatic symptoms have no organic basis. In an era when medical opinions are increasingly challenged, patients having somatoform disorders are more likely to exaggerate their symptoms and to insist on a medical explanation for their perceived infirmity. When workers' compensation claims are at stake, patients have an even greater incentive to secure a medical explanation for their complaints.

When treating such patients, it remains a challenge for the orthopaedic surgeon to remain objective. Some surgeons may be biased, consciously or otherwise, to view this population as malingering, inventing or magnifying symptoms for the purposes of secondary gain. Other surgeons represent the opposite extreme, uncomfortable with uncertainty and craving a medical explanation. Such surgeons are apt to assign a specific diagnosis despite a relative lack of objective clinical criteria.

Neither extreme is beneficial to the patient, and care must be taken to ensure that diagnoses are neither missed nor inappropriately assigned.

Much of the debate surrounding work-related musculoskeletal disorders centers on the relative lack of evidence supporting the notion that such disorders are actually caused or aggravated by conditions at work. Most studies supporting a relationship between activity at work and the development of musculoskeletal pathology are epidemiologic studies by design. Many of these studies have been criticized for their failure to include accepted diagnostic criteria in the identification of upper extremity disorders.[10] Furthermore, with the exception of age and gender, most studies have failed to control for confounding variables.[10] Epidemiologic studies may identify that a population exposed to a supposedly injurious agent (for example, repetitive wrist motion) demonstrates a higher incidence of a known disease or disorder (for example, carpal tunnel syndrome). From this finding, an association may be inferred between the agent and the disorder. However, such an association does not establish a causal link.[3,11]

Carpal Tunnel Syndrome

Work-related carpal tunnel syndrome (compressive neuropathy of the median nerve at the wrist) has received particular attention. Forceful grip has been postulated a biologically plausible mechanism to produce increased pressure on the median nerve. This finding has been corroborated by MRI studies showing that when the wrist is flexed, the median nerve becomes compressed between the flexor tendons and the flexor retinaculum.[12] Also, direct measurements of hydrostatic pressures in the carpal tunnel show that the pressure increases with wrist flexion and extension.[13] However, the evidence linking carpal tunnel syndrome to potentially harmful workplace exposures is limited, and the potential role for repetitive activity in the development of carpal tunnel syndrome continues to be a topic of debate.

It has been observed that the rate of carpal tunnel syndrome in the general population is the same whether or not people perform repetitive activities.[14] Previous studies linking carpal tunnel syndrome to workplace exposure have been criticized for poor methodology, lack of clinical data, and failure to control confounding variables.[15] Many early studies lack documentation of objective baseline data before workplace exposure, so it is difficult to prove a causal link to workplace exposure even if objective clinical disease is subsequently observed. Measuring workplace exposure is likewise difficult if not impossible when said exposure is estimated retrospectively at the time of diagnosis.

Two recent longitudinal studies with objective preexposure data including electrodiagnostic studies have been published.[16,17] Both studies show positive associations between the development of carpal tunnel syndrome and well-known patient-specific (intrinsic) factors. For example, female gender and obesity were both found to have a positive correlation with carpal tunnel

t6sd367asdaoeu

syndrome.[17] Also, the presence of preexisting subclinical median nerve mononeuropathy was found to have a positive correlation with the subsequent development of clinical carpal tunnel syndrome.[16] Neither study demonstrates a significant correlation between workplace activity and the development of carpal tunnel syndrome. One study shows a trend between carpal tunnel syndrome and occupations characterized by higher upper extremity demand, although this trend does not reach statistical significance.[16] The other study shows an inverse relationship, with carpal tunnel syndrome developing less frequently in those occupations requiring higher upper extremity repetitions and heavy lifting.[17]

The notion that computer use, or keyboard activity, may lead to the development of carpal tunnel syndrome is a popular misconception. In a society where up to one half of the workforce uses a computer station for a significant portion of the day, it is no surprise that this topic should receive such attention by the lay press. This topic has received particular scrutiny; however, computer use does not appear to be related to the development of carpal tunnel syndrome.[18] Still, a significant number of workers report symptoms of upper extremity pain and discomfort related to computer use. Although no well-established musculoskeletal disease has been associated with computer use, the idea that employees may experience upper-extremity symptoms as a result of keyboard activity has been broadly accepted by society.

Ergonomics

In an effort to decrease the rate of work-related musculoskeletal disorders, several ergonomic interventions, or workplace modifications, have been investigated. Modifications in keyboard design have been suggested, but there appears to be little evidence to support their effectiveness. Various postural changes have been recommended to reduce the rate of musculoskeletal symptoms in computer users. One randomized study evaluating two recommended postural interventions failed to demonstrate any reduction in the rate of neck and shoulder symptoms.[19] Another recent randomized study suggests that the rate of computer-related musculoskeletal symptoms may be reduced by equipping computer terminals with a broad forearm support.[20] Overall, ergonomic data remain limited. When it comes to the design of computer workstations, there is insufficient evidence to support the broad application of any specific intervention. Furthermore, different employees may respond differently to the same intervention.

Some authors criticize the popular emphasis on ergonomic modifications in the workplace. Given the relative lack of evidence to support a causal relationship between workplace activity and the development of musculoskeletal disorders, it has been suggested that ergonomic intervention cannot lower the prevalence of clinical musculoskeletal disease. It is argued that ergonomic intervention may improve employee comfort,

but it does not reduce the rate of objective musculoskeletal pathology.[4] Even so, it is difficult to understand why employee comfort should not be a priority in its own right. Some have suggested that a broad emphasis on ergonomics has the potential to place employers at undue financial and legal risk.[2] However, it has been demonstrated in multiple industries that formal ergonomic intervention has the potential to decrease reported musculoskeletal symptoms and to reduce time lost from work. Furthermore, these benefits have been associated with an overall cost savings to employers.[21]

It is possible that the institution of formal ergonomic policies may reduce the incidence of work-related musculoskeletal disorders for reasons beyond the prevention of actual tissue injury. For example, employees satisfied with the environment may be more tolerant of symptoms than employees who view their work environment as less hospitable. Workers' perception of the workplace environment and organizational climate has been shown to correlate with the incidence of reported symptoms and frequency of sickness absence.[22] When a company devotes resources to evaluate and implement ergonomic policies, this may represent managerial priorities that promote employee satisfaction in addition to safety. It is possible that the tendency of employees to report work-related illness is reduced when it is perceived that a company has conspicuous policies in place for the purposes of protecting workers.

Treating Injured Workers

The treatment of a work-related injury should be essentially no different than the treatment of a similar injury sustained outside of work. However, when care is provided within the context of a workers' compensation system, the treating physician takes on several roles not otherwise assumed in the care of patients. The treating physician becomes the gatekeeper for the provision of benefits, including ongoing disability payments as well as final settlements. In the care of an injured worker, a doctor's treatment recommendations translate into work restrictions and time off from work. Given the potential for considerable expense, recommendations are scrutinized with every clinic visit. The employer or insurance carrier may request an independent medical evaluation, especially if surgery or prolonged therapy is part of the recommended treatment plan. In this way, the traditional doctor-patient relationship is modified somewhat, as the patient yields a portion of confidentiality to qualify for workers' compensation benefits.

Documentation

In the care of an injured worker, obtaining a detailed history is of paramount importance. As the details of an injury may become the subject of a subsequent dispute at the time of settlement hearings, it is important to record these details at the time of the first clinic visit or consultation. For an employee to receive workers' compensation benefits, a physician's statement is required to establish that the injury is, indeed, related to work. In addition to clarifying the details surrounding the mechanism of injury, the treating physician should inquire into the patient's preinjury level of function. Any preexisting medical conditions or previous injuries should be documented at the time of initial evaluation. With the passage of time, it becomes increasingly difficult for a patient to recall the exact details of his or her injury. After a prolonged or painful recovery, a patient's estimation of preinjury status may be especially unreliable.

Throughout the course of treatment and recovery, the physician will be expected to correspond with the insurance company and/or employer regarding disability status and expected return to work. Often, this documentation may be provided by forwarding a copy of the relevant clinic notes. Some companies have specific forms to be filled out by the attending physician at every clinic visit. At times, providing requested documentation may seem to be an especially laborious task. It should be understood that communication regarding patient progress is essential for a successful workers' compensation system. A physician who is reluctant to provide appropriate and timely documentation may delay the administration of benefits and impede patient recovery.

Rehabilitation and Return to Work

Until full recovery or MMI is reached, a patient is considered to be partially or totally disabled. During recovery, treatment recommendations translate into work restrictions. If the workplace cannot accommodate specific work restrictions, then return to work may be postponed until such time that work restrictions can be modified. It may be difficult for a physician, unfamiliar with an employee's workplace or usual activity, to recommend specific modifications to the workplace routine. Often, generic light duty or specific lifting restrictions are suggested, and specific modifications are avoided. On-site evaluation and modification of workplace characteristics by nurse case managers trained in ergonomic intervention has been suggested as a possible solution to this dilemma. When this so-called integrated case management has been used, it has been shown not only to improve worker satisfaction, but to decrease the time spent away from work.[23,24]

Barriers to Recovery

Patients treated for work-related injuries have been noted to have poorer results than patients treated for similar injuries sustained outside of the workplace. This topic has received considerable attention and has been the subject of a recent meta-analysis.[25] It seems clear that compensation status is an independent risk factor for poor functional outcomes following surgery, and orthopaedic surgeons treating injured workers should be aware of this information. It has been suggested that injured workers may tend to exaggerate symptoms to validate workers' compensation claims or to strengthen their case for planned litigation. It is possible that the

reporting of symptoms may be influenced by coaching from lawyers, but it seems equally plausible that those who are more severely injured are more likely to retain the services of a lawyer. It remains a challenge for the surgeon to maintain an objective perspective, for compensation status provides a convenient opportunity to blame the patient for poor surgical results.

Disparities in the delivery of health care are known to be associated with race and socioeconomic status. As alarming as this fact may be, it is especially troubling that such trends should be observed in a workers' compensation system designed to guarantee equal access to care for all injured employees. A recent study evaluating workers' compensation claimants with low back injuries demonstrates that African Americans and claimants of lower socioeconomic status have significantly poorer outcomes when compared with Caucasian claimants or those of higher socioeconomic status.[26] Two potential explanations or trends are offered: African Americans and patients with lower socioeconomic status face greater obstacles to their recovery; or different standards are used in the diagnosis and treatment of patients according to their race or socioeconomic status. Physicians may not be able to change the former trend, but they are in a prime position to diminish, if not eliminate, the latter trend.

Patients who seek treatment of a work-related musculoskeletal disorder can be expected to show anxiety regarding their work demands, the potential for prolonged disability, and their ability to return to work. It has been shown that patient expectations may predict outcomes following treatment and rehabilitation.[27] With this factor in mind, the importance of communication between the patient and the physician is paramount. Surgeons may be hesitant to explore the psychological aspects of an injury. However, an inquiry regarding patient expectations may identify those patients who could benefit from psychological support or additional education before surgery. Postoperatively, dialogue with patients should include a discussion of anxiety regarding return to work and expectations regarding disability. In this way, patients with unrealistic expectations can be identified and educated accordingly. With realistic expectations, patients may be less likely to become frustrated with their rehabilitation and more likely to adhere to treatment recommendations.

Patients with chronic disabling work-related musculoskeletal disorders pose a particular challenge. Often, the goal of returning to work is delayed while multiple therapeutic interventions fail to return the patient to a productive status. Many such patients demonstrate a lack of belief in their diagnosis, and they are unwilling or unable to accept their physician's advice or explanations. When patients continue to seek the advice of additional physicians or specialists, they may become labeled as "doctor shopping." This type of behavior has been criticized because it increases direct health care costs without providing obvious benefit to the patient. The tendency for patients to pursue additional medical advice after the completion of a tertiary rehabilitation program has been identified as a risk factor for poor outcomes.[28] While patients continue to seek additional opinions, their return to productivity is delayed. Meanwhile, workers' compensation settlements are postponed, final disability status remains unresolved, and disability payments continue.

Work Hardening

The concept of work hardening is meant to address those patients who have failed to return to work after initial treatment and therapy have been completed. The goal is return to work or productivity, not relief of pain. The proposed work environment is evaluated, and the anticipated occupational routine is detailed. In this way, the therapist can tailor therapy so that the injured worker develops the ability to tolerate specific activities that will be expected upon return to work. It has been shown that work-hardening programs including a cognitive-behavioral approach are more effective at reducing the time off work than programs focusing specifically on physical conditioning.[29] With this in mind, the therapy is as much about developing psychological coping skills as it is about regaining muscular strength, range of motion, or endurance.

Independent Medical Evaluation and Impairment Ratings

When a patient reaches the point where no additional treatment is recommended and no additional therapy is anticipated, they are said to have reached MMI. When MMI is reached, some patients may have recovered completely, with no significant lasting disability. However, some patients will be left with a degree of permanent disability. MMI marks the end of treatment and the end of ongoing disability payments. The assignment of permanent partial disability allows for patients to reach a final settlement and, hopefully, to move on with their lives.

The assignment of permanent disability status in the workers' compensation system is especially problematic. In an effort to limit costs, the opinions of an outside physician are often sought to settle disputes. If the treating physician is considered to be the patient's advocate in the workers' compensation system, then he or she must be expected to take the side of the patient in disability proceedings. In this way, the treating physician is necessarily biased. Independent medical evaluations (IMEs) have been established as a means of avoiding this expected (and appropriate) bias. Whereas the treating physician is charged to act in the best interests of his or her patient, the IME physician must act as an impartial observer. The IME doctor is considered to be more of a scientist than a physician. However, the fact that most IME physicians are paid by insurance companies or employers means it is possible that IME opinions may not be entirely free from bias. If an IME physician develops a track record showing no tendency to favor one side over the other, then his or her opinions may be considered more credible.

Table 1

Waddell's Nonorganic Physical Signs in Low Back Pain

1. Tenderness	Tenderness related to physical disease should be specific and localized to specific anatomic structures. Superficial: tenderness to pinch or light touch over a wide area of lumbar skin. Nonanatomic: deep tenderness over a wide area, not localized to a specific structure
2. Simulation tests	These tests should not be uncomfortable. Axial loading — reproduction of low back pain with vertical pressure on the skull. Rotation — reproduction of back pain when shoulders and pelvis are passively rotated in the same plane
3. Distraction tests	Findings that are present during physical examination and disappear at other times, particularly while the patient is distracted
4. Regional disturbances	Findings inconsistent with neuroanatomy. Motor — nonanatomic voluntary release or unexplained giving way of muscle groups. Sensory — nondermatomal sensory abnormalities
5. Overreaction	Disproportionate verbal or physical reactions

(Reproduced from Moy OJ, Ablove RH: Work-related illnesses, cumulative trauma, and compensation, in Vaccaro AR (ed): Orthopaedic Knowledge Update, ed 8. Rosemont, IL, American Academy of Orthopaedic Surgeons, 2005, pp 143-148.)

The setting of an IME examination has the potential to be somewhat tense, and it is understandable that a patient may view the IME physician with distrust. The relationship between patient and IME physician is almost adversarial by definition. With this in mind, the physician should make every effort to maintain a neutral bearing and a straightforward manner. The potential for an uncooperative patient to exaggerate symptoms has received a fair amount of attention. Waddell's nonorganic physical signs, categorized into five groups, are a well-accepted measure of this tendency (Table 1). It is suggested that if patients demonstrate multiple positive signs from three or more of the five types there may be a high likelihood of nonorganic pathology.[30] The authors note that nonorganic signs are common in the general population, and they caution against giving too much significance to the isolated positive sign as false-positive results may occur. Accusations of malin-

1: Principles of Orthopaedics

gering are difficult to prove, and should be avoided if possible. Instead, neutral language such as "the symptoms are not entirely explained by physical findings" may be most useful.[31]

The process of performing impairment ratings and completing disability evaluations is characterized by a unique interface between the medical and legal professions. The physician who completes IMEs and performs impairment ratings should be familiar with several legal terms. Apportionment is the process of determining the degree to which each of several exposures or injuries has contributed to a specific disability. Impairment is the loss of function resulting from an anatomic or physiologic derangement. As such, impairment is understood to be a medical designation, and it forms the basis for determining disability status. Disability is defined as a limitation of an individual's capacity to meet certain personal, social, or occupational demands. As such, disability is not an objective medical designation. Rather, the definition of any given disability is subject to change according to the sociologic and political forces that shape public policy and opinion. In the context of work-related injury, causation refers to the effect of a proposed injurious agent toward the development of an illness or injury. Whether or not the alleged agent could have caused the illness is a medical question. Whether or not the alleged agent did cause the illness is a legal question.[32]

The American Medical Association has published a series of guidelines (*Guides to the Evaluation of Permanent Impairment*) to standardize the determination of permanent impairment.[33] Whereas the determination of impairment ratings is known to be an imperfect science, the criteria set forth in the *Guides* has been shown to be reliable and accurate when compared with other measures of musculoskeletal function.[34] Despite an explicit caveat in the introduction to the *Guides* that the criteria are not intended to be used for the determination of workplace disability, no other reliable system has been established for this purpose. The criteria of the *Guides* have been broadly accepted, and these criteria are commonly used to establish impairment ratings and associated disability in most workers' compensation systems.

Summary

Work-related illness is characterized by a variety of psychological and sociologic challenges not common to injuries sustained outside the workplace. Therefore, the orthopaedic surgeon who undertakes the care of injured workers should expect to provide services beyond the usual evaluation and treatment of an injury. For patients to receive timely treatment and therapy, the treating physician must provide accurate documentation regarding the injury, the diagnosis, and the expected treatment. To facilitate the distribution of disability benefits, timely updates are required, and the input of an outside physician in the form of an IME should be expected. A physician who understands the unique problems facing an injured worker is most likely to tailor therapy when indicated and to return a worker to productivity in the shortest time possible.

Annotated References

1. Gochfeld M: Occupational medicine practice in the United States since the industrial revolution. *J Occup Environ Med* 2005;47:115-131.

   This article discusses the history of occupational medicine.

2. AAOS Committee on Occupational Health: Workers' compensation systems. *A Physician's Primer on Worker's Compensation*. Rosemont, IL, American Academy of Orthopaedic Surgeons, 1992, pp 5-13.

3. Hooper G, Sher JL, Mulligan PJ: Work-related disorders of the upper limb. *J Bone Joint Surg Br* 2002;84:322-323.

4. Szabo RM, King KJ: Repetitive stress injury: Diagnosis or self-fulfilling prophecy? *J Bone Joint Surg Am* 2000;82:1314-1322.

5. Miller MH, Topliss DJ: Chronic upper limb pain syndrome (repetitive strain injury) in the Australian workforce: A systematic cross sectional rheumatological study of 229 patients. *J Rheumatol* 1988;15:1705-1712.

6. Barsky AJ, Borus JF: Functional somatic syndromes. *Ann Intern Med* 1999;130:910-921.

7. Ireland DCR: Psychological and physical aspects of occupational arm pain. *J Hand Surg Br* 1985;13:5-10.

8. Ryall C, Coggon D, Peveler R, Reading I, Palmer KT: A case-control study of risk factors for arm pain presenting to primary care services. *Occup Med (Lond)* 2006;56:137-143.

   This case-control study showed that patients with upper extremity pain are more likely to have a greater somatizing tendency compared with other patients. This tendency was found to be no greater among individuals with vague pain compared with those with a discrete diagnosis. Level of evidence: III.

9. Ring D, Kadzielski BA, Malhotra L, Sang-Gil PL, Jupiter JB: Psychological factors associated with idiopathic arm pain. *J Bone Joint Surg Am* 2005;87:374-380.

   This prospective cohort study compared patients with idiopathic upper extremity pain with patients with known upper extremity pathology. Those with idiopathic pain demonstrated greater anxiety, helplessness, and pain magnification, and they demonstrated a greater tendency to report somatic symptoms. Level of evidence: III.

10. Vender MI, Kasdan ML, Truppa KL: Upper extremity disorders: A literature review to determine work-relatedness. *J Hand Surg Am* 1995;20:534-541.

11. Melhorn JM: Repetitive strain injuries: Fact or fiction. *Curr Opin Orthop* 2004;15:226-233.

    The authors reviewed the literature regarding three diagnoses frequently described as repetitive strain injuries: carpal tunnel syndrome, lateral epicondylitis, and shoulder impingement. The evidence for and against repetition as an etiologic factor is presented. Level of evidence: V.

12. Skie M, Zeiss J, Ebraheim NA, Jackson WT: Carpal tunnel changes and median nerve compression during wrist flexion and extention seen by magnetic resonance imaging. *J Hand Surg Am* 1990;15:934-939.

13. Szabo RM, Chidgey LK: Stress carpal tunnel pressures in carpal tunnel patients and normal patients. *J Hand Surg Am* 1989;14:624-627.

14. Atroshi I, Gummesson C, Johnsson R, Ornstein E, Ranstam J, Rosen I: Prevalence of carpal tunnel syndrome in a general population. *JAMA* 1999;282:153-158.

15. Szabo RM: Carpal tunnel syndrome as a repetitive motion disorder. *Clin Orthop Relat Res* 1998;351:78-89.

16. Gell N, Werner RA, Franzblau A, Ulin SS, Armstrong TJ: A longitudinal study of industrial and clerical workers: Incidence of carpal tunnel syndrome and assessment of risk factors. *J Occup Rehabil* 2005;15:47-55.

    This study followed 432 clerical workers over an average of 5.4 years. Predictors of developing carpal tunnel syndrome included abnormal baseline nerve conduction velocity studies and a history of hand numbness or dysesthesia. There was a trend for those with repetitive hand and wrist activities to develop carpal tunnel syndrome, but this did not reach statistical significance.

17. Nathan PA, Istvan JA, Meadows KD: A longitudinal study of predictors of research-defined carpal tunnel syndrome in industrial workers: Findings at 17 years. *J Hand Surg Br* 2005;30:593-598.

    This study presents data for 166 industrial workers followed for 17 years. Predictors of carpal tunnel syndrome included obesity and female gender. Occupations with repetitive motions and heavy lifting were shown to have a decreased rate of carpal tunnel syndrome. Use of vibratory tools was correlated with an increased rate of carpal tunnel syndrome.

18. Andersen JH, Thomsen JF, Overgaard E, et al: Computer use and carpal tunnel syndrome: A 1-year follow-up study. *JAMA* 2003;289:2963-2969.

19. Gerr F, Marcus M, Monteilh C, Hannan L, Ortiz D, Kleinbaum D: A randomized controlled trial of postural interventions for prevention of musculoskeletal symptoms among computer users. *Occup Environ Med* 2005;62:478-487.

    This randomized controlled study evaluated two recommended postural interventions for computer users. Neither intervention was shown to have a significant effect.

20. Rempel DM, Krause N, Goldberg R, Benner D, Hudes M, Goldner GU: A randomised controlled trial evaluating the effects of two workstation interventions on upper body pain and incident musculoskeletal disorders among computer operators. *Occup Environ Med* 2006; 63:300-306.

    This randomized controlled trial tested the effects of four different ergonomic interventions for computer operators. Use of a large forearm support combined with ergonomic training was associated with a significant decrease in reports of upper extremity pain.

21. Melhorn JM, Gardner P: How we prevent prevention of musculoskeletal disorders in the workplace. *Clin Orthop Relat Res* 2004;419:285-296.

    This review of the literature supports ergonomic interventions and workplace modifications. Several case studies are presented to show that such intervention programs can decrease workers' compensation claims and result in overall cost savings.

22. Piirainen H, Rasanen K, Kivimaki M: Organizational climate, perceived work-related symptoms and sickness absence: A population-based survey. *J Occup Environ Med* 2003;45:175-184.

23. Bernacki EJ, Tsai SP: Ten years' experience using an integrated workers' compensation management system to control workers' compensation costs. *J Occup Environ Med* 2003;45:508-516.

24. Feuerstein M, Huang GD, Ortiz JM, Shaw WS, Miller VI, Wood PM: Integrated case management for work-related upper-extremity disorders: Impact of patient satisfaction on health and work status. *J Occup Environ Med* 2003;45:803-812.

25. Harris I, Mulford J, Solomon M, van Gelder JM, Young J: Association between compensation status and outcome after surgery: A meta-analysis. *JAMA* 2005;293: 1644-1652.

    The authors present a meta-analysis reviewing the literature that has reported workers' compensation claim status in relation to surgical intervention. The presence of workers' compensation claims is shown to be an independent risk factor for poor outcome. Level of evidence: III.

26. Chibnall JT, Tait RC, Andresen EM, Nortin M: Race and socioeconomic differences in post-settlement outcomes for African American and Caucasian workers' compensation claimants with low back injuries. *Pain* 2005;114:462-472.

    This study describes results of a population-based telephone survey evaluating the outcomes for workers' compensation claimants in Missouri. Functional outcomes as well as financial variables were compared among Caucasian and African Americans and patients with low socioeconomic status. African American race and low socioeconomic status are risk factors for poor functional outcomes and predictors of financial struggle. In this study, the effect of race appears to be independent of socioeconomic status. Level of evidence: III.

1: Principles of Orthopaedics

27. Cole DC, Mondloch MV, Hogg-Johnson S: Early Claimant Cohort Prognostic Modelling Group: Listening to injured workers. How recovery expectations predict outcomes: A prospective study. *CMAJ* 2002;166: 749-754.

28. Proctor TJ, Mayer TG, Gatchel RJ, McGeary DD: Unremitting health-care-utilization outcomes of tertiary rehabilitation of patients with chronic musculoskeletal disorders. *J Bone Joint Surg Am* 2004;86:62-69.

    In this study, a group of patients is identified on the basis that they continue to seek the input of additional health care providers after completing a tertiary rehabilitation program. Compared with patients who do not seek the advice of additional providers, these patients are more likely to have poor outcomes, less likely to return to work, and less likely to have settled their legal disputes by 1 year following completion of therapy. Level of evidence: III.

29. Scholnstein E, Kenny DT, Keating J, Koes BW: Work conditioning, work hardening and functional restoration for workers with back and neck pain. *The Cochrane Database of Sytematic Reviews*, 2007. Available at www.interscience.wiley.com/cochrane/clsysrev/ articles/CD001822/frame.html. Accessed October 1, 2007.

    The authors concluded that back pain management programs that included features such as a cognitive-behavioral approach are better than usual care at reducing sick days for some workers with back and neck pain.

30. Waddell G, McCulloch JA, Kummel E, Verner RM: Non-organic physical signs in low-back pain. *Spine* 1980;5:117-125.

31. Mandell PJ: Malingering and somatization, in Grace TG (ed): *Independent Medical Evaluations*. Rosemont, IL, American Academy of Orthopaedic Surgeons, 2001, pp 71-79.

32. Melhorn JM: Impairment and disability evaluations: Understanding the process. *J Bone Joint Surg Am* 2001; 83:1905-1911.

33. Cocchiarella L, Andersson GBJ (eds): *Guides to the Evaluation of Permanent Impairment*, ed 5. Chicago, IL, AMA Press, 2000.

34. McCarthy ML, McAndrew MP, MacKenzie EJ, et al: Correlation between the measures of impairment according to the modified system of the American Medical Association, and function. *J Bone Joint Surg Am* 1998; 80:1034-1042.

Chapter 14

Outcomes Assessment and Evidence-Based Practice Guidelines in Orthopaedic Surgery

Michael W. Keith, MD

Introduction

The communication of ideas, opinion, and measurement of clinical outcomes and indicators of quality of practice is currently more common and timely in the field of orthopaedic surgery. The day-to-day practice of surgery is open to greater external scrutiny, analysis, comparison for continued improvement, legislation, and leveraged performance assessment by patients, organizations, payers, and government entities. The standards of practice are increasingly set by stakeholders and social engineers.

The prudent surgeon needs to understand the complexity of this interaction and requires the ability to respond to these market-economic, ethical-professional, and practical-regulatory forces to chart a surgical practice strategy. This chapter describes the changes in recent years in the quest for quality in orthopaedic surgical practice and the means to achieve it that are under development. Of primary importance is the idea that the control over setting standards of practice is no longer only in the hands of the scientist or medical author. Many of the origins of evidence-based medicine and the key studies are coming from professional management and policy literature. Many of the decisions in health care policy are coming from studies of outcome not originated by the treating physicians.

Quality as the Guiding Principle

The current definition of quality in health care began with the Institute of Medicine (IOM) report *Crossing the Quality Chasm: A New Health System for the 21st Century*, in which the staggering financial and social impact of hospital and clinical practice errors were revealed. This report led to reevaluation of ways to improve quality in health care and patient safety and better promote patient-centered medicine. Table 1 presents a comprehensive listing of current resources and electronic access to sources and documents.

Measures to improve patient safety include elimination of preventable adverse outcomes. The American Academy of Orthopaedic Surgeons (AAOS) has conducted a safety campaign through the widely familiar "Sign Your Site" program. The Leapfrog Group has promoted the implementation of electronic medical records because of their ability to improve legibility and detect errors before they are committed. In addition, the efforts of the Centers for Medicare and Medicaid Services (CMS) through the Doctor's Office Quality–Information Technology initiative (commonly known as DOQ-IT) and the US Department of Veterans Affairs' development of electronic medical record software (Veterans Health Information System and Technology, commonly known as VistA) are noteworthy. Safety campaigns for legibility of records, laterality (right or left side of the body), identification of the patient for surgery using unique characteristics such as birth date or phone number, and simple "time-outs" (a halt in surgical procedures to obtain concurrence of nursing, anesthesia, and surgical teams on patient and procedure) during surgical preparation have shown that changing the culture of surgery is as important as its practice.

Not all patients receive the quality and quantity of health care the medical profession in the United States believes they need. One study showed that approximately 50% of indicated care was provided.[1] Despite the shortfall, national costs of health care have almost doubled over a 5-year period and the proportion of gross domestic product devoted to health care rises annually. Others have found that the existence of quality care and reporting does not change the practice preferences of practitioners.[2]

For the financial stakeholder, it is "value" (benefit/cost) that is the quality objective. For the health care regulator, it is value or "efficiency" (outcomes/cost). For CMS, the fixed total cost of health care as a fraction of gross domestic product is a key indicator of successful management. For the practitioner, the best clinical practices, including elimination of disparate care distribution and the delivery of patient-centered care, are believed to be quality objectives.

Table 1

Internet Resources for Health Care Quality*

American Academy of Orthopaedic Surgeons (AAOS)
"Clinical Guidelines are valuable tools that will allow you to advance the physician-patient communications process and enhance the diagnosis and treatment of musculoskeletal conditions. The guidelines not only support referrals when working with managed care companies, but they can also be used as an educational tool when interacting with patients."
http://www.aaos.org/Research/guidelines/guide.asp
AAOS is the leading developer of guidelines and performance measures for musculoskeletal disorders.

Agency for Healthcare Research and Quality (AHRQ)
"The Agency for Healthcare Research and Quality (AHRQ) is the lead Federal agency charged with improving the quality, safety, efficiency, and effectiveness of health care for all Americans. As one of 12 agencies within the Department of Health and Human Services, AHRQ supports health services research that will improve the quality of health care and promote evidence-based decision making." http://www.ahrq.gov/
AHRQ is a national support agency for research into quality assessment and implementation.

National Guideline Clearinghouse (NGC)
"The National Guideline Clearinghouse™ (NGC) is a comprehensive database of evidence-based clinical practice guidelines and related documents. NGC is an initiative of the Agency for Healthcare Research and Quality (AHRQ), US Department of Health and Human Services."
http://www.ngc.gov/
The NGC is a resource for published Clinical Practice Guidelines. AAOS has two current guidelines on the Website.

American Medical Association Physician Consortium
"The American Medical Association (AMA)-convened Physician Consortium for Performance Improvement® (Consortium) is committed to enhancing quality of care and patient safety by taking the lead in the development, testing, and maintenance of evidence-based clinical performance measures and measurement resources for physicians. The Consortium is comprised of over 100 national medical specialty and state medical societies; the Council of Medical Specialty Societies; American Board of Medical Specialties and its member-boards; experts in methodology and data collection; the Agency for Healthcare Research and Quality; and Centers for Medicare and Medicaid Services."
http://www.ama-assn.org/
This group will prepare performance measures for national implementation by government and likely by payers.

Institute of Medicine (IOM) of the National Academies
"The nation turns to the Institute of Medicine (IOM) of the National Academies for science-based advice on matters of biomedical science, medicine, and health. A nonprofit organization specifically created for this purpose as well as an honorific membership organization, the IOM was chartered in 1970 as a component of the National Academy of Sciences." The IOM has issued an important report supporting pay-for-performance strategies for quality improvement. This endorsement paves the way for further efforts to tie the overall budget for national health care to quality improvement and proof of quality practice. A mechanism to achieve this objective has not been completed and is under discussion. Government leaders have called for hundreds of guidelines to be created and implemented.
http://www.iom.edu/
This group of highly qualified leaders evaluates health care status and technology and makes policy recommendations to the US government and public. Periodic assessments of topics include expert opinion and evidence analysis.

Pay for Performance
"The Institute of Medicine released on September 21, 2006 a report by the Committee on Redesigning Health Insurance Performance Measures, Payment, and Performance Improvement Programs called 'Rewarding Provider Performance: Aligning Incentives in Medicare.' The report analyzes the risks and potential benefits of instituting a pay-for-performance program within Medicare and also provides recommendations for implementing such a program."
http://www.iom.edu/Object.File/Master/37/236/11723_report_brief.pdf
This brief report, available on the Website noted above, is a roadmap for implementation of pay for performance.

Dartmouth Atlas
"The Dartmouth Atlas Project works to accurately describe how medical resources are distributed and used in the United States. The project offers comprehensive information and analysis about national, regional, and local markets, as well as individual hospitals and their affiliated physicians, in order to provide a basis for improving health and health systems."
http://www.dartmouthatlas.org/
The Dartmouth Atlas provides graphical comparisons of disparities of care and variations across the country.

Table 1

Internet Resources for Health Care Quality* (continued)

CMS Physician Voluntary Reporting Program
"As part of its overall quality improvement efforts, CMS is launching the Physician Voluntary Reporting Program (PVRP). This new program builds on Medicare's comprehensive efforts to substantially improve the health and function of our beneficiaries by preventing chronic disease complications, avoiding preventable hospitalizations, and improving the quality of care delivered. Under the voluntary reporting program, physicians who choose to participate will help capture data about the quality of care provided to Medicare beneficiaries, in order to identify the most effective ways to use the quality measures in routine practice and to support physicians in their efforts to improve quality of care. Voluntary reporting of quality data through the PVRP will begin in January 2006."
http://www.cms.hhs.gov/
This program assesses compliance with new preoperative antibiotic administration guidelines, for example.

National Committee for Quality Assurance
"The National Committee for Quality Assurance (NCQA) is the leading independent organization providing information that allows employers and consumers of health care to distinguish among health plans and physicians based on quality of care."
http://www.ncqa.org/
NCQA is a national reference for health care groups, health maintenance organizations, preferred provider organizations, and eventually practitioner-level quality.

National Quality Forum
"The National Quality Forum (NQF) is a not-for-profit membership organization created to develop and implement a national strategy for health care quality measurement and reporting. A shared sense of urgency about the impact of health care quality on patient outcomes, workforce productivity, and health care costs prompted leaders in the public and private sectors to create the NQF as a mechanism to bring about national change."
http://www.qualityforum.org/
NQF is an influential national stakeholder policy making group.

The Leapfrog Group
"The Leapfrog Group is a voluntary program aimed at mobilizing employer purchasing power to alert America's health industry that big leaps in health care safety, quality, and customer value will be recognized and rewarded. Among other initiatives, Leapfrog works with its employer members to encourage transparency and easy access to health care information and rewards hospitals that have a proven record of high quality care."
http://www.leapfroggroup.org/

Premier Pay for Performance Health Initiative
"The CMS/Premier Pay-for-Performance Demonstration (or Hospital Quality Incentive Demonstration) is the first national pay-for-performance project of its kind, designed to determine if financial incentives are effective at improving the quality of inpatient hospital care. The three-year project is conducted by the Centers for Medicare and Medicaid Services (CMS) and Premier Inc. More than 260 hospitals are voluntarily participating. The project's foundation for tracking a hospital's performance is Premier's Perspective™ database, the largest clinical comparative database in the nation."
http://www.premierinc.com/quality-safety/tools-services/p4p/hqi/index.jsp
This program is an example of process-based quality improvement, providing incentives to hospitals for reporting and achieving care improvements.

Institute for Work and Health
"We are an independent, not-for-profit research organization whose mission is to conduct and share research with workers, labour, employers, clinicians and policy-makers to promote, protect and improve the health of working people. Since 1990, we have been providing research and producing evidence-based products to inform and assist clinicians, researchers, policy-makers, employers, labour and workers. We also train and provide mentorship for the next generation of work and health researchers."
http://www.iwh.on.ca/
The Canadian Institute is a key partner in the development and maintenance of health care outcomes measures and instruments. Many of the currently used outcomes measures are a result of the efforts of this group.

RAND Corporation
This research and development group assesses clinical practice guidelines, outcomes measures, and guidelines created by health organizations.
http://www.rand.org/
The RAND Assessment of Guidelines for Worker's Compensation is available at
http://www.rand.org/pubs/monographs/MG400/index.html

Table 1

Internet Resources for Health Care Quality* (continued)

Pacific Business Group on Health (PBGH)
"The Pacific Business Group on Health is a nonprofit association of many of the nation's largest purchasers of health care, based in California. PBGH represents both public and private purchasers who cover over 3 million Americans, seeking to improve the quality of health care while moderating costs. The members of PBGH range from large public and private purchasers such as Bank of America, CalPERS, FedEx, Target, the University of California and Wells Fargo, to thousands of small businesses in California that we serve through our small employer purchasing pool, PacAdvantage. For fifteen years, PBGH has been a catalyst promoting performance measurement and public reporting at every level of the health care system to improve performance and to help consumers make better choices."
http://www.pbgh.org/news/eletters/documents/PBGH-Medicare-WaysMeans-03-15-05-Att.pdf
http://www.pbgh.org
PBGH is a strong advocate of pay for performance. The Congressional testimony available at the above cited Website is a summary of the organization's many efforts in the private sector.

World Health Organization (WHO) International Classification of Functioning, Disability and Health (ICF)
"As a new member of WHO Family of International Classifications, ICF describes how people live with their health condition. ICF is a classification of health and health related domains that describe body functions and structures, activities and participation. The domains are classified from body, individual and societal perspectives. Since an individual's functioning and disability occurs in a context, ICF also includes a list of environmental factors. ICF is useful to understand and measure health outcomes. It can be used in clinical settings, health services or surveys at the individual or population level. Thus ICF complements ICD-10, The International Statistical Classification of Diseases and Related Health Problems and therefore is looking beyond mortality and disease."
http://www.who.int/classifications/icf/en/
WHO believes that health quality is not merely an expression of disease and treatment but should include the context of life events and forces that shape decisions and perceptions regarding medical care. This is a better explanation for how patients choose their care.

Ambulatory Care Quality Alliance
"In September 2004, the American Academy of Family Physicians (AAFP), the American College of Physicians (ACP), America's Health Insurance Plans (AHIP), and the Agency for Healthcare Research and Quality (AHRQ), joined together to lead a collaborative effort for determining, under the most expedient timeframe, how to most effectively and efficiently improve performance measurement, data aggregation and reporting in the ambulatory care setting.
The mission of this effort—named the Ambulatory Care Quality Alliance (ACQA)—is to improve health care quality and patient safety through a collaborative process in which key stakeholders agree on a strategy for measuring performance at the physician level; collecting and aggregating data in the least burdensome way; and reporting meaningful information to consumers, physicians and other stakeholders to inform choices and improve outcomes."
http://www.aqaalliance.org/
Ambulatory Quality Alliance (AQA) is a leading voice in this quest for practicality. These interest groups represent physicians in the debate and evolution of quality standards.

* Quoted descriptions are from the organizations' Websites.

The user model for "value-based purchasing" of health care is a well-informed patient who is able to choose to purchase cost-effective, high-quality care, including performance information about the individual providers.

The Physician Quality Assessment Paradigm

Fundamental to an assessment of individual practitioner quality is the notion that the measurement is of an attributable action. Any performance measure must be applied to something that the surgeon is responsible for and can influence, or it will reflect system or process rather than physician activity. The search for inexpensive methods to achieve this goal continues. Additional mandatory reporting without incentive has stalled these programs because of the time and, implicitly, cost associated with reporting aimed at reducing compensation. Although many incentive formulae for these programs can exist and leaders of national quality agencies and organizations such as National Quality Forum, American Medical Association, American College of Surgeons, CMS, and IOM have consistently recommended them, most payers have chosen zero-sum formulae in which all providers compete for the same budget and pay discounts and penalties for deviating from local health standards.

Single-payer economies with collectivized decision-making leverage are becoming more common. In most metropolitan areas, through mergers and acquisitions, patient access and therefore reimbursement rules are

Table 2

Levels of Evidence for Primary Research Question*

Types of Studies

	Therapeutic Studies Investigating the results of treatment	Prognostic Studies Investigating the effect of a patient characteristic on the outcome of disease	Diagnostic Studies Investigating a diagnostic test	Economic and Decision Analyses Developing an economic or decision model
Level I	• High-quality randomized trial with statistically significant difference or no statistically significant difference but narrow CIs • Systematic review[†] of level I RCTs (and study results were homogeneous[‡])	• High-quality prospective study[§] (all patients were enrolled at the same point in their disease with ≥ 80% follow-up of enrolled patients) • Systematic review[†] of level I studies	• Testing of previously developed diagnostic criteria on consecutive patients (with universally applied reference "gold" standard) • Systematic review[†] of Level I studies	• Sensible costs and alternatives; values obtained from many studies; with multiway sensitivity analyses • Systematic review[†] of level I studies
Level II	• Lesser quality RCT (eg, < 80% follow-up, no blinding, or improper randomization) • Prospective[§] comparative study[‖] • Systematic review[†] of level II studies or level I studies with inconsistent results	• Retrospective[¶] study • Untreated controls from a RCT • Lesser quality prospective study (eg, patients enrolled at different points in their disease or < 80% follow-up) • Systematic review[†] of level II studies	• Development of diagnostic criteria on consecutive patients (with universally applied reference "gold" standard) • Systematic review[†] of level II studies	• Sensible costs and alternatives; values obtained from limited studies; with multiway sensitivity analyses • Systematic review[†] of level II studies
Level III	• Case control study[#] • Retrospective[¶] comparative study[‖] • Systematic review[†] of level III studies	• Case control study[#]	• Study of nonconsecutive patients; without consistently applied reference "gold" standard • Systematic review[†] of level III studies	• Analyses based on limited alternatives and costs; and poor estimates • Systematic review[†] of level III studies
Level IV	• Case series**	• Case series	• Case-control study • Poor reference standard	• Analyses with no sensitivity analyses
Level V	• Expert opinion	• Expert opinion	• Expert opinion	• Expert opinion

*A complete assessment of quality of individual studies requires critical appraisal of all aspects of the study design.
[†]A combination of results from two or more prior studies.
[‡]Studies provided consistent results.
[§]Study was started before the first patient enrolled.
[‖]Patients treated one way (eg, cemented hip arthroplasty) compared with a group of patients treated in another way (eg, cementless hip arthroplasty) at the same institution.
[¶]The study was started after the first patient enrolled.
[#]Patients identified for the study based on their outcome, called cases (eg, failed total arthroplasty are compared with those who did not have outcome, called controls, eg, successful total hip arthroplasty).
**Patients treated one way with no comparison group of patients treated in another way.
CI= confidence interval; RCT= randomized clinical trial
Data for this table are from http://www.ejbjs.org/misc/public/instrux.shtml and http://cebm.net/levels_of_evidence.asp.

determined by a few competing payers, multispecialty groups, or federal programs. Providers have decreasing control and leverage, which results in lower payments and more regulations.

Public reporting has been a fundamental part of the movement toward influencing surgeon performance. This has taken the form of report cards, publication of rank ordering, classification of practitioners based on performance measures, comparisons of mortality, and other outcomes.

Business principles may be the guiding force needed for future medical decision making, including factors such as competition, patient purchasing power, negotiated pricing, and creation of larger geographic medical hierarchies of quality.[3]

Role of Guidelines

By current standards, the best evidence is unbiased, the studies are well designed to produce unambiguous conclusions, and the studies themselves are powerful

1: Principles of Orthopaedics

Table 3

Example of Grades of Recommendation for Summaries or Reviews of Orthopaedic Surgical Studies Used by the AAOS Guidelines Committee

A	Good evidence (Level I studies with consistent findings) for or against recommending intervention
B	Fair evidence (Level II or III studies with consistent findings) for or against recommending intervention
C	Poor-quality evidence (Level IV or V studies with consistent findings) for or against recommending intervention
I	There is insufficient or conflicting evidence not allowing a recommendation for or against intervention

(Adapted with permission from Wright JG, Einhorn TA, Heckman JD: Grades of recommendation. J Bone Joint Surg Am 2005;87:1909-1910.)

Table 4

Formal Processes of Surgical Care

Needs Assessment
Determination of patient requirements for satisfaction by standard instrument, such as the Canadian Occupational Performance Measure.

Expectations Training
Education regarding alternative forms of medical care, outcomes achievable, and informed consent, which includes not only risks but limited benefits.

Choice of Intervention
Personal decisions and other issues including external factors above and beyond the evidence base (such as World Health Organization [WHO], International Classification of Functioning, Disability and Health [ICF]).

Outcomes
Measurement of results; values by stakeholders based on treatment selection.

Guidelines
Derived from outcomes studies, they provide decision support for the clinician.

Performance Measures
Accountability, outcomes compared with guidelines, medical care incentivization through pay for performance.

Efficiency
Analysis for the treatment; outcome/cost influences payer benefit determination.

Quality Improvement
Continuous assessment of the impact of the quality review process and subsequent medical progress. (Information on how studies are designed can be found at http://www.ahrq.gov/clinic/outcosum.htm.) The American College of Surgeons has supported a collaboration with surgeons and medical physicians to express a balanced view of the pace and intensity of quality review.

enough to discourage simple criticism. In other words, the necessary methodology is better defined. Perhaps more importantly, the consumers and payers know what the standards (such as quality indicators, performance measures, and needed outcomes) should be. It is no longer ethically possible to rely on expert opinion alone to justify a procedure or course of management that results in poor quality outcomes by some providers.

Guideline Development

Guideline development has become a structured and methodology-driven activity. The AAOS Guidelines Committee uses a standard model. Two guidelines have been completed and two more are under development. The diagnosis of carpal tunnel syndrome and the prevention of pulmonary embolism in hip and knee surgery have been published by the National Guideline Clearinghouse (available at www.ngc.com). New guidelines for carpal tunnel syndrome treatment and knee arthritis are under development. The first and most difficult task is to choose a topic for the guideline. The existence of previous high-quality studies on a topic makes guideline creation easier. It is often the importance of the topic, either a common disorder or controversial treatment alternatives, that makes the guidelines on a subject most valuable. The deficiencies described in the rigorous analysis of the evidence base can spur new studies in the area.

The committee develops important questions to be answered by the literature search. Typically four or five questions are addressed. Evidence is extracted from the literature after defining criteria for restrictions on date range, language, and indexing sources. This filter specification makes the search reproducible as an audit trail for subsequent revisions and to set an example for others. Evidence tables array the papers by strength of study design. Current methodology restricts papers to those of level I and II evidence (**Table 2**). The papers are read and a consensus is reached by panel members regarding the strength of recommendations supported by the evidence (**Table 3**). Consensus development is governed by normative group technique. The guidelines are published, typically by the National Guideline Clearinghouse (NGC), and disseminated to practitioners, payers, and government agencies. Performance standards and measures are derived from the guidelines and regulators.

A general model of formalized medical care by addition of measurements and judgments of each step is presented in **Table 4**.

AAOS Activity

The AAOS has solidified its commitment to guiding the process of quality health care for patients with musculoskeletal disorders and developing the capability to respond to payers, government agencies such as CMS, and other entities that examine orthopaedic practice quality.

Clinical practice guideline committees have been created to formulate processes for examining the evidence base, creating usable guidelines for practitioners, and setting standards for others to use in review of insurance benefits and practitioner performance measurement.

Performance measures will be developed that represent achievable quality performance standards regarding the treatment of orthopaedic disorders. These performance measures will be conveyed through a series of professional organizations that endorse them. Legislative representation and lobbying responsiveness is needed to guide the implementation of and restriction of payer and governmental initiatives.

Summary

Quality assessment and public performance measurement are not likely to disappear. Many have anticipated that the true costs of quality measurement, the complexity and legitimacy of quality reporting, its cost, and the difficulty of reaching consensus on the price for higher quality may temper the pace and enthusiasm for this process. Many individuals and groups stand to gain financially from the professionalization of quality consulting, health policy writing, regulatory activity, certification of providers, and contentious advocacy. These costs are yet to be added to the cost of medical care.

Consumer demand for medical care and the unwillingness or inability of the consumer or employer to pay higher health care costs are the most powerful forces that will confront the rising demand for the health budget. Challenges include the shift toward an older, health-focused population; increasing numbers of residents without citizenship, entitlement, or health care planning; decreasing medical manpower; and lower provider effectiveness because of regulation. The rising rate at which providers are opting out of federal, indigent, and overregulated payer programs as well as patient care as a career is testimony of the strength of provider dissent.

It is recommended that subspecialty surgical societies continue writing the guidelines, performance measures, and payment initiatives.

Annotated References

1. McGlynn EA, Asch SM, Adams J, et al: The quality of health care delivered to adults in the United States. *N Engl J Med* 2003;348:2635-2645.

2. Curtin CM, Gater DR, Chung KC: Upper extremity reconstruction in the tetraplegic population: A national epidemiologic study. *J Hand Surg Am* 2005;30:94-99.

   Underutilization of evidence-based proven treatment is common. Demonstrated quality influence referral, overcoming regional disparities, and payer-controlled access are discussed.

3. Porter ME, Teisberg EO: *Redefining Heath Care*. Boston, MA, Harvard Business School Press, 2006.

   This excellent summary of the business view of competitive forces, limits, and strategies for health care provides a compendium of recent health controversies and data.

1: Principles of Orthopaedics

Chapter 15

Orthopaedic Research: Clinical Epidemiology and Biostatistics

Regis J. O'Keefe, MD, PhD   G. Russell Huffman, MD, MPH   Susan V. Bukata, MD

The Role of the Orthopaedic Clinician-Scientist in Orthopaedic Research

Musculoskeletal diseases are the most common reason patients seek medical care and rank among the most important causes of morbidity. It is in part for this reason that President George W. Bush declared 2002–2011 as the United States Bone and Joint Decade.

Orthopaedic clinician-scientists play a critical role in orthopaedic research, serving as an essential bridge between basic science discoveries and the development of novel therapies to improve patient care. In addition to enhancing translational research, the orthopaedic clinician-scientist also assists in defining critical problems and questions in orthopaedic care. Moreover, the clinician-scientist also helps to phrase the questions so that scientific discovery is more likely to positively impact patient care.

Several important discoveries have changed the practice of orthopaedics over the years. Advances in the development, use, and fabrication of biomaterials, coupled with improved understanding of joint kinematics and biomechanics, have resulted in the development of total joint arthroplasty as a procedure to ameliorate the morbidity of arthritis. Urist's insight regarding the presence of stimulating factors within the bone matrix has resulted in the development of bone morphogenetic proteins as agents to enhance bone repair and improve outcomes for patients with fractures and those who have undergone spinal fusion. Application of imaging and fiberoptic technologies for orthopaedic procedures resulted in minimally invasive arthroscopic techniques for the diagnosis and treatment of joint abnormalities. Advances in imaging and the application of computerized approaches are leading to the development of computer navigation surgery. All of these advances are dependent on the efforts and expertise of orthopaedic clinician-scientists.

The Orthopaedic Scientist as an Endangered Species

There is a general concern regarding an ongoing decline over the past several decades in the number of clinicians dedicating most of their time to research efforts. Compared with PhD scientists, the number of MD or MD/PhD scientists applying for and receiving grants from the National Institutes of Health (NIH) has been in sharp decline across the field of medicine. Moreover, the number of MD graduates seeking training in either basic or clinical research also has been declining.[1] Although there is some suggestion that the trend is improving and that increasing numbers of medical students are interested in research, it is not yet clear that the improvements involve the surgical specialties.[2]

Compared with medical specialties, surgical subspecialties have additional challenges for clinician-scientist development. Surgical training is extremely rigorous and requires a highly focused and concentrated effort. The field of orthopaedics is very dynamic, and constant innovations in surgical techniques and devices demand attention and continuous practice to maintain surgical proficiency. The practice of orthopaedics is highly demanding even for surgeons who dedicate complete efforts to orthopaedic surgical and nonsurgical care. In this context, the challenges facing clinician-scientists are obvious. Clinician-scientists are expected to provide outstanding clinical care and at the same time are required to compete with full-time scientists for funding and academic standing while conducting part-time research.

In understanding the status of the orthopaedic clinician-scientist, an important consideration is what criteria are used in this definition. In most disciplines, the clinician-scientist is defined by the ability to act as the principal investigator and leader of a highly competitive extramurally funded research program.[3,4] Funding sources typically considered consistent with a clinician scientist designation include funding through the NIH, National Science Foundation, Centers for Disease Control and Prevention, and Shriners Research Foundation. Clinician-scientists typically dedicate 40% or more of their time to research activities.

A recent survey of the Orthopaedic Research Society determined the number of orthopaedic surgeons who had received more than $1 million in NIH funding in the decade between 1992 and 2001. This is a figure consistent with a single NIH grant for a principal investigator. The survey indicated that only 22 orthopaedic surgeons received this degree of funding, consistent with a 0.14% rate of NIH funding for American Academy of Orthopaedic Surgeons (AAOS) members.[3]

Moreover, the survey found that the amount of NIH funding going to support research conducted by or with orthopaedic surgeon coinvestigators declined over the decade and that orthopaedic departments received less than 1% of NIH funds.[3] Using this standard metric, the investment in orthopaedic research and number of orthopaedic clinician-scientists has lagged behind that of other medical specialties.

Orthopaedic surgeons in both academic medical centers and private practice settings contribute through clinical studies that define the natural history of orthopaedic diseases and treatments and as part of research teams that include PhD scientists as lead investigators. Orthopaedic surgeons play an important role in advancing industry-sponsored research programs that frequently involve preclinical trials. Similarly, these investigators also face the challenge of balancing clinical and research activities.

Response of the Orthopaedic Community to Clinician-Scientist Development

The orthopaedic community has realized the importance of the clinician-scientist and has been extremely responsive to this need. The orthopaedic surgeon's credibility with the public and within the medical field requires an ongoing commitment to the improvement of patient care through excellence in educational activities and research. The orthopaedic surgeon's responsibility to patients requires not only care for immediate health issues, but a commitment to improved understanding and management of orthopaedic diseases.

Several organizations have taken an active role in promoting the development of the clinician-scientist. The AAOS has developed mentoring programs to identify potential clinician-scientists and to foster their development. The American Orthopaedic Association has similarly developed programs to enhance clinician-scientist development. Several orthopaedic subspecialty organizations provide grant support for research projects for orthopaedic surgeons. The Orthopaedic Research Society has also created mentoring programs, traveling fellowships, and other awards to support research by clinician-scientists.

The Orthopaedic Research and Education Foundation (OREF) is a nonprofit organization that for the past 50 years has raised money to support orthopaedic research and to stimulate scientific discovery in orthopaedics. The OREF provides more than $3 million in funding each year to orthopaedic surgeons across the United States. Most of the funding comes from industry support, but orthopaedic surgeons also contribute through personal donations. The OREF is celebrating its 50th anniversary and one of the goals is to increase the rate of donation to a level higher than the traditional 14% rate observed in recent years. The OREF has begun a partnership with the National Institute of Arthritis, Musculoskeletal, and Skin Diseases to co-fund a research fellowship program in which orthopaedic surgeons can obtain support for clinical research programs and development. The OREF also works with the specialty societies to raise funds for their research programs.

Support and Infrastructure Required for Clinician-Scientist Development

Similar to surgical training, research training requires concentrated effort. Typically, clinician-scientist investigators in either basic or clinical scientific areas have at least 1 and often 2 or more years of scientific training at some point during medical school, residency, or later.[4] Often clinician-scientists have obtained additional degrees, such as doctor of philosophy or master of public health. A survey of 64 surgeons with more than $100,000 in funding from the NIH over a 10-year period showed that 95% believed that 30% or more time dedicated to research was ideal. However, most of these individuals were able to dedicate only 20% or less of their time to research.[4]

Thus, development of a research program takes considerable time and is expensive. For basic science investigators, the salary support required to offset a 2-day-per-week commitment is in the range of $100,000 per year. Technical support, supplies, and equipment represent an additional commitment of $100,000 or more per year, for a total of $200,000 per year. Development costs related to clinical research are similarly expensive in that data collection requires considerable infrastructure and support staff, and time is required for oversight of the process.

One disturbing trend is that the time required for development of research programs has increased over the past decade. According to NIH data, the age at which scientists with MD degrees achieve their first grant has trended upward to 44 years, compared with 38 years two decades ago. This trend suggests that the duration of support necessary for scientific development is prolonged at a time when reimbursement of academic departments for procedures has diminished.

Summary of Key Components for the Development of the Clinician-Scientist

Although there are many important components necessary for the development of a clinician-scientist as an independently funded investigator, one that stands out is a passion for contributing to and advancing the field of orthopaedics. The clinician-scientist should have significant scientific training and should have 30% or more of their time "protected" for research activities. The clinician-scientist should have access to a team of outstanding investigators that include PhD scientists who can act as mentors and collaborators. Adequate funding must be available for salary support, supplies, and equipment and should be sustained for 5 years or longer.

It is also essential to recognize the extraordinary efforts of orthopaedic surgeons who commit to research activities as coinvestigators of extramurally funded programs. These surgeon-scientists contribute substantially to the field through the role they play as collaborators in clinical studies or as part of basic science research teams. The entire orthopaedic community and the patients stand to benefit from these activities and scientific advances by orthopaedic surgeons.

Clinical Epidemiology

Introduction and Relevance

The systematic approach to accruing biomedical knowledge and accurately incorporating this knowledge into the "best" surgical practice involves the fields of epidemiology, biostatistics, and evidenced-based medicine. Methodologies from each of these studies are applied to the routine decisions concerning patient care, but these principles are also applied to the incremental advancement of orthopaedic surgery. Familiarity with quantitative clinical science allows one to more accurately and critically assess the existing evidence that justifies the assessment of at-risk populations, allows correct diagnosis of injury and illness, and appropriate treatment of musculoskeletal diseases. Biostatistics may be defined as the application of mathematical methods to the collection, organization, and interpretation of biologic or medical data. Inference is the act of deriving logical conclusions from the existing knowledge regarding a condition. Biostatistical methods allow inferences to be made with a quantifiable degree of certainty. Epidemiology is the study of the distribution and determinants of disease frequency and incorporates the tools of inference and the mathematical principles of biostatistics to methodically examine clinical occurrences and test hypotheses. Evidence-based medicine incorporates the conscientious, explicit, and judicious use of the "current best evidence" in making decisions about the care of individual patients. This evidence is acquired through epidemiologic studies analyzed with biostatistical methods from which inferences (conclusions) have been made. The more rigorously designed the study and the more carefully a study's authors have analyzed data to minimize error, the more confident one can be in the meaningfulness and applicability of a given study.

Errors in Inference

The purpose of a well-designed research study is to provide insight into the "truth" regarding a clinical problem. In statistical assessment, conclusions are drawn about the population as a whole based on information gathered from a sample, whether or not the sample accurately represents the whole. The ability to determine the "truth," or to infer from a limited sample of the whole, is compromised by a systematic or study design flaw in the form of bias and/or confounding. Alternatively, chance or random occurrence may influence whether the results of a study accurately reflect the "truth." The validity with which trust is placed in a study's results, therefore, depends largely on the authors' ability to minimize errors in design and their ability to minimize chance.

Bias is a nonrandom, systematic error in the design or conduct of a study that may result in mistaken infer-

ence about association or causation. In the orthopaedic literature, common types of bias include recall bias, or potential error introduced in a retrospective study in which patients or clinicians are asked to relay an exposure that previously occurred and about which imperfect records may exist. For example, if one is to examine an association between antibiotics and the risk of subsequent Achilles tendon rupture, the researcher may wish to first identify patients with Achilles tendon ruptures. Once these patients are identified, the researcher then assesses exposure to antibiotics by asking these patients about history of antibiotic use before the tendon rupture. In a similar group of patients without tendon rupture, the exposure risk to antibiotics over the same time period is assessed in a similar fashion. The drawback with using this methodology is that patients may not perfectly remember their history of antibiotic exposure. Similarly, patients may be influenced by the manner in which a question is asked. This type of error is inherent in retrospective studies assessing exposure risk (antibiotics) to an outcome of interest (tendon rupture). A method to avoid recall bias is to enroll a cohort of persons without Achilles tendon rupture in a prospective study in which the use of antibiotics is carefully monitored. As each new case of tendon rupture is identified, the researchers are readily, and without bias, able to determine whether the person was exposed to antibiotics. In contrast to retrospective studies, longitudinal, prospective studies are extremely time consuming and costly, particularly for events that occur rarely.

In addition to recall bias, other types of bias common in orthopaedic literature include selection bias, measurement bias, sampling bias, and publication bias. Selection bias may occur when comparisons are made between groups of patients who differ in important ways other than the main factor under consideration. For instance, healing rates after lumbar spinal fusion are compared using two different devices at two different treatment centers all performed by a single surgeon with privileges at both centers. If one device is used exclusively in one setting and the other in a different location, then factors such as education, smoking rates, and median income between the two treatment centers may be associated with healing rates and be different between the two treatment locations. Measurement bias occurs when quantitative or qualitative data collected on one treatment group differ from that of another treatment group—that is, in a retrospective study more complete data have been collected on patients treated surgically compared with patients treated nonsurgically. Measurement bias is possible when patients in one subgroup are more likely to have their outcome or exposure detected than another subgroup. This factor may be minimized by blinding researchers to the type of treatment when determining exposure, establishing strict definitions of exposure or risk, and seeking to determine outcome events in all patient subgroups with equal vigor. However, in retrospective studies, measurement bias may occur without the knowledge of the study author. In addition to blinding, prospective assessment of outcomes and having an independent assessment

1: Principles of Orthopaedics

Table 1

Demographic Table

Factor	Implant A	Implant B	P-value
Age (mean)	67	66	0.48
Gender (% male)	56	54	0.45
BMI	40	31	0.04

Factors that may be associated with both the dependent variable of interest and independent variables should be assessed to control for any confounding. A less stringent P-value for association (P < 0.01) should be used to determine whether confounding variables (such as BMI in this example) need to be accounted for using multivariate statistical analyses. BMI = body mass index

Table 2

Criteria for Causality

Term	Meaning
Temporality	Cause precedes effect
Strength	Large relative risk
Dose-Response	Larger exposures are associated with higher rates of disease or more severe disease
Reversibility	Reduction in exposure is followed by lower rates of disease
Consistency	Repeatedly observed by different researchers, in different places, times
Biologic Plausibility	Is reasonable based upon current scientific understanding
Specificity	One cause leads to one effect
Analogy	Cause-and-effect relationship already established for a separate, but similar exposure or disease

(Reproduced with permission from Hill AB: The environment and disease: Association and causation. Proc R Soc Med, 1965;58:295-300.)

Confounding occurs when a variable has an association with both the independent (either treatment being evaluated or a risk factor under assessment) and dependent variables (the outcome of interest) of a study. The confounding variable need not have a causal association with the outcome of interest to lead to an error in inference. Simply, a confounding variable has a statistical association with both independent and dependent factors. Common examples of confounders include age, gender, socioeconomic status, and medical comorbidities. For example, if one wishes to determine the longevity of implant A against implant B, then the researcher should account for each patient's activity level, body mass index, and age. If it can be shown through preliminary or historical data that young age is associated with accelerated implant wear, then it is vital that the researcher demonstrate that there is no statistical difference in the central tendency (mean or median) age of those treated with implant A compared with those treated with implant B. For this reason every comparative study should have a clearly demarcated demographic table (Table 1) showing a value of central tendency (mean or median) for each variable that might possibly be related to both outcome (implant longevity) and exposure (implant A versus B). Randomization that occurs in prospective clinical trials may eliminate the potential for confounding if the sample size is adequately large, making the probability distribution equal within each treatment arm unless differences occur by chance alone. For example, in a randomized study, as the sample size increases, the probability of confounding by chance diminishes. In short, if study groups differ with respect to potential confounders (identified during preliminary data analysis or from prior studies), then the confounding variables should be accounted for with appropriate statistical measures including multivariate statistical analysis.

Chance is the probability that two unrelated events will appear associated by random occurrence rather than through a causal association. The criteria for causality have been established in the literature[5] (Table 2). Studies that fail to adequately control for chance occurrences may lead to invalid conclusions based on the probability (α) of type I error (concluding a causal association exists between risk factors and an outcome when in truth there is no association) and type II error (β, the probability of failing to find a true association when one in fact does exist) (Figure 1). The most common level of chance accepted in the published literature is an uncertainty that a true association exists of 1 in 20 (5% of the time), or $\alpha = 0.05$. The most common level of chance of failing to find a true association in the literature is 1 in 5 or $\beta = 0.2$. The power of a study is the researchers' ability to detect a true association if one exists. Power is defined as probability equal to $1 - \beta$, typically a probability of 0.8. The more stringent the β error, the narrower the confidence intervals will be, and the more certain one may be of the results in representing the "truth." Thus, inference is improved with increasing certainty, or an increasing power. For this reason, β is better set at 0.1 to yield a power ($1 - \beta$) or

of outcome help minimize this type of bias. Sampling bias occurs when patients selected for a study differ systematically from the population to which the results are generalized. In addition to the potential for erroneous conclusions, this systematic error may lead to a lack of external validity, or inability to extrapolate the study's findings to populations in different geographic regions. Publication bias is the tendency for published studies to differ systematically from other completed but unpublished studies. The most common example is that more favorable (or statistically significant) results are more likely to reach formal publication irrespective of the quality of the study.

Study Conclusion	Reality (Truth)	
	Treatments not different	Treatments are different
Treatments not different	Correct decision	Type II error (Probability = β)
Treatments are different	Type I error (Probability = α)	Correct decision (Probability = 1 − β)

Figure 1 Hypothesis testing.

certainty of 90%. Other means of increasing a study's power include increasing the sample size evaluated.[6]

In short, a researcher may minimize systematic errors in inference (bias, confounding, and chance) both before a study is started and after a study is completed, respectively, through study design and statistical analysis.

Study Design and Level of Evidence

Clinical studies are categorized as observational or experimental. In observational studies no allocation of treatment groups is assigned and data may be collected prospectively or retrospectively. Observational studies are either descriptive or analytic in design. Examples of descriptive studies include case reports, case series, and cross-sectional studies in which simple associations may be assessed. During the analysis of descriptive observational data, one is unable to demonstrate causality; however, these studies are typically inexpensive and are informative for obtaining background information in the planning and preparation of more sophisticated studies and for reporting unusual or newly discovered occurrences.

Alternatively, an observational study may be analytic in which the author quantitatively explores the association between a given outcome and potentially related variables. Examples of analytic, observational studies include case-control studies, cohort studies, and meta-analyses. Analytic observational studies are powerful in determining the natural history of a disease, determining causality, and for obtaining background information for designing more expensive experimental or longitudinal prospective observational studies.

In contrast to an observational study design, an experimental design is poorly suited to determine risk factors associated with rare events or outcomes. An experimental clinical trial is best suited to examine the efficacy of distinct treatment options with respect to a defined, quantifiable clinical outcome. The double-blind, prospective, randomized clinical trial based on preliminary data from observational studies and prior experimental studies is the gold standard of an experimental design in clinical medicine.

In either observational or experimental studies, greater validity is placed on studies that are able to minimize systematic error. Methods to control systematic error can occur at the design phase of a prospective study or during data analysis of retrospective studies (Table 3). Systematic error is diminished before study initiation by ensuring adequate sample size to test the hypothesis, applying rigid study inclusion and exclusion criteria, and collecting data consistently throughout the course of a study without respect to disease occurrence or to observed risk factors. In therapeutic studies, randomization with blinded assessment with respect to treatment is the best means of minimizing confounding and bias. Adequate sample size will minimize chance occurrences and type I error.

In observational and occasionally experimentally designed studies, data analysis may be necessary to account for observed systematic error at the conclusion of a study. Quantitative tools to accomplish this include matching of subjects with respect to demographic or other variables to minimize confounding, stratification of subgroups, and multivariate statistical analysis.

Table 3

Methods for Minimizing Errors in Inference

Design Phase of Study

Term	Meaning
Randomization	Assign patients into treatment groups in a manner that affords an equal probability of a particular patient being given each treatment
Restriction	Limit the characteristics of patients studied; also referred to by inclusion and exclusion criteria
Matching	Select control patients with similar characteristics to the group of interest with respect to potentially confounding characteristics save for the exposure or characteristic of interest to the study

Statistical Analysis Phase of Study

Term	Meaning
Stratification	Compare rates within subgroups (strata) with otherwise similar probability of the outcome. An example would be a comparison of outcomes after either surgical or nonsurgical treatment of a given fracture type. A logical stratification of outcomes would be according to fracture classification (severity).
Simple Adjustment	Mathematical adjustment of crude rates for a given characteristic(s) so that equal weight is assigned to strata of similar risk
Multivariable Analysis	Mathematical modeling that adjusts the risk assigned to a given factor based on the influence or association of this factor to other characteristics

1: Principles of Orthopaedics

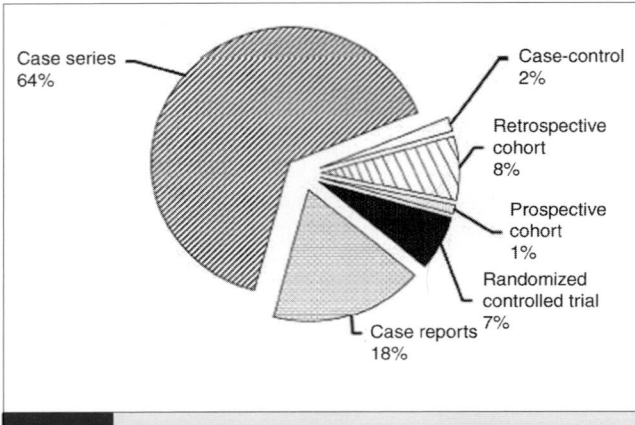

Figure 2 Distribution of study type in the orthopaedic literature. (*Reproduced with permission from Freedman KB, Back S, Bernstein J: Sample size and statistical power of randomised, controlled trials in orthopaedics. J Bone Joint Surg Br 2001;83:397-402.*)

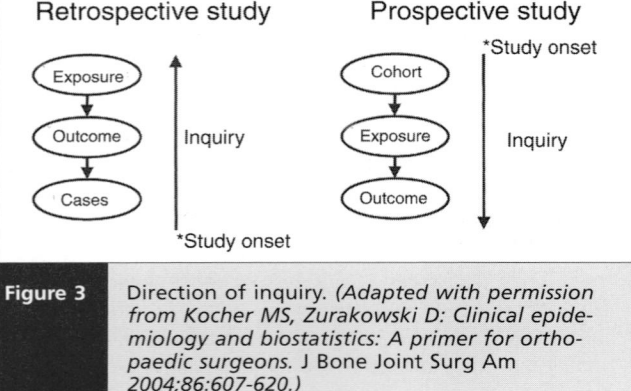

Figure 3 Direction of inquiry. (*Adapted with permission from Kocher MS, Zurakowski D: Clinical epidemiology and biostatistics: A primer for orthopaedic surgeons. J Bone Joint Surg Am 2004;86:607-620.*)

A study is endorsed with a level of evidence based on its designer's ability to minimize systematic error and to make correct inferences regarding the data obtained. The application of this assessment into clinical practice is evidence-based medicine. Evidence-based medicine incorporates the conscientious, explicit, and judicious use of the "current best evidence" in making decisions about the care of individual patients.[7,8] This evidence is acquired through epidemiologic and scientific studies analyzed with biostatistical methods and from which inferences (conclusions) have been made. The more rigorously designed the study and the more carefully a study's authors have analyzed data to minimize error, the more confident one can be in the meaningfulness of a given study. A systematic assessment of the levels of evidence for clinical studies has been established. In short, one may more confidently draw inferences about a study that has adequately accounted for bias, confounding, and chance. Most orthopaedic surgery literature is observational in design (**Figure 2**); however, there is support that publication preference in the orthopaedic literature is currently placed on studies with higher levels of evidence than was previously done.

Observational studies may further be categorized as retrospective or prospective, depending on the line of inquiry (**Figure 3**). In a retrospective study, the direction of inquiry begins with the outcome of interest and attempts to determine a risk factor or exposure that led to the observed outcome. The classic example of a retrospective study design is the case-control design. This type of study is most efficient when dealing with rarely observed events or outcomes. In contrast, the direction of inquiry begins with defining an exposure or risk factor and waiting to observe the outcome of interest to occur in a prospective study. This is more efficient with a predictable rate of outcome or event to more quickly determine associated risk factors with the incidence of an outcome as it occurs.

Clinical Study Designs

Case series are descriptive observational studies detailing observations of a group of patients sharing an interesting or unique set of characteristics (undergoing the same injury or treatment). The usefulness of this type of information lies in describing potential complications or successes in a given cohort. An example of a case series is the description of the successful use of methylmethacrylate in securing components used in total hip arthroplasty to inform the orthopaedic community of its safety and potential success. The strengths of this type of report include the ease of data collection, low cost, the description of novel treatments, background information when performing power calculations in the planning of more sophisticated study designs, and the possibility of alerting the orthopaedic community to previously unknown adverse effects or complications. The weaknesses of any case series is susceptibility to bias, confounding, and chance in leading to erroneous conclusions if statistical assessment is applied. There is no hypothesis, no comparison group, and often little external validity outside of the precise group described in the report. Case series provide level IV evidence.

Cross-sectional surveys are observational descriptive studies that provide a snapshot of a population at a given time. One may ascertain the epidemiology of an outcome or of a risk factor. Alternatively, population-based normative data are derived from such surveys (of median household income, body mass index, intelligence quotient, bone mineral density) that provide necessary information in the design of experimental and prospective studies. The strengths of this study design include the relative speed of data collection at a single point; generalizability to a larger population if sampling is representative of the population from which the sample was derived; analysis of demographic associations; and determination of disease prevalence (number of cases divided by the number of individuals at risk within a single given time period) within a population. Limitations of cross-sectional studies include sampling bias limiting the external validity or general applicability of findings observed in the study group, and inability to provide disease incidence, which requires a temporal association.

Case-control studies are observational and analytic in design. Patients with a given outcome (cases) are compared with patients without the outcome of interest (controls) and risk factors are statistically assessed for strength of association. This scenario allows one to draw inferences regarding the causality of rare or uncommon occurrences. Typically, results are reported as an odds ratio or the odds of a case being exposed to a factor of interest compared with the odds of a control being exposed to the same factor. Both groups are retrospectively examined for the exposure of interest before event occurrence. The advantages of case-control design includes its efficiency in assessing risk-outcome associations when assessing rare occurrences at a relatively low cost. Weaknesses of the case-control design include the difficulty in defining an appropriate control group; the lack of access to complete, thorough medical records; and the susceptibility to confounding and bias. Confounding may be minimized by matching cases and controls with respect to similar attributes not directly related to the exposure of interest or by performing a multivariate analysis. Recall, reporting, and sampling bias may all be limited, but never completely eliminated, through careful study design or nesting a case-control analysis within a prospective cohort study. Case-control studies typically support level III evidence, although nested case-control studies within a prospective cohort design may provide level II evidence.

Cohort studies are observational analytic studies in which a population of interest is identified at study inception and followed over time to determine the incidence of a disease or outcome of interest. In this example, exposure data are collected before event occurrence. Statistical associations with known (and potentially unknown) risk factors may be examined and are reported as the relative risk of disease occurrence with respect to given exposures. In clinical medicine, the most widely recognized cohort study is the Framingham Heart Study, which has prospectively collected information on the incidence of heart disease and examined risk factors associated with this occurrence. The strengths of the prospective cohort design are that the incidence (rate of occurrence over a given period of time) of an outcome may be defined for a population; one may observe the natural history of disease; risk factors are identified in an unbiased fashion with respect to recall, information, and selection bias; and the statistical power increases with increasing disease frequency. Longitudinal prospective cohorts are limited by their tremendous expense in observation and complete data acquisition; their labor-intensive nature; the need for a stable population; and their inefficiency with rare occurrences. Multiyear funding including support staff is necessary to sustain these endeavors. Well-designed, prospective cohort studies provide level II evidence while retrospective cohorts and prospective cohorts with design flaws or poor follow-up provide level III evidence.

Clinical trials are experimental clinical studies that use concurrent (randomized clinical trial), sequential (crossover trial), or, less preferably, historical controls. In effect, the exposure of interest is controlled and the outcome of interest is prospectively observed. The old standard is the double-blind (both patient and examiner are unaware of the treatment assigned), placebo controlled, randomized clinical trial. Additionally, in surgical research a sham procedure is not always ethical.[9] A randomized clinical trial requires strict enforcement of a protocol establishing patient eligibility, adequate sample size, informed consent, the method of randomization, blinding of independent examiners and of study subjects, rules for study cessation, approval by an institutional review board, compliance monitoring, periodic safety assessment, and prospectively determined methods of data analysis. Additional clearance and regulation of a study may be required from the federal government for new, experimental, or off-label treatments.

To make correct inferences from experimental clinical trials, the same principles mentioned previously for observational studies apply. Adequate sample size will ensure a study's ability to detect a true difference in treatments if one truly exists, thereby minimizing type II error. Randomization minimizes selection bias as well as known and unknown confounding variables. Blinding minimizes performance, detection, and interviewer bias. During data analysis, the use of an intention-to-treat analysis will minimize nonresponder bias, that is, minimize systematic error introduced as individuals or groups switch from one group to another in nonrandom ways (such as by selecting treatment A over treatment B, to which they were randomized). The quality of these studies is improved and more valid when patient compliance to study completion remains greater than 90%. Well-conducted and designed clinical trials result in excellent assessment of a treatment's efficacy or effect under ideal circumstances. These results, however, may not truly represent a treatment's effectiveness in general applications—for example, with less well-controlled and compliant patients or less knowledgeable clinicians. An excellent study may be valid under the test circumstances (internal validity), but lack external validity or generalizability to the population at large. External validity depends on whether the sample (experimental group) is truly representative of all patients with the given condition or disease and whether the standard of care applied in the study is available to other populations of interest.

Experimental studies are expensive, timely, and logistically difficult to implement. For success, they require adequate patient accrual as well as physician acceptance of the treatment alternatives rendered. This ethically requires equipoise, or that there is no known or perceived advantage to one treatment over the alternative treatment with respect to safety and patient benefit. Equipoise must exist for the study designer, general medical community, and all participating clinicians. Experimental clinical trials, in general, have no use for determining cause and effect of rare conditions and are not always methodologically appropriate to examine some associations.[10,11] The strength of experimental

1: Principles of Orthopaedics

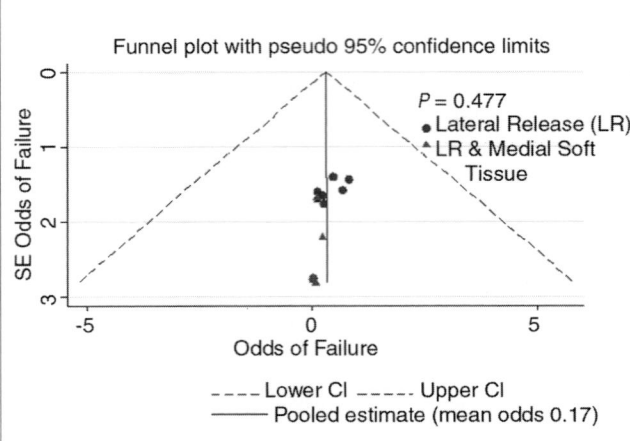

Figure 4 Funnel plots are used to detect publication bias in the literature when one conducts a systematic review or meta-analysis. On the y-axis the size of each study is compared to the outcome of interest. A significant correlation between the outcome of interest, in this case "failure," and the size of published studies (represented by the standard error (SE) in this graph), indicates that publication bias exists. With a funnel plot, one may also detect outliers in the literature, which may not be representative of the other literature meeting study inclusion criteria. *(Reproduced with permission from Ricchetti E, Mehta S, Sennett BJ, Huffman GR: Comparison of lateral release versus lateral release with medial soft-tissue realignment for the treatment of recurrent patellar instability: A systematic review. Arthroscopy 2007;23:463-468.)*

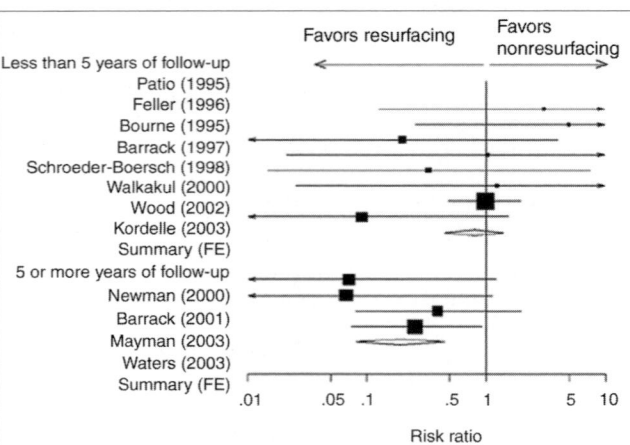

Figure 5 Forest plot. The effect size (risk ratio) with 95% confidence intervals is plotted for each study that meets inclusion criteria. A summary effect size may be calculated for each treatment type (represented by rhomboids). In this example, the existing literature clearly favors patellar resurfacing in total knee arthroplasty for both 5-year and greater than 5-year follow-up. *(Reproduced with permission from Pakos EE, Ntzani EE, Trikalinos TA: Patellar resurfacing in total knee arthroplasty: A meta-analysis. J Bone Joint Surg Am 2005;87:1438-1445.)*

clinical studies lies in the researcher's ability to minimize chance, bias, and confounding and to equitably distribute the exposure (treatment) of interest. Additionally, this design is ideal for determining and for comparing treatment efficacy. Experimental clinical studies have a level of evidence of I or II depending on sample size, randomization technique, blinding, appropriate nontreatment (placebo) control, and percentage of retained subjects (> 90%).

Literature Reviews

A review may range in sophistication from a summary of expert opinion (level V evidence) to a meta-analysis, which is a well-organized, systematic, and quantitative analysis of randomized clinical trial from which one may draw valid statistical inferences (level I evidence). Without the systematic selection of studies based on quality criteria from all available published data, a review is simply an assimilation by an author of his or her knowledge of the existing literature. A systematic review is an evidence-based summary of the entire literature—published and unpublished when possible—that uses explicit methods to perform a complete literature search and critical appraisal of the studies with a priori inclusion and exclusion criteria established during study design. Often the quality of published data on a given subject does not allow rigorous statistical analysis (much of the data are from retrospective studies) and a systematic description with limited quantitative analysis is possible (level of evidence is reflective of included studies, typically levels II to V).[12,13] In contrast, a meta-analysis entails the quantitative assessment of data gathered from a systematic review of prospective studies, preferably randomized controlled trials with similar inclusion criteria, outcomes assessed, and treatment regimens. In the design and analysis of studies to be examined by meta-analysis, one must quantifiably test prospective studies for homogeneity with respect to clinical treatment, methodology, and measured effect (outcome of interest) using a Q-test or other validated statistical means. Publication bias may be assessed using a funnel plot (**Figure 4**) and is tested using either parametric (Egger's linear regression model) or nonparametric (Begg's test) methods. Because the successful results are more likely to be published, meeting abstracts and other nonpublished materials should be reviewed to further minimize publication bias. A summary estimate of treatment efficacy across trials may then be created and represented by the use of a forest plot (**Figure 5**).

Hypothesis Testing and Biostatistics
Types of Data
Data are factual information, especially information organized for analysis or used to reason or make decisions. This information may or may not be numerical. Biomedical data may be broadly characterized as one of three types: continuous, ordinal, or categorical. The type of data determines the appropriateness of given statistical methods to analyze a set of data. Information acquired for a given characteristic is defined as a variable. Each of

these defined characteristics about which the researcher inquires and stores as data is a variable. Statistical methods may subsequently be used to find the likelihood of an association between the outcome of interest and each variable or combination of variables.

An independent variable is one whose value determines the value of other variables. In an experimental trial, this variable would be controlled by the researcher as one of the treatment arms. In a cohort study this would be the exposure of interest. A dependent variable is the observed variable in an experiment or study whose changes are determined by the presence or degree of one or more independent variables. The dependent variable is the outcome of interest.

A continuous variable describes numerical information that can be any given value within a range of values. Common examples of continuous variables used in medical research include age and body mass index. An ordinal variable is one in which the data are represented in an ordered fashion. For example, a researcher wishes to examine factors potentially associated with the severity of osteonecrosis of the femoral head. The researcher may use a common grading scale with a severity scale ranging from 1 to 4. For the purposes of statistical analysis, each number would represent a discrete increase in the radiographic severity of the disease. A categorical (nominal) variable is one in which the primary data are best described qualitatively rather than quantitatively. An example would be an epidemiologic study designed to examine different manufacturers of total hip arthroplasty implants. Each of these companies is distinctly different from the other, and may be assigned a numerical representation for the purposes of data analysis only. However, there is no clear ordering of these variables.

Data Distribution

Continuous data may be parametric or nonparametric. Parametric data may be represented in a distribution explained by a single mathematical equation. The most widely recognized distribution of continuous, parametric data is Gaussian or normally distributed data (Figure 6). The y-axis represents the probability of observing a given value. The x-axis represents the range of possible continuous values. The area under the curve is 1.0, or the sum of probability of observing all given values. For a value to fall within "normal" limits, the value must fall within the mean plus or minus 2 standard deviations (SDs). With a normal distribution, 95% of the values will fall within 2 SDs of the mean; 69% of values will fall within ± 1 SD, 95% within ± 2 SD, and 99% within ± 3 SD of the mean. In a normal distribution, the mean, median, and mode are all equal. Each of these terms is a measurement of a data's central tendency, that is, the value that is most representative of the typical (or most predictable) value for an entire group. The mean is the sum of all observed measurements divided by the number of observations (for example, the average value). The median is the 50th percentile, or the value below which half of the values fall.

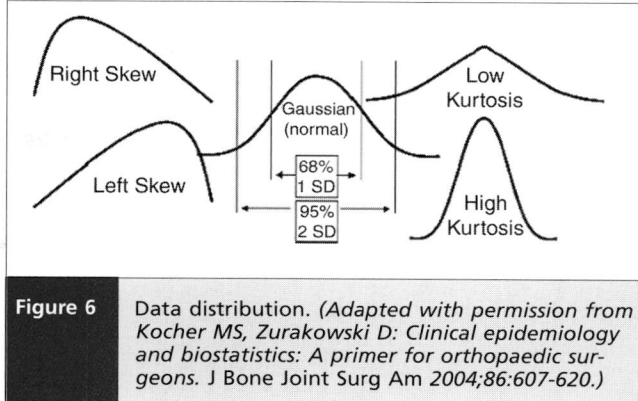

Figure 6 Data distribution. *(Adapted with permission from Kocher MS, Zurakowski D: Clinical epidemiology and biostatistics: A primer for orthopaedic surgeons. J Bone Joint Surg Am 2004;86:607-620.)*

For nonparametric data, the median is a more robust measurement of the central tendency than the mean. The mode is the most frequently occurring observation. Continuous data may be skewed, or asymmetric about the mean (Figure 6). Skewness is a statistical measure of the symmetry of the distribution of values about the mean for a given variable. For a normal distribution, the skewness = 0. In general, a right skew means that the median and mean have a smaller value than the mode. A left skew indicates that the mean and mode have a greater value than the median. Kurtosis is a measure of the peakedness of a unimodal distribution of data. Statistical tests for data skewness and kurtosis may be used to determine whether parametric means testing is appropriate.

Hypothesis Testing

Hypothesis testing entails an assessment of the statistical significance of findings. It involves comparing observed findings from a data sample with expected findings (the hypothesis). This comparison allows computation of the probability that the observed outcome could have been due to chance alone. The comparison also determines if a null hypothesis (there is no difference between treatments or there is no association between a risk factor and a given outcome) is correct or may be rejected.

Classic methods of hypothesis testing will not help determine statistical significance compared with clinical significance. For example, an investigator wants to determine whether one anterior cruciate ligament reconstruction is superior to another. The null hypothesis is that the two are the same. Clinically, a failure is defined as 3 mm of side-to-side (anterior cruciate ligament reconstructed to contralateral normal knee) anterior tibial displacement with KT-1000 arthrometer testing. Patients are randomized to group A and group B with significance set at 0.05 and adequate power to detect a real difference with 90% certainty given at least a 1-mm side-to-side difference. Group A patients and group B patients do equally well clinically. However, a 1.2-mm side-to-side difference favors group A with a *P* value of 0.02. The result is that group A is statistically superior to group B, but this difference may have no

1: Principles of Orthopaedics

Table 4

Common Statistical Tests

Type of Data	No. of Groups	Independent	Paired
Continuous			
Normal	2	Student's t test	Paired t test
Non-normal	2	Mann-Whitney U test	Wilcoxon's signed rank test
Normal	> 2	ANOVA test	Repeated measures ANOVA test
Non-normal	> 2	Kruskal-Wallis test	Friedman's test
Proportions	2 (large number of observations)	Chi square test	
	2 (small number of observations)	Fisher's exact test	
Ordinal	2	Mann-Whitney U test	Wilcoxon's signed rank test
	> 2	Kruskal-Wallis test	Friedman's test
Nominal	2	Fisher's exact test	McNemar's test
	> 2	Pearson chi square test	Cochran's Q test
Survival	2 / > 2	Log-rank test	Conditional logistic regression

practical or clinical relevance. In other words, findings may show statistical significance for clinically unimportant parameters.

The P value is the probability of an occurrence or association by chance alone and is determined through the use of statistical testing. In itself this probability has no practical significance, but is the measure of the strength of evidence in favor of the alternative hypothesis.[14-17] It is the probability of determining an association is true when in fact it has been observed by chance alone. Thus, the P value is measured against a predetermined level of certainty or acceptance of chance explaining the findings. This probability is known as the α-level or the probability of making a type I error (concluding an association exists when in fact it occurs by chance alone). For most clinical studies a probability of 1 in 20 or $P < 0.05$ is determined an acceptable certainty for rejecting the null hypothesis. More rigorous studies lower this certainty to 1 in 100 ($\alpha < 0.01$). The probability value has no strength of association or units. In contrast, confidence intervals do provide practical significance with a magnitude of values ascribed a unit of measurement. Additionally, confidence intervals are precise as a range of values are given and are seen as significant at either 95% or 99% levels if values do not overlap between treatment groups.

The probability of concluding an association does not exist, when in truth it does, is known as type II error, or β. A studies power is $1 - \beta$, or the probability of detecting a difference between treatments or an association that in truth does exist. When a study demonstrates significant association, then the potential error is type I. However, when a study demonstrates no significant association, then the potential error is type II and it may be that with increased number of subjects or less variation a significant association would become apparent.

When no statistically significant association is detected, then the power of a study should be routinely reported by the authors to indicate the study's ability to actually detect a difference.[18] The elements of a power calculation include α, β, variance (standard deviation about the mean), the sample size, and estimated values or effect size in each group. These elements will help determine the ability of a study to detect a statistically significant difference if one truly exists. Each component of the power calculation may be determined from the other elements. In prospective study design the power calculation is conducted in the planning of the study. In retrospective, observational studies, a post hoc power calculation will determine the ability of the given observations to allow appropriate inferences and will determine sample sizes for future hypothesis-driven studies.

Statistical tests of inference require assumptions about data type and distribution. A brief summary of commonly used statistical tests is listed in Table 4. Means testing entails comparison of central tendency values. To perform means testing, the data are assumed to be parametric and normally distributed. If the data do not meet those criteria, then alternate central tendency tests are applied. Mathematical modeling of continuous data are possible using regression models. The simplest form of this is linear regression modeling in which $Y = a + bX$, where X is the explanatory variable (exposure or risk factor), Y is the dependent variable (outcome of interest), b is the slope of the line, and a is the y-intercept (the value of y when x = 0) (Figure 7). Time-to-event analysis is when the probability of event occurrence is a product of time, and the rate of occurrence probability over time becomes the outcome of interest. Survival analysis with the use of the Kaplan-Meier probability plot is commonly used in the orthopaedic literature to determine survival or fre-

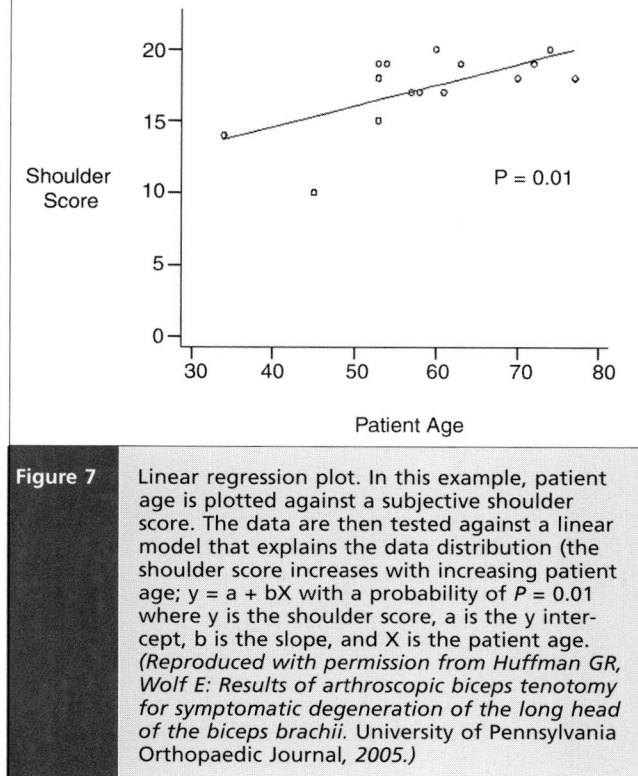

Figure 7 Linear regression plot. In this example, patient age is plotted against a subjective shoulder score. The data are then tested against a linear model that explains the data distribution (the shoulder score increases with increasing patient age; y = a + bX with a probability of P = 0.01 where y is the shoulder score, a is the y intercept, b is the slope, and X is the patient age. *(Reproduced with permission from Huffman GR, Wolf E: Results of arthroscopic biceps tenotomy for symptomatic degeneration of the long head of the biceps brachii.* University of Pennsylvania Orthopaedic Journal, *2005.)*

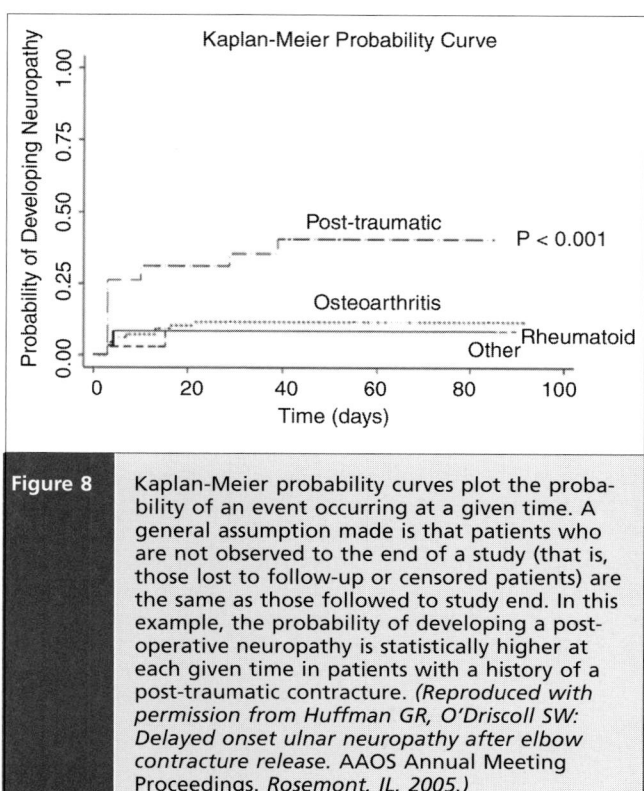

Figure 8 Kaplan-Meier probability curves plot the probability of an event occurring at a given time. A general assumption made is that patients who are not observed to the end of a study (that is, those lost to follow-up or censored patients) are the same as those followed to study end. In this example, the probability of developing a postoperative neuropathy is statistically higher at each given time in patients with a history of a post-traumatic contracture. *(Reproduced with permission from Huffman GR, O'Driscoll SW: Delayed onset ulnar neuropathy after elbow contracture release.* AAOS Annual Meeting Proceedings. *Rosemont, IL, 2005.)*

quency of event occurrence at each time an event occurs (Figure 8). This model requires the assumption that individuals lost to follow-up do not differ in event probability over time compared with those who are followed to the eventual outcome of interest (for example, death or implant failure).

Diagnostic Test Performance
The determination of disease and correct diagnosis depends on clinical evaluation and specific diagnostic tests to confirm or exclude the diagnosis suspected. A test will either yield a positive result when in fact the disease is present (true positive); a positive result when in fact the disease is not present (false positive), a negative result when in fact the disease is present (false negative), or a negative result when the disease is not present (true negative). The sensitivity of a test lies in its ability to detect disease when present. The specificity of a test is its ability to exclude a disease when not present (Figure 9). From sensitivity and specificity, the predictive value of a given test can be calculated. Positive predictive value (PPV) is defined as the probability of a patient having a disease when a test result is positive (PPV = [(prevalence)(sensitivity) / [(prevalence)(sensitivity) + (1 − prevalence) (1 − specificity)]).

Negative predictive value (NPV) is defined as the probability of patient not having a disease when a test result is negative (NPV = (1-prevalence)(specificity) / [(1 − prevalence)(specificity) + (prevalence) (1 − sensitivity)]).

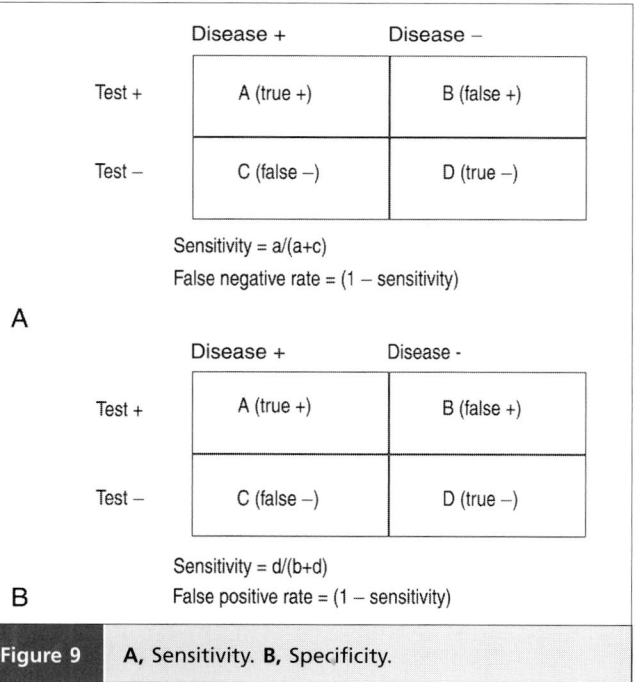

Figure 9 A, Sensitivity. B, Specificity.

Health Outcomes Research
The AAOS and other organizations have developed instruments designed to collect standardized patient-respondent data for use in clinical practice settings to assess the effectiveness of treatment regimens and in

musculoskeletal research to study the clinical outcomes of treatment. These instruments have been validated (they measure what they are intended to measure) and are reliable (similar results are obtained for a given respondent at a given time when the outcomes assessment is repeated). Population-based normative values have been published and are readily available for AAOS-sponsored musculoskeletal outcome instruments.[19] Examples of region-specific outcomes instruments include the Hip Society Score, Knee Society Score, Disabilities of the Arm, Shoulder, and Hand, Pediatric Outcomes Data Collection Instrument, International Knee Documentation Committee Subjective Knee score, and the American Shoulder and Elbow Surgeons subjective shoulder scale. In contrast, general health outcomes instruments are used to determine an individuals overall health and well-being. Examples of general outcomes assessments include the Medical Outcomes Society 36-Item Short Form and Western Ontario and McMaster Universities Osteoarthritis Index. For each outcomes assessment to be useful, it must be valid, reliable, and have published normative data from a sample of the population of interest.[20-23]

Annotated References

1. Rosenberg L: Physician-scientists: Endangered and essential. *Science* 1999;283:331-332.

2. Ley TJ, Rosenberg LE: The physician-scientist career pipeline in 2005: Build it, and they will come. *JAMA* 2005;294:1343-1351.

3. Brand RA, Chaw ES, Karam MD: The number and the scope of activity of orthopaedic clinician-scientists in the United States. *J Bone Joint Surg Am* 2003;85-A:374-379.

4. Brand RA, Hannafin JA: The environment of the successful clinician-scientist. *Clin Orthop Relat Res* 2006;449:67-71.

   Fifty-eight orthopaedic clinician-scientists were surveyed to assess environmental factors that might lead to success and obstacles faced. Demands on clinical time were a major impediment.

5. Hill AB: The environment and disease: Association and causation. *Proc R Soc Med* 1965;58:295-300.

6. Bernstein J, McGuire K, Freedman KB: Statistical sampling and hypothesis testing in orthopaedic research. *Clin Orthop Relat Res* 2003;413:55-62.

7. Kaska SC, Weinstein JN: Historical perspective: Ernest Amory Codman, 1869-1940: A pioneer of evidence-based medicine: The end result idea. *Spine* 1998;23:629-633.

8. Bernstein J: Evidence-based medicine. *J Am Acad Orthop Surg* 2004;12:80-88.

   The author reviewed the concept of evidence-based medicine and commented that evidence-based medicine requires its users to embrace uncertainty in medical decision making because information that is simultaneously true and complete cannot be attained. Recognizing medicine's inherent uncertainty, proponents of evidence-based medicine advocate using a five-step process for sound decision making: formulate answerable questions, gather evidence, appraise the evidence, implement the valid evidence, and evaluate the process.

9. Mehta S, Myers TG, Lonner JH, Huffman GR, Sennett BJ: The ethics of sham surgery in clinical orthopaedic research. *J Bone Joint Surg Am* 2007;89:1650-1653.

   This article discusses the methodology, feasibility, and ethics of performing sham surgery for the purposes of providing a double-blinded control in orthopaedic surgery research.

10. Abel U, Koch A: The role of randomization in clinical studies: Myths and beliefs. *J Clin Epidemiol* 1999;52:487-497.

11. Benson K, Hartz AJ: A comparison of observational studies and randomized, controlled trials. *N Engl J Med* 2000;342:1878-1886.

12. Spindler KP, Kuhn JE, Freedman KB, Matthews CE, Dittus RS, Harrell FE Jr: Anterior cruciate ligament reconstruction autograft choice: Bone-tendon-bone versus hamstring: Does it really matter? A systematic review. *Am J Sports Med* 2004;32:1986-1995.

    This is a systematic applied to randomized clinical trials comparing two different anterior cruciate ligament reconstruction techniques. This article serves as an excellent example of a rigorously-conducted systematic review of the literature.

13. Wright RW, Brand RA, Dunn W, Spindler KP: How to write a systematic review. *Clin Orthop Relat Res* 2007;455:23-29.

    This article identifies systematic reviews and meta-analyses as the highest level of evidence. The rationale and methodology for performing a systematic review is explained in a standard format.

14. Goodman SN: Toward evidence-based medical statistics: 1. The P value fallacy. *Ann Intern Med* 1999;130:995-1004.

15. Goodman SN: Of P-values and Bayes: A modest proposal. *Epidemiology* 2001;12:295-297.

16. Goodman S: Commentary: The P-value, devalued. *Int J Epidemiol* 2003;32:699-702.

17. Goodman SN: Toward evidence-based medical statistics: 2. The Bayes factor. *Ann Intern Med* 1999;130:1005-1013.

18. Freedman KB, Back S, Bernstein J: Sample size and statistical power of randomised, controlled trials in orthopaedics. *J Bone Joint Surg Br* 2001;83:397-402.

19. Hunsaker FG, Cioffi DA, Amadio PC, Wright JG, Caughlin B: The American Academy of Orthopaedic Surgeons outcomes instruments: Normative values from the general population. *J Bone Joint Surg Am* 2002;84: 208-215.

20. Briggs KK, Kocher MS, Rodkey WG, Steadman JR: Reliability, validity, and responsiveness of the Lysholm knee score and Tegner activity scale for patients with meniscal injury of the knee. *J Bone Joint Surg Am* 2006; 88:698-705.

   This article provides application of validated, joint-specific outcome measures, the Lysholm knee score and Tegner activity scale, to a particular set of patients (those with meniscal injury). An appreciation for assessment of reliability, validity, and responsiveness to change that tests for a given outcome measure within a well-defined patient population will be gained.

21. Crawford K, Briggs KK, Rodkey WG, Steadman JR: Reliability, validity, and responsiveness of the IKDC score for meniscus injuries of the knee. *Arthroscopy* 2007;23: 839-844.

   The psychometric properties of the International Knee Documentation Committee (IKDC) score for meniscus injuries of the knee were studied.

22. Kocher MS, Horan MP, Briggs KK, Richardson TR, O'Holleran J, Hawkins RJ: Reliability, validity, and responsiveness of the American Shoulder and Elbow Surgeons subjective shoulder scale in patients with shoulder instability, rotator cuff disease, and glenohumeral arthritis. *J Bone Joint Surg Am* 2005;87:2006-2011.

   The psychometric properties of the American Shoulder and Elbow Surgeons subjective shoulder scale were studied in patients with shoulder instability, rotator cuff disease, and glenohumeral arthritis. The responsiveness, reliability, and validity of this joint-specific outcomes measurement and its usefulness in examining a specific patient population was assessed.

23. Kocher MS, Steadman JR, Briggs KK, Sterett WI, Hawkins RJ: Reliability, validity, and responsiveness of the Lysholm knee scale for various chondral disorders of the knee. *J Bone Joint Surg Am* 2004;86:1139-1145.

   The psychometric properties of the Lysholm knee scale for various chondral disorders of the knee are discussed.

1: Principles of Orthopaedics

Section 2

Systemic Disorders

SECTION EDITORS:

TUSHAR PATEL, MD
SUKEN A. SHAH, MD

Chapter 16

Bone Metabolism and Metabolic Bone Disease

Mathias P. G. Bostrom, MD

Introduction

The fundamental understanding of bone metabolism has changed dramatically over the past 10 years. Although the three critical basic functions of the skeleton: (1) mechanical support and locomotion, (2) protection of the internal organs, and (3) metabolic activities related to calcium homeostasis remain, the fundamental mechanism of how bone successfully achieves these functions is gradually being understood at the molecular level.[1] Traditionally the study of bone metabolism and disease has focused on the role of osteoblasts, osteocytes, and osteoclasts; however, with modern molecular biologic analysis methods, a very precise regulation of bone metabolism can be determined, allowing a better understanding of the pathophysiologic abnormalities involved so that new targeted therapeutic approaches can be devised.

Bone Formation

Osteoblasts are primarily responsible for bone formation. These cuboid cells are aligned in layers along osteoid and synthesize the organic bone matrix that is subsequently mineralized to form bone. A subpopulation of these cells becomes embedded in the matrix and develops into osteocytes, whose function includes calcium homeostasis and serving as mechanoreceptors of the skeleton.

Osteoblasts and osteocytes are derived from pluripotential mesenchymal stem cells, which are present in many adult tissues but primarily in bone marrow stroma. Depending on the precise molecular signaling, these stem cells differentiate and proliferate into cells that form bone, cartilage, and adipose and fibrous tissue.

The regulation of osteoblastogenesis and bone formation is quite complex, involving several transcriptional regulators, growth factors, hormones, and other signal molecules[2-4] (Table 1). It is these factors that determine the sequence of differentiation and proliferation from mesenchymal stem cell, osteoprogenitor cell, preosteoblast, and finally to mature osteoblast. Each of these stages has defined phenotypic cell markers, allowing for the ability to modulate the differentiation into different cell lineages. Once differentiated, mature osteoblasts begin to synthesize bone matrix, which is primarily composed of primarily type I collagen along with other collagen proteins and critical noncollaginous proteins.

Table 1

Factors Associated With the Regulation of Osteoblastogenesis and Bone Formation

Transcriptional regulators
  Shock protein factors
  Activating transcription factors
  Runt homology domain
Growth factors
  Insulin-like growth factor-1 and -2
  Platelet-derived growth factor
  Epidermal growth factor
  Endothelin
Hormones
  Parathyroid hormone
  1,25-dihydroxyvitamin D
  Glucocorticoids
  Sex steroids
    Progesterone
    Estrogen
    Androgen
  Growth hormone
  Thyroid stimulating hormone
Signaling molecules
  Prostaglandin E_2
  Oncostatin 2
  Leptin
  Sclerostin
Osteoprogenitor cell commitment and expansion
  Bone morphogenetic proteins 2 through 7
  Indian hedgehog
  Interleukin-18
  Pleiotropin

(Data from Favus MJ (ed): Primer on the Metabolic Bone Diseases and Disorders of Mineral Metabolism, ed 6. Washington, DC, ASBMR, 2006.)

2: Systemic Disorders

Table 2

Factors Influencing Renal Absorption of Calcium

Decreased Renal Calcium Resorption	Increased Renal Calcium Resorption
Increased calcium intake	Parathyroid hormone
Increased sodium intake	Parathyroid hormone-related protein
Metabolic acidosis	1,25-dihydroxyvitamin D
Phosphate depletion	Calcitonin
Glucocorticoids	Increased phosphate intake
Furosemides	Chronic thiazide diuretic use

Bone Resorption

Whereas the osteoblasts are responsible for bone formation, the osteoclasts are responsible for bone resorption through enzymatic degradation. Osteoclasts are located on the calcified bone as multinucleated cells in resorption cavities known as Howship's lacunae. The characteristic feature of the osteoclast is its ruffled border. This membrane secretes lysosomal enzymes, which degrade the organic matrix of bone, and a low pH causes dissolution of the calcium of the mineralized bone.

Osteoclasts are derived from hematopoietic monocyte cell precursors, which are present in several tissues; osteoclast differentiation and proliferation are tightly regulated by stromal and osteoblastic cells.[5] Specifically, the regulation of osteoclast differentiation and maturation is dependent on the receptor activator of nuclear factor-kappa B ligand (RANKL) pathway, with the RANKL present on the osteoblasts stimulating RANK on precursor osteoclasts to differentiate into active osteoclasts. Thus, bone formation and resorption are tightly coupled. Both of these cell lineages are important because their regulation is critical in the maintenance of normal calcium homeostasis as well as maintenance of the structural integrity of the skeleton. The complex cell-to-cell interactions involve several transcriptional factors. Several treatment modalities (antiresorptive agents such as the bisphosphonates and anabolic agents such as parathyroid hormone [PTH]) are now available for the treatment of osteoporosis and may have applicability in orthopaedics.[6]

In addition to the complex signaling involved in bone homeostasis, the importance of a mechanical response of the bone cell populations and maintaining the biologic function of the skeleton has emerged. These pathways are critical in understanding bone healing and bone regeneration. Over the next decade, understanding these pathways will allow changes to the local osseous environments through both local and systemic agents to enhance the bone repair process. This should prove useful not only in the field of traumatology but arthroplasty and spine surgery as well.

Regulation of Cell Differentiation and Calcium and Phosphorus Metabolism

Bone is a critical component of calcium homeostasis. Calcium is a critical regulator of muscle contraction, coagulation, intracellular signal transaction, and control of cell membrane potentials. Calcium levels are tightly regulated by intestinal absorption of dietary intake, excretion by the kidneys, and storage in the skeleton. Normal serum calcium levels range from 8.5 to 10 mg/dL, and circulation calcium exists approximately equally in free ionized form and protein-bound form, with albumin as the major binding protein. A small portion of the body's total calcium is bound to ions, such as phosphate. The skeleton acts a reserve for calcium that can be metabolized to maintain circulating concentrations. All calcium for the body is obtained from the diet, and its absorption from the intestines is regulated according to perceived body needs.

Dietary calcium absorption in the intestine occurs in the duodenum and the jejunum and is a function of active transport using a calcium-binding protein regulated by vitamin D and passive gradient-dependent transport. Calcium absorption is regulated by 1,25-dihydroxyvitamin D concentration and by calcium intake. Increases in calcium intake and in 1,25-dihydroxyvitamin D serum concentration act to increase intestinal calcium absorption.

Calcium is excreted in the kidneys at an approximate rate of 150 to 200 mg/day, an amount that balances the calcium absorbed in the intestine. Most of the calcium is absorbed in the proximal tubule through solvent gradient, although active transfer occurs in the distal portions by a sodium-calcium exchange pump. Some calcium is also absorbed in the loop of Henle through an electrochemical gradient. Factors that influence renal resorption of calcium are outlined in **Table 2**.

Recommended dietary calcium intake varies by age (**Table 3**). Several calcium supplements are available; although no single product is better than another, some are better tolerated than others. In general, calcium supplements should be taken several times a day with the maximum dose not exceeding 500 mg at any one time so as to maximize absorption. Care should be exercised when these supplements are taken with other medications, because certain antibiotics such as tetracycline interact with the calcium. In addition, iron supplements should not be taken at the same time as a calcium supplement. Calcium carbonate is better absorbed when taken with food, whereas calcium citrate can be taken on an empty stomach. Combination products are not necessary as long as adequate intake of vitamin D is achieved through diet.

An increase in calcium is required during growth, pregnancy, and lactation, and calcium intake must be increased in older individuals to counteract the effect of calcium loss caused by increased bone resorption. Because dietary intake of calcium is usually not adequate in elderly people, supplementation is usually indicated.

As with calcium, phosphorus is also critical for proper mineralization of bone, with 85% of all phosphorus present in the crystalline form in the skeleton and the remaining 15% largely present in either the extracellular fluid or as intracellular phosphorylated intermediates. Serum concentrations of phosphorus are tightly regulated between 2.5 to 4.5 µg/dL in adults. Passive transport is directly related to the intestinal concentration of phosphate after eating.

Vitamin D

The principal regulators of calcium metabolism are vitamin D and PTH. Vitamin D is a fat-soluble steroid that is derived from cholesterol and undergoes hydroxylation in the liver and kidney to its biologically active form vitamin 1,25-dihydroxyvitamin D. Normal serum calcium levels are maintained by increasing intestinal absorption of calcium and maturation of osteoclasts to mobilize calcium from bone when needed. In addition, vitamin D affects cell differentiation and proliferation and enhances insulin secretion that regulates the renin-angiotensin system. Vitamin D is produced in the skin during exposure to sunlight and is absorbed from dietary intake.

Sunscreen severely impairs the production of vitamin D by sunlight. Dietary sources of vitamin D are limited to oily fish (such as salmon, mackerel, or sardines); however, many foods are fortified with vitamin D, such as milk and orange juice. Multivitamins are also a source of vitamin D. In fair-skinned individuals, exposure of the hands and face to bright sunlight for approximately 15 minutes is adequate for production of vitamin D; however, in darker-skinned individuals, more exposure is necessary. The recommended daily requirement is between 400 and 800 IU in individuals who do not have adequate sunlight exposure. Vitamin D levels decrease with age and impaired renal function, and these two factors can combine to affect vitamin D levels and calcium absorption in elderly people.

Parathyroid Hormone

PTH is used to maintain serum calcium levels; its synthesis and release is stimulated by low extracellular ionized calcium levels. PTH binds to osteoblasts where it stimulates bone formation and the production of factors (such as interleukin-6) that stimulate osteoclasts to resorb bone. PTH-stimulated osteoclasts secrete neutral proteases that degrade osteoid and initiate bone remodeling. Parathyroid hormone-related protein (PTHrP) increases osteoblast expression of RANKL and decreases production of osteoprogerin in the development and progression of bone metastases in breast carcinoma.

Intermittent PTH clearly seems to be anabolic in bone formation and, in preclinical animal studies, it stimulates increased bone formation and acceleration of healing.[8] Thus, PTH plays a central role in calcium regulation and the coupling of bone resorption and formation.

Sex Steroids and Estrogen

There is a clear association between decreased estrogen levels and increased rates of bone resorption, as indicated by the rapid acceleration of bone loss following meno-

Table 3

Recommended Calcium Intake

Age	Amount (mg/d)
Birth to 6 months	210
6 months to 1 year	270
1 to 3 years	500
4 to 8 years	800
9 to 13 years	1,300
14 to 18 years	1,300
19 to 30 years	1,000
31 to 50 years	1,000
51 to 70 years	1,200
71 or older	1,200
Pregnant and lactating	
14 to 18 years	1,300
19 to 50 years	1,000

pause, during which bone loss accelerates to 2% to 3% per year for the first 6 to 8 years of the postmenopausal period, returning to the normal age-related loss of 0.3% to 0.5% per year. Estrogen receptors are found on osteoblasts and osteoclasts and may work through the interleukin-6 as well as the RANKL pathway.

The exact role of androgens in retaining skeletal mass in men is not clear. Men with idiopathic hypogonadotropic hypogonadism have reduced levels of cortical and trabecular bone loss, and delayed puberty is also associated with osteopenia in men. Androgens prevent bone resorption and may stimulate an increase in bone mass, but the mechanism is not known. Corticosteroids are known to inhibit calcium absorption in the intestine by decreasing the production of calcium-binding proteins, increasing calcium excretion in the kidneys, and inhibiting bone formation and resorption. In addition, corticosteroids may slow bone healing and can also indirectly stimulate secondary hyperparathyroidism.

Thyroid Hormone

Hyperthyroidism is associated with osteoporosis. Thyroid hormones T4 and T3 circulate bound to plasma proteins. They interact with specific cell receptors and bind to nuclear DNA, increase thyroid hormone, and stimulate bone resorption and formation; however, resorption occurs at a slightly greater rate, eventually resulting in bone loss. Thus, chronic hyperthyroidism and thyroid supplementation can contribute to osteoporosis.

Clinical Evaluation of Bone and Mineral Disorders

Despite the plethora of sophisticated biochemical and diagnostic modalities, a through medical history and

Table 4

Absolute Fracture Risk Versus Age

Age (Years)	T Score	Absolute Risk
50	0	0.2%
	−1	0.4%
	−2	1.1%
60	0	0.4%
	−1	1.0%
	−2	2.7%
70	0	0.7%
	−1	1.9%
	−2	5.3%

(Reproduced with permission from Blake GM, Knapp KM, Fogelman I: Absolute fracture risk varies with bone densitometry technique used: A theoretical and in vivo study of fracture cases. J Clin Densitom 2002;5:109-116.)

physical examination remain essential in evaluating any patient with metabolic bone disorders. The initial assessment includes the patient's age, sex, race, menopausal status, and a complete medical, pharmacologic, nutritional, and family history. Although the diagnosis of postmenopausal osteoporosis or age-related osteoporosis seems straightforward, other metabolic bone disorders must be ruled out with the appropriate medical history, physical examination, and diagnostic tests.

Of particular importance in the medical history are questions regarding dietary and lifestyle issues, specifically whether or not adequate calcium, phosphorus, and vitamin D are being consumed. The use of tobacco and caffeine as well as potential alcohol abuse needs to be documented. Similarly, the patient's medication history is of value, as many medications predispose patients to metabolic bone disorders. Questions regarding other endocrine, renal, or gastrointestinal diseases are important, and in women menstrual history is essential, especially questions regarding amenorrhea, time of onset of menses, and menopause. Family history also remains important as many metabolic bone disorders are heritable, and many genetic disorders including osteogenesis imperfecta, Ehlers-Danlos syndrome, Marfan syndrome, X-linked hypophosphatemic rickets, and vitamin D-dependent rickets are associated with reduced bone mass, fractures, or osteomalacia.

During the physical examination, height and weight must be documented along with an evaluation for bony deformities and ligamentous laxity. In addition, examination for neuromuscular irritability associated with hypocalcemia may be done, and characteristic skeletal changes associated with Paget's disease as well as the findings of established osteoporosis including dorsal kyphosis (or dowager's hump) and loss of height should be noted. Secondary causes of osteoporosis such as Cushing syndrome and hypogonadism should be noted.

Initial laboratory studies should include assessment of appropriate serum calcium levels as well as determination of total and free calcium. Phosphorus levels

should also be measured along with magnesium levels. Serum bone formation markers include bone-specific alkaline phosphatase, osteocalcin, C-terminal propeptide of type I collagen, and N-terminal propeptide of type I collagen. Similarly, there are a number of bone resorption markers including free and total pyridinolines, free and total deoxypyridinolines, N-telopeptide of collagen at cross-links, and C-telopeptides at collagen cross-links. In the serum, similar N- and C-telopeptides of collagen cross-links, tartrate-resistant acid phosphatase, and cross-linked C-telopeptide of type I collagen can be measured.[9]

Of these markers, urine and serum assays of N-telopeptides are commercially available and are important for establishing the nature of the metabolic bone disorder and also are of value in terms of monitoring effectiveness of any treatment, selection of patients for therapy, prediction of response to therapy, and prediction of fracture risk, bone loss, and bone mass. Of these clinical uses, currently the most appropriate is monitoring effectiveness of any treatment.

In terms of imaging studies for metabolic bone disorders, standard radiographic techniques such as plain skeletal radiography, CT, MRI, and nuclear medicine as well as ultrasound have value specifically in the diagnosis of osteogenesis imperfecta, osteomalacia, and rickets. They can also be of value in the diagnosis of primary hyperparathyroidism, renal osteodystrophy, scurvy, hypothyroidism, hyperthyroidism, hypophosphatemia, hyperphosphatemia, osteopetrosis, Paget's disease, and fibrous dysplasia.

Although all of these modalities are important in the diagnosis of unique metabolic bone disorders, the mainstay of diagnosis is the use of bone mass measurements in the assessment and management of osteoporosis, primarily the use of bone mineral density (BMD) for fracture risk.[10] The clinical indications for use of bone mass measurements include women age 65 years and older, postmenopausal women younger than 65 years with risk factors, men age 70 years or older, adults with a fragility fracture, adults with a disease or condition associated with low bone mass, adults taking medications associated with low bone mass or bone loss, anyone being considered for pharmacologic therapy, anyone being treated to monitor treatment effect, and anyone not receiving therapy and in whom evidence of bone loss would lead to treatment based on International Society for Clinical Densitometry standards (www.iscd.org).

The result of BMD measurements are given in terms of a T score, which is a standard deviation below or above a young adult mean value. For example, a patient with a T score of -2.5 has a BMD that is 2.5 times below the mean of a young adult population. A patient with a T score below -2.5 is considered to have osteoporosis by World Health Organization standards and treatment is usually recommended. A patient with a T score between -1.0 and 2.5 is considered to have osteopenia based on World Health Organization criteria. These relationships are important, as outlined in **Table 4**, where the T scores clearly correlate with the absolute risk of fracture and age.

Although not used on a routine clinical basis, bone biopsies and histomorphology remain important as research tools and in patients with metabolic bone disorders with unclear diagnoses. If an iliac crest bone biopsy is considered, then appropriate antibiotic labeling must be performed to maximize diagnostic information.

The use of modern molecular biologic approaches such as polymerase chain reaction and direct DNA sequencing in combination with genetic information will be important in the future for the diagnosis and clinical management of patients with bone and mineral disorders.

Osteoporosis and Osteoporotic Fractures

The most prevalent metabolic bone disorder is osteoporosis, specifically postmenopausal osteoporosis. It is estimated that 10 million Americans older than age 50 years have osteoporosis; 1.5 million of these patients experience fragility fractures each year. Another 34 million Americans are at risk for osteoporosis.[11]

The cost of treatment of fragility fractures has increased exponentially over the past several decades and this increase is projected to continue. As the world population ages, the number of these fractures will continue to increase in parallel with the requirements of health care systems for the treatment of these fractures.

Most fragility fractures are fractures of cancellous bone as opposed to diaphyseal cortical bone. They occur either in metaphyseal regions of long bones such as the proximal femur, distal forearm, proximal humerus, and proximal tibia, or are vertebral fractures.

The overall fracture incidence in the developed world is bimodal, with peaks in childhood and early adulthood and in the elderly population. In young people, fractures of long bones predominate, usually secondary to significant trauma, and occur more frequently in males than females. In women older than 35 years, the fracture incidence increases steeply so that fracture rates become twice those of men, with fractures of the distal forearm, hip, and vertebral body occurring most often.[12]

It has been estimated that in the United Kingdom the lifetime risk of a hip fracture for a 50-year-old is approximately 14% for women and 3% for men, with these fractures requiring hospitalization. These fractures have a significant degree of morbidity and mortality. Universally these patients lose one level of function after any hip fracture.

Although most if not all hip fractures require some medical intervention, vertebral body fractures may be asymptomatic and initially remain undiagnosed. If vertebral fractures are correctly diagnosed, the incidence is probably much higher than previously suspected, with a 28% lifetime risk in women and a 12% lifetime risk in men. Most of these fractures occur as a result of normal activities such as lifting rather than a fall, which is the mechanism most often associated with hip fractures. Few of these fractures require hospitalization but they are associated with significant pain and disability.

Patients with significant pain after a fracture may benefit from either vertebroplasty or kyphoplasty.

The incidence of distal forearm fractures is higher in women between the ages of 45 and 60 years than in the elderly population. This may be secondary to altered neuromuscular reflexes associated with aging. As aging progresses, individuals tend to fall sideways or backward and thus are not able to break the fall with an outstretched upper extremity. Data from the United Kingdom show that women have a 13% lifetime risk of wrist fracture, whereas the lifetime risk in men is 2%. Fortunately, these fractures rarely affect longevity and if treated properly should not lead to significant disability.

The most important determinants of postmenopausal osteoporosis are those factors that determine peak bone mass. Thus, postmenopausal osteoporosis can also often be viewed as the sequela of childhood and adolescence factors because there is little increase in bone mass after menarche. Resultant peak bone mass is achieved by age 20 to 30 years and subsequently there is a steady decline in bone mass, with an accelerated rate of bone loss in the postmenopausal period.

There are numerous genetic factors that determine peak bone mass. Heritability seems to account for 50% to 80% of the variance in bone mass depending on skeletal site. Several related genes seem to regulate bone mass, including genes for type I collagen, lipoprotein receptor-related protein-5, and vitamin D receptors. Bone loss in the postmenopausal period is the result of increased rate of bone remodeling and imbalance between activity of osteoclasts and osteoblasts. One major cause of bone loss and imbalance of this coupled mechanism is estrogen deficiency associated with the postmenopausal period. Aging has also been associated with bone loss specifically related to such factors as increased levels of PTH and to osteoblast senescence. Several diseases and drugs are clearly important in the acceleration of bone loss such as glucocorticoid therapy.

Bone strength is not only related to BMD. The role of other factors, including bone geometry, fatigue damage, and loss of trabecular connectivity is currently being studied. In addition to the risk factors noted above, there are several other clinical risk factors for fractures (Table 5).

Patients recommended for osteoporosis screening with bone densitometry include patients who have experienced low trauma fractures, men with significant risk factors, and women older than 65 years or those who are postmenopausal or have other fracture risks such as maternal/paternal history of fracture, substantial weight loss, and long-term use of benzodiazepines and anticonvulsants. At minimum, any patient treated for a fragility fracture should be referred for evaluation and secondary prevention therapy.

Treatment

The mainstay of treatment of osteoporosis in addition to calcium and vitamin D supplementation is antiresorptive agents. These agents include calcitonin and the bisphosphonates. Although the number of currently

2: Systemic Disorders

Table 5

Clinical Risk Factors for Fracture

Female sex
Advanced age
Caucasian
Prior fragility fracture
Medications
  Glucocorticoids
  Anticonvulsants
  Benzodiazepines
  Antidepressants
Medical conditions
  Diabetes
  Hyperparathyroidism
  Hyperthyroidism
  Inflammatory arthritis
  Hypercortisolism
  Neuromuscular conditions
Eating disorders
Family history
Low body mass index
Smoking

Table 6

Causes of Drug-Induced Rickets/Osteomalacia

Drugs resulting in hypocalcemia
  Inhibitors of vitamin D formation or intestinal absorption
    Suncreens
    Cholestyramine
  Increased catabolism of vitamin D or its metabolites
    Anticonvulsants
Drugs resulting in hypophosphatemia
  Inhibitors of intestinal phosphate reabsorption
    Aluminum containing antacids
  Impaired renal phosphate reabsorption
    Cadmium
    Ifosfamide
    Saccharated ferric oxide
  Direct impairment of mineralization
    Parental aluminum
    Fluoride
    Etidronate

(Reproduced from Pettifor JM: 2003 Nutritional and Drug-Induced Rickets and Osteomalacia, in Favus MJ (ed): The Primer on the Metabolic Bone Diseases and Disorders of Mineral Metabolism, ed 5. American Society for Bone and Mineral Research, Washington, DC, pp 399-407 with permission of the American Society for Bone and Mineral Research.)

available bisphosphonates has increased, overall the treatment approach has not changed. The oral bisphosphonates in the United States for which the most clinical data has been compiled are alendronate, risedronate, and ibandronate. Newer, more potent intravenous forms of bisphosphonates such as zoledronic acid are appealing because the dosing can be as infrequent as every 12 months. Whether these newer agents pose a higher risk for the development of osteonecrosis of the jaw remains to be determined.

In addition to the antiresorptive agents, the use of intermittent PTH (teriparatide) has been shown to be effective in the treatment of osteoporosis. This anabolic agent alone has been shown to stimulate significant increases in cancellous BMD and decrease fracture risk. The combination of PTH with antiresorptive agents has solid theoretic justification but has not yet been demonstrated clinically.

Other Metabolic Bone Diseases

Paget's Disease of Bone

Paget's disease is a localized disorder of bone remodeling that initially involves an increase in osteoclast-mediated bone resorption followed by compensatory increase in bone formation. The result is that of a disorganized mosaic of woven and lamellar bone at the affected sites.

A combination of environmental and genetic factors is required for the disease to develop. Multiple studies have demonstrated a genetic predisposition for Paget's disease, and recently gene mutations in specific genes involved in bone remodeling have been mapped in these familial cases. Specifically, mutations of the *p62/ZIP* gene have been documented but genetic predisposition is not enough to cause the disease. Many believe that paramyxoviral infection may also be required. Why paramyxoviral infections, such as measles, which occur worldwide, only affect individuals in certain geographic distributions and why these viruses, which generally affect children, lead to a disease that is primarily diagnosed in patients older than age 55 years are questions about the viral etiology of Paget's disease that remain unanswered.

Treatment for Paget's disease has evolved from the 1970s, when bisphosphonates were first introduced, to newer bisphosphonates such as pamidronate, alendronate, and zoledronic acid. The rationale behind treatment is to avoid complications. Calcitonin is also used in the treatment of Paget's disease. Other agents such as nonsteroidal anti-inflammatory drugs have a role in relieving pain related to Paget's disease but do not modify the underlying disease process.

Surgery on pagetoid bone may be necessary for an established or impending fracture and occasionally total joint arthroplasties are necessary when associated with osteoarthritis. It is strongly suggested that a potent bisphosphonate be used before elective surgery on pagetoid bone with the goal being to reduce the hypervascularity associated with the moderate active disease, thus diminishing the amount of blood loss during surgery.

Osteomalacia and Rickets

Osteomalacia results from failure of mineralization at newly formed osteoid sites either periosteal or endosteal, whereas rickets is failure of or delay in the mineralization of new bone formation at growth plates. Rickets is a disease of childhood whereas osteomalacia tends to occur in adults, although children also may have areas of osteomalacic bone.

Although vitamin D supplementation and fortification of foods have dramatically decreased the worldwide incidence of osteomalacia and rickets, some patients are still affected by these metabolic bone disorders; vitamin D dietary deficiencies in combination with calcium deficiencies often is the causative factor. There are several drug-induced causes of rickets and osteomalacia (Table 6). Several medications that result in hypophosphatemia such as inhibitors of intestinal phosphate absorption and those that impair renal phosphate reabsorption also lead to osteomalacia.

Rickets and osteomalacia may also be caused by impaired vitamin D activation and hormone resistance. Pseudovitamin D-deficient rickets and hereditary vitamin D-resistant rickets both have specific gene mutations, with pseudovitamin D-deficient rickets having a mutation in one α hydroxylase, and hereditary vitamin D-resistant deficiencies having a gene mutation of the vitamin D receptor gene. Another form of osteomalacia is hypophosphatemic vitamin D-resistant rickets, which is caused by a mutation in the phosphate regulating gene with homologies to endopeptidase on the X chromosome (*Phex*). Rarer forms of osteomalacia occur such as tumor-induced osteomalacia and high turnover renal osteodystrophy have not been completely eliminated.

Summary

The bone healing and repair process involves not merely recruiting stem cells and allowing them to proliferate and differentiate, but also allows the skeleton to repair itself to achieve its normal architecture and material properties. The process of fracture healing involves a complex cascade of growth factors, cytokines, and signaling molecules with many of the same regulatory mechanisms for bone turnover, formation, and resorption that are also involved in the regulation of bone homeostasis.[13] Similarly, hematopoietic and inflammatory mediators are involved in fracture healing as is the process of angiogenesis.[7] These same mediators and processes also play a role in the development of osteoporosis and other bone disorders. An understanding of how these morphogenetic factors play a role in skeletal development and bone metabolism may

also further understanding of bone healing and repair. The future of enhanced bone healing and repair and other orthopaedic applications therefore lies within the arena of bone metabolism and understanding these processes.

Annotated References

1. Favus MJ (ed): *Primer on the Metabolic Bone Diseases and Disorders of Mineral Metabolism*, ed 6. Washington, DC, American Society of Bone and Mineral Research, 2006.

   An overview of metabolic bone diseases and bone metabolism is presented, written by experts in the field.

2. Bennett CN, Longo KA, Wright WS, et al: Regulation of osteoblastogenesis and bone mass by Wnt 10b. *Proc Natl Acad Sci USA* 2005;102:3324-3329.

   In this comprehensive study, the importance of wnt as an endogenous regulator of bone formation is demonstrated. The authors present convincing evidence that wnt10b stimulates osteoblastogenesis and inhibits adipogenesis in mesenchymal stem cells.

3. Canalis E, Economdies AN, Gazzerro E: Bone morphogenetic proteins, their antagonists and the skeleton. *Endocr Rev* 2003;24:218-235.

4. Janssens K, Ten DP, Janssens S, Van HW: Transforming growth factor beta 1 to the bone. *Endocr Rev* 2005;26:743-774.

   Transforming growth factor-beta is a ubiquitous protein involved in embryogenesis, angiogenesis, inflammation, and wound healing. It also plays a critical role in bone development, homeostasis, and repair; this article describes its role as it pertains to bone.

5. Xing L, Boyce BF: Regulation of apoptosis in osteoclasts and osteoblastic cells 2005. *Biochem Biophys Res Commun* 2005;328:709-720.

   The regulation of osteoblasts and osteoclasts is becoming increasingly clear. This article describes the role of apoptosis in the regulation of these two cell lineages and how this affects bone homeostasis.

6. Rogers MJ: From molds and macrophages to mevalonate: A decade of progress in understanding the molecular action of bisphosphonates. *Calcif Tissue Int* 2004;75:451-461.

   Bisphosphonates are a class of one of the most commonly used pharmacologic agents currently available for the treatment of osteoporosis. The molecular action of this class of molecules is described, along with the difficulties associated with determining the pathway of action of these agents.

7. Simon AM, Manigrasso MB, O'Connor JP: Cyclooxygenase 2 function is essential for bone fracture healing. *J Bone Miner Res* 2002;17:963-976.

8. Rubin MR, Bilezikian JP: The anabolic effects of parathyroid hormone therapy. *Clin Geriatr Med* 2003;19: 415-432.

9. Sarkar S, Reinster JY, Frans GG, Diez-Perez A, Pinette KV, Delmas PD: Relationship between changes in biochemical markers of bone turnover and BMD to predict vertebral fracture risk. *J Bone Miner Res* 2004;19:394-401.

   Changes in osteocalcin, a marker of bone turnover, was found to be a better predictor of vertebral fracture risk than lumbar BMD in a large multicenter trial of an oral selective estrogen receptor modulator that is used in the prevention of osteoporosis in postmenopausal women.

10. Kanis JA, Borgstrom F, DeLaet C, et al: Assessment of fracture risk. *Osteoporos Int* 2005;16:581-589.

    Risk factors other than BMD such as age, prior fragility fracture, parental history of hip fracture, smoking, use of systemic corticosteroids, excess alcohol intake, and rheumatoid arthritis are important in the determination of fracture risk. Once the probability of fracture has been determined, proper treatment can be instituted.

11. Melton JL III, Chrisschilles EA, Cooper C, Lane AW, Riggs BL: How many women have osteoporosis? *J Bone Miner Res* 2005;20:886-892.

    This article is an update of the classic article describing the prevalence of osteoporosis in women.

12. Johnell O, Kanis JA: Epidemiology of osteoporotic fractures. *Osteoporos Int* 2005;16(suppl2):S3-S7.

    This article reviews the most current epidemiology of osteoporotic fractures worldwide and provides accurate data on this growing public health issue.

13. Lehmann W, Edgar CM, Wang K, et al: Tumor necrosis factor alpha coordinately regulates the expression of specific matrix metalloproteinases and angiogenetic factors during fracture healing. *Bone* 2005;36:300-310.

    Tumor necrosis factor alpha is an important regulator of a variety of immune functions. It also plays a role in bone homeostasis, specifically in osteoclastogenesis as well as bone healing and repair through both matrix metalloproteinases and angiogenetic pathways.

Chapter 17

Musculoskeletal Oncology

Mihir M. Thacker, MD

Epidemiology

Cancer is the second leading cause of death among Americans. According to American Cancer Society data, cancer will be diagnosed in approximately 1.44 million Americans in 2007 and approximately 560,000 will die of their disease. These numbers are expected to double over the next 50 years. Bone and soft-tissue sarcomas are not common; the National Cancer Institute estimates that sarcoma will be diagnosed in 11,590 Americans in 2007 (2,370 bone sarcomas and 9,220 soft-tissue sarcomas) and 4,890 of them will die of their disease. The incidence rates of bone and soft-tissue sarcomas have remained fairly constant over the past 30 years at approximately 0.8 to 1 per 100,000 people.

Tumor Biology

As the understanding of mechanisms involved in tumorigenesis has improved, certain syndromes that predispose individuals to musculoskeletal malignancy have been identified. Genetic alterations have been identified in many tumors, and current research is focused on identification of genetic abnormalities in patients with musculoskeletal tumors and the mechanisms by which these affect cell proliferation and differentiation. Balanced translocations have been identified in several tumors (Table 1). Balanced translocations may result in abnormal gene fusions, which in turn result in the formation of chimeric proteins (transcription factors and tyrosine kinases). This results in deregulation of gene expression and cell signaling. Unbalanced translocations may result in either gain of an oncogene or loss of tumor suppressor genes, leading to disinhibition of growth of cells. Some syndromes in which these processes are involved are retinoblastoma gene alterations, Li-Fraumeni syndrome, Rothmund-Thomson syndrome, and Bloom syndrome.

The *RB1* gene is a tumor suppressor gene found on chromosome 13. It regulates the cell cycle, and its absence in hereditary retinoblastoma predisposes the affected children to development of multiple retinoblastomas and other primary tumors including osteosarcoma.

Li-Fraumeni syndrome is an autosomal dominant inherited syndrome that is associated with a mutation in the *p53* (tumor suppressor) gene. Patients with this syndrome have a high incidence of multiple primary malignancies including osteosarcoma, soft-tissue sarcomas, premenopausal breast carcinoma, and gastrointestinal malignancies.

Rothmund-Thomson syndrome is a rare autosomal recessive syndrome that occurs as a result of mutations in the *RECQL4* gene on chromosome 8q24. It is associated with skin rashes (poikiloderma), photosensitivity, juvenile cataracts, skeletal dysplasias, osteosarcoma, and cutaneous malignancies.

Bloom syndrome is characterized by growth deficiency, telangiectasis, photosensitivity, and increased risk of malignancy. Similar to Rothmund-Thomson syndrome, this condition is inherited in an autosomal recessive fashion. The gene defect, which has been traced to the 15q26.1 locus, results in increased sister chromatid exchange and chromosomal instability.

Diagnosis of Musculoskeletal Tumors

The diagnosis of a musculoskeletal tumor is made based on correlation of the patient's clinical, radiographic, and pathologic information.

Clinical

Diagnosis begins with a thorough patient history and examination. Pain not related to activity, while at rest, and pain that awakens the patient from sleep and prevents return to sleep warrants a detailed evaluation. A large, rapidly growing mass or recent change in a previously stable lesion also are suggestive of an aggressive

Table 1

Translocations Associated With Commonly Seen Tumors

Neoplasm	Translocation
Dermatofibrosarcoma protuberans	t(17;22)(q22;q13)
Ewing's sarcoma/peripheral primitive neuroectodermal tumor	t(11;22)(q24;q12) t(21;22)(q22;q12)
Extraskeletal myxoid chondrosarcoma	t(9;22)(q22-31;q12)
Myxoid/round cell liposarcoma	t(12;16)(q13;p11)
Synovial sarcoma	t(X;18)(p11.2;q11.2)

2: Systemic Disorders

Table 2

Commonly Seen Tumors in Different Locations

Location	Commonly Seen Tumors
Spine: anterior elements	Metastatic, myeloma, Paget disease, vascular malformation, GCT
Spine: posterior elements	Osteoid osteoma, osteoblastoma; ABC
Pelvis	Metastatic, myeloma, chondrosarcoma, GCT, ABC, Paget disease, EWS
Sacrum	Chordoma (midline), chondrosarcoma, GCT, ABC, lymphoma
Tibia	Adamantinoma, chondromyxoid fibroma
Ribs	Metastatic, myeloma, fibrous dysplasia, chondrosarcoma
Small bones of the hands and feet	Enchondroma, exostosis
Calcaneus	UBC and lipoma (under the angle of Gissane), chondroblastoma, osteosarcoma
Surface lesions	Exostosis, parosteal osteosarcoma (posterior distal femur), periosteal osteosarcoma (proximal tibia or anterior distal femur), periosteal chondroma or chondrosarcoma, myositis ossificans.

GCT = giant cell tumor, ABC = aneurysmal bone cyst, EWS = Ewing's sarcoma, UBC = unicameral bone cyst

Table 3

Commonly Seen Tumors According to Their Location in Bone

Location in Bone	Commonly Seen Lesions
Epiphysis	Chondroblastoma, clear cell chondrosarcoma, GCT, infection, dysplasia epiphysealis hemimelica (DEH)
Metaphysis	Most common site of involvement by most tumors
Diaphysis (HEALOF)	H-Histiocytosis (LCH) E-Ewing's sarcoma A-Adamantinoma L-Leukemia/lymphoma O-Osteoid osteoma, osteoblastoma F-Fibrous dysplasia

GCT = giant cell tumor, LCH = Langerhans cell histiocytosis

process. Age is an important consideration in formulating an appropriate differential diagnosis. The most likely differential diagnosis for a destructive round blue cell lesion, for example, is neuroblastoma in a patient 0 to 5 years of age, Ewing's sarcoma in patients 5 to 15 years of age, lymphoma in those age 15 to 40 years, and myeloma in patients older than 40 years. Some tumors have a gender predilection; for example, giant cell tumors are more common in females and osteosarcomas in males. Race rarely helps confirm the diagnosis, although Ewing's sarcoma is uncommon in African Americans.

Size and depth of the lesion per se do not predict aggressive behavior (many atypical lipomatous tumors may be large and deep but not aggressive), but larger and deeper tumors are often more aggressive. Most tumors are solitary; however, multiple bone involvement may occur in certain conditions such as fibrous dysplasia, enchondromas (Ollier disease, Maffucci's syndrome), osteochondromas (multiple hereditary exostoses), and Langerhans cell histiocytosis (LCH).

Most laboratory tests are not specific for the diagnosis of bone tumors. Serum chemistry is often useful in determining cellular turnover (lactate dehydrogenase [LDH] level) or the degree of bone destruction and formation (calcium, alkaline phosphatase). There are tumor markers that can aid in the diagnosis and are also useful in the surveillance of various tumors; for example, prostate-specific antigen levels aid in the diagnosis and monitoring of prostate carcinoma; rising levels after an initial response to treatment indicate residual/recurrent disease.

Imaging

Radiographs form the cornerstone for the diagnosis of osseous tumors. Radiographs not only reflect the underlying pathology but also are useful in predicting the clinical behavior (growth rate and biologic potential) of the tumor. Certain tumors (such as most osteochondromas and nonossifying fibromas) have a characteristic radiographic appearance and may not need additional imaging studies to confirm the diagnosis.

Analysis of radiographs of the tumor should be systematic and should include the following questions: (1) Where is the tumor—in which bone (Table 2) and in which part of the bone (Table 3)? (2) What is the tumor doing to the bone (clinical behavior)? (3) What is the bone doing to the tumor (biologic response)? (4) Are there any intrinsic clues to the histology (matrix pattern)?

The margin is the junction between the tumor and the host bone (Figure 1). The margin between the tumor and the host bone is a good indicator of the biologic aggressiveness of the tumor.[1] Periosteal reaction is a biologic measure of the inherent aggressiveness of the inciting process and the ability of the bone to respond to it. Certain tumors are associated with characteristic periosteal reaction patterns such as onion skinning or a lamellated periosteal response seen in Ewing's sarcoma. This reaction pattern is not pathognomonic of Ewing's sarcoma nor universally seen in patients with Ewing's sarcoma; however, when seen, they suggest the possibility of Ewing's sarcoma. Matrix is the acellular interstitial substance produced by tumor cells. The different types of matrix patterns that are commonly seen are shown in Figure 2.

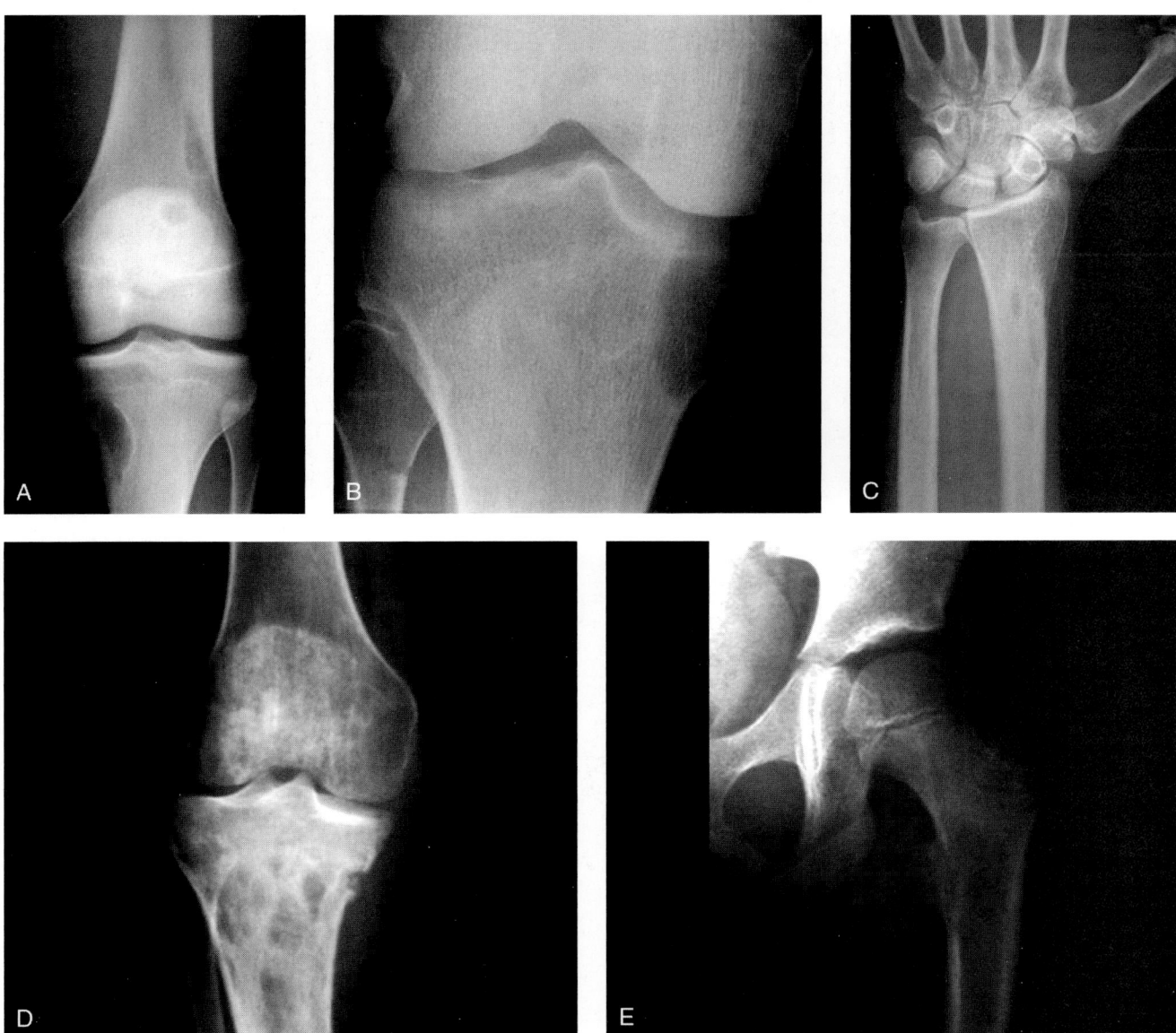

Figure 1   Lodwick classification of margins. Type I, geographic margins, which are further subclassified as IA: geographic with a rind of surrounding sclerosis **(A)**, IB: geographic without surrounding sclerosis **(B)** and IC: ill defined **(C)**. Type II (motheaten) **(D)** and type III (permeative) margin **(E)** are usually seen in aggressive processes (infection, malignancy).

Computed Tomography

CT is less useful than MRI for evaluating the local extent of disease. However, CT scans show cortical detail better than MRI and therefore are useful for showing nondisplaced fractures and the degree of endosteal scalloping, as well as subtle matrix mineralization. CT scans of the chest are important for staging and surveillance of malignant tumors because most of these tumors usually metastasize to the lungs. CT also is useful for biopsy of certain tumors, especially deep-seated pelvic lesions.

Magnetic Resonance Imaging

MRI has become the imaging modality of choice for most tumors (the notable exception being osteoid os-

teomas, for which CT is preferred). MRI is useful for determining marrow involvement, intraosseous as well as extraosseous extension of the tumor, and tumor size and proximity to neurovascular structures. The entire length of the involved bone should be scanned in patients with suspected osseous malignancies to look for skip lesions.

Nuclear Imaging

Technetium Tc 99m bone scans are the method of choice to localize a suspected lesion with no changes on radiographs and for multifocal lesions (except myeloma, for which bone scans often fail to show increase in radiotracer uptake and a skeletal survey is required). They are also important for staging malignant tumors

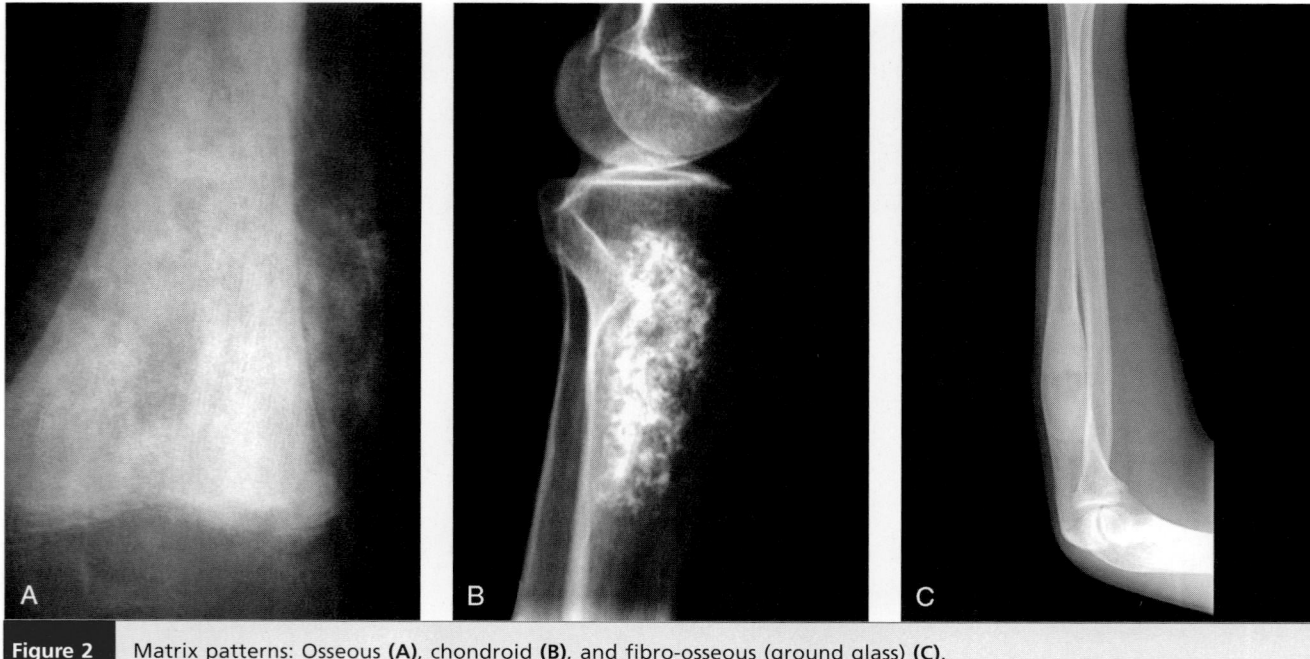

| Figure 2 | Matrix patterns: Osseous (A), chondroid (B), and fibro-osseous (ground glass) (C). |

and for postoperative surveillance. Technetium Tc 99m bone scans are nonspecific and have a high false-positive rate. As a result of the advances in MRI techniques, bone scans may be replaced by whole-body MRI in the future. Positron emission tomography (PET) has proved to be useful in identifying certain tumors such as lymphoma and lung cancer, but its role in the imaging of bone tumors needs to be better defined. The high cost of PET continues to limit its use.

Angiography

Angiography is an extremely useful adjunct in highly vascular tumors such as metastatic renal cell and thyroid carcinoma as well as melanoma. With these tumors, preoperative embolization may be performed to minimize intraoperative blood loss. Embolization may be used as therapeutic treatment or aneurysmal bone cysts and giant cell tumors.

Biopsy of Musculoskeletal Lesions

The biopsy is the final step in the diagnosis of a musculoskeletal lesion.[2,3] A thorough analysis of the clinical and radiographic findings before the biopsy is essential. The biopsy findings are always interpreted in light of the clinical and radiographic appearance of the tumor. Although technically a minor procedure, a biopsy that is poorly conceived or executed may lead to alteration in treatment and an adverse outcome. It has therefore been recommended that the biopsy be performed by the surgeon providing the definitive treatment.

The biopsy may be performed as an open procedure or with a needle. Needle biopsy is currently preferred at most centers whenever possible. It is an outpatient procedure that minimizes the morbidity to the patient as well as decreases cost. An open biopsy may be indicated

in difficult locations such as the axilla and the popliteal fossa, where the proximity of vital structures may make needle placement difficult. Open biopsy provides more tissue for diagnosis and research purposes and its diagnostic accuracy is somewhat better than needle biopsy, which may be limited by the amount of tissue obtained and sampling error. Image-guided biopsies (guided by CT or ultrasonography) can help reduce sampling error by accurate placement of the needle into the desired portion of the tumor. This type of biopsy is especially useful in pelvic or retroperitoneal lesions. Some of the principles of biopsy are outlined in Table 4.

Pathology

Analysis of the lesional tissue includes standard hematoxylin and eosin preparations as well as special stains, immunohistochemistry, and other special tests (such as fluorescent in situ hybridization or flow cytometry) as indicated. In a patient with a suspected Ewing's sarcoma, for example, the tissue is sent for chromosomal translocation studies to look for the characteristic 11-22 translocation; if lymphoma is suspected, flow cytometry helps confirm the diagnosis and immunohistochemistry helps to further categorize the tumor subtype.

An analysis of the predominant cell type and the pattern of arrangement help in the diagnosis of the tumor. Spindle cell lesions are characterized by cells with elongated nuclei. These include fibrosarcoma and fibromatosis, leiomyosarcoma, synovial sarcoma, nerve sheath tumors (benign and malignant), and vascular tumors. Epithelioid (polygonal cell) lesions include metastatic carcinomas, epithelioid sarcoma, alveolar soft-part sar-

Table 4

Principles of Biopsy of Musculoskeletal Tumors

Review the clinical and radiographic findings with the radiologist and pathologist before the biopsy.

The biopsy should be performed at the site of definitive treatment by appropriately trained personnel or in consultation with them if the former is not feasible.

Use a tourniquet whenever possible. Avoid expressive exsanguination (Esmarch bandage).

Use the shortest possible incision, longitudinally placed, along the line of the eventual resection.

Minimize soft-tissue dissection and contamination of tissue planes. Dissect through and not in between muscles to minimize contamination and need for eventual resection.

Choose the best site for the biopsy—usually the advancing edge of the tumor or the extraosseous component of a bone tumor and not the central portion, which may often be necrotic. A thorough analysis of MRI scans helps in planning.

Obtain an adequate amount of tissue for diagnosis and ancillary tests. Minimize distortion of the specimen and send it fresh to the pathologist for appropriate tests (eg, flow cytometry in suspected lymphomas).

Achieve hemostasis and use a drain (brought out in line with the incision and close to it), if needed.

Sutures should be placed close to the wound edges to minimize the amount of skin to be excised at the time of definitive resection.

Culture what you biopsy and biopsy what you culture.

Table 5

Histologic Growth Patterns in Tumors

Alveolar	Alveolar rhabdomyosarcoma, alveolar soft-part sarcoma
Biphasic	Synovial sarcoma, mesothelioma, round cell liposarcoma
Fascicular	Fibrous lesions, cellular schwannoma, peripheral nerve sheath tumors
Storiform (cartwheel)	Dermatofibrosarcoma protuberans, neurofibroma, fibrous histiocytoma, malignant fibrous histiocytoma

coma, clear cell sarcoma, and melanoma. Round blue cell lesions include leukemia, lymphoma, neuroblastoma, Ewing's sarcoma/primitive neuroectodermal tumor, rhabdomyosarcoma, and myeloma. Myxoid lesions are characterized by a myxoid or faintly basophilic stroma. These include myxoma, myxoid liposarcoma, myxofibrosarcoma, and extraskeletal myxoid chondrosarcoma. Pleomorphic lesions contain cells of different shapes and sizes, usually with high nucleus to cytoplasm ratio and hyperchromatism. These include pleomorphic liposarcoma and malignant fibrous histiocytoma (MFH), which is now called high-grade undifferentiated pleomorphic sarcoma. Certain tumors exhibit characteristic growth patterns; some of these are outlined in Table 5.

Immunohistochemistry

A major advance has been made in the diagnosis, classification, and understanding of the lineage of several (primarily soft-tissue) tumors. Several useful immunohistochemical markers are available. Keratins are typically seen in epithelial cells and therefore are the hallmark of carcinomas. Although usually not seen in sarcomas, they may be present in sarcomas with epithelioid components, such as epithelioid sarcoma, synovial sarcoma, and adamantinomas.

Muscle tumors are typically desmin positive. If there is a skeletal muscle differentiation (rhabdomyosar-

coma), then the cells will have myogenin or Myo-D immunoreactivity. If there is a tendency for smooth muscle differentiation (leiomyosarcoma), the cells show smooth muscle actin immunoreactivity. Smooth muscle actin may also be positive in myofibroblastic lesions such as fibromatosis. Vascular tumors typically show CD 31 and 34 immunoreactivity. They may also demonstrate immunoreactivity to factor VIII-related antigen and von Willebrand factor.

Neural tumors typically are S-100 positive, although this by no means is diagnostic of neural differentiation because S-100 is commonly seen in a host of other tissues such as fat, cartilage, or melanocytic cells. CD 99 is typically seen in Ewing's sarcoma, but may also be seen in some rhabdomyosarcomas, synovial sarcomas, small cell osteosarcoma, and mesenchymal chondrosarcoma.

Grading

An analysis of the histology of the lesion determines the tumor grade, which is an important prognostic factor. Tumor grade is decided based on the degree of cellularity, pleomorphism or anaplasia, mitotic activity (frequency and abnormality of mitotic figures), degree of necrosis, and infiltrative or invasive growth pattern. There are various grading systems with a different number of grades (two, three, or four) in each. The histologic type and subtype may provide an idea about the grade of the tumor. Well-differentiated liposarcoma and dermatofibrosarcoma protuberans, for example, are low-grade lesions whereas alveolar rhabdomyosarcoma, Ewing's sarcoma, and neuroblastoma are all high-grade lesions. The grade of the tumor helps decide tumor staging. Both grading and staging systems have their limitations and different histologic parameters vary in significance as well as predictive value, especially in soft-tissue sarcomas that have a wide biologic range of activity.

Staging Systems

Staging of a tumor involves determination of the extent of the tumor and its biologic behavior. Tumor stage de-

2: Systemic Disorders

Table 6	
Musculoskeletal Tumor Society Staging of Bone Sarcomas	
Stage	Description
IA	Low-grade intracompartmental lesions
IB	Low-grade extracompartmental lesions
IIA	High-grade intracompartmental lesions
IIB	High-grade extracompartmental lesions
III	Metastatic disease

Reproduced with permission from Enneking WF, Spanier SS, Goodman MA: A system for the surgical staging of musculoskeletal sarcoma. Clin Orthop Relat Res 1980; 153:106-120.

termines both the treatment and prognosis. Staging is also useful for comparison of outcomes. The most commonly used staging system for bone sarcomas is the Musculoskeletal Tumor Society (MSTS) staging system[4] (Table 6). An alternative, but less commonly used, staging system is the American Joint Committee on Cancer system, which is based on the local extent of the tumor (T), grade (G1-4), nodal involvement (N), and distant spread (M).

Bone-Forming Tumors

Osteosarcoma

Osteosarcoma, the most common primary malignant tumor of bone, is characterized by formation of neoplastic osteoid. Osteosarcomas are classified as surface or intramedullary (conventional), depending on their site in bone. Conventional osteosarcomas are histologically divided according to the predominant cell type as osteoblastic, chondroblastic, fibroblastic, telangiectatic, round cell, and MFH-like. They typically show a bimodal age distribution with most tumors occurring in the second decade of life. There is a smaller peak beyond the fourth decade; these tumors are mostly secondary osteosarcomas that develop in abnormal tissue, for example, in bone affected by Paget's disease or in previously irradiated beds. See chapter 65 for a detailed discussion of conventional osteosarcoma. Some variants of osteosarcomas that occur in adults are described in the next paragraphs.

Parosteal Osteosarcoma

Parosteal osteosarcomas are low-grade surface lesions typically seen in women in the third through fifth decades of life. The posterior distal femoral metaphysis is a favored location (**Figure 3**). Tumors are usually seen as lesions "pasted on" to the cortex of the underlying bone. Invasion of the medullary canal may occur in up to one third of patients. These tumors have very low metastatic potential, unless there is a higher grade (dedifferentiated) component.

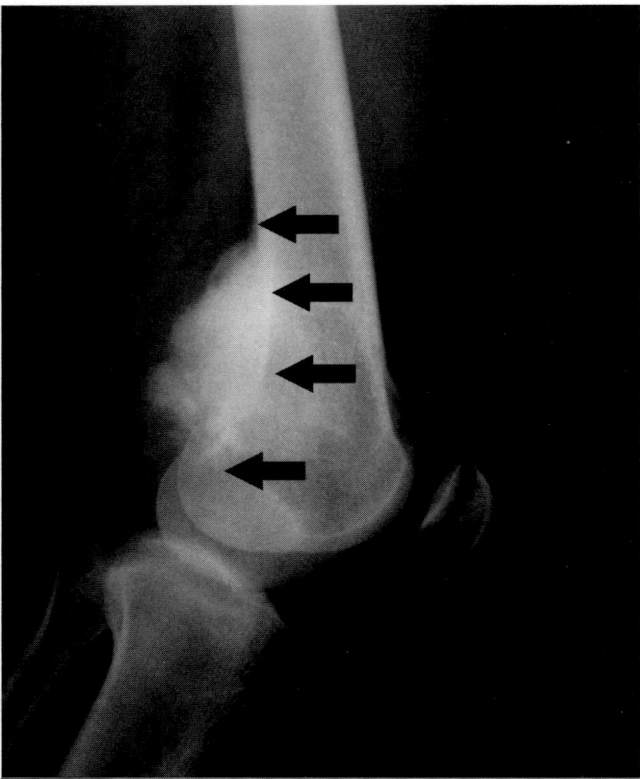

Figure 3 Sclerotic surface lesion (*arrows*) over the posterior distal femur with a "pasted on" appearance suggests a parosteal osteosarcoma.

Chemotherapy is not indicated unless the lesion is dedifferentiated. Wide surgical excision and reconstruction is the treatment of choice. Histologically, these tumors have a fairly bland fibrous stroma; however, unlike fibrous dysplasia, they have prominent osteoblastic rimming.

Periosteal Osteosarcoma

This rare form of osteosarcoma is usually seen in the proximal tibia or distal femur (often the anterior surface). Periosteal osteosarcoma is an intermediate-grade lesion on the surface of the bone and is typically chondroblastic on histology, although with less atypia than a conventional chondroblastic osteosarcoma. Imaging shows a radiolucent lesion with scalloping of the underlying cortex, often with a spiculated periosteal reaction (sunburst appearance). Treatment of low- and intermediate-grade lesions is wide surgical excision. The rare high-grade periosteal osteosarcoma may be treated similarly to a conventional osteosarcoma.

Low-Grade Central Osteosarcoma

Low-grade central osteosarcomas are rare variants (< 1% incidence) of osteosarcomas, commonly occurring in the third and fourth decades of life. Most lesions occur around the knee. Radiographically, these lesions are sclerotic and poorly margined with extensive involvement of the medullary trabeculae. These tumors often

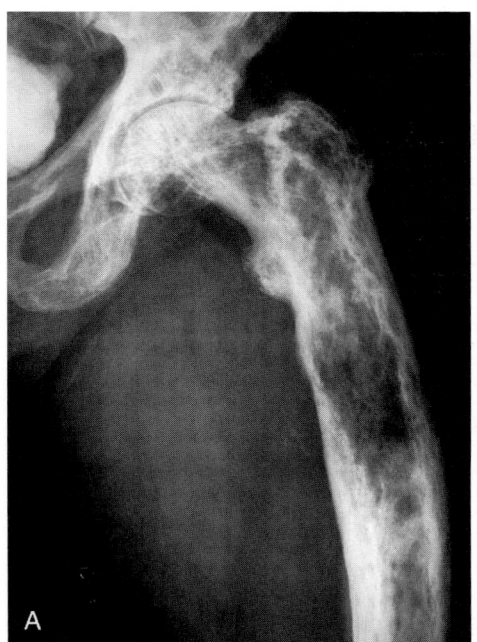
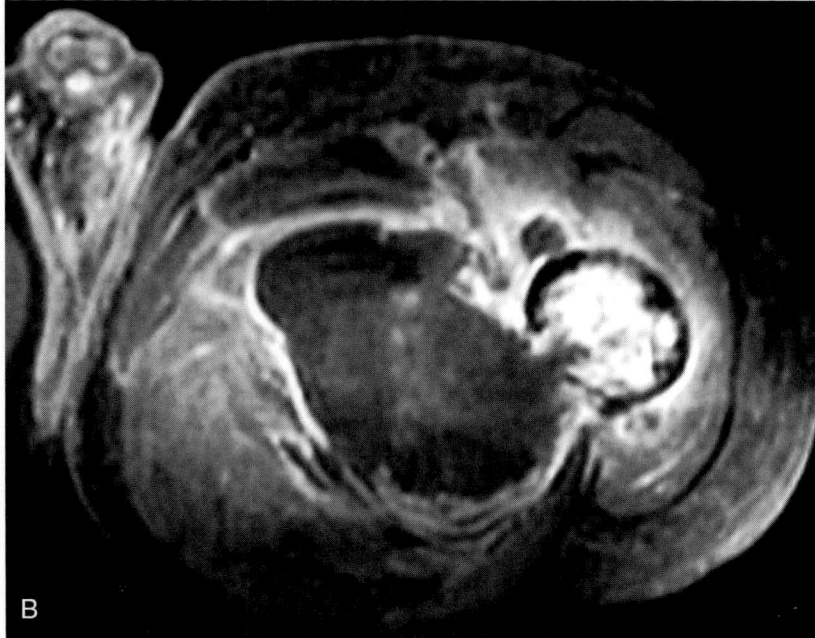

Figure 4 **A,** Lytic area in pagetic bone with recent onset of symptoms suggests a malignant lesion, most commonly osteosarcoma. **B,** Axial cut of the postcontrast fat-suppressed T1-weighted sequence shows loss of normal fatty signal in the bone marrow. There is destruction of the cortex and a large soft-tissue extension in shadow is noted.

disrupt the cortex and extend into the surrounding soft tissues without inciting a periosteal reaction. Treatment is surgical and the prognosis is excellent, with 85% to 90% 5-year survival.

Paget's Sarcoma
Paget's sarcoma is a rare but feared complication of Paget's disease that occurs in approximately 1% of patients with Paget's disease. The most common tumor to develop is an osteogenic sarcoma, although fibrosarcoma, chondrosarcoma, and MFH have all been described. Sarcomatous degeneration is more common in polyostotic forms of Paget's disease. The pelvis is most commonly affected but the tumor can develop in the extremities (humerus and femur) and the spine as well as the skull. Presenting features are usually increasing pain, neurologic symptoms, or pathologic fractures. Radiographs show osteolytic areas, and MRI characteristically show low signal intensity on T1-weighted sequences with loss of the normal fatty marrow signal (**Figure 4**). A bone scan is essential because some of these lesions may be multifocal. Because these patients are old and the vascularity of the pagetic bone is increased, there may be an increased predisposition to development of metastatic carcinomas in the involved bone; accordingly, biopsy is essential to establish the diagnosis.

The treatment of Paget's sarcoma is primarily surgical. Advanced age of the patient and existent comorbidities often limit the use of chemotherapy in this population. Radiation may be used postoperatively if surgical margins are inadequate.

The prognosis is dismal. The median survival of 13 patients with Paget's sarcoma of the spine in a recent study was 4.22 months.[5] An older study of 41 patients with Paget's sarcoma primarily involving the pelvis and extremities showed a 5-year survival of 8%.[6]

Radiation-Induced Sarcoma
With improving prognosis of patients with malignant bone and soft-tissue tumors, the long-term consequences of treatment are being seen with increasing frequency. Development of a radiation-induced sarcoma is one of the feared complications of radiation therapy. The criteria for diagnosis include: (1) histology distinct from the original lesion, (2) development of a sarcoma in the irradiated field, and (3) an adequate latent period (3 to 5 years) between radiation and development of the sarcoma.

Women are affected more often than men, as carcinomas of the breast and cervix account for a large portion of the primary lesions. These tumors most frequently are osteosarcomas, although chondrosarcoma, fibrosarcoma, and MFH also can develop. Some studies suggest that aggressive treatment with a combination of chemotherapy and surgery is associated with better outcomes. The prognostic effect of response to chemotherapy is not as well established as it is in conventional osteosarcoma. Metastatic disease at presentation and onset of the radiation-induced sarcoma within 10 years are poor prognostic factors.

Ewing's Sarcoma
Ewing's sarcoma is a tumor of uncertain lineage. It is the second most common primary bone tumor in the

2: Systemic Disorders

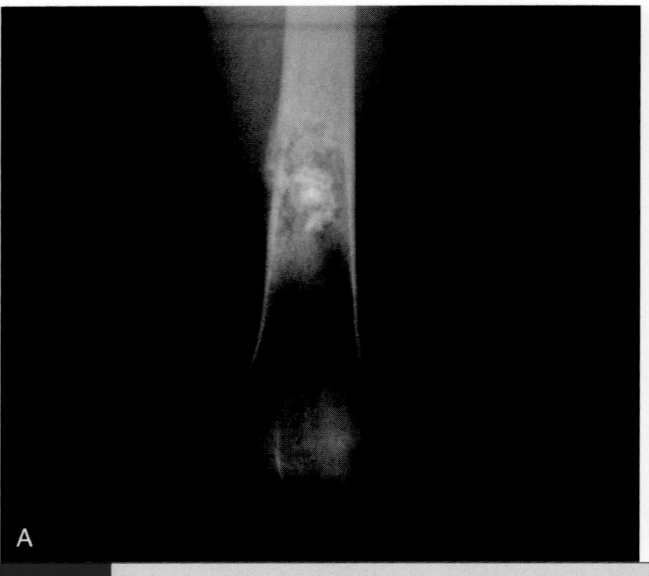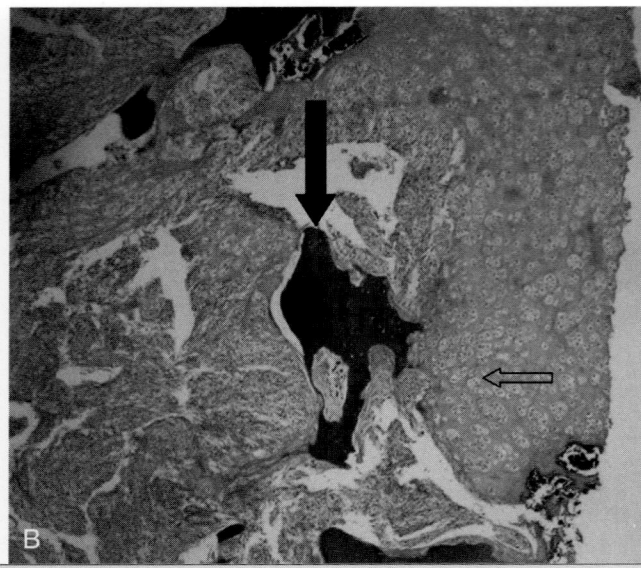

Figure 5 **A,** Radiograph of the distal femur shows a lytic lesion in the metadiaphysis with a chondroid matrix, cortical penetration, and a periosteal reaction—a chondrosarcoma. **B,** Photomicrograph showing typical histologic features of a chondrosarcoma—hypercellularity, binucleate lacunae (*hollow arrow*), and entrapment of native bone by malignant cartilage (*solid arrow*). (Hematoxylin and eosin, ×40.)

skeletally immature population and rarely occurs in patients older than 30 years. Males are more frequently affected than females, and this tumor is rare in African Americans. It has a propensity to involve the axial skeleton and the diaphysis of long bones. Extraskeletal involvement may also be seen. A lamellated or "onion skin" periosteal reaction is often associated with these tumors. A large soft-tissue extension from the primary bone tumor may be seen frequently. Histology reveals a small round blue cell tumor with sheets of uniform cells with CD99 immunoreactivity. The cells show a characteristic t(11-22) translocation in most instances. Staging may include a bone marrow biopsy in addition to a bone scan to identify distant disease. Ewing's sarcoma is both chemosensitive and radiosensitive. Treatment usually consists of multiagent neoadjuvant chemotherapy (vincristine, cyclophosphamide, doxorubicin, ifosfamide, etoposide), followed by restaging and surgery and/or radiation therapy for local control followed by adjuvant chemotherapy. Five-year survival rates as high as 80% to 85% have been reported in patients with localized disease with good response to chemotherapy and negative margins. Radiation is primarily used in the spine and pelvis (surgically inaccessible locations) or in patients with positive margins. Surgical excision with negative margins, when possible, in the pelvis may offer better results than radiation.[7]

Cartilage-Forming Tumors

Chondrosarcomas

Chondrosarcomas are the third most common primary bone malignancies (after osteosarcoma and Ewing's sarcoma) and are characterized by formation of neoplastic cartilage. They can be classified according to site as intramedullary or surface lesions. Histologically, these may either be conventional (hyaline, myxoid), clear cell, mesenchymal, or dedifferentiated. They may also be primary or secondary (developing in preexistent lesions such as exostoses or enchondromas).

Conventional chondrosarcomas are the most common type and typically occur in older patients (age 40 years or older). Men are more commonly affected than women. These tumors are frequently seen in the central skeleton—pelvic and shoulder girdles and ribs. Radiographically, these lesions are characterized by the typical chondroid matrix mineralization (arc and rings or popcorn calcifications) and an aggressive growth pattern (**Figure 5**). MRI shows the typical lobular growth pattern and the high water content of these lesions (low signal on T1-weighted sequences and high signal on T2-weighted sequences). There is considerable controversy regarding the differentiation of low-grade chondrosarcomas from active enchondromas[8] (**Table 7**).

Clear cell chondrosarcoma and mesenchymal chondrosarcoma occur in younger patients (second to fifth decades of life). Clear cell chondrosarcomas are rare (1% to 2% of chondrosarcomas) low-grade lesions that often affect the epiphyses. These tend to metastasize late and therefore require prolonged follow-up, beyond the usually recommended 5 years.[9] Histologically, clear cell chondrosarcomas are characterized by sheets of large malignant chondrocytes with abundant clear cytoplasm. Numerous osteoclast-like giant cells and reactive new bone formation within the lesion may also be seen. Mesenchymal chondrosarcomas (2% to 13% of all chondrosarcomas) are aggressive high-grade lesions characterized by well-differentiated hyaline cartilage surrounded by small round cells (biphasic pattern). The facial skeleton is the most frequently involved. The pelvic and scapular girdles are frequently involved as well. Dedifferentiated chondrosarcomas have areas of low-grade chondrosarcoma with areas of a second higher-grade component immediately adjacent, which may be an osteosarcoma, fibrosarcoma, or MFH, among others.

Extraskeletal Myxoid Chondrosarcoma

Extraskeletal myxoid chondrosarcoma is a rare but well-recognized soft-tissue neoplasm. It is usually seen in the deep soft tissues in the proximal extremities, with the lower extremities being the most commonly involved site. Imaging studies show a lobular deep soft-tissue mass with extracompartmental spread and with invasion of the surrounding bones and vessels. Clinically, these are aggressive lesions that have a greater tendency to metastasize than skeletal myxoid chondrosarcomas.

Treatment of Chondrosarcomas

Chondrosarcoma cells usually are not chemosensitive or radiosensitive. Surgery remains the mainstay of treatment of malignant chondroid lesions. The choice of surgical procedure for low-grade chondrosarcomas, intralesional or wide excision, remains a topic of controversy. For high-grade lesions, wide or radical resection with or without reconstruction is the treatment of choice. Pelvic and, to a lesser extent, scapular chondrosarcomas have a high recurrence rate, largely because of the difficulty in obtaining adequate margins. Chemotherapy was used in the past to treat patients with dedifferentiated chondrosarcomas; however, recent studies have shown that the addition of adjuvant chemotherapy does not significantly affect survival rates for patients with this condition.[10]

Fibrous Lesions of Bone

Desmoplastic Fibroma

Desmoplastic fibroma is an extremely rare locally aggressive tumor that was first described by Jaffe in 1958. It is usually seen in adolescents and young adults. The mandible and long bones (femur, pelvis, radius, and tibia) are commonly affected. Radiographs show a metadiaphyseal lytic, geographic lesion with a soap bubble appearance (internal pseudotrabeculations) and endosteal scalloping. Histologically, the condition has a striking resemblance to desmoid tumors of the abdominal wall or aggressive fibromatosis of soft tissue. The tumor consists of monotonous, bland-appearing fibroblasts that are evenly distributed. Broad bundles of collagen are characteristically seen. Wide excision is recommended to avoid local recurrence.

Malignant Fibrous Histiocytoma of Bone

MFH of bone is a rare aggressive tumor typically seen in the metadiaphysis of long bones with a distribution similar to that of osteosarcoma. It is sometimes seen in previously abnormal bone (for example, nonossifying

Table 7
Features Suggestive of Malignancy in Chondroid Lesions
Persistent pain and night pain
Radiographic features:
Endosteal scalloping > two thirds of cortical thickness
Cortical penetration; periosteal reaction or soft-tissue extension
Increased radiotracer uptake on bone scans (compared with anterior superior iliac spine)
Histologic features:
Hypercellularity
Cellular atypia
Pleomorphism
Binucleate forms
Myxoid intercellular matrix
Entrapment of native bone

Adapted with permission from Murphey MD, Flemming DJ, Boyea SR, Bojescul JA, Sweet DE, Temple HT: Enchondroma versus chondrosarcoma in the appendicular skeleton: Differentiating features. Radiographics 1998; 18:1213-1237.

fibromas and bone infarcts). Radiographs show an aggressive destructive lesion, usually with a soft-tissue extension. Histologically, there is lack of neoplastic osteoid formation that distinguishes MFH of bone from an osteosarcoma. There is a variable proportion of fibroblastic and myofibroblastic elements as well as histiocytes. Multinucleated giant cells and mitotic figures are common. Treatment is similar to that of osteosarcoma. Prognosis in secondary MFH is worse than in primary lesions.

Malignant Vascular Tumors

Hemangioendothelioma

Hemangioendothelioma is an intermediate-grade malignant neoplasm that arises from the vascular endothelium. The epithelioid variant is the one most commonly seen in bone. Long bone involvement (tibia, femur, and humerus) is common. Radiographs usually show a metadiaphyseal lytic lesion without matrix mineralization, often with a soap bubble appearance. A periosteal reaction usually is not seen in the absence of a pathologic fracture. Histologically, the tumor consists of small nests or cords of eosinophilic cells in a basophilic myxoid stroma. The degree of vasoformative activity, atypia in the endothelial cells, and mitotic figures determines the malignant potential. A skeletal survey is indicated because 20% to 50% of lesions may be multifocal. Curettage for low-grade lesions and wide excision for high-grade lesions are the recommended forms of treatment. Radiation may be useful in multifocal lesions.

Hemangiopericytoma

Hemangiopericytoma is an uncommon tumor that is usually seen in middle-aged or elderly males and has an

2: Systemic Disorders

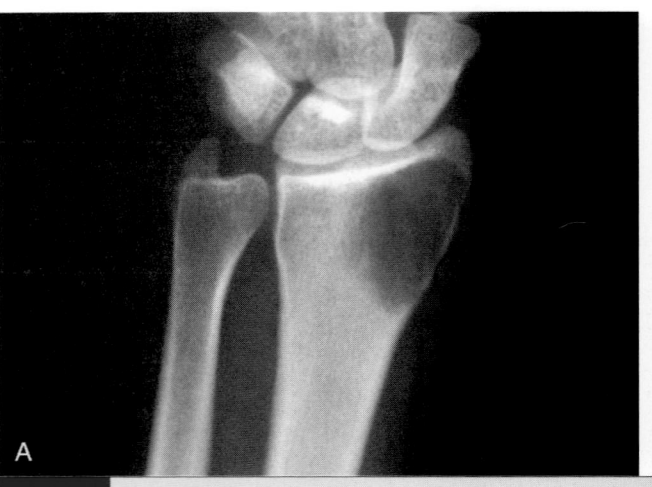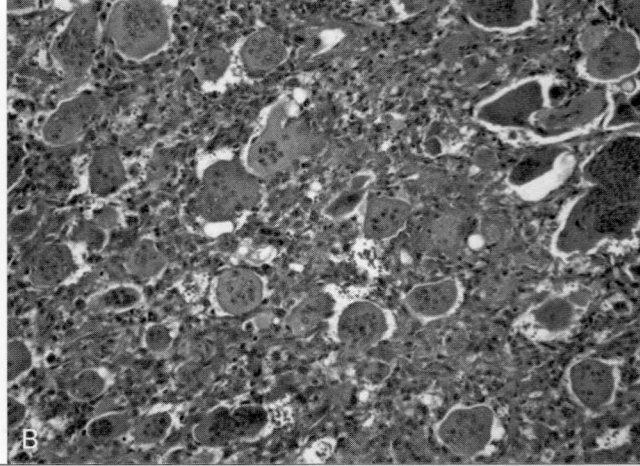

Figure 6 **A,** Eccentric, epiphyseal lytic lesion in the distal radius with a Lodwick type IB margin effacing subchondral bone—a giant cell tumor. **B,** Photomicrograph shows many multinucleate giant cells with nuclei identical to those of the stromal cells, characteristic of giant cell tumor. (Hematoxylin and eosin, ×100.)

unpredictable pattern of behavior. It preferentially involves the axial skeleton and proximal long bones. Unlike hemangioendotheliomas, hemangiopericytoma is usually a solitary lesion. Histologically, these tumors are characterized by slit-like, branching vascular spaces (staghorn appearance). The tumor cells resemble pericytes or cells of Zimmerman (cells normally seen adjacent to capillaries) and show immunoreactivity to CD-34. Wide excision is the treatment of choice. This tumor usually occurs in the soft tissue and bone involvement is rare.

Angiosarcoma of Bone

Angiosarcoma is a rare vascular malignancy of intermediate or high aggressiveness that is usually seen in elderly males. Osseous involvement is seen in a minority of cases (< 10%); long bones are involved in 60% of patients with osseous involvement. Histologically, the tumors are characterized by the presence of vascular channels and a variable degree of anaplasia. Wide excision is the treatment of choice. Radiation may be used in multifocal lesions or surgically inaccessible locations.

Other Tumor Types

Giant Cell Tumor of Bone

Giant cell tumor of bone is a tumor of uncertain etiology that is commonly seen in women 20 to 40 years of age. Pain and pathologic fracture (in approximately 15% of patients) are the most common presenting symptoms. Radiographically, these are eccentric, epimetaphyseal lytic lesions that efface subchondral bone (**Figure 6, A)**. They may also occur in skeletally immature patients (2% of all giant cell tumors) and usually begin in the metaphysis in these patients. The margins are usually well defined without a rind of scle-

rosis around them (Lodwick type IB margin). The knee, distal radius, proximal humerus, and pelvis are favored sites of involvement. Histologically, they show the presence of multinucleate giant cells (osteoclastic) and mononuclear stromal cells (**Figure 6, B)**. These mononuclear stromal cells may either be round cells (nonneoplastic, belonging to the monocyte-macrophage family) or spindle cells (neoplastic component). The nuclei of the giant cells characteristically resemble the nuclei of the spindle-shaped stromal cells. The histologic grade does not predict the biologic behavior of giant cell tumors.

These tumors, although benign, can metastasize to the chest in 1% to 3% of primary cases; imaging studies of the chest should be obtained at presentation as well as during follow-up. Late local recurrences and development of chest metastases are well known. Histologically, these are similar to the primary tumor. Long-term survival after development of metastatic disease is well described. A malignant counterpart, primary malignant giant cell tumor, also has been described and has a poor prognosis.

Treatment of giant cell tumors is with curettage and extension of the margins by a high-speed burr (10% to 15% recurrence).[11] Recurrence rates are high with simple curettage (15% to 55%). The use of adjuvants (cryosurgery, phenol, polymethylmethacrylate [PMMA]) may help decrease recurrence rates.[12,13] The use of a high-speed burr to extend the margins of curettage yields similar recurrence rates (10% to 15%). Wide or en bloc excision may be required in patients with pathologic fractures and extensive soft-tissue extension. Radiation may be used in tumors that are relatively inaccessible surgically, or when surgery would be associated with significant morbidity. Bisphosphonates have been shown to induce apoptosis in the stromal as well as the giant cells in these tumors, and this treatment is currently being tested in patients with giant cell tumors.

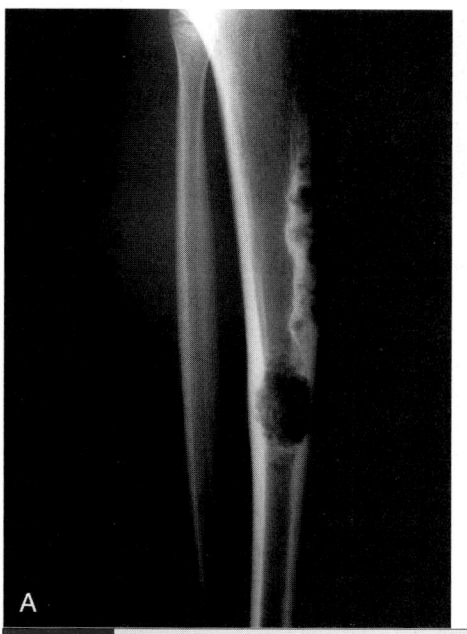
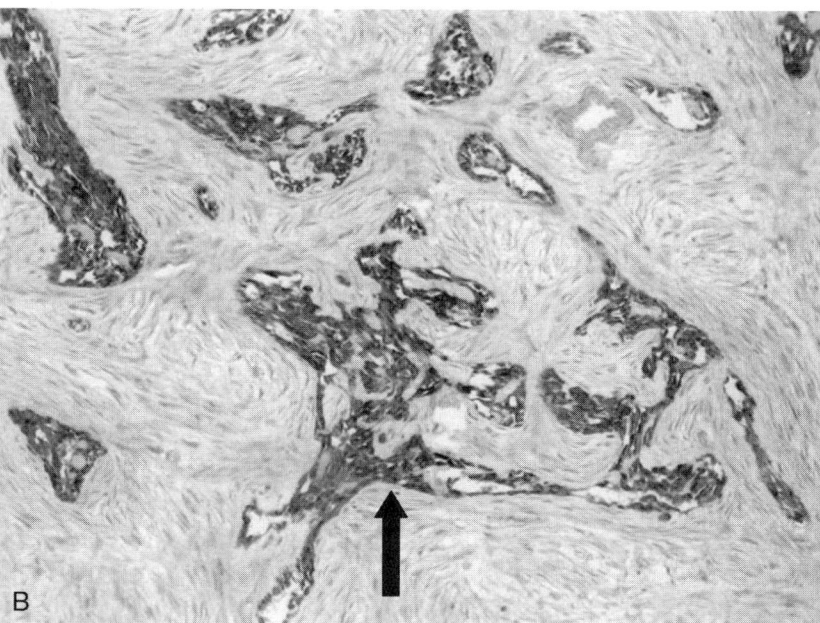

Figure 7 **A,** A lytic area in the medullary cavity in the setting of osteofibrous dysplasia (sclerosis and soap bubble appearance of the anterior tibial cortex) should arouse suspicion for adamantinoma. **B,** Immunoreactivity to the epithelial marker keratin (*arrow*) helps confirm the diagnosis of adamantinoma.

Osteofibrous Dysplasia and Adamantinoma

Osteofibrous dysplasia or cortical fibrous dysplasia, also known as ossifying fibroma, is a peculiar condition seen most often in young males in the first and second decades of life. This condition is characterized by involvement of the tibial diaphysis, typically the anterior cortex, with a characteristic soap bubble appearance. It is usually diagnosed incidentally, although patients may present with pain and/or deformity of the tibia. Histologically, the findings resemble those in fibrous dysplasia; however, prominent osteoblastic rimming is seen. Its relationship with adamantinoma is controversial, but some people believe cortical fibrous dysplasia to be a precursor.

Adamantinomas are low-grade malignancies capable of metastasis. These are almost exclusively seen in the tibia and/or fibula (**Figure 7,** *A)* and occur in both males and females, in contrast with osteofibrous dysplasia, which almost always occurs in boys. The presence of epithelioid cells (cytokeratin immunoreactivity) in the background of an osteofibrous dysplasia suggests a diagnosis of adamantinoma (**Figure 7,** *B).* Histologic appearance is variable, and adamantinomas may show a tubular, basaloid, squamoid, or spindled pattern.

The treatment of osteofibrous dysplasia is watchful monitoring; these tumors become quiescent at maturity. Careful monitoring is necessary because of their controversial relationship with adamantinomas. Bowing deformities may require bracing or surgery. The treatment of adamantinoma is with wide surgical excision and reconstruction with allograft or fibular autograft or bone transport.

Primary Lymphoma of Bone

Primary lymphoma of bone is defined as malignant lymphoid infiltrate within bone with or without soft-tissue involvement and without concurrent involvement of regional lymph nodes or distant viscera. They account for 2% to 7% of all neoplasms of bone and 5% of all extranodal lymphomas. Histologically, diffuse large B cell lymphomas are the most common. Long bones are more frequently affected than the spine. The peak age of occurrence is in the fifth decade, and males are more commonly affected than females. Treatment is usually multimodal, with a combination of chemotherapy and radiation. Surgery may be required for stabilization of pathologic fractures or impending pathologic fractures. The prognosis is excellent, with 5-year survival rates approaching 85% in young patients with good performance status and multimodal treatment. Five- and 10-year survival in patients with primary lymphoma of bone is approximately 61% and 42%, respectively.[14]

Chordoma

Chordoma is a rare tumor arising in the midline from notochordal rests at either end of the spine (sacrum more commonly than clivus). Chordomas are typically seen in middle-aged to older males and usually present late with bladder and bowel symptoms or seating discomfort. Imaging typically shows a destructive lesion with a large soft-tissue mass (**Figure 8,** *A)* that is hyperintense on T2-weighted sequences (**Figure 8,** *B).* Histologically, it is an epithelioid lesion with cells arranged in cords in a loose myxoid background (**Figure 8,** *C).* The characteristic cell is a vacuolated physaliferous cell. Treatment is

2: Systemic Disorders

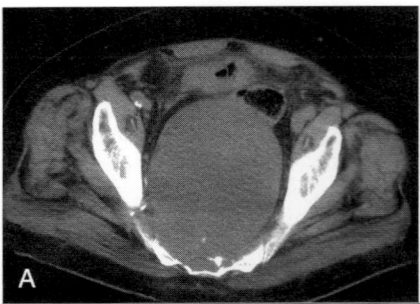 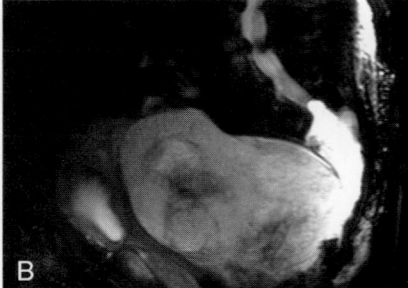 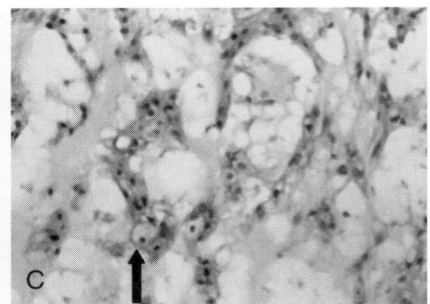

Figure 8 **A,** Destructive midline sacral lesion with a large soft-tissue extension anteriorly. **B,** The lesion is uniformly hyperintense on the T2-weighted sequence, suggestive of a chordoma. **C,** Photomicrograph shows an epithelioid lesion (*arrow*) with cells arranged in strands or cords, in a loose myxoid background, diagnostic of a chordoma. (Hematoxylin and eosin, ×100.)

surgical, with tumors below S2 managed with posterior approach. Tumors extending above the body of S2 require both an anterior and posterior approach, and muscle (gluteus maximus) and omental flaps and a mesh are often used for reconstruction. There is a significant incidence of loss of bladder and bowel control with these lesions and urinary diversion and colostomy may be needed. There is a high local recurrence rate; the use of adjuvant radiation may improve local disease control, especially in primary lesions.[15]

Multiple Myeloma

Myeloma is the most common primary bone malignancy. It is a monoclonal proliferative disorder of B cells, characterized by (1) infiltration of the bone marrow by malignant plasma cells (> 10%; if < 10%, monoclonal gammopathy of undetermined significance), (2) evidence of monoclonal protein (M protein) in the serum and/or urine, and (3) evidence of end organ damage (hypercalcemia, renal insufficiency, anemia, or bone disease).[16]

A solitary lesion in bone with the characteristic laboratory findings is known as a plasmacytoma. Bone disease in myeloma may range from bone pain and diffuse osteopenia to focal lytic lesions with or without pathologic fractures and hypercalcemia. These are the major causes of morbidity and mortality in patients with myeloma.

The pathogenesis of bone disease in myeloma has been better understood recently. Myeloma cells produce macrophage inflammatory protein 1-alpha, which directly stimulates osteoclast formation and differentiation. Myeloma cells release hepatocyte growth factor and parathyroid hormone-related peptide, and also induce the stromal cells in the bone marrow to release osteoclast activating factors. These in turn increase the expression of receptor activator of nuclear factor κB ligand (RANKL) on the surface of stromal cells in the bone marrow. RANKL binds to the receptor activator of the RANK receptor on the osteoclast precursors and induces osteoclast differentiation and activation. This process also stimulates the growth of myeloma cells and sets up a self-perpetuating cycle of bone destruction. Also, the inhibitory effects of osteoprotegerin

(OPG) on RANKL in myeloma are blunted as a result of decreased OPG messenger RNA expression and increased OPG destruction induced by the myeloma cells. Moreover, even when the osteoblastic activity is inhibited by bisphosphonate treatment, myeloma cells secrete substances that inhibit osteoblast differentiation and activity; as a result, there is impairment of new bone formation and healing of the bone lesions.

The workup of a patient with suspected myeloma includes serum and urine electrophoresis to detect the M protein, which is also useful for monitoring disease activity. The bone marrow is evaluated for the percentage of malignant plasma cells. Laboratory studies should include complete blood cell count, erythrocyte sedimentation rate, calcium levels, renal function assessment, and β-2-microglobulin levels (which are useful for prognosis because they indicate the tumor burden and renal function, but are not useful for monitoring disease activity). Skeletal evaluation should include a skeletal survey (because bone scans may show a false negative result in more than two thirds of patients) and a dual energy x-ray absorptiometry scan (baseline).

Treatment of plasmacytoma is usually with radiation (45 Gy) to the involved field with or without stabilization of the affected bone. Treatment of myeloma is primarily chemotherapy and peripheral blood stem cell transplantation, either autogenous or allogenic. Chemotherapy consists of an induction phase followed, if possible, by peripheral blood stem cell transplantation and then by maintenance-phase chemotherapy (usually prednisone or single-agent thalidomide) to maximize the benefit of induction chemotherapy. Radiation therapy is indicated in patients with bone pain and impending fractures or large soft-tissue masses. The usual dose of radiation is approximately 3,000 cGy delivered in 10 to 15 fractions. Radiation carries a risk of bone marrow suppression; this condition needs to be looked for in patients with an already compromised bone marrow reserve.

Surgery has been underutilized in patients with myeloma. Many patients (50% to 70%) with myeloma have or go on to develop a vertebral compression fracture. These fractures typically involve the lower thoracic or upper lumbar vertebrae and may be treated with surgery and/or radiation. Kyphoplasty has been shown to be extremely useful in providing pain relief in this situation, with or without associated radiation therapy. The risk of cement extravasation and related complications are lower with kyphoplasty compared with vertebroplasty. Surgery for spinal lesions is indicated if there is instability of the spine or if there is neural compression that does not respond to radiation. Surgical stabilization of impending or pathologic long bone fractures along with radiation of the affected bone help to restore stability and aid in fracture healing and resumption of a pain-free active lifestyle. Supportive therapy includes lifestyle modifications such as weight-bearing exercise programs, vaccination to prevent infections, and the use of erythropoietin for the treatment of anemia (Hgb < 10 g/dL). The use of bisphosphonates (intravenous pamidronate or zoledronic acid every 4 weeks in stage II and III disease) to decrease the osteoclastic activity in these patients has resulted in improvement of bone pain, decreased fracture risk, and improvement of bone mass.

Soft-Tissue Tumors

Soft-tissue sarcomas are more common than primary bone sarcomas, with approximately 9,000 new cases occurring every year. These tumors are more common in older adults than in children and often may be painful. The patient may have a history of antecedent trauma that is not usually a causative factor, but draws attention to the mass. Soft-tissue tumors may arise from a histologically diverse population of cells, and their biologic behavior is accordingly different. Soft-tissue tumors in the thigh or the pelvis often grow to a large size before becoming symptomatic. There may consequently be a considerable delay in their diagnosis. Lesions in the foot are often symptomatic early and may be diagnosed when they are relatively small in size. Care must be taken to carefully evaluate these tumors before definitive treatment is undertaken so as not to inadvertently treat a malignant lesion as a benign one and adversely affect outcome.

Evaluation of Soft-Tissue Tumors

Ultrasonography is a quick and inexpensive test that may help differentiate solid from cystic lesions and assist in further evaluation of these lesions. MRI is the gold standard for evaluation of soft-tissue tumors. Soft-tissue sarcomas grow in a centrifugal fashion and usually have well-defined margins. They tend to push normal tissue rather than invade it, resulting in a plane between the tumor and the surrounding soft tissues. Tumors are most often hypointense in comparison with skeletal muscle on T1-weighted sequences and hyperintense on T2-weighted and short tau inversion recovery sequences. Postcontrast imaging helps to differentiate cysts or abscess cavities from solid tumors. Few tumors can be diagnosed based on their imaging characteristics alone (for example, lipomas); for most tu-

mors, biopsy is needed to establish the diagnosis. The principles of biopsy of soft-tissue tumors are similar to those for the biopsy of bone lesions.

Lymph node metastases are present in approximately 5% of patients with soft-tissue sarcoma. Tumors that have a predilection to spread to lymph nodes include epithelioid sarcoma, rhabdomyosarcoma, clear cell sarcoma, and less frequently, angiosarcoma and synovial sarcoma.

Aggressive Fibromatosis or Extra-Abdominal Desmoid

Aggressive fibromatosis is one of the deep fibromatoses and occurs in adolescents and young adults. The extremities are involved in approximately 70% of patients, and multifocal involvement may be seen in 10% to 15%. These tumors are more aggressive in younger patients and have a tendency for local recurrence. Histologically, these tumors show an infiltrative pattern, with bland-appearing spindle-shaped fibroblasts arranged in a uniform fashion surrounded by variable amounts of collagen. MRI shows an infiltrative mass, and signal characteristics are variable depending on the relative amounts of cells and collagen. The highly cellular areas show hyperintense signal on T2-weighted sequences, whereas the collagenized areas show decreased signal intensity on both the T1- and the T2-weighted sequences. Extra-abdominal desmoids are locally aggressive and are treated with wide excision. If the margins are positive or close, adjuvant radiation therapy has been used to minimize recurrences. Chemotherapeutic regimens using vinblastine and methotrexate have been used with some success, particularly in children.

Liposarcoma

Liposarcomas account for up to one third of all soft-tissue sarcomas in adults. There are several subtypes, including well-differentiated liposarcoma (atypical lipomatous tumor of the extremity), dedifferentiated, myxoid or round cell liposarcoma, and pleomorphic.

Atypical lipomatous tumors or well-differentiated liposarcoma (50% of all liposarcomas) are well-differentiated lesions seen in the extremities, more commonly in the lower than upper extremity. These tumors often present as large painless masses, usually in the sixth or seventh decade of life. They have no metastatic potential unless they dedifferentiate. On MRI scans, they differ from lipomas because they have thick (> 2 mm) septations that enhance with contrast.[17] Histologically, they are characterized by well-differentiated, mature fat with interspersed lipoblasts; some may have broad bands of collagen (sclerosing subtype) (**Figure 9,** *A)* and still others have an inflammatory lymphocytic or plasma cell infiltrate (retroperitoneal lesions). Treatment with wide excision is usually adequate and no adjuvants are needed. The CT or MRI evidence of a nonlipomatous area larger than 1 cm in a well-differentiated liposarcoma is suggestive of a dedif-

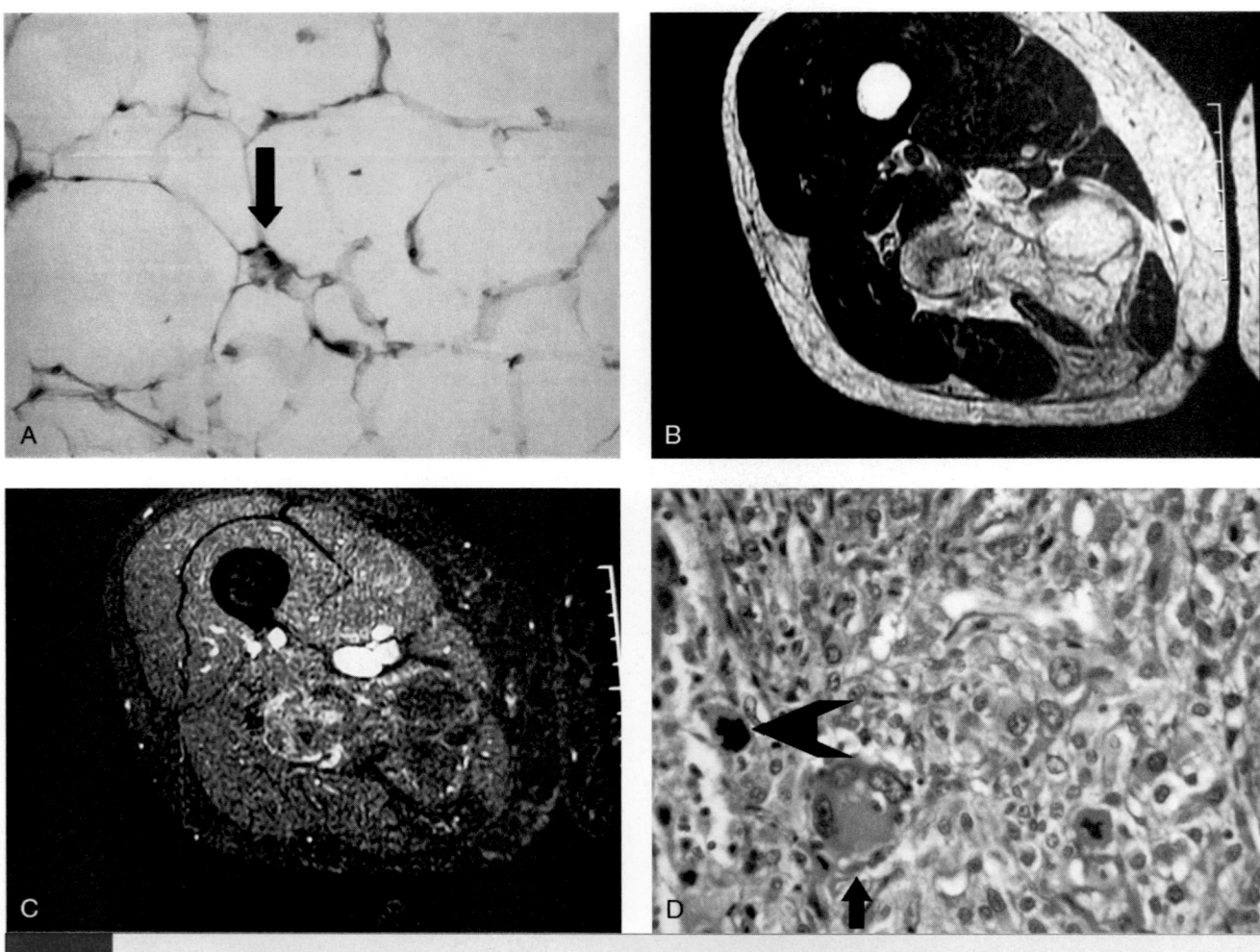

Figure 9 **A,** Photomicrograph shows well-differentiated fat cells with a plump lipoblast (*arrow*) in a patient with a lipoma-like, well-differentiated liposarcoma or atypical lipomatous tumor. (Hematoxylin and eosin, ×400.) **B,** Axial T1-weighted MRI shows a mass in the posterior thigh with signal intensity similar to subcutaneous fat with mild heterogeneity. **C,** Fat-suppressed sequence demonstrating an area of hyperintensity with otherwise uniform fat suppression within the mass, suggestive of a focus of dedifferentiation. **D,** Photomicrograph shows a high-grade neoplasm with giant cells (*arrow*) and mitotic figures (*arrowhead*) in the dedifferentiated focus. (Hematoxylin and eosin, ×400.)

ferentiated liposarcoma (**Figure 9,** *B* through *D*). Myxoid/round cell liposarcomas (20% to 50% of liposarcoma) are characterized by small foci of liposarcoma in a predominant myxoid background. This variant is more common in younger patients (fourth and fifth decades of life) and is the most common liposarcoma in children. Myxoid liposarcomas have a propensity to develop extrapulmonary metastases (**Figure 10**). The degree of round cell component correlates with metastatic risk. Pleomorphic liposarcomas (5% to 15% of liposarcomas) are high-grade lesions affecting older patients (> 50 years of age) and have an aggressive course. Mixed liposarcomas (5% to 10% of liposarcomas) have features that are a combination of the above.

Synovial Sarcoma
Synovial sarcoma accounts for 10% to 15% of all soft-tissue sarcomas in adults. The lower extremity is the most common location for these tumors. Synovial sar-

comas are the most common soft-tissue sarcomas of the foot and ankle (**Figure 11,** *A*). They are intermediate-to high-grade lesions and are commonly seen in close proximity to joints, but rarely in the joint. The X:18 translocation with fusion of the *SYT* and *SSX* genes is characteristic and may help establish the diagnosis. Clinical presentation is a mass, usually painful, in a young adult. Large, high-grade lesions have a high incidence of distant metastases, most frequently to the lung. Radiographs may show calcification in up to 30% of patients. MRI may show a "triple density sign" on T2-weighted sequences with high signal representing viable tumor, intermediate to low signal representing fibrosis, and low signal accounted for by the hemosiderin resulting from acute or subacute bleeding. Histologically, these tumors may either be monophasic (spindled or epithelioid), biphasic (with both spindled and epithelioid cells), or undifferentiated (**Figure 11,** *B)*. Although spread to lymph nodes may occur in a

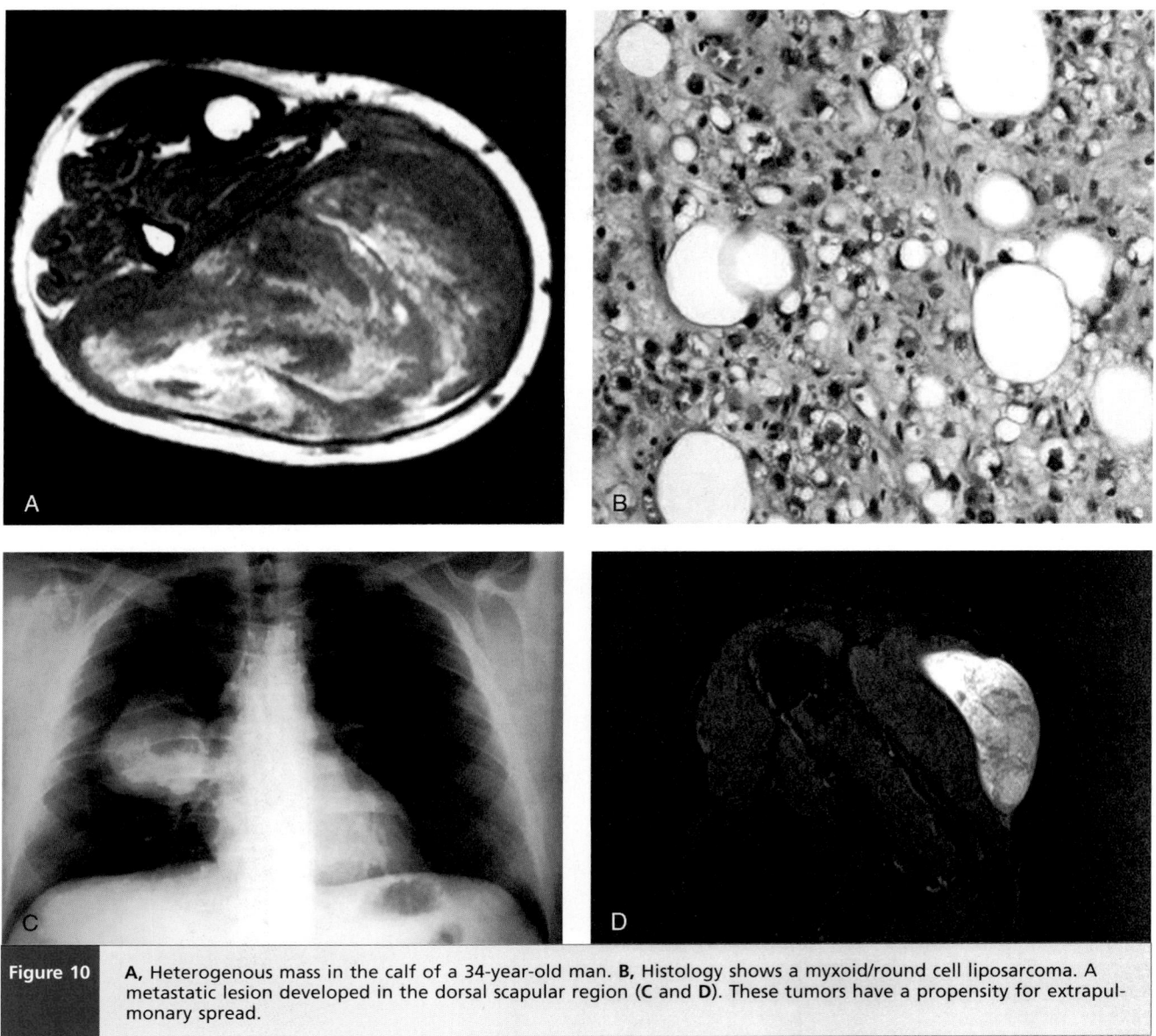

Figure 10 **A,** Heterogenous mass in the calf of a 34-year-old man. **B,** Histology shows a myxoid/round cell liposarcoma. A metastatic lesion developed in the dorsal scapular region (**C** and **D**). These tumors have a propensity for extrapulmonary spread.

small number of patients, the lung is the most common site of distant metastasis. Metastases are common in high-risk lesions (> 5 cm, deep to the fascia, and high grade) and may develop late; consequently, these patients need to be monitored for at least 10 years.

Malignant Fibrous Histiocytoma

The term "malignant fibrous histiocytoma" is falling out of favor, and these tumors are now being referred to as high-grade pleomorphic undifferentiated sarcomas. Careful histologic evaluation may result in some of these tumors being reclassified as pleomorphic liposarcomas. High-grade pleomorphic undifferentiated sarcomas are the most common soft-tissue sarcomas in adults. Unlike synovial sarcomas, these lesions occur more frequently in older adults. The lower extremities are the most commonly affected, with the thigh being a

favored location. Two thirds of these tumors are intramuscular. MRI shows a heterogeneous mass that may have some hemorrhage and/or necrosis. There are several histologic subtypes, including storiform (most common), myxoid, giant cell, inflammatory (usually retroperitoneal), and angiomatoid (usually superficial). All of these lesions are characterized by a variable proportion of spindle cells and histiocytic cells; giant cells and bizarre mitotic figures are common. These are often aggressive lesions and mostly metastasize to the lungs, although bone involvement occurs in up to 10% of patients. The prognosis in high-grade lesions is poor, with a 10% to 20% 5-year survival.

Epithelioid Sarcoma

Epithelioid sarcoma is an aggressive, high-grade, deep dermal or subcutaneous sarcoma of the distal extremi-

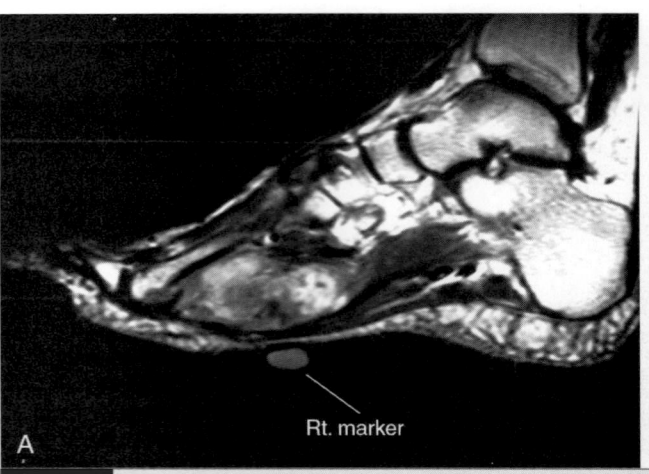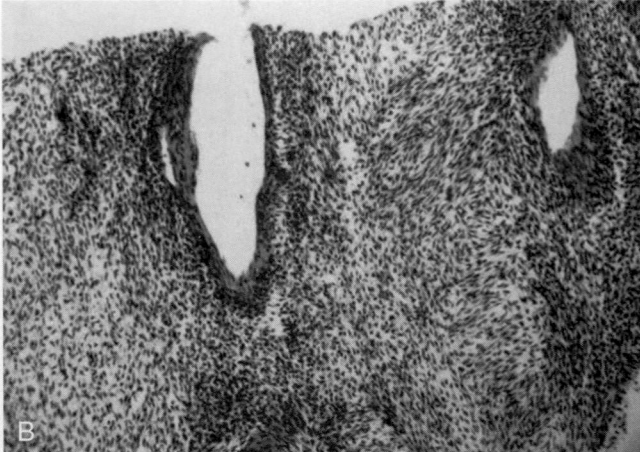

Rt. marker

Figure 11 **A,** Sagittal cut of the MRI scan of the foot shows a heterogenous mass on the plantar aspect of the foot. Synovial sarcoma is the most common soft-tissue malignancy of the foot and ankle in young adults. **B,** Photomicrograph from the needle biopsy of the mass shows a monophasic synovial sarcoma. (Hematoxylin and eosin, ×40.)

ties and is the most common soft-tissue sarcoma of the hand. It is commonly seen in young adult males and usually presents as a subcutaneous mass or a nonhealing ulcer. Histologically, these tumors are characterized by epithelioid cells arranged in a nodular fashion with central necrosis. The tumor may show a biphasic tendency with epithelioid cells and spindled areas that merge into each other. Metastases to lymph nodes may occur in up to one third of patients. There is a high rate of local recurrence and the tumor tends to be multifocal at initial presentation or recurrence. Proximal lesions have a worse prognosis than distal lesions. The mean 5-year survival rate is close to 70% and 10-year survival is approximately 45%, indicating there is significant disease activity even beyond 5 years.

Treatment of Bone and Soft-Tissue Tumors

Treatment of bone and soft-tissue sarcomas involves a multidisciplinary effort—usually a combination of chemotherapy, surgery, and/or radiation. Staging studies, local and distant, are usually repeated after neoadjuvant therapy and before surgical excision. Multiple studies have established the need for neoadjuvant chemotherapy for most pediatric bone sarcomas. Chondrosarcomas are neither chemosensitive nor radiosensitive and surgery is the primary mode of treatment of this condition. Ewing's sarcoma of the extremities is commonly treated with neoadjuvant chemotherapy, surgery, and adjuvant chemotherapy. However, Ewing's sarcoma of the spine or pelvis may be treated with a combination of chemotherapy and surgery and/or radiation for local control. Soft-tissue sarcomas have been traditionally treated with a combination of surgery and radiation. Treatment needs to be individualized according to the histopathologic diagnosis as well as its location.

Treatment of bone tumors depends on the inherent aggressiveness of the disease and its location. Treatment

has been classified as intralesional procedures, marginal resection, wide resection, and radical resection.

Intralesional procedures include curetting the lesion with or without the use of bone graft or any other synthetic fillers. These procedures are best suited for benign lesions such as nonossifying fibromas or unicameral bone cysts. Lesions with a higher potential for local recurrence such as aneurysmal bone cysts or giant cell tumors may need a more aggressive approach with thorough curetting of the walls, extension of the margins with a high-speed burr with or without the use of adjuvants such as PMMA, phenol, or liquid nitrogen (extended intralesional treatment).

Marginal resection refers to resection of the lesion through the reactive zone around the tumor. This is typically done for soft-tissue tumors such as lipomas, which must be resected with their pseudocapsule to avoid recurrence.

Wide resection is the preferred treatment of highly aggressive benign conditions as well as malignant tumors. This entails removal of the tumor with a cuff of normal tissue all around it.

Radical resection consists of resection of the tumor with the entire compartment it involves. Bone is considered to be a separate compartment as are rays of the foot. If the tumor extends out of bone into the surrounding muscles, a radical resection would entail removal of the affected bone and the entire compartment of muscle that is involved by the tumor.

The biopsy track with a bridge of normal tissue (and skin) around it is typically included in the resection of malignant lesions. Wide and radical margins are usually considered to be adequate for malignant tumors. A radical amputation used to be the most common form of treatment 20 to 30 years ago. Amputation is still indicated in approximately 10% of patients. The indications for amputation include tumors surrounding the neurovascular bundle (although vascular grafts are being done in some instances) and tumors with a large soft-tissue component that render the residual extremity nonfunctional. Sciatic nerve involvement was believed to be an absolute indication for amputation in the past, but this concept has been challenged recently. Advances in imaging have improved preoperative planning and decision making and neoadjuvant therapies provide the advantage of decreasing the vascularity and the size of the tumor, making it more amenable to limb salvage. Moreover, better reconstructive options are now available with the availability of modern modular prostheses; this has led to limb-salvage procedures in almost 80% to 90% of patients. Although there is no significant difference in oncologic outcomes in patients undergoing amputation and limb salvage, local recurrences may be somewhat more frequent in patients undergoing limb salvage.

There are many options for reconstruction once adequate tumor resection has been performed. These options include biologic measures, nonbiologic measures, or a combination of the two (alloprosthetic composites). The biologic measures include autografts (vascularized or nonvascularized) and allografts. The nonbiologic options include endoprosthetic replacement. Autografts are limited by size and donor-site morbidity. Vascularized fibular autograft is an excellent biologic reconstruction material, especially for intercalary defects where it may be used with allograft to improve the union rates. Allografts can be used for reconstruction of osteoarticular or intercalary defects, with better results with the latter.[18] The results of osteoarticular allograft reconstruction are site-specific, with the best results being in the distal femur and the worst in the proximal tibia. Allografts have the advantage of being biologic and provide the opportunity to preserve the unaffected side of the joint. However, they have a high rate of infection within the first year and a high rate of fracture (usually within the first 3 years) and nonunion. With improvements in technology and metals, there is a trend toward using endoprosthetic replacement more often. Endoprostheses have the advantage of immediate mobilization (cemented prostheses) and low rates of infection and fracture. Disadvantages include suboptimal soft-tissue attachment, and loosening and polyethylene wear in the long term, making revision necessary (in up to one third of patients at 10 years).[19,20] Children younger than 10 years of age require specialized reconstruction techniques to maintain limb-length equality. In young patients, there is a bias toward more biologic reconstruction; options include rotationplasty and expandable prostheses. The use of muscle flaps (such as medial gastrocnemius flaps) has resulted in improved soft-tissue coverage of the endoprostheses or allograft and decreased wound complications.

The treatment of soft-tissue sarcomas is surgical, with wide excision preferred for most tumors. Postoperative radiation may be used in patients with large (> 5 cm), high-grade tumors deep to the fascia, especially if the margins are close or positive. Preoperative radiation therapy may be used in large tumors in an attempt to induce fibrosis and decrease vascularity. Preoperative radiation has been consistently shown to increase wound complication rates. The role of chemotherapy in patients with soft-tissue sarcomas is controversial. A clear benefit has been shown in patients with metastatic disease. There is some evidence to suggest that there may be a benefit to ifosfamide-based chemotherapy in high-risk patients with nonmetastatic synovial sarcomas and liposarcomas of the extremities. Studies have shown a slight increase in disease-specific survival but not local recurrence-free survival in this select group of patients.[21]

Table 8

Steps Involved in Development of Metastatic Lesions

Tumor growth (lack of contact inhibition)
Detachment from adjacent cells (lack of cohesiveness)
Invasion of adjacent tissues and capillaries (matrix metalloproteinase, gelatinase)
Attachment to basement membrane
Secretion of proteolytic enzymes
Migration through the basement membrane
Migration, chemotaxis
Adhesion of cells to host tissue (cell adhesion molecules: cadherin, laminin, integrins, etc)

Metastatic Bone Disease

Metastatic bone disease is a source of considerable morbidity. It is much more common than primary bone malignancies. Bone is the third most common site for metastatic disease after the lung and liver. Cancers that commonly metastasize to bone are breast, prostate, lung, thyroid, and kidney. These collectively account for more than 75% of all metastatic lesions in bone. Metastatic bone disease may be the initial presentation in up to 23% of patients with carcinomas.

In patients older than 40 years of age, metastatic disease and myeloma are statistically the most common lesions in bone. The most common site of involvement is the axial skeleton and proximal ends of long bones. Acral (distal to the knee and elbow) metastases are rare but most commonly occur with bronchogenic and renal cell carcinomas. Similarly, cortical-based or "cookie cutter" metastases often are seen in bronchogenic carcinoma.

The unique characteristics of malignant cells enable them to detach themselves from one location and set up a metastatic focus at a distant site. The steps involved in metastasis are outlined in Table 8.

Workup of a patient with suspected metastatic disease to bone should include studies to localize the primary tumor and estimate the local and distant extent of the disease. Studies to localize the primary focus include CT of chest, abdomen, and pelvis; mammography; tumor markers (for example, prostate-specific antigen); serum and urine electrophoresis (M band); and PET scans (especially for head and neck primaries or lymphoma). Studies to assess bone turnover and distant spread include pyridinoline cross-links in urine, N- and

2: Systemic Disorders

Table 9

Mirels Scoring System for Predicting the Risk of Pathologic Fracture*

Variable	1	2	3
Site	Upper extremity	Lower extremity	Peritrochanteric
Pain	Mild	Moderate	Functional
Lesion	Blastic	Mixed	Lytic
Size	< 1/3	1/3-2/3	> 2/3

*Prophylactic internal fixation was recommended at a score of 8 or more.
Reproduced with permission from Mirels H: Metastatic disease in long bones: A proposed scoring system for diagnosing impending pathologic fractures. Clin Orthop Relat Res 1989;249:256-264.

C-terminal telopeptides, alkaline phosphatase (bone-specific), radiographs (if lesion > 1 cm or if > 30% to 50% mineral washed out), bone scans (false negative in myeloma, leukemia, and highly anaplastic tumors), and PET scans.

Treatment of Patients With Metastatic Disease

Because patients with cancer often have longer survival rates and a better quality of life, it is important to identify potential weakness in the bone and treat it before a pathologic fracture occurs. The treatment of bone metastasis is multidisciplinary. It includes the use of systemic and/or local treatment measures. Systemic measures that have been successfully used include symptomatic treatment with analgesics, chemotherapy, hormonal therapy (breast, prostate carcinoma), radioactive isotopes (strontium 89, phosphorus 32, samarium 153, rhenium 186), and the use of bisphosphonates to inhibit osteoclastic resorption of bone. The use of bisphosphonates has been one of the most significant advances in the treatment of metastatic disease and has significantly decreased the number of pathologic fractures and impending fractures and thus the intervention required for them. Local measures include radiation to the affected bone and surgical stabilization of impending or pathologic fractures.

Endosteal defects larger than 50% of cortical thickness at the site of maximum bending stress decrease the strength of the bone by almost 90%. Similarly, stress risers (open defects in the cortex less than one third the circumference of the bone) and open segment defects (more than one third the circumference of the bone at the level of the defect) decrease the structural integrity of the bone by 60% and 90%, respectively. When bone destruction by the metastatic process reaches this level, the risk of a pathologic fracture increases significantly, especially with trivial torsional stress. Many studies have looked at methods of predicting the risk of a pathologic fracture and recommending an appropriate time for intervention; however, each has its shortcomings. The most commonly used classification system is the one proposed by Mirels[22] (Table 9).

Surgery in patients with metastatic disease is usually palliative and does not significantly improve survival. The goals are pain relief and re-establishing stability to facilitate mobilization. Surgery should be performed in all patients except those whose condition is terminal (< 6 weeks of life expectancy) or whose comorbidities place them at an extreme risk with the use of anesthesia.

Stabilization of an impending fracture is easier than stabilization of a pathologic fracture. The modes of stabilization of metastatic lesions depend on the site involved, location within bone, and the underlying etiology. Several guidelines have been proposed for the use of an appropriate surgical procedure.[23] Adequate preoperative planning and optimizing the medical condition of the patient before surgery are crucial. The surgery should be timed appropriately so that it does not coincide with the nadir of the white blood cell count in patients on chemotherapy. All patients undergoing lower extremity stabilization should have their upper extremities evaluated for a potential lesion; if present, this may need to be treated at the same time as the lower extremity lesion to avoid a pathologic fracture with the use of crutches. The technique of stabilization depends on the location of the lesion within bone as well as the underlying diagnosis and the prognosis.

Diaphyseal lesions are curetted out (intralesional) and stabilized with plates or intramedullary nails (Figure 12, A and B) with or without PMMA supplementation (reinforced internal fixation). Adequate imaging of the entire length of the bone before surgery is essential to ensure adequate purchase proximal and distal to the lesion. Metaphyseal lesions in the distal femur may be stabilized with curettage, cement, and a retrograde nail. A periarticular lesion, especially in the presence of renal cell carcinoma, is best stabilized with resection and prosthetic reconstruction (Figure 12, C and D). Epiphyseal lesions may be stabilized with curettage and cementation, if not involving the subchondral bone, or with endoprosthetic reconstruction. Pathologic fractures through the epiphysis are usually treated with resection and endoprosthetic reconstruction. In the pelvis, a cavitary defect may be stabilized with curettage and cementation with the use of Steinmann pins if the defect is large. If the lesion extends into the acetabulum and there is sufficient bone stock on the medial wall, a cemented acetabular component with or without a mesh may be used. If there is insufficient bone stock medially, an antiprotrusio cage with augmentation of the medial wall may be required (Figure 13). If there is laxity as a result of resection of the soft tissues around the hip, a constrained acetabular liner may be needed to prevent dislocation. A detailed discussion of reconstructive options in metastatic disease can be found in the literature.[24]

First Osseous Lesion in a Patient With a Known Carcinoma

This lesion should be evaluated carefully to determine if it is a metastatic lesion or a new primary malignancy.

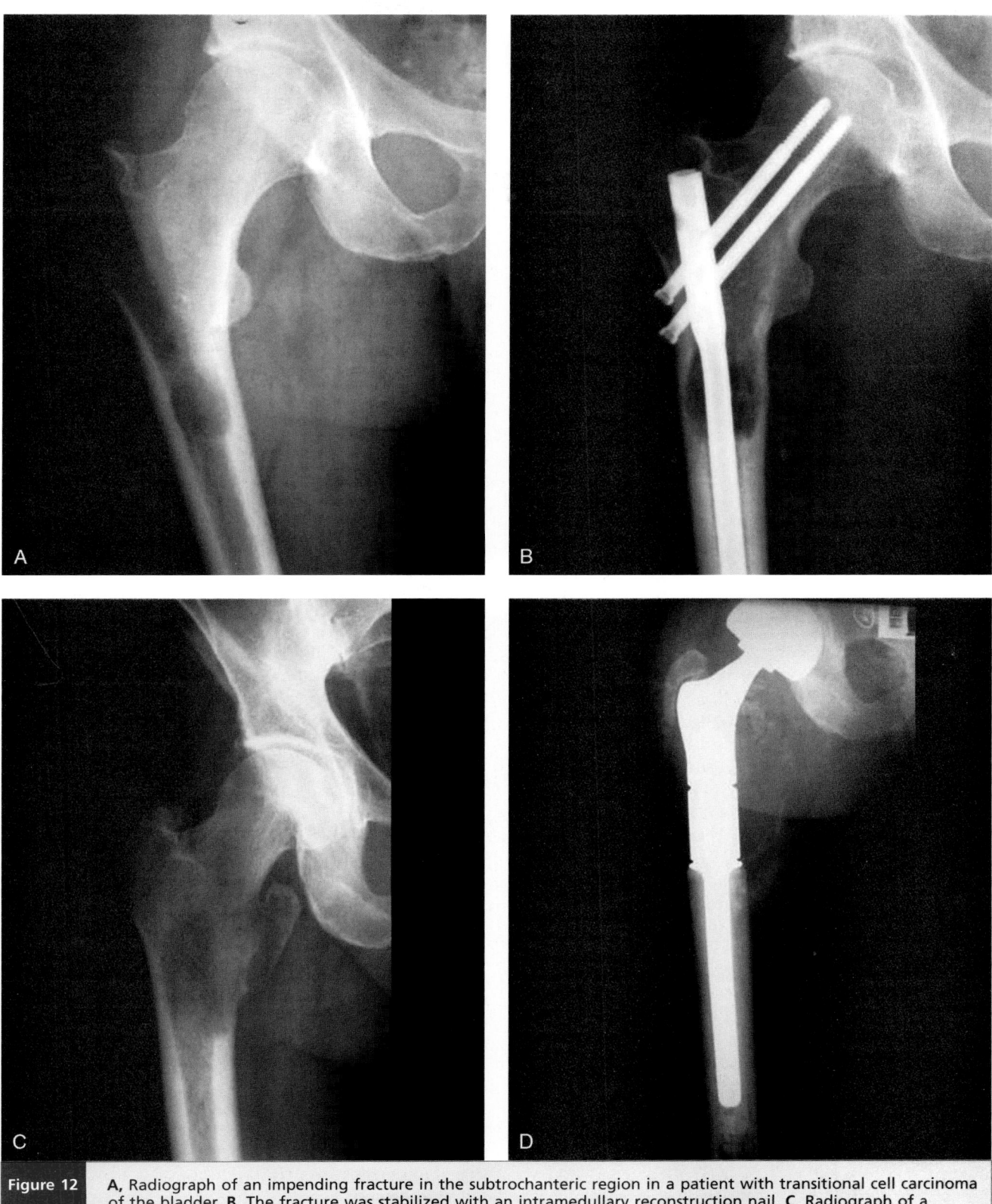

Figure 12 **A,** Radiograph of an impending fracture in the subtrochanteric region in a patient with transitional cell carcinoma of the bladder. **B,** The fracture was stabilized with an intramedullary reconstruction nail. **C,** Radiograph of a pathologic fracture through the lesser trochanter in a patient with a metastatic renal cell carcinoma. **D,** The fracture was treated with wide resection and cemented proximal femoral replacement. Preservation and reattachment of the greater trochanter provides better attachment of the abductors to the prosthesis.

2: Systemic Disorders

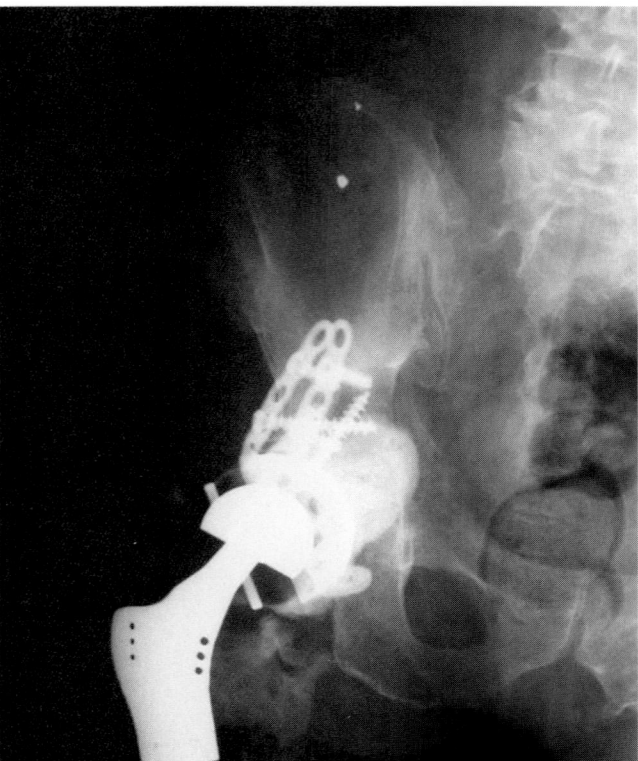

Figure 13 Reconstruction of the medial wall of the pelvis with cement and antiprotrusio cage in a patient with metastatic disease of the acetabulum. A cemented total hip arthroplasty with a constrained acetabular liner was used to decrease the risk of dislocation.

A recent study examining this question found that development of a new lesion in patients with renal or lung carcinomas was metastatic disease.[25] However, in patients with breast and prostate carcinoma, the lesion was likely to be a distinct malignancy different from the index diagnosis. It was recommended that a biopsy be done for all new lesions, especially in patients with breast or prostate carcinomas. It is important to rule out development of another primary bone malignancy in a patient with an underlying cancer with a new solitary bone lesion.

Skeletal Metastasis of Unknown Origin

Skeletal metastasis may be the initial presenting symptom in up to 23% of patients with underlying carcinomas. In patients presenting with a skeletal lesion without a prior diagnosis of cancer, a strategy was recommended that included a history and physical examination, chest radiographs, CT of the chest and abdomen, and a biopsy of the lesion.[26] This diagnostic strategy resulted in identification of the primary lesion in 85% of patients studied. It was also noted that biopsy of the lesion alone would have led to identification of the primary lesion in only approximately one third of patients studied.

Metastatic Disease to the Spine

Metastases to the spine are common, with 10% to 30% of patients with newly diagnosed cancer presenting with symptomatic spinal metastases.[27] The vertebral bodies are most commonly involved, although the typical "winking owl" sign is seen as a result of pedicular destruction by the tumor. Thoracic lesions tend to be the most symptomatic because of the relatively small size of the thoracic canal. Most patients with spinal metastases present with axial, nonmechanical pain. Symptoms of night pain and rest pain should prompt a workup for malignant etiology. Patients may also have mechanical back pain because of instability secondary to bone destruction by the tumor. Patients may also present with neurologic symptoms secondary to direct compression of the neuroelements by the tumor or secondary to instability or progressive deformity. Early lesions may be asymptomatic and the diagnosis is made incidentally.

Evaluation

Assessment includes a thorough history and physical examination to determine the etiology of the pain and to identify the potential primary focus of malignancy (thyroid, prostate, or breast examination). Biplanar radiographs should be obtained and the degree of vertebral destruction and collapse should be noted. Radiographs may be negative early in the disease process and advanced imaging in the form of MRI may be indicated in these patients. MRI typically shows hypointense signal on T1-weighted sequences and hyperintense signal on T2-weighted sequences. The hypointense signal on T1 with loss of normal marrow fat suggests a diagnosis of pathologic fracture secondary to a malignant process rather than an osteoporotic compression fracture. MRI is also superior to CT for evaluation of neurologic structures and to assess the degree of cord compression and intracordal signal abnormality.

In a patient with known or suspected malignancy, a bone scan should be obtained to look for other foci of metastatic disease. A biopsy is usually required to establish the histologic diagnosis and rule out any primary neoplasms (especially for solitary lesions). The biopsy is often done under CT guidance to ensure that the needle tip is appropriately placed; this maximizes the yield of diagnostic tissue. The accuracy of CT-guided biopsies in lytic lesions of the spine is close to 90%, whereas the diagnostic accuracy with this procedure in sclerotic lesions is approximately 25%.

Spinal Stability

Collapse with more than 50% loss of vertebral body height or progressive angular deformities suggests instability. The Kostuik system for evaluation of spinal instability uses the three-column classification of Denis and then further subdivides each column into right and left halves, thus dividing each vertebral body into six segments. If there is destruction of one or two segments, the spine is considered stable; three- or four-segment destruction is classified as an unstable spine; and destruction of five or six segments makes the spine markedly unstable.

Treatment of Spinal Metastases

Once spinal metastasis is diagnosed, patients need multidisciplinary care. The team usually includes a medical oncologist, a radiation oncologist, radiologist, pathologist, and a spine surgeon trained in the treatment of these lesions. Treatment of metastatic spinal lesions needs to be individualized depending on the primary lesion, the degree of osseous destruction and neurologic compromise, as well as patient comorbidities and expectations. The various treatment modalities include: (1) nonsurgical measures, including pain management and use of bisphosphonates to minimize risk of further osteoclastic destruction of bone; (2) chemotherapy; (3) radiation therapy; and (4) surgery.

Radiation therapy may be used for treatment of bone pain or neurologic deficits in the absence of mechanical compromise. Conventional radiation doses are usually between 2,500 and 4,000 cGy delivered over 8 to 20 daily fractions; as a result, the surrounding structures (including the spinal cord) are at risk for radiation-induced damage. Newer, more conformal radiation techniques (intensity modulated radiation therapy, CyberKnife [Accuray Inc, Sunnyvale, CA]), which are capable of delivering a larger dose in a better focused area, help improve the tumor kill and minimize side effects and damage to the surrounding normal tissues. Response to radiotherapy depends on the radiosensitivity of the primary tumor (for example, metastasis from breast, prostate, myeloma, and lymphoma are extremely sensitive, but renal and thyroid metastases are much less sensitive to radiation). Adjuvant radiation therapy following surgical decompression and stabilization tends to improve outcomes compared with radiation alone.[28]

Surgery is indicated in patients with mechanical instability or in those with advanced destruction and progressive neurologic compromise. Surgical treatment is generally indicated in patients with at least 3 months of expected survival. The goals of surgery are to decompress the neurologic structures, correct deformities, and stabilize the vertebral column to provide pain relief and the best environment for neurologic recovery and function.

Surgical treatment involves an adequate decompression of the dural elements and stabilization of the spine using instrumentation that is expected to outlive the patient. Anterior vertebral body reconstruction using an anterior or a posterolateral approach (costotransversectomy) has significantly improved results of spinal stabilization from the back alone. Anterior reconstruction can be achieved with the use of autograft, allograft, or a combination of the two, as well as PMMA. In patients with a good prognosis for long-term survival, a more biologic approach using bone graft is preferred. This approach, however, is associated with complications with healing in an unfavorable radiation or surgical bed, and other complications, primarily infection. PMMA provides immediate stability and allows

faster rehabilitation but is generally used in patients with a shorter life expectancy.

Emerging Concepts and Future Directions

Tremendous strides are being made in the fields of genomics and proteomics, which will improve the understanding of the underlying processes involved in the development of tumors (for example, studies looking at the role of transforming growth factor-β in the regulation of gene expression). Advances in pathologic diagnostic techniques (immunohistochemistry, fluorescent in situ hybridization) will enable better and more precise diagnosis and subtyping of tumors. Advances in imaging are aimed at predicting tumor necrosis in patients treated with neoadjuvant chemotherapy to enable potential modification of therapeutic regimens in patients with a poor response. Significant improvements continue to be made with the development of better targeted radiation delivery systems (CyberKnife), which are able to deliver high doses of radiation in an extremely narrow, precise area to kill tumor cells but not damage surrounding normal tissue. The role of chemotherapy in soft-tissue tumors continues to evolve, with several phase II and phase III trials evaluating various chemotherapeutic agents and regimens (such as temozolomide, gemcitabine, and docetaxel). Improvements in design and metallurgy to improve soft-tissue attachment and reduce loosening and wear are under development, which will ultimately improve the survival of endoprostheses and improve function.

There is a push toward more specific targeted therapies for various tumors, such as the use of imatinib for gastrointestinal stromal tumors. The use of immunotherapy with monoclonal antibodies such as trastuzumab in the treatment of *HER2*-positive metastatic breast cancer has led to significant improvement in survivorship. Targeted chemotherapy is available for several tumors (bortezomib, an inducer of apoptosis, is approved by the US Food and Drug Administration for treatment of refractory myeloma). Biologic approaches to anticancer therapy including the use of adenovirus-based therapies, use of monoclonal antibodies, and use of antiangiogenic agents are also being investigated.

Annotated References

1. Lodwick GS, Wilson AJ, Farrell C, Virtama P, Smeltzer FM, Dittrich F: Estimating rate of growth in bone lesions: Observer performance and error. *Radiology* 1980;134:585-590.

2. Mankin HJ, Lange TA, Spanier SS: The hazards of biopsy in patients with malignant primary bone and soft-tissue tumors. *J Bone Joint Surg Am* 1982;64:1121-1127.

3. Mankin HJ, Mankin CJ, Simon MA: The hazards of the

biopsy, revisited: Members of the Musculoskeletal Tumor Society. *J Bone Joint Surg Am* 1996;78:656-663.

4. Enneking WF, Spanier SS, Goodman MA: A system for the surgical staging of musculoskeletal sarcoma. *Clin Orthop Relat Res* 1980;153:106-120.

5. Sharma H, Mehdi SA, MacDuff E, Reece AT, Jane MJ, Reid R: Paget sarcoma of the spine: Scottish Bone Tumor Registry experience. *Spine* 2006;31:1344-1350.

   This was a study of 13 patients with Paget's sarcoma of the spine. The sacrum was the most common site of involvement (7 of 13 patients). The prognosis was dismal, with a mean survival of 4.2 months. Level of evidence: IV.

6. Greditzer HG III , McLeod RA, Unni KK, Beabout JW: Bone sarcomas in Paget disease. *Radiology* 1983;146: 327-333.

7. Murphey MD, Flemming DJ, Boyea SR, Bojescul JA, Sweet DE, Temple HT: Enchondroma versus chondrosarcoma in the appendicular skeleton: Differentiating features. *Radiographs* 1998; 18:1213-1237.

8. Itälä A, Leerapun T, Inwards C, Collins M, Scully SP: An institutional review of clear cell chondrosarcoma. *Clin Orthop Relat Res* 2005;440:209-212.

   This retrospective study of 16 patients with clear cell chondrosarcomas demonstrated that the prognosis was good with a 10-year survival rate of 89%. The authors found that metastatic disease developed late (mean, 8.1 years) and recommended long-term follow-up beyond the usual 5 years in this group of patients.

9. Thacker MM, Temple HT, Scully SP: Current treatment for Ewing's sarcoma. *Expert Rev Anticancer Ther* 2005; 5:319-331.

   A review of current treatment of Ewing's sarcoma and future directions are presented.

10. Staals EL, Bacchini P, Bertoni F: Dedifferentiated central chondrosarcoma. *Cancer* 2006;106:2682-2691.

    This retrospective study of 123 patients with dedifferentiated chondrosarcomas demonstrated no benefit to adjuvant chemotherapy in these patients. Metastatic disease at presentation, MFH dedifferentiation, and a higher percentage of dedifferentiated tumor were associated with a poor prognosis. Level of evidence: III.

11. Blackley HR, Wunder JS, Davis AM, White LM, Kandel R, Bell RS: Treatment of giant-cell tumors of long bones with curettage and bone-grafting. *J Bone Joint Surg Am* 1999;81:811-820.

12. Lackman RD, Hosalkar HS, Ogilvie CM, Torbert JT, Fox EJ: Intralesional curettage for grades II and III giant cell tumors of bone. *Clin Orthop Relat Res* 2005;438: 123-127.

    This study showed excellent outcomes and a low recurrence rate (6%) in 63 patients with Campanacci grade II and II giant cell tumors of bone treated with curettage,

burring, phenolization, and use of PMMA. Level of evidence: III.

13. Malawer MM, Bickels J, Meller I, Buch RG, Henshaw RM, Kollender Y: Cryosurgery in the treatment of giant cell tumor: A long-term followup study. *Clin Orthop Relat Res* 1999;359:176-188.

14. Beal K, Allen L, Yahalom J: Primary bone lymphoma: Treatment results and prognostic factors with long-term follow-up of 82 patients. *Cancer* 2006;106:2652-2656.

    This study demonstrated significantly better 5-year overall survival and disease-specific survival in 82 patients with primary lymphoma of bone treated with multimodal therapy compared with one modality alone. Level of evidence: III.

15. Park L, Delaney TF, Liebsch NJ, et al: Sacral chordomas: Impact of high-dose proton/photon-beam radiation therapy combined with or without surgery for primary versus recurrent tumor. *Int J Radiat Oncol Biol Phys* 2006;65:1514-1521.

    This study highlighted the poor results of treatment (surgery and radiation) in recurrent chordomas. Level of evidence: III.

16. Yeh HS, Berenson JR: Myeloma bone disease and treatment options. *Eur J Cancer* 2006;42:1554-1563.

    This article is a good review of bone disease in myeloma and current treatment strategies. Level of evidence: V.

17. Kransdorf MJ, Bancroft LW, Peterson JJ, Murphey MD, Foster WC, Temple HT: Imaging of fatty tumors: Distinction of lipoma and well-differentiated liposarcoma. *Radiology* 2002;224:99-104.

18. Mankin HJ, Gebhardt MC, Jennings LC, Springfield DS, Tomford WW: Long-term results of allograft replacement in the management of bone tumors. *Clin Orthop Relat Res* 1996;324:86-97.

19. Torbert JT, Fox EJ, Hosalkar HS, Ogilvie CM, Lackman RD: Endoprosthetic reconstructions: Results of long-term followup of 139 patients. *Clin Orthop Relat Res* 2005;438:51-59.

    This was a retrospective review of 139 patients treated with endoprosthetic reconstruction. They found 69% prosthetic survival at 10 years. The best results were seen in the proximal femur and the worst results in the distal humerus. Level of evidence: IV.

20. Unwin PS, Cannon SR, Grimer RJ, Kemp HB, Sneath RS, Walker PS: Aseptic loosening in cemented custom-made prosthetic replacements for bone tumours of the lower limb. *J Bone Joint Surg Br* 1996;78:5-13.

21. Eilber FC, Tap WD, Nelson SD, Eckardt JJ, Eilber FR: Advances in chemotherapy for patients with extremity soft tissue sarcoma. *Orthop Clin North Am* 2006;37: 15-22.

    The authors present a good review of the current status

of treatment with chemotherapy for soft-tissue sarcomas of the extremities. Level of evidence: V.

22. Mirels H: Metastatic disease in long bones: A proposed scoring system for diagnosing impending pathologic fractures. *Clin Orthop Relat Res* 1989;249:256-264.

23. Capanna R, Campanacci DA: The treatment of metastases in the appendicular skeleton. *J Bone Joint Surg Br* 2001;83:471-481.

24. Damron TA, Sim FH: Surgical treatment for metastatic disease of the pelvis and the proximal end of the femur. *Instr Course Lect* 2000;49:461-470.

25. Clayer M, Duncan W: Importance of biopsy of new bone lesions in patients with previous carcinoma. *Clin Orthop Relat Res* 2006;451:208-211.

    This study highlights the need for a biopsy of the first osseous lesion in a patient with a known primary carcinoma, especially if the primary lesion is a breast or pros-

tate carcinoma. Level of evidence: II.

26. Rougraff BT, Kneisl JS, Simon MA: Skeletal metastases of unknown origin: A prospective study of a diagnostic strategy. *J Bone Joint Surg Am* 1993;75:1276-1281.

27. Tatsui H, Onomura T, Morishita S, Oketa M, Inoue T: Survival rates of patients with metastatic spinal cancer after scintigraphic detection of abnormal radioactive accumulation. *Spine* 1996;21:2143-2148.

28. Patchell RA, Tibbs PA, Regine WF, et al: Direct decompressive surgical resection in the treatment of spinal cord compression caused by metastatic cancer: A randomised trial. *Lancet* 2005;366:643-648.

    This was a prospective randomized study that demonstrated improved pain scores as well as functional outcomes in patients treated with a combination of surgery and adjuvant radiation compared with patients treated with radiation alone. Level of evidence: I.

Chapter 18

Arthritis

David Borenstein, MD   Shari Diamond, MD

Introduction

Arthritis is a term that encompasses a variety of inflammatory and noninflammatory disorders affecting synovial joints. Patients with arthritis have significant pain, loss of motion, and joint deformity. When left untreated, these disorders cause severe disability and increased mortality. Over the past decade, advances in basic science have resulted in a better understanding of the mechanisms of disease progression. Based on this information, specific therapies have been developed that normalize these destructive processes. This chapter will concentrate on the three most common forms of rheumatic disorders in adult patients: rheumatoid arthritis (RA), spondyloarthritis, and osteoarthritis (OA). In addition, fibromyalgia, a nonarthritic central pain syndrome characterized by increased generalized musculoskeletal discomfort, is discussed.

Rheumatoid Arthritis

RA is a chronic, inflammatory, autoimmune disease that targets the synovial joints. It affects approximately 75 of every 100,000 persons, and is more common in women than men. RA manifests as a polyarthritis that is symmetric, erosive, and deforming. Patients develop joint inflammation and early morning stiffness typically lasting longer than 1 hour. Classic joint involvement includes the wrists and the metacarpophalangeal (MCP), proximal interphalangeal (PIP), and metatarsophalangeal (MTP) joints.

RA is diagnosed in individuals with symmetrical inflammatory polyarthritis affecting the small joints of the hands, feet, and wrists persisting for more than 6 weeks with characteristic laboratory abnormalities. The most specific laboratory finding for rheumatoid arthritis is the presence of anticyclic citrullinated peptide antibodies (in two thirds of patients). Anticyclic citrullinated antibody may be present before rheumatoid factor is detected. A less specific but more sensitive finding is the presence of rheumatoid factor, an immunoglobulin M antibody directed against the constant portion of immunoglobulin G, in 90% of patients. Antinuclear antibody with a homogenous pattern is found in 30% to 40% of patients with RA. Other laboratory findings that are compatible but not diagnostic of RA include elevated erythrocyte sedimentation rate (ESR), elevated C-reactive protein, decreased hematocrit level, and/or elevated platelet count.

Joint damage occurs early in the course of disease, with radiographic evidence of bony erosions in many patients by the time of diagnosis. Bony erosions and deformities are irreversible once they have occurred. Until as recently as 10 years ago, little could be done to prevent the long-term consequences of disease. However, over the past decade, improved understanding of the pathophysiology of RA has led to new treatments and therapeutic strategies. Evidence is mounting that early diagnosis and treatment with combination therapy that includes disease-modifying antirheumatic drugs (DMARDs) and anticytokine medications to achieve tight control of the disease is more effective in preventing joint damage.[1]

In the past, standard treatment of RA began with nonsteroidal anti-inflammatory drugs (NSAIDs). DMARDs, which most commonly included hydroxychloroquine, intramuscular gold, and sulfasalazine, and more recently methotrexate and leflunomide, were reserved only for patients with radiographic bony erosions. Recent studies have shown that early intervention with DMARDs and more effective disease control produce better outcomes.[1,2] Aggressive initial treatment of early RA with a combination of three different DMARDs for the first 2 years has been shown to limit peripheral joint damage and improve radiologic outcome for at least 5 years.[1] A strategy of intensive management improves disease activity, radiographic disease progression, and physical function in patients with RA. Frequent assessment and escalation of therapy on the basis of disease activity has been effective in retarding disease progression.[2] The irreversible joint damage of RA is becoming less common with the availability of new treatments (Table 1).

An understanding of the role of cytokines in the pathogenesis of RA will lead to greater appreciation of current targeted therapies. Cytokines are produced by activated immune cells, and either enhance or inhibit the immune response. Th1 cells, a subset of T helper lymphocytes, act as inflammatory cells and secrete proinflammatory cytokines, which include interleukin-2 (IL-2), interferon gamma (IFN-γ), and tumor necrosis factor α (TNF-α). TNF-α and interleukin-1b (IL-1b) are also secreted by synovial macrophages. They are considered to be the major proinflammatory cytokines in the pathogenesis of RA and other chronic inflammatory diseases. When TNF-α and IL-1b are secreted, they

2: Systemic Disorders

Table 1

Treatments for Rheumatoid Arthritis

	Dose and Route of Administration	Mechanism of Action	Efficacy	Side Effects
Infliximab	5 mg/kg IV one time on weeks 0, 2, 6; then every 6 weeks	Chimeric monoclonal antibody binds to TNF-α, interfering with endogenous TNF-α activity	In combination with MTX; ACR50 in 50% at 1 year	Infusion reaction Infection Malignancy Demyelination ?CHF
Etanercept	50 mg SC every week or 25 mg SC biweekly	Recombinant TNF receptor binds TNF and blocks its interaction with cell surface receptors	In combination with MTX; ACR50 in 69% at 1 year	Injection site reaction Infection Malignancy Demyelination ?CHF
Adalimumab	40 mg SC every other week	Recombinant monoclonal antibody that binds to TNF-α, interfering with binding to TNF-α receptor	In combination with MTX; ACR50 in 62% at 1 year	Injection site reaction Infection Malignancy Demyelination ?CHF
Anakinra	100 mg SC every day	Recombinant human IL-1ra binds to the IL-1 receptor	In combination with MTX; ACR50 in 24% at 24 weeks	Injection site reaction Infection
Abatacept	< 60 kg* = 500 mg 60-100 kg* = 750 mg > 100 kg* = 1,000 mg; IV one time on weeks 0,2,4; then every 4 weeks	Selective costimulation modulator; inhibits T cell activation by binding to CD80 and CD86 on APC, blocking the CD28 interaction between APCs and T cells	In combination with MTX; ACR50 in 40% at 1 year	Infusion reaction Infection Malignancy
Rituximab	1,000 mg IV on day 1 and day 15	Chimeric monoclonal antibody directed against the CD20 antigen on B-lymphocytes	In combination with MTX; ACR50 in 43% at 24 weeks	Infusion reaction Infection
Corticosteroid	Low dose; 5-10 mg PO every day	Anti-inflammatory, decreases production of matrix metalloproteinases	Reduces radiographic progression at 6 months and 2 years in low dose	Dermatologic Gastrointestinal Musculoskeletal Endocrine central Nervous system Cardiovascular Hematologic Metabolic
Doxycycline	100 mg PO twice a day	Unknown; inhibits matrix metalloproteinases, immunomodulatory	In combination with MTX; ACR50 in 40% at 2 years	Photosensitivty

* patient's weight; IV = intravenous; MTX = methotrexate; CHF =congestive heart failure; ACR50 = A 50% improvement in symptoms according to American College of Rheumatology criteria. SC = subcutaneous; APC = antigen-presenting cells; PO = by mouth

stimulate synovial cells to proliferate and synthesize collagenase, causing cartilage degradation, bone resorption, and inhibition of proteoglycan synthesis. They also cause induction of other inflammatory cytokines and matrix metalloproteinases, all components needed to sustain the inflammatory cascade. Contemporary available treatments target cytokines and attempt to downregulate or inhibit the effector functions of these cytokines. Targeting specific receptors or cytokines may selectively suppress or modulate the immune

dysfunction that contributes to the pathogenesis of RA (Table 2).

TNF-α Antagonists

Three TNF-α antagonists are currently approved for the treatment of RA in the United States: infliximab, etanercept, and adalimumab. Infliximab is a chimeric (mouse/human) immunoglobulin G (IgG) monoclonal anti-TNF-α antibody administered in regular intravenous infusions. It has been shown in multiple clinical

Table 2			
Cytokines in RA			
Cytokine	**Source**	**Effect**	**Targeting Drug**
IL-1	T cells, macrophages, neutrophils, endothelial cells Found in rheumatoid synovium	Stimulates synovial cells to proliferate and synthesize collagenase and metalloproteinases, induction of other inflammatory cytokines, activates T and B cells	Anakinra
TNF	T cells, macrophages, neutrophils Found in rheumatoid synovium	Stimulates synovial cells to proliferate and synthesize collagenase and metalloproteinases, induction of other inflammatory cytokines, activates T and B cells, upregulates macrophages and neutrophils, tumor cytotoxicity	Infliximab Etanercept Adalimumab
IFN-γ	T cells, natural killer cells Found in rheumatoid synovium	Activates T cells and other inflammatory cytokines	

trials to improve symptoms while reducing radiographic progression of joint erosions.[3,4] Although approved for use in combination with methotrexate, some patients do receive infliximab alone.[3] However, patients started on a combination of infliximab and methotrexate early on in the disease course (less than 3 years duration) have significantly more improvement than patients started on methotrexate alone.[4] Patients who receive initial combination therapy with infliximab, rather than progressive or "step-up" combination therapy or sequential monotherapy, have better functional improvement and less joint structural damage as evidenced on plain radiographs, ultrasound, and MRI.[4] When infliximab is used in combination with methotrexate at the beginning of treatment, patients have better outcomes.[5]

Etanercept, a soluble TNF-α receptor fusion protein, has proved to be as effective as infliximab.[6] As a soluble receptor molecule it binds to free cytokine, inhibiting the cytokine's ability to bind to cell surface receptors. It is given as a weekly (50 mg) or biweekly (25 mg) subcutaneous injection. When combined with traditional DMARDs, etanercept and infliximab offer similar protection against progressive joint structural damage.[5] In combination with methotrexate, etanercept also significantly reduces disease activity, improves function, and retards radiographic progression of disease.[7]

The newest anti-TNF-α agent is adalimumab, a fully human monoclonal TNF-α antibody. It is administered subcutaneously every other week. As with etanercept and infliximab, clinical trials have established adalimumab's efficacy in preventing the irreversible joint structural damage of RA.[8] Combination therapy with adalimumab plus methotrexate is superior to either medication alone in improving signs and symptoms of disease and inhibiting radiographic progression, as seen with infliximab and etanercept.[8]

The adverse effect profiles for these three TNF-α an-

tagonists are similar.[9] The most common adverse events reported are injection site reactions seen with etanercept and adalimumab, and infusion reactions with infliximab. Although generally well tolerated, there is evidence of an increased risk of serious infection, particularly tuberculosis reactivation.[9] Patients should be screened with a purified protein derivative for latent tuberculosis before any of the anti-TNF-α agents are administered. Other significant infections that have been found include *Pneumocystis carinii*, candidiasis, histoplasmosis, listeriosis, nocardiosis, aspergillosis, *Cytomegalovirus*, cryptococcosis, and coccidioidomycosis. The presence of demyelinating disease in patients receiving these agents is cause for concern because its incidence seems to be higher than in the general population. No definitive causal relationship has been established. However, it is reasonable to avoid use of anti-TNF-α agents in patients with preexisting demyelinating disease and discontinue treatment in any patient with suspected demyelination. Data on the risk of anti-TNF-α therapy in patients who have experienced heart failure are inconclusive. Because some studies suggest a possible exacerbation of heart failure, these agents should be avoided in patients with risk factors for heart failure. Results from a recent study of more than 13,000 patients showed no increased incidence of heart failure in RA patients treated with anti-TNF-α when compared with other RA patients.[10]

The risk of developing malignancy in patients receiving anti-TNF-α therapy is still uncertain. Studies have suggested an increased risk of hematologic malignancies in patients treated with anti-TNF-α agents. Differences in neoplasm occurrence between the treatment groups have not been statistically significant.[9] It has also been difficult to assess whether the elevated risk is caused by the immunosuppressant medications or RA itself, which is known to predispose patients to malignancy. A recent meta-analysis of nine clinical trials found a statistically significant increased incidence of

2: Systemic Disorders

neoplasm in RA patients treated with anti-TNF-α agents. However, inferences regarding the risk of malignancy should be made with caution because of several important limitations of the study.[9] Because these medications are still fairly new, more time and additional studies are needed to determine actual risk.

Perioperative Management of TNF-α Therapy

Currently, there are no established guidelines regarding perioperative use of anti-TNF-α agents. The concern for increased risk of infection caused by immunosuppression from treatment has led some to suggest that perioperative treatment be discontinued. RA is an independent risk factor for postoperative orthopaedic infection, with an infection rate two to four times higher than in patients who do not have RA, and anti-TNF-α agents are known to enhance the risk of infection with mycobacteria and other opportunistic organisms.[9,11] However, withholding treatment in some patients could induce a disease flare, complicating wound healing after surgery. Maintaining the balance between disease control while minimizing the postoperative risk of infection is the clinical dilemma. There are few data to support either withholding or continuing treatment perioperatively. The available data are limited to retrospective and observational studies in a small number of patients with conflicting results regarding the effects of anti-TNF-α agents on surgical outcomes.[12-15] Generally, infliximab was withheld 4 weeks before surgery and etanercept and adalimumab were withheld for 2 weeks before surgery. When deciding whether to discontinue treatment, the physician should consider the patient's individual medical history and disease course as well as the surgical procedure and its potential risks. Similarly, there are no data regarding reinitiation of therapy after surgery. Thus, the decision to restart therapy should be guided by the patient's individual course, balancing the concerns for adequate wound healing with the level of RA disease activity.

Anakinra

IL-1 receptor antagonist (IL-1Ra) is a naturally-occurring protein secreted by macrophages that inhibits IL-1 by binding to the IL-1 receptor. Anakinra is recombinant human IL-1Ra and is approved for the treatment of RA. It is administered in daily subcutaneous doses. Several clinical trials have shown anakinra to be moderately effective in slowing radiographic progression and improving disease activity.[16] The most frequent adverse effects were injection site reactions and serious infections similar to those seen with the anti-TNF-α agents. The addition of anakinra to etanercept and methotrexate has not been found to be any more effective in treating RA and is associated with a higher rate of serious infection.[16] Because of its modest efficacy and daily subcutaneous dosing, anakinra is more commonly started in patients in whom anti-TNF-α therapy has failed.

Abatacept

The important role the T cell plays in the pathogenesis of RA has led to the development of T cell targeted therapy for the treatment of RA. Once T cells are activated, macrophages and B cells are stimulated to release cytokines (TNF-α and IL-1). Thus, the goal is the inactivation of pathogenic T cells by directing therapy at specific sites in the activation pathway. Antigen-presenting cells (APC) present antigen (Ag)-derived peptides bound to the class II major histocompatibility complex (MHC) to CD+4 T cells. The binding complex consists of the MHC class II molecules, Ag, and the T cell receptor (TcR). T cell activation then requires two signals. The first signal is between the MHC on the APC and the TcR. The second is a costimulatory signal. There are several costimulatory pathways on T cells, including the CD80/86 on the APC with the CD28 and/or cytotoxic T lymphocyte-associated antigen 4 (CTLA-4) on the T cell. CD28 provides an activating signal whereas CTLA-4 provides an inhibitory signal. Abatacept is a selective costimulation modulator and works by selectively targeting the CD80/86:CD28 costimulation pathway. It is a soluble fusion protein of CTLA-4 and IgG; therefore, it interferes with the ability of CD28 to bind to its receptor, thereby preventing the costimulatory signal from occurring and keeping the T cell inactive. Thus, abatacept results in immunomodulation rather than complete immunosuppression by reducing T cell proliferation and other downstream markers of inflammation.[17]

Abatacept is given as an intravenous infusion every 4 weeks. Its efficacy has been shown in several studies and, importantly, efficacy has been demonstrated for patients who have active RA and have not responded to methotrexate and/or anti-TNF-α agents. Significant reductions have been seen in disease activity and radiographic progression.[17] Abatacept should not be used concurrently with TNF-α antagonists or anakinra because of a higher rate of serious infections.[17] Similar to the anti-TNF-α agents, the most serious adverse reactions reported were infection and malignancy. Patients should be screened for tuberculosis before beginning treatment. The most common adverse effects include infusion reactions in about 10% of patients, nausea, and headache.

Rituximab

Although the role of the T cell in the pathogenesis of RA has been evident for years, the role of the B cell has been more controversial. It is known that antigen-specific B cells are important for autoantibody production as well as presentation of antigen to T cells. The idea of using B cell targeted therapy for treating RA is based on the hypothesis that B cells are needed to renew autoantibody-secreting plasma cells, to present antigen to synovial T cells and thereby activating the T cells to release cytokines, and possibly themselves producing proinflammatory cytokines. Depletion of synovial B cells using B cell targeted therapy with rituximab has led to a decrease in production of TNF-α.[18]

Rituximab is a chimeric monoclonal antibody that was originally developed for the treatment of B cell lymphomas. It is directed against the CD20 cell surface molecule. CD20 is a membrane protein that is present only on B cells, and is expressed initially at the immature B cell stage, remaining until the final differentiation into plasma cells. Treatment with rituximab results in prolonged depletion of B cells from peripheral blood.[18]

Since its approval for treatment of lymphoma in 1997, rituximab has been used to treat a variety of autoimmune diseases, often with success. The most extensive data has been published for the treatment of RA, for which rituximab recently obtained Food and Drug Administration approval. In several trials, the addition of rituximab to methotrexate significantly reduced the signs and symptoms of RA.[18] These results have been confirmed, and one trial showed benefits even in patients in whom anti-TNF-α treatment had previously failed.[19] The recommended protocol being used for treatment of RA consists of two intravenous infusions of 1,000 mg of rituximab separated by 2 weeks, with the administration of glucocorticoid premedication before each infusion. Infusion reactions are serious and most common with the first infusion, occurring in approximately 30% of patients. The severity and frequency of these reactions is significantly reduced when patients are premedicated with glucocorticoids. As with the anti-TNF-α agents, infection is a serious concern.[18] Rituximab appears to be well tolerated overall, although data on its long-term effects in patients with RA are limited.

Glucocorticoids

Glucocorticoids have been used in the treatment of active RA for several decades. The fast-acting anti-inflammatory effects of glucocorticoids are well established. A possible disease-modifying effect of glucocorticoids causing decreased disease activity and inhibition of radiographic damage also has been postulated. However, their extensive adverse effect profile has rendered long-term use of glucocorticoids an unattractive option. Recent investigation into the disease-modifying properties and clinical efficacy of very low-dose prednisone in patients with early active RA receiving concomitant treatment with a DMARD found significantly less radiographic progression and disease activity.[20] The improvement in the rate of disease progression appears to be greatest in the first 6 months of treatment with low-dose prednisolone. The glucocorticoid is useful and effective early in the course of disease, and the DMARD maintains the benefit.[20] Hence, the strategy of early administration of glucocorticoids and DMARDs together followed by reduction and eventual cessation of prednisolone can provide sustained joint protection. Early use of glucocorticoids retards disease progression, but there is little to be gained and adverse effects will occur if glucocorticoids are continued for more than 6 months, even in low doses.[20] On occasion, some patients continue low-dose prednisone for extended periods of time.

Doxycycline

Although the mechanism of action of tetracyclines in RA is poorly understood, in addition to their antibacterial effects, tetracyclines inhibit matrix metalloproteinases and are immunomodulatory. Tetracyclines were originally used in the treatment of RA because *Mycoplasma* was believed to be a potential cause of RA. It is now evident that tetracyclines are useful in RA because of their anti-inflammatory effects rather than their antimicrobial effects. Early trials studying the efficacy of tetracyclines have had mixed results. Some studies have shown improvement in patients treated with tetracyclines whereas other trials have not been able to reproduce those same benefits. A recent trial studied the effects of doxycycline in combination with methotrexate in the treatment of early RA and found that initial therapy with the combination of the two drugs was superior to treatment with methotrexate alone.[21] Because this is only one trial, additional studies are needed to confirm these findings and further define the mechanism of action of tetracyclines in treating RA before adopting doxycycline as an established treatment of RA. Photosensitivity was the most common adverse effect of doxycycline.[21]

Statins

Statins are inhibitors of 3-hydroxy-3-methylglutaryl-coenzyme A. Statins lower serum cholesterol levels and are widely used in the prevention and treatment of atherosclerotic cardiovascular disease. These drugs also seem to have anti-inflammatory properties. Statins have been reported to inhibit interactions between leukocytes and endothelial cells, to reduce the production of inflammatory cytokines, and to decrease T cell activation.[22] Several animal models have demonstrated success with statins in treating inflammatory diseases, but only a small number of trials have been performed to evaluate the benefits of statins in human rheumatic diseases and in particular RA.[22] Current data on efficacy of statins for treatment of RA are mixed.[22] Statins clearly have anti-inflammatory properties. However, the data are still preliminary and more studies are needed to assess whether their anti-inflammatory capabilities are clinically relevant for the treatment of rheumatic diseases.

Seronegative Spondyloarthritis

The term spondyloarthritis encompasses a heterogeneous group of inflammatory diseases characterized by spinal and peripheral joint oligoarthritis and enthesitis. They often have associated mucocutaneous, ocular, and/or cardiac manifestations. This family of diseases includes ankylosing spondylitis (AS), psoriatic arthritis, enteropathic arthritis (associated with inflammatory bowel diseases), reactive arthritis, and undifferentiated spondyloarthropathy.

2: Systemic Disorders

Ankylosing Spondylitis

AS is a chronic inflammatory disease of the axial skeleton manifested by back pain and progressive stiffness of the spine. The prevalence of AS varies from 0% to 1.4%, depending on the ethnic group. It characteristically affects young adults, males more than females, with a peak age of onset between 20 to 30 years. Patients present with back pain with prolonged morning stiffness (for greater than 1 hour) and progressive loss of motion of the axial spine. In addition to the spine, sacroiliac involvement, arthritis of the hips, peripheral arthritis, and enthesitis are common. As the disease progresses, increasing flexion of the neck, increased thoracic kyphosis, and loss of normal lumbar lordosis lead to a stooped posture. On plain radiographs, squaring of the vertebral bodies as a result of anterior and posterior spondylitis will be seen early and bridging syndesmophytes, ankylosis of the facet joints and calcification of the anterior longitudinal ligament, and anterior atlantoaxial (C1-C2) subluxation occur later in the disease process.

Laboratory tests add little in the diagnosis of AS. ESR is increased in 80% of patients with active disease. C-reactive protein levels may be elevated if ESR is normal. Rheumatoid factor and antinuclear antibody are characteristically absent in these patients. Genetic and environmental factors play important roles in the pathogenesis of AS. The only locus definitively linked to the spondyloarthritis is HLA-B27 allele. HLA-B27 is present in at least 95% of AS patients and the prevalence of HLA-B27 among the general population is between 5% and 8%. Only certain subtypes of HLA-B27 predispose to AS. No general agreement exists on how HLA-B27 contributes to disease susceptibility; the presence of HLA-B27 is not needed to confirm a diagnosis of AS.

The goals of therapy for patients with AS are not only to provide symptomatic relief, but as in the treatment of RA, to prevent permanent irreversible joint damage. However, progress in identifying disease-modifying medications for the treatment of AS has been hampered by the still limited understanding of the pathologic processes involved in spinal inflammation and fusion. The same DMARDs that have proved effective in the treatment of RA have not all shown the same efficacy in AS. For example, although sulfasalazine and methotrexate are somewhat effective in treating the peripheral arthritis associated with AS, they have not shown the same benefits in treating the axial symptoms of AS. TNF-α has been identified as an important cytokine mediating inflammation in AS and the same anti-TNF-α treatments useful in RA have been used successfully for AS.[23]

Nonsteroidal Anti-Inflammatory Drugs

NSAIDs are among the most frequently prescribed medications for AS and numerous studies in patients with AS have demonstrated improvement in back pain and stiffness with use of these drugs. Many physicians recommend patients with AS take NSAIDs only as necessary because of the significant risk of adverse effects, particularly on the gastrointestinal system. Continuous use of NSAIDs, regardless of symptoms, is another approach. Evidence exists that continuous use is associated with a decrease in disease progression on radiographs. When continuous celecoxib is compared with on-demand treatment, a significant reduction in disease progression radiographically in symptomatic patients with AS has been seen.[24] This finding suggests that NSAIDs may have disease-modifying properties in addition to being just symptom modifiers. Additional studies are needed to confirm these results.

TNF-α Antagonists

Until recently, treatment options for patients with AS have been limited to NSAIDs; however, the role of anti-TNF-α in patients with AS is becoming more established. As discussed, anti-TNF-α therapy is accepted as an important and effective therapy in RA. It is becoming clear that anti-TNF-α therapy in treatment of AS is at least as effective as or more effective than for RA.[25] Although the pathologic process is not completely understood and seems to be different from RA, TNF-α still appears to be important in the inflammatory response observed in AS. TNF-α, messenger RNA, and protein have been found in the sacroiliac joints of patients with AS. Thus, therapeutic agents that target the proinflammatory cytokine TNF-α are currently the most effective treatment options for patients with AS.

The three available anti-TNF-α agents, infliximab, etanercept, and adalimumab have been effective in the treatment of AS in clinical trials.[26] Patients treated with infliximab have been shown in several studies to have significant improvement in disease activity in both peripheral and spinal manifestations.[26] In one recent large study, patients receiving infliximab as monotherapy exhibited significant improvement in the signs and symptoms of AS. The patients in this trial had shorter disease durations than those in the previous randomized controlled trial of infliximab. Shorter disease duration has recently been shown to be a strong predictor of clinical response to anti-TNF-α therapy in patients with AS, presumably because irreversible structural damage occurs as the disease progresses. These results together suggest that earlier treatment with anti-TNF-α therapy may provide a better overall prognosis for patients with AS. However, additional studies should be conducted in patients in whom AS was recently diagnosed to more accurately determine the appropriate time to initiate anti-TNF-α therapy.

Treatment of AS with etanercept has also been studied and found to be effective in several clinical trials.[25] The response has typically been rapid, within the first 6 weeks of treatment, and etanercept appears to have continued efficacy for at least 2 years. Most recently, the therapeutic efficacy of adalimumab for the treatment of active AS has been demonstrated. Patients have exhibited a significant improvement in clinical signs and symptoms, similar to that observed with the other anti-TNF-α agents.[27]

Physicians should be aware that the same adverse effect profile applies to AS and RA patients treated with anti-TNF-α therapy. Infusion/injection reactions, infections, malignancy, demyelinating disorders, and possibly congestive heart failure are of serious concern. As in patients with RA, tuberculosis screening with purified protein derivative skin testing should be done before therapy with anti-TNF-α is initiated.

Psoriatic Arthritis

Psoriatic arthritis is a chronic inflammatory rheumatic disease that affects peripheral joints and, in approximately one third of patients, the spine. Psoriatic arthritis affects approximately 20% to 30% of patients with psoriasis, with women and men being affected equally. The arthritis appears after the onset of a skin lesion in most patients. However, the arthritis can precede the skin disease in approximately 13% to 17% of patients. Patients often experience nail pitting and onycholysis as do patients with uncomplicated skin psoriasis. Several clinical patterns of joint involvement in psoriatic arthritis have been identified: distal arthritis, characterized by involvement of the distal interphalangeal joints; asymmetric oligoarthritis in which less than five small and/or large joints are affected in an asymmetric distribution; symmetric polyarthritis, similar to and at times indistinguishable from RA; arthritis mutilans, characterized by deforming and destructive arthritis; and spondyloarthritis, including both sacroiliitis and spondylitis.

Patients are often treated with NSAIDs for psoriatic arthritis, but to date evidence supporting the use of NSAIDs for psoriatic arthritis is scarce. DMARDs such as methotrexate and cyclosporine are also commonly used for patients with psoriatic arthritis. Recently, strong evidence has emerged supporting the use of anti-TNF-α agents for the treatment of psoriatic arthritis.[28] The importance of T cells and of TNF-α in the pathogenesis of psoriasis and psoriatic arthritis appears to be well established, and TNF-α is found at high levels in the joint fluid and tissue of patients with psoriatic arthritis. Sustained benefits for patients with skin and joint disease were seen at 1 year in a trial using infliximab.[28] Etanercept was also found to reduce joint symptoms, improve psoriatic lesions, and inhibit radiographic progression of disease at 1 year. Adalimumab showed similar efficacy with significantly improved joint and skin manifestations and a reduction in irreversible structural damage on radiographs. All three agents have proven efficacy in preventing and retarding joint damage and are approved by the Food and Drug Administration for use in the treatment of psoriatic arthritis.[28] As in both RA and AS, before initiating anti-TNF-α therapy for psoriatic arthritis, patients should be screened for tuberculosis with purified protein derivative skin testing. Physicians should be aware of the adverse effects profile.

Enteropathic Arthritis, Reactive Arthritis, and Undifferentiated Spondyloarthropathy

Enteropathic arthritis is the spondyloarthropathy associated with ulcerative colitis and Crohn's disease. This spondyloarthropathy follows a pattern similar to AS. Characteristically, the spinal disease of these individuals progresses independent of activity of bowel lesions. Patients with enteropathic arthritis have good responses to the TNF-α inhibitors. Patients with reactive arthritis with HLA B27 develop axial disease after an exposure to an infectious agent, such as *Salmonella*, *Shigella*, or *Chlamydia*. Disease patterns mirror those associated with psoriatic arthritis. Therapy used for psoriatic arthritis may be just as effective for reactive arthritis. Patients with undifferentiated spondyloarthropathy do not have an adequate number of symptoms or signs to designate a specific form of axial arthritis. These patients are treated as symptoms dictate until a specific diagnosis is identified.

Osteoarthritis

OA is a common age-related disorder characterized by damage to hyaline articular cartilage and associated bony remodeling. Variable degrees of synovitis are present in some patients as well as thickening of the joint capsule.[29] Advanced disease will be visible on plain radiographs as narrowing of the joint space, osteophytes, and sometimes changes in the subchondral bone. OA can arise in any synovial joint in the body, but occurs most commonly in the hands, feet, knees, hips, and spine. Clinically, OA manifests as joint pain related to use and short-lasting joint stiffness after inactivity. In addition to age, the main risk factors for the development of OA include female sex, prior joint injuries, family history, and obesity.

In response to stress, chondrocytes release degradative proteolytic enzymes, which result in the changes of the cartilage seen in OA. OA has traditionally been regarded as a purely mechanical and noninflammatory arthritis. Improved understanding of the pathogenesis shows that inflammatory pathways are upregulated as well with release of inflammatory cytokines by the cartilage.[29] The goals of management of patients with OA are to control pain and swelling, minimize disability, and maintain quality of life. Initial treatment should be with acetaminophen or NSAIDs as appropriate. Exercise to strengthen the muscles and improve flexibility, as well as weight loss, should be implemented immediately. In some patients with knee OA, intra-articular hyaluronic acid (HA) may help to improve short-term pain and function. The ability to significantly alter the progression of joint damage with a currently available pharmacologic agent has not been clearly shown.

Nonsteroidal Anti-Inflammatory Drugs

NSAIDs are effective pain relievers in patients with OA.[30] These medications are intended to reduce pain and inflammation associated with OA by inhibiting the

2: Systemic Disorders

production of prostaglandins in the cyclooxygenase (COX) pathway. The demonstration of prostaglandin E_2 in human OA cartilage suggests that prostaglandin E_2 may contribute to the local inflammation and provides a rationale for the use of NSAIDs in treatment of OA. A 2004 meta-analysis of randomized controlled trials showed that NSAIDs can reduce short-term pain in OA of the knee better than placebo.[29] The efficacy of acetaminophen at doses of up to 4 g per day also has been demonstrated to be superior to placebo in relief of pain resulting from OA, but is less effective than NSAIDs.

The potential for gastrointestinal toxicity, including dyspepsia, ulcer, perforation, and hemorrhage, is an important concern for patients taking NSAIDs. One strategy to decrease the potential gastric toxicity of NSAIDs has been the use of COX-2 inhibitors. These medications have been designed to selectively inhibit the COX-2 enzyme, which limits inflammation without interfering with the normal production of protective prostaglandins and thromboxane. Studies have shown the COX-2 inhibitors to be as effective as the nonspecific NSAIDs in treating OA, although there is a decreased incidence of gastric toxicity.[30] It is important to note that all NSAIDs and COX-2 inhibitors may cause cardiovascular and renal side effects to varying degrees. In 2004, two COX-2 inhibitors, rofecoxib and valdecoxib, were withdrawn from the worldwide market because of concern for an increase in serious cardiovascular events. No statistically significant difference has been shown for celecoxib compared with NSAIDs in the number of serious cardiovascular events.[31] Other selective COX-2 inhibitors that are being actively investigated include etoricoxib and lumircoxib. In studies to date, these two medications have been shown to have similar efficacy to nonspecific NSAIDs with fewer gastrointestinal complications and without a significant increase in the rate of serious cardiac events.

Exercise and Weight Loss

Exercise is a valuable and commonly prescribed intervention for lower limb OA.[32] By improving flexibility and strengthening muscles supporting the affected joints, patients improve functional outcome and pain scores.[32] In patients with OA of the knee, weakness of the quadriceps muscles is caused by disuse and by inhibition of muscle contraction in the presence of adjacent capsular swelling. Strengthening the muscles improves the stability of the joints and lessens pain. Low-impact exercises to avoid excessive joint loading are preferable, including isokinetic and isotonic strengthening. Not only is moderate exercise effective in improving joint symptoms and function but an improvement in the cartilage glycosaminoglycan content in vivo also has been found.

Obesity is strongly associated with OA. Weight loss reduces the symptoms of OA in weight-bearing joints. In addition to reducing the risk of progression of OA, moderate weight loss may produce improvement in joint pain and function. The relationship between the amount of weight lost and the reduced incidence of OA appears to be linear, suggesting that even modest weight loss may be beneficial. Each pound of weight loss results in a fourfold reduction in the load exerted on the knee per step during daily activities. The combination of diet and exercise is the most effective strategy and is associated with decreased knee pain and improved self-reported and measured function.[33]

Intra-Articular Hyaluronans

HA forms the backbone of aggrecan, the large macromolecule that makes up the cartilage matrix. HA has viscous and elastic properties that are critical to normal joint function. At low load speeds it acts as a lubricant and during faster movements as a shock absorber. In OA, the concentration of HA is reduced by one half to one third of normal, which leads to decreased effectiveness and increased wear rates. Several articular injectable variations of HA have been approved for OA with the aim of decreasing the symptoms of OA by supplementing the HA, which is deficient in degenerative cartilage. Data regarding the efficacy of HA injections have been mixed. Overall, HA injections appear to moderately improve short-term pain but not function.[34]

Few adverse effects have been reported with HA injections. Those that have occurred are usually mild pain at the injection site. More severe reactions have been described and are known as pseudoseptic reactions. They are characterized by increased pain, swelling, and an inflammatory joint effusion and are seen in 1.5% to 5% of injected knees. Joint fluid analysis reveals elevated white blood cell counts (possibly up to 100,000 per mm^3) but sterile cultures.[34]

Glucosamine and Chondroitin Sulfate

Glucosamine sulfate is the monosaccharide precursor to glycosaminoglycans, which makes up proteoglycan, the macromolecule that constitutes 5% to 10% of articular cartilage. Chondroitin sulfate is composed of repeating units of galactosamine sulfate and glucuronic acid and is the predominant glycosaminoglycan found in articular cartilage. It is postulated that oral supplementation with glucosamine and/or chondroitin sulfate can slow cartilage breakdown by stimulating cartilage to synthesize glycosaminoglycan and proteoglycans and by inhibiting degradative proteolytic enzymes.[35] Current dosing is weight dependent, with the recommended daily average of 1,500 mg glucosamine and 1,200 mg chondroitin taken in combination.

Although some data show an improvement in pain and function and possibly a decreased incidence of radiographic changes with the combination of glucosamine and chondroitin sulfate, other studies, including the largest randomized placebo controlled study to date, did not find glucosamine alone or the combination to be more effective in relieving pain or improving function than placebo.[35] For those patients whose symptoms do improve with glucosamine sulfate, the optimal treatment duration is uncertain. There is some evidence that suggests regular use for more than 6 months is no more effective than placebo. Adverse effects reported with use of glucosamine and chondroitin sulfate include hypersensitivity in patients who are allergic to shellfish, gastrointestinal discomfort, and skin reactions.[35]

Doxycycline

Matrix metalloproteinases are a group of proteolytic enzymes that includes collagenases, stromelysins, and gelatinases. They degrade all components of articular extracellular matrix and can cause destruction of articular cartilage. Tetracyclines appear to be potent inhibitors of two major matrix metalloproteinases, collagenase and gelatinase. In OA, the activities of collagenase, gelatinase, and stromelysin are increased in articular cartilage. Doxycycline may slow the rate of progression of OA. A recent study of patients with symptomatic unilateral knee OA found that the patients treated with 100 mg doxycycline twice daily had significantly less joint space narrowing but not less pain than the placebo group.[36] Additional studies are needed to confirm these findings and assess the benefits of doxycycline in treating OA.

Topical Products

Many over-the-counter topical products for OA contain capsaicin, the active ingredient of hot chili pepper, that is believed to decrease pain by depleting the stores of substance P and other neurotransmitters from nerve endings. Topical NSAIDs recently have become available in some countries (not the United States). A topical preparation of diclofenac was found to be effective for short-term pain relief in the treatment of OA of the knee. Topical NSAIDs offer the theoretic advantage of decreasing pain locally without the gastrointestinal and renal toxicities of oral NSAIDs. Local skin irritation is a relatively frequent adverse effect in patients receiving topical NSAIDs.

Fibromyalgia

Fibromyalgia is now recognized as one of the central pain syndromes that occur commonly in the population. The prevalence of fibromyalgia in the general population of industrialized countries has been reported to range from 0.5% to 4%. Patients with fibromyalgia experience augmented central pain processing, so they feel more pain than other individuals when exposed to the same stimuli. Although a complete understanding of the pathophysiology of fibromyalgia is still lacking, evidence now suggests that a combination of neurobiologic abnormalities interact with psychosocial and behavioral factors to contribute to symptom expression in fibromyalgia.

Both genetic and environmental influences have been found to confer an increased risk for fibromyalgia. Polymorphisms in the genes encoding for the serotonin 5-HT2A receptor, the serotonin transporter, the dopamine-4 receptor and catecholamine *o*-methyl transferase occur at a higher frequency in patients with fibromyalgia. These monoamines play a critical role in both sensory processing and the human stress response. Studies also have shown that some individuals who are exposed to various external stressors such as physical trauma, certain infections, and emotional stress subsequently develop fibromyalgia.[37]

The most consistent objective findings in patients with fibromyalgia involve the sensory processing system. These patients have enhanced nociceptive sensation caused by central neural activation in the absence of peripheral input. The antinociceptive serotonergic-noradrenergic pathways are abnormal. Patients with fibromyalgia have higher levels of substance P, a pronociceptive compound, in their cerebrospinal fluid, reduced levels of the principal metabolite of norepinephrine in their cerebrospinal fluid, as well as low serum serotonin levels. These abnormalities are based in the central nervous system. The recommended medications to treat fibromyalgia are, therefore, agents that affect sensory processing, such as tricyclic antidepressants and serotonin/norepinephrine reuptake inhibitors rather than NSAIDs or opioids used to treat peripheral pain. Additionally, behavioral and psychological factors play an important role in symptoms expression and functional decline of patients with fibromyalgia. Pain can lead to distress, which can lead to more pain and further exacerbate symptoms. A reduction in activity levels and poor sleep because of symptoms can lead to further pain and worsen feelings of depression. The physician should recognize patients will be more likely to have a flare-up of pain symptoms during periods of increased stress, such as surgery. In these situations adjusting the dose of tricyclic antidepressants rather than opioids would likely be more helpful in controlling symptoms.

In making the diagnosis of fibromyalgia the physician must first rule out other disorders. All routine laboratory and radiographic testing will be normal, including serum inflammatory markers. Patients not only report chronic pain, but will also often experience fatigue, nonrestorative sleep, paresthesias, memory difficulties, and other nondefining symptoms. The American College of Rheumatology classification criteria for fibromyalgia require chronic widespread pain and the finding of tenderness at 11 or more of 18 anatomically defined points on examination.[38] Therapeutic options for patients in whom fibromyalgia has been diagnosed should consist of both pharmacologic and nonpharmacologic therapies. Nonpharmacologic therapies include exercise and cognitive behavioral therapy. For example, swimming can be an aerobic exercise that generates endorphin response without stress to the musculoskeletal system. A number of drug therapies that affect the central nervous system processing of pain have beneficial effects on fibromyalgia. New directions in pharmacotherapy include dual reuptake inhibitors (duloxetine and milnacipran) and anticonvulsants (pregabalin).[39]

2: Systemic Disorders

Summary

New therapies are available for the treatment of arthritis and fibromyalgia. With arthritis, early diagnosis and aggressive treatment with DMARDs and TNF-α inhibitors has changed the destructive course of these conditions. The need for surgical intervention should diminish for patients who have access to these agents. Fibromyalgia is a pain condition that may complicate the clinical improvement of surgical patients. New pharmacologic agents in combination with increased physical activity have the potential to control generalized pain and malaise.

Annotated References

1. Korpela M, Laasonen L, Hannonen P, et al: Retardation of joint damage in patients with early rheumatoid arthritis by initial aggressive treatment with disease-modifying antirheumatic drugs: Five year experience from the FIN-RACo study. *Arthritis Rheum* 2004;50: 2072-2081.

   This study provides strong evidence that treatment of early RA with a combination of 3 DMARDs for the first 2 years provides improved long-term radiologic outcome.

2. Grigor C, Capell H, Stirling A, et al: Effect of a treatment strategy of tight control for rheumatoid arthritis (the TICORA study): A single-blind randomized controlled trial. *Lancet* 2004;364:263-269.

   This study shows that intensive management of RA rather than routine care improves disease activity and radiologic outcome at no additional cost.

3. St Clair EW, van der Heijde DM, Smolen JS, et al: Combination of infliximab and methotrexate therapy for early rheumatoid arthritis: A randomized, controlled trial. *Arthritis Rheum* 2004;50:3432-3433.

   This study showed strong evidence that patients with early active RA have better outcomes when treated with combination of methotrexate and infliximab in early stages of disease.

4. Goekoop-Ruiterman YP, de Vries-Bouwstraa JK, Allaart CF, et al: Clinical and radiographic outcomes of four different treatment strategies in patients with early rheumatoid arthritis (the BeSt study): A randomized, controlled trial. *Arthritis Rheum* 2005;52:3381-3390.

   This study shows that in patients with early RA, initial combination therapy resulted in earlier functional improvement and less radiographic damage after 1 year than did sequential monotherapy.

5. Finckh A, Simard JF, Duryea J, et al: The effectiveness of anti-tumor necrosis therapy in preventing progressive radiographic joint damage in rheumatoid arthritis: A population-based study. *Arthritis Rheum* 2006;54:54-59.

   This study shows that both etanercept and infliximab offer similar therapeutic advantages. Combination therapy with either agent and a DMARD is more effective than treatment with etanercept alone.

6. Moreland LW, Schiff MH, Baumgartner SW, et al: Etanercept therapy in rheumatoid arthritis: A randomized, controlled trial. *Ann Intern Med* 1999;130:478-486.

7. Klareskog L, van der Heijde D, de Jager JP: Therapeutic effect of the combination of etanercept and methotrexate compared with each treatment alone in patients with rheumatoid arthritis: Double-blind randomised controlled trial. *Lancet* 2004;363:675-681.

   This study shows that combination of etanercept and methotrexate is superior than either treatment alone in patients with RA.

8. Breedveld FC, Weisman MH, Kavanaugh AF, et al: The PREMIER study: A multicenter, randomized, double-blind clinical trial of combination therapy with adalimumab plus methotrexate versus methotrexate alone or adalimumab alone in patients with early, aggressive rheumatoid arthritis who had not had previous methotrexate treatment. *Arthritis Rheum* 2006;54:26-37.

   Combination therapy with adalimumab plus methotrexate was superior to either therapy alone in effecting clinical remission and inhibiting radiographic progression.

9. Bongartz T, Sutton AJ, Sweeting MJ, et al: Anti-TNF antibody therapy in rheumatoid arthritis and the risk of serious infections and malignancies: Systematic review and meta-analysis of rare harmful effects in randomized controlled trials. *JAMA* 2006;295:2275-2285.

   An important review and meta-analysis of the side effects of anti-TNF antibody therapy.

10. Wolfe F, Michaud K: Heart failure in rheumatoid arthritis: Rates, predictors, and the effect of anti-tumor necrosis factor therapy. *Am J Med* 2004;116:305-311.

    Heart failure occurs more commonly in RA than OA patients but less frequently in RA patients receiving anti-TNF-α therapy.

11. Poss R, Thornhill TS, Ewald FC, et al: Factors influencing the incidence and outcome of infection following total joint arthoplasty. *Clin Orthop Relat Res* 1984;182: 117-126.

12. Wendling D, Balbanc JC, Brousse A, et al: Surgery in patients receiving anti-tumour necrosis factor α treatment in rheumatoid arthritis: An observational study on 50 surgical procedures. *Ann Rheum Dis* 2005;64: 1378-1379.

    A retrospective observational study evaluating the safety of patients on anti-TNF-α therapy at time of surgery did not find increased risk of infection when therapy was discontinued.

13. Talwalkar SC, Grennan DM, Gray J, et al: Tumour necrosis factor α antagonists and early postoperative complications in patients with inflammatory joint disease undergoing elective orthopaedic surgery. *Ann Rheum Dis* 2005;64:650-651.

A retrospective study on postoperative outcomes in RA and psoriatic arthritis patients did not find increased risk of infection when anti-TNF-α therapy was discontinued.

14. Giles JT, Bartlett SJ, Gelber AC, et al: Tumor necrosis factor inhibitor therapy and risk of serious postoperative orthopedic infection in rheumatoid arthritis. *Arthritis Rheum* 2006;55:333-337.

    A chart review evaluating the safety of patients on anti-TNF-α therapy at time of surgery found a statistically significant increased risk for infection in patients who continued therapy perioperatively.

15. Bibbo C, Goldberg JW: Infectious and healing complications after elective orthopedic foot and ankle surgery during tumor necrosis factor-alpha inhibition therapy. *Foot Ankle Int* 2004;25:331-335.

    A prospective study evaluated the risk of healing and infectious complications in 31 RA patients perioperatively, one half of whom were on anti-TNF-α therapy versus patients not treated with anti-TNF therapy. Infectious and healing complications were similar between the two groups.

16. Jiang Y, Genant HK, Watt I, et al: A multicenter, double-blind, dose-ranging, randomized, placebo-controlled study of recombinant human IL-1 receptor antagonist in patients with rheumatoid arthritis: Radiologic progression and correlation of Genant and Larsen scores. *Arthritis Rheum* 2000;43:1001-1009.

17. Genovese MC, Becker JC, Schiff M, et al: Abatacept for rheumatoid arthritis refractory to tumor necrosis factor alpha inhibition. *N Engl J Med* 2005;353:1114-1123.

    This study provides strong evidence that abatacept is an effective treatment for patients with RA who had an inadequate response to anti-TNF-α therapy.

18. Edwards JC, Szczepanski L, Szechinski J, et al: Efficacy of B-cell-targeted therapy with rituximab in patients with rheumatoid arthritis. *N Engl J Med* 2004;350:2572-2581.

    This study shows that patients with active RA despite treatment with methotrexate, have significant improvement after treatment with rituximab alone or in combination with cyclophosphamide or methotrexate.

19. Cohen SB, Emery P, Greenwald MW, et al: Rituximab for rheumatoid arthritis refractory to anti-tumor necrosis factor therapy: Results of a multicenter, randomized, double-blind, placebo-controlled, phase III trial evaluating primary efficacy and safety at twenty-four weeks. *Arthritis Rheum* 2006;54:2793-2806.

    Rituximab is an efficacious treatment in RA patients in whom anti-TNF-α therapy has failed.

20. Svensson B, Boonen A, Albertsson K, et al: Low-dose prednisolone in addition to the initial disease-modifying antirheumatic drug in patients with early active rheumatoid arthritis reduces joint destruction and increases the remission rate: A two-year randomized trial. *Arthritis Rheum* 2005;52:3360-3370.

This study provides strong evidence that prednisolone 7.5 mg in combination with a DMARD slowed the radiographic progression after 2 years in patients with early RA.

21. O'Dell JR, Elliott JR, Mallek JA, et al: Treatment of early seropositive rheumatoid arthritis: Doxycycline plus methotrexate versus methotrexate alone. *Arthritis Rheum* 2006;54:621-627.

    This study shows that in patients with early seropositive RA, initial therapy with doxycycline and methotrexate was superior to treatment with methotrexate alone.

22. Abeles AM, Pillinger MH: Statins as antiinflammatory and immunomodulatory agents: A future in rheumatologic therapy? *Arthritis Rheum* 2006;54:393-407.

    An important review of the anti-inflammatory and immunomodulatory effects of statins and its mechanism of action is presented.

23. Heiberg MS, Nordvag BY, Mikkelsen K, et al: The comparative effectiveness of tumor necrosis factor-blocking agents in patients with rheumatoid arthritis and patients with ankylosing spondylitis: A six month, longitudinal, observational, multicenter study. *Arthritis Rheum* 2005;52:2506-2512.

    This study provides strong evidence that effects of treatment with anti-TNF therapy in patients with AS is comparable to and sometimes greater than that in RA patients.

24. Wanders A, Heijde D, Landewe R, et al: Nonsteroidal anti-inflammatory drugs reduce radiographic progression in patients with ankylosing spondylitis: A randomized clinical trial. *Arthritis Rheum* 2005;52:1756-1765.

    A 2-year study demonstrates the slowing of disease progression with daily NSAID therapy without increased toxicity in comparison with intermittent NSAID use.

25. Braun J, Baraliakos X, Brandt J, et al: Persistent clinical response to the anti-TNF-alpha antibody infliximab in patients with ankylosing spondylitis over 3 years. *Rheumatology (Oxford)* 2005;44:670-676.

    This study provides strong evidence that patients with AS treated with infliximab for 3 years had a durable clinical response without loss of efficacy.

26. Baraliakos X, Davis J, Tsuji W, Braun J: Magnetic resonance imaging examinations of the spine in patients with ankylosing spondylitis before and after therapy with the tumor necrosis factor alpha receptor fusion protein etanercept. *Arthritis Rheum* 2005;52:1216-1223.

    This study shows that treatment with etanercept of patients with AS results in improved spinal inflammation on MRI scans.

27. van der Heijde D, Kivitz A, Schiff M, et al: Efficacy and safety of adalimumab in patients with ankylosing spondylitis. *Arthritis Rheum* 2006;54:2136-2146.

    This study provides strong evidence that patients with AS treated with adalimumab for 24 weeks had improve-

2: Systemic Disorders

ment in disease activity. The treatment was well tolerated.

28. Antoni CE, Kavanaugh A, Kirkham B, et al: Sustained benefits of infliximab therapy for dermatologic and articular manifestations of psoriatic arthritis: Results from the infliximab multinational psoriatic arthritis controlled trial (IMPACT). *Arthritis Rheum* 2005;52: 1227-1236.

This study provides strong evidence that patients with psoriatic arthritis treated with infliximab had improvement in both dermatologic and articular signs and symptoms.

29. Dieppe PA, Lohmander LS: Pathogenesis and management of pain in osteoarthritis. *Lancet* 2005;365: 965-973.

An excellent review of the pathogenesis, risk factors, and management of OA is presented.

30. Bjordal JM, Ljunggren AE, Klovning A, Slordal L: Non-steroidal anti-inflammatory drugs, including cyclooxygenase-2 inhibitors, in osteoarthritic knee pain: Meta-analysis of randomised placebo controlled trials. *BMJ* 2004;329:1317.

A meta-analysis of 23 trials showed that NSAIDs can reduce short-term pain in OA of the knee.

31. Singh G, Fort JG, Goldstein JL, et al: Celecoxib versus naproxen and diclofenac in osteoarthritis patients: SUCCESS-I Study. *Am J Med* 2006;119:255-266.

This study shows that celecoxib is as effective as the naproxen and diclofenac in the treatment of OA, but had fewer serious upper gastrointestinal events.

32. Roddy E, Zhang W, Doherty M, et al: Evidence-based recommendations for the role of exercise in the management of osteoarthritis of the hip or knee: The MOVE consensus. *Rheumatology (Oxford)* 2005;44:67-73.

This study provides evidence-based recommendations for exercise for patients with hip and knee OA.

33. Messier SP, Loeser RF, Miller GD, et al: Exercise and dietary weight loss in overweight and obese older adults with knee osteoarthritis: The arthritis, diet, and activity promotion trial. *Arthritis Rheum* 2004;50:1501-1510.

The combination of weight loss and exercise has a better overall effect on knee OA than either intervention alone.

34. Arrich J, Piribauer F, Mad P, et al: Intra-articular hyaluronic acid for the treatment of osteoarthritis of the knee: Systematic review and meta-analysis. *CMAJ* 2005;172: 1039-1043.

A review and meta-analysis of randomized controlled trials of HA for treatment of knee OA did not find it a clinically effective treatment.

35. Clegg DO, Reda DJ, Harris CL, et al: Glucosamine chondroitin sulfate, and the two in combination for painful knee osteoarthritis. *N Engl J Med* 2006;354: 795-808.

This large trial did not find that glucosamine and chondroitin sulfate alone or in combination were effective treatment in patients with knee OA. But subgroup analysis may show the combination effective for patients who have moderate to severe knee pain.

36. Brandt KD, Mazzuca SA, Katz BP, et al: Effects of doxycycline on progression of osteoarthritis: Results of a randomized, placebo-controlled, double-blind trial. *Arthritis Rheum* 2005;52:2015-2025.

This study shows that patients with knee OA treated with doxycycline have a slower rate of joint space narrowing and less increase in knee pain.

37. Clauw DJ, Chrousos GP: Chronic pain and fatigue syndromes: Overlapping clinical and neuroendocrine features and potential pathogenic mechanisms. *Neuroimmunomodulation* 1997;4:134-153.

38. Wolfe F, Smythe HA, Yunus MB, et al: The American College of Rheumatology 1990 criteria for the classification of fibromyalgia: Reports of the multicenter criteria committee. *Arthritis Rheum* 1990;33:160-172.

39. Rooks DS: Fibromyalgia treatment update. *Curr Opin Rheumatol* 2007;19:111-117.

This article summarizes results from recent studies discussing a multimodal treatment approach for patients with fibromyalgia.

Chapter 19

Neurology and Electromyography
Robert N. Kurtzke, MD

Neuromuscular Evaluation

Most patients present to an orthopaedic surgeon reporting pain. The sensory examination is typically guided by the patient's specific complaint. Relevant to this discussion, nerve root injury or irritation causes pain and sensory disturbance that is more difficult to localize than focal nerve injury. C5 root involvement causes scapular pain with vague sensory change along the shoulder and upper arm. C6 and C7 root involvement also can cause retroscapular pain; C6 radiculopathy more reliably causes discomfort and numbness in the thumb and often the index finger, whereas C7 root involvement generally causes pain and numbness in the long and middle fingers. C8 and T1 radiculopathies are less common and produce pain and numbness in the medial forearm and ring and pinky fingers. In contrast to the vague sensory report of nerve root origin, focal peripheral nerve injury generally causes a more defined area of paresthesia, pain, and sensory loss. There is substantial sensory overlap of the various nerves and nerve roots, so that the area of greatest sensory involvement generally provides the most localizing information. The territory of pain and numbness described by the patient is often disassociated from the area of sensory loss demonstrated by the examiner. For example, a patient with carpal tunnel syndrome may report pain and numbness involving the entire hand radiating up the forearm, while the objective sensory loss is generally confined to the thumb, index, and middle fingers, and sometimes the ring finger. A simplified version of cervical and lumbosacral myotomes and the principal disorder to be differentiated is provided in Table 1. There is substantial overlap in the myotomes.

The reflex examination provides additional clues to the level of dysfunction. The familiar reflexes are easily tested and in this context are most informative when asymmetry is present.

Nerve Conduction Velocity Study and Electromyography

Nerve conduction velocity studies and electromyography (EMG) are important aids in clarifying the clinical conditions of pain, numbness, and weakness.

Nerve conduction is performed by stimulating a major nerve over accessible locations on the arm or leg and measuring a response using surface electrodes over the muscle or skin in the distribution of the nerve under

Table 1		
Cervical and Lumbosacral Myotomes and the Principal Differential		
Spinal Segment	**Myotome**	**Principal Disorder to Be Differentiated**
C5	Supraspinatus, infraspinatus, deltoid	Upper brachial plexopathy or isolated mononeuropathies (suprascapular, axillary nerves)
C6	Biceps, brachioradialis, pronator teres	Brachial plexopathy
C7	Triceps, wrist, finger extensors and flexors	Brachial plexopathy and isolated mononeuropathies (radial or median nerve)
C8/T1	Finger extensors and flexors, intrinsic hand muscles	Lower brachial plexopathy and focal neuropathy (radial, median, or ulnar)
L2/L3	Hip flexion and thigh adduction	Lumbar plexopathy
L4	Vastus lateralis, vastus medialis, rectus femoris, anterior tibialis, thigh adduction	Femoral neuropathy and lumbar plexopathy
L5	Anterior tibialis, peroneus longus, extensor hallucis longus, posterior tibialis, gluteus medius	Sciatic neuropathy principally involving the peroneal fascicle or isolated peroneal neuropathy
S1	Hamstrings, gastrocnemius	Sciatic neuropathy

2: Systemic Disorders

study (**Figure 1**). The most useful information includes the amplitude of the response and how quickly the response travels down the nerve measured by conduction velocity, distal motor latency, or, for the sensory nerves, distal latency. Motor nerve conduction velocity needs to be calculated because motor nerve impulses traverse the neuromuscular junction; this action requires additional time and does not reflect conduction along the nerve. Thus for motor nerves, the nerve is stimulated in a distal location (such as the median nerve over the wrist) and then at a proximal location (such as the median nerve at the elbow). The terminal or distal motor latency is subtracted from the proximal latency, providing the time it takes for the stimulus to travel from the proximal to the distal location (in this example, from the elbow to the wrist). The distance is measured by a tape measure in centimeters or millimeters and divided by the time it takes for the impulse to travel from the elbow to the wrist, providing the conduction velocity for that segment.

Because sensory nerves have no neuromuscular junctions, calculating conduction velocity is not necessary nor does it provide additional information over the distal latency. Sensory conduction velocities are still reported as another means of describing sensory nerve function (**Figure 2**).

Conduction velocity, sensory latency, and distal motor latencies all reflect the speed with which the impulse travels down the nerve and this generally reflects the integrity of the insulating myelin sheath. Focal conduction slowing implies focal pathology and can help localize the lesion. The most common clinical scenario using focal conduction slowing is the prolongation of the sensory and motor latencies at the wrist in persons with carpal tunnel syndrome. The other important datum provided by nerve conduction velocity studies is the amplitude of the response, which reflects the integrity of the axons. Low-amplitude sensory or motor responses usually imply axon loss. In some situations, low-amplitude response can be seen with disturbance of the insulating myelin; this is typified by focal neuropathy, such as ulnar neuropathy at the elbow. In this situation, the motor response has a robust amplitude when the nerve is stimulated distally (for example, at the wrist); however, with stimulation above or proximal to the site of compression (for example, at the elbow), the amplitude of the response drops by more than 40%. This finding is called conduction block and implies sufficient damage to the nerve to cause focal de-

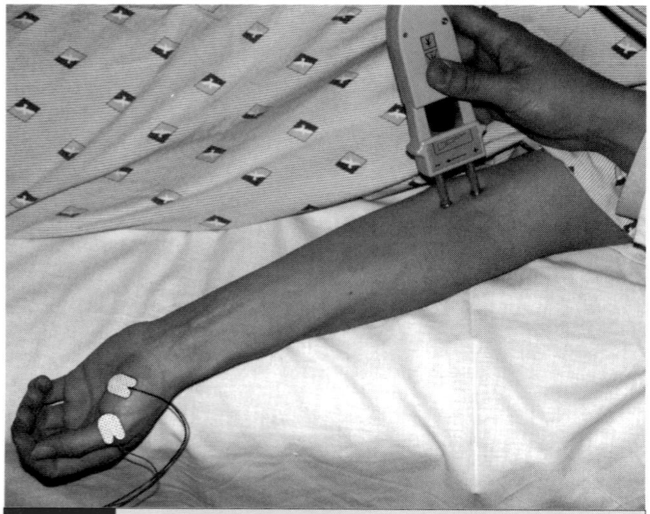

Figure 1   Setup for median nerve motor study: recording electrode (wire on the right) over abductor pollicis brevis; reference electrode (wire on the left) over tendon; ground electrode on dorsum of the hand (wire not clearly visible). Stimulating electrode is over the median nerve at elbow. *(Courtesy of American Association of Neuromuscular and Electrodiagnostic Medicine.)*

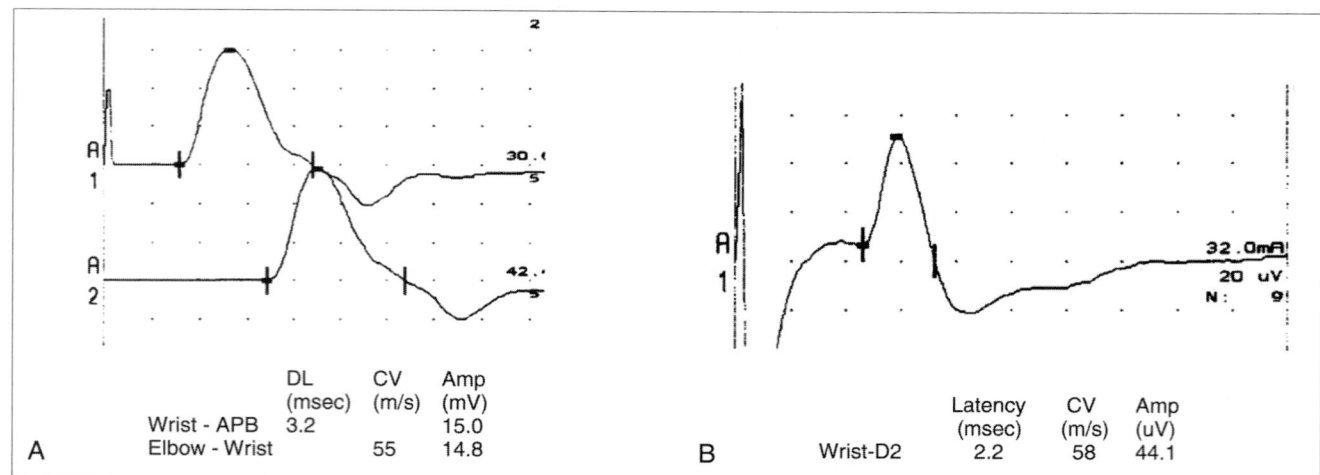

	DL (msec)	CV (m/s)	Amp (mV)
Wrist - APB	3.2		15.0
Elbow - Wrist		55	14.8

	Latency (msec)	CV (m/s)	Amp (uV)
Wrist-D2	2.2	58	44.1

Figure 2   **A,** Normal responses recorded over abductor pollicis brevis. A1 (top trace) response, stimulating median nerve at the wrist; A2 (bottom trace) response, stimulating median nerve at the elbow. **B,** Normal sensory response for median nerve stimulating the nerve over the wrist, recording over D2 (index finger). *(Courtesy of American Association of Neuromuscular and Electrodiagnostic Medicine.)*

myelination, but not necessarily axon loss. Conduction block is generally readily reversible, whereas axon loss typically requires axon regeneration, a slower and less complete process.

EMG involves placing a small needle electrode in the belly of the muscle. Normal muscle is electrically quiet at rest; when activated, the muscle produces electrical activity that is picked up by the needle. Early investigators determined the nature of nerve supply to the muscle and constructed the concept of the motor unit. The motor unit is composed of the motor neuron/anterior horn cell, the exiting motor nerve axon, and the muscle fibers it supplies. Anatomic and physiologic studies reveal that there are different numbers of motor units in various muscles, but the number of motor units per muscle is of an order of magnitude in the hundreds. Additionally, the number of muscle fibers belonging to a specific motor unit varies from muscle to muscle. One axon might supply only a small number of muscle fibers in muscles requiring finely graded control (such as extraocular and laryngeal muscles) compared with one axon supplying hundreds of muscle fibers in larger muscles such as the vastus or gastrocnemius muscles. Muscle fibers of adjacent motor units intermingle, and individual motor unit territory is in the range of 5 to 10 mm.

In healthy muscle, the motor unit action potential recorded by the needle electrode has typical shape, duration, and amplitude that can be quantitated. Duration is the most informative feature of the motor unit action potential, a concept proposed in the early 1950s and confirmed by computer-assisted studies.[1,2] Amplitude is another important feature, but is more dependent on how close the needle electrode is to the muscle fibers in the motor unit generating the potential. Some motor unit action potentials appear serrated or polyphasic in disease state in both myopathies and neuropathies; when polyphasic potentials appear in excessive numbers, that finding is considered abnormal. The other major electromyographic finding of interest is how the motor units are brought to work, or recruited. Recruitment tends to be a more subjective assessment of the numbers of motor unit action potentials active for a given level of muscular effort provided by the patient (**Figure 3**).

On the EMG screen, with increasing levels of effort, more motor unit action potentials are seen and heard and at a high level of effort produce an interference pattern, where so many units are firing that the individual units cannot be distinguished—analogous to a forest of trees. In neurogenic illness, there is a dropout of motor units and by necessity, the ones remaining will fire more rapidly to compensate for the reduced numbers available for work. Consequently, fewer motor unit action potentials are heard and seen during EMG, producing a reduced recruitment pattern or incomplete interference pattern of fast-firing motor unit action potentials. In severe neurogenic illness, the interference pattern can be so diminished as to produce what is termed a discrete interference pattern, in which individual motor unit action potentials can be discerned.

In nerve disease and some muscle diseases, EMG ab-

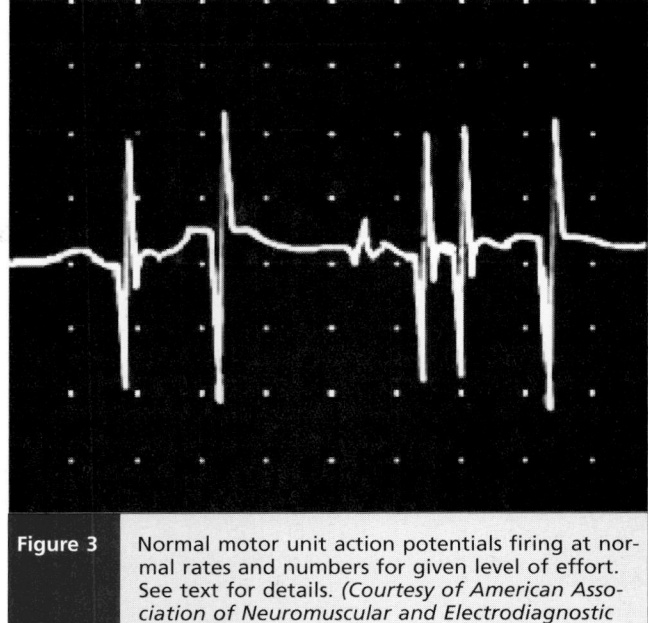

Figure 3 | Normal motor unit action potentials firing at normal rates and numbers for given level of effort. See text for details. *(Courtesy of American Association of Neuromuscular and Electrodiagnostic Medicine.)*

normalities include muscle membrane instability that manifests as spontaneous muscle fiber discharges called insertional positive waves and fibrillation potentials. Because they are produced by single muscle fibers, fibrillation potentials have short durations, 1 to 5 ms, and a crisp high-pitched sound with regular discharge rate. Positive sharp waves also originate from individual muscle fibers and generally have the same significance as fibrillation potentials. Positive sharp waves have a downward or positive deflection that looks like shark teeth on the EMG screen; the appearance is believed to be the result of depolarization of the electrode-damaged segment of the muscle fiber. Fibrillation potentials and insertional positive waves typically appear several weeks after an injury (**Figure 4**).

As previously stated, with nerve disease or focal nerve injury, dropout of anterior horn cells or nerve fibers may occur and EMG will record reduced numbers of active motor unit action potentials or reduced recruitment. The remaining motor unit action potentials change over time, becoming longer in duration and larger in amplitude as reinnervation occurs (**Figure 5**).

In muscle disease, membrane instability may also manifest as fibrillation potentials and insertional positive waves, but the recruitment and motor unit action potential changes are different. Whereas in nerve disease there is dropout of motor units, in muscle disease there is random dropout of individual muscle fibers, which produce motor unit action potentials of shorter duration and typically smaller amplitude. Because individual motor unit action potentials represent fewer muscle fibers, which generate less force, individual units need to be recruited earlier at lower levels of effort and a full interference pattern may be seen even with mild to moderate levels of effort.

2: Systemic Disorders

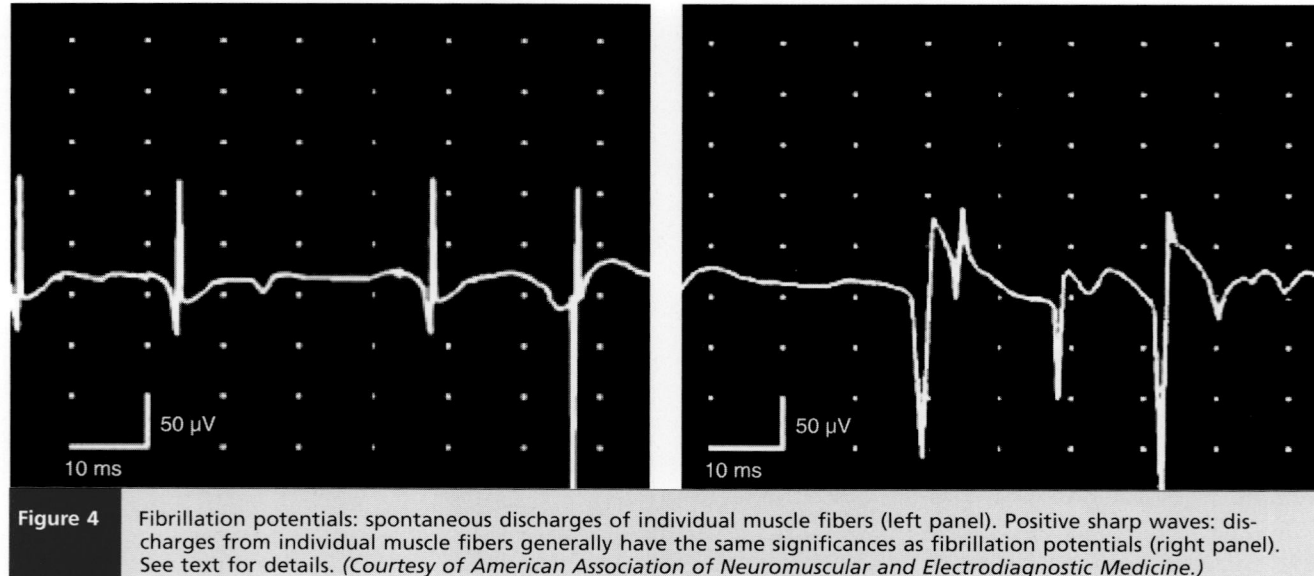

Figure 4 Fibrillation potentials: spontaneous discharges of individual muscle fibers (left panel). Positive sharp waves: discharges from individual muscle fibers generally have the same significances as fibrillation potentials (right panel). See text for details. *(Courtesy of American Association of Neuromuscular and Electrodiagnostic Medicine.)*

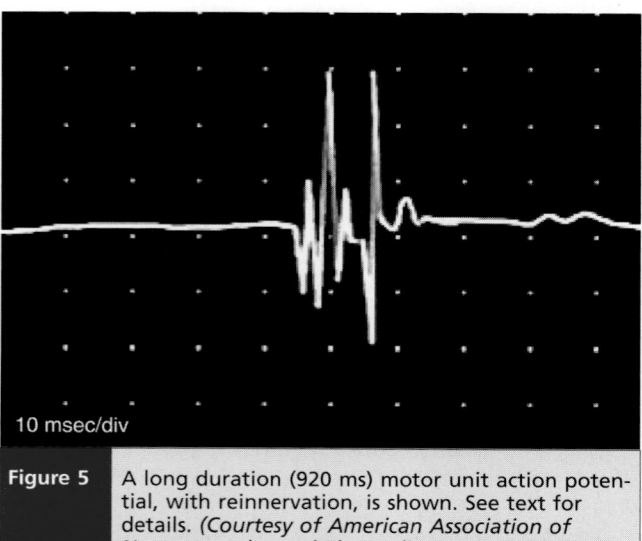

Figure 5 A long duration (920 ms) motor unit action potential, with reinnervation, is shown. See text for details. *(Courtesy of American Association of Neuromuscular and Electrodiagnostic Medicine.)*

EMG can readily distinguish between nerve and muscle disease and can typically determine whether the pattern of abnormal muscles belongs to an individual nerve or nerve root or whether the representative abnormalities suggest plexus involvement or a generalized neuropathy. Nerve conduction velocity studies can help determine whether there is focal or generalized neuropathy, and a combination of nerve conduction velocity studies and EMG can distinguish focal neuropathy from radiculopathy.

Disorders Associated With Neuropathy

Neuropathy refers to nerve disease but implies a generalized dysfunction, usually in length-dependent fashion so that the longest nerves are affected first and have the greatest degree of dysfunction. The nerve bundles are composed of hundreds of individual nerve fibers, varying in size from small unmyelinated or thinly myelinated fibers to large, thickly myelinated fibers. Neuropathy can be clinically and electrically segregated into axonal neuropathy or demyelinating neuropathy. Demyelinating polyneuropathy is characterized electrically by slow conduction velocity, prolonged sensory and motor latencies, and generally preserved amplitudes. EMG may reveal reduced recruitment and a paucity of spontaneous activity unless there is concomitant axonal damage. In contrast, axonal neuropathy typically is characterized by reduced sensory and motor amplitudes on nerve conduction velocity studies, with normal latencies and velocities. EMG in axonal neuropathy reveals fibrillation potentials and positive waves, generally in distal muscles, with reduced recruitment and features of reinnervation—large-amplitude, long-duration motor unit action potentials. Reinnervation typically means that the neuropathy has been present for some time, at least 6 to 12 months. Axonal neuropathy is often idiopathic, but may be caused by a metabolic disturbance such as the neuropathy of diabetes or a toxic disturbance that can occur with alcoholism or cisplatin-induced neuropathy.

Demyelinating neuropathy is grouped into inherited and acquired forms. The most common inherited demyelinating neuropathy is Charcot-Marie-Tooth disease type 1A. In most inherited demyelinating polyneuropathies, conduction velocities are uniformly slow; for example, if the velocity in the median nerve is 25 m/s, it is similarly slow in the ulnar and peroneal nerves in contrast to acquired demyelinating neuropathy, in which conduction velocities may vary from nerve to nerve.[3] Another feature of acquired neuropathy, which generally distinguishes it from inherited neuropathies, is conduction block, in which compound muscle action potential amplitude drops by more than 40% on proximal stimulation in comparison with distal stimulation. Conduction block is highly suggestive of acquired demyelinating neuropathy. The most common acquired demyelinating neuropathy is Guillain-Barré syndrome and its chronic counterpart, chronic inflammatory demyelinating polyneuropathy (CIDP).

The patient's history provides the first clues in formulating the differential diagnosis of neuropathy; the symptoms are numbness, tingling, and pain or weakness alone or in combination. The tempo of progression of the symptoms provides additional information. Acute neuropathy is usually either toxin or immune-mediated, whereas an indolent progressive neuropathy can be inherited, toxic, or diabetic. Physical examination may disclose muscular wasting and weakness, loss of reflexes, and sensory loss in a stocking-glove distribution. Reduced vibratory sensation and joint position sensation suggest demyelinating neuropathy, as does reflex loss with weakness disproportionate to muscular atrophy.

Delayed or reduced cold sensation over the feet, preserved reflexes, and preserved proximal strength in a patient with burning feet are features typical of small fiber axonal neuropathy. History and physical examination can generally differentiate peripheral neuropathy from lumbosacral polyradiculopathy or cervical myelopathy, but nerve conduction velocity studies and EMG are more sensitive and also better distinguish between a generalized sensorimotor neuropathy and less common disorders such as mononeuritis multiplex or multifocal demyelinating neuropathy.

Diabetic Neuropathy

Diabetes is considered to be the most common cause of peripheral neuropathy in the United States and other developed countries. Because of a trend of increased body fat observed in recent years that has often been associated with dyslipidemia and insulin resistance, type 2 diabetes may become an increasingly frequent cause of neuropathy in the United States. Neuropathy in patients with diabetes is often a relatively symmetric, nerve length-dependent process causing stocking-glove sensory disturbance, pain, and numbness with distal weakness. Because nerve cells are the longest cells in the body, it is not surprising that these metabolically active cells should suffer accelerated breakdown and an impaired repair process in the diabetic state. It is somewhat surprising that impaired glucose tolerance, to a level not generally considered to cause diabetes, is also associated with peripheral neuropathy. Idiopathic neuropathy should now be evaluated not only with fasting blood glucose but also a 2-hour glucose tolerance test.[4] In addition to the generalized neuropathy that affects many patients with diabetes, there is also an increased incidence of focal neuropathy, including carpal tunnel syndrome and ulnar neuropathy at the elbow or wrist. Focal and regional neuropathy can occur in patients with diabetes on a compressive, ischemic, or inflammatory basis alone or in combination. Diabetic radiculop-

athy, plexopathy, or proximal neuropathy may occur on an inflammatory or ischemic basis, causing proximal pain and weakness that can mimic compressive radiculopathy.[5] The most common example of this is diabetic amyotrophy, characterized by severe pain in the hip girdle and thigh, usually associated with pronounced wasting and weakness of the thigh muscles, loss of the knee jerk, and often with pronounced weight loss, sometimes of 20 to 40 pounds (diabetic cachexia). This syndrome often affects older adults with type 2 diabetes that is often well controlled, without the typical complications of advanced diabetes. It is believed that ischemia from microvasculitis is the principal cause of this proximal radicular plexopathy.[6] The course of diabetic amyotrophy is progression of severe pain, asymmetric thigh-wasting, and weakness for several weeks, but pain and weakness may last for many months and recovery may take several years. Intractable pain often requires narcotic analgesia. Neurologic evaluation, lumbar and pelvic imaging, nerve conduction velocity studies, and EMG often distinguish this condition from malignancy, compressive radiculopathy, or canal stenosis.

Guillain-Barré Syndrome

Guillain-Barré syndrome is caused by an immune-mediated attack on the peripheral nerve causing segmental demyelination, which causes conduction slowing on nerve conduction velocity studies and conduction block, where the compound muscle action potential amplitude drops more than 40% when the nerve is stimulated proximal to the site of demyelination. The clinical characteristics include loss of tendon reflexes, vague numbness and tingling, and progressive weakness disproportionate to sensory complaints. A good number of patients report aching muscular back pain; these patients may present to the orthopaedic surgeon for their first medical encounter. The diagnosis is complicated by the fact that loss of tendon reflexes takes time and so the patient may have preserved reflexes when first examined. Many patients experience upper respiratory or gastrointestinal infection in the weeks preceding examination by the physician. A diarrheal illness from *Campylobacter* infection can be associated with severe Guillain-Barré syndrome. Weakness may progress over hours or days and typically hits its nadir after several weeks, sometimes leading to complete paralysis. These patients should be hospitalized and their vital capacity monitored, as many of them require ventilatory support. The diagnosis remains clinical, but is supported by elevated spinal fluid protein without pleocytosis. Nerve conduction velocity studies and EMG can provide early diagnostic information by demonstrating evidence of acquired acute demyelinating polyneuropathy before spinal fluid abnormalities are evident and reflexes are lost. As noted earlier, the features of an acute acquired demyelinating polyneuropathy include prolonged sensory and distal motor latencies, conduction slowing in nerves to variable degrees, and conduction block. Another feature typical of Guillain-Barré syndrome is the preservation of sural nerve responses, when median and ulnar sensory nerve action potentials are abnormal either in latency or amplitude; this finding is called sural sparing. Nerve conduction velocity studies also provide early prognostic information. Preserved compound muscle action potential amplitudes are a favorable feature and bode well for ultimate motor function and ambulation. Plasmapheresis and intravenous immunoglobulin therapy shorten the duration of the illness, the time of hospitalization, ventilator dependence, and time to ambulation.[7] Despite the autoimmune basis, steroid therapy does not benefit patients with Guillain-Barré syndrome.[8]

A small group of patients initially suspected to have Guillain-Barré syndrome will ultimately exhibit symptoms of CIDP, a chronic disorder with progressive weakness or a relapsing course. In other patients with CIDP a subacute or insidiously progressive neuropathy develops; nerve conduction velocity studies disclose demyelinating features. Spinal fluid protein is generally elevated. CIDP is also amenable to intravenous immunoglobulin therapy or plasmapheresis, and these patients generally benefit from steroid therapy, in contrast to patients with Guillain-Barré syndrome.

Hereditary Sensorimotor Neuropathy/Charcot-Marie-Tooth Disease

This group of neuropathies was originally classified according to clinical characteristics and inheritance patterns but will be increasingly refined and sometimes redefined by genetic testing. Charcot-Marie-Tooth disease is a clinical disorder of progressive wasting and weakness in the distal leg, especially peroneal-innervated muscles associated with high arched feet and hammer toes, that was first described in the late 1880s. Clinical heterogeneity and variable inheritance patterns led to classifications that will likely be supplanted by molecular genetic identification of the culpable gene and abnormal protein. Nerve conduction velocity studies and EMG facilitated classification into primarily demyelinating versus axonal neuropathies, and this classification still holds value. Genetic confirmation of suspected inherited neuropathies is now available for more than a dozen conditions, and that number will grow as genetic testing sophistication increases. Patients with Charcot-Marie-Tooth disease are often evaluated for foot deformity or foot pain; the orthopaedic surgeon recognizes the potential neuropathic process and often discovers a family history of similar foot deformity or neuropathy. Nerve conduction velocity studies show significant nerve conduction slowing, often in the range of 20 m/s, and EMG may show evidence of reinnervation in distal muscles. The nerve conduction abnormalities are generally uniform in Charcot-Marie-Tooth disease type 1A, but in a related disorder, hereditary neuropathy with predisposition to pressure palsy (HNPP), some nerves may be more affected than others. Both conditions are caused by abnormalities of the peripheral myelin protein 22 (PMP-22) coded on chromosome 17. In Charcot-Marie-Tooth disease type 1A, there is duplication of the *PMP-22* gene, whereas in HNPP, the *PMP-22* gene is deleted.[9] In either situation, the duplication or the deletion leads to dysfunction in the compact myelin sheath laid down by the Schwann cell and the myelin disruption accounts for the conduction slowing evident on nerve conduction velocity studies. The clinical disability is not caused by the slow conduction, but rather subsequent axonal degeneration secondary to interruption in Schwann cell/axon interaction. Patients with HNPP may have symptoms suggesting carpal tunnel syndrome, ulnar neuropathy, or foot drop suspected to be caused by peroneal neuropathy. A thorough patient history may disclose previous episodes of similar symptoms but these patients may not show the typical features of inherited neuropathy, such as the high arched feet. Nerve conduction velocity studies reveal abnormalities of demyelinating polyneuropathy, more prominent at sites of common compression, such as the ulnar nerve at the elbow, the peroneal nerve at the fibular head, or the median nerve in the carpal tunnel.

Multiple Sclerosis

Multiple sclerosis (MS) is a disease of the central nervous system with an autoimmune component clinically expressed by relapses and remission of inflammation and demyelination of the brain and spinal cord. The cause is unknown but it may be an environmental trigger that produces the disease in those who are genetically susceptible. Epidemiologic studies suggest a specific trigger, perhaps a virus.[10] The myelin of the central nervous system is laid down by the oligodendroglia and is distinct from peripheral nerve myelin, which is laid down by Schwann cells. In MS attacks, symptoms depend on the specific site in the brain or spinal cord involved in the inflammatory response. Common symptoms include numbness and tingling, band-like sensations, urinary frequency and urgency, double vision, visual loss, and ataxia. When the lesion of MS involves the spinal cord, it can cause the syndrome of acute transverse myelitis with progressive numbness and weakness below the site of the lesion, often with a sensory level. Although the diagnosis is still clinical, it has been greatly facilitated by MRI, which shows high signal lesions in a characteristic periventricular distribution in the brain or in the spinal cord. Spinal fluid analysis reveals scant white blood cells, mild elevation in protein, and an increase in immunoglobulin synthesis with oligoclonal banding. Clinically, there are not many conditions that mimic MS; although uncommonly, lupus can involve the nervous system as can sarcoidosis. Patients with suspected MS and cervical spondylosis can present a diagnostic and therapeutic conundrum. When the cardinal symptoms and signs are those of progressive spastic paraparesis and MRI discloses spondylosis with severe canal stenosis in patients with prior neurologic symptoms suggesting MS, these patients may benefit from neurologic consultation, cerebral MRI, and visual-evoked potentials to investigate otherwise subclinical involvement of the optic nerves and sometimes spinal fluid analysis. In some patients with both MS and spondylosis, surgical decompression can be offered after due consideration in an effort to minimize cord injury from progressive canal stenosis. Disease-modifying treatment is now available for MS, chiefly beta-interferons and glatiramer acetate. These agents reduce the severity of attacks and their frequency by one third; the number of MRI lesions and degree of long-term disability are also reduced.[11] These agents are currently injectable. Alternative immunotherapy has been attempted with more potent immunosuppressants such as cyclophosphamide and more recently mitoxantrone. These agents have significant potential toxicity and are currently not viewed as first-line therapy for patients with relapsing remitting disease, but are considered in patients with recalcitrant, severe relapsing, or progressive disease. In recent years, the natalizumab Tysabri (Biogen Idec, Cambridge, MA) was approved by the Food and Drug Administration for use in clinical practice. Tysabri is a monoclonal antibody that binds α-4-integrin on the surface of white blood cells and selectively inhibits adhesion and prevents lymphocytes from crossing the blood brain barrier into the inflamed brain and spinal cord.[12] Shortly after Food and Drug Administration approval, two patients being treated for MS developed progressive multifocal leukoencephalopathy, generally a fatal disorder, and a third patient who took the medication for Crohn's disease also developed progressive multifocal leukoencephalopathy. All three patients were recently or concomitantly receiving immunomodulating therapy. The medication is currently available under a supervised program developed in consultation with the Food and Drug Administration, and long-term results are not yet known.[13]

Amyotrophic Lateral Sclerosis

Amyotrophic lateral sclerosis (ALS), also known as Lou Gehrig's disease, is a disorder causing relentlessly progressive muscular wasting and weakness and ultimately paralysis of limb, oropharyngeal, and respiratory muscles leading to death from respiratory failure in just a few years. The etiology of the disease is unknown and the disease is generally sporadic; although about 5% of patients with ALS have a familial form, with some of these patients mapping to the gene for superoxide dismutase on chromosome 21.[14] The diagnosis is based on clinical findings with signs of disease of the upper motor neuron (whose cell body lives in the motor cortex and whose fiber track runs through the white matter of the brain to the lateral column of the spinal cord), and the lower motor neuron (whose cell body lives in the anterior horn of the spinal column and whose process runs through the peripheral nerve to the muscle). Upper motor neuron dysfunction leads to spasticity, exaggerated reflexes, Hoffman and Babinski signs, and spastic dysarthria. Lower motor neuron dysfunction produces muscular atrophy, weakness, and clinical fasciculations. The diagnosis is generally secure when lower motor and upper motor neuron signs are present in the same

limb and cranial nerve findings are present (dysarthria with wasting and twitching of the tongue). Nerve conduction velocity studies are generally normal in the early stages of the disease but as muscular atrophy progresses, the compound muscle action potential amplitude declines. Sensory nerve conduction velocity studies are normal. EMG discloses fasciculation potentials, fibrillation potentials, and positive waves with reduced recruitment of motor unit action potentials. Generally, there are signs of reinnervation with large-amplitude long-duration motor unit action potentials. Fasciculation potentials are spontaneous discharges of single motor units. Fasciculation potentials may be generated at a variety of sites from the anterior horn cell through axonal branches. When associated with other features of denervation (fibrillations, positive waves) and reinnervation, these fasciculation potentials are suggestive of ALS. Fasciculation potentials can be seen in other conditions with chronic denervation and in the syndrome of benign fasciculations and muscular cramps. In isolation, fasciculations can be a benign finding and they do not in and of themselves imply the presence of ALS. This is particularly important because some patients and physicians observe occasional fasciculations without other symptoms and can needlessly suspect ALS. EMG can bolster the clinical suspicion of ALS by revealing fibrillation potentials, positive waves, and long-duration large-amplitude motor unit action potentials with reduced recruitment in cranial and limb muscles of a patient presenting with spasticity and weakness. Currently, there is no satisfactory treatment for ALS. Riluzole is prescribed, but provides only modest benefits with studies suggesting prolongation of life or time to ventilator by a few months.[15,16] The major thrust of treatment is supportive medical and emotional care. Severe cervical spondylosis can sometimes mimic ALS by causing cord compression from canal stenosis and multilevel radiculopathy from foraminal stenosis. In these patients, there may be wasting and weakness in arm muscles from nerve root compression and spasticity of the legs from spinal cord compression. Sensory symptoms may be minimal and urinary frequency or incontinence can be late features. Again, EMG is quite useful when it reveals evidence of lower motor neuron involvement in the spastic legs, or when it reveals abnormalities in the face or tongue, cranial innervated muscles that would be normal in cervical spondylosis. If clinical fasciculations are present in the legs of a person with suspected cervical spondylosis, ALS should be considered.

Summary

Nerve conduction velocity studies and EMG help clarify neuromuscular conditions for orthopaedic surgeons and neurologists, confirm suspected diagnoses, offer alternative diagnoses, and assist in formulating prognoses. The American Association of Neuromuscular and Electrodiagnostic Medicine provides educational material to physicians involved in the care of patients

2: Systemic Disorders

with neuromuscular and musculoskeletal conditions, and their Website offers links to other relevant Websites as well as educational materials in the form of monographs, slides, and articles.[17]

Annotated References

1. Buchthal F, Pinelli P, Rosenfalck P: Action potential parameters in normal human muscle and their physiological determinants. *Acta Physiol Scand* 1954;32:219-229.

2. Dorfman L, McGill K: AAEE minimonograph 29: Automatic quantitative electromyography. *Muscle Nerve* 1988;11:804-818.

3. Lewis RA, Sumner AJ, Shy ME: Electrophysiological features of inherited demyelinating neuropathies: A reappraisal in the era of molecular diagnosis. *Muscle Nerve* 2000;23:1472-1487.

4. Hoffman-Snyder C, Smith BE, Ross MA, Hernandez J, Bosch EP: Value of the oral glucose tolerance test in the evaluation of chronic idiopathic axonal polyneuropathy. *Arch Neurol* 2006;63:1075-1079.

   This report highlights the importance of the oral glucose tolerance test in patients with idiopathic neuropathy. It is recognized that many of those affected by small fiber axonal neuropathy have impaired glucose tolerance.

5. Dyck PJ, Kratz KM, Karness JL, et al: The prevalence by staged severity of various types of diabetic neuropathy, retinopathy, and nephropathy in a population-based cohort: The Rochester Diabetic Neuropathy Study. *Neurology* 1993;43:817-824.

6. Dyck PJ, Windebank AJ: Diabetic and nondiabetic lumbosacral radiculoplexus neuropathies: New insights into the pathophysiology and treatment. *Muscle Nerve* 2002;25:477-491.

7. Plasma Exchange/Sandoglobulin Guillain-Barré Trial Group: Randomized trial of plasma exchange, intravenous immunoglobulin, and combined treatments in Guillain-Barré syndrome. *Lancet* 1997;349:225-230.

8. Hughes RA, van der Meche FG: Corticosteroids for treating Guillain-Barré syndrome. *Cochrane Database Syst Rev* 2000;3:CD001446.

9. Chance PF, Alderson MK, Leppig KA, et al: DNA deletion associated with hereditary neuropathy with liability to pressure palsies. *Cell* 1993;72:143-151.

10. Kurtzke JF, Heltberg A: Multiple sclerosis in the Faroe Islands: An epitome. *J Clin Epidemiol* 2001;54:1-22.

11. Goodin DS, Frohman EM, Garmany GP Jr, et al: Disease-modifying therapies in multiple sclerosis: Report of the Therapeutics and Technology Assessment Subcommittee of the American Academy of Neurology and the MS Council for Clinical Practice Guidelines. *Neurology* 2002;58:169-178.

12. Polman CH, O'Connor PW, Havrdova E, et al: A randomized, placebo-controlled trial of natalizumab for relapsing multiple sclerosis. *N Engl J Med* 2006;354:899-910.

    Natalizumab is a potentially powerful treatment for multiple sclerosis, but is complicated by the development of progressive multifocal leukoencephalopathy in two of the patients studied.

13. Kappos L, Bates D, Hartung HP, et al: Natalizumab treatment for multiple sclerosis: Recommendations for patient selection and monitoring. *Lancet Neurol* 2007;6;431-441.

    This article provides a summary of the current position on recommendations for patient selection and monitoring of Tysabri and progressive multifocal leukoencephalopathy.

14. Siddique T, Nijhawan D, Hentati A, et al: Molecular genetic basis of familial ALS. *Neurology* 1996;47(suppl 2): S27-S31.

15. Bensimon G, Lacomblez L, Meininger V, et al: A controlled trial of riluzole in amyotrophic lateral sclerosis: ALS/Riluzole Study Group. *N Engl J Med* 1994;330: 585-591.

16. Lascomblez L, Bensimon G, Leigh PN, Guillet P, Meininger V: Dose-ranging study of riluzole in amyotrophic lateral sclerosis: Amyotrophic Lateral Sclerosis/Riluzole Study Group II. *Lancet* 1996;347:1425-1431.

17. American Association of Neuromuscular and Electrodiagnostic Medicine Website. Available at: www.aanem.org/education/education.cfm. Accessed July 2, 2007.

Chapter 20

Infection

Kenneth O. Cayce IV, MD   Marc T. Galloway, MD

Introduction

Infections in orthopaedic surgery have been associated with considerable morbidity and mortality. Recognition of these infections, along with prevention and treatment, is crucial in providing optimal patient care. With the continued use of antibiotics, emerging bacterial resistance demonstrates the importance of diligence in treating these infections appropriately. Over the past 5 to 10 years, the development of new antibiotics has been extremely limited, which further emphasizes the importance of prevention and proper treatment of infections. New techniques in diagnosis and surgical procedures have helped decrease the incidence of infections, but much work needs to be done in this area.

Pathogenesis and Pathophysiology of Musculoskeletal Infections

Bacteria form a large and diversified group of organisms that is further divided into two large classification systems, gram-positive and gram-negative bacteria. Unlike gram-positive bacteria, gram-negative bacteria have an outer lipopolysaccharide layer and display proteinaceous structures called pili and fimbriae. These groups can be further divided into aerobic (living in an oxygen-rich environment), anaerobic, and facultative (living in more than one specific environment) organisms. Therefore, some bacteria have acquired a glycosylated cell wall that makes them resistant to antibiotics and allows them to live in more than one specific environment. Destroying the architecture and mechanical strength of this wall renders the bacteria much more susceptible to treatment by antibiotics.[1]

Well-known pathogens such as *Staphylococcus aureus*, which is the most common organism present in musculoskeletal infections, have recently shown resistance to antibiotics because of plasmid-mediated resistance. Approximately 50% of the *Staphylococcus* strains studied exhibit plasmid-mediated resistance to antibiotics. It also has been shown that adherence to biomaterials is specific for certain bacteria, which indicates specificity for certain *Staphylococcus* species, *Pseudomonas* species, and gram-negative bacteria to adhere to certain polymeric and metallic surfaces. With the addition of a membrane, the adherence has increased by one order of magnitude and is a major cause

of nosocomial infections. This adhesion and development of plasmids makes the bacteria resistant to many antibiotics in current use.[2]

Homeostasis, the equilibrium/stability in the normal body states, is an important factor in the management of infection. Once the homeostasis of the body has been altered, bacteria can enter the body through various portals. The simplest way bacteria can enter the body is through a wound or surgical site. Under these conditions, bacteria can spread easily because the environment has been compromised by diminished blood flow and oxygen tension, as well as the presence of foreign bodies such as debris, plates, screws, or prostheses; therefore, the infection must be contained before hematogenous or contiguous spread occur.[3]

One of the most important factors in homeostasis is blood supply to the surrounding tissues. Many studies have demonstrated that reduced blood flow to an extremity results in lower tissue concentrations of antibiotics. According to a recent study, it was proposed that warming an extremity would increase blood flow by vasodilation of the underlying arteries, and thus increase the amount of absorption of antibiotics in the tissues. This study showed that an increase in microcirculatory blood flow to an extremity did increase the maximum concentration of an antibiotic to the tissue, and concluded that warming an extremity increases blood flow and thus increases the antibiotic's ability to penetrate the soft tissue and decrease bacterial virulence.[4]

Traumatic injury and the presence of implants increase the risk of infection. Osseous trauma results in periosteal injury and ensuing microvascular and macrovascular compromise. In addition, trauma to bone exposes the collagen matrix and acellular crystal faces, making it easier for bacteria to adhere to these structures. The ligands that allow bacteria to adhere to bone are sialoprotein, collagen, fibrinogen, laminin, von Willebrand factor, osteoponsatin, thrombospondin, vitronectin, and fibronectin. These ligands are found on the membrane of certain bacteria and bind to the surface of bone or implants in a receptor-ligand fashion. The most common bacteria that adhere to implants are the *Staphylococcus* species found in a glycocalyx capsule. This capsule is composed of fibrous exopolysaccharides within a thick biofilm. The properties of the capsule impair normophysiologic immune function as well as antibiotic penetration, thereby creating a "barrier" for the bacteria. Bacterial adhesion to the implant

Table 1

Surgical Prophylaxis for Orthopaedic Surgery

Procedure	Drug	Dose/Route	Comments
Hip arthroplasty	Cefazolin Cefuroxime Vancomycin	1-2 g/IVPB 1.5 g 1 g	Initiate dose no more than 1 h before incision. All drugs only require one-time dose preoperatively. If surgical time exceeds 3 h, redose is required. Reserve vancomycin for patients with MRSA colonization, or institutions with a high MRSA rate. Consider intranasal mupirocin ointment.
Spinal fusion	Cefazolin Cefuroxime Vancomycin	1-2 g/IVPB 1.5 g/IVPB 1 g/IVPB	Initiate dose no more than 1 h before incision. All drugs only require one-time dose preoperatively. If surgical time exceeds 3 h, redose is required. Reserve vancomycin for patients with MRSA colonization, or institutions with a high MRSA rate Consider intranasal mupirocin ointment.
Total joint arthroplasty (except hip)	Cefazolin Vancoymcin	1-2 g/IVPB 1 g/IVPB	Duration not to exceed 24 h if prescribing therapy for more than one-time dose.
Open reduction of closed fracture with internal fixation	Ceftriaxone	2 g/IV or IM	IV preferred, IM absorption unpredictable in some patients. IM injection extremely painful.

MRSA = methicillin-resistant *Staphylococcus aureus*; IVPB = intravenous piggyback; IV=intravenous; IM = intramuscular.
Adapted with permission from The Sanford Guide to Antimicrobial Therapy. Sperryville, VA, Antimicrobial Therapy, Inc, *2006, p 161.*

or devitalized bone surfaces is facilitated by charged properties and van der Waals forces between the bacteria and tissue or implant surfaces. Once the adhesion has occurred, replication begins, which is dependent on the genetics and metabolism of the specific bacteria. As the infection proliferates, the bacteria can spread to the surrounding tissue and possibly into the circulatory system, causing sepsis.[1]

Many factors can increase the host's susceptibility to infections. When bacteria are introduced into the host organism, the complement system is activated (chemotaxis) and a systemic inflammatory reaction occurs. This in turn enhances immune adherence and signals polymorphonuclear (PMN) cells to the affected area. PMN cells then cause bacterial lysis and cell death via phagocytosis. Factors decreasing the local immune response include decreased blood flow (as a result of peripheral arterial disease, venous stasis, smoking, irradiation, and the presence of scar tissue), neuropathy, trauma, and implants, as well as medications such as nonsteroidal anti-inflammatory drugs, aspirin, disease-modifying antirheumatic drugs, and steroids. Other factors that may decrease the systemic immune response include renal and liver disease, malignancy, diabetes mellitus, alcoholism, malnutrition, rheumatologic diseases, and an immunocompromised state (associated with human immunodeficiency virus [HIV], hepatitis, or immunosuppressive therapy).[1,3] Table 1 summarizes surgical prophylaxis for the most common orthopaedic procedures.

The effect of exercise on the immune system is controversial. Some studies have shown that exercise can make athletes more susceptible to bacterial infection whereas other studies have found greater resistance to infections in individuals after exercise. Many studies have shown that exercise helps the immune system by increasing natural killer cells, macrophage count, cytokines, neutrophil count, and lymphocyte count. There is a small time frame (open window) when athletes are immunosuppressed after an intense physical activity, when ciliary action, immunoglobulin A levels, natural killer cells, T lymphocyte count, and CD4/CD8 ratio are decreased. This susceptibility to infections in athletes in the past was called the "J-curve," but has been recently updated and termed the "S-curve."[5]

Diagnostic Modalities in Musculoskeletal Infections

Clinical

The diagnosis of musculoskeletal infections is established through physical examination and laboratory studies. The gold standard of diagnosis is culture of the suspected fluid or tissue. Patients often present with pain, warmth, swelling, and redness as clinical signs of an infection. Other symptoms that are consistent with infection are fever, chills, night sweats, nausea, vomiting, and loss of motion in a joint.

Serology

Standard tests to perform when infection is suspected are complete blood count (CBC) with differential, erythrocyte sedimentation rate (ESR), C-reactive protein (CRP), blood cultures, and Gram stain. The ESR will rise first (within 2 days) and will continue to rise for the next 3 to 5 days after appropriate therapy has started. The CRP level will rise within 6 hours, peak in about 48 hours, and return to normal 1 week after the appropriate therapy has started. Studies have shown that CRP is more sensitive than ESR for an infection and is the best indicator for diagnosis and monitoring treatment. The Gram stain can help the physician determine the most appropriate antibiotic for initial therapy.[3] Recently, evidence has been presented supporting an elevation in serum interleukin-6 (IL-6) to be indicative of a periprosthetic infection in patients who have recently had either total hip or knee arthroplasty.[6]

Radiology

When infection is suspected, radiographs of the infected area and blood tests should be obtained during the patient's initial visit. Soft-tissue swelling and loss of tissue planes are the earliest radiographic changes. Bony abnormalities with bone loss of 30% to 40% can be seen 1 to 2 weeks after the onset of the infection. If there are no changes seen on the initial radiographs, but infection is still suspected, then a three-phase bone scan using technetium Tc 99m (^{99m}Tc) diphosphonate should be performed. Other scans can be helpful in determining infection if the three-phase bone scan is inconclusive, such as a gallium citrate Ga 67 scan (70% to 80% sensitivity), indium-111 leukocyte-labeled nuclear imaging study (83% to 85% sensitivity and 75% to 94% specificity), indium-111-labeled immunoglobulin (90% to 93% sensitivity and 85% to 89% specificity), and ^{99m}Tc ciprofloxacin (70% to 85% sensitivity and 91% to 96% specificity). Positron emission tomography (PET) with F-18 fluorodeoxyglucose can be used with approximately 99% sensitivity and 88% specificity for the diagnosis of any musculoskeletal infections. Because these scans are more expensive and time-consuming, their frequent use is discouraged. MRI also can be used to determine infection with the advantages of high sensitivity (100%), specificity, and no radiation exposure. Limitations include expense and the inability to use the modality in patients with a prosthetic device or internal fixation. Bone marrow normally exhibits high-signal intensity on the T1-weighted images; therefore, low signal on the T1-weighted images could be indicative of infection. In addition, MRI can identify abscess formation or sinus tracts. These areas of infection can be mapped and needle aspiration done to obtain a culture to identify the organism.[3,7,8]

Identification of bacteria by genomic markers is another option, expanding the scope of antibacterials and improving the mode of action and targets of antibiotics. Polymerase chain reaction techniques can determine the types of bacteria, leading to early diagnosis and treatment. As resistant bacteria are formed, newer antibiotics are made to target new areas of the genome. With continued research, new antibiotics can be made that will also be safe, well tolerated, and efficacious.[9]

Musculoskeletal Infections in Adults

Adult Osteomyelitis

Adult osteomyelitis most commonly occurs in patients with open fractures or diabetic foot infections, or during surgery. Osteomyelitis can be classified as either hematogenous (originated or transported by blood) or caused by a prior infection, which is termed contiguous-focus osteomyelitis. Two types of hematogenous osteomyelitis are vertebral osteomyelitis and pyogenic vertebral osteomyelitis. Contiguous-focus osteomyelitis can be further subdivided based on the presence or absence of vascular insufficiency. Both hematogenous and contiguous-focus osteomyelitis are further classified as acute, subacute, or chronic. Other classification systems include descriptions of the host, anatomic bone involvement, treatment, and prognosis using four stages: (1) medullary, (2) superficial, (3) localized, and (4) diffuse, as well as the three host categories: normal (A), compromised (B), and treatment worse than disease (C). Using this system, there are 12 types of osteomyelitis, each with a designated clinical stage.[10]

Hematogenous osteomyelitis occurs in approximately 20% of all patients with adult osteomyelitis. It is more common in males and the vertebrae is the most common site of infection, followed by long bones, pelvis, and clavicle. S aureus is the most common bacteria that causes adult osteomyelitis, but other types of organisms can be found in intravenous drug users and immunocompromised individuals. Patients usually present with pain and constitutional symptoms (fever, chills, swelling, and erythema) either acutely or lasting up to 3 months.[11]

Vertebral osteomyelitis occurs mostly in patients older than 50 years of age, but 1% to 2% of patients are children (mean age, 7.5 years). The incidence increases with each decade of life and men are affected twice as often as women. Death is rare, but if the disease is not diagnosed early, excessive morbidity or mortality will ensue. Pyogenic vertebral osteomyelitis is an infection that is commonly contracted hematogenously from an arterial route that may involve two adjacent vertebrae and the intervertebral disk (diskitis). The lumbar region is most commonly affected (45%), but the infection also can be seen in the thoracic (35%) and cervical (20%) regions. S aureus is the most common organism isolated, but in intravenous drug users Pseudomonas aeruginosa is commonly found. Patients present with fever and increasing pain over the affected area, lasting from 3 weeks to 3 months. Meningitis and abscesses can result in prolonged infection, with motor and sensory deficits occurring in 15% of patients.[12,13]

Contiguous-focus osteomyelitis without generalized vascular insufficiency can be caused by trauma with direct contact to bone, infection spread from soft tissue, or by nosocomial infection. Causes of this type of osteomyelitis include open reduction and internal fixation of fractures, prosthetic devices, open fractures, and chronic soft-tissue infections. S aureus is the most com-

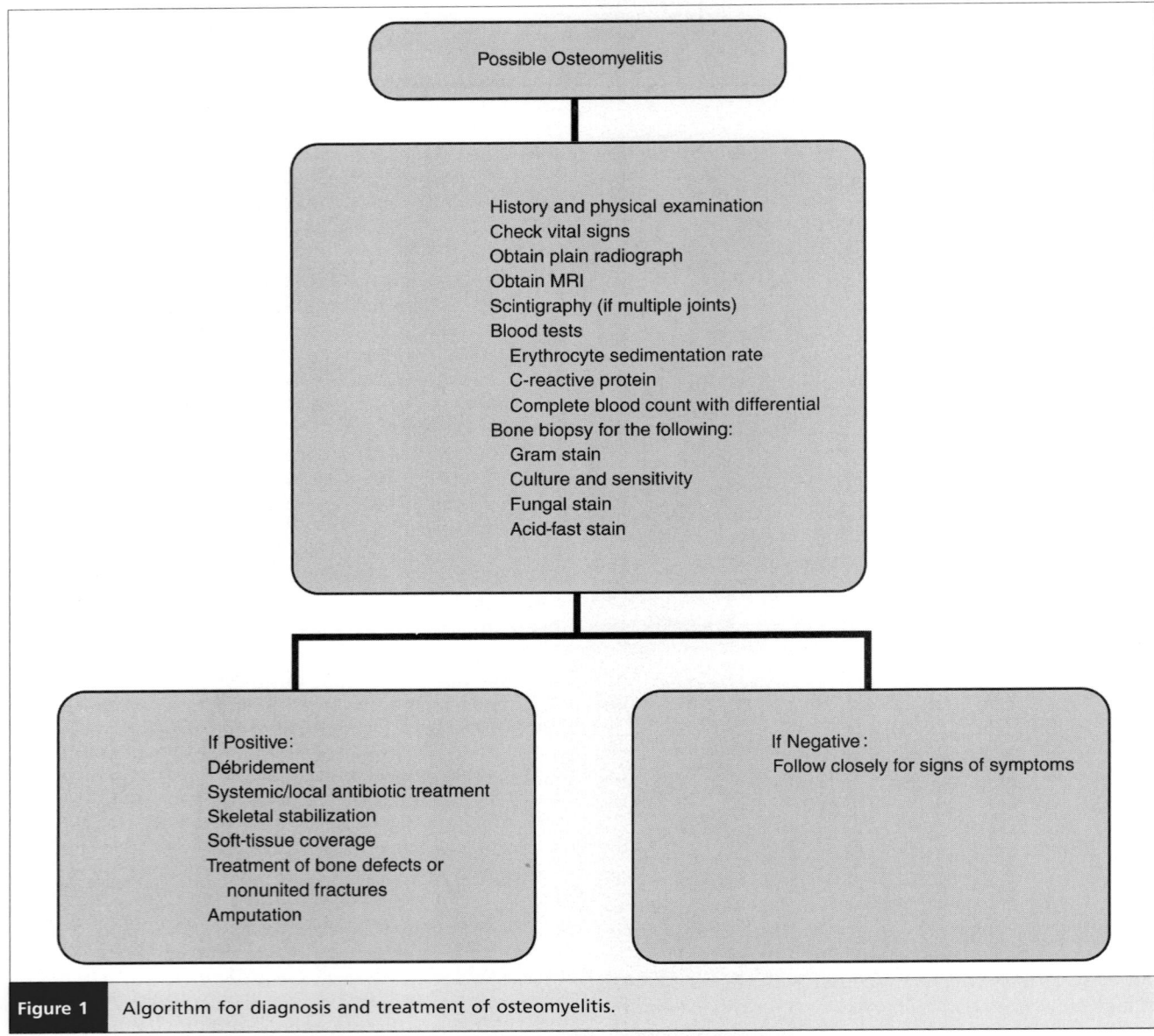

Figure 1 Algorithm for diagnosis and treatment of osteomyelitis.

mon organism found, but studies have also found gram-negative bacilli and anaerobic organisms by culture. This type of infection occurs about 1 month after the trauma, surgery, or primary cause of the infection. Patients report pain and fever, with drainage of the area leading to decreased bone stability, necrosis, and soft-tissue damage.[10]

Contiguous-focus osteomyelitis with generalized vascular insufficiency is most often seen in patients with diabetes mellitus and commonly occurs in the small bones of the feet. The most common pathogens include *Staphylococcus* species, *Streptococcus* species, *Enterococcus* species, gram-negative bacilli, and anaerobic bacteria. Patients present with a variety of unsuspected diagnoses such as ingrown toenails, cellulitis, foot ulcers, or deep space infections because of the peripheral neuropathy associated with decreased vasculature.[10]

Chronic osteomyelitis occurs in patients with a prior history of osteomyelitis—most commonly hematogenous or contiguous-focus osteomyelitis—who have a recurrence of pain, fever, drainage, erythema, and swelling. Antibiotic therapy alone is usually insufficient; therefore, the nidus of the infection must be removed. If the infection ensues, squamous cell carcinoma (Marjolin's ulcer) or amyloidosis can be found at the drainage site.[10,14]

Diagnosis
Diagnosis of osteomyelitis is often difficult because the pathology itself can affect the testing process (**Figure 1**). Anaerobic and aerobic culture is the best method for diagnosis, and the antibiotics used are based on the culture and sensitivities. Other tests can include ESR, CRP, Gram stain, blood cultures, acid-fast staining, and CBC

with differential. Imaging studies are also helpful in the diagnosis and can include plain radiographs, ^{99m}Tc polyphosphate scans, gallium scans, CT, and MRI. In hematogenous osteomyelitis, bone loss must be at least 30% to 40% in order for it to be evident on plain radiographs; therefore, a 2-week lag time between identification of the condition and confirmation with plain radiographs is common. Osteomyelitis is sometimes called the "great mimic" because of its similarity in radiographic appearance to healing fractures, cancers, and benign tumors.[10]

Treatment

Osteomyelitis is treated with antibiotics and surgery (consisting of adequate drainage, débridement, dead space management, maintenance of adequate blood supply, and wound care). Smoking, diabetes, tumors, vascular compromise, and poor nutrition have an adverse effect on the healing process; therefore, every effort to improve these conditions is prudent. Antibiotics are administered for 4 to 6 weeks. This determination is based on animal studies demonstrating a 4- to 6-week interval for long bone revascularization after débridement. Antibiotic therapy longer than 6 weeks has not proven more efficacious. Treatment with antibiotics depends on the stage of osteomyelitis. Stage 1 osteomyelitis is treated with 4 weeks of antibiotics (from initiation of treatment or last débridement) and surgical intervention (bone or soft-tissue débridement). Failure of surgical intervention or antibiotics requires more bone or soft-tissue débridement with another 4 weeks of antibiotics. Stage 2 osteomyelitis requires a shorter course of antibiotic administration (2 weeks) followed by débridement of bone and soft tissue. This treatment is effective in 100% of A hosts and 79% of B hosts. In stage 3 and 4 osteomyelitis, antibiotics are administered for 4 to 6 weeks after adequate débridement surgery. This treatment is effective in 98% of A hosts and 80% (stage 4) and 92% (stage 3) of B hosts. Suppressive antibiotic therapy should be initiated when surgical treatment is not an option. This therapy consists of rifampin with a fluoroquinolone or trimethoprim-sulfamethoxazole for a period of 6 months. If this therapy fails, then lifelong suppressive therapy is considered.[10] Surgical treatment is a mainstay in the treatment of osteomyelitis. Débridement is complete when punctuate bleeding, known as the "paprika sign," is present at the tissue base.[15] The degree of tissue resection must take into account the degree of bacterial contamination as well as host factors, normal or compromised. Bony defects following tissue débridement can be filled with autogenous bone, and soft-tissue voids may require vascularized tissue flaps.

Antibiotic-impregnated beads containing vancomycin, tobramycin, and gentamicin are commonly used to sterilize and fill the dead space. These beads are usually removed in 2 to 4 weeks and replaced with cancellous bone graft, and are effective in 55% to 96% of patients.[16] Biodegradable antibiotic beads also have been shown to be effective.[17] The use of antibiotic-impregnated cancellous bone grafts has demonstrated 95% efficacy in one clinical trial.[18] Clindamycin and amikacin pumps have been used with good results in patients with osteomyelitis.[19] For some patients, such as those with vascular compromise, amputation of the affected limb may be indicated.[10]

Infections in the presence of fractures represent a significant clinical complication. When infections are associated with fractures, osseous stabilization is essential. Stabilization is often accomplished with rods, screws, and fixators; external fixation (Ilizarov technique) is preferred over internal fixation because of the possibility of secondary infection. External fixation is preferable because it allows the reconstruction of difficult segments and infected nonunions that can help with stabilization and bone lengthening. This technique requires the patient to be in the device for approximately 8.5 months for adequate reconstruction to be achieved. The rate of reoccurrence of osteomyelitis is low using this technique, with an overall cure rate of 75% to 100%.[20,21]

Soft-tissue coverage is used to help with wound healing and to prevent the spread of osteomyelitis. This can be accomplished by using split-thickness skin grafts or local muscle grafts that may be done in one or two stages 3 to 7 days after débridement. Muscle flaps allow for adequate closure of dead space, provide soft-tissue coverage, decrease contamination, help maintain homeostasis, increase concentration of antibiotics, and provide a basis for healing. Antibiotics may be used in combination with the muscle grafts and débridement, with success rates ranging from 90% to 100%.[22] Healing by second intention (not closing the wound surgically, leaving the wound open to allow it to heal itself) should not be used because scar tissue that encompasses the defect is avascular, thereby precluding successful healing.[10]

Hyperbaric oxygen therapy has been shown to be a useful treatment strategy in chronic osteomyelitis. It has been used in patients with recurring chronic osteomyelitis and with infection persisting longer than 1 month, at least one surgical débridement, and prior treatment with hyperbaric oxygen therapy, surgery, and antibiotics. Hyperbaric oxygen therapy promotes collagen formation, angiogenesis, and healing of ischemic or infected wounds by providing oxygen to the area.[10] The results of one study showed an 85% remission of osteomyelitis;[23] another study reported 34 of 38 patients were free of infection at 1-year follow-up.[24]

Special situations occur in patients with other clinical conditions making treatment more challenging. In hemodialysis patients with indwelling catheters, *S aureus* and *Staphylococcus epidermidis* are the most common bacteria found. The ribs and thoracic vertebral column are the most common sites of infection. The diagnosis can be made 12 to 72 months after hemodialysis is started because the symptoms may be mistaken for renal osteodystrophy. Sickle cell disease may mimic thrombotic marrow crisis, with a history of bone pain, fever, chills, and leukocytosis. Early cultures and treatment, which includes antibiotics effective against *Sal-*

monella species, *S aureus*, and streptococci, are needed because of the multiple sites of infection. Intravenous drug users usually have hematogenous osteomyelitis and are afebrile; the only symptom may be localized pain. In these patients, osteomyelitis is found in the vertebrae, pubis, and clavicles and is usually caused by *S aureus*, *S epidermidis*, gram-negative rods, *P aeruginosa*, and *Candida* species. Multiple radiographs are usually taken along with blood cultures and, if needed, bone cultures to make the correct diagnosis and guide treatment.[8] Brodie's abscess (sclerotic bone surrounding dense fibrous tissue) is found in chronic osteomyelitis, most commonly along the distal part of the tibia near the metaphysis. Patients are usually younger than 25 years of age and present with fever, pain, and periosteal elevation, but patients with chronic disease can be afebrile and have dull pain. Débridement and antibiotics based on the cultures are the mainstay of treatment in these patients.[25,26]

Adult Septic Arthritis

Septic arthritis can occur by many different mechanisms, which include a hematogenous route from a different infection or intravenous drug use, direct route from trauma or joint aspiration, contiguous spread from an area close to the joint (cellulitis, abscess, septic bursitis, or tenosynovitis), and contamination from prior osteomyelitis. Predisposing patient factors leading to septic arthritis include diabetes, rheumatoid arthritis, lupus, HIV, steroid use, malignancy, intravenous drug use, and old age.[27] The incidence of septic arthritis is believed to be 0.034% to 0.13% for nongonococcal arthritis in urban medical centers. As the bacteria disseminate throughout the joint, they destroy the cell lining by breaking down the glycosaminoglycan found in the cartilage. This layer is composed of chrondroitin-4 sulfate, chrondroitin-6 sulfate, keratan sulfate, and marrow dermatan sulfate. These subsets of the glycosaminoglycan molecule give the cartilage its properties of fluid retention. With the breakdown of this layer and the inflammatory response (release of IL-1) that is found in the joint, the cartilage is broken down and damaged.[3]

Neisseria gonorrhoeae was formerly noted to be the most common organism causing septic arthritis, but recent studies have found that *S aureus* may be the most common organism in septic arthritis, possibly because of the increase in intravenous drug use. *S aureus* is the most common organism found in nongonococcal septic arthritis.[28] A study of 28 patients with nongonococcal arthritis found that intravenous drug use was the most common factor; methicillin-sensitive *S aureus* was the bacteria found in 25% of patients, whereas methicillin-resistant *S aureus* (MRSA) was implicated in 39% of patients. Other common organisms found in patients with septic arthritis include streptococci and gram-negative bacteria such as *Escherichia coli*, *Pseudomonas*, *Clostridium* and other anaerobes.[29] Fungal septic arthritis has been found in many in patients with acquired immunodeficiency syndrome. In one case study, a patient who was HIV-positive and an intravenous drug user was positive for *Candida* septic arthritis in the sternoclavicular joint; this patient also had contiguous-focus osteomyelitis caused by fungemia.[30]

Diagnosis

The knee is the joint most commonly affected in patients with septic arthritis (50% to 54% of patients), followed by the hip (20% to 25%), shoulder (10% to 15%), ankle (10% to 15%), elbow (10% to 15%), and wrist (10%) (**Figure 2**). Patients present with a warm, swollen, and painful joint. Blood studies should be obtained and include ESR, CRP, blood cultures, and CBC with differential. Aspiration of the joint should always be done and it should be sent for Gram stain, anaerobic and aerobic culture, sensitivity testing, white blood cell (WBC) count with differential, acid-fast staining, and crystal analysis. A WBC count greater than 80,000 cells/mm³ with 75% more polymorphonuclear leukocytes is indicative of septic arthritis, but lower counts (55,000 cells/mm³) may also indicate septic arthritis.[31] The pathophysiology may become evident in patients after the second day of inoculation. Glycosaminoglycan degradation starts by the fifth day after the start of disease, with cartilage destruction by day 7. Pannus overgrowth starts by day 11 and erosion of the joint capsule begins by day 17. Complete destruction of the joint that occurs with fibrous ankylosis can be seen as early as 5 weeks.[27]

Treatment

Treatment of septic arthritis includes sterilization; decompression; removal of inflammatory cells, foreign material, and pannus; and complete restoration of the joint.[32] Antibiotics, arthrotomy, or arthroscopy are the standards of treatment in septic arthritis. The choice of antibiotic is critical and is based on the cultures and sensitivity of the aspirate from the infected joint. The treatment can last from 14 days to 6 weeks, depending on the route of administration of antibiotic and patient history. Recently, it has been proposed that concurrent treatment with nonsteroidal anti-inflammatory drugs can help decrease cartilage loss in the affected joint. It was shown that animals treated with naproxen and antibiotics lost 38% of the glycosaminoglycans, whereas those treated with antibiotics alone lost 51%. This resulted in a cartilage loss of 19% and 30%, respectively, in animal studies.[27]

Septic arthritis occurs in about 0.1% to 0.9% in patients 4 to 6 weeks after ligament surgery. These patients should be distinguished as those with and without positive cultures. Antibiotics should be started immediately, before culture results, if the physician suspects septic arthritis. The orthopaedic surgeon should perform an arthroscopic débridement and lavage in all patients with positive culture results and patients not improving 24 to 48 hours after parenteral therapy. The antibiotics used are based on the cultures and should be continued for a minimum of 6 weeks.[33]

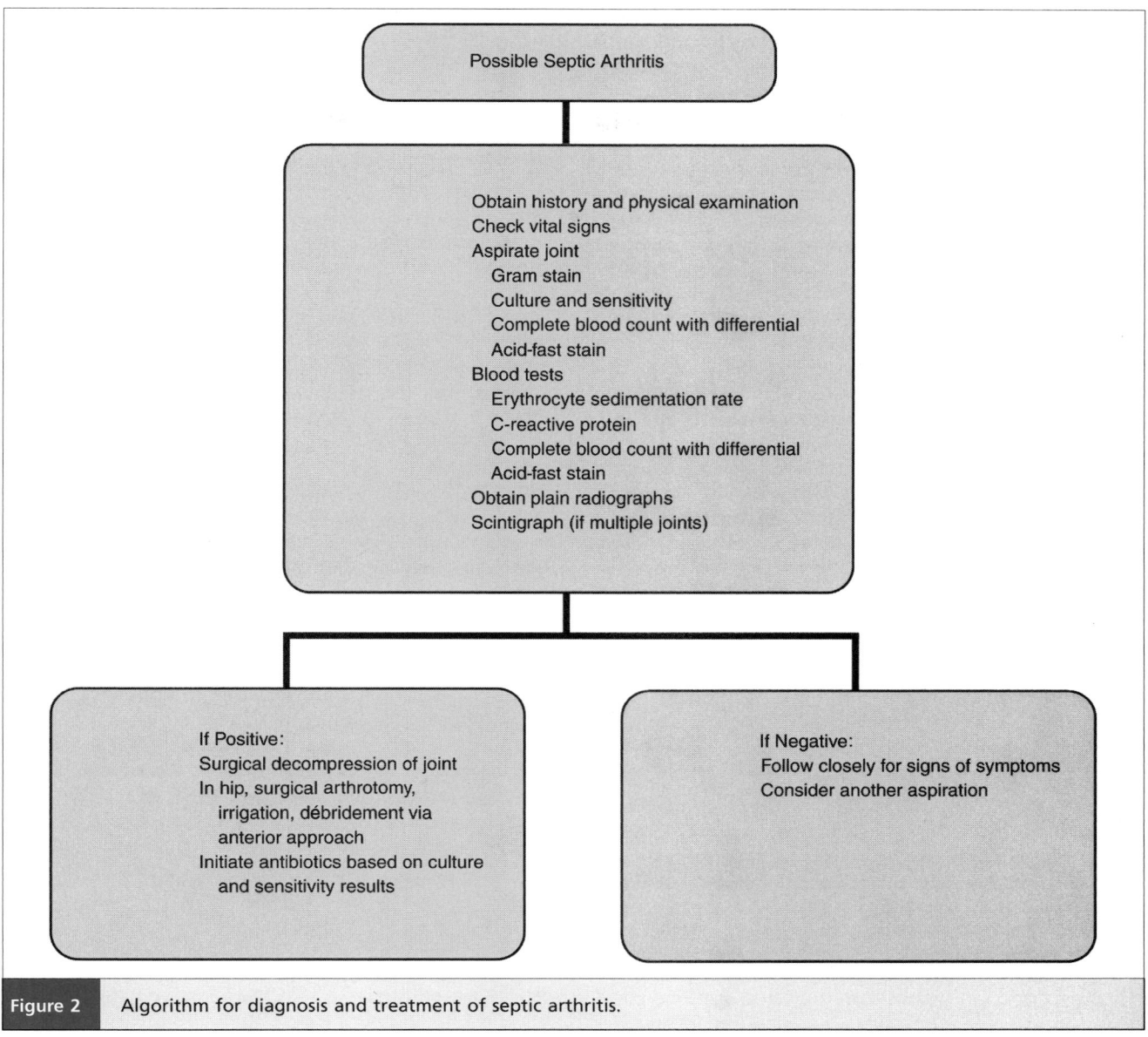

Obtain history and physical examination
Check vital signs
Aspirate joint
   Gram stain
   Culture and sensitivity
   Complete blood count with differential
   Acid-fast stain
Blood tests
   Erythrocyte sedimentation rate
   C-reactive protein
   Complete blood count with differential
   Acid-fast stain
Obtain plain radiographs
Scintigraph (if multiple joints)

If Positive:
Surgical decompression of joint
In hip, surgical arthrotomy,
   irrigation, débridement via
   anterior approach
Initiate antibiotics based on culture
   and sensitivity results

If Negative:
Follow closely for signs of symptoms
Consider another aspiration

Figure 2   Algorithm for diagnosis and treatment of septic arthritis.

Lyme Disease

Lyme disease is the most common vector-borne infection in the United States. It is caused by the spirochete, *Borrelia burgdorferi*, which is transmitted by the bite of an infected tick. It occurs most commonly in the Northeast, Midwest, and Northwest regions of the United States where there are many wooded or rural areas. This disease begins with a skin lesion, erythema migrans, that expands on the skin (stage 1, localized infection). After several days, the infection spreads hematogenously to other sites and may include meningitis, neuritis, carditis, atrioventricular node block, or musculoskeletal pain (stage 2, disseminated infection). Months to years after the initial infection, patients report intermittent or chronic arthritis, encephalopathy, or acrodermatitis (stage 3, persistent infection). Most patients have these localized symptoms in the summer, but the infection may not be noticed until it progresses to stage 2 or 3. Diagnosis may be negative during the first several weeks, but a positive result in both immunoglobulin M and immunoglobulin G may be seen during the first month of infection. The Centers for Disease Control and Prevention recommends a two-stage approach for diagnosis that includes enzyme-linked immunosorbent assay and Western blot testing. The spirochete can be cultured from synovial fluid or skin lesions, because other cultures have shown low yields in prior studies. The arthrocentesis may closely resemble septic arthritis. Antibiotic prophylaxis is not routinely indicated, and treatment is based on the amount of infection and history of the patient. If the infection is localized to the skin, a 20-day course of antibiotics is needed; in contrast, if the infection is disseminated, a 30-day course of antibiotics is sufficient. The treatment

2: Systemic Disorders

needs to be sustained for a longer period for Lyme arthritis (30 to 60 days) and treatment may include anti-inflammatory agents or even synovectomy. Intravenous antibiotics may be needed for neurologic or cardiac-related symptoms and for patients who live in specific areas; a vaccination may be offered with a booster each year.[34]

Mycobacterium Tuberculosis

Mycobacterium tuberculosis occurs in about one third of patients throughout the world and is second to HIV as a leading cause of death. It should be considered in all patients with septic arthritis and chronic osteomyelitis and is found in 1% to 4% of patients with tuberculosis. It most commonly occurs in patients with the following demographics: homeless, intravenous drug users, migratory dwelling patterns, noncompliance with tuberculosis medications, use of immunosuppressive medications (for example, tumor necrosis factor inhibitors), and HIV.[35] The onset is insidious, with monoarticular swelling and pain and most often is found in the hip, knee, and ankle. Aspiration, synovial biopsy, acid-fast staining, and cultures may be positive in approximately 90% of patients and can be determined in 24 to 48 hours with DNA amplification. Radiographs show peripheral erosions, osteopenia, and joint-space narrowing. Pott's disease is defined as tuberculosis spondylitis and can be seen in patients with kyphosis and neurologic deficits. Therapy includes the same treatment as that used for tuberculosis pulmonary disease with the use of many agents for 6 to 9 months and even longer for immunocompromised patients.[36]

Musculoskeletal Infections in Children

Pediatric Osteomyelitis

Pediatric osteomyelitis occurs mainly in highly vascular bones at the metaphyseal-epiphyseal vascular supply. The most common type is hematogenous osteomyelitis, which occurs in about 1 in 5,000 children. There are three routes through which an infection can be contracted: hematogenous, contiguous, and direct implantation (trauma, fractures, foreign body). Almost 50% of the documented cases are in children younger than 5 years of age, with 25% younger than age 1 year; males are twice as likely as females to be affected. There is no racial difference, and 68% of cases occur in the long bones (femur, tibia, and humerus). In most patients, the condition is seen in one site, but in 10% of patients it can be found in multiple sites.[37-39] *S aureus* is the most common organism seen in pediatric hematogenous osteomyelitis and accounts for 61% to 89% of cases,[37] followed by group A beta-hemolytic streptococci (GABHS) (10%) and *Haemophilus influenzae* (3% to 7%), with immunization almost eliminating this latter pathogen as a cause of osteomyelitis.[40] Other causes of pediatric osteomyelitis include *Kingella kingae* (seen in late summer to early winter and presents with a prior upper respiratory tract infection or stoma-

titis);[41] *Salmonella* species (found in sickle cell patients); *Bartonella henselae* (found in patients with cat-scratch disease; and *P aeruginosa* (common in patients with puncture wounds of the feet).[42,43]

Pediatric osteomyelitis usually occurs in the metaphysis of long bones because of their highly vascular nature. In neonates, the periosteum is thin and thus can perforate and allow the bacteria to spread to the surrounding structures and other joints. Spread to the epiphysis can lead to septic arthritis and growth plate abnormalities that are most commonly found in the hips and shoulders. In infants, the risk for epiphyseal and soft-tissue spread decreases because the cortex begins to thicken and metaphyseal capillaries start to atrophy, but abscesses can still form in the subperiosteal layer. In children and adolescents, the cortex continues to thicken so that the infection cannot travel beyond it.[37]

Diagnosis

Any child presenting with a fever and limb pain for 3 days needs to be evaluated for osteomyelitis. Several features found in certain age groups can help lead to the diagnosis of osteomyelitis. In neonates, symptoms may include pseudoparalysis, pain with palpation at the affected site or multiple sites, local swelling, concomitant joint infection, decreased appetite, and inconsolable crying.[44] Infants, toddlers, and young children typically present with fever of unknown origin, irritability, limp, an inability to bear weight, swelling, warmth of the extremity, and erythema. Older children and adolescents report constant pain that is well localized and a fever that has been present for days to weeks.[37] Diagnosis of pediatric osteomyelitis is similar to that of adult osteomyelitis, which can be obtained by aspiration and ordering CBC with differential, anaerobic and aerobic culture and sensitivity, acid-fast staining, and Gram stain. Serology includes CBC with differential, ESR, CRP, and blood cultures. A diagnosis is made with needle aspiration in 66% of patients and with blood cultures in 36% to 55% of patients. The ESR and CRP are elevated in 90% of patients and peak 2 to 5 days after treatment. These tests are used to follow response to treatment and results return to normal in 1 week (CRP) to 3 weeks (ESR).[45] Plain radiographs have limited value in diagnosis; they may show localized soft-tissue swelling after 3 days, swelling of the surrounding structures after 7 days, and osteolytic lesions after 50% disruption of normal bone (usually after 14 days). MRI is the modality of choice in the detection of pediatric osteomyelitis, with 97% sensitivity that can increase with the use of gadolinium.[37]

Treatment

Treatment is a combination of antibiotics and diagnostic needle aspiration, with possible decompression and drainage of the infected area. Some physicians recommend a conservative approach with surgical intervention indicated in only 50% of patients. Antibiotics should be started that cover *S aureus* and GABHS; however, in communities where MRSA is prevalent, vancomycin should be considered.[46] Once results from the cultures and sensitivities have been determined, the route of administration and dosage of antibiotics should be modified to reflect these results. Antibiotics given intravenously should be administered for 4 to 6 weeks and can be changed to an oral antibiotic if the patient can be compliant, and the organism is sensitive to antibiotic and clinical improvement (the patient is afebrile and normal inflammatory markers are present).[47,48] These oral antibiotics are usually two to three times the normal dose for other infections and the patient needs to be followed closely with blood tests for adverse reactions and/or drug levels.[49]

Special situations occur in pediatric patients with chronic osteomyelitis. Chronic osteomyelitis occurs in 19% of patients with acute hematogenous osteomyelitis and is characterized by suppurative symptoms and acute exacerbations. It can occur after inadequate treatment or open fracture when the infectious site is not adequately drained. Treatment lasts for 6 to 12 months with extensive débridement. Débridement is considered if subperiosteal or soft-tissue abscesses, sequestra, or intramedullary purulence can be identified on imaging studies. Surgical intervention is needed in approximately 50% of patients because the infection is contained with antibiotics.[50]

Children with different types of osteomyelitis require special consideration because of the different types of bacteria present. In sickle cell disease, patients may have fever, chills, bone pain, and tenderness. Needle aspiration along with biopsy is required and antibiotic therapy should cover both *S aureus* and *Salmonella* species. Therapy for 6 to 8 weeks is required for adequate treatment.[51] Osteochondritis caused by *Pseudomonas* is found in 2% of patients and is usually the result of a puncture wound to the foot. Treatment includes intravenous antibiotics for 10 to 14 days and surgical débridement for cultures.[52] Spinal osteomyelitis can be classified as diskitis or vertebral osteomyelitis. Diskitis usually occurs in the lumbar disk and can be caused by an infection or trauma to the spine. It is most commonly found in patients younger than 5 years of age (mean age, 2.8 years) who have a backache, limp, or pain with ambulation. Plain radiographs may show some narrowing of the disk space. Treatment includes intravenous antibiotics that cover *S aureus* and GABHS for a duration of 5 to 7 days, which can be followed by oral antibiotics for an additional 7 to 14 days. Chronic recurrent multifocal osteomyelitis occurs in children and adolescents with a mean age of 14 years. These patients have pain, fever, and recurrent episodes of inflammation and remission. Cultures are usually negative and antibiotics do not alleviate symptoms. This syndrome can be associated with Sweet's syndrome, which is defined as psoriasis and pustulosis palmaris or plantaris. Plain radiographs show multiple areas of inflammation and sclerosis, most commonly on the long bones and clavicle. Treatment consists of glucocorticoids, immune modulators, antimetabolites, calcium modulators, colchicine, hyperbaric oxygen therapy, and nonsteroidal anti-inflammatory drugs.[37]

Pediatric Septic Arthritis

Septic arthritis has an estimated incidence of 5.5 to 12 cases per 100,000 children, with its peak in patients younger than 3 years of age. Males are affected twice as often as females, and the lower extremity (hip) is affected in 80% of patients. Polyarticular joint septic arthritis occurs in fewer than 10% of patients, but can occur in 50% of patients with arthritis caused by *N gonorrhoeae*. Septic arthritis can be caused by seeding of the synovial membrane by contiguous spread by trauma, surgery, or osteomyelitis. The bacteria enter the joint rapidly because of the highly vascular nature of the synovium and lack of a basement membrane. Once the bacteria enter the joint, proteolytic enzymes cause articular cartilage degeneration, which results in release of endotoxins and cytokines such as tumor necrosis factor and IL-1. This degeneration causes a loss of proteoglycans 5 days after the bacteria enter the joint and collagen 9 days after the bacteria enter the joint.[37,53] The most common bacteria isolated in all age groups are *S aureus*. Other bacteria found can include GABHS and *S pneumoniae*, *H influenzae* type B, *K kingae*, *P aeruginosa*, *Neisseria meningitidis*, *N gonorrhoeae*, and *Salmonella* species. In the neonate, group B streptococci and gram-negative bacilli have also been found.

Diagnosis

Patients can present with edema, fever, anorexia, irritability, erythema, joint effusion, and pain at the site of the infection. The child usually refuses to ambulate or use the joint because of pain (pseudoparalysis) and keeps the joint in one position to alleviate pain, thereby increasing joint fluid and decreasing tension on the capsule. Septic arthritis of the hip can occur during external rotation, abduction, and mild flexion. Patients usually present within 72 hours of the time of the infection. The condition may be more difficult to detect in neonates, who may have hip pain during diaper changing. The gold standard for detecting septic arthritis is aspiration of the infected joint. The aspirate should be sent for Gram stain, CBC with differential, aerobic and anaerobic cultures, acid-fast staining, and sensitivity. Blood work should also be performed and can include blood cultures, CBC with differential, CRP, and ESR. Culture of the aspirate can lead to identification of an organism that can direct antibiotic treatment in 60% of patients. A WBC count greater than 12,000/mm^3 with 40% to 60% polymorphonuclear leukocytes and an ESR greater than 55 mm/h is indicative of a septic joint. The CRP and ESR are helpful in the diagnosis, but both tests are nonspecific and levels are elevated in 90% of children with any infection peaking after 48 hours and normalizing after treatment.[54] An aspirate WBC count greater than 50,000/mm^3 with 75% polymorphonuclear leukocytes and Gram stain are helpful in 30% to 50% of patients with septic arthritis. Plain radiographs can be useful for ruling out other diagnoses such as fractures, Legg-Calvé-Perthes disease, and slipped capital femoral epiphysis; widened joint spaces are found in septic joints as a result of effusion. MRI, CT, and ultrasound can also be used for diagnosis and aiding in the aspiration of the hip, but require more time.[55]

Treatment

Treatment of pediatric septic arthritis is similar to that for adult septic arthritis. Antibiotics must be started immediately and the joint surgically drained and irrigated. Arthroscopic treatment of septic arthritis has been shown to be an excellent choice for surgical drainage and irrigation in a study of 10 patients with 5-year follow-up.[56] Total duration of antibiotic therapy is at least 3 weeks, with intravenous therapy for at least 1 week. If inflammatory markers (such as ESR, CRP) are normal and the patient is asymptomatic, therapy can be switched to oral antibiotics for the final 2 weeks of treatment. Antibiotics can be chosen based on the results of the Gram stain and should be tailored after cultures and susceptibilities have been reported. Close follow-up with physical therapy and appropriate blood testing for adverse reactions and drug levels are needed. However, even after correct management, the pediatric patient may still have significant morbidity such as growth plate damage and loss of function.[37]

Infections Associated With Internal Fixation

Internal fixation presents a complicated situation in which physicians must consider the status of fracture healing, location of the infection, and chronicity. During the acute postoperative period, if internal fixation is needed and the construct is stable, it should be kept in place. If the fracture is not united but fixation is stable, the internal fixation device should be left in place. In these instances, irrigation, débridement, and 6 weeks of antibiotic therapy are needed. During the surgery, cultures need to be obtained to determine sensitivity and antibiotic coverage. If the fracture is stable and has united, or if the internal fixation device is not providing stability or is loose, then the device should be removed. If the internal fixation device is removed, then an external fixation device should be used if necessary. If the internal fixation device is a rod, the rod should be removed and either replaced with another rod or an external fixation device after extensive surgical débridement. Intra-articular fixations should not be removed unless the fixation is loose or not providing adequate stability.[57]

Infections Associated With Arthroplasty

Arthroplasty infection can occur in 1% to 2% of patients with a total joint arthroplasty. S aureus and S epidermidis are the most common organisms found after surgery. These infections occur either by direct contact with the arthroplasty during the surgery, after the surgery, or by hematogenous inoculation. A classification system based on symptoms, clinical presentation, and timing of the infection has been proposed.[58] Type 1 infection has positive cultures after surgical revision, type 2 has positive cultures 30 days after arthroplasty, type 3 is by hematogenous spread and with an otherwise well-functioning prosthesis, and type 4 is known as chronic or late infection.[58]

Pain in the joint is the first indicator of infection and usually occurs at night or when the patient is at rest. This pain is not aggravated by weight bearing or caused by loosening of the implant; however, loosening may be caused by the infection. Persistent pain, stiffness, or wound drainage is strongly suggestive of an infection and should be managed appropriately. The diagnosis is established by an arthrocentesis of the joint or tissue biopsy, but other laboratory tests that can be used for the diagnosis include ESR, CRP, IL-6, blood cultures, purified protein derivative (tuberculin), and CBC with differential. The aspirate from the arthrocentesis should be sent for aerobic and anaerobic culture, sensitivity, Gram stain, acid-fast staining, and CBC with differential. A leukocyte count greater than 1.7 × 10^9/L in synovial fluid or greater than 65% of leukocytes in the blood is 94% to 97% sensitive and 88% to 98% specific for prosthetic joint infection. Blood tests (ESR, CRP) are nonspecific and should be considered positive only if levels continue to rise 48 hours after surgery. Plain radiographs may show progressive radiolucencies, osteopenia or osteolysis, and periosteal new bone formation. Other screening techniques, such as ^{99m}Tc study or indium-111 leukocyte scanning, can increase the accuracy to 95% for detecting infection, but can produce false-positive results. Other tests such as molecular genetic testing (polymerase chain reaction techniques) may be useful in the future, but are still in the experimental stage. A diagnosis can be established if the patient has any one of the following conditions: (1) growth of the same organism discovered via two or more diagnostic methods (aspiration, biopsy), (2) acute inflammation on histology, (3) gross purulence, or (4) actively discharging sinus tract.[59]

Treatment is based on whether the infection is deep or superficial, time between the arthroplasty and infection, host factors, the condition of tissue surrounding the joint, looseness of the implant, the pathogen present, the physician's ability to clear infection, and the patient's expectations. Treatment methods for infection following arthroplasty are antibiotic therapy, open débridement, arthroscopy, exchange arthroplasty (one stage or delayed), resection arthroplasty, arthrodesis, and amputation.[59] Antibiotics alone are not a good alternative to surgery for the treatment of deep infections and in patients with other joint prostheses. Antibiotic therapy alone should be reserved for patients in whom the prosthesis cannot be removed because of a medical condition that prevents the patient from undergoing surgery, in situations in which the pathogen has low virulence or is susceptible to oral antibiotics, the antibiotic to be used causes few adverse reactions, and the prosthesis is not loose. In one multicenter study, antibiotics alone were successful in only 40 of 225 knees

Table 2

Most Common Diagnoses and Treatments of Musculoskeletal Infections

Diagnosis	Causative Organisms	Initial Treatment	Alternative Treatment
Cellulitis nondiabetic	Group A, B, C, G streptococci *Staphylococcus*	Nafcillin 2 g IV q4h cefazolin 1 g IV q8h	Cefazolin 1 g IV q6h; azithromycin 500 mg IV; 250 mg PO q24h; amoxicillin/clavulanic acid extended release 1,000 mg/62.5 mg PO bid
Cellulitis diabetic	Group A streptococcus, *Staphylococcus aureus*; *Enterobacteriaceae*	Mild: TMP/SMX 2 tabs PO bid + rifampin 300 mg PO bid	Severe: Imipenem 500 mg IV q6h or Etrapenem 1 g IV q24hr + vancomycin 1 g IV q12h
Infected wound posttrauma	Polymicrobic; MRSA, MSSA *Streptococcus, Enterobacteriaceae, Clostridium tetani, perfringens* +/– *Pseudomonas*	Mild: TMP/SMX DS 2 tabs PO bid Severe: Ampicillin/sulbactam 3 g IV q6h or Piperacillin/tazobactam 3.375 g IV q6h Plus Vancomycin 1 g IV q12h	Mild: Clindamycin 450 mg PO q6h Severe: Vancomycin 1 g IV q12h + ciprofloxacin 400 mg IV q12h
Infected wound postsurgical	*Staphylococcus aureus*, Group A, B, C, G streptococcus	Mild: TMP/SMX DS 2 tabs PO bid Severe: Vancomycin 1 g IV q12h	Mild: Clindamycin 450 mg PO q6h Severe: Daptomycin 6 mg/kg IV q24h
Infected wound human bite	*Streptococcus viridans, Staphylococcus epidermidis, Staphylococcus aureus, Bacteroides, Peptostreptococcus*	Early onset no sign of infection: Irrigation and débridement in addition to amoxicillin/clavulanic acid 875 mg PO bid x 5 days	Delayed, signs of infection present: Ampicillin/sulbactam 1.5 g IV q6h or cefoxitin 2 g IV q8h
Infected wound, nail puncture through shoe	*Pseudomonas aeruginosa*	Débridement and tetanus prophylaxis	Osteomyelitis occurs in 1% to 2% of all plantar puncture wounds Treat as directed for osteomyelitis
Necrotizing fasciitis	Group A, C, G streptococcus, *Clostridium*, polymicrobic, community acquired MRSA	Immediate surgical débridement in addition to antibiotic therapy. *Streptococcus* or *Clostridium*, use penicillin G Polymicrobial-imipenem MRSA-vancomycin	
Whirlpool folliculitis	*Pseudomonas sp*	Self–limiting; generally no treatment necessary	Must decontaminate hot tub and any associated reusable products
Hematogenous osteomyelitis (newborn to 4 months)	*Staphylococcus aureus, Group B streptococcus,* gram-negative bacilli	MSSA suspected: Nafcillin dose based on age and weight + ceftazidime dose based on age and weight	MRSA suspected: Vancomycin dose based on age and weight + ceftazidime dose based on age and weight
Hematogenous osteomyelitis (age 4 months to adult)	*Staphylococcus aureus,* Group A streptococcus, gram-negative bacilli (infrequent)	MRSA suspected: Vancomycin 60 mg/kg/d divided q6h If gram-negative bacilli suspected add cefotaxime 100 to 200 mg/kg/d divided q8h Or Ceftazidime 100 to 200 mg/kg/d divided q8h	MRSA suspected: Linezolid 10 mg/kg IV/PO q8h
Hematogenous osteomyelitis (adult age 21 years or older); vertebral osteomyelitis +/– epidural abscess	Multiple causative organisms, *Staphylococcus aureus* most common	MRSA suspected: Vancomycin 1 g IV q12h MRSA not a concern: Nafcillin 2 g IV q4h	Linezolid 600 mg IV/PO q12h Or TMP/SMX 8 to 10 mg/kg /qd TMP component divided q8h

Table 2

Most Common Diagnoses and Treatments of Musculoskeletal Infections (Cont.)

Diagnosis	Causative Organisms	Initial Treatment	Alternative Treatment
Selected therapies based on culture and sensitivity results	MSSA	Nafcillin 2 g IV q4h Cefazolin 2 g IV q8h	Vancomycin 1 g IV q12h, clindamycin 600 mg IV q8h. Be aware of inducible clindamycin resistance.
Selected therapies based on culture and sensitivity results	MRSA	Vancomycin 1 g IV q12h	Linezolid 600 mg IV/PO q12h +/– rifampin 300 mg PO /IV bid
Hematogenous osteomyelitis; Sickle cell/ thalassemia	*Salmonella sp.*, gram-negative bacilli	Ciprofloxacin 400 mg IV q12h	Levofloxacin 750 mg IV q24h
Contiguous osteomyelitis without vascular insufficiency (foot)	*Pseudomonas aeruginosa*	Mild: Ciprofloxacin 750 mg PO bid	Severe: Ceftazidime 2 g IV q8h Or Cefepime 2 g IV q12h
Contiguous osteomyelitis without vascular insufficiency (long bone, post internal fixation)	*Staphylococcus aureus*, gram-negative bacilli, *Pseudomonas sp.*	Vancomycin 1 g IV q12h Plus Ceftazidime 2 g IV q8H Or Cefepime 2 g IV q12h	Linezolid 600 mg IV/PO q12h Plus Ceftazidime 2 g IV q8h Or Cefepime 2 g IV q12h
Contiguous osteomyelitis without vascular insufficiency (prosthetic joint)	Group A, B, G streptococcus, *Streptococcus viridans/ pyrogenes*	Débridement and prothesis retention in addition to ceftriaxone 2 g IV q24h ×4 weeks	Highest cure rate for the following: remove infected prosthesis and leave spacer, provide antibiotic therapy, then reimplant new prosthesis
Contiguous osteomyelitis without vascular insufficiency (prosthetic joint)	MSSA/MSSE	Nafcillin 2 g IV q4h + rifampin 300 mg PO bid x 6 weeks	Vancomycin 1 g IV q12h + rifampin 300 mg PO bid x 6 weeks
Contiguous osteomyelitis without vascular insufficiency (prosthetic joint)	MRSA/MRSE	Vancomycin 1 g IV q12h + rifampin 300 mg Po bid x 6 weeks	Ciprofloxacin 750 mg PO/IV bid or Linezolid 600 mg PO/IV + rifampin 300 mg PO bid x 6 weeks. Therapy based on culture sensitivities
Contiguous osteomyelitis without vascular insufficiency (prosthetic joint)	*Pseudomonas aeruginosa*	Ceftazidime 2 g IV q8h + ciprofloxacin 750 mg PO bid	
Contiguous osteomyelitis with vascular insufficiency	Polymicrobic, gram + cocci, MRSA, gram-negative bacilli, aerobic and anaerobic	Débridement and culture, antibiotic therapy targeted to culture results. Empiric therapy not recommended unless patient is acutely ill	
Chronic osteomyelitis	*Staphylococcus aureus*, *Enterobacteriaceae*, *Pseudomonas aeruginosa*	Culture, antibiotic therapy targeted to culture results. Empiric therapy not recommended	Removal of hardware, débridement, vascularized muscle flaps. Antibiotic impregnated bone cement and hyperbaric oxygen may be beneficial.
Septic arthritis Children younger than 3 months	*Staphylococcus aureus*, *Enterobacteriaceae*, *Neisseria gonorrhoeae*, gram-negative bacilli	MSSA is suspected Nafcillin dose based on age and weight + ceftazidime dose based on age and weight	MRSA suspected Vancomycin dose based on age and weight + ceftazidime dose (based on age and weight)

Table 2

Most Common Diagnoses and Treatments of Musculoskeletal Infections (Cont.)

Diagnosis	Causative Organisms	Initial Treatment	Alternative Treatment
Septic arthritis (children 3 months-14 years)	*Staphylococcus aureus, Streptococcus pyogenes/pneumoniae, Hemophilus influenzae,* gram-negative bacilli	Vancomycin 60 mg/kg/d divided q6h + Ceftazidime 150 mg/kg/d divided q8h	
Septic arthritis, (adults) monoarticular, at risk for sexually transmitted disease	*Neisseria gonorrhoeae*	Gram stain negative: Ceftriaxone 1 g IV q24h or Cefotaxime 1 g IV q8h	Gram stain positive: vancomycin 1 g IV q12h
Septic arthritis, adults not at risk for sexually transmitted disease	*Staphylococcus aureus, Streptococcus,* gram-negative bacilli	Vancomycin 1 g IV q12h + ceftazidime 2 g IV q8h	Vancomycin 1 g IV q12h + ciprofloxacin 750 mg IV/PO q12h
Septic arthritis, adults, chronic monoarticular	*Mycobacteria sp.*	Mycobacteria: Azithromycin 500 mg IV/250mg PO qd Or ciprofloxacin 750 mg IV/PO qd	Doxycycline 100 mg IV/PO bid
	Brucella sp.	Doxycycline 100 mg PO/IV bid + gentamicin 1.5 mg/kg IV q8h	Doxycycline 100 mg IV/PO bid or ciprofloxacin 750 mg IV/PO bid + rifampin 300 mg IV/PO bid
	Nocardia sp.	TMP/SMX 8 to10 mg/kg/d (trimethoprim component) divided q8h	Minocycline 100 mg PO bid
Septic arthritis, polyarticular	*Neisseria gonorrhoeae,* acute rheumatic fever, viruses	Gram stain negative for gonorrhea and chlamydia; if sexually active, culture throat, cervix, urethra, blood and joint aspirate, then ceftriaxone 1 g IV q24h	
Septic arthritis, post intra-articular injection	MSSA MSSE, MRSA, MRSE, *Pseudomonas sp.*	No empiric therapy, arthroscopy for culture and sensitivity in addition to washout, antibiotic therapy based on culture and sensitivity results	Treat 14 days with culture targeted therapy
Septic arthritis, Lyme disease	*Borrelia burgdorferi*	Doxycycline 100 mg PO bid or amoxicillin 500 mg PO qid ×30 to 60 days	Ceftriaxone 2 g IV q24h or penicillin G 20 to 24 million units/d IV x 14 to 28 days
Abscess	MSSA, MRSA, community-acquired MRSA	Afebrile, immunocompetent: TMP/SMX DS 2 tabs PO bid or doxycycline 100 mg PO bid or minocycline 100 mg PO bid for 10 days, with irrigation and drainage	Febrile: TMP/SMX DS 2 tabs PO bid and rifampin 300 mg PO bid or linezolid 600 mg PO/IV bid or 1 dose of dalbavancin 1,000 mg, 500 mg IV 8 days later × 10 days, with irrigation and drainage

Adapted with permission from *The Sanford Guide to Microbial Therapy. Sperryville, VA, Antimicrobial Therapy, Inc, 2006, pp 4-50.*

IV = intravenous; q = every; h = hours; bid = twice daily; qid = four times a day; PO = by mouth; MSSE = methicillin-sensitive *Staphylococcus epidermidis*; MRSE = methicillin-resistant *Staphylococcus epidermidis*; MSSA = methicillin-sensitive *Staphylococcus aureus*; MRSA = methicillin-resistant *Staphylococcus aureus*; TMP/SMX = trimethoprim/sulfamethoxazole; DS = dry swallow

(18%) and another study reported success in only 62 of 261 knees (24%).[59-61] Systemic antibiotics are given for 4 to 6 weeks and may be changed to oral antibiotics after 4 weeks if the patient is asymptomatic. Other types of delivery systems have been used for antibiotics, including an implantable pump and spacers with antibi-

2: Systemic Disorders

otic bone cement that may aid local drug delivery.[62] The type of surgery depends on the type of infection that is found in the prosthetic joint. Open débridement is indicated in the acute postoperative time frame (type 2) or by hematogenous spread (type 3). Criteria for this type of surgery include symptoms of less than 2 weeks duration, gram-positive organisms, no sinus tract or drainage, and no loosening of the prosthesis.[63] One multicenter study of 154 knees demonstrated success in 30 (19%), and another study showed success in 140 of 445 knees (31.5%).[60,61] Another study concluded that arthroscopic débridement is a reasonable treatment and was shown to be as effective as open débridement, with 28% of the prostheses retained.[64] Reimplantation is the treatment preferred by most patients, which is performed as a one- or two-stage procedure. Delayed reimplantation after intravenous antibiotics for 6 weeks or 3 to 4 weeks with antibiotic-impregnated cement offers the best method of treatment. This delayed treatment involves removal of the prosthesis and all cement, débridement of bone and surrounding tissue, 4 to 6 weeks of antibiotics, and implantation of a new prosthesis. Prior to the reimplantation of the prosthesis, a spacer is used to deliver antibiotics and maintain ligament length while awaiting implantation of the prosthesis. The two-stage reconstruction with antibiotic-loaded cement is the most effective treatment of the final fixation of the prosthesis.[59] Resection arthroplasty is recommended for patients with polyarticular rheumatoid arthritis and low demands for ambulation. The three stages of this surgery are débridement, temporary fixation to maintain the alignment, and immobilization in a weight-bearing cast for 6 months. This type of treatment has satisfactory results, and patients most commonly report pain with ambulation, instability, and decreased walking tolerance. Arthrodesis has historically been an accepted option for patients with recalcitrant infections following total knee replacement. Indications for arthrodesis include high functional demands, single joint infection, young patient age, loss of extensor mechanism, soft-tissue reconstruction, an immunocompromised patient, and the presence of pathogens resistant to most antibiotics. Contraindications to arthrodesis include infection in more than one joint, segmental bone loss, and prior amputation in the other extremity.[59] Many studies have compared arthrodesis and two-stage revision, and showed equal Oxford scores for both procedures.[65] Amputation is another approach to the infected prosthesis and is only recommended for life-threatening sepsis, after multiple revision procedures, and with pain or persistent infection with major bone loss. Because of hematogenous spread of infection to the prosthesis, prophylaxis for 2 years after total joint arthroplasty with antibiotics before any dental procedure (lasting longer than 45 minutes) or surgery is recommended. This can be provided as a single dose of amoxicillin, cephalosporin, or clindamycin (in penicillin-allergic patients). Table 2 presents appropriate antibiotic therapy of the most common diagnoses and treatments of musculoskeletal infections.

Infections Associated With Bone and Soft-Tissue Allografts

In 2001, more than 875,000 allografts were used by orthopaedic surgeons in reconstructive surgery. Infection resulting from an allograft may be viral (hepatitis B and C, HIV) or bacterial (*Clostridium* species, *S aureus*, GABHS, *Pseudomonas*, fungi, or *Enterococcus* organisms). After the death of a 23-year-old-man with *Clostridium sordellii* sepsis as a result of allograft transplantation, there have been many changes in testing to prevent allograft-associated infections. Aseptic processing of allografts has evolved but will not completely sterilize the tissue of organisms or spores. Some tissue banks submerge the tissue in antimicrobial solutions, but this process does not ameliorate the spores. To destroy the spores, gamma radiation and treatment with ethylene oxide or a low-temperature chemical sterilization at the time of implantation showed a success rate of 99% in one study, but these treatments may decrease the integrity of the graft and may cause synovitis.[66] Irradiation reduces bacterial transmission and may inactivate HIV; the success rate has not yet been reported in published literature. Because of the number of infections with allografts, the Centers for Disease Control and Prevention, the American Medical Association, and the US Food and Drug Administration (FDA) have recommended guidelines to reduce allograft-associated infections. All tissue banks should be accredited by the American Association of Tissue Banks (AATB). The FDA requires each tissue bank to have written procedures to reduce contamination and must follow strict guidelines for processing and testing. The AATB reports quality standards for screening donors and for procuring, processing, preserving, sterilizing, preparing, evaluating, and labeling of tissue. These standards include testing for aerobic and anaerobic organisms and fungi as well as reporting of infections. In 2002, 90% of the tissue banks were accredited by the AATB. There needs to be more research and improved guidelines for tissue processing, monitoring, and testing (tissue, donor) for allograft-associated infections.[66-68]

Summary

Timely diagnosis and appropriate drug therapy are essential to the successful treatment of orthopaedic infections. The ability to obtain adequate drug concentrations at the affected site and the presence of resistant bacteria are limitations to successful treatment. With pathogens evolving faster than new drug production, diligence in aseptic technique and prophylaxis must be optimized. Culture and sensitivity results from the site of infection are keys to guiding therapy. Selection and duration of drug therapy in combination with invasive interventions require the surgeon to be skilled in prevention and treatment methods.

Annotated References

1. Gristina AG, Naylor PT, Myrvik QN: Molecular mechanisms of musculoskeletal sepsis, in Esterhai JL, Gristina AG, Poss R (eds): *Musculoskeletal Infection.* Rosemont, IL, Amerian Academy of Orthopaedic Surgeons, 1992, pp 13-25.

2. Ug A, Ceylan O: Occurrence of resistance to antibiotics, metals, plasmids in clinical strains of *Staphylococcus* spp. *Arch Med Res* 2003;34:130-136.

3. Gavin KL, Luck JV, Rupp ME, Fey PD: Infections in orthopaedics, in Buckwalter JA, Einhorn TA, Simon SR (eds): *Orthopaedic Basic Science: Biology and Biomechanics of the Musculoskeletal System*, ed 2. Rosemont, IL, American Academy of Orthopaedic Surgeons, 2000, pp 239-259.

4. Joukhadar C, Dehghanyar P, Traunmuller F, et al: Increase of microcirculatory blood flow enhances penetration of ciprofloxacin into soft tissue. *Antimicrob Agents Chemother* 2005;49:4149-4153.

   Improved blood flow to an extremity allows the antibiotic to penetrate soft tissue and is linked to an improved antimicrobial effect.

5. Malm C: Susceptibility to infections in elite athletes: The S-curve. *Scand J Med Sci Sports* 2006;16:4-6.

   It is suggested that there is an S-shaped relationship between elite athletes (exercise load) and risk of infections.

6. Di Cesare PE, Chang E, Preston CF, Liu CJ: Serum interleukin-6 as a marker of periprosthetic infection following total hip and knee arthroplasty. *J Bone Joint Surg Am* 2005;87:1921-1927.

   A rise in serum IL-6 correlated with the presence of a periprosthetic infection in patients who are treated with revision surgery for a total knee or hip arthroplasty.

7. Palestro CJ: Nuclear medicine, the painful prosthetic joint, and orthopedic infection. *J Nucl Med* 2003;44:927-929.

8. Concia E, Prandini N, Massari L, et al: Osteomyelitis: Clinical update for practical guidelines. *Nucl Med Commun* 2006;27:645-660.

   This article discusses the current types, symptoms, diagnosis, and treatment of osteomyelitis. It also gives guidelines for treatment and outcomes of certain treatments.

9. Payne DJ, Gwynn MN, Holmes DJ, Rosenberg M: Genomic approaches to antibacterial discovery. *Methods Mol Biol* 2004;266:231-259.

   The authors discuss strategies in the discovery of new antibiotics and the role of genomics in the discovery of antibacterial agents.

10. Calhoun JH, Manring MM: Adult osteomyelitis. *Infect Dis Clin North Am* 2005;19:765-786.

    This review article of adult osteomyelitis includes classification, diagnosis, treatment, and cases involving special patient populations.

11. Lew DP, Waldvogal FA: Osteomyelitis. *Lancet* 2004; 364:369-379.

    The authors discuss the epidemiology, diagnosis, and treatment of osteomyelitis with emphasis on hematogenous osteomyelitis.

12. Sapico FL, Montgomerie JZ: Pyogenic vertebral osteomyelitis: Report of nine cases and review of the literature. *Rev Infect Dis* 1979;1:754-756.

13. Batson OV: The function of the vertebral veins and their role in the spread of metastases. *Clin Orthop Relat Res* 1995;312:4-9.

14. Gruber HE: Bone and the immune system. *Proc Soc Exp Biol Med* 1991;197:219-225.

15. Cierny G, Mader JT: The surgical treatment of adult osteomyelitis, in Evarts CMC (ed): *Surgery of the Musculoskeletal System.* New York, NY, Churchill Livingstone, 1983.

16. Cho SH, Song HR, Koo KH, Jeong ST, Park YJ: Antibiotic-impregnated cement beads in the treatment of chronic osteomyelitis. *Bull Hosp Jt Dis* 1997;56: 140-144.

17. Liu SJ, Weng-Neng Ueng S, Lin SS, Chan EC: In vivo release of vancomycin from biodegradable beads. *J Biomed Mater Res* 2002;63:807-813.

18. Chan YS, Ueng SW, Wang CJ, Lee SS, Chen CY, Shin CH: Antibiotic-impregnated autogenic cancellous bone grafting is an effective and safe method for the management of small infected tibial defects: A comparison study. *J Trauma* 2000;48:246-255.

19. Perry CR, Davenport K, Vossen MK: Local delivery of antibiotics via implantable pump in the treatment of osteomyelitis. *Clin Orthop Relat Res* 1988;226:222-230.

20. Cattaneo R, Catagni M, Johnson EE: The treatment of infected nonunions and segmental defects of the tibia by the methods of Ilizarov. *Clin Orthop Relat Res* 1992; 280:143-152.

21. Morandi M, Zembo MM, Ciotti M: Infected tibial pseudarthrosis: A 2-year follow up on patients treated by the Ilizarov technique. *Orthopedics* 1989;12:497-508.

22. May JW, Gallico GG, Lukash FN: Microvascular transfer of free tissue for closure of bone wounds of the distal lower extremity. *N Engl J Med* 1982;306:253-257.

23. Morrey BF, Dunn JM, Heimbach RD, Davis J: Hyperbaric oxygen and chronic osteomyelitis. *Clin Orthop Relat Res* 1979;144:121-127.

2: Systemic Disorders

24. Davis JC, Heckman JD, DeLee JC, Buckwold FJ: Chronic non-hematogenous osteomyelitis treated with adjuvant hyperbaric oxygen. *J Bone Joint Surg Am* 1986;68:1210-1217.

25. Dunn EC, Singer L: Operative treatment of Brodie's abscess. *J Foot Surg* 1991;30:443-445.

26. Miller WB, Murphy WA, Gilula LA: Brodie abscess: Reappraisal. *Radiology* 1979;132:15-23.

27. Esterhai JL, Ruggiero V: Adult septic arthritis, in Esterhai JL, Gristina AG, Poss R (eds): *Musculoskeletal Infection*. Rosemont, IL, Amerian Academy of Orthopaedic Surgeons, 1992, pp 409-419.

28. Cooper C, Cawley MI: Bacterial arthritis in an English health district: A 10 year review. *Ann Rheum Dis* 1986; 45:458-463.

29. Ang-Fonte GZ, Rozboril MB, Thompson GR: Changes in nongonococcal septic arthritis: Drug abuse and methacillin-resistant Staphylococcus aureus. *Arthritis Rheum* 1985;28:210-213.

30. Edelstein H, McCabe R: Candida albicans septic arthritis and osteomyelitis of the sternoclavicular joint in a patient with HIV. *J Rheumatol* 1991;18:110-111.

31. Brinker MR, Miller MD: *Fundamentals of Orthopaedics*. Philadelphia, PA, WB Saunders, 1999, p 26.

32. Goldenberg DL, Cohen AS: Acute infections agent arthritis: A review of patients with nongonococcal joint infections (with emphasis on therapy and prognosis). *Am J Med* 1976;60:369-377.

33. Musso AD, McCormack RG: Infection after ACL reconstruction: What happens when cultures are negative? *Clin J Sport Med* 2005;15:381-384.

   The authors examined an outbreak of nine cases that occurred after anterior cruciate ligament reconstruction and developed a treatment algorithm for patients with negative and coagulase-negative *Staphylococcus*.

34. Steere AC: Lyme borreliosis, in Braunwald E, Fauci AS, Kasper DL, Hauser SL, Longo DL, Jameson L (eds): *Principles of Internal Medicine*. New York, NY, McGraw-Hill, 2001, pp 1061-1065.

35. Colmegna I, Koehler JW, Garry RF, Espinoza LR: Musculoskeletal and autoimmune manifestations of HIV, syphilis and tuberculosis. *Curr Opin Rheumatol* 2006; 18:88-95.

   The pandemic of HIV has caused an increase in opportunistic infections that have occurred in patients, including syphilis and tuberculosis. This article reviews the musculoskeletal and autoimmune manifestations of HIV, syphilis, and tuberculosis, and treatments.

36. Thaler SJ, Maguire JH: Infectious arthritis, in Braunwald E, Fauci AS, Kasper DL, Hauser SL, Longo DL, Jameson L (eds): *Principles of Internal Medicine*. New York, NY, McGraw-Hill, 2001, pp 1998-2003.

37. Frank G, Mahoney HM, Eppes SC: Musculoskeletal infections in children. *Pediatr Clin North Am* 2005;52: 1083-1106.

   This is a review article of the epidemiology, pathogenesis, diagnosis, clinical presentation, evaluation, and treatment of pediatric osteomyelitis, septic arthritis, pyomyositis, and necrotizing fasciitis.

38. Schmit P, Glorion C: Osteomyelitis in infants and children. *Eur Radiol* 2004;14(Suppl 4):44-54.

   This article discusses the radiographic analysis of pediatric osteomyelitis with different modalities and procedures. Patients with underlying disease are also discussed.

39. Steer AC, Carapetis JR: Acute hematogenous osteomyelitis in children: Recognition and management. *Paediatr Drugs* 2004;6:333-346.

   The article is a review of acute hematogenous osteomyelitis, covering recognition with epidemiology, clinical presentation, diagnosis, and treatment.

40. Ibia EO, Imoisili M, Pikis A: Group A beta-hemolytic streptococcal osteomyelitis in children. *Pediatrics* 2003; 112:22-26.

41. Yagupsky P, Dagan R, Howard CB, et al: Clinical features and epidemiology of invasive *Kingella kingae* infections in southern Israel. *Pediatrics* 1993;92:800-804.

42. Raz R, Miron D: Oral ciprofloxacin for treatment of infection following nail puncture wounds of the foot. *Clin Infect Dis* 1995;21:194-195.

43. Mirakhur B, Shah S, Ratner A, et al: Cat scratch disease presenting as orbital abscess and osteomyelitis. *J Clin Microbiol* 2003;41:3991-3993.

44. Asmar BI: Osteomyelitis in the neonate. *Infect Dis Clin North Am* 1992;6:117-132.

45. Unkila-Kallio L, Kallio MJ, Eskola J, et al: Serum C-reactive protein, erythrocyte sedimentation rate, and white blood count in acute hematogenous osteomyelitis of children. *Pediatrics* 1994;93:59-62.

46. Dich VQ, Nelson JD, Haltalin KC: Osteomyelitis in infants and children. *Am J Dis Child* 1975;129:1273-1278.

47. Vazquez M: Osteomyelitis in children. *Curr Opin Pediatr* 2002;14:112-115.

48. Bryson YJ, Conner JD, LeClerc M, et al: High-dose oral dicloxacillin treatment of acute staphylococcal osteomyelitis in children. *J Pediatr* 1979;94:673-676.

49. Vaughan PA, Newman NM, Rosman MA: Acute hematogenous osteomyelitis in children. *J Pediatr Orthop* 1987;7:652-655.

50. Ramos OM: Chronic osteomyelitis in children. *Pediatr Infect Dis J* 2002;21:431-432.

51. Mallouh A, Talab Y: Bone and joint infection in sickle cell disease. *J Pediatr Orthop* 1985;5:158-162.

52. Jarvis JG, Skipper J: Pseudomonas osteochondritis complicating puncture wounds in children. *J Pediatr Orthop* 1994;14:755-759.

53. McCarthy JJ, Dormans JP, Kozin SH, Pizzutillo PD: Musculoskeletal infections in children: Basic treatment principles and recent advancements. *Instr Course Lect* 2005;54:515-528.

    This article reviews the etiology, diagnosis, treatment, and recent advances in many pediatric infections. Osteomyelitis, septic arthritis, cellulitis, necrotizing fasciitis, diskitis, and soft-tissue hand infections are discussed.

54. Unkila-Kallio L, Kallio MJ, Peltola H: The usefulness of C-reactive protein levels in the identification of concurrent septic arthritis in children who have acute hematogenous osteomyelitis: A comparison with the usefulness of the erythrocyte sedimentation rate and the white blood-cell count. *J Bone Joint Surg Am* 1994;76:848-853.

55. Greenspan A, Tehranzadeh J: Imaging of musculoskeletal and spinal infections. *Radiol Clin North Am* 2001;39:267-276.

56. Kim SJ, Choi NH, Ko SH, et al: Arthroscopic treatment of septic arthritis of the hip. *Clin Orthop Relat Res* 2003;407:211-214.

57. Patzakis MJ: Microorganisms in nature and disease: The surgeon's perspective, in Esterhai JL, Gristina AG, Poss R (eds): *Musculoskeletal Infection.* Rosemont, IL, American Academy of Orthopaedic Surgeons, 1992, pp 29-33.

58. Segawa H, Tsukayama DT, Kyle RF, Becker DA, Gustilo RB: Infection after total knee arthroplasty: A retrospective study of the treatment of eighty-one infections. *J Bone Joint Surg Am* 1999;81:1434-1445.

59. Leone JM, Hanssen AD: Management of infection at the site of a total knee arthroplasty. *J Bone Joint Surg Am* 2005;87:2335-2348.

    This review article discusses the diagnosis and treatment of infections that occur in patients with total knee arthroplasty.

60. Bengtson S, Knutson K: The infected knee arthroplasty: A 6 year follow up of 357 cases. *Acta Orthop Scand* 1991;62:301-311.

61. Tsukayama DT, Goldberg VM, Kyle R: Diagnosis and management of infection after total knee arthroplasty. *J Bone Joint Surg Am* 2003;85:75-80.

62. Hanssen AD, Spangehl MJ: Practical application of antibiotic-loaded bone cement for treatment of infected joint replacements. *Clin Orthop Relat Res* 2004;427:79-85.

    Many physicians use antibiotic-loaded bone cement for infected joint prostheses. The authors discuss the difference between low-dose and high-dose cement with the use of spacers, static or articulating, in the treatment of infected arthroplasties.

63. Brandt CM, Sistrunck WW, Duffy MC, et al: Staphylococcus aureus prosthetic joint infection treated with debridement and prosthesis retention. *Clin Infect Dis* 1997;24:914-919.

64. Dixon P, Parish EN, Cross MJ: Arthroscopic debridement in the treatment of the infected total knee replacement. *J Bone Joint Surg Br* 2004;86:39-42.

    This study showed that in certain patients, arthroscopic débridement can allow retention of the prosthesis and may be an alternative to open débridement or revision in the treatment of infected prostheses.

65. Blom AW, Brown J, Taylor AH, et al: Infection after total knee arthroplasty. *J Bone Joint Surg Br* 2004;86:688-691.

    This study of 13 patients with deep infection compared the patient outcomes of arthrodesis and two-stage revision procedures using the Oxford scale.

66. Kainer MA, Linden JV, Whaley DN, et al: Clostridium infections associated with musculoskeletal-tissue allografts. *N Engl J Med* 2004;350:2564-2571.

    The authors discuss the *Clostridium* infections traced to allografts, and provide recommendations for physicians and tissue banks to follow in sterilization methods to prevent allograft-related infections.

67. Kwong FNK, Ibrahim T, Power RA: Incidence of infection with the use of non-irradiated morcellised allograft bone washed at the time of revision arthroplasty of the hip. *J Bone Joint Surg Br* 2005;87:1524-1526.

    This article discusses the implication of allograft bone washed using pulsed irrigation before implantation. The deep infection rate was 0.7% at 1-year follow-up and thus achieved a low risk of allograft-related bacterial infection.

68. Patel R, Trampuz A: Infections transmitted through musculoskeletal-tissue allografts. *N Engl J Med* 2004;350:2544-2546.

    This article provides further discussion of the need for guidelines and testing methods for allograft-related infections.

2: Systemic Disorders

Chapter 21

Pain Management in Orthopaedics

Kamran Majid, MD

Introduction

The first documented attempt to understand pain was by Rene Descartes with his *Treatise of Man* published in 1664. Acute postoperative pain from inpatient and ambulatory surgery is often undertreated, the consequences of which add to the already huge burden of pain management on patients and society. Inadequate relief of postoperative pain can delay recovery, necessitate rehospitalization, increase the duration of the hospital stay, increase health care costs, and reduce patient satisfaction.

Inadequately treated acute pain can result in sensitization of the peripheral and central nervous system, which may ultimately lead to the development of chronic pain. Acute pain results in various physiologic changes that have important effects on the patient's clinical course. Unrelieved pain is likely to cause adverse effects on more than one body system, particularly in high-risk surgical patients, and the development of chronic pain.

Orthopaedic procedures may induce more intense pain than other surgical procedures because bone injury is more painful than soft-tissue injury; this increased pain occurs because the periosteum has the lowest pain threshold of the deep somatic structures. Many factors, such as patient age, health status, medications taken on a regular basis, medical history, chronic pain history, use of analgesics, type of surgery, and inpatient/outpatient setting influence the choice of anesthesia and technique of acute pain management.

Basic Science of Pain

The processing of pain takes place in an integrated matrix at peripheral, spinal, and supraspinal nerve sites (Figure 1). Basic strategies of pain control use the concept of pain integration by attenuation or blockade of pain through an intervention at the peripheral nerve, by activation of inhibitory processes that gate pain at the spinal cord and brain, and by interference with the perception of pain.[1]

At the peripheral level, there are two types of axons that conduct impulses caused by pain and inflammation. The myelinated A delta and beta fibers conduct cold and well-localized pain sensations whereas unmyelinated C fibers signal pain that is poorly localized or caused by heat or mechanical stimuli. Tissue damage can sensitize these nociceptors, causing release of various analgesic mediators. Synapse of these fibers occurs in the dorsal horn of the spinal cord, where spinal modulation occurs. Synaptic transmission between nociceptors and dorsal horn neurons is mediated by chemical neurotransmitters (such as γ-aminobutyric acid [GABA], adenosine, glycine, calcitonin gene-related peptide, glutamate) released from central sensory nerve endings. In conditions of persistent injury, C fibers fire repetitively and the response of the dorsal horn neurons increases. This phenomenon is termed "wind-up," and is dependent on the release of glutamate, which acts on both gated N-methyl-D-aspartate receptors and non-N-methyl-D-aspartate receptors. Glutamate also plays a major role in the process of central sensitization. The ascending pathways and, in particular, the spinothalamic tract carry messages to these higher modulatory centers. Descending inhibitory pathways, which are mainly noradrenergic or serotoninergic modulated, function to inhibit the release of substance P in the substantia gelatinosa (lamina II) of the dorsal horn.

Morphine is considered the gold standard of analgesia because of its potent action against pain. Its mechanism of action involves selectively inhibiting the release of neurotransmitters, including substance P, and mimicking the action of endogenous opioids. Postsynaptically, opioid receptors decrease neuronal excitability by opening potassium channels. Presynaptically, opioids inhibit neurotransmitter release by inactivating voltage-gated calcium channels.

Chronic neuropathic and radicular pain is typically resistant to opioids and systemic nonsteroidal anti-inflammatory drugs (NSAIDs). Cyclooxygenase-2 (COX-2) inhibitors are being used to alleviate acute and chronic pain, but several were removed from the market after a report of increased risk of heart attacks and strokes. Although psychological factors rarely cause pain, these factors may trigger or exacerbate pain experienced with chronic pain disorders.

Mechanism of Action

Acute pain results from mechanically, chemically, or thermally induced damage to tissue integrity. Several chemicals (such as histamine, bradykinin, prostaglandins, serotonin, substance P, acetylcholine, leukotrienes) are released by damaged cells in response to tissue injury and local inflammation. Sensitization

2: Systemic Disorders

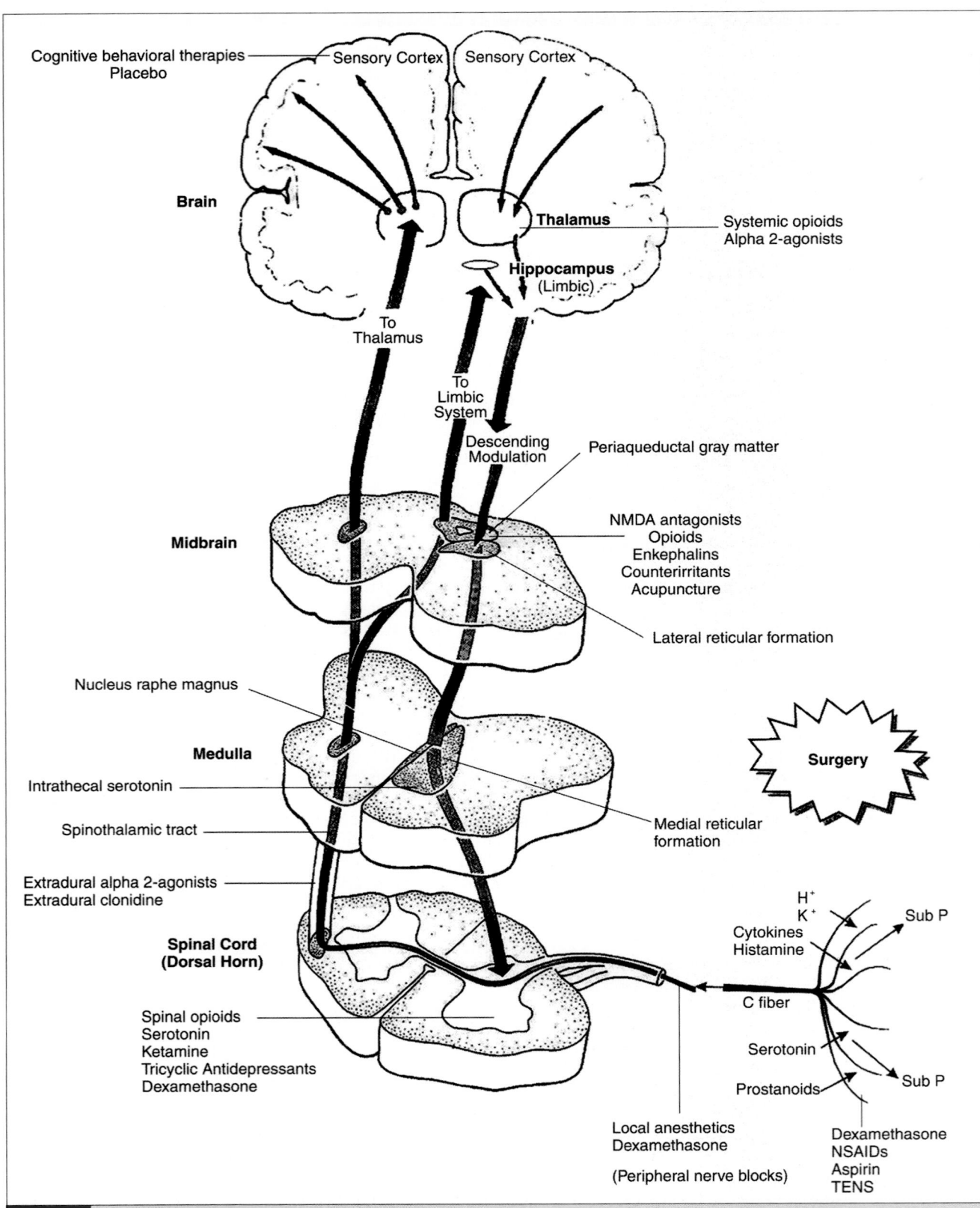

Figure 1   Pain transmission, modulation, and sites of action. NMDA = N-methyl-D-aspartate. H = hydrogen; K = potassium; Sub P = substance P; TENS = transcutaneous electrical nerve stimulation. *(Reproduced with permission from Salerno A, Hermann R: Efficacy and safety of steroid use for postoperative pain relief: Update and review of the medical literature.* J Bone Joint Surg Am *2006;88:1361-1372.*

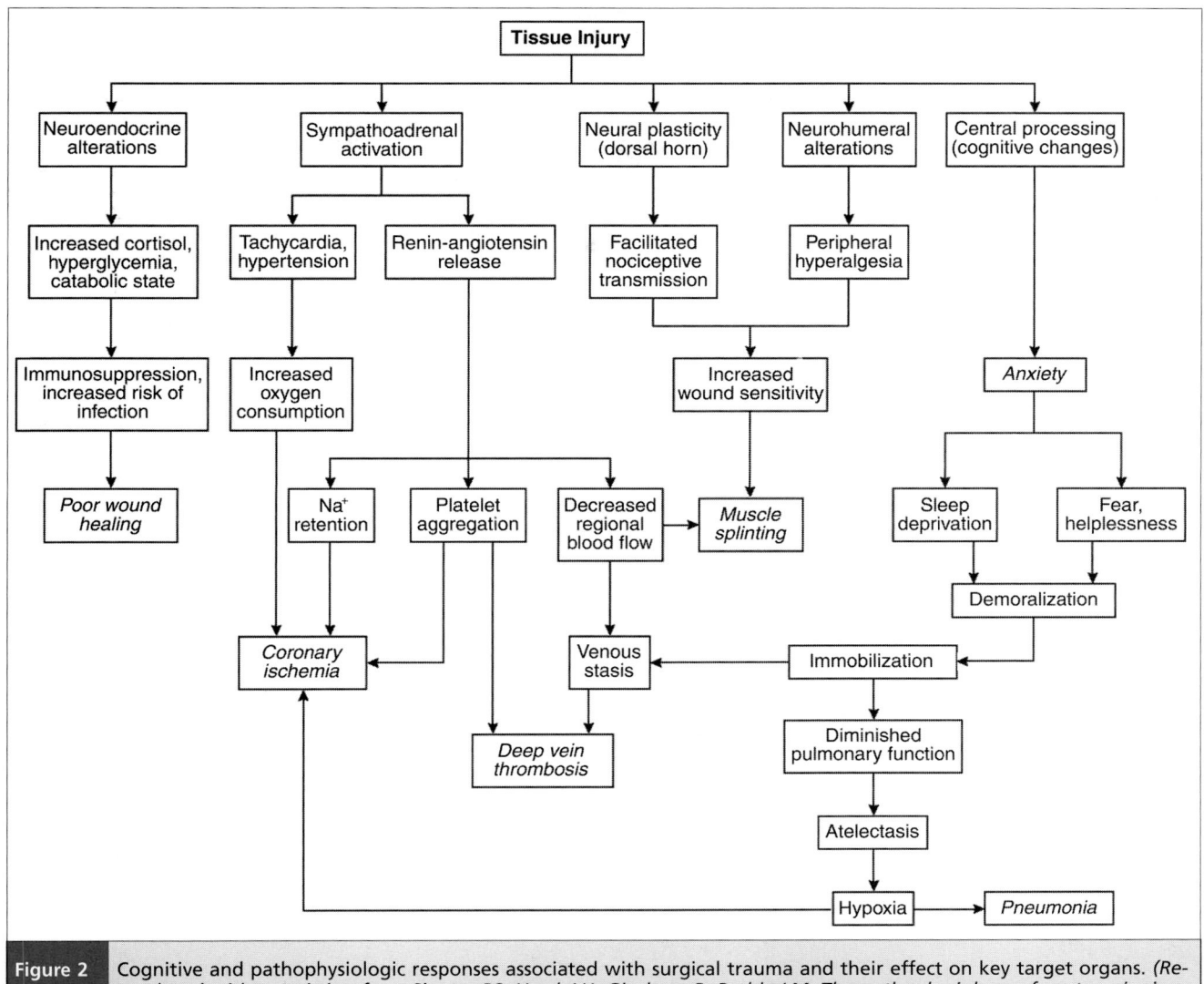

Figure 2 Cognitive and pathophysiologic responses associated with surgical trauma and their effect on key target organs. *(Reproduced with permission from Sinatra RS, Hord AH, Ginsberg B, Preble LM: The pathophysiology of acute pain, in Sinatra RS, Hord AH, Ginsberg B, Preble LM: Acute Pain: Mechanisms and Management. St Louis, MO, Mosby-Year Book, 1992, p 54.)*

lowers the nociceptive threshold to painful stimuli and can result in repeated afferent input in the nervous system that leads to activation-dependent neuronal plasticity.[2]

There are three types of plasticity: activation, modulation, and modification. Increased and persistent afferent input to the dorsal horn leads to increased neurotransmitter release, activating signaling cascades in postsynaptic neurons. This increased signaling causes posttranslational changes (modulation) in secondary sensory neurons, which results in increased sensitivity to neurotransmitter activity. These changes in neuronal sensitivity enhance activity in pain transmission neurons, which is termed central sensitization. These processes lead to amplified responses to all sensory input and result in allodynia, or pain evoked by a normally innocuous stimulus, and hyperalgesia, an exaggerated, prolonged pain response. Modification occurs in both

peripheral and central neurons and involves induced expression of normally dormant genes that encode ion channels, receptors, and neurotransmitters.

Disinhibition of spinal inhibitory mechanisms also occurs. Sensitization of the peripheral and central nervous systems, if improperly treated, can result in neuronal plasticity such that hypersensitive pain responses persist even after the initial injury has resolved.

Pain is recognized not only as a sensory experience but also as a phenomenon with affective and cognitive components (**Figure 2**). The general stress response to surgical and other trauma results in endocrine and metabolic changes that affect respiratory, cardiovascular, gastrointestinal, and musculoskeletal systems. The general stress response may be caused by nociceptive impulses and by factors including anxiety, hemorrhage, and infection as well as local tissue factors. Anxiety and fear resulting from unrelieved, severe, acute pain

2: Systemic Disorders

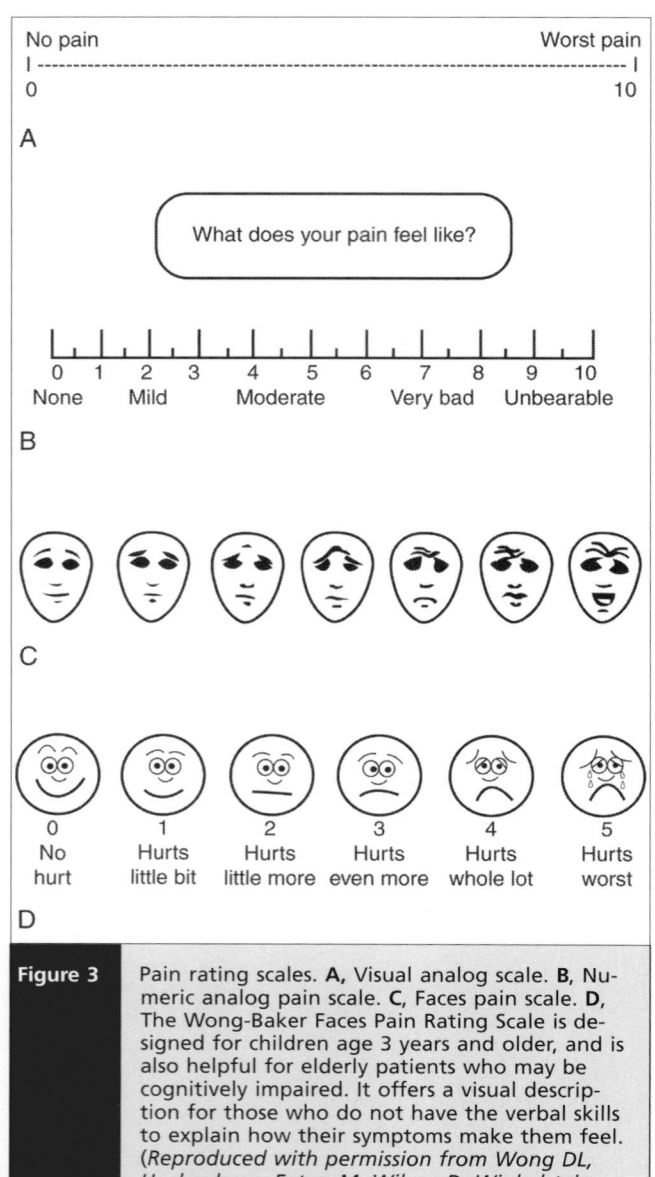

No pain   Worst pain

|---|
0   10

A

What does your pain feel like?

0   1   2   3   4   5   6   7   8   9   10
None   Mild   Moderate   Very bad Unbearable

B

C

0   1   2   3   4   5
No   Hurts   Hurts   Hurts   Hurts   Hurts
hurt   little bit little more even more whole lot   worst

D

Figure 3   Pain rating scales. **A,** Visual analog scale. **B,** Numeric analog pain scale. **C,** Faces pain scale. **D,** The Wong-Baker Faces Pain Rating Scale is designed for children age 3 years and older, and is also helpful for elderly patients who may be cognitively impaired. It offers a visual description for those who do not have the verbal skills to explain how their symptoms make them feel. (*Reproduced with permission from Wong DL, Hockenberry-Eaton M, Wilson D, Winkelstein ML, Schwartz P:* Wong's Essentials of Pediatric Nursing, *ed 6. St Louis, MO, 2001, p 1301.*)

can exacerbate the perception of pain and lead to behavioral changes, including depression.

Pain also can cause sleeplessness, which can further compound the vicious cycle of acute pain. Acute pain also has been associated with decreased peripheral blood flow, which can have deleterious effects on wound repair. Segmental and suprasegmental motor activity in response to pain results in muscle spasm.

Pain Assessment

In 1995, the American Pain Society developed standards that recommended that patients be assessed for pain every time pulse, blood pressure, core tempera-

ture, and respiration are measured. An important concept in these standards is that patients are entitled to appropriate assessment and management of their pain.[3] According to the guidelines of the American Society of Anesthesiologists, pain assessment and reassessment should take place during preoperative, intraoperative, and postoperative pain management. Once the patient has recovered from anesthesia, the mainstay of pain assessment should be the patient's self-report. It should be recognized that a patient's behavior and self-report of pain may show discrepancies as a result of excellent coping skills.

Common pain assessment measures include pain intensity, pain relief, and function. The visual analog scale and the McGill Pain Questionnaire are also commonly used to measure pain intensity and relief. The goal of pain management in orthopaedics is to meet the humanitarian need for pain relief and to facilitate rehabilitation and return to normal function by reducing pain and inflammation at the peripheral and central levels.

Pain measurement instruments are used to evaluate and document pain and are useful for studying pain mechanisms and assessing methods for controlling pain. Clinicians also use pain end points as sensitive surrogates to demonstrate how a method of pain relief mediates postoperative responses, such as clinical course or recovery time.

Pain instruments (**Figure 3**) rely on verbal assessments of pain because the correlation between physical abnormalities and patients' reports of pain has been found to be poor and ambiguous. Intensity is considered to be the most salient dimension of pain, and many procedures for quantifying this dimension have been validated. However, because pain is a complex, multidimensional, subjective experience, the use of a single dimension, such as intensity, does not capture the other qualities and dimensions of the pain experience.

The visual analog scale measures pain intensity and pain relief. It consists of a 10-cm horizontal line with the descriptors "no pain" and "worst pain" at the two ends. The patient places a mark at the point between the two ends that best represents pain intensity. This scale has the advantage of being easy to administer and minimally obtrusive, but it does not take into account the subjective and multidimensional characteristics of pain, including affective qualities. It is, however, widely accepted and validated, and it is easily added to any existing medical record.[4]

In addition to the visual analog scale, the McGill Pain Questionnaire (**Figure 4**) is the most frequently used self-rating instrument.[5] It was designed to assess the multidimensional nature of the pain experience with use of sensory, affective, and evaluative words, and it has been shown to be a reliable, valid, and consistent measurement tool. The McGill Pain Questionnaire evolved into components of the American Pain Society Patient Outcome Questionnaire. It uses small groups of descriptive words to assess the sensory, subjective, and affective qualities of pain. The questionnaire is often used to assess chronic pain. Its purpose is

McGill Pain Questionnaire

Patient's Name _____ Date _____ Time _____ am/pm

PRI: S _____ A _____ E _____ M _____ PRI(T) _____ PPI _____
    (1-10)   (11-15)   (16)   (17-20)   (1-20)

1 FLICKERING / QUIVERING / PULSING / THROBBING / BEATING / POUNDING	11 TIRING / EXHAUSTING
2 JUMPING / FLASHING / SHOOTING	12 SICKENING / SUFFOCATING
3 PRICKING / BORING / DRILLING / STABBING / LANCINATING	13 FEARFUL / FRIGHTFUL / TERRIFYING
4 SHARP / CUTTING / LACERATING	14 PUNISHING / GRUELLING / CRUEL / VICIOUS / KILLING
5 PINCHING / PRESSING / GNAWING / CRAMPING / CRUSHING	15 WRETCHED / BLINDING
6 TUGGING / PULLING / WRENCHING	16 ANNOYING / TROUBLESOME / MISERABLE / INTENSE / UNBEARABLE
7 HOT / BURNING / SCALDING / SEARING	17 SPREADING / RADIATING / PENETRATING / PIERCING
8 TINGLING / ITCHY / SMARTING / STINGING	18 TIGHT / NUMB / DRAWING / SQUEEZING / TEARING
9 DULL / SORE / HURTING / ACHING / HEAVY	19 COOL / COLD / FREEZING
10 TENDER / TAUT / RASPING / SPLITTING	20 NAGGING / NAUSEATING / AGONIZING / DREADFUL / TORTURING

BRIEF / MOMENTARY / TRANSIENT — RHYTHMIC / PERIODIC / INTERMITTENT — CONTINUOUS / STEADY / CONSTANT

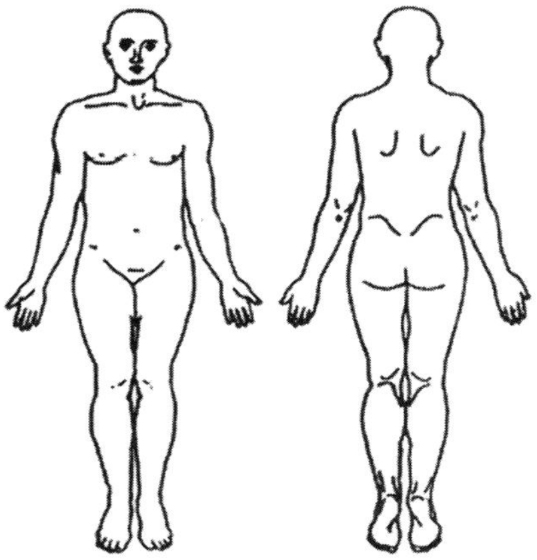

E = EXTERNAL
I = INTERNAL

PPI
0 NO PAIN
1 MILD
2 DISCOMFORTING
3 DISTRESSING
4 HORRIBLE
5 EXCRUCIATING

COMMENTS:

Figure 4 McGill Pain Questionnaire. The descriptors fall into four major groups: sensory, 1 to 10; affective, 11 to 15; evaluative, 16; and miscellaneous, 17 to 20. The rank value for each descriptor is based on its position in the word set. The sum of the rank values is the pain rating index (PRI). The present pain intensity (PPI) is based on a scale of 0 to 5. (Reproduced with permission from R. Melzack. Copyright R. Melzack, 1970.)

to examine the level of disability and interference caused by pain.

Treatment of Acute Pain

Preoperative Acute Pain Management

When discussing the various aspects of preoperative acute pain management, treatment options are varied and often tailored to the patient's level of pain, location of pain, and duration of symptoms. Opioids, NSAIDs, and steroids have classically been offered as first-line treatments of acute pain. Acute pain management starts with the use of preemptive, preoperative techniques, including COX-2 inhibitors and nerve blocks.

Preemptive analgesia refers to the concept that blocking neuronal pathways, before or during injury (surgery), can reduce or eliminate the hyperexcitability of these pathways and pain memory during recovery.[6] Preemptive analgesia can be achieved by infiltration of local anesthetic into surgical wounds. This technique improves postoperative pain relief and decreases the total opioid requirement.[7]

NSAIDs

The primary mechanism of action of NSAIDs is inhibition of prostaglandin production by the COX enzyme. Analgesia and the anti-inflammatory activity of NSAIDs are produced by inhibition of the COX-2 isoenzyme. COX-2 is inducibly expressed only in the central nervous system, kidney, tracheal epithelium, and testicles. COX-2 specific agents were developed with a bulky side chain that binds to the catalytic binding site of COX-2 with substantially greater affinity than the binding site of COX-1, allowing selective inhibition. COX-2 specific inhibitors are at least as effective as nonspecific NSAIDs for managing pain associated with chronic conditions such as osteoarthritis and rheumatoid arthritis. COX-2 specific inhibitors have also been shown as effective as hydrocodone or acetaminophen in relieving postoperative pain following various ambulatory orthopaedic procedures, including anterior cruciate ligament repair, laminectomy, open reduction and internal fixation of long bone fractures, and osteotomy. The results of multiple clinical trials have shown that treatment with COX-2 specific inhibitors is associated with significantly fewer ulcer-related complications than is treatment with nonspecific NSAIDs. Other studies have shown that even short-term use of COX-2 specific inhibitors is significantly less toxic to the upper gastrointestinal mucosa than is short-term use of nonspecific NSAIDs.

On September 30, 2004, the manufacturer of rofecoxib announced that the drug was being withdrawn from the worldwide market. This decision was based on data from a study of rofecoxib in the prevention of adenomatous colonic polyps (APPROVe) trial in which 2,586 patients were randomly assigned to rofecoxib (25 mg/day) or placebo with a planned follow-up of 3 years.[8] Safety monitoring indicated a significant difference in the incidence of thrombotic cardiovascular events (such as myocardial infarction or stroke). In summary, all of the COX-2 inhibitors appear to have some potential cardiovascular risk that may be dose dependent. The magnitude of the risk may differ between agents. Patients with known coronary heart disease or cerebrovascular disease who require concomitant therapy with low-dose aspirin should only receive a selective COX-2 inhibitor after full disclosure of their possible risks. The safety of nonselective NSAIDs in this patient group has not been established. Such patients may require prophylaxis to prevent gastroduodenal damage.

NSAIDs are considered the drug of choice for mild to moderate postoperative pain after many minor and ambulatory procedures when there is no contraindication to their use. They are known to decrease the opioid requirement and enhance the quality of analgesia produced by opioid medications, but provide insufficient coverage for severe pain when used alone. NSAIDs are frequently indicated for inflammation and pain associated with arthritis, which is common in the elderly population; because of known interference with platelet function, these drugs are normally discontinued 7 to 10 days preoperatively.[9]

Inflammation is an essential component of the healing process for bone injuries and fracture repair. Therefore, there is a concern that because NSAIDs are frequently used to manage pain associated with fractures, they may also delay the healing of bone injuries. A reasonable body of preclinical evidence shows that both nonselective and COX-2 selective NSAIDs do delay fracture union, especially during early stages of healing. However, there are few high-quality published randomized, controlled trials to verify the effects of NSAIDs on fracture healing.

Acetaminophen

The antipyretic and analgesic effects of acetaminophen are centrally mediated. Acetaminophen exerts its analgesic effects by increasing the pain threshold, possible by means of central inhibition of prostaglandin production. Its antipyretic properties have been attributed to its action on the hypothalamic heat center. Acetaminophen or aspirin, when compounded with narcotics, effectively relieves moderate to severe acute postoperative pain.

Although acetaminophen is remarkably safe when used at usual therapeutic doses (325 to 650 mg every 4 to 6 hours or 1,000 mg three to four times/day; not to exceed 4 g/day), overdoses have been recognized to cause fatal and nonfatal hepatic necrosis. Given its widespread availability and its combined use with other oral opioid medications (for example, acetaminophen and hydrocodone bitartrate combinations), acetaminophen accounts for more overdoses and deaths from overdose each year in the United States than any other pharmaceutical agent. Acetaminophen poisoning, particularly among alcoholics, has likely become the most common cause of acute liver failure in the United States. Symptoms of an overdose include hepatic necrosis, transient azotemia, renal tubular necrosis, anemia, and gastrointestinal disturbances. The treatment for an overdose includes the use of either acetylcysteine or activated charcoal.

Opioids

Opioids include all endogenous and exogenous compounds that possess morphine-like analgesic properties. Opioids are commonly used to treat moderate to severe pain that is usually acute in nature. Opioids produce their analgesic effect by mimicking the actions of endogenous opioid peptides. There are three major classes of opioid receptor, mu (to which morphine binds), kappa, and delta. Mu subtype 1 produces supraspinal analgesia and mu subtype 2 affects respiratory, cardiovascular, and gastrointestinal function.

Opioid analgesics are also an option in pain management. Codeine is a weak opioid derived from morphine that must be metabolized for analgesic effects. Approximately 5% to 10% of the Caucasian population in the United States is deficient in the enzyme CYP2D6, and are unable to convert codeine to morphine. Codeine is effective against mild to moderate pain and can be combined with acetaminophen and NSAIDs. The strong opioid analgesics, with morphine being the gold standard, are generally reserved for severe pain arising from deep structures. Major side effects include nausea, vomiting, constipation, and respiratory depression. Tolerance may occur with repeated dosage, but is unlikely with use in the acute setting. Methadone hydrochloride differs from the other agents because it is well absorbed after being taken by mouth, and is slowly metabolized by the liver, which makes it more suitable for treatment of chronic pain. Fentanyl citrate is used predominantly for intraoperative analgesia because of its short duration of action.

Oxycodone is an oral opioid used to relieve moderate to severe pain. Taking oxycodone daily can result in physical dependence. The Food and Drug Administration has recently strengthened the warnings and precautions sections in the labeling of oxycodone tablets. There have been numerous reports of oxycodone abuse in several states.

Tramadol Hydrochloride

Tramadol, a synthetic analog of codeine, has a dual mode of action: as a centrally acting analgesic agent with a weak affinity for the mu, omega, and opioid receptors, and as an inhibitor of norepinephrine and serotonin uptake. Tramadol hydrochloride has proven to be a weak opioid with analgesic potency similar to that of meperidine hydrochloride but without the adverse effects of sedation, respiratory depression, gastrointestinal stasis, or abuse potential. The combination of tramadol hydrochloride and acetaminophen has been used successfully to treat moderate to moderately severe acute and chronic pain. The advantages are the rapid onset of analgesia caused by the acetaminophen, and the long duration of analgesia caused by the tramadol hydrochloride.

Corticosteroids

Glucocorticoids (corticosteroids) have the most powerful anti-inflammatory characteristics of all steroids. Corticosteroids are divided into short, intermediate, and long-acting groups. Many of the unwanted side effects of corticosteroids are caused by their mineralocorticoid properties. Factors that influence both the therapeutic and the adverse effects of corticosteroids include pharmacokinetic properties of the glucocorticoid, the daily dosage and timing of doses, individual differences in steroid metabolism, and the duration of treatment.

Corticosteroids have adverse effects on many organ systems and thus numerous potential side effects (**Table 1**). Potential side effects include impaired wound healing, skin thinning, and cushingoid features. They are also known to dampen the febrile response to infection, increase intraocular pressure, increase risk of a number of gastrointestinal events, increase blood pressure, have numerous effects on bone and mineral metabolism, exacerbate affective disorders, and can lead to hyperglycemic events.

Studies have been conducted to assess the efficacy of corticosteroid administration for analgesic control after total hip arthroplasty, with contradicting results. One reason for the differences in findings between the two studies may be because corticosteroids do not produce changes in the pain parameters when there is not enough pain, edema, and trauma.[10] Even with contradicting results in orthopaedic studies, neurosurgeons and podiatrists regularly administer corticosteroids for reduction of pain and inflammation after surgery. However, treatment of overall pain relief after surgery is with multimodal analgesia, with a combination of NSAIDs and weak opioids.

Corticosteroid toxicity is one of the most common causes of iatrogenic illness associated with chronic inflammatory disease. It has been demonstrated that side effects from corticosteroid use are proportional to the duration and intensity of therapy and that long-term, low-dose corticosteroid use is an independent predictor of numerous serious side effects. The literature clearly reflects the safety of short-term use of corticosteroids for acute postoperative analgesia in relatively healthy individuals. Adverse effects associated with the use of steroids can be attributed to high mineralocorticoid activity and/or long-term dosing. Some surgeons have concerns about steroids masking the clinical signs of infection. No detrimental side effects in terms of wound healing were demonstrated in various studies. Although the ideal dose and mode of administration has yet to be determined, there is overwhelming evidence that corticosteroids increase the efficacy of pain reduction following surgery in a manner that does not significantly compromise patient safety.

Perioperative Acute Pain Management

The American Society of Anesthesiologists Task Force on Pain Management has produced practice guidelines for acute pain management in the perioperative setting. Several recommendations were developed to assist the

Table 1

Potential Side Effects Associated With Corticosteroid Therapy

Dermatologic and Soft Tissue	Gastrointestinal	Muscle
Skin thinning and purpura	Gastritis	Myopathy
Cushingoid appearance	Peptic ulcer disease	**Neuropsychiatric**
Alopecia	Pancreatitis	Euphoria
Acne	Steatohepatitis	Dysphoria/depression
Hirsutism	Visceral perforation	Insomnia/akathisia
Striae	**Renal**	Psychosis
Hypertrichosis	Hypokalemia	Pseudotumor cerebri
Eye	Fluid volume shifts	**Endocrine**
Posterior subcapsular cataract	**Genitourinary and Reproductive**	Diabetes mellitus
Elevated intraocular pressure/glaucoma	Amenorrhea/infertility	Hypothalamic-pituitary-adrenal insufficiency
Exophthalmos	Intrauterine growth retardation	**Infectious Disease**
Cardiovascular	**Bone**	Heightened risk of typical infections
Hypertension	Osteoporosis	Opportunistic infections
Perturbations of serum lipoproteins	Osteonecrosis	Herpes zoster
Premature atherosclerotic disease		
Arrhythmias with pulse infusions		

(Reproduced with permission from Saag KG, Furst D. Major side effects of glucocorticoids, in Bose BD (ed): UpToDate. Wellesley, MA, UpToDate, 2004.)

practitioner and the patient in making decisions about pain control. This task force has produced several guidelines including proactive planning, patient education about pain control, 24-hour availability of anesthesiologists, and use of standardized institutional policies. They also recommend a multimodal, organized interdisciplinary approach to perioperative pain management and have recognized the special needs of geriatric, pediatric, and ambulatory surgery patients.[11]

Local anesthetics may block peripheral nerve function and are used primarily during surgery. The primary mode is through sodium channel and axonal conductive blockade. When administered as an epidural infusion, local anesthetics such as ropivacaine or bupivacaine are effective analgesics. Analgesic effects of neuraxial blocks only partially inhibit pain responses and do not affect any humoral component, for example, the activity of inflammatory cytokines such as IL-I. These agents should be used in conjunction with other forms of pain control.

Regional anesthesia has been shown to help prevent the development of deep venous thrombosis in this population. Prophylaxis against deep venous thrombosis with low molecular weight heparin in patients treated with spinal and epidural neuraxial analgesia is associated with a risk of epidural hematoma.

Evidence supports the concept that regional anesthesia may be preferable to general anesthesia in elderly patients. Elderly patients typically present preoperatively with more complex medical histories than younger patients. Neuraxial blocks and lumbar plexus blocks have been shown to decrease blood loss during hip surgery.

Anesthetic options include general anesthesia, neuraxial blocks, and peripheral nerve blocks, alone or in combination. Regional techniques for anesthesia are not contraindicated in patients who require an anticoagulant postoperatively. Regional techniques are performed safely in patients who are scheduled to receive an anticoagulant after surgery as long as there is an appropriate interval between removal of the epidural catheter and the start of the anticoagulant therapy. The advantages to regional techniques include the ability to adjust the intensity and prolong the duration of the sensory block, thus creating excellent pain control for an extended postoperative period. Evidence indicates that neuraxial blocks and peripheral blocks reduce blood loss in patients undergoing hip surgery. Similarly, interscalene blocks reduce bleeding during arthroscopic surgery.[12] Peripheral nerve blocks provide adequate anesthesia for upper and lower extremity surgery; however, they can provide postoperative analgesia for only a few hours. In many instances, a few hours is not enough time to provide sustained postoperative analgesia or effective analgesia to initiate active physical therapy, which is essential to optimize functional recovery. However, peripheral nerve blocks may not perform consistently, possibly resulting in delays in preparing the patient for surgery. Lumbar plexus blocks provide anesthesia for hip surgery in only a small percentage of patients, but the combination of femoral and sciatic nerve blocks provides adequate anesthesia for most surgeries performed in the thigh, leg, ankle, and foot.

Epidural anesthesia, as opposed to general anesthesia, is associated with reduced morbidity and mortality in patients undergoing general and orthopaedic procedures.[13] Epidural anesthesia/analgesia reduces perioperative bleeding and the incidence of pulmonary and cardiac complications and improves recovery of gastrointestinal and cognitive functions. Other evidence suggests that epidural anesthesia/analgesia reduces the risk for venous thromboembolism.[14] However, to avoid the complication of epidural hematoma, the use of epidural analgesia requires the strict observance of guidelines for neuraxial blockade in patients receiving thromboprophylaxis.

Regional anesthesia including neuraxial and peripheral nerve blocks offers effective alternatives to general anesthesia in orthopaedics. The ultimate choice of anesthesia technique depends on the patient preference and type and duration of surgery, patient positioning, and blood loss. Effective postoperative management is based on a multimodal approach including COX-2 inhibitors and peripheral nerve blocks, especially continuous nerve block techniques.

Preemptive analgesia may have less of an effect in patients with preoperative pain who undergo orthopaedic procedures, as was demonstrated in a study showing a definitive preemptive effect on postoperative pain following hardware removal and mass excision but less of an effect after fracture and arthritis-related surgery. It also has been suggested that the timing of preemptive analgesia, coordinated so that the analgesic reaches peak levels in the peripheral and central nervous system as a surgical procedure begins, may influence the effectiveness of postoperative pain relief.

Postoperative Acute Pain Management

Postoperative pain, whether after ambulatory surgery or major inpatient procedures, can cause significant patient suffering and delay recovery and discharge from the hospital. One of the goals of effective postoperative pain management is to suppress the development of the acute postoperative stress syndrome. When taking the relative effectiveness of analgesics into account, opioids are ineffective in preventing the development of the acute postoperative stress syndrome and minimally affect functional recovery when used as a patient-controlled analgesia technique. Additionally, preoperative patient education is essential and includes identifying options, setting realistic goals, and reassuring the patient that pain issues will be adequately addressed. The degree of tissue trauma plays a major role in the intensity of postoperative pain.[15]

Postoperative pain varies in its intensity and duration according to the degree of bony versus soft-tissue damage, as well as the requirement for postoperative physical therapy. The requirement of active versus passive physical therapy influences the postoperative pain management regimen. Active mobilization requires a preferential sensory block with motor sparing, whereas passive therapy does not. The use of low-concentration local anesthetics (particularly ropivacaine, which is motor sparing) produces preferential sensory block when active physical therapy is required. Continuous peripheral nerve block techniques also eliminate the concern of anticoagulation therapy and the risk of epidural hematoma.

Treatment of Chronic Pain

When considering the treatment of chronic pain, the physician must understand that its pathophysiology and treatment varies greatly from that of acute pain. Various treatment modalities, including multimodal anesthesia, selective serotonin receptor uptake inhibitors, tricyclic antidepressants, and nonpharmacologic therapies are used to provide symptomatic relief to those suffering from chronic pain. Depression and anxiety are two of the most common psychologic correlates of chronic pain and greatly complicate the patient's condition and treatment. Sleep disturbance, loss of appetite, lack of energy, and diminished physical activity all contribute to an increasingly debilitated state and amplify the patient's pain symptoms. Patients commonly describe a lack of pleasure and an absence of control in their lives; ultimately, as they continue to seek assistance in desperation, they become increasingly vulnerable to treatments that may be highly suspect or even dangerous.

Multimodal Anesthesia

The term multimodal analgesia refers to the simultaneous use of multiple analgesic methods or drugs. Because pain is an integrated process that is mediated by activation of numerous biochemical and anatomic pathways, a multimodal approach typically deploys interventions such as local anesthesia, NSAIDs, or an opioid to achieve combination analgesic chemotherapy. The integration of pain modulation at multiple foci affords the clinician an opportunity to address peripheral, spinal, and supraspinal mechanisms of pain transmission. By effectively targeting each site, decreased doses of individual agents may be used to diminish the side effects. Synergistic action can also be expected through this approach (Table 2).

Antiepileptic Medications

The efficacy and safety of gabapentin in treating a variety of chronic pain states has renewed interest and enthusiasm in its use. The precise mechanism of action of gabapentin is unknown. It is structurally related to the inhibitory neurotransmitter, GABA, and postulated to increase the level of GABA in the nervous system. However, gabapentin does not interact with any of the GABA receptors, nor is it converted to GABA, and it does not affect the metabolism of GABA in neurons. The most common adverse effects include somnolence, diarrhea, mood swings, ataxia, fatigue, nausea, and dizziness.

Pregabalin is an $\alpha2$-δ ligand that is structurally related to gabapentin but without known activity at GABA or benzodiazepine receptors. It appears to act as a presynaptic inhibitor of the release of excitatory neu-

Table 2

Recommendations for Postoperative Pain Management in Bone and Joint Surgery

Intervention	Grade of Recommendation*	Comment/Application
Nonsteroidal anti-inflammatory drugs		
Oral (alone)	A (against)	Mild pain only
Oral (with opioid)	A	Moderate/severe pain
Paracetamol		
Oral (alone)	A (against)	Mild pain only
Oral (with opioid)	A	Moderate/severe pain
Opioid		
Oral	A	
Intramuscular	A	Painful; unreliable absorption
Subcutaneous (infusion device)	A	
Intravenous	A	Choice in major surgery
Patient-controlled anesthesia (systemic)	A	
Epidural/intrathecal	A	
Local anesthetics		
Epidural/intrathecal	A	
Peripheral nerve block	A	
Corticosteroids		
Subcutaneous (with local anesthesia)	A	
Intravenous (with patient-controlled anesthesia)	A	
Intra-articular (with local anesthesia)	A	
Nonpharmacologic methods		
Transcutaneous electrical nerve stimulation	A (against)	
Psychological therapies	A	
Acupuncture	I	

A = good evidence (Level I studies with consistent findings) for or against recommending intervention; I = insufficient evidence or conflicting evidence not allowing a recommendation for or against intervention.
(Reproduced with permission from Salerno A, Hermann R: Efficacy and safety of steroid use for postoperative pain relief: Update and review of the medical literature. J Bone Joint Surg Am 2006;88:1361-1372.)

rotransmitters including glutamate, substance P, and calcitonin gene-related peptide. Pregabalin can cause sedation and confusion. It is classified as a schedule V drug and therefore may be habit forming. It is generally held that more clinical experience with the drug will determine if its efficacy outweighs its potential habit-forming classification.

Tricyclic Antidepressants

None of the tricyclic antidepressants (TCAs) carries an indication for pain management. Nevertheless, they remain a pharmacologic mainstay in a variety of chronic pain states, with or without coexisting depression. Amitriptyline has been the most widely studied TCA in the management of chronic pain, although a number of others, including doxepin, imipramine, nortriptyline, and desipramine also have been used with success. TCAs are believed to have independent analgesic effects as well as an ability to relieve the depressive symptoms associated with chronic pain. The mechanism of their analgesic action is uncertain; it has been theorized that the analgesic properties are associated with their action as serotonin and norepinephrine reuptake inhibitors. Consistent with this theory is the observation that TCAs with the greatest effect on serotonin seem to have the greatest analgesic effect. TCAs prescribed for chronic pain have typically been given at doses somewhat lower than those used in depression, although higher doses have provided superior analgesia in some studies. Some patients respond only as the dose is steadily increased. TCAs can cause wide-ranging adverse effects. In addition to anticholinergic effects (strong for amitriptyline, imipramine, and doxepin, and minimal for nortriptyline and desipramine), most of the more troubling or serious side effects involve the gastrointestinal, cardiovascular, and neurologic systems.

Selective Serotonin Receptor Uptake Inhibitors

The mechanism of analgesia with selective serotonin receptor uptake inhibitors is less well documented and less well understood than with the TCAs, but may be associated with the primary relief of depression, especially in somatically expressive instances of depression. Such cases, sometimes referred to as "masked" depression, may be characterized by the patient's tendency to deny or minimize sad mood and dysphoric ideation, while mobilizing somatization as a defense against depression. In many of these patients, effective treatment of the primary depression can ameliorate or even resolve the complaint of chronic pain. In other patients, for whom the symptoms of depression are a complicating feature and sometimes natural consequence of chronic pain, favorable response to a selective serotonin receptor uptake inhibitor will greatly relieve the subjective experience of distress and, therefore, the affective and emotional intensity with which physical pain is experienced.

The serotonin norepinephrine reuptake inhibitor venlafaxine may also be useful in the treatment of chronic pain. A randomized trial of venlafaxine in patients with painful polyneuropathy found that venlafaxine was superior to placebo and was similar in efficacy to imipramine.[16]

Nonpharmacologic Pain Control

Pain is determined by an interaction between sensorineural factors and nonnociceptive factors that comprise both organic and psychological processes. Nonpharmacologic approaches to pain relief are cognitive behavioral therapies, that change the way that people perceive and react to their pain. These approaches include behavioral interventions and physical agents. Physical agents provide comfort, correct physical dysfunction, alter physiologic responses, and reduce fears associated with pain-related immobility or restriction of activity. Examples of physical modalities to control pain include superficial heat or cold, massage, exercise, acupuncture, and electroanalgesia.[17]

Transcutaneous electrical nerve stimulation and acupuncture are peripheral stimulatory techniques that appear effective for certain patients. Transcutaneous electrical nerve stimulation might work by stimulating A-beta fibers to "close the gate" to incoming pain signals on C and A-delta fibers. Acupuncture may also work by the gate mechanism, or by activating opioidergic, serotonergic, or noradrenergic modulatory systems.

There is a wealth of anecdotal experience suggesting that when chosen carefully and applied properly, adjunctive therapies enhance the efficacy of pharmacologic and interventional therapies. However, supporting data are lacking. One meta-analysis considering the role of adjunctive therapies in the management of chronic nonmalignant pain reported that the combination of exercise and psychoeducational approaches can lead to a significant reduction in pain and improvement in functional status for a number of musculoskeletal

conditions.[18] It was concluded that as chronic pain is a summation of physical and psychologic derangements, managing it successfully requires addressing all of its aspects. This begins with making patients aware of what is available therapeutically and explaining what each component therapy offers. There is evidence that combination therapies are more effective than any single approach for maintaining long-term gains. Consideration is also given to the issue of relapse prevention through the integration of behavioral work.

Summary

Despite the great advances made over the past several decades in the diagnosis and treatment of most common orthopaedic disorders, the source of musculoskeletal pain is often an enigma to the treating physician. Appropriate pain management in orthopaedic surgery can be obtained through a multimodal approach, proper education, appropriate expectations, and a comprehensive treatment plan.

Annotated References

1. DeLeo JA: Basic science of pain. *J Bone Joint Surg Am* 2006;88:58-62.

   A review article is presented on the history of pain management, supraspinal modulation of pain transmission, mechanism of actions of analgesics, recent animal model studies, and neuroimmune activation in chronic pain states.

2. Ekman EF, Koman LA: Acute pain following musculoskeletal injuries and orthopaedic surgery: Mechanisms and management. *J Bone Joint Surg Am* 2004;86:1316-1327.

   The authors present a review article on the basic science, current strategies, and novel approaches for acute pain management.

3. Sinatra RS, Torres J, Bustos A: Pain management after major orthopaedic surgery: Current strategies and new concepts. *J Am Acad Orthop Surg* 2002;10:117-129.

4. Bodian CA, Freedman G, Hossain S, Eisenkraft JB, Beilin Y: The visual analog scale for pain: Clinical significance in postoperative patients. *Anesthesiology* 2001;95:1356-1361.

5. Melzack R: The short-form McGill Pain Questionnaire. *Pain* 1987;30:191-197.

6. Kissin I: Preemptive analgesia. *Anesthesiology* 2000;93:1138-1143.

7. Aida S, Fujihara H, Taga K, Fukuda S, Shimoji K: Involvement of presurgical pain in preemptive analgesia for orthopedic surgery: A randomized double blind study. *Pain* 2000;84:169-173.

2: Systemic Disorders

8. Bresalier RS, Sandler RS, Quan H, et al: Cardiovascular events associated with rofecoxib in a colorectal adenoma chemoprevention trial. *N Engl J Med* 2005;352: 1092-1102.

This article reported on the cardiovascular outcomes associated with the use of the selective COX-2 inhibitor rofecoxib in a long-term, multicenter, randomized, placebo-controlled, double-blind trial designed to determine the effect of 3 years of treatment with rofecoxib on the risk of recurrent neoplastic polyps of the large bowel in patients with a history of colorectal adenomas. There were 1,287 patients who were assigned to receive 25 mg of rofecoxib daily and 1,299 who received a placebo. Forty-six patients in the rofecoxib group had a confirmed thrombotic event during 3,059 patient-years of follow-up (1.50 events per 100 patient-years), compared with 26 patients in the placebo group during 3,327 patient-years of follow-up (0.78 event per 100 patient-years). Among patients with a history of colorectal adenomas, the use of rofecoxib was associated with an increased cardiovascular risk. Level of evidence: I.

9. Buvanendran A, Kroin JS, Tuman KJ, et al: Effects of perioperative administration of a selective cyclooxygenase 2 inhibitor on pain management and recovery of function after knee replacement: A randomized controlled trial. *JAMA* 2003;290:2411-2418.

10. Salerno A, Hermann R: Efficacy and safety of steroid use for postoperative pain relief: Update and review of the medical literature. *J Bone Joint Surg Am* 2006;88: 1361-1372.

This review article covers the latest debate on corticosteroids and their role in postoperative pain relief. The discussion covers the basic science, pathophysiology, potential side effects, and mechanism of action.

11. American Society of Anesthesiologists Task Force on Acute Pain Management: Practice guidelines for acute pain management in the perioperative setting: An updated report by the American Society of Anesthesiologists Task Force on Acute Pain Management. *Anesthesiology* 2004;100:1573-1581.

This article presents updated guidelines on pain management.

12. Reuben SS, Skylar J: Pain management in patients who undergo outpatient arthroscopic surgery of the knee. *J Bone Joint Surg Am* 2000;82:1754-1766.

13. Gonano C, Leitgeb U, Sitzwolh C, Ihra G, Weinstabl C, Kettner SC: Spinal versus general anesthesia for orthopedic surgery: Anesthesia drug and supply costs. *Anesth Analg* 2006;102:524-529.

This review article studies the economic aspects associated with spinal anesthesia versus general anesthesia in patients undergoing hip or knee arthroplasty.

14. Sharrock NE, Go G, Williams-Russo P, Haas SB, Harpel PC: Comparison of extradural and general anesthesia on the fibrinolytic response to total knee arthroplasty. *Br J Anaesth* 1997;79:29-34.

15. Chelly JE, Ben-David B, Williams BA, Kentor ML: Anesthesia and postoperative analgesia: Outcomes following orthopedic surgery. *Orthopedics* 2003;26: S865-S871.

16. Sindrup SH, Bach FW, Madsen C, et al: Venlafaxine versus imipramine in painful polyneuropathy: A randomized, controlled trial. *Neurology* 2003;60: 1284-1289.

17. Brodke DS, Ritter SM: Nonoperative management of low back pain and lumbar disc degeneration. *J Bone Joint Surg Am* 2004;86:1810-1818.

This review article covers natural history and treatment options for the nonsurgical management of low back pain. A back pain treatment algorithm included medicines, bed rest, physical therapy, chiropractics, orthotics, and injections.

18. Allegrante JP: The role of adjunctive therapy in the management of nonmalignant pain. *Am J Med* 1996; 101:33S-39S.

Section 3

Upper Extremity

SECTION EDITOR:

SCOTT P. STEINMANN, MD

Chapter 22

Shoulder and Elbow Injuries in the Athlete

Jay D. Keener, MD   Christopher S. Ahmad, MD   *Neal S. ElAttrache, MD   *Ken Yamaguchi, MD

Shoulder

Throwing Mechanics and Adaptive Changes

The mechanics of the baseball pitch can be divided into discrete phases with unique demands placed on the shoulder joint (Figure 1). The phases of the pitch that place the shoulder at greatest risk of injury are late cocking, acceleration, and deceleration. In late cocking the glenohumeral joint abducts, extends, and assumes a maximally externally rotated position. The posterior cuff and the subscapularis muscles are active to assume the externally rotated position and to create a buttress against anterior humeral subluxation, respectively.[1] During acceleration, kinetic energy is transferred upward from the legs and torso, the scapula is stabilized, and the powerful internal rotators create a rapid internal rotation moment at the shoulder producing angular velocities of the humerus approaching 7,000 to 8,000°/s. In the deceleration phase, the energy not transferred to the ball is dissipated by controlled deceleration of the arm. High eccentric forces in the rotator cuff are responsible for decelerating the upper extremity.[2] The repetitive performance of the throwing motion leads to fatigue of the rotator cuff and, potentially, microtrauma and tensile failure over time. Postpitching muscle strength testing has shown significant decreases in shoulder flexion, internal rotation, and adduction strength compared with baseline values.[3]

Overhead throwers, particularly pitchers, have well recognized adaptive changes that occur at the glenohumeral joint. Altered mobility patterns for internal and external rotation range of motion have consistently been reported in the throwing shoulder. Pitchers display increased external rotation and decreased internal rotation of the throwing shoulder with the total arc of motion re-

maining similar to the opposite shoulder. This shift in motion arc may result from adaptive changes of the soft tissues; lengthening of the anterior capsular restraints, and tightening of the posterior capsular restraints. One recent study examined the change in rotational motion of the dominant shoulder in overhead athletes as a function of age. The authors noted that the adaptive shift in shoulder rotational range of motion begins and progresses through adolescence.[4] Another factor implicated in the shift of rotational range of motion in pitchers is increased humeral retroversion from adaptive changes that occur at the proximal humeral physis during development.[5,6] Results from a recent ultrasound study examining the amount of humeral retroversion in the dominant and nondominant shoulders of skeletally immature competitive baseball players have suggested that the increased retroversion seen in throwing shoulders is caused by a decrease in the normal derotation of the proximal humeral physis that occurs with age.[7] The authors theorize that the repetitive stress of throwing alters the normal remodeling process of the proximal humerus that occurs with skeletal maturation.

Although the increased external rotation range of motion likely enhances throwing performance, speculation exists whether these adaptive changes compromise the static stability of the joint or predispose the shoulder to other types of soft-tissue injuries. It has been demonstrated that posterior capsular tightness results in in-

*Neal S. ElAttrache, MD or the department with which he is affiliated has received research or institutional support and royalties from Arthrex and is a consultant or employee for Arthrex. Ken Yamaguchi, MD or the department with which he is affiliated has received research or institutional support from Zimmer, Arthrex, and Tornier and has received royalties from Zimmer and Tornier.

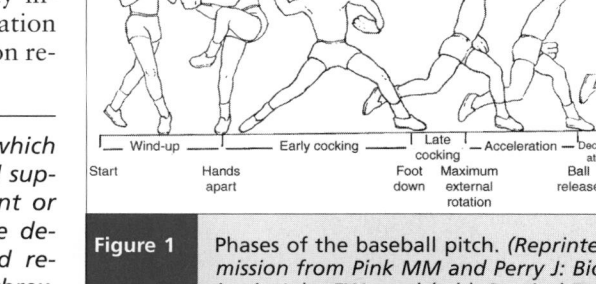

| Figure 1 | Phases of the baseball pitch. (Reprinted with permission from Pink MM and Perry J: Biomechanics, in Jobe FW, et al (eds): Surgical Techniques in Upper Extremity Sports Injuries. St. Louis, MO: Mosby-Year Book, 1996.) |

3: Upper Extremity

creased posterosuperior humeral head migration in the late cocking phase, possibly reducing impingement of the greater tuberosity against the posterior glenoid and allowing increased external rotation range of motion.[8] One potential consequence of increased external rotation range of motion is greater torsional stress of the biceps anchor and predisposition to the development of superior labral anterior to posterior (SLAP) tears.[9,10] Although rotational range-of-motion adaptations are common in overhead athletes, no difference in passive glenohumeral translation and joint stiffness has been demonstrated between the dominant and nondominant shoulders of professional baseball pitchers.[11,12]

History and Physical Examination

A thorough history in the overhead athlete should include the exact nature of the symptoms, onset and duration, response to treatment, and the location of pain. The location of pain and its relationship to the phase of throwing clue the clinician to the etiology of the symptoms. Often throwers will report loss of control or velocity and ease of fatigue, in addition to pain. Dead arm symptoms are the result of loss of dynamic stability of the throwing shoulder. The athlete or training staff may report a change in throwing mechanics, which may contribute to or signal an underlying problem.

Physical examination should include evaluation of the cervical spine and elbow joints to rule out associated pathology or referred pain. Inspection is performed to assess for asymmetries in scapular posture or muscle development. Atrophy of the posterior rotator cuff can be a sign of suprascapular neuropathy. Asymptomatic isolated atrophy of the infraspinatus muscles has been reported in 4.4% of professional baseball pitchers, compared with 0.2% of position players.[13] Observation of scapular mechanics during active range of motion of the shoulder should be assessed. Scapular dyskinesia and winging not only reflects weakness but also may suggest underlying glenohumeral instability. Active range of motion is assessed in all planes, with particular attention given to pain generation and asymmetry. Assessment of capsular mobility in throwers is important to identify and quantify adaptive changes and potential candidates for injury prevention strategies such as posterior capsular stretching. External and internal rotation range of motion is quantified with the scapula stabilized and the shoulder in 90° of abduction and compared with the nonthrowing shoulder. Strength of the rotator cuff muscles and scapular stabilizers are carefully assessed. Specific examination tests are described in later sections.

Imaging

Standard radiographic evaluation includes an AP, true AP, axillary, and outlet views of the shoulder. Calcifications at the posterior labrum and cystic changes in the greater tuberosity are common in throwers. Mineralization of the posteroinferior glenoid is known as a Bennett lesion and is believed to occur in response to traction of the capsule from the repetitive stresses of throwing. The clinical significance of a Bennett lesion is unknown. Recently these lesions have been reported in 22% of asymptomatic professional pitchers.[14]

MRI remains the modality of choice for soft-tissue imaging of the shoulder. Intra-articular contrast improves accuracy for detection of labral pathology, articular cartilage damage, biceps tendon abnormalities, and partial thickness rotator cuff tears. Despite the enhanced definition of anatomy afforded by the addition of contrast, the reported accuracy of MRI arthrogram for the detection of SLAP tears is quite variable.

Instability

Anterior Instability

In the late cocking phase, the position of extreme horizontal abduction and external rotation imparts significant stretch on the anterior glenohumeral stabilizers, particularly the anterior band of the inferior glenohumeral ligament.[15] The repetitive nature of overhead throwing can lead to gradual elongation of these tissues. With increasing laxity, displacement of the humeral head from the glenoid may occur, especially with fatigue of the rotator cuff and scapular stabilizers. Frank anterior instability is rare, because detachment of the anteroinferior labrum (Bankart lesion) is unlikely without a history of trauma. Those athletes with a trauma history or who are involved in collisions sports are more likely to have a true Bankart lesion and/or a bony defect involving the anteroinferior glenoid.

Overhead throwers with anterior instability usually report looseness or shifting of the shoulder with the arm in the cocked position. In the absence of frank instability, the athlete will often note sudden pain with loss of control of the arm. Tingling in the arm or dead arm symptoms suggest anterior instability. The apprehension test is helpful in identifying anterior instability. The arm is positioned in abduction and external rotation while an anteriorly directed force is applied to the proximal humerus. A positive test will elicit the sensation of instability. The relocation test is performed by applying a posterior force to the shoulder and confirms the diagnosis.

Treatment is based on the severity of the instability and the timing in the competitive season. For those with laxity from repetitive microtrauma, rehabilitation focused on strengthening of the rotator cuff and scapular stabilizers, and proprioception of the shoulder is initiated. Return to sports is dictated by successful completion of a throwing progression with emphasis on proper throwing mechanics. Surgery is reserved for those who fail conservative treatment or have a history of traumatic recurrent instability. The goals of correcting the underlying pathology while preserving range of motion of the shoulder can be accomplished with either open or arthroscopic techniques. The potential advantages of arthroscopic repair include evaluation of associated intra-articular pathology, preservation of external rotation range of motion, and decreased morbidity to the subscapularis tendon. Young athletes who participate in contact sports represent a high-risk group for recurrent instability following both open and arthroscopic Bankart lesion repair, with recurrent instability rates historically between 10% and 25%. Acceptable outcomes using contemporary arthroscopic techniques have been reported in 89% to 93% of contact and overhead throwing athletes in two recent studies.[16,17] Ninety percent of nonthrowing athletes and 68% percent of overhead throwing athletes were able to return to full competition. Recurrence rates for contact and noncontact athletes was 9.5% and 6%, respectively.[16] The highest rates of recurrent instability in contact athletes following arthroscopic anterior stabilization have been reported in those with significant osseous defects of the glenoid.[18]

Posterior Instability

Posterior instability can be classified as unidirectional or multidirectional. Unidirectional instability is often traumatic, resulting in detachment of the posterior glenoid labrum with avulsion of the posterior capsuloligamentous restraints. These injuries occur when a posterior directed force is applied to the forward flexed extremity, resulting in dislocation or subluxation of the humeral head. Atraumatic posterior instability results from progressive stretching of the posterior stabilizers and rotator interval tissues and is often seen in the context of multidirectional (MDI) instability.

Without a history of trauma, unidirectional posterior instability of the shoulder is uncommon in overhead throwing athletes. Instability symptoms usually occur with loading of the flexed and adducted extremity such as occur in football lineman and linebackers. Pain rather than instability may be the primary symptom. The athlete may be able to recreate the sensation of instability by circumducting the extremity from an abducted and externally rotated position to a horizontally adducted, flexed, and internally rotated position. The posterior load and shift test and jerk test help to quantify the degree of posterior laxity and recreate symptoms of instability. A sulcus test should be performed and compared with the opposite shoulder to rule out MDI.

The initial treatment of patients with posterior instability of the shoulder should be conservative and focused on strengthening the rotator cuff and scapular stabilizers and proprioception of the shoulder. Surgery is indicated for those patients with recurrent instability in whom conservative treatment has failed. Both open and arthroscopic techniques have been successful in restoring shoulder stability in patients with unidirectional posterior instability. Repair of the avulsed posterior labrum creating a posterior labral bumper is combined with a shift of the posterior capsule. Recent arthroscopic reports have demonstrated restoration of stability in 88% to 100% of shoulders and a high rate of return to preinjury sporting activities (67% to 90%) in those with unidirectional posterior instability.[19-22]

Multidirectional Instability

MDI of the shoulder is defined as symptomatic instability in more than one direction. By convention, this condition is usually defined as anterior and/or posterior instability combined with symptomatic inferior glenohumeral joint hyperlaxity. MDI is classified as either primary anterior or posterior based on the most symptomatic direction of instability. Repetitive activities causing the arm to be raised over the head, such as swimming and volleyball, can lead to gradual elongation of the glenohumeral joint stabilizers in young patients with compliant soft tissues. Hyperlaxity of the rotator interval tissues contributes to inferior joint subluxation and increased posterior translation. Frank labral detachments are less common than with traumatic unidirectional instability; however, hidden detachment of the deep posterior labrum is common in shoulders with posterior MDI.[23] In addition, loss of the normal chondrolabral containment from partial detachment of the posterior labrum and gradual erosion of the posterior glenoid articular cartilage has been described in patients with multidirectional posterior shoulder instability.[24]

MDI is more common in younger athletes and females. Often there is no discrete history of trauma or frank dislocations. MDI can be difficult to diagnose because the primary symptom may be pain. Early fatigue, weakness, and dead arm symptoms are common with activity. Stability examination shows increased inferior translation of the humeral head (sulcus sign). Anterior and posterior instability tests along with the patient's history help to classify the primary direction of instability. Inflammation of the rotator cuff is common secondary to compensatory overuse. Careful assessment of scapular mechanics is important as scapular dyskinesia with overhead motions is common. Often, voluntary subluxation of the humeral head can be demonstrated. Hyperlaxity of other joints should be assessed as a sign of generalized ligamentous hyperlaxity.

The cornerstone of treatment of athletes with MDI is dedicated rehabilitation. Therapy should focus on strengthening and endurance of the rotator cuff and scapular stabilizer muscles. Successful rehabilitation is more likely in patients with MDI in comparison with traumatic unidirectional instability. Surgical indications include a failed course of rest and rehabilitation of 6 months' duration. Surgery should be avoided in those with habitual voluntary instability or abnormal collagen synthesis. Results of surgery are poor but many have surgery because of incapacitating symptoms. Both open and arthroscopic techniques have been successful in treating patients with MDI. The open capsular shift procedure decreases the glenohumeral joint volume by imbrication of the joint capsule and remains the gold standard for surgical treatment. Arthroscopic stabilization involves repair of labral detachments, capsular imbrication and, in those with posterior MDI, rotator interval closure. Recent outcomes following arthroscopic stabilization for those with MDI have rivaled those of open stabilization in properly selected patients.[25,26]

3: Upper Extremity

Internal Impingement

Internal impingement is defined as abnormal contact of the posterosuperior labrum and the undersurface of the rotator cuff tendons that occurs in the abducted and externally rotated position. Although contact between these tissues is likely physiologic, repetitive forces can lead to damage of the rotator cuff and posterosuperior labrum. Adaptive changes that occur in the throwing shoulder may contribute to the pathogenesis of internal impingement. Extremes of external rotation and hyperabduction range of motion increase the contact of the undersurface of the rotator cuff against the posterosuperior glenoid rim. Increased anterior translation of the humeral head resulting from attritional anterior hyperlaxity may exacerbate these phenomena. It has been theorized that increased horizontal abduction of the shoulder occurs with fatigue of the throwing shoulder resulting in greater contact of the greater tuberosity to the posterosuperior glenoid. Excessive posterior capsular tightness and internal rotation range-of-motion deficit is more common in throwers with pathologic internal impingement compared with throwers with no shoulder pain.[27]

Athletes report pain in the posterior aspect of the shoulder during the early acceleration phase of throwing. Posterior shoulder pain is reproduced with the anterior apprehension test and is relieved with the relocation test. The shoulder should be carefully examined for signs of excessive anterior translation and posterior capsular tightness. Initial treatment is focused on rehabilitation. Stretching of the posterior capsule and strengthening of the rotator cuff and scapular stabilizing muscles is emphasized. Radiographs frequently show cystic changes and sclerosis of the greater tuberosity. Common MRI findings include posterosuperior labral fraying and glenoid sclerosis, undersurface rotator cuff tendon fraying/partial thickness tears involving both the supraspinatus and infraspinatus tendons, and humeral head edema with articular erosion near the greater tuberosity.

Surgery is indicated for the thrower in whom a dedicated rest and rehabilitation program fails. The type of treatment is based on the severity of rotator cuff and labral damage noted at the time of surgery and the degree of anterior hyperlaxity and posterior capsular contracture. Arthroscopy allows débridement of partial thickness rotator cuff tears and labral fraying. For those believed to have an abnormal amount of anterior hyperlaxity, suture plication allows tightening of the anterior capsuloligamentous restraints. Posterior capsular release may be necessary for those with excessive tightness (loss of glenohumeral internal rotation of 20° to 25°).

Rotator Cuff Disease

Overhead athletes place significant demands on the rotator cuff; however, full thickness tendon tears are relatively uncommon. The rotator cuff is actively stabilizing the humeral head during late cocking and acceleration of the arm and is under tremendous tensile load during the deceleration phase of throwing. Repetitive loads can lead to microdamage, inflammation, and, ultimately, loss of tendon integrity. Pathogenesis of the tears likely relates to high local tensile and shear forces, deficient vascularity, and mechanical contact of the articular side of the tendon with the posterosuperior labrum. Most of the pathology is seen in the supraspinatus and infraspinatus tendons and manifests as activity-related shoulder pain. Nonthrowing overhead athletes with increased glenohumeral joint laxity, such as swimmers, are prone to overuse tendinitis or secondary impingement as the cuff works to provide increased dynamic stability to the shoulder.

Treatment is dictated by the severity of tendon injury. Rehabilitation focuses on posterior capsular stretching and rotator cuff and scapular stabilizer strengthening and endurance. The addition of intra-articular contrast improves the accuracy of MRI in characterizing cuff tendon injury and allows more accurate identification of associated pathology in the painful throwing shoulder. Treatment of partial thickness tendon tears is controversial. Partial thickness tears involving less than 25% to 50% of the tendon thickness are treated with arthroscopic débridement and posterior capsule release if significant loss of internal rotation is present. Higher-grade partial thickness and full thickness tendon tears are treated with repair. Successful return to high-level throwing, such as pitching, is uncommon following rotator cuff repair.[28]

SLAP Lesions

SLAP lesions involve detachment of the superior labrum and biceps root from the superior glenoid attachment. Overhead athletes are prone to these injuries because of the extremes of motion of the shoulder combined with increased torsional and eccentric loads that occur at the biceps anchor. There are three proposed mechanisms for the development of SLAP lesions in the athlete: increased external rotation of the shoulder in the late cocking phase of throwing increases the torsional force of the biceps root that can result in a dynamic "peel-back" load to the posterosuperior labrum;[9] posterior capsular contracture may increase stress to the labrum by increasing posterosuperior migration of the humeral head; and degenerative fraying may result from repetitive mechanical contact of the posterosuperior labrum with the undersurface of the rotator cuff. Cadaver studies have shown the greatest strains on the superior labrum with the biceps loaded in the late cocking phase of throwing.[29] The ultimate strength of the biceps anchor is less in the late cocking phase (posterior biceps vector) in comparison with the deceleration phase (eccentric load) of throwing in a cadaver model.[30] Finite element analysis has shown that the greatest stress at the superior labrum glenoid interface may occur during the deceleration phase of throwing because of the large eccentric forces of the biceps tendon.[31]

SLAP tears often occur in association with other injuries, making the diagnosis difficult. A combination of patient history, physical examination, and MRI arthrography is often used to assist in making the diagnosis. Throwing athletes will often report deep shoulder pain in the late cocking position and loss of velocity. Because of overlapping symptoms from other pathology, symptoms are often nonspecific. Many provocative tests have been described for the diagnosis of SLAP tears. The accuracy of a variety of SLAP-specific physical examination tests has been quite variable, with most of these tests lacking specificity.[32] Commonly used provocative tests include those that assess biceps tendon pathology and the O'Brien's (active compression) test. O'Brien's test is performed by positioning the shoulder in 90° of flexion, slight horizontal adduction, and internal rotation. The test is positive if the patient experiences deep or anterior shoulder pain with resisted forward flexion that is relieved with external rotation. MRI arthrogram is the preferred modality for detecting SLAP tears and identifying associated pathology. However, the reported accuracy of MRI in comparison with surgical findings is variable. The most accurate method of diagnosis is arthroscopy.

Because the etiology of shoulder pain in the overhead athlete is often not known, the initial treatment focuses on rest and rehabilitation. Treatment is focused on improving the strength of the dynamic stabilizers of the shoulder. For those in whom conservative treatment has failed and the suspicion of a SLAP tear is evident, arthroscopic evaluation is warranted. Four basic types of SLAP tears have been described. Type I has superior labral fraying and a stable biceps anchor. Type II has superior labral detachment and an unstable biceps anchor. Type III has a superior labral tear and a stable biceps anchor. Type IV has a superior labral tear with intrasubstance biceps tendon extension. Treatment is based on the type of SLAP tear, the age of the patient, and associated biceps tendon pathology. Most type II SLAP tears are repaired arthroscopically by reattaching the labrum and biceps root to the superior glenoid with suture anchors or absorbable tacks.

Rehabilitation following SLAP repair focuses on restoring range of motion while allowing 6 to 8 weeks for tissue healing. Extremes of rotational motion are avoided during this period. Motion and strength are the focus of treatment until 3 to 4 months after surgery when sports-specific training is initiated. A throwing progression is initiated at 5 to 6 months following surgery. The results of arthroscopic SLAP repair in athletes show 86% to 90% good to excellent results, with approximately 75% of athletes returning to their preinjury level of competition.[33,34]

Acromioclavicular Joint Pathology

Repetitive throwing and overhead activity can produce irritation and microtrauma of the acromioclavicular (AC) joint. For some athletes, a hyperemic response occurs in the distal clavicle that results in inflammation, bone resorption, and secondary arthritic changes of the AC joint. The athlete will report local pain with terminal overhead motions and when reaching across the body. A history of trauma should alert the clinician to possible AC joint injury or distal clavicle fracture. Low-grade AC joint separations can lead to secondary osteoarthritis. Physical examination will show local tenderness to palpation. Localized pain is reproduced with horizontal adduction and the active compression test. The AC joint is best visualized with the Zanca view, which may show osteolysis of the distal clavicle or arthritic changes in the AC joint. Injection of local anesthetic with steroid is helpful for diagnosis and treatment. For patients in whom conservative treatment has failed, distal clavicle excision is recommended. Diagnostic arthroscopy is performed to define associated pathology. Removal of 5 to 10 mm of the distal clavicle is adequate. Restoration of motion and strength generally allows return to sports activity within 3 months.

Suprascapular Neuropathy

Clinically significant injuries to the suprascapular nerve may be more common in overhead throwing athletes in comparison with the general population. The suprascapular nerve is most likely to be compressed at the suprascapular and the spinoglenoid notches. The extremes of range of motion required during sports that require the arm to be raised over the head can result in traction or compression injury at these points. In the abducted and externally rotated position, the medial tendinous margin of the supraspinatus and infraspinatus tendons impinge against the scapular spine, thereby compressing branches of the suprascapular nerve supplying the infraspinatus. In addition, paralabral cysts that result from labral tears can extend into the spinoglenoid notch, compressing the motor branches to the infraspinatus. Proximal compression at the suprascapular notch results in denervation of both the supraspinatus and infraspinatus muscles.

Athletes with suprascapular nerve injuries often report aching pain and weakness of the shoulder, similar to rotator cuff tendinitis. Careful inspection will reveal atrophy of the infraspinatus or both the infraspinatus and supraspinatus muscles. Weakness of the posterior rotator cuff is typically dramatic. An MRI arthrogram is helpful in identifying the presence of a paralabral cyst and labral tears, quantifying the degree of muscle atrophy, and assessing the rotator cuff tendons. Paralabral cysts are usually located medial to the posterosuperior glenoid within the spinoglenoid notch and have high signal intensity on T2-weighted images. Electrodiagnostic studies confirm the diagnosis and help to localize the site and severity of nerve compression.

Conservative treatment is indicated initially for athletes without anatomic cause for nerve compression. Most patients will improve over time.[35] For those with early atrophy, focal compression, or an anatomic lesion, surgical decompression is indicated. Paralabral cysts can be treated arthroscopically with indirect sublabral decompression of the cysts and labral repair. Open removal of spinoglenoid cysts is generally not indicated. Compression of the nerve at the level of the suprascapular notch is usually treated with open nerve exploration and release of the transverse scapular ligament. Most patients with suprascapular nerve lesions resulting from spinoglenoid cysts will improve with arthroscopic treatment.[36] The likelihood of successful surgery is related to the severity and duration of nerve compression.

Vascular Injuries

Vascular injuries in overhead athletes are rare but must be considered in certain circumstances. Pathology includes digital vessel thrombosis, proximal thrombosis with distal embolization, aneurysms, and vessel compression such as thoracic outlet syndrome and quadrilateral space syndrome.

Proximal aneurysms have been described in the subclavian, axillary, and posterior humeral circumflex vessels. These vessels can be partially occluded by the pectoralis minor or the humeral head during throwing. Turbulent blood flow can lead to local thrombosis formation with distal embolization. The athlete will report symptoms caused by ischemia, including fatigue, arm heaviness, cold intolerance, and numbness in the fingers. The diagnosis can be difficult to confirm and requires a high index of suspicion. Physical examination should include assessment of pulses and change of pulse in the abducted and externally rotated position. Auscultation for bruits in the axilla should be performed. Signs of distal embolization include petechia in the nail beds. A chest radiograph should be obtained to identify a cervical rib. Vascular studies are necessary to confirm the diagnosis and include duplex Doppler scans and arteriograms. Differential diagnosis includes valvular heart disease, vasculitis, and cardiac arrhythmias. Treatment of aneurysms starts with rest and rehabilitation. Surgery is reserved for those patients in whom conservative treatment has failed.[37]

Quadrilateral space syndrome is a condition unique to throwers. The quadrilateral space is bounded by the teres minor superiorly, teres major inferiorly, the long head of the triceps medially, and the humeral shaft laterally. In the late cocking position the posterior humeral circumflex artery and axillary nerve can become compressed, leading to posterior shoulder pain and fatigue. It is generally believed that symptoms are related to compression of the axillary nerve. Local fascial bands can exacerbate compression. Physical examination includes point tenderness locally, especially along the teres minor insertion. Neurologic findings are rare. Pain and paresthesias may be provoked when the shoulder is held in the late cocking position. The diagnosis is made by excluding other pathology, especially thoracic outlet syndrome. Subclavian arteriography may reveal obstruction of the posterior humeral circumflex vessels but may also be seen in normal shoulders. MRI may be helpful in ruling out associated shoulder pathology. Treatment includes rest and rehabilitation with focus on stretching the posterior soft tissues of the shoulder. Surgical exploration and decompression has proved to be beneficial when conservative measures are unsuccessful.[38]

Elbow

Elbow Anatomy and Throwing Biomechanics

In the acceleration phase, the elbow reaches an angular velocity of 3000°/s as it extends from 110° to 20° flexion. This corresponds to 64 N-m valgus torque during throwing. The combination of the valgus torque and rapid extension generates three major stresses: a tensile stress along the medial side (ulnar collateral ligament [UCL], flexor pronator mass, medial epicondyle apophysis), a shear stress in the posterior compartment (posteromedial tip of the olecranon and trochlea/olecranon fossa), and compression stress as high as 500 N laterally in the radiocapitellar joint.

On the medial side, these estimated forces during throwing exceed the known ultimate tensile strength of cadaver UCL specimens (33 N-m), creating an obvious risk for injury from repetitive throwing. Muscle dynamic stabilization has been suggested as a factor involved in protecting the UCL. A cadaver model has demonstrated that the flexor carpi ulnaris is a primary dynamic contributor to valgus stability and the flexor digitorum superficialis is a secondary stabilizer.[39] These muscular dynamic forces must be emphasized in prevention, nonsurgical treatment, and protected from undue injury during surgical exposure.

In the posterior compartment, the olecranon is repeatedly and forcefully driven into the olecranon fossa. Shear forces on the medial aspect of the olecranon tip and olecranon fossa may cause injury and development of osteophytes. The posterior compartment shear and medial compartment tension causes a constellation of injuries and has earned the term "valgus extension overload syndrome." The relationship between the posterior compartment of the elbow and the UCL is becoming clearer. In a study of professional baseball players who underwent olecranon débridement, 25% developed valgus instability and eventually required UCL reconstruction.[40] This observation suggests that both the olecranon and the UCL contribute to valgus stability. A cadaver biomechanical study demonstrated that sequential partial resection of the posteromedial aspect of the olecranon caused increases in elbow valgus angulation.[41] Another cadaver study confirmed that strain in the UCL is increased with increasing posteromedial olecranon resection beyond 3 mm. These studies suggest that aggressive olecranon resection to treat posteromedial impingement places the UCL at risk for injury.[42]

An alternative concept has been proposed that subtle valgus instability may lead to symptomatic posteromedial impingement. A cadaver study demonstrated that UCL injury results in contact pressure alterations in the posterior compartment, which explains the formation of osteophytes on the posteromedial olecranon.[43] Patients with posteromedial impingement pain should

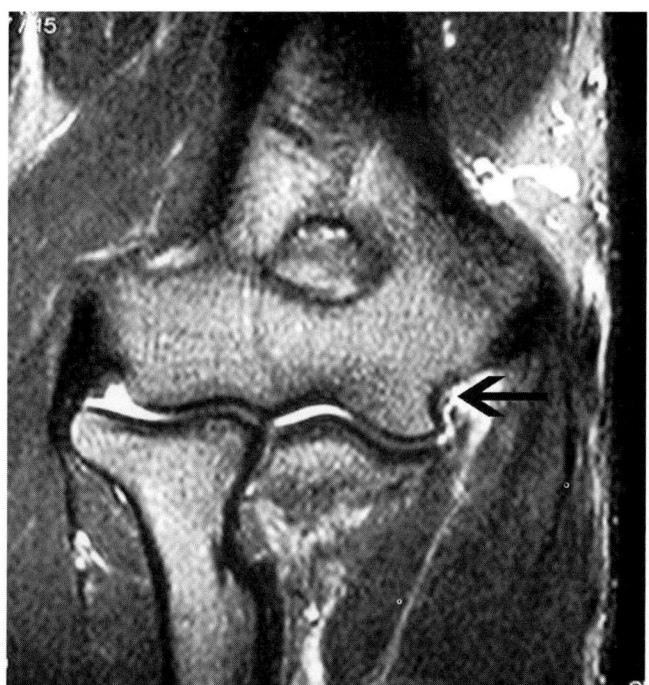

Figure 2 MRI indicating tear of the medial collateral ligament from attachment to epicondyle. *(Reproduced with permission from Ahmad CS, ElAttrache NS: MUCL reconstruction in the overhead athlete, in Browner BD: Techniques in Orthopedics: Surgical Management of Complex Elbow Problems: Update. Philidelphia, PA, Lippincott Williams & Wilkins, 2006, vol 21, pages 290-298.)*

therefore be critically evaluated for suspected concomitant UCL pathology.

Different pitches can also produce more or less torque on the elbow. The fastball and slider produce the highest forces on the shoulder and elbow. The curveball generates the highest elbow valgus stress whereas the change-up produces less torque on the elbow and is thus safer than either the curveball or the fastball.[44]

History and Physical Examination
Physical examination of the medial elbow focuses on the UCL, medial epicondyle, and flexor pronator mass. Examination features indicating UCL injury include point tenderness directly over the UCL or toward its insertion sites. Valgus instability is tested with the patient's elbow flexed between 20° and 30° to unlock the olecranon from its fossa as valgus stress is applied. The milking maneuver is performed by either the patient or the examiner pulling on the patient's thumb to create valgus stress, with the patient's forearm supinated and elbow flexed beyond 90°. The moving valgus stress test is a modification of the milking maneuver. Valgus torque is applied to the elbow until the shoulder reaches its limit of external rotation. The elbow is then flexed and extended with the constant valgus torque. The test is considered positive if the medial elbow pain is reproduced maximally be-

tween 70° and 120°. Medial epicondylitis can be confused with and may coexist with medial collateral ligament injury. Patients demonstrate tenderness at the common flexor origin just distal to the medial epicondyle and pain with resisted pronation and/or flexion of the wrist. The ulnar nerve is assessed for subluxation and irritation with Tinel's sign.

The posterior compartment examination focuses on the olecranon. Pain may be elicited in the posterior compartment with pronation, valgus, and extension forces indicating valgus extension overload. Tenderness and crepitus over the posteromedial olecranon should also be evaluated. Lateral elbow examination assesses the radial head, capitellum, and presence of a synovial plica. Crepitus may be appreciated in the radiocapitellar joint and signify capitellar osteochondritis dissecans (OCD). Pain localized in the lateral aspect of the elbow that is reproduced during flexion-extension of the pronated forearm suggests a synovial plica in the radiocapitellar joint.

Imaging
Elbow imaging begins with standard radiographs, including AP, lateral, and oblique views; these images are assessed for joint space narrowing, osteophytes, and loose bodies. Valgus stress radiographs may be used to quantify medial joint line opening. Greater than 3 mm of opening on side-to-side comparison views is considered diagnostic of valgus instability. It should be noted, however, that mild increased valgus elbow laxity exists in the uninjured, asymptomatic dominant elbow of professional baseball pitchers when compared with the nondominant elbow.[45] Conventional MRI is capable of identifying thickening within the ligament from chronic injury or more obvious full thickness tears (Figure 2). MRI is also helpful in determining if a traumatic tear of the flexor-pronator origin has occurred. Magnetic resonance arthrography enhanced with intra-articular gadolinium improves the diagnosis of partial undersurface tears. Dynamic ultrasonography is a noninvasive, inexpensive method to evaluate the UCL and is capable of detecting increased laxity with valgus instability.[46] Dependence on operator experience can be seen as a drawback to the use of dynamic ultrasonography.

Medial Elbow Pain
UCL Injury
Nonsurgical treatment includes a 6- to 12-week period of rest from throwing and flexor pronator strengthening. If the patient becomes asymptomatic and physical examination is normal, then return to throwing with optimizing throwing mechanics is begun. A study has shown that 42% of athletes return to their previous level of competition with nonsurgical treatment of UCL injuries.[47] No patient factors were found that could predict the success of nonsurgical treatment.

Jobe's original UCL reconstruction technique used a tendinous transection and reflection of the flexor-pronator mass, submuscular transposition of the ulnar

3: Upper Extremity

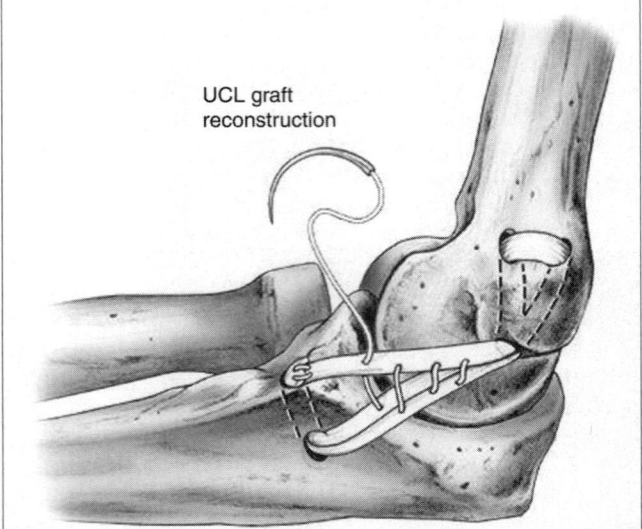

Figure 3 Jobe UCL reconstruction demonstrating figure-of-8 graft pattern. *(Reproduced with permission from Safran MR: Injury to the ulnar collateral ligament: Diagnosis and treatment.* Sports Med Arthrosc *2003;11:15-24.)*

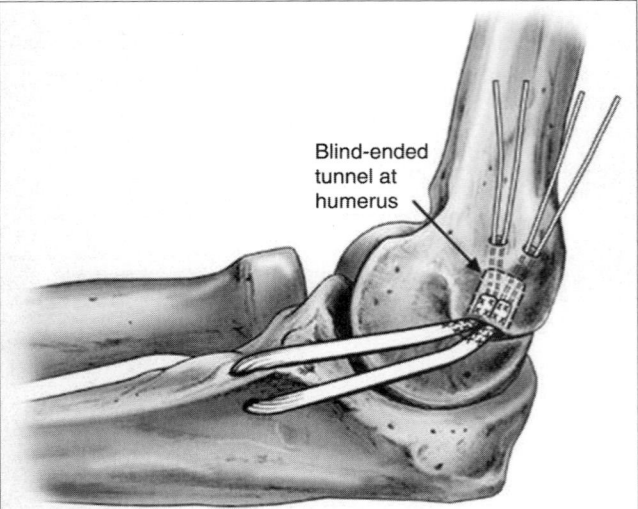

Figure 4 Docking UCL reconstruction with sutures tensioning graft into humeral tunnel. *(Reproduced with permission from Safran MR: Injury to the ulnar collateral ligament: Diagnosis and treatment.* Sports Med Arthrosc *2003;11:15-24.)*

nerve, and creation of humeral tunnels that penetrated the posterior humeral cortex[48] (Figure 3). This technique provided excellent exposure but at the expense of morbidity to the flexor-pronator mass and ulnar nerve. Several modifications in surgical technique have been made to ease technical demands and decrease soft-tissue morbidity. A muscle-splitting approach has been developed to avoid detachment of the flexor-pronator mass with or without subcutaneous transposition of the ulnar nerve. Modifications in bone tunnel creation have also been made that direct the suture tunnels anteriorly on the humeral epicondyle, avoiding risk of ulnar nerve injury. The modified Jobe technique is considered the gold standard, with success rates reportedly as high as 93% in returning throwing athletes to competition.[49]

Docking Technique
The docking technique is another modification of the Jobe technique that simplifies graft passage, tensioning, and fixation. The docking technique uses the muscle-splitting approach with tunnel creation on the ulna similar to that of the Jobe technique. The 15-mm deep humeral tunnel is created for the proximal graft. Two small exit tunnels separated by 5 mm to 1 cm are created to allow suture passage from the primary humeral tunnel. The graft is then passed through the ulnar tunnel from anterior to posterior. The posterior limb of the graft is passed into the humeral tunnel. The length of the anterior limb of the graft is adjusted, creating appropriate tension. The sutures tensioning the graft into the humeral "docking" tunnel are tied over bony the bridge (Figure 4).

A review of 100 consecutive overhead throwing athletes who underwent the docking reconstruction tech-

nique found 90% were able to compete at the same or a higher level for more than 12 months.[50] A further modification of the docking technique using a four-strand palmaris longus graft instead of the two-strand graft for reconstruction has been reported in 25 athletes, and 92% were able to return to their preinjury level of competition.[51]

Interference Screw Fixation Technique
A new technique of UCL reconstruction has been developed that reconstructs the central isometric fibers of the native ligament and achieves fixation with interference screws. This technique is less technically demanding because the required number of drill holes is reduced. Less dissection through a muscle-splitting approach is afforded because only a single central tunnel is required rather than two tunnels with an intervening bony bridge on the ulna. With a single tunnel, the posterior ulnar tunnel, which is in closest proximity to the ulnar nerve, is avoided. Finally, graft passage is less difficult with an interference screw in a single tunnel. The graft fixation strength was found to be 95% that of control intact UCLs under valgus load. Reconstruction of the UCL also restored valgus stability to within less than one degree of the intact elbow throughout flexion and extension. A hybrid technique uses interference screw fixation on the ulna and docking fixation on the humeral epicondyle (Figure 5).

Posterior Elbow Pain
For isolated valgus extension overload, elbow pain is localized to the posterior and medial aspects of the olecranon and is present in the deceleration phase of throwing as the elbow reaches terminal extension. Patients may report limited extension that results from

impinging posterior osteophytes or locking and catching resulting from loose bodies. Examination will elicit pain localized to the posterior compartment by snapping the elbow into extension.

Radiographs of the elbow may reveal posteromedial olecranon osteophytes and/or loose bodies within the articulation. CT and MRI may further define loose bodies and osteophytes. Nonsurgical treatment consists of activity modification, intra-articular cortisone injections, and nonsteroidal anti-inflammatory drugs (NSAIDs). Patients require a period of rest from throwing followed by a progressive throwing program. Pitching instruction should be instituted to correct flaws that may be contributing to the injury. Surgical options include arthroscopic débridement or limited incision arthrotomy to decompress the posterior compartment. Arthroscopy offers the advantages of limited morbidity and complete diagnostic assessment of the elbow. Surgical treatment is indicated for those patients who maintain symptoms of posteromedial impingement despite nonsurgical management.

A relative contraindication to performing isolated olecranon débridement is the presence of UCL insufficiency. Biomechanical studies in cadavers have demonstrated that olecranon resection increases both valgus angulation of the elbow and strain on the UCL during valgus stress.[41,42] In addition, existing UCL insufficiency causes contact alterations in the posteromedial compartment that may be the cause of symptomatic chondrosis and osteophyte formation that manifest as valgus extension overload syndrome. This finding suggests that valgus extension overload with symptomatic posteromedial impingement may occur in the setting of valgus instability because of UCL insufficiency. The UCL insufficiency may then become symptomatic following posteromedial decompression. Therefore, a careful patient history, physical examination, and advanced imaging must be performed to avoid missed UCL injuries or valgus instability.

Olecranon Stress Fracture

The triceps contracts forcefully on the olecranon during the acceleration phase of throwing. In children with open physes, the strong triceps contractions to the olecranon apophysis cause shear and distraction forces. Repeated triceps contractions can ultimately result in olecranon apophysitis. In adolescents with closed physes, stress fractures of the olecranon apophysis can occur. Patients will report pain, weakness, decreased range of motion, and swelling over the posterior elbow. Symptoms are worse during the acceleration and follow-through phases of throwing. Physical examination findings include tenderness over the olecranon and pain with resisted extension. A common radiographic finding is widening or fragmentation of the olecranon physis and sclerosis in comparison with the normal contralateral side. Technetium bone scan or MRI may help confirm the diagnosis. Initial treatment of olecranon apophysitis should be conservative. Activity modification, NSAIDs, ice application, and physical therapy

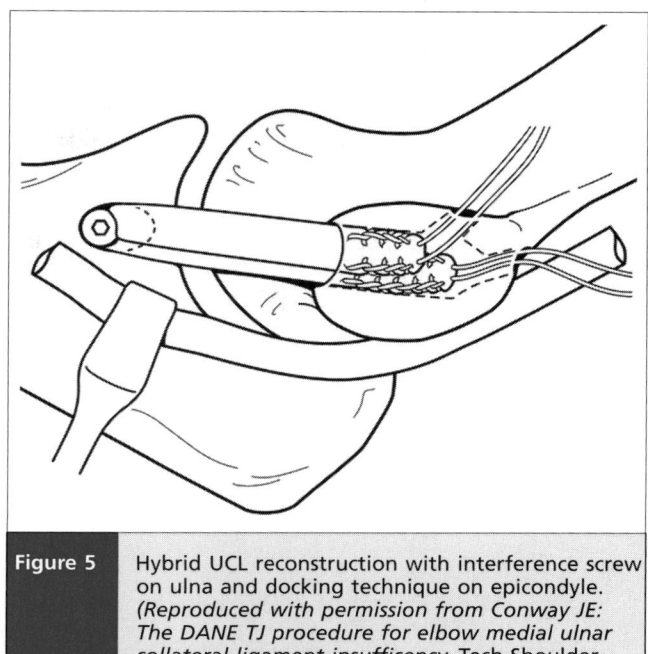

Figure 5 Hybrid UCL reconstruction with interference screw on ulna and docking technique on epicondyle. *(Reproduced with permission from Conway JE: The DANE TJ procedure for elbow medial ulnar collateral ligament insufficency. Tech Shoulder Elbow Surg 2006;7:36-43.)*

usually help resolve symptoms by 4 to 6 weeks. If chronic apophysitis develops, surgical treatment may be warranted. Surgical treatment is indicated for patients with refractory symptoms and a documented failure of olecranon apophyseal closure after 3 to 6 months of conservative treatment. A single cancellous 6.5-mm or 7.3-mm cannulated screw is placed down the intramedullary canal crossing the fracture site or unfused apophysis.

Lateral Elbow Pain
Capitellar Osteochondritis Dissecans
OCD is more common in the skeletally immature athlete than in the adult. In addition to the lateral compression incurred during throwing, risk factors include genetic predisposition and the tenuous end-artery vascular supply to the capitellum. The capitellum is supplied by two end arteries coursing from posterior to anterior (the radial recurrent and interosseous recurrent arteries.)

Patients with OCD report lateral elbow pain and stiffness and locking over time because of intra-articular loose bodies. Physical examination is remarkable for capitellar tenderness and limited range of motion. Capitellar OCD lesions have been classified based on status and stability of the overlying cartilage. Initial treatment of all lesions consists of activity modification, avoidance of throwing or other related sports, NSAIDs, and occasionally a short period of bracing for acute symptoms. For lesions that do not demonstrate detachment or frank loose bodies, throwing and sports are restricted for 4 weeks. Physical therapy, proper pitching instruction, and a progressive throwing program may allow athletes to return to preinjury performance. Surgery is indicated for patients in whom

3: Upper Extremity

nonsurgical treatment has failed. Surgical treatment includes diagnostic arthroscopy confirming the stability of the overlying cartilage followed by drilling of the lesion with a 2-mm smooth pin.

For patients with lesions that are partially or fully detached, surgery is indicated immediately. Loose bodies are removed and the cartilage is contoured to a stable rim. Antegrade drilling of the lesion is then performed to introduce marrow elements and create a fibrocartilage healing response. Mosaicplasty is a technique of multiple osteochondral autograft transfer and is an alternative option for large OCD lesions of the capitellum.[52] Advantages of mosaicplasty include ready availability of donor cartilage-bone plugs, ability to cover defects of varying size, and use of native hyaline cartilage containing active, mature chondrocytes.

Radiocapitellar Plica
Recently, lateral synovial plica in the elbow has been identified as a cause of lateral elbow pain. A report on the arthroscopic treatment of posterolateral elbow impingement resulting from synovial plicae involved 12 patients who were either throwers or golfers. All patients had posterolateral elbow pain, often with clicking or catching. All patients demonstrated a thickened, hypertrophic lateral synovial plica. Most patients had associated adjacent synovitis and capitellar and/or radial head chondromalacia. After a mean follow-up of 34 months, 11 patients reported an excellent outcome following resection of the plicae.[53]

Annotated References

1. DiGiovine NM, Jobe FW, Pink M, Perry J: An electromyographic analysis of the upper extremity in pitching. *J Shoulder Elbow Surg* 1992;1:15-25.

2. Fleisig GS, Andrews JR, Dillman CJ, Escamilla RF: Kinetics of baseball pitching with implications about injury mechanisms. *Am J Sports Med* 1995;23:233-239.

3. Mullaney MJ, McHugh MP, Donofrio TM, Nicholas SJ: Upper and lower extremity muscle fatigue after a baseball pitching performance. *Am J Sports Med* 2005;33:108-113.

   The authors report the effects of fatigue following a pitching performance on the strength of a variety of muscle groups as compared to baseline values. Decreased strength with shoulder internal rotation, flexion and adduction were noted. Minimal fatigue was seen with the empty can test and scapular stabilizers.

4. Levine WN, Brandon ML, Stein BS, Gardner TR, Bigliani LU, Ahmad CS: Shoulder adaptive changes in youth baseball players. *J Shoulder Elbow Surg* 2006;15:562-566.

   The change in glenohumeral range of motion in the dominant arm of 298 throwers stratified by age was studied. The authors noted a significant loss of internal rotation and gain in external rotation of the shoulder that begins in adolescence and progresses with age.

5. Crockett HC, Gross LB, Wilk KE: Osseous adaptation and range of motion at the glenohumeral joint in professional baseball pitchers. *Am J Sports Med* 2002;30:20-26.

6. Osbahr DC, Cannon DL, Speer KP: Retroversion of the humerus in the throwing shoulder of college baseball players. *Am J Sports Med* 2002;30:347-353.

7. Yamamoto N, Itoi E, Minagawa H, et al: Why is the humeral retroversion of throwing athletes greater in dominant shoulders than in nondominant shoulders? *J Shoulder Elbow Surg* 2006;15:571-575.

   In this clinical study, ultrasound was used to assess the degree of proximal humeral retroversion in 66 youth overhead throwing athletes. Increased proximal humeral retroversion was noted on the dominant side that was influenced by age. The authors theorize that the normal loss of retroversion with skeletal maturation is decreased in the dominant arm of throwers.

8. Grossman MG, Tibone JE, McGarry MH, Schneider DJ, Veneziani S, Lee TQ: A cadaveric model of the throwing shoulder: A possible etiology of superior labrum anterior-to-posterior lesions. *J Bone Joint Surg Am* 2005;87:824-831.

   Humeral head position in the late cocking phase of throwing was examined in a cadaver study. After creation of anterior capsular laxity and posterior contracture, increased external rotation and decreased internal rotation range of motion of the shoulder was noted. Slight posterosuperior migration of the humeral head was seen in the late cocking phase.

9. Burkhart SS, Morgan CD: The peel-back mechanism: Its role in producing and extending posterior type II SLAP lesions and its effect on SLAP repair rehabilitation. *Arthroscopy* 1998;14:637-640.

10. Burkhart SS, Morgan CD, Kibler WB: The disabled throwing shoulder: Spectrum of pathology. Part I: Pathoanatomy and biomechanics. *Arthroscopy* 2003;19:404-420.

11. Borsa PA, Wilk KE, Jacobsen JA, et al: Correlation of range of motion and glenohumeral translation in professional baseball pitchers. *Am J Sports Med* 2005;33:1392-1399.

    In a clinical study of 43 professional baseball pitchers demonstrating adaptive changes in rotational range of motion, there was no difference in passive humeral head translation between dominant and nondominant shoulders. The authors suggest that factors other than the glenohumeral capsule may create the observed altered rotational range of motion.

12. Borsa PA, Dover GC, Wilk KE, Reinhold MM: Glenohumeral range of motion and stiffness in professional baseball pitchers. *Med Sci Sports Exerc* 2006;38:21-26.

    In a clinical study of 34 professional baseball pitchers,

there was increased external rotation and decreased internal rotation range of motion of the dominant shoulder in comparison with the nondominant shoulder. There was no difference in the stiffness of the glenohumeral joint as measured by humeral head translation.

13. Cummins CA, Messer TM, Schafer MF: Infraspinatus muscle atrophy in professional baseball players. *Am J Sports Med* 2004;32:116-120.

    In a retrospective study of 1,491 asymptomatic professional baseball players, 4.4% of pitchers and 0.2% of position players were noted to have infraspinatus muscle atrophy on clinical examination.

14. Wright RW, Paletta GA: Prevalence of the Bennett lesion of the shoulder in major league pitchers. *Am J Sports Med* 2004;32:121-124.

    The authors report a series of 55 professional baseball pitchers evaluated with shoulder radiographs. Twenty-two percent were noted to have the presence of a Bennett lesion. There was no correlation to age or pitching history with the presence of the radiographic finding.

15. Kuhn JE, Bey MJ, Huston LJ, Blasier RB, Soslowsky LJ: Ligamentous restraints to external rotation of the humerus in the late-cocking phase of throwing: A cadaveric biomechanical investigation. *Am J Sports Med* 2000;28:200-205.

16. Ide J, Maeda S, Takagi K: Arthroscopic Bankart repair using suture anchors in athletes. *Am J Sports Med* 2004; 32:1899-1905.

    The authors present the results of a prospective study of 55 athletes with recurrent anterior instability treated with arthroscopic Bankart repair. Rowe score improved from 30 to 92 points. Four (7%) patients had recurrent instability. The recurrence rate for contact and noncontact athletes was similar. Sixty-eight percent of throwing athletes returned to previous sports activity, compared with 90% of nonoverhead throwing athletes. Level of evidence: IV.

17. Mazzocca AD, Brown FM, Carreira DS, Hayden J, Romeo AA: Arthroscopic anterior shoulder stabilization of collision and contact athletes. *Am J Sports Med* 2005;33:52-60.

    Outcomes following arthroscopic stabilization for anterior shoulder instability in 18 contact and collision athletes were retrospectively reviewed. Initial restoration of stability and return to sport rate was 100%. Two patients (11%) suffered recurrent instability.

18. Burkhart SS, DeBeer JF: Traumatic glenohumeral bone defects and their relationship to failure of arthroscopic Bankart repairs: Significance of the inverted-pear glenoid and the humeral engaging Hill-Sachs lesion. *Arthroscopy* 2000;16:677-694.

19. Kim SH, Ha KI, Park JH, et al: Arthroscopic posterior labral repair and capsular shift for traumatic unidirectional recurrent posterior subluxation of the shoulder. *J Bone Joint Surg Am* 2003;85:1479-1487.

20. Provencher MT, Bell SJ, Menzel KA, Mologne TS: Arthroscopic treatment of posterior shoulder instability: Results in 33 patients. *Am J Sports Med* 2005;33:1463-1471.

    Thirty-three patients were retrospectively reviewed following arthroscopic posterior stabilization at 39 months follow-up. There were seven failures (21%), four due to persistent pain and three patients with recurrent instability. Outcomes were worse in patients with voluntary instability and with revision surgery. Level of evidence: IV.

21. Bottoni CR, Franks BR, Moore JH, DeBerardino TM, Taylor DC, Arciero RA: Operative stabilization of posterior shoulder instability. *Am J Sports Med* 2005;33: 996-1002.

    Thirty-one patients were retrospectively reviewed following arthroscopic or open treatment of posterior shoulder instability. Good outcomes were noted in both groups in multiple outcome scales. The authors provide a good description of surgical technique and review the literature. Level of evidence: IV.

22. Bradley JP, Baker CL III, Kline AJ, Armfield DR, Chhabra A: Arthroscopic capsulolabral reconstruction for posterior instability of the shoulder. *Am J Sports Med* 2006;34:1061-1071.

    One hundred patients with unidirectional posterior instability were prospectively followed for 27 months after arthroscopic capsulolabral reconstruction. American Shoulder and Elbow Surgeons scores improved from 50 to 85 points. The results of athletes involved in contact sports were similar to those of other athletes, with 89% of athletes able to return to sports activity. Level of evidence: IV.

23. Kim SH, Ha KI, Yoo JC, Noh KC: Kim's lesion: An incomplete and concealed avulsion of the posteroinferior labrum in posterior or multidirectional posteroinferior instability of the shoulder. *Arthroscopy* 2004;20:712-720.

    The authors report a series of 15 patients with posterior shoulder instability with variable pathology of the posterior labrum. In all patients, hidden lesions of the posterior labrum were evident on careful inspection. These lesions appear as flattening of the posterior glenoid and loss of the normal labral height. Fourteen of 15 patients were successfully treated arthroscopically.

24. Kim SH, Noh KC, Park JS, Ryu BD, Oh I: Loss of chondrolabral containment of the glenohumeral joint in atraumatic posterior multidirectional instability. *J Bone Joint Surg Am* 2005;87:92-98.

    MRI evaluation of the osseous and chondrolabral anatomy of 33 patients with posteroinferior MDI of the shoulder was performed. Increased retroversion of the osseous and chondrolabral glenoid was noted in the middle and inferior glenoid compared with uninjured shoulders. Level of evidence: IV.

25. Gartsman GM, Roddey TS, Hammerman SM: Arthroscopic treatment of multidirectional glenohumeral instability: 2- to 5-year follow-up. *Arthroscopy* 2001;17: 236-243.

3: Upper Extremity

26. Kim SH, Kim HK, Sun J, Park JS, Oh I: Arthroscopic capsulolabroplasty for posterior multidirectional instability of the shoulder. *Am J Sports Med* 2004;32:594-607.

    The authors reported the results of 31 patients with posterior MDI of the shoulder treated with arthroscopic capsulolabroplasty. Variable posterior labral pathology was noted. Thirty of 31 patients had stable shoulders and good or excellent results (Rowe score). Level of evidence: IV.

27. Myers JB, Laudner KG, Pasquale MR, Bradley JP, Lephart SM: Glenohumeral range of motion deficits and posterior shoulder tightness in throwers with pathologic internal impingement. *Am J Sports Med* 2006;34:385-391.

    Eleven throwers with internal impingement were compared with 11 throwers without shoulder pain. The athletes with internal impingement were noted to have greater loss of internal rotation range of motion but similar external rotation motion compared with the throwers who did not have pain.

28. Mazoue CG, Andrews JR: Repair of full-thickness rotator cuff tears in professional baseball players. *Am J Sports Med* 2006;34:182-189.

    Results from a study of 16 professional baseball players were reviewed retrospectively following miniopen rotator cuff repair using double-row cuff fixation. Three of 16 (1 of 12 pitchers) were able to return to competitive play. Level of evidence: IV.

29. Pradhan RL, Itoi E, Hatakeyama Y, Urayama M, Sato K: Superior labral strain during the throwing motion: A cadaveric study. *Am J Sports Med* 2001;29:488-492.

30. Shepard MF, Dugas JR, Zeng N, Andrews JR: Differences in the ultimate strength of the biceps anchor and the generation of type II superior labral anterior posterior lesions in a cadaveric model. *Am J Sports Med* 2004;32:1197-1201.

    The strength of the superior labrum in the late cocking and deceleration phases of throwing was evaluated in a cadaver study. The biceps anchor/superior labrum was significantly weaker with a posterior directed load (late cocking) compared with in-line loading.

31. Yeh ML, Lintner D, Luo ZP: Stress distribution in the superior labrum during throwing motion. *Am J Sports Med* 2005;33:395-401.

    A finite element analysis of stress at the superior labrum and glenoid interface at various stages of throwing was performed. The stress magnitudes were greatest during the deceleration phase of throwing.

32. Parentis MA, Glousman RE, Mohr KS, Yocum LA: An evaluation of the provocative tests for superior labral anterior posterior lesions. *Am J Sports Med* 2006;34:265-268.

    A series of 132 patients were examined preoperatively and a final diagnosis was made arthroscopically. The most sensitive diagnostic tools for type II SLAP tears were the O'Brien, Hawkins, Speed, Neer, and Jobe relocation tests. The authors' results contradict the current literature regarding provocative testing SLAP tears. They conclude that there is no single test for accurate diagnoses of SLAP tears and arthroscopy remains the standard for diagnosis. Level of evidence: II.

33. Rhee YG, Lee DH, Lim CT: Unstable isolated SLAP lesion: Clinical presentation and outcome of arthroscopic fixation. *Arthroscopy* 2005;21:1099.

    The authors retrospectively reviewed the results of 44 patients following arthroscopic SLAP repair with suture anchors or absorbable tacks. Thirty-eight of 44 patients had good or excellent results (UCLA score) with 76% of athletes able to return to sports activities. Throwing athletes had better outcomes than nonthrowers. Level of evidence: IV.

34. Ide J, Maeda S, Takagi K: Sports activity after arthroscopic superior labral repair using suture anchors in overhead-throwing athletes. *Am J Sports Med* 2005;33:507-514.

    Forty athletes with a mean age of 24 years were reviewed 41 months following arthroscopic SLAP repairs using suture anchors. Ninety percent good and excellent results (Rowe score) were seen with 75% of athletes returning to previous sports activity. Sixty percent to 75% of baseball players returned to full sports activity. Level of evidence: IV.

35. Martin SD, Warren RF, Martin TL, Kennedy K, O'Brien SJ, Wickiewicz TL: Suprascapular neuropathy: Results of non-operative treatment. *J Bone Joint Surg Am* 1997;79:1159-1165.

36. Youm T, Matthews PV, El Attrache NS: Treatment of patients with spinoglenoid cysts associated with superior labral tears without cyst aspiration, debridement, or excision. *Arthroscopy* 2006;22:548-552.

    Results from a study of 10 patients with SLAP tears and spinoglenoid cysts treated with arthroscopic cyst decompression and labral repair were retrospectively reviewed. Successful results were seen in all patients. Suprascapular nerve recovery was seen in all patients with abnormal electrodiagnostic examinations preoperatively. Postoperative MRI showed cyst resolution in 80% of patients. Level of evidence: IV.

37. Schneider K, Kasparyan NG, Altchek DW, Fantini GA, Weiland AJ: An aneurysm involving the axillary artery and its branch vessels in a major league baseball pitcher: A case report and review of the literature. *Am J Sports Med* 1999;27:370-375.

38. Lester B, Jeong GK, Weiland AJ, Wickiewicz TL: Quadrilateral space syndrome: diagnosis, pathology, and treatment. *Am J Orthop* 1999;28:718-722.

39. Park MC, Ahmad CS: Dynamic contributions of the flexor-pronator mass to elbow valgus stability. *J Bone Joint Surg Am* 2004;86-A:2268-2274.

    Cadaver elbows were tested after creation of UCL insufficiency. Muscle forces were simulated based upon physiologic cross-sectional area. The flexor carpi ulnaris is the primary stabilizer and the flexor digitorum superficialis is a secondary stabilizer. The pronator teres provides the least dynamic stability.

40. Andrews JR, Timmerman LA: Outcome of elbow surgery in professional baseball players. *Am J Sports Med* 1995;23:407-413.

41. Kamineni S, Hirahara H, Pomianowski S, et al: Partial posteromedial olecranon resection: A kinematic study. *J Bone Joint Surg Am* 2003;85-A:1005-1011.

42. Kamineni S, ElAttrache NS, O'Driscoll SW, et al: Medial collateral ligament strain with partial posteromedial olecranon resection: A biomechanical study. *J Bone Joint Surg Am* 2004;86-A:2424-2430.

An electromagnetic tracking device was used to investigate the strain in the anterior bundle of the UCL following posteromedial resection of the olecranon in cadaveric elbows. The strain in the anterior bundle of the UCL was found to increase with olecranon resection beyond 3 mm, suggesting local bone resection may jeopardize the anterior UCL.

43. Ahmad CS, Park MC, Elattrache NS: Elbow medial ulnar collateral ligament insufficiency alters posteromedial olecranon contact. *Am J Sports Med* 2004;32:1607-1612.

Cadaver elbows were tested with tears of the medial UCL. Pressure-sensitive film was placed in the posteromedial elbow compartment. UCL insufficiency was found to alter contact area and pressure between the posteromedial trochlea and olecranon, which helps explain the development of posteromedial osteophytes.

44. Fleisig GS, Kingsley DS, Loftice JW, et al: Kinetic comparison among the fastball, curveball, change-up, and slider in collegiate baseball pitchers. *Am J Sports Med* 2006;34:423-430.

Twenty-one healthy collegiate pitchers were studied with a high-speed automated digitizing system. Elbow varus torque was greater in the fastball and curveball than in the change-up, suggesting that the change-up poses the least risk of injury.

45. Ellenbecker TS, Mattalino AJ, Elam EA, Caplinger RA: Medial elbow joint laxity in professional baseball pitchers: A bilateral comparison using stress radiography. *Am J Sports Med* 1998;26:420-424.

46. Sasaki J, Takahara M, Ogino T, Kashiwa H, Ishigaki D, Kanauchi Y: Ultrasonographic assessment of the ulnar collateral ligament and medial elbow laxity in college baseball players. *J Bone Joint Surg Am* 2002;84-A:525-531.

47. Rettig AC, Sherrill C, Snead DS, Mendler JC, Mieling P: Nonoperative treatment of ulnar collateral ligament injuries in throwing athletes. *Am J Sports Med* 2001;29:15-27.

48. Conway TE, Jobe FW, Glousman RE, Pink M: Medial instability of the elbow in throwing athletes: Treatment by repair or construction of the ulnar collateral ligament. *J Bone Joint Surg Am* 1992;74:67-83.

49. Thompson WH, Jobe FW, Yocum LA, Pink MM: Ulnar collateral ligament reconstruction in athletes: Muscle-splitting approach without transposition of the ulnar nerve. *J Shoulder Elbow Surg* 2001;10:152-157.

50. Dodson CC, Thomas A, Dines JS, Nho SJ, Williams RJ 3rd, Altchek DW: Medial ulnar collateral ligament reconstruction of the elbow in throwing athletes. *Am J Sports Med* 2006;34:1926-1932.

One hundred consecutive overhead throwing athletes were treated with UCL reconstruction using the docking technique. The ulnar nerve was transposed in 22 patients. The mean follow-up was 36 months. Ninety of 100 patients (90%) were able to compete at the same or a higher level. Level of evidence: IV.

51. Paletta GA Jr, Wright RW: The modified docking procedure for elbow ulnar collateral ligament reconstruction: 2-year follow-up in elite throwers. *Am J Sports Med* 2006;34:1594-1598.

The authors retrospectively reviewed 25 elite baseball players who underwent UCL reconstruction using the modified docking procedure with a four-strand palmaris graft. Twenty-three of 25 (92%) returned to their preinjury levels of competition. Complications included one transient postoperative ulnar nerve neurapraxia and one stress fracture of the ulnar bone bridge. Level of evidence: IV.

52. Nakagawa Y, Matsusue Y, Ikeda N, Asada Y, Nakamura T: Osteochondral grafting and arthroplasty for end-stage osteochondritis dissecans of the capitellum: A case report and review of the literature. *Am J Sports Med* 2001;29:650-655.

53. Kim DH, Gambardella RA, Elattrache NS, Yocum LA, Jobe FW: Arthroscopic treatment of posterolateral elbow impingement from lateral synovial plicae in throwing athletes and golfers. *Am J Sports Med* 2006;34:438-444.

Twelve patients with lateral synovial plica and posterolateral elbow pain with a mean age of 21.6 years were reviewed. Fifty-eight percent reported clicking or catching, whereas only 25% experienced effusion. At arthroscopy, a thickened synovial lateral plica was débrided. Ninety-two percent reported an excellent outcome with a mean elbow score of 92.5 points. Return to competitive play averaged 4.8 months. Level of evidence: IV.

3: Upper Extremity

Chapter 23

Shoulder Trauma: Bone

Kenneth C. Lin, MD   *Sumant G. Krishnan, MD

Clavicle Fractures

Mechanism of Injury

The clavicle is the bony "strut" connecting the appendicular upper extremity to the axial skeleton. As such, the bony morphology of the clavicle provides minimal ability to deform under supraphysiologic stress. Clavicle fractures in the adult are most commonly caused by a fall on an outstretched arm or by a direct blow. Because neurovascular structures (brachial plexus, subclavian vessels) run in close proximity, displaced fractures of the clavicle can lead to injury to these structures.

Presentation

Patients with acute clavicle fractures classically present with ecchymosis surrounding the clavicle and proximal shoulder girdle, often demonstrate bony deformity or prominence, sometimes present with skin abrasions from the incipient trauma, and nearly always demonstrate ptosis of the involved shoulder in the acute setting. Because this injury typically is associated with high-energy trauma (and because of the protective mechanism that the clavicle provides to the underlying brachial plexus and subclavian vessels), associated injuries, including other injuries to the shoulder girdle, must be assessed during initial evaluation. Assessment of neurovascular status as well as skin compromise or impending compromise should also be performed. The presence of such concomitant injuries may indicate the need for surgical intervention

Radiographic Evaluation and Classification

The diagnosis of a clavicle fracture is typically apparent on AP radiographs of the shoulder or even of the chest (Figure 1). For complete evaluation, a true AP view of the clavicle plus a 30° cephalic tilt view allow for biplanar assessment of the bony deformity. A shoulder girdle view is often helpful in determining shortening of the clavicle. Similarly, a serendipity view (as described by Rockwood) can be used to evaluate medial clavicular injuries and concomitant displacement of the sternoclavicular articulation. Though not routinely used, CT may be useful in special situations, such as for evalua-

tion of medial clavicular physeal fractures and sternoclavicular fracture-dislocations. The commonly used Allman classification broadly groups such fractures by location in the proximal, middle, or distal thirds of the clavicle, with middle third fractures being the most common.

Treatment

The treatment of clavicle fractures continues to evolve. Most of these fractures are treated nonsurgically; however, the role of surgery in preventing the not-insignificant potential morbidity associated with these fractures continues to expand.

Middle Third (Midshaft) Clavicle Fractures

Fractures of the middle third of the clavicle are the most common (up to 81% of all clavicle fractures), and bony union is usually achieved uneventfully without surgery. A prospective observational cohort study found the nonunion rate of diaphyseal fractures of the clavicle to be 4.5%, which is consistent with previous reports.[1] Significant risk factors for nonunion were age, female gender, fracture displacement, and comminution.

Recent literature has examined not only bony union of these fractures, but also malunion and its associated morbidity. Most clavicle fractures treated nonsurgically will heal with some degree of malunion. In a study of

*Sumant G. Krishnan, MD, or the department with which he is affiliated has received research or institutional support and royalties from Tornier.

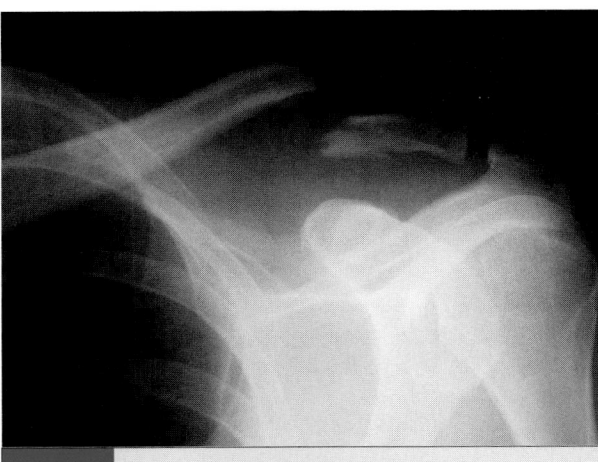

Figure 1   AP radiograph of a clavicle fracture. (Courtesy of Sumant G. Krishnan, MD, The Carrell Clinic.)

3: Upper Extremity

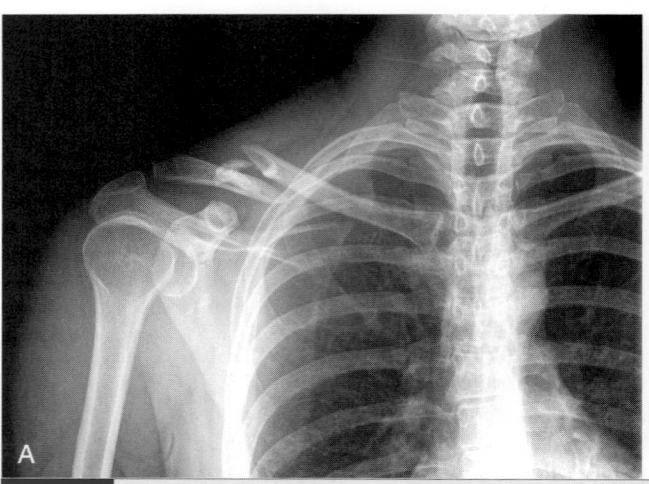
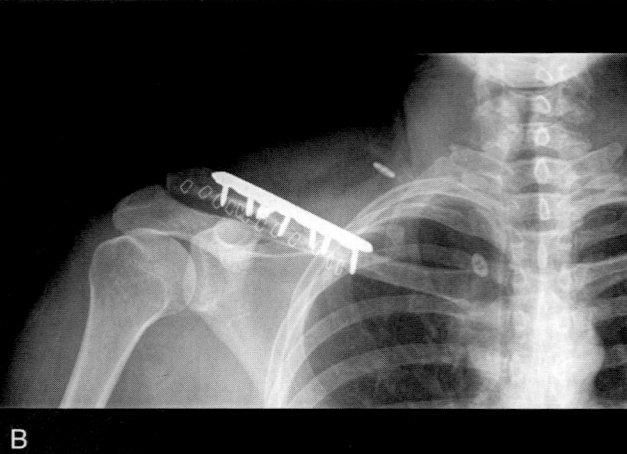

Figure 2   **A,** Preoperative AP radiograph of a clavicle fracture. **B,** Postoperative AP radiograph of a clavicle fracture treated with plate fixation. *(Courtesy of Sumant G. Krishnan, MD, The Carrell Clinic.)*

1,430 adult skeletons, 73 fractures of the clavicle were noted; 54 of these were malunited.[2] Thirty-six of the 73 fractured clavicles had shortening greater than 1 cm.

Clavicle malunions previously were believed to be clinically insignificant. However, recent literature has challenged this concept and the conventional wisdom that nonsurgical therapy with likelihood of malunion and/or nonunion yields universally good results. Although nonunion is relatively rare, the incidence of morbidity secondary to malunion is more significant than previously believed. In a recent study, 208 patients with clavicle fractures treated nonsurgically were prospectively evaluated. At follow-up 9 to 10 years after initial injury, 46% of patients still did not consider themselves fully recovered from their fracture.[3] Nine percent of patients had pain at rest whereas 29% had pain with activity. Fracture displacement without bony contact was found to be the most predictive indicator of fracture sequelae.

In another recent study, 30 patients who had been treated nonsurgically for a displaced midshaft clavicle fracture were retrospectively reviewed. Constant scores and disabilities of the arm, shoulder, and hand (DASH) scores for these patients continued to show significant residual disability even at a mean of 55 months after injury.[4] A higher prevalence of patient dissatisfaction was reported when shortening was greater than 2 cm than when shortening was less than 2 cm. This finding corroborates with previous reports that fractures with more than 2 cm of shortening are associated with poorer outcomes. Objective strength and endurance deficits in the shoulders of patients treated nonsurgically for displaced clavicle fractures were also found when comparisons were made with the uninjured, contralateral shoulder.

The literature continues to expand the understanding of midshaft clavicle fractures and the risk factors for not only nonunion but also disability with malunion. A multitude of surgical fixation techniques

exist, each with reported good results. However, because most clavicle fractures are treated nonsurgically with good to excellent results, the challenge is identifying those fractures at risk for poor results. Increased shortening of the fractured clavicle has been correlated with an increased risk of poor results and the few studies in the peer-reviewed literature appear to support consideration for surgical reduction and fixation for fractures with more than 2 cm of shortening, minimal bony contact, segmental fracture, and/or a transversely displaced butterfly fragment. Classic surgical management for middle third clavicle fractures has been plate fixation for open reduction and internal fixation (ORIF) of clavicle fractures. Standard dynamic compression plates have now progressed to locking plate variations. Either standard 3.5-mm locking dynamic compression plates or specific precontoured clavicle locking plates are currently available and have been used with success. Because the clavicle lies in a subcutaneous position, the least prominent position for a plate is the superior aspect of the clavicle (Figure 2). Plates placed anterior require greater contouring and negatively affect the deltoid and pectoralis muscle origins.

Intramedullary fixation of the acute clavicle fracture has continued to gain popularity. Such fixation is less invasive than plate fixation and involves less periosteal stripping to obtain reduction and fixation. Special differentially threaded pins have been developed for clavicle fixation. However, simplified surgical techniques using a 6.5-mm cannulated screw have been used with success (Figure 3).

Risk factors for malunion and nonunion have been described previously. Surgical management usually involves plate fixation with autologous (either local or iliac crest) bone graft. In a 2003 study, a clavicular osteotomy along with internal fixation and local bone graft were used to treat symptomatic, shortened clavicle nonunions.[5] Of 15 patients studied, high satisfac-

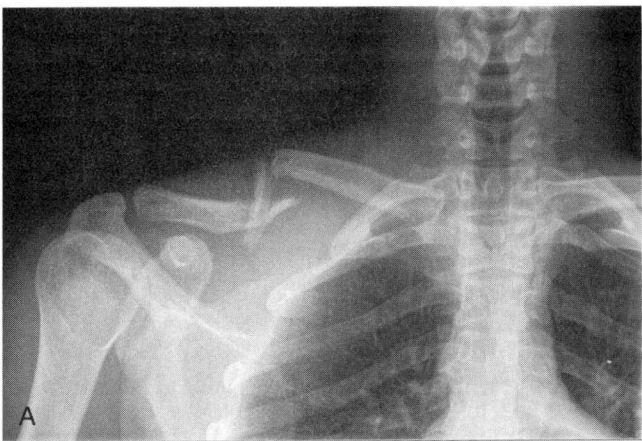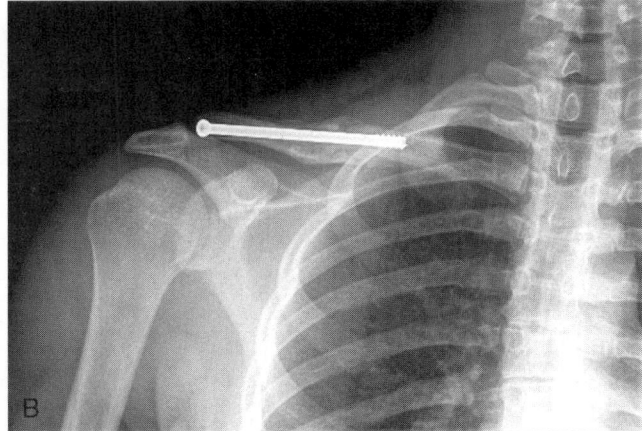

Figure 3 **A,** Preoperative AP radiograph of a clavicle fracture. **B,** Postoperative AP radiograph of a clavicle fracture treated with intramedullary fixation with a 6.5-mm cannulated screw. *(Courtesy of Sumant G. Krishnan, MD, The Carrell Clinic.)*

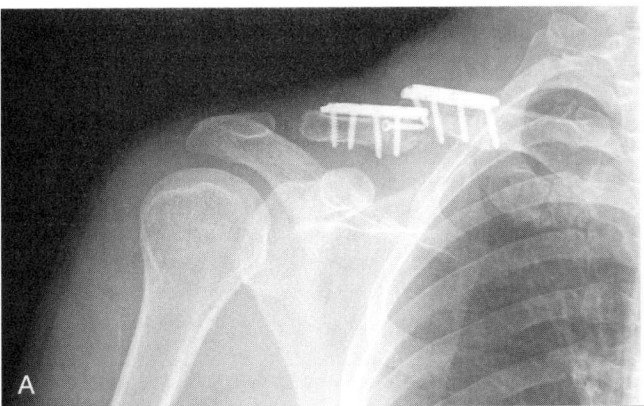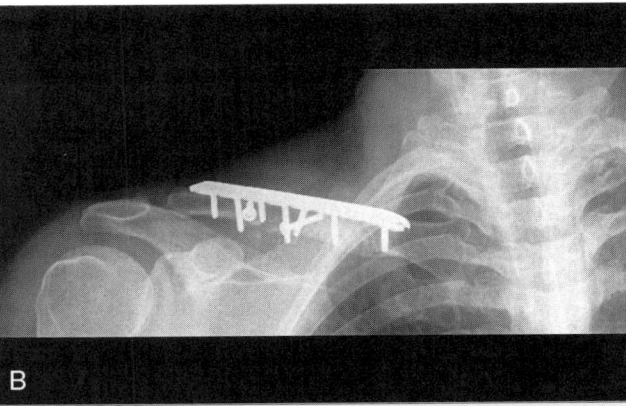

Figure 4 **A,** Preoperative AP radiograph of a clavicle fracture nonunion. **B,** Postoperative AP radiograph of a clavicle fracture nonunion treated with plate fixation and intercalary iliac crest bone graft. *(Courtesy of Sumant G. Krishnan, MD, The Carrell Clinic.)*

tion rates were reported, with 100% of those who had preoperative weakness and pain having some improvement of their symptoms and 66% of the patients having complete resolution of their symptoms at a mean of 20 months follow-up. Mean DASH scores also showed improvement, dropping from a preoperative score of 32 to 12 postoperatively.

Intercalary iliac crest grafts with plate fixation for severe shortening have been successful (Figure 4). Although intramedullary fixation holds promise for the treatment of nonunions, restoration and maintenance of clavicular length is more difficult with intramedullary devices. Vascularized bone transfer from the medial femoral condyle has been used as a salvage procedure for recalcitrant nonunions.

Distal Third Clavicle Fractures
Distal third clavicle fractures represent approximately 15% of all clavicle fractures. The Neer classification of distal clavicle fractures takes into account fracture loca-

tion relative to the coracoclavicular ligaments and the acromioclavicular (AC) joint and is indicative of fracture stability. Type I fractures are interligamentous and are therefore only minimally displaced as both the proximal and distal fragments continue to be stabilized by the coracoclavicular ligaments. Type II fractures occur medial to the coracoclavicular ligaments. They are subdivided into type IIA and type IIB fracture patterns. In type IIA fractures, both the conoid and trapezoid remain attached to the distal fragment. In type IIB, either the conoid is torn or both the conoid and trapezoid are torn. In both instances, the end result is that the proximal fragment is no longer stabilized by the coracoclavicular ligaments and the distal fragment tends to be displaced inferiorly by the downward pull of the arm. These are the fracture patterns that tend to be displaced and are associated with delayed union and nonunion rates of 30% to 45%. Type III fractures extend into the articular surface of the AC joint with no ligamentous injury and tend to be stable.

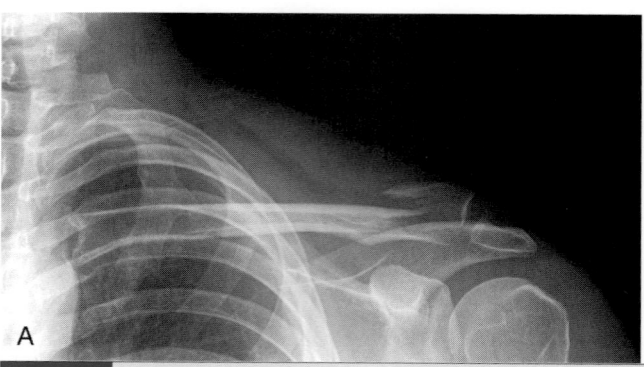
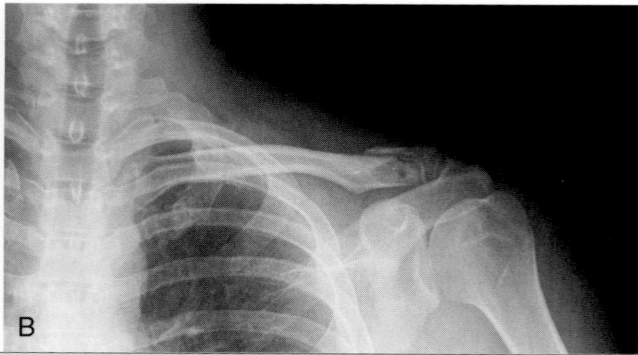

Figure 5 **A,** Preoperative AP radiograph of a distal clavicle fracture. **B,** Postoperative AP radiograph of a distal clavicle fracture stabilized with coracoclavicular and AC reconstruction using autologous hamstring tendon graft. *(Courtesy of Sumant G. Krishnan, MD, The Carrell Clinic.)*

Fractures of the distal clavicle that are displaced are associated with higher rates of nonunion and delayed union. Although nondisplaced fractures can be treated nonsurgically with a sling and early mobilization, displaced fractures have typically been candidates for surgical intervention. One recent study, however, has reported good results with primary nonsurgical treatment of displaced distal clavicle fractures.[1] One hundred twenty-seven patients who had been treated nonsurgically for their distal clavicle fracture were retrospectively identified; 86 of 127 were available for assessment at an average of 6.2 years after injury. This cohort included 57 type IIA fractures, 33 type IIB fractures, and 11 type III fractures. Most patients had good results with an average Constant score of 93 points (range, 82 to 98 points), although 14% of patients eventually required surgery for significant symptoms. This study also found equally good Constant scores in those treated nonsurgically in comparison with those whose surgery was delayed. Nevertheless, surgical fixation of displaced distal clavicle fractures should be considered given their propensity for nonunion, delayed union, and residual disability.

Many methods of surgical stabilization have been described, such as plate fixation, trans-AC joint wire fixation, and coracoclavicular screw fixation. However, the often comminuted nature of these fractures as well as the subcutaneous position of the distal clavicle can lead to prominence of and discomfort with metallic implants. Primary suture fixation of the fracture fragments with absorbable suture as well as suture stabilization to the coracoid and/or acromion have been successful. New techniques using autologous hamstring tendon grafts to "bypass" the fracture via coracoclavicular and AC stabilization have also demonstrated promise in the surgical management of these challenging injuries (Figure 5).

Medial Third Clavicle Fractures

The medial clavicular physis is the final physis to close in the bony skeleton, usually between the ages of 18 to 25 years. Often, medial third clavicle fractures are actually physeal fracture-dislocations, usually in a posterior direction. Although these injuries are quite rare (2% to 3% of all clavicle fractures), airway and great vessel compromise must be assessed during the management considerations for this injury. Serendipity radiographic views (as described by Rockwood) and CT evaluation can be helpful aids in decision making. Posteriorly displaced fractures should be managed surgically. Closed reduction under anesthesia is often unsuccessful. If surgical stabilization of the fracture is required, at minimum a thoracic surgeon should be on standby for assistance if significant interference with the vasculature occurs. Fixation methods usually include suture fixation of the fracture to the rhomboid (costoclavicular ligament) ligament with sternoclavicular joint stabilization and/or autologous graft reconstruction of the sternoclavicular joint after fracture reduction.

Scapula Fractures

Mechanism of Injury

Because of the relative protection afforded by the soft tissue and muscle envelope surrounding the scapula, as well as its position against the posterior thoracic cage, fractures of the scapula are relatively uncommon and represent only 3% to 5% of all shoulder girdle fractures. When these fractures do occur, they often result from significant, high-energy trauma. Consequently, there should be a high index of suspicion for associated injuries, such as pulmonary injury, ipsilateral rib fractures, and ipsilateral upper extremity injury, that can occur from 85% to 90% of the time.

Presentation

As previously mentioned, most patients with scapular fractures present to the emergency department after high-energy trauma. Full physical evaluation for associated injury (especially head, chest, abdominal, and pelvic injury) is mandatory. Because of the high incidence of associated ipsilateral rib fracture, physical examina-

3: Upper Extremity

tion of the involved shoulder can be extremely difficult in patients with an acute scapular fracture. Nevertheless, a complete neurovascular examination must not be ignored, because of the extent of injuries from high-energy trauma.

Radiographic Evaluation and Classification

Although plain radiographs from a standard trauma series are mandatory, the most important radiographic examination after scapular fracture is a CT scan. CT evaluation can help determine displacement and angulation, which are important considerations in the management of these fractures.

Scapular fractures are usually divided first according to location: scapular body, glenoid neck, glenoid fossa, coracoid process, and acromion. Glenoid fossa fractures are further subclassified via the modified Ideberg classification depending on location within the fossa and associated scapular body involvement. Type I fractures involve the glenoid rim. Type II fractures involve the superior 30% to 50% of the glenoid surface with the coracoid. Types III, IV, and V fractures involve the lateral border of the scapula, and type VI fractures are severely comminuted. This classification scheme can be useful in determining nonsurgical versus surgical management.

Treatment

Generally, good results can be expected with nonsurgical care. The long-term results of fractures of the scapular body, scapular neck, and scapular spine treated nonsurgically have been studied.[6] At 10- to 20-year follow-up, 25% of patients had some residual disability, although it was reported to be slight to moderate. When fracture types were examined independently, patients with scapular neck fractures had 32% fair or poor results; patients with scapular body fractures had 22% fair to poor results. This difference in outcomes may be because the scapulothoracic articulation is more tolerant of deformity than the glenohumeral articulation.

Glenoid Neck Fractures

Fractures of the glenoid neck usually occur as a result of direct trauma. Although these fractures are extra-articular, they can cause morbidity as the mechanics of the glenohumeral joint are altered. The deforming force is typically the long head of the triceps, which tends to displace the glenoid inferiorly and laterally. In a 2005 study, nine patients who had been treated nonsurgically for their extra-articular glenoid neck fractures were clinically evaluated 1 year after their initial injury; all had some degree of pain.[7] In an older study, 50% of patients with displaced scapular neck fractures treated nonsurgically had residual pain, 40% had weakness, and 20% had decreased range of motion.[8] Based on these results, surgery was recommended for patients with greater than 40° of angulation and greater than

1 cm of medial translation; however, these recommendations were theoretically based. In the 2005 study, it was noted that all patients studied fell below the criteria established in the older study and therefore would have been recommended for nonsurgical management. Nonetheless, 100% of these patients had residual pain and 33% had residual weakness. Surgical stabilization requires large surgical approaches that will result in scarring and loss of motion. Hence, the indications for surgery and the results of surgery versus nonsurgical treatment remain poorly defined.

In general, ORIF of the glenoid neck and/or scapular body will likely involve some sort of posterior approach to the shoulder to apply plate fixation (usually 3.5-mm reconstruction plate fixation) (Figure 6). If the fracture is an isolated glenoid neck fracture, a modified posterior approach using the subdeltoid plane is quite helpful. The skin incision for this approach is an extended posterior axillary fold incision, usually performed with the patient in the lateral decubitus position. With the arm abducted 90°, the deltoid relaxes and can be retracted superiorly. The interval between the infraspinatus and teres minor can now be developed and used. If further inferior extension is necessary, the interval between teres minor and teres major can also be exploited—taking care to avoid the quadrangular space and the axillary nerve and posterior humeral circumflex artery.

For complex glenoid neck and/or scapular body fractures, a Judet approach is most utilitarian. In this approach, the skin incision parallels the scapular spine and the medial border of the scapula. The deltoid can be detached from the scapular spine, and the infraspinatus is reflected laterally on its neurovascular pedicle. This muscle "take-down" approach provides excellent access to the entire scapula and may avoid the incidence of heterotopic ossification that often accompanies muscle splitting approaches to the scapula. The morbidity of this approach is, however, not insignificant and will result in scarring and permanent alteration of rotator cuff muscle function. Use of this exposure should be undertaken with caution.

Glenoid Fossa Fractures

Intra-articular glenoid fractures are believed to result from an impaction of the humeral head against the glenoid from a medially directed force. As described previously, glenoid fractures are classified by location of the fracture on the glenoid face and resultant extension into the scapular body. As in other joints, articular incongruity with such fractures raises concerns about posttraumatic degenerative arthrosis and associated pain and disability. Subluxation and articular step-off are cited as indications for surgical reduction and fixation. Good results were reported for 10 displaced intra-articular fractures treated with ORIF.[9] (Nondisplaced fractures with displacement less than 2 mm were treated with immobilization and early physical therapy.) In the surgically treated patients, at an average of

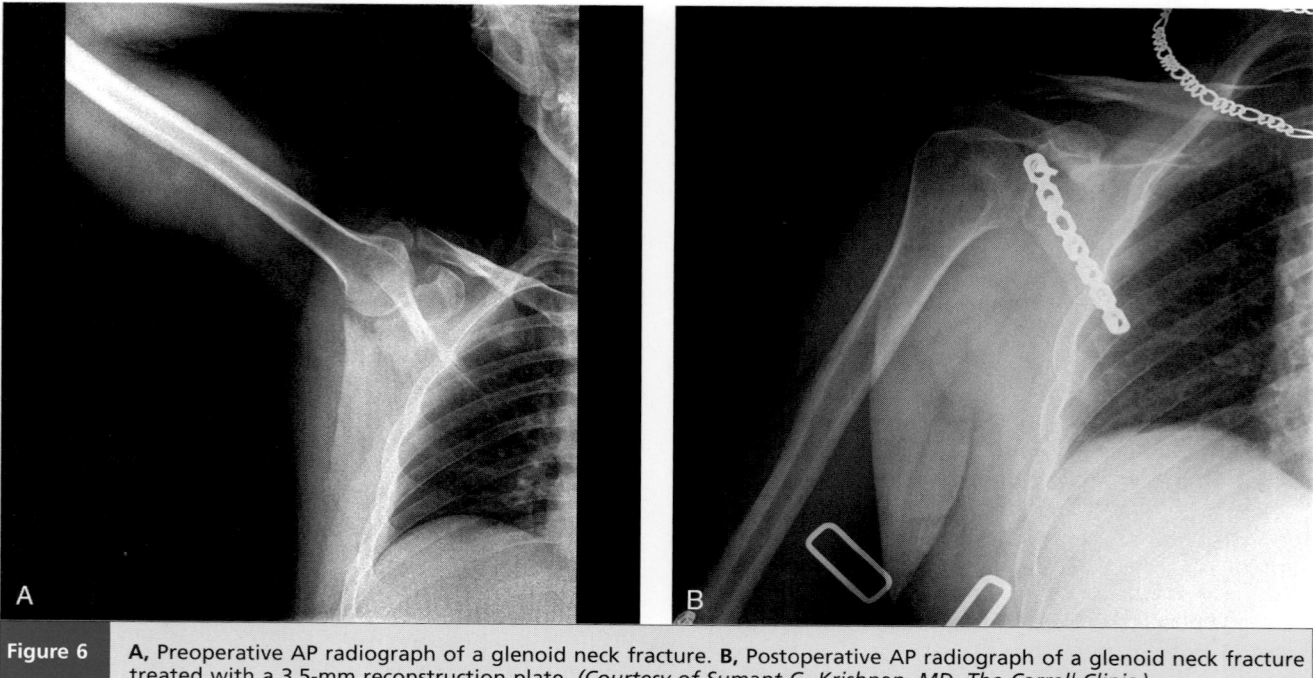

Figure 6 **A,** Preoperative AP radiograph of a glenoid neck fracture. **B,** Postoperative AP radiograph of a glenoid neck fracture treated with a 3.5-mm reconstruction plate. *(Courtesy of Sumant G. Krishnan, MD, The Carrell Clinic.)*

4 years after initial injury, there was no radiographic evidence of osteoarthritis in any of the patients. None of the patients had pain with daily activities and range of motion and strength were only mildly affected. Despite these good results, the authors of the study noted that the approach used for this procedure involved extensive dissection, and postoperative physical therapy was prolonged, making careful patient selection paramount.

Depending on location, intra-articular glenoid fractures can be surgically managed with percutaneous fluoroscopically assisted and/or arthroscopically assisted methods or with conventional open plate and/or screw fixation. The surgical approach is dictated by location, with anterior fractures approached (if done with open surgery) through a deltopectoral approach and posterior fractures fixed through a modified axillary-based intermuscular interval approach as described previously. Percutaneous methods, while attractive, remain technically challenging in the treatment of these complex injuries.

Combined Injuries and Floating Shoulder Injuries

Although shoulder injuries may occur in isolation, combined injuries present a special challenge. The clavicular shaft with associated ipsilateral scapular neck fracture (or "floating shoulder") is one such combination that has received special attention. Whereas separately these injuries can be treated nonsurgically with expectation of good results, this pattern of injury in combination has been traditionally believed to be un-

stable and surgical treatment is recommended. The superior shoulder suspensory complex may help conceptualize this injury.[10] The shoulder is described as a ring of stability created by both soft tissue and bony elements. The superior shoulder suspensory complex includes the glenoid, coracoid, distal clavicle, acromion, and coracoclavicular and AC ligaments. A double disruption of this ring is considered unstable. The floating shoulder injury pattern represents one such double disruption. Fixation of at least one component of the double disruption (often the clavicle injury) may stabilize the other element.

Management of Floating Shoulder Injuries

The clinical results of surgically and nonsurgically treated floating shoulder injuries were retrospectively evaluated at an average of 35 months after injury.[11] Good results were noted with both surgical as well as nonsurgical treatment, with Constant scores of 76 and 71, respectively. Of 28 patients treated nonsurgically, 6 had fracture displacement caudally at the end of treatment that correlated with a substantially lower average Constant score of 42 in these patients. It was concluded that although fracture displacement does correlate with inferior outcomes, floating shoulders are not all inherently unstable and some can be successfully treated nonsurgically. Ideally, those fractures with a propensity to displace would be treated with surgical fixation.

The underlying biomechanics of instability in floating shoulder injuries were studied in a cadaver model.[12] The combination of a scapular neck fracture with a clavicle fracture resulted in a 31% decrease in shoulder stability. It was not until both the coracoacromial ligaments and the AC capsular ligaments were sectioned that complete instability resulted. Complete instability resulted only when both coracoacromial and coracoclavicular ligaments were sectioned in combination with scapular neck and clavicle fractures. The ability to diagnose these ligamentous injuries would therefore be helpful in predicting which of these injuries are unstable and will displace with nonsurgical treatment. However, diagnostic parameters either by physical examination or radiographic examination of such ligamentous disruption remains to be established.

Proximal Humerus Fractures

Mechanism of Injury

Proximal humerus fractures represent 4% to 5% of all fractures and are the most common fractures of the shoulder girdle. In a review of all fractures treated in a single hospital over a 1-year period, proximal humerus fractures accounted for 53% of all significant shoulder girdle injuries.[13] Most of these fractures are the result of a fall. There is a 2:1 female-to-male distribution, and increasing age has been shown to correlate with increasing fracture risk in women, suggesting an association with osteoporosis. Fractures of the humerus represent the third most common fracture in the elderly, with only hip fractures and Colles fractures being more common. According to a study of patients age 60 years and older who were treated primarily for a proximal humerus fracture from 1970 to 2002, the incidence of proximal humeral fractures in the elderly has been increasing in recent decades, although the underlying cause for this trend is not clear.[14]

Presentation

The shoulder is often extremely swollen after a proximal humeral fracture. Often, ecchymosis tracks down the arm and into the chest. Because most patients with proximal humeral fractures are elderly, assessment for concomitant injuries is paramount. Head injuries from the fall, cardiac or neurologic reasons for the fall, and other fractures are often first diagnosed at the initial evaluation for the shoulder injury.

Electromyographic evaluation has demonstrated that approximately 67% of all patients with proximal humeral fractures suffer acute neurologic injury.[15] Most commonly, either the axillary nerve and/or the suprascapular nerve is involved. Appreciation and documentation of this finding is important for both prognostic evaluation as well as appropriate management of the injury.

Radiographic Evaluation and Classification

Initial radiographic evaluation consists of a Neer trauma series with AP, scapular Y, and axillary views. Because of the anatomy of the proximal humerus it may be difficult to appreciate fracture lines and fragment displacement. If plain radiographs do not offer adequate visualization, a CT scan with reconstructions may be necessary.

Neer's four-part classification system of proximal humerus fractures has endured by virtue of its simplicity. It allows for a conceptual understanding of the fracture pattern by defining the fracture into separate parts. Interobserver reliability and intraobserver reproducibility, however, has been reported to be only poor to fair. A "comprehensive binary" description of fractures based on Codman's original concept of fracture planes rather than fracture parts was described in a recent study.[16] These fracture planes run along the old physeal lines of the proximal humerus. The system results in 12 possible fracture patterns: 6 patterns resulting in 2 fracture fragments, 5 patterns resulting in 3 fracture fragments, and 1 pattern resulting in 4 fracture fragments. This system has demonstrated improved interobserver reliability as well as better intraobserver reproducibility.

Treatment

Fracture treatment has been traditionally guided by Neer's concept of fracture parts with treatment tailored to the characteristics of each individual fracture. Nondisplaced or Neer one-part fractures represent 85% of fractures of the proximal humerus. For these fractures, nonsurgical management with initial immobilization (usually for 3 to 6 weeks) followed by early passive then active range of motion is the gold standard of treatment. Treatment of displaced fractures is more controversial. With significant fracture displacement the risk of nonunion, malunion, and avascularity significantly increases. Anatomic recreation of the native anatomy is certainly the ideal of treatment. When the native anatomy is not salvageable, primary shoulder arthroplasty is considered.

When considering ORIF versus arthroplasty for proximal humeral fractures, the question of humeral head viability is paramount. One hundred intracapsular fractures of the proximal humerus were prospectively evaluated for perfusion.[16] Perfusion was assessed intraoperatively by observation of backflow through a centrally placed borehole in the humeral head as well as by intraosseous laser Doppler. This assessment was then correlated with preoperative radiographs. The results of this study demonstrated that ischemia of the humeral head correlated with posteromedial metaphyseal extension of less than 8 mm and disruption of the medial hinge defined as displacement of the humeral shaft greater than 2 mm. These two preoperative findings in combination with an anatomic neck fracture resulted in a 97% positive predictive value for humeral head ischemia.

Surgical Techniques for Fixation

When the humeral head is deemed viable and fracture fixation is attempted, many methods of fracture fixation are available, each with inherent advantages and disadvantages. Percutaneous fixation can be performed with minimal soft-tissue stripping and devascularization (Figure 7). Twenty-seven three- and four-part

3: Upper Extremity

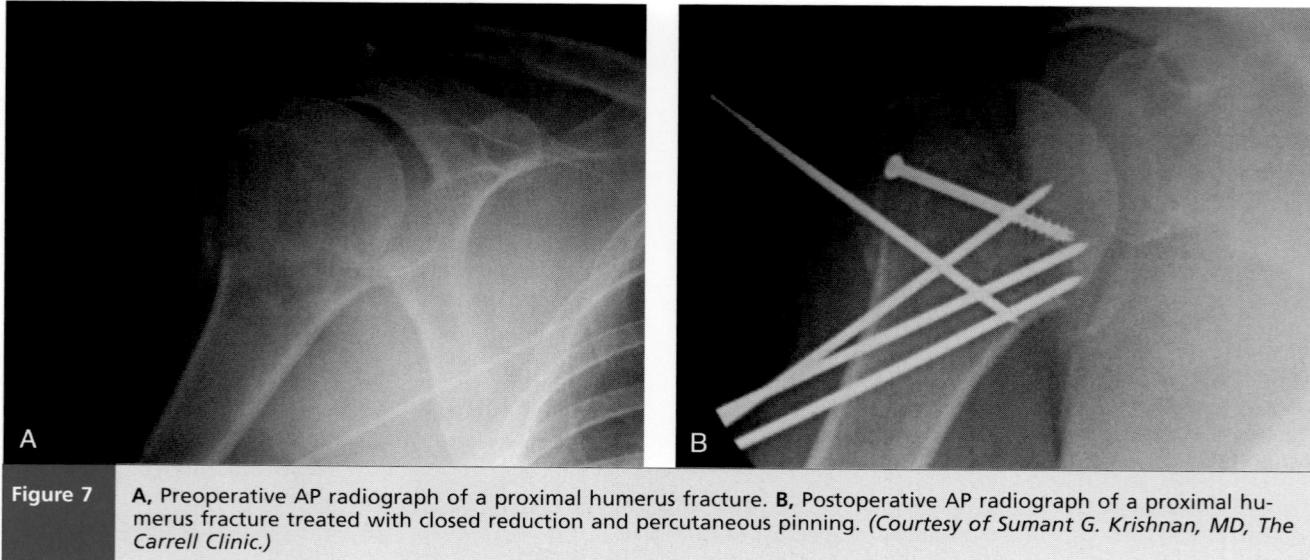

Figure 7   **A,** Preoperative AP radiograph of a proximal humerus fracture. **B,** Postoperative AP radiograph of a proximal humerus fracture treated with closed reduction and percutaneous pinning. *(Courtesy of Sumant G. Krishnan, MD, The Carrell Clinic.)*

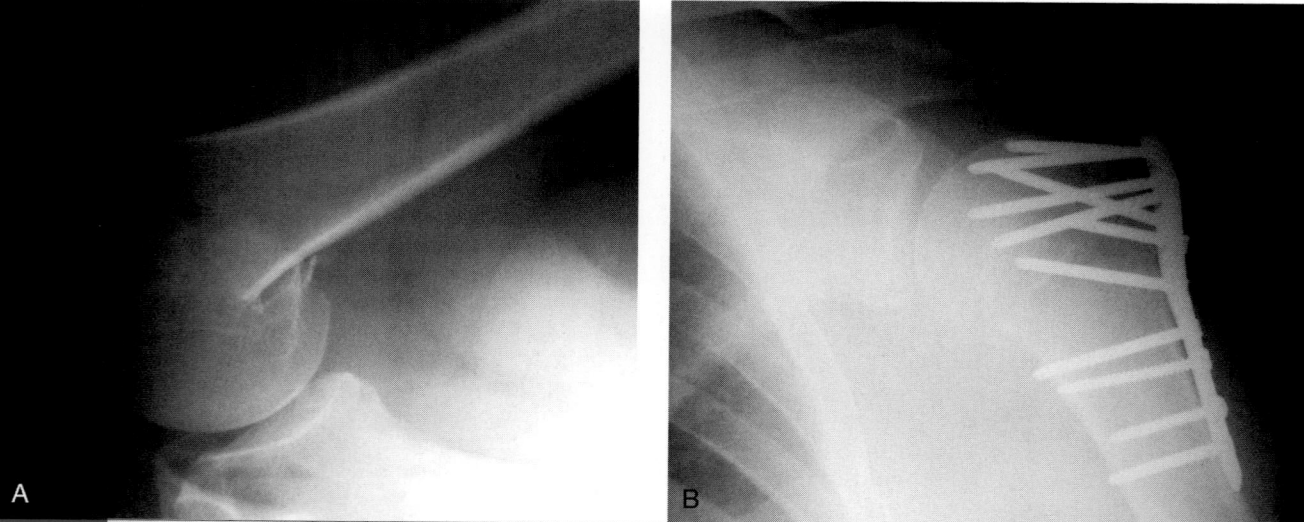

Figure 8   **A,** Preoperative AP radiograph of a proximal humerus fracture. **B,** Postoperative AP radiograph of a proximal humerus fracture treated with locked plating technique. *(Courtesy of Sumant G. Krishnan, MD, The Carrell Clinic.)*

proximal humerus fractures were treated with percutaneous pin fixation, with good to very good results in all three-part fractures at an average 24-month follow-up.[17] Results from the patients with four-part fractures were not as good, with 2 of the 18 patients eventually requiring revision to a prosthesis, one patient because of osteonecrosis and another because of displacement. The direct exposure used for proximal humeral plating allows for potentially greater control of and ability to manipulate individual fracture fragments into anatomic alignment (Figure 8). This direct exposure comes at the cost of soft-tissue stripping, which may lead to complications, and in osteoporotic bone adequate fixation may be difficult. Recent advances in plate designs such

as the proximal humeral locking plates have renewed interest in this treatment option. In a cadaver study, improved resistance to torsion in locking plate constructs was shown when compared with fixed-angle blade plates in fixation of three-part proximal humerus fractures.[18] These differences were particularly pronounced in osteoporotic specimens. Intramedullary nails designed for proximal humeral fixation remain enticing but current designs still demonstrate higher postoperative dissatisfaction rates with reports of rotator cuff pain and dysfunction. Hence, no single technique can be universally applied.

Primary hemiarthroplasty for fractures of the proximal humerus can result in good patient satisfaction and

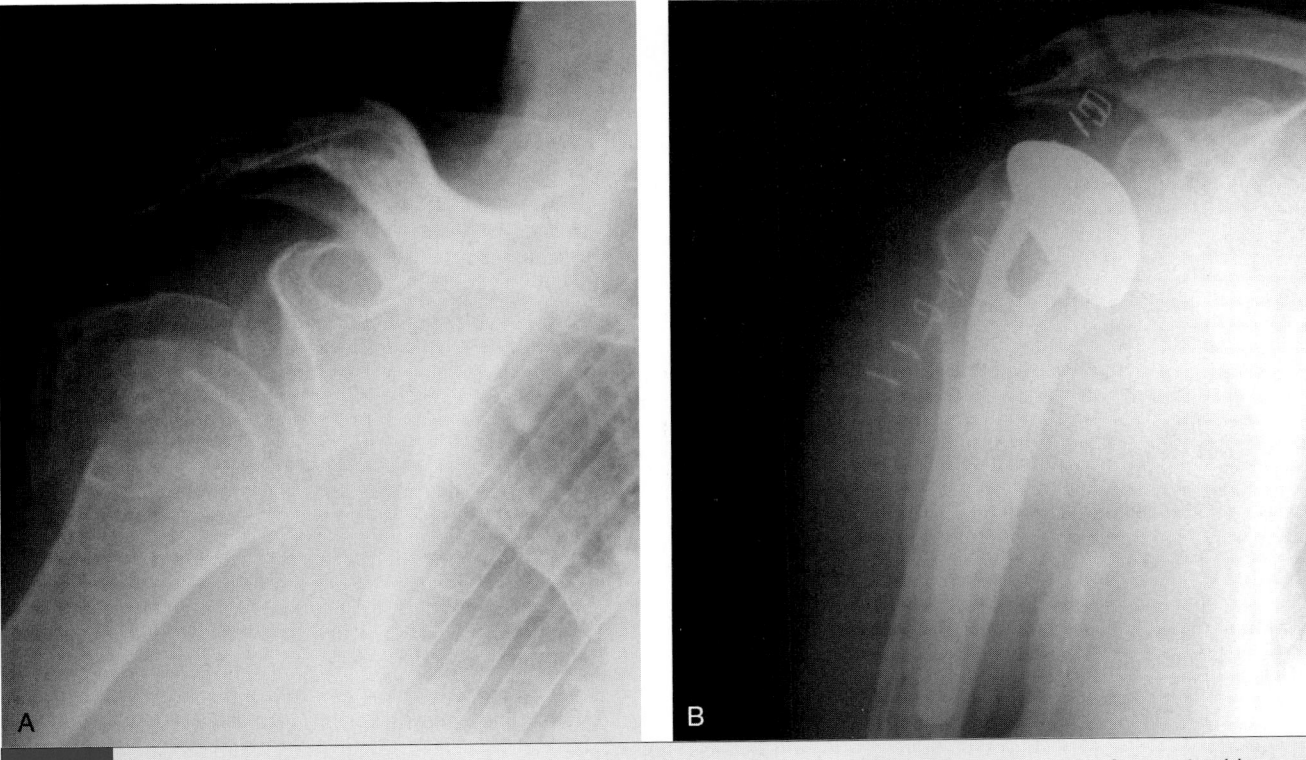

Figure 9 **A,** Preoperative AP radiograph of a proximal humerus fracture. **B,** Postoperative AP radiograph of a proximal humerus fracture treated with proximal humeral hemiarthroplasty. *(Courtesy of Sumant G. Krishnan, MD, The Carrell Clinic.)*

pain relief when ORIF is not possible (Figure 9). In one study, 66 patients were reviewed, with minimum 2-year follow-up after hemiarthroplasty for a proximal humerus fracture.[19] Ninety-three percent of patients were pain free and satisfied with their results. Similarly, other authors have also demonstrated successful pain relief but poorer functional outcomes when compared with replacement arthroplasty performed for osteoarthritis.

Recent work has highlighted the importance of intraoperatively restoring anatomic humeral height, humeral version, and tuberosity reconstruction to improve outcomes after arthroplasty for shoulder fracture. The importance of anatomic repositioning of the tuberosities when performing hemiarthroplasty for proximal humeral fracture was demonstrated in a cadaver study.[20] In cadaver shoulder specimens, four-part proximal humerus fractures were created and repaired with a shoulder hemiarthroplasty in which the tuberosities were intentionally positioned either anatomically or nonanatomically. The biomechanical effects of this tuberosity positioning demonstrated that anatomic repositioning of the tuberosities around a shoulder hemiarthroplasty produced external rotation kinematics identical to the native shoulder. When the tuberosities were malpositioned, however, an eightfold increase in torque was required to achieve the same degree of external rotation. Another study of 66 patients documented that failure to recreate proximal humeral anatomy when treating proximal humerus fractures with hemiarthroplasty can have negative clinical consequences.[21] In this retrospective study of patients treated with hemiarthroplasty, radiographic evidence of final tuberosity malpositioning correlated with poor functional results. Malpositioning of the prosthesis itself in turn correlated with tuberosity malposition. The "unhappy triad," defined as when a prosthesis not only has excessive height but also is in excessive retroversion and the greater tuberosity has been positioned too low, was identified. This combination of findings was associated with poor functional results, persistent pain, and stiffness. It is clear from these studies that careful attention to the recreation of proximal humeral anatomy is critical in shoulder fracture arthroplasty.

Current surgical techniques emphasize that, after standard deltopectoral exposure and identification of the fracture planes and tuberosities, the humeral prosthetic head should be placed approximately 3 to 5 mm above the tip of the anatomically reduced greater tuberosity fragment. Humeral version is selected via the technique of Neer: the forearm is pointed straight ahead in neutral position and the humeral head is turned to face the glenoid (approximately 20° of retroversion relative to the transepicondylar axis of the elbow). The tuberosities are rigidly fixed with horizontal cerclage suture fixation around the medial neck of the prosthetic stem as well as with vertical tension-band suture fixation through drill holes in the humeral shaft.

This reproducible technique allows for recreation of the "gothic arch" of the shoulder girdle and minimizes potential technical errors in prosthetic placement and tuberosity osteosynthesis.

After arthroplasty for fracture, pejorative factors associated with poor outcomes include tuberosity malpositioning/malunion/nonunion, and surgery more than 3 weeks after injury. According to a study of 39 consecutive hemiarthroplasties performed for proximal humerus fractures, the best predictor of outcome was time to surgery.[22] Outcomes were inversely proportional to length of time to surgery with early surgery (< 4 weeks) resulting in much better outcomes when compared to late surgery (> 4 weeks). In patients with chronic shoulder arthroplasty, results were inferior compared with acute fracture management.[23]

Role of Arthroscopy

In a series of 80 fractures and fracture-dislocations of the proximal humerus, arthroscopy was performed to evaluate soft-tissue injuries.[24] Significant soft-tissue injury to the rotator cuff, labrum, and capsuloligamentous structures is often underappreciated. Others have described arthroscopically assisted treatment of greater tuberosity fractures and even arthroscopically assisted reduction of four-part fracture-dislocations with percutaneous fixation in case reports. No large studies are available and the role of arthroscopy continues to be defined in the minimally invasive treatment of these injuries.

Proximal Humeral Nonunion and Malunion

Nonunion of the proximal humerus is relatively uncommon but when it does occur tends to involve the surgical neck or the greater tuberosity. The deforming forces acting on the fragments contribute to this tendency toward nonunion. Malunion is another difficult complication of proximal humerus fractures that can result from failure of either primary surgical or nonsurgical treatment. Shoulder arthroplasty for the treatment of late sequelae of proximal humerus fractures has been used with caution because of high complication rates and unpredictable results.[25] These concerns were first noted by Neer and have subsequently been confirmed by other authors.

Given the poor results of arthroplasty with surgical neck nonunions and greater tuberosity severe malunion/nonunions, shoulder arthroplasty is not recommended in these cases. The successful treatment of surgical neck nonunions with an intramedullary peg bone graft and ORIF has been described in the literature.[26] A low-profile fracture stem is added if humeral head replacement is necessary because of severe osteoarthritis or head cavitation. For severe tuberosity nonunions, a reverse total shoulder arthroplasty is currently recommended, although the indications for this implant in fracture sequelae situations are still being defined.

Humeral Shaft Fracture

Mechanism of Injury

Humeral shaft fractures are relatively rare and represent approximately 3% of all fractures. They can be isolated injuries or occur in multiple-trauma patients. When associated with multiple-trauma, a thorough examination based on Advanced Trauma Life Support protocols should be performed along with a thorough examination of the injured extremity. The mechanism and associated energy of the trauma should help guide the assessment.

Presentation

Patients may present with obvious deformity and pain of the extremity. Careful evaluation including evaluation of the skin and neurovascular status should be performed. Radial nerve palsies occur in up to 18% of closed injuries. Actual transection of the radial nerve is uncommon and is associated with open injuries. In closed injuries (90% of all injuries), radial nerve palsies are most commonly the result of a neurapraxia with anticipated recovery in 3 to 4 months. A retrospective review of 24 patients with radial nerve palsies associated with a high-energy diaphyseal fracture of the humerus was done.[27] Eleven patients had open fractures that were explored immediately; at surgery, six were found to have a transected radial nerve, and five of these patients had primary repair. None of these patients had recovery of radial nerve function. Of the remaining patients (both those with explored and unexplored injuries) all but one experienced recovery of nerve function. Given the low probability with closed injuries of transection, and the poor results of primary repair, routine exploration of radial nerve palsies is not recommended.

Radiographic Evaluation

Two views of the humerus allow for biplanar evaluation of the fracture. Dedicated views of the shoulder as well as the elbow should be obtained for appropriate evaluation of the joints both proximal and distal to the fracture. Transverse fracture patterns have been associated with higher rates of nonunion because of the potential development of angular deformity.

Management

Nonsurgical, functional bracing remains the gold standard of treatment with high success rates and low complication rates. In a 2000 study, 620 patients were identified who had sustained a humeral shaft fracture between 1978 and 1990.[28] Nonunion rates of less than 2% for closed injuries and 6% for open injuries were noted. Varus malunion is a potential complication, but 87% of patients went on to heal with less than 16° of varus. Eighty-one percent of patients had healing with less than 16° of anterior angulation. Ultimately, in 98% of the patients, the degree of limitation in their shoulder function was less than 25%. In a later study of 67 fractures, 58 were successfully treated with functional bracing, with 95% good to excellent results.[29] A slightly higher rate of treatment failure was observed; 13.4% required subsequent surgical intervention. Alignment is considered acceptable with approximately 20° of anterior angulation, 30° of varus angulation, and/or 3 cm of shortening.

Despite the high success rate of functional bracing, indications for surgical treatment include pathologic fracture, fracture with associated vascular or neurologic injury, multiple-trauma and/or associated ipsilateral upper extremity fracture, and failure of nonsurgical treatment. Any patient who will require nursing care that would be severely compromised by nonsurgical management should be considered for surgery. Surgical treatment options include external fixation, plate fixation, and intramedullary fixation. Intramedullary fixation has been associated with higher rates of nonunion and functional disability because of persistent subacromial and rotator cuff related symptoms, although conclusive studies directly comparing plate and intramedullary fixation are still unavailable.

Surgical Techniques for Fixation

Osteosynthesis with locking plate fixation has become the most widely accepted method for surgical treatment of acute humeral shaft fractures, with union rates exceeding 95%. Controversy exists regarding the surgical approach (posterior, lateral, and/or anterolateral) and is largely determined by both fracture location and surgeon comfort. Fixation with both 4.5 mm large-fragment plates as well as 3.5 mm small-fragment plates have been described. Plate fixation necessitates more soft-tissue dissection although radial nerve complications are less than with intramedullary approaches.

Closed intramedullary nailing of humeral shaft fractures via either antegrade or retrograde approaches has appeal from the standpoint of less invasive handling of the traumatized tissues. Unfortunately, the incidence of nonunion and even radial nerve injury has been reported to be equal to (5% to 6%) or even higher with intramedullary nailing techniques. Antegrade devices that violate the rotator cuff for insertion have an unacceptably larger proportion of patients (16% to 37%) with persistent subacromial symptoms even after nail removal. Locking flexible nails for humeral shaft fractures have been described. Implants such as these attempt to reduce complications related to violation of the rotator cuff either by their lateral antegrade insertion entry point or by virtue of a retrograde insertion. In one study, 5 complications in 4 of 41 patients at mean 22-month follow-up treated with such a device were reported.[30] These complications included two nonunions, two hardware failures, and one wound infection. Closed nailing appears to have greatest merit in the treatment of pathologic fractures, segmental fractures, and for those with severe skin compromise.

Nonunion

Nonunion rates in both surgically and nonsurgically treated humeral shaft fractures have been reported to be from 8% to 12%. Appropriate treatment requires an understanding of the mechanical and biologic factors involved. Good results in 15 patients with atrophic nonunions of the humeral shaft with wave-plate osteosynthesis and cancellous autograft were described.[31] In this study, at 30 months, only one fracture failed to unite. Good results were also reported in a study of 6 patients treated in this manner who had previously undergone fixation with intramedullary nailing.[32] The use of wave-plate osteosynthesis with commercially available demineralized bone matrix instead of autograft showed comparable results while avoiding associated iliac crest donor site morbidity.[33] Successful treatment of four atrophic nonunions of the humeral shaft with an anterior plate, iliac crest bone graft, and a vascularized fibular bone graft was reported.[34] The patients in this study had one to five previous unsuccessful surgical attempts to achieve union. All achieved union with this procedure at an average of 27 months' follow-up. In another study, either fresh frozen allograft fibula or autograft fibula placed within the intramedullary canal and a compression plate were used.[35] Eight of nine patients healed at an average of 3.5 months. Allograft fibula placed as an additional "bone plate" combined with metallic plate fixation and autologous cancellous bone graft continues to show good results. Newer techniques of vascularized and bone graft from the medial femoral condyle also show promise.

Annotated References

1. Robinson CM, Court-Brown CM, McQueen MM, Wakefield AE: Estimating the risk of nonunion following nonoperative treatment of a clavicular fracture. *J Bone Joint Surg Am* 2004;86:1359-1365.

   In this case series of 127 patients with displaced lateral clavicle fracture, 120 were treated nonsurgically and 7 treated surgically. Of the patients contacted, 14% had delayed surgical intervention for significant symptoms and 21% had fracture nonunion. No significant differences in Constant scores or Medical Outcomes Study 36-Item Short Form were found between those patients who had union of their fracture, those patients who experienced nonunion of their fracture, and those who had delayed or primary surgery for their fracture.

2. Edelson JG: The bony anatomy of clavicular malunions. *J Shoulder Elbow Surg* 2003;12:173-178.

3. Nowak J, Holgersson M, Larsson S: Can we predict long-term sequelae after fractures of the clavicle based on initial findings? A prospective study with nine to ten years of follow-up. *J Shoulder Elbow Surg* 2004;13: 479-486.

   In this prospective study of 245 clavicle fractures treated nonsurgically, 208 were available for examination at 9- to 10-year follow-up. Forty-six percent of patients did

3: Upper Extremity

not consider themselves recovered from their fracture. (This defined the primary end point of "sequelae.") Nonunion had occurred in 7% of patients. The factor most predictive for sequelae was lack of bony contact.

4. McKee MD, Pedersen EM, Jones C, et al: Deficits following nonoperative treatment of displaced midshaft clavicular fractures. *J Bone Joint Surg Am* 2006;88: 35-40.

Thirty patients with displaced midshaft distal clavicle fractures were retrospectively identified and examined at a minimum of 12 months (mean, 55 months) after their injury. Significant residual disability was detected on patient-based Constant and DASH scores. Although range of motion was well maintained, residual deficits in strength and endurance were found on objective measurement.

5. McKee MD, Wild LM, Schemitsch EH: Midshaft malunions of the clavicle. *J Bone Joint Surg Am* 2003; 85:790-797.

6. Nordqvist A, Petersson C: Fracture of the body, neck, or spine of the scapula: A long-term follow-up study. *Clin Orthop Relat Res* 1992;283:139-144.

7. Pace AM, Stuart R, Brownlow H: Outcome of glenoid neck fractures. *J Shoulder Elbow Surg* 2005;14:585-590.

A clinical evaluation was performed 1 year after injury for 9 patients with extra-articular glenoid fractures treated nonsurgically. Although patient satisfaction was high, 100% residual pain as well as 33% residual weakness was observed.

8. Ada JR, Miller ME: Scapular fractures: Analysis of 113 cases. *Clin Orthop Relat Res* 1991;269:174-180.

9. Kavanagh BF, Bradway JK, Cofield RH: Open reduction and internal fixation of displaced intra-articular fractures of the glenoid fossa. *J Bone Joint Surg Am* 1993;75:479-484.

10. Goss TP: Double disruptions of the superior shoulder suspensory complex. *J Orthop Trauma* 1993;7:99-106.

11. van Noort A, te Slaa RL, Marti RK, van der Werken C: The floating shoulder: A multicentre study. *J Bone Joint Surg Br* 2001;83:795-798.

12. Williams GR Jr , Naranja J, Klimkiewicz J, Karduna A, Iannotti JP, Ramsey M: The floating shoulder: A biomechanical basis for classification and management. *J Bone Joint Surg Am* 2001;83:1182-1187.

13. Nordqvist A, Petersson CJ: Incidence and causes of shoulder girdle injuries in an urban population. *J Shoulder Elbow Surg* 1995;4:107-112.

14. Palvanen M, Kannus P, Niemi S, Parkkari J: Update in the epidemiology of proximal humeral fractures. *Clin Orthop Relat Res* 2006;442:87-92.

Data from the National Hospital Discharge Register of all patients 60 years of age and older admitted to Finnish hospitals between 1970 and 2002 and treated primarily for proximal humeral fractures were reviewed. Overall there was an increasing age-adjusted incidence of proximal humerus fractures.

15. Visser CP, Coene LN, Brand R, Tavy DL: Nerve lesions in proximal humeral fractures. *J Shoulder Elbow Surg* 2001;10:421-427.

16. Hertel R, Hempfing A, Stiehler M, Leunig M: Predictors of humeral head ischemia after intracapsular fracture of the proximal humerus. *J Shoulder Elbow Surg* 2004;13: 427-433.

One hundred intracapsular fractures of the proximal humerus were evaluated intraoperatively for humeral head perfusion and then correlated with preoperative radiographic findings. Good predictors of humeral head ischemia included medial metaphyseal head extension less than 8 mm and loss of integrity of the medial hinge (as measured by greater than 2 mm medial or lateral displacement). The presence of these two findings in the presence of an anatomic neck fracture gave a 97% positive predictive value for humeral head ischemia.

17. Resch H, Povacz P, Frohlich R, Wambacher M: Percutaneous fixation of three- and four-part fractures of the proximal humerus. *J Bone Joint Surg Br* 1997;79:295-300.

18. Weinstein DM, Bratton DR, Ciccone WJ II, Elias JJ: Locking plates improve torsional resistance in the stabilization of three-part proximal humeral fractures. *J Shoulder Elbow Surg* 2006;15:239-243.

Torsional strength of a proximal locking plate construct was compared with that of a blade plate construct in a cadaver model.

19. Mighell MA, Kolm GP, Collinge CA, Frankle MA: Outcomes of hemiarthroplasty for fractures of the proximal humerus. *J Shoulder Elbow Surg* 2003;12:569-577.

20. Frankle MA, Greenwald DP, Markee BA, Ondrovic LE, Lee WE III: Biomechanical effects of malposition of tuberosity fragments on the humeral prosthetic reconstruction for four-part proximal humerus fractures. *J Shoulder Elbow Surg* 2001;10:321-326.

21. Boileau P, Krishnan SG, Tinsi L, Walch G, Coste JS, Mole D: Tuberosity malposition and migration: Reasons for poor outcomes after hemiarthroplasty for displaced fractures of the proximal humerus. *J Shoulder Elbow Surg* 2002;11:401-412.

22. Bosch U, Skutek M, Fremerey RW, Tscherne H: Outcome after primary and secondary hemiarthroplasty in elderly patients with fractures of the proximal humerus. *J Shoulder Elbow Surg* 1998;7:479-484.

23. Antuna SA, Sperling JW, Sanchez-Sotelo J, Cofield RH: Shoulder arthroplasty for proximal humeral nonunions. *J Shoulder Elbow Surg* 2002;11:114-121.

24. Schai PA, Hintermann B, Koris MJ: Preoperative arthroscopic assessment of fractures about the shoulder. *Arthroscopy* 1999;15:827-835.

25. Boileau P, Trojani C, Walch G, Krishnan SG, Romeo A, Sinnerton R: Shoulder arthroplasty for the treatment of the sequelae of fractures of the proximal humerus. *J Shoulder Elbow Surg* 2001;10:299-308.

26. Walch G, Badet R, Nove-Josserand L, Levigne C: Nonunions of the surgical neck of the humerus: Surgical treatment with an intramedullary bone peg, internal fixation, and cancellous bone grafting. *J Shoulder Elbow Surg* 1996;5:161-168.

27. Ring D, Chin K, Jupiter JB: Radial nerve palsy associated with high-energy humeral shaft fractures. *J Hand Surg Am* 2004;29:144-147.

    A review of 24 patients with radial nerve palsy associated with high-energy diaphyseal fracture of the humerus is presented. Radial nerve transection was associated with open fractures only and primary repair was associated with universally poor results.

28. Sarmiento A, Zagorski JB, Zych GA, Latta LL, Capps CA: Functional bracing for the treatment of fractures of the humeral diaphysis. *J Bone Joint Surg Am* 2000;82: 478-486.

29. Koch PP, Gross DF, Gerber C: The results of functional (Sarmiento) bracing of humeral shaft fractures. *J Shoulder Elbow Surg* 2002;11:143-150.

30. Stannard JP, Harris HW, McGwin G Jr, Volgas DA, Alonso JE: Intramedullary nailing of humeral shaft fractures with a locking flexible nail. *J Bone Joint Surg Am* 2003;85:2103-2110.

31. Ring D, Jupiter JB, Quintero J, Sanders RA, Marti RK: Atrophic ununited diaphyseal fractures of the humerus with a bony defect: Treatment by wave-plate osteosynthesis. *J Bone Joint Surg Br* 2000;82:867-871.

32. Gerber A, Marti R, Jupiter J: Surgical management of diaphyseal humeral nonunion after intramedullary nailing: Wave-plate fixation and autologous bone grafting without nail removal. *J Shoulder Elbow Surg* 2003;12: 309-313.

33. Hierholzer C, Sama D, Toro JB, Peterson M, Helfet DL: Plate fixation of ununited humeral shaft fractures: Effect of type of bone graft on healing. *J Bone Joint Surg Am* 2006;88:1442-1447.

    Delayed unions or nonunions of humeral shaft fractures treated with plate fixation and bone grafting were retrospectively reviewed. The use of autologous iliac crest bone graft or demineralized bone matrix gave equivalent healing rates and time to healing. However, the use of demineralized bone matrix avoided the complications of donor site morbidity.

34. Jupiter JB: Complex non-union of the humeral diaphysis: Treatment with a medial approach, an anterior plate, and a vascularized fibular graft. *J Bone Joint Surg Am* 1990;72:701-707.

35. Wright TW, Miller GJ, Vander Griend RA, Wheeler D, Dell PC: Reconstruction of the humerus with an intramedullary fibular graft: A clinical and biomechanical study. *J Bone Joint Surg Br* 1993;75:804-807.

3: Upper Extremity

Chapter 24

Shoulder Instability

*Joseph P. Burns, MD   *Stephen J. Snyder, MD

Natural History

Although many attempts have been made to clarify the natural history of traumatic anterior shoulder instability, several questions and philosophical differences of opinion remain. Patients age 22 years or younger with a first-time traumatic shoulder dislocation have a high rate of recurrent dislocation, ranging from 60% to 90%. The rate of recurrent dislocation decreases for patients in their 30s and 40s, but it is still significant, ranging from 50% to 64%. As patient age increases, the rate of associated rotator cuff tearing increases significantly, reaching approximately 15% for patients in their 40s and climbing to approximately 40% in patients older than 60 years.

Historically, rates of redislocation and resubluxation have been the primary measure of treatment failure or success—and therefore have been the primary mode of describing the natural history of shoulder instability. Because patient health status is affected by factors other than frank dislocation/subluxation, more attention is now being given to the impact that shoulder instability may have on the overall quality of life and participation in recreational activities. In a recently published analysis of the quality of life and postoperative sports activity of athletes with shoulder instability who were treated with open stabilization surgery, even though the clinical scoring results were good to excellent in all patients, quality of life and sports activity measures were significantly lower than they were at the preinjury state, suggesting that the degree of overall morbidity may be significantly greater than traditional outcome measures have described.[1] The true natural history of shoulder instability will be more accurately defined as future outcome measures evaluate effects on quality of life, sports activity, and patient satisfaction.

Joseph P. Burns, MD or the department with which he is affiliated has received miscellaneous nonincome support, commercially derived honoraria or other nonresearch-related funding from Mitek. Stephen J. Snyder, MD or the department with which he is affiliated has received royalties from Linvatec Wright Medical Technologies, Arthrex, Smith & Nephew, and DJ Ortho and is a consultant or employee for Linvatec Wright Medical Technologies and OBI.

Biomechanics

Several elements work together to create shoulder stability: the osseous concave/convex structures of the glenoid and humerus, the circumferential labrum, the capsuloligamentous complex, a slight negative intra-articular pressure, and an adhesive-cohesive relationship between the articular surfaces and synovial fluid. These combined elements allow the shoulder to maximize stability while providing a wide range of motion.

In patients with traumatic anteroinferior shoulder instability, avulsion of the labrum off the anteroinferior glenoid (Bankart lesion) is a common finding. It is still unknown whether this avulsion injury itself is sufficient to cause recurrent instability. Cadaver studies have been unsuccessful in reproducibly creating true Bankart lesions by inducing dislocations, and specimens in which isolated Bankart lesions have been manually created tend to maintain a high degree of stability. Complete excision of the labrum does decrease the depth of the glenoid socket by 50% and reduces resistance to instability by 20% in cadavers,[2] but there is likely some degree of capsular stretching that contributes to instability in patients with Bankart lesions of the labrum. Each subsequent traumatic anterior dislocation likely causes progressive damage to not only the soft tissues, but to osseous structures as well in the form of progressive glenoid rim erosion and enlarging humeral Hill-Sachs lesions.[3] Stability tends to decrease as these lesions worsen with multiple dislocations.

Patient Evaluation

History

When evaluating a patient for shoulder instability, the concepts of laxity and instability should be differentiated. Laxity is an objective measurement of joint mobility, whereas instability is the subjective symptomatology associated with excessive joint motion. Patients with hyperlaxity do not necessarily have instability. Without symptoms of discomfort, joint mobility should not necessarily be considered pathologic.

In patients who report symptoms of instability, the direction of the symptoms should be identified by history and physical examination. Patients will often be able to describe or demonstrate the position(s) of instability or injury, providing information about the direc-

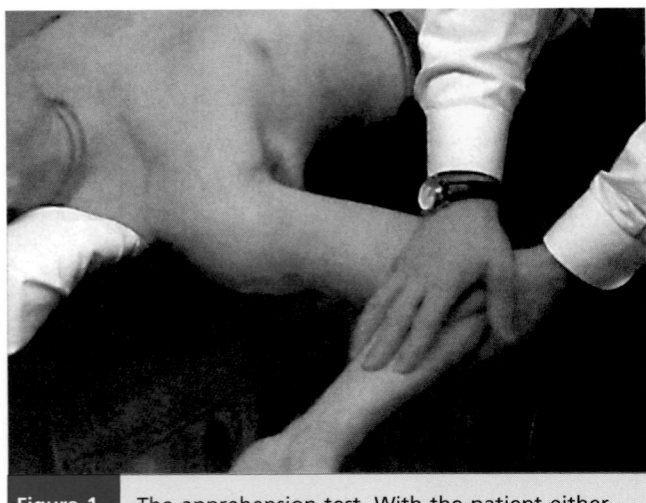

Figure 1 | The apprehension test. With the patient either supine or upright, the examiner gently externally rotates the humerus in 90° of abduction. Apprehension of subluxation signifies a positive test and is suggestive for anterior instability.

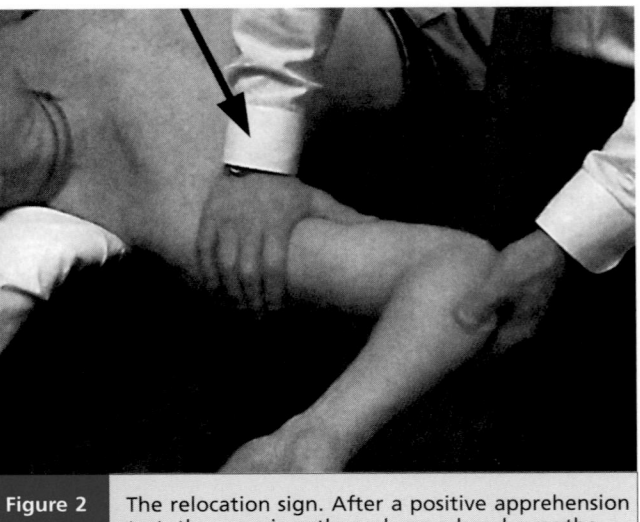

Figure 2 | The relocation sign. After a positive apprehension test, the examiner then places a hand over the proximal humerus and applies a firm posterior stabilizing force (arrow). The apprehension test is then repeated with gentle humeral external rotation. If the patient's apprehension improves, this is a positive test and is suggestive of anterior instability.

tion of excess motion and the location of capsulolabral pathology.

The number of episodes of instability is important because research has suggested that, for traumatic anteroinferior dislocations, the severity of soft-tissue and bony injury can increase with each subsequent dislocation.[4] There also seems to be some degree of capsuloligamentous stretching that occurs over the course of several dislocations. For patients with multidirectional instability who have general ligamentous laxity, however, there is often much less cumulative trauma to bone and soft tissues with multiple dislocations. This instability is usually less traumatic, and it is likely related to intrinsic differences in the collagen, joint volume, and possibly patient proprioception.

Physical Examination

Physical examination will provide important information about the direction of instability as well as the degree of instability. Active range of motion often will be normal. Fixed posterior dislocations commonly are missed because the AP radiographs of patients with this type of injury may appear nearly normal. Without a good axillary radiograph, the next best method to diagnose shoulder instability is to determine whether the patient lacks normal external rotation. The function of the axillary nerve and the rotator cuff should always be evaluated because associated injuries to these structures are relatively common after dislocation.[5]

Specific tests enable the physician to identify the pattern of instability, and the results of tests of the symptomatic shoulder and the asymptomatic shoulder are compared. The anterior apprehension test is used to evaluate anterior stability. Gentle, passive external rotation is performed with the patient's arm in 90° of abduction and the elbow flexed. Feelings of apprehension or instability signify a positive test result (Figure 1).

The diagnosis of anterior instability is then supported with a positive relocation test result. With the patient in the supine position, the examiner places a hand anteriorly on the patient's shoulder and provides a posterior stabilizing force to the humeral head as the arm is again externally rotated. If this support improves or relieves the patient's apprehension, it signifies a positive test result (Figure 2).

Posterior instability is evaluated by the jerk test. With the patient in the lateral position and the scapula stabilized, the affected shoulder is flexed forward, internally rotated, and then slowly retracted (not actually jerked) through the axial plane into abduction, applying a posterior force to the humerus. Apprehension or frank instability as the arm is retracted signifies a positive test result (Figure 3).

The sulcus sign evaluates inferior shoulder laxity and instability. With the arm at the side and the patient as relaxed as possible, a firm gradual downward force is applied to the humerus, and the gap between the acromion and humeral head is measured for laxity while the patient is monitored for symptoms of instability (Figure 4). The competence of the tissues of the rotator interval may be estimated by the effect of humeral external rotation on the sulcus sign. If the sulcus sign fails to improve with the arm in external rotation, the rotator interval may be incompetent and should be closely evaluated at surgery.

Patients should also be evaluated for the degree of generalized ligamentous laxity by checking the ability to touch the ipsilateral forearm with the thumb, place the palms of the hands on the floor with knees locked, and hyperextend the elbow, knee, and metacarpophalangeal joints.

Imaging

Radiographs are mandatory in the evaluation of shoulder instability. The axillary radiograph is of paramount importance because it may be the only view to confirm an obvious locked posterior dislocation. It will also provide information regarding the version and contour of the glenoid. Bony Bankart lesions may be better identified with a West Point view and Hill-Sachs lesions may be better identified with a Stryker notch view. A Zanca view of the acromioclavicular joint should also be obtained in the evaluation of acromioclavicular separations.

MRI is valuable in assessing labral and rotator cuff pathology, capsular volume, and even bony defects. Arthrography is not always necessary if the radiologist and surgeon are experienced, but it may provide a clearer understanding of the pathology in the evaluation of glenohumeral instability. Although CT may be beneficial for precise evaluation of bone loss, erosions, and version, better quality MRI scans are often sufficient.

Examination Under Anesthesia

Once the patient is in the operating room, a carefully planned examination under anesthesia should be performed on both the affected and unaffected shoulders. Laxity should be graded in anterior, posterior, and inferior directions. Because pathologic anatomy can often be difficult to identify during surgery, the examination under anesthesia can provide valuable decision-making information before the first incision is made.

Anterior Instability

Nonsurgical Treatment

Managing in-season athletes with traumatic anterior shoulder dislocations can be challenging because they need to minimize their time away from their sport but maximize their performance on the field. A recent study found that nonsurgical treatment of dislocation and subluxation allowed 26 of 30 athletes to return and complete their seasons after an average of 10.2 days.[6] Ten of the 26 (38%) had at least one additional episode of instability during the season, and 16 (61.5%) elected to have surgical stabilization in the subsequent off-season. In general, patients should have full strength and range of motion comparable with the contralateral side before returning to athletic participation. They should also be informed of the risks and possible sequelae of reinjury. Braces that prevent abduction and external rotation may help some athletes return to competition.

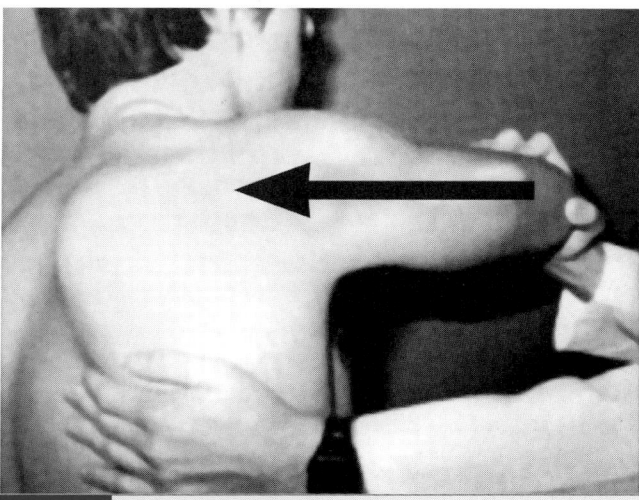

| Figure 3 | The jerk test. While stabilizing the scapula, the examiner applies a posterior force (arrow) to the elbow with the patient's arm flexed and internally rotated. Posterior subluxation may be appreciated by a palpable shift from a subluxated to a reduced state as the examiner moves the arm from a flexed to an abducted position. |

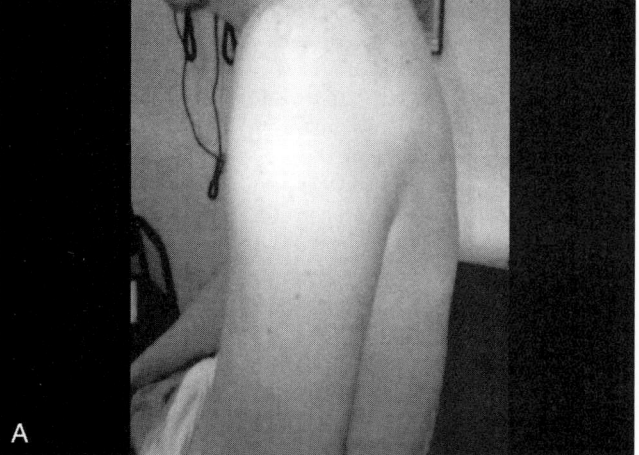
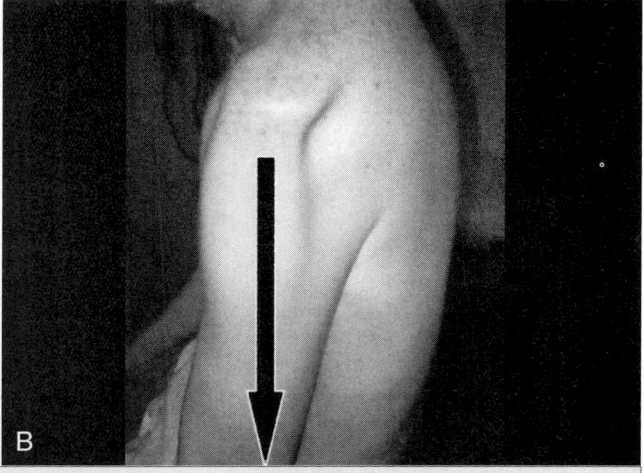

| Figure 4 | A and B, The sulcus sign. Inferior laxity can be measured by applying a firm downward pull (arrow) on the humerus and evaluating the displacement of the proximal humerus from beneath the acromion. |

3: Upper Extremity

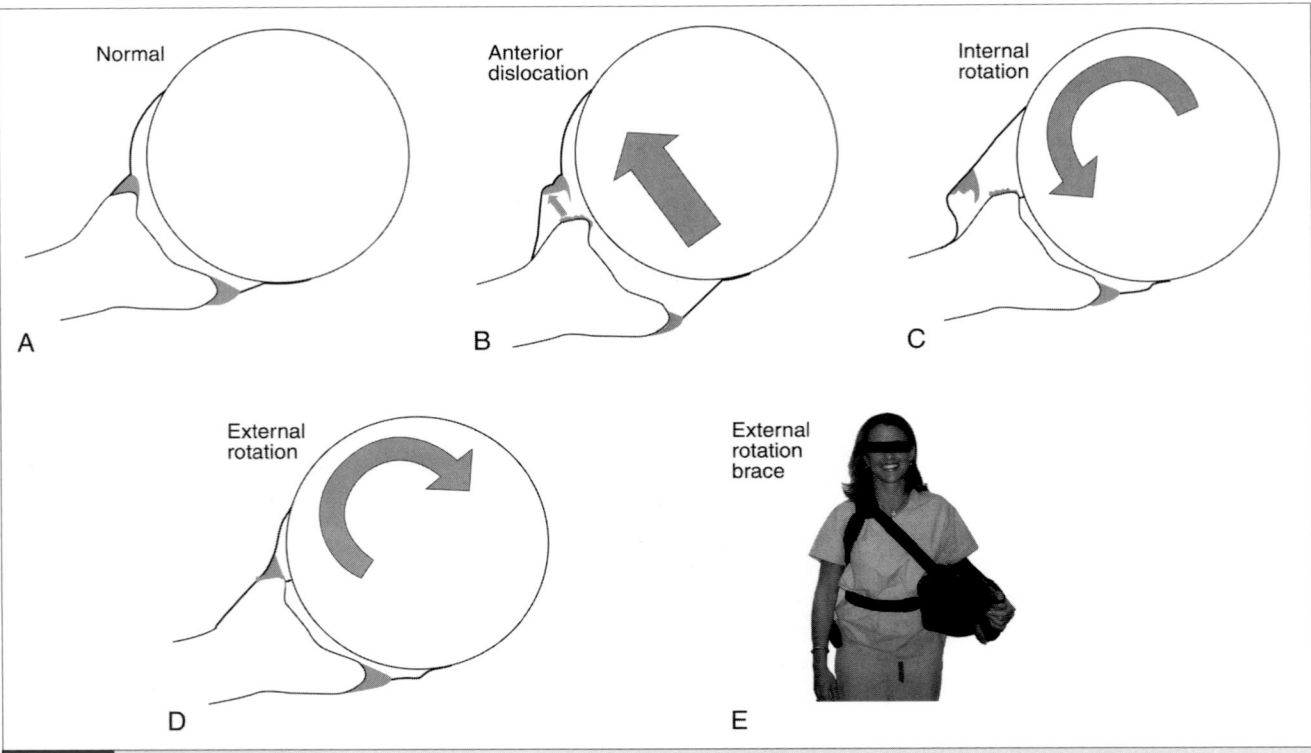

Figure 5 **A,** The normal position of the labrum on the anterior glenoid. **B,** With anterior dislocation (*arrow*), the labrum is often torn from the glenoid. **C,** Subsequent immobilization in internal rotation (*curved arrow*) allows the injured labrum to heal in a suboptimal position down on the glenoid neck. **D,** Immobilization in external rotation (*curved arrow*) pulls the labrum back to the glenoid rim where it has a chance to heal more anatomically. **E,** Photograph of a patient in an external rotation brace.

For nonsurgical treatment, the position of shoulder immobilization after first-time dislocation has been recently studied more closely. When immobilized with the shoulder in internal rotation (as is the common position of the arm in a sling), Bankart lesions have a tendency to reapproximate and heal nonanatomically down on the glenoid neck, rather than back to the glenoid edge (**Figure 5**). Results from a 2003 study showed that the rates of redislocation can be significantly decreased, at least in the short term, by initially immobilizing the shoulder in external rotation.[7] MRI follow-up suggests that this positioning may allow the labrum to heal in a more anatomic position on the glenoid edge. At a mean follow-up of 15.5 months, the authors reported a 30% recurrence rate for the 20 patients immobilized in internal rotation, and no recurrent instability for those immobilized in external rotation. For patients younger than 30 years, the difference was even greater, with a 45% recurrence rate in the internal rotation group and no recurrent instability in the external rotation group. Other studies have been similarly promising in the short term.[8,9]

Arthroscopic Surgery

Arthroscopic management of traumatic shoulder instability has evolved from transglenoid drilling to the use of staples to the use of suture anchors. Transglenoid drilling necessitated a posterior approach to the shoulder and put posterior extra-articular shoulder structures at risk of injury. Arthroscopic staple capsulorrhaphy resulted in significant complications related to staple loosening, breakage, migration, chondrolysis, and subscapular bursitis. With the development of suture anchors, a low-profile, stable anatomic reconstruction can be achieved while sparing the healthy surrounding subscapularis and deltoid tissues.

The results of arthroscopic Bankart repair have been steadily approaching those of traditional open repair as technology, technique, and the learning curve all have progressed. In a recently published prospective study of 72 arthroscopic Bankart repairs using suture anchors with nonabsorbable sutures, at a minimum 2-year follow-up the authors reported a 10% failure rate, which is similar to the results of traditional open repair.[10] In another study, it was reported that there was no significant difference between open and arthroscopic outcomes of Bankart repair, with each group demonstrating 10% recurrence rates.[11]

In collision and contact athletes, most surgeons still opt to use an open approach to shoulder stabilization. Recent evidence suggests that modern arthroscopic technique can yield similar results. In one study, 13 collision (football) and 5 contact (soccer and wrestling) athletes with traumatic anterior instability underwent arthroscopic repair using a suture anchor technique.[12] At a mean 37-month follow-up, only 2 of the 18 patients (11%) experienced treatment failure (1 subluxation and 1 dislocation). Although the cohort is small, this failure rate is similar to that for open surgery, and this finding suggests that arthroscopic technique is a viable option, even in contact and collision athletes. It should be noted that collision athletes can be expected to have a higher rate of recurrence than noncollision athletes because of the nature of their activities. Pending more definitive long-term data, use of the stabilization technique should be based on surgeon experience and comfort level.

Open Surgery

As surgeons have gained experience with instability surgery, they have learned that procedures that involve nonanatomic reconstruction of the anterior shoulder (Putti-Platt and Magnuson-Stack procedures) may be fairly effective in preventing dislocation, but they may lead to significant loss of motion or development of osteoarthritis. A purely open technique also makes a complete glenohumeral evaluation difficult because posterior structures cannot be easily evaluated or treated. As a result, the open Bankart procedure is still considered by many to be the gold standard for patients with recurrent posttraumatic anterior shoulder instability. The Bankart procedure seeks to address the pathologic lesion (the anteroinferior labral avulsion) of anteroinferior instability, while making an attempt to minimize iatrogenic injury to normal surrounding tissues.

Two long-term studies recently reviewed the results of open Bankart reconstructions. Of 83 patients in one study, the recurrence rate (dislocation and subluxation) was found to be 12% at a mean 9-year follow-up.[13] The average patient lost nearly 20° of external rotation, and the authors admitted to being somewhat disappointed in terms of patient stability and function. The other study had 30 patients with a mean 29-year follow-up.[14] The patients lost an average of 43° of rotatory motion (24° of external rotation and 19° of internal rotation); three patients (10%) had recurrent dislocation, and five patients (17%) went on to require shoulder arthroplasty after developing osteoarthritis. Overall, osteoarthritis developed in more than 23% of the patients.

Dislocation arthropathy after surgical treatment of recurrent anterior dislocation has been a subject of debate for years. The development of glenohumeral osteoarthritis has been noted after both nonsurgical and surgical management of shoulder instability. In 1996, a study of prospective data revealed a 9% rate of moderate to severe arthropathy in patients treated nonsurgically for primary dislocation at 10-year follow-up.[15] In 2005, the same lead author published prospective data on patients treated surgically with open Bristow-Latarjet procedures and found a 14% rate of moderate to severe osteoarthritis at 15-year follow-up.[16] Although the development of arthritis did not ap-

pear to be related to the degree of any postoperative motion loss, it seemed to be minimized in patients with well-placed coracoid transfers (2 to 4 mm medial to the glenoid lip) and parallel screw/coracoid/glenoid orientation. The findings of this study also suggested that the subcoracoid projection radiograph (angled inferiorly 45° from above) was the most accurate view for revealing osteoarthritis, whereas true AP views tended to minimize or miss the presence of arthritic changes. Other long-term studies have also approximated a 1% to 1.5% per year rate of moderate to severe arthritis after open coracoid transfer procedures.[17,18]

A long-term study of Navy midshipmen reported a 15% rate of recurrence (dislocation or subluxation) at a mean 26-year follow-up after primary Bristow procedures, with approximately 70% good to excellent results.[19] Similarly, a 14% recurrence rate at 15-year follow-up was reported in the previously cited 118 patients who underwent primary Bristow-Latarjet procedures; 98% of these patients were either very satisfied or satisfied on subjective questioning.[20]

Multidirectional Instability

Most instances of multidirectional instability are atraumatic or minimally traumatic in origin. Symptoms usually result from a combination of generalized ligamentous laxity, muscular dyskinesia, and activity-related demands. Occasionally, glenoid anatomy will contribute to the condition because a lack of adequate glenoid size, concavity, or labral support may allow excessive humeral translation.[21] Symptoms of instability (not just laxity) in more than one direction constitute multidirectional instability, and patients with multidirectional instability will often have symptoms in all directions. Because there is often a generalized collagenous predisposition to the excessive joint mobility in these patients, treatment of multidirectional instability can be challenging. The first line of treatment should focus on patient education and activity modification. It is also important to maximize strength and balance of the dynamic shoulder stabilizers (rotator cuff, deltoid, and periscapular stabilizers) through an aggressive physical therapy program.

If the previously mentioned treatment modalities fail, the most common surgical options include arthroscopic capsular plication, thermal capsular shrinkage, and open capsular shift. In recent years, thermal capsular shrinkage has received a lot of attention and has generally fallen out of favor because of reports of severe tissue necrosis, chondrolysis, and clinical failures. Although most of these reports have been anecdotal,[22] the difficulty of predicting complications and the subsequent revision surgery to treat such complications has led many shoulder specialists away from the use of thermal treatment. A recent study evaluated the state of the capsule and outcomes of open suture plication after failed thermal capsular shrinkage in 14 patients.[23] Capsular thinning was the most common finding, and one patient was noted to have a completely ablated capsule.

3: Upper Extremity

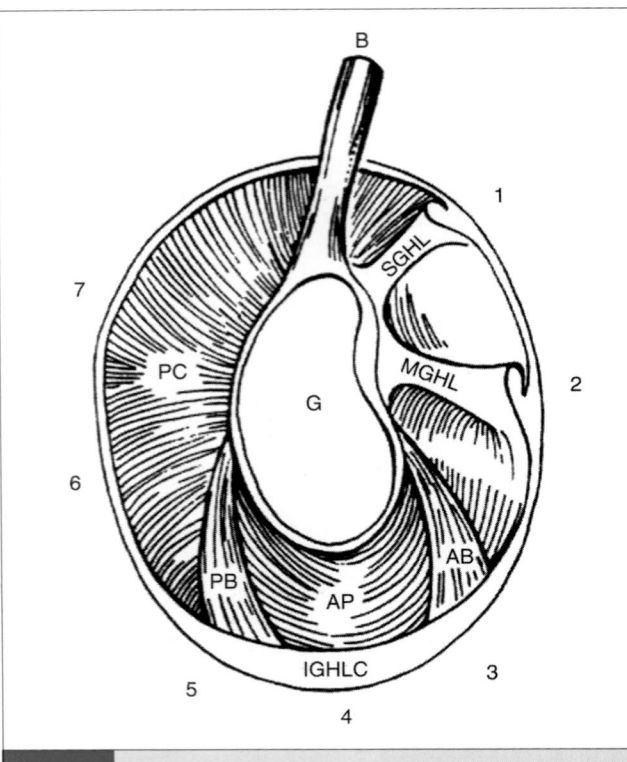

Figure 6 The glenohumeral ligaments as they attach to the glenoid (G). B, biceps tendon; PC, posterior capsule; PB, posterior band; AP, axillary pouch; IGHLC, inferior glenohumeral ligament complex; AB, anterior band; MGHL, middle glenohumeral ligament; SGHL, superior glenohumeral ligament.

At a mean 35-month follow-up, most patients (86%) had good results after the revision surgery with open capsular plication, with no further episodes of subluxation.

In young, athletic patients, a recent long-term outcome study evaluated the results of the nonsurgical treatment of 59 patients with multidirectional instability at 7- to 10-year follow-up. Approximately one third (20 patients) required surgery, one third (17 patients) had generally good outcomes (good/excellent Rowe scores), and one third (19 patients) had poor outcomes (poor Rowe scores). Only eight patients (14%) reported their shoulders to be free of any pain or instability. Of the 39 patients treated with activity modification and physical therapy, 19 (53%) were rated as having poor results and only 5 (13%) had excellent results.[24] This study suggests generally poor long-term outcomes despite rehabilitation and activity modification for patients with multidirectional instability.

Posterior Instability

Posterior instability is significantly less common than anteroinferior instability, occurring in only 2% to 5% of patients with shoulder instability.[25] In patients with

posterior shoulder instability, the diagnosis can be challenging to make and is often missed. Traumatic posterior shoulder instability is often unidirectional, whereas patients with posterior instability as part of a multidirectional instability syndrome tend to have more atraumatic presentations and often present with pain only.

Posterior glenohumeral stability primarily depends on the static capsulolabral structures of the shoulder (Figure 6). With the arm in abduction, the posterior band of the inferior glenohumeral ligament complex is primarily responsible for resisting posterior translation of the humeral head. With the arm flexed, adducted, and internally rotated, it is the superior glenohumeral ligament and the coracohumeral ligament that primarily maintain posterior stability. Traumatic unidirectional posterior instability can occur as a single event, often with the shoulder in a flexed, adducted, and internally rotated position. Football offensive linemen are classically predisposed to recurrent posterior subluxation because of the position of their arms during blocking.

When nonsurgical treatment such as activity modification and strengthening of the dynamic muscular stabilizers fails, surgical intervention can be considered. A recent study followed 100 athletes whose shoulders were treated with arthroscopic capsulolabral reconstruction for unidirectional posterior instability.[26] At a mean follow-up of 27 months, 89% of the athletes had returned to athletic participation and 67% had returned to their prior level of participation. Collision and noncollision athletes had similar results. Another study retrospectively reviewed the results of both open and arthroscopic management of unidirectional posterior instability and found that although both methods had acceptable results (29 of 31 shoulders with good or excellent ratings), the arthroscopically managed shoulder had statistically superior outcomes in terms of both the Western Ontario Shoulder Instability Index scores and Rowe scores.[27] Mean Simple Shoulder Test scores and Single Assessment Numeric Evaluation scores were also better in the arthroscopically managed group, but the difference between the groups did not quite reach statistical significance ($P = 0.06$ and $P = 0.057$, respectively).

When bony pathology exists, an open approach can be used to either restore the concavity of an eroded glenoid with a bone graft or correct excessive posterior retroversion with an opening wedge glenoid osteotomy.[28]

Failed Instability Surgery

Patients with traumatic glenohumeral bone defects are at high risk for recurrence of instability. Purely arthroscopic intervention has had poor results, and open Bankart repair without addressing the bony loss has not fared much better. Inverted pear glenoids, where the normally pear-shaped glenoid has lost enough bone inferiorly to take the shape of an inverted pear, and engaging Hill-Sachs lesions, where the humeral head defect contacts and engages with the glenoid when the arm is abducted and externally rotated, have been shown to significantly increase the failure rate of arthroscopic Bankart repairs.[29]

Risk factors for recurrence after arthroscopic Bankart repair were evaluated in a prospective study of 91 patients. There was an overall failure rate of 15% (six dislocations, eight subluxations) at mean 3-year follow-up. The presence of a bone defect on the glenoid side or the humeral side (Hill-Sachs lesion), generalized ligamentous hyperlaxity or especially the combination of both, were again noted to be significant predictors of postoperative instability recurrence. Patients with both glenoid bone loss and inferior hyperlaxity had a recurrence rate as high as 75%.[30]

For those patients in whom standard open or arthroscopic Bankart repair has failed, attention should be directed toward determining the cause of failure. Were there bony defects or a generalized laxity that was not addressed? Was a thermal device used that may have damaged the capsule? Or was the patient just "unlucky" and the repair failed because of a new injury? As tempting as it may be for a surgeon to assume the latter option, a detailed evaluation must be made of the patient's anatomy (including ligamentous status, radiographs, MRI, and often CT scans), prior surgical technique, the circumstances around the failure episode, and their condition before the episode (presence of prodromal feelings of instability).

Failed primary anteroinferior instability is often treated with an open Bristow-Latarjet repair, transferring the coracoid to the anterior glenoid rim to provide bony reinforcement as well as a soft-tissue sling of support as the conjoined tendons cross the humeral head with the arm in abduction and external rotation. When done correctly, this procedure can be an excellent option for patients in whom other types of stabilization surgery has failed. The procedure is technically demanding and may lead to glenohumeral arthritis if the transferred coracoid is not placed precisely, ideally 2 to 4 mm medial to the glenoid edge (**Figure 7**).

Tricortical bone grafting is another option for patients with significant glenoid bone loss in whom surgery has failed. Anatomic bony reconstruction from the iliac crest may produce stability in these patients.[31]

Chronic Dislocations

Chronic fixed anterior shoulder dislocations are often associated with excessive bone loss on the humeral head and glenoid, making stable maintenance of reduction difficult. For these patients, arthroplasty (total shoulder or hemiarthroplasty) may be necessary, often requiring osseous reconstruction of the glenoid. These patients may have reliable improvement in pain scores, but complications are common, most notably postoperative instability and loosening of glenoid components in shoulders treated with total shoulder arthroplasty.[32]

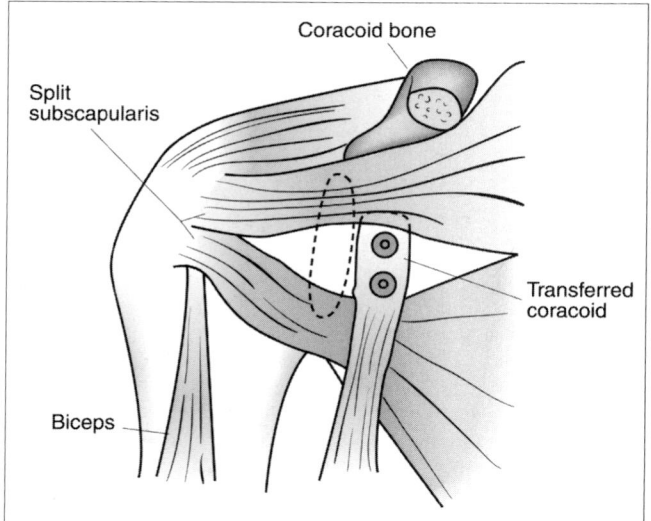

| Figure 7 | The Latarjet procedure transfers the coracoid to the medial glenoid through a subscapularis split. The bone provides mechanical stability while the conjoint tendon provides a stabilizing sling over the humeral head when the arm is in a position of abduction and external rotation. |

Acromioclavicular Separations

Acromioclavicular separations typically occur as a result of direct trauma to the superior shoulder, causing a disruption to the acromioclavicular ligaments, and often to the coracoclavicular ligaments. The injuries have been classified by Rockwood into six types: type I injury represents a nondisplaced sprain of the acromioclavicular ligaments; type II injuries represent tears to the acromioclavicular ligaments with partial tearing of the coracoclavicular ligaments and partial clavicular displacement; type III injuries represent complete acromioclavicular and coracoclavicular ligament disruption with approximately 100% superior clavicular displacement above the acromion; type IV injuries are characterized by significant posterior displacement of the clavicle into the muscle tissue of the trapezius; type V injuries are a more severe form of type III where the clavicle is displaced 100% to 300% superiorly; and type VI injures are characterized by significant inferior displacement and locking of the clavicle under the coracoid process or acromion.

Type I separations are managed nonsurgically, whereas types IV through VI generally require surgical fixation. The controversy involves the treatment of type II and III separations. Prospective studies in the 1980s failed to show a significant difference between surgical and nonsurgical treatment of the type III injury. Because nonsurgical treatment is not successful in all patients, there is interest in developing stronger and more anatomic reconstructive techniques. Allograft reconstruction of the coracoclavicular trapezoid and conoid ligaments has been shown to have less translation than

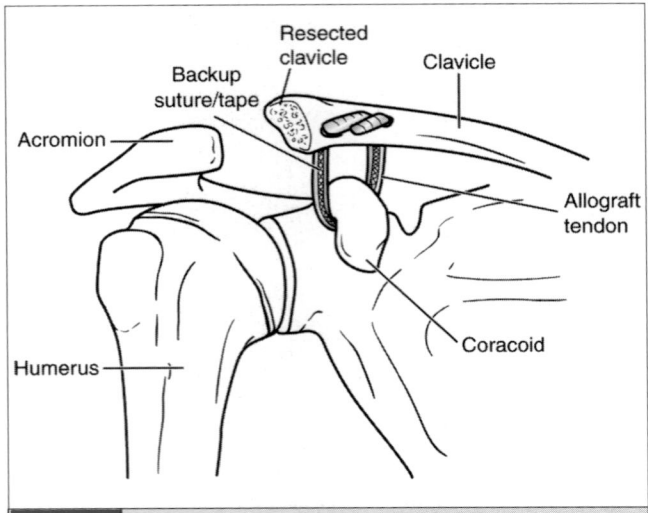

Figure 8	An example of an acromioclavicular reconstruction. After resecting 10 mm from the distal clavicle, the trapezoid (lateral) and conoid (medial) ligaments can be more anatomically reconstructed with a graft placed around the coracoid. The graft is stabilized into the clavicle with interference screws and reinforced with strong suture or tape while the biologic graft incorporates.

and the surgeon should be prepared to perform an open reduction. The shoulder should then be immobilized in a sling for 6 to 8 weeks to allow the ligaments to heal.

Anterior injuries are generally more benign, but can become chronically unstable. Traditional treatment of this condition has been as symptoms dictate, with an emphasis on pain control and activity modification. When this treatment fails, surgical intervention may be required. For those patients with well-maintained articular surfaces, ligament reconstruction has been advocated, whereas for those patients with signs of joint arthrosis, medial clavicular excision has been the procedure of choice. Semitendinosus, fascia lata, subclavius tendon, sternocleidomastoid fascia, and suture anchors all have been used in repair or reconstructions. A recent study reviewed the results of 15 patients (age 12 to 23 years) who underwent surgical intervention for chronic anterior instability. Eleven patients had ligament reconstruction with autograft and four had clavicular head excision. Although no patients needed revision surgery, only 60% reported stable, pain-free joints, and 87% had limitations on athletic or recreational activity.[34] Although this study suggests that pain may be improved with surgery, return to unrestricted activities will likely be limited.

traditional Weaver-Dunn reconstructions in controlled cadaver models.[33] A more anatomic reconstruction using a free tendon graft of both the trapezoid and conoid ligaments may provide a stronger, permanent biologic solution for dislocation of the acromioclavicular joint, although long-term clinical data are still necessary (Figure 8).

Sternoclavicular Instability

Sternoclavicular instability is generally characterized as anterior or posterior, depending on the position of the clavicular head in relation to the sternum. The condition usually results from trauma, often secondary to motor vehicle crashes or athletic injuries causing a direct blow or significant indirect compression on the shoulder girdle. Anterior instability is much more common than posterior instability and can often be differentiated on physical examination by palpating the position of the clavicle. Radiographs taken with a 40° cephalic tilt (serendipity view) may also be helpful in confirming the diagnosis, but CT is accepted as the study of choice.

Posteriorly displaced injuries may lead to significant complications because of compression of vital thoracic structures by the displaced clavicle. Vascular insufficiency, respiratory distress, brachial plexus injury, and even death have all been reported as a result of posterior injuries. Acute dislocations should be managed with an attempt at closed reduction under general anesthesia. This course of action is not often successful

Annotated References

1. Meller R, Krettek C, Gosling T, Wahling K, Jagodzinski M, Zeichen J: Recurrent shoulder instability among athletes: Changes in quality of life, sports activity, and muscle formation following open repair. *Knee Surg Sports Traumatol Arthrosc* 2007;15:295-304.

   The authors retrospectively reviewed 19 patients with recurrent posttraumatic shoulder instability that was treated with open stabilization. At a minimum 2-year follow-up, the authors concluded that despite good-to-excellent clinical results, there was significant impairment of quality of life and sports activity in these patients, and muscle activity and muscle strength were diminished. Level of evidence: IV.

2. Lippitt S, Madsen F: Mechanisms of glenohumeral joint stability. *Clin Orthop Relat Res* 1993;291:20-28.

3. Habermeyer P, Gleyze P, Rickert M: Evolution of lesions of the labrum-ligament complex in posttraumatic anterior shoulder instability: A prospective study. *J Shoulder Elbow Surg* 1999;8:66-74.

4. Habermeyer P, Gleyze P, Rickert M: Evolution of lesions of the labrum-ligament complex in posttraumatic anterior shoulder instability: A prospective study. *J Shoulder Elbow Surg* 1999;8:66-74.

5. Hawkins RJ, Mohtadi NG: Clinical evaluation of shoulder instability. *Clin J Sports Med* 1991;1:59-64.

6. Buss DD, Lynch GP, Meyer CP, Huber SM, Freehill

MQ: Nonoperative management for in-season athletes with anterior shoulder instability. *Am J Sports Med* 2004;32:1430-1433.

The authors followed 30 athletes who were treated non-surgically after traumatic shoulder dislocations, with emphasis on early return to sport. Recurrent instability episodes, additional injuries, subjective ability to compete, and ability to complete their season or seasons of choice were all followed. The authors reported that 26 of 30 athletes returned to athletic activity for the complete season, with an average time missed of 10.2 days (range, 0 to 30 days); 10 athletes experienced sport-related recurrent instability episodes (range, 0 to 8 years). Level of evidence: IV.

7. Itoi E, Hatekeyama Y, Kido T, et al: A new method of immobilization after traumatic anterior dislocation of the shoulder: A preliminary study. *J Shoulder Elbow Surg* 2003;12:413-415.

8. Seybold D, Gekle C, Fehmer T, Pennekamp W, Muhr G, Kalicke T: Immobilization in external rotation after primary shoulder dislocation. *Chirurg* 2006;77:821-826.

    The authors evaluated a new method of immobilization with the arm in external rotation to improve the position of the displaced labrum on the glenoid rim and the use of control MRI before and after immobilization. The authors concluded that after primary shoulder dislocation, immobilizing the arm in 10° to 20° of external rotation provided stable fixation of Bankart lesions in an anatomic position.

9. Miller BS, Sonnabend DH, Hatrick C, et al: Should acute anterior dislocations of the shoulder be immobilized in external rotation? A cadaveric study. *J Shoulder Elbow Surg* 2004;13:589-592.

    The authors studied the contact pressures of the glenoid labrum to the glenoid bone in 10 cadavers with the arm in varying degrees of rotation and noted no contact pressure in neutral or internal rotation and increased contact pressure in up to 45° of external rotation. Level of evidence: III.

10. Carreira DS, Mazzocca AD, Oryhon J, Brown FM, Hayden JK, Romeo AA: A prospective outcome evaluation of arthroscopic Bankart repairs: Minimum 2-year follow-up. *Am J Sports Med* 2006;34:771-777.

    The authors prospectively followed 85 patients treated with arthroscopic repair of traumatic Bankart lesions and reported 90% good or excellent results (Rowe scores) and a 10% recurrence rate, which is similar to historic open stabilization outcomes. Level of evidence: IV.

11. Kim SH, Ha KI, Kim SH: Bankart repair in traumatic anterior shoulder instability: Open versus arthroscopic technique. *Arthroscopy* 2002;18:755-763.

12. Mazzocca AD, Brown FM Jr, Carreira DS, Hayden J, Romeo AA: Arthroscopic anterior shoulder stabilization of collision and contact athletes. *Am J Sports Med* 2005;33:52-60.

In this case series, the authors retrospectively collected data on the outcomes of arthroscopically reconstructed Bankart lesions in 18 contact and collision athletes. They found that the failure rate was similar to that for traditional open repairs at 2-year follow-up. Level of evidence: IV.

13. Strahovnik A, Fokter SK: Long-term results after open Bankart operation for anterior shoulder instability: A 3- to 16-year follow-up. *Wien Klin Wochenschr* 2006;118 (suppl 2):58-61.

    The authors retrospectively reviewed the long-term results (mean follow-up, 9 years) of 83 patients with anterior shoulder instability that was managed with open Bankart repair. After evaluating the postoperative recurrence rate including subluxations (12%), mean Constant score (77), mean Rowe score (63), and average loss of external rotation in 90° of abduction (19°), the authors concluded that the results were disappointing in terms of stability and function. Level of evidence: IV.

14. Pelet S, Jolles BM, Farron A: Bankart repair for recurrent anterior glenohumeral instability: Results at twenty-nine years' follow-up. *J Shoulder Elbow Surg* 2006;15:203-207.

    The authors retrospectively reviewed the long-term results of 39 open Bankart reconstructions. At an average 29-year follow-up, the recurrence rate was 10% and osteoarthritis developed in 40% of the patients. Level of evidence: IV.

15. Hovelius L, Augustini BG, Fredin H, Johansson O, Norlin R, Thorling J: Primary anterior dislocation of the shoulder in young patients: A ten-year prospective study. *J Bone Joint Surg Am* 1996;78:1677-1684.

16. Hovelius L, Sandstrom B, Saebo M: One hundred eighteen Bristow-Latarjet repairs for recurrent anterior dislocation of the shoulder prospectively followed for fifteen years: Study II. The evolution of dislocation arthropathy. *J Shoulder Elbow Surg* 2006;15:279-289.

    This was a large, long-term prospective study of 118 Bristow-Latarjet repairs with special attention given to assessing the development of arthropathy; independent examinations were conducted. At 2- and 15-year follow-up, the AP radiographs of 115 of the 118 shoulders were reviewed; dislocation arthropathy was found in 46 of 115 shoulders (mild in 39, moderate in 5, and severe in 2). The authors stress using a subcoracoid view, angled 45° from above, for the best assessment of osteophyte formation. Level of evidence: III.

17. Allain J, Goutallier D, Glorion C: Long-term results of the Latarjet procedure for the treatment of anterior instability of the shoulder. *J Bone Joint Surg Am* 1998;80:841-852.

18. Singer GC, Kirkland PM, Emery R: Coracoid transposition for recurrent anterior instability of the shoulder. *J Bone Joint Surg Br* 1995;77:73-76.

19. Schroder DT, Provencher MT, Mologne TS, Muldoon MP, Cox JS: The modified Bristow procedure for anterior shoulder instability: 26-year outcomes in Naval

3: Upper Extremity

Academy midshipmen. *Am J Sports Med* 2006;34:778-786.

The authors retrospectively reviewed 52 Bristow procedures and found a 70% rate of good and excellent results and a recurrent instability rate comparable with that of other long-term follow-up studies of open instability procedures. Level of evidence: IV.

20. Hovelius L, Sandstrom B, Sundgren K, Saebo M: One hundred eighteen Bristow-Latarjet repairs for recurrent anterior dislocation of the shoulder prospectively followed for fifteen years: Study I. Clinical results. *J Shoulder Elbow Surg* 2004;13:509-516.

    The authors of this large, long-term, prospective study with independent examinations and no patient dropouts followed 118 Bristow-Latarjet repairs (111 of which were primary reconstructions) with special attention to assessing clinical outcome. At 15-year follow-up, 76% of patients reported being "very satisfied" with the outcome, and the redislocation/resubluxation rate was 15.5%. Level of evidence: III.

21. Matsen FA III, Lippitt SB, Sidles JB, Harryman DT II : Stability, in Matsen FA III (ed): *Practical Evaluation and Management of the Shoulder.* Philadelphia, PA, WB Saunders, 1994, pp 59-111.

22. Levine WN, Clark AM Jr, D'Alessandro DF, Yamaguchi K: Chondrolysis following arthroscopic thermal capsulorrhaphy to treat shoulder instability: A report of two cases. *J Bone Joint Surg Am* 2005;87:616-621.

    The authors discuss the treatment and outcomes of two young athletes with severe chondrolysis after undergoing thermal capsulorrhaphy for shoulder instability. The authors conclude that the effects of thermal capsulorrhaphy are of concern not only because of its previously described high rate of complications, but also because of the unknown effects that it may have on chondrocytes.

23. Park HB, Yokota A, Gill HS, El Rassi G, McFarland EG: Revision surgery for failed thermal capsulorrhaphy. *Am J Sports Med* 2005;33:1321-1326.

    The authors of this article report the anatomic findings and revision surgery outcomes for 14 patients with failed thermal capsulorrhaphy. Five shoulders were believed to have thin capsules and one had necrosis. All were managed with open capsular plication after diagnostic arthroscopy. Two patients (14%) had recurrence by a mean 35-month follow-up. Level of evidence: IV.

24. Misamore GW, Sallay PI, Didelot W: A longitudinal study of patients with multidirectional instability of the shoulder with seven- to ten-year follow-up. *J Shoulder Elbow Surg* 2005;14:466-470.

    The authors retrospectively reviewed the results of 56 patients with multidirectional instability that was treated nonsurgically. At 7- to 10-year follow-up, 21 patients had required surgery, 17 had generally good outcomes (good/excellent Rowe scores), and 19 had poor outcomes (poor Rowe scores). Only eight patients (14%) reported that their shoulders were free of any pain or instability. Level of evidence: IV.

25. Arciero RA, Mazzocca AD: Traumatic posterior shoulder subluxation with labral injury: Suture anchor technique. *Tech Shoulder Elbow Surg* 2004;5:13-24.

    The authors describe the etiology and mechanism of injury, pertinent pathomechanics, clinical presentation, and evaluation of patients with traumatic, recurrent posterior shoulder subluxation. They also describe the arthroscopic technique of repair and reconstruction of the posterior capsulolabral complex for the treatment of recurrent posterior shoulder subluxation in patients in whom a rehabilitation program has failed.

26. Bradley JP, Baker CL 3rd, Kline AJ, Armfield DR, Chhabra A: Arthroscopic capsulolabral reconstruction for posterior instability of the shoulder: A prospective study of 100 shoulders. *Am J Sports Med* 2006;34:1061-1071.

    The authors prospectively followed 100 shoulders that were arthroscopically managed for unidirectional posterior instability. At a mean 27-months follow-up, contact athletes had outcomes similar to those of noncontact patients, with overall significant improvements in American Shoulder and Elbow Surgeons scores, stability, pain, and function. Level of evidence: II.

27. Bottoni CR, Franks BR, Moore JH, DeBerardino TM, Taylor DC, Arciero RA: Operative stabilization of posterior shoulder instability. *Am J Sports Med* 2005;33:996-1002.

    Patients with traumatic unidirectional posterior shoulder instability were retrospectively reviewed after either open or arthroscopic management of symptomatic, traumatic posterior shoulder instability. At an average 40-month follow-up, the authors reported that both groups did well; however, the arthroscopic group tended to have better outcomes. Level of evidence: IV.

28. Millett PJ, Clavert P, Hatch GF III, Warner JJ: Recurrent posterior shoulder instability. *J Am Acad Orthop Surg* 2006;14:464-476.

    For optimal results in patients with posterior shoulder instability, the authors recommend accurate definition of the pattern of instability with care taken to address all soft-tissue and bony injuries present at the time of surgery. Level of evidence: V.

29. Burkhart SS, De Beer JF: Traumatic glenohumeral bone defects and their relationship to failure of arthroscopic Bankart repairs: Significance of the inverted-pear glenoid and the humeral engaging Hill-Sachs lesion. *Arthroscopy* 2000;16:677-694.

30. Boileau P, Villalba M, Héry JY, Balg F, Ahrens P, Neyton L: Risk factors for recurrence of shoulder instability after arthroscopic Bankart repair. *J Bone Joint Surg Am* 2006;88:1755-1763.

    In this study, the authors followed 91 patients who were treated arthroscopically with suture anchor technique. At a mean 36-month follow-up, the overall recurrence rate was 15% (14 patients), which was significantly correlated with large Hill-Sachs lesions, glenoid bone loss, the number of suture anchors (fewer than four), and the presence of underlying hyperlaxity. Bony Bankart glenoid separation fractures did not seem to correlate with recurrence.

31. Warner JJ, Gill TJ, O'Hollerhan JD, Pathare N, Millett PJ: Anatomical glenoid reconstruction for recurrent anterior glenohumeral instability with glenoid deficiency using an autogenous tricortical iliac crest bone graft. *Am J Sports Med* 2006;34:205-212.

   The authors assessed 11 patients with traumatic recurrent anterior instability that required bony reconstruction for severe anterior glenoid bone loss; all patients underwent surgical reconstruction using an intra-articular tricortical iliac crest bone graft contoured to reestablish the concavity and width of the glenoid. At a mean 33-month follow-up, the mean American Shoulder and Elbow Surgeons score was 94 postoperatively (65 preoperatively). The mean University of California Los Angeles score was 33 postoperatively (18 preoperatively). The mean Rowe score was 94 postoperatively (28 preoperatively). The authors concluded that anatomic reconstruction of the glenoid with autogenous iliac crest bone graft is an effective treatment for this condition. Level of evidence: IV.

32. Matsoukis J, Tabib W, Guiffault P, et al: Primary unconstrained shoulder arthroplasty in patients with a fixed anterior glenohumeral dislocation. *J Bone Joint Surg Am* 2006;88:547-552.

   In this study, the authors retrospectively reviewed 11 patients who were managed with either total shoulder arthroplasty or hemiarthroplasty. At a mean 24-month follow-up, pain scores improved significantly from the preoperative state; however, complications such as glenoid loosening and recurrent instability were common.

33. Mazzocca AD, Santangelo SA, Johnson ST, Rios CG, Dumonski ML, Arciero RA: A biomechanical evaluation of an anatomical coracoclavicular ligament reconstruction. *Am J Sports Med* 2006;34:236-246.

   This cadaveric study was conducted to evaluate the biomechanical performance of acromioclavicular joint reconstructions. The authors report that anatomic coracoclavicular reconstruction has less anterior and posterior translation and more closely approximates the intact state than arthroscopic reconstruction or reconstruction using a modified Weaver-Dunn procedure. Level of evidence: III.

34. Bae DS, Kocher MS, Waters PM, Micheli LM, Griffey M, Dichtel L: Chronic recurrent anterior sternoclavicular joint instability. *J Pediatr Orthop* 2006;26:71-74.

   This study was conducted to determine the functional outcome of surgical treatment in adolescent and young adult patients with chronic recurrent anterior sternoclavicular joint instability. Fifteen patients with chronic recurrent anterior sternoclavicular joint instability underwent joint reconstruction or medial clavicular resection. At an average 55-month follow-up, the mean American Shoulder and Elbow Surgeons score was 85 and the mean Simple Shoulder Test score was 10.9. The authors concluded that surgical treatment of chronic anterior sternoclavicular joint instability in adolescents and young adults can provide near-complete pain relief and return of shoulder and upper extremity function. Level of evidence: IV.

3: Upper Extremity

Chapter 25

Shoulder Reconstruction

*John W. Sperling, MD   Robert H. Cofield, MD

Introduction

To successfully treat the patient with shoulder arthritis, it is important to understand the patient's functional demands, severity of symptoms, and the patient's capacity to comply with postoperative restrictions. Appropriate imaging studies together with a careful history and examination will allow the physician to outline a proper treatment plan for the patient.

Patient Evaluation

History

An accurate history allows the surgeon to obtain a clear understanding of the severity of the patient's symptoms as well as functional demands. It is critical to understand the patient's primary complaint—is it pain, weakness, or loss of motion?

The patient should be asked about the duration of shoulder pain, specific alleviating and aggravating factors, and whether a specific traumatic event brought on the discomfort. Typically, patients are asked to localize and rate their shoulder pain (at night, with activities, and at rest) on a scale of 1 to 10, with 10 being the highest pain rating. It is important to know whether the pain occurs in the typical anterior or superolateral aspect of the shoulder. Pain that occurs in a radicular pattern down the arm is cause for concern because it is indicative of a possible neurologic disorder.

Prior evaluations and treatment, including physical therapy, cortisone injection, and surgical procedures should be assessed, along with complications with wound drainage or skin healing.

Review of Systems

Evaluation of the shoulder requires a focused review of systems. In patients with a history of metabolic or rheumatologic disease, other joints may be involved and a decision will need to be made regarding the specific order in which reconstructive procedures should be performed. It is also important to determine if there is a history of neurologic symptoms or neck pain (which may indicate cervical radiculopathy), cough, or shortness of breath.

John W. Sperling, MD is a consultant or employee for Biomet.

Physical Examination

The upper extremities are examined for signs of muscle atrophy and prior incisions are carefully inspected. Atrophy may be associated with long-standing rotator cuff disease. In addition, careful attention must be paid to the integrity of the deltoid, particularly among patients who have undergone prior surgery. Cervical range of motion is assessed as well as midline and paraspinal palpation. A Spurling test is routinely performed to evaluate for possible cervical radiculopathy. The examination is performed bilaterally and includes the shoulder, elbow, and wrist.

A standard shoulder evaluation also includes assessment of range of motion, reflexes, and strength, recording both active and passive shoulder abduction. In patients with rotator cuff deficiency, it is important to determine whether there is a component of anterosuperior humeral head escape. Scapulothoracic motion is evaluated and evidence of scapular winging is noted. Shoulder strength is graded on a 1 to 5 scale for internal rotation, external rotation, flexion, extension, and abduction.

Radiographic Studies

At minimum, three radiographic shoulder views are obtained: an axillary view and 40° posterior oblique views with internal and external rotation. The posterior oblique views are used to evaluate both the superoinferior and the mediolateral acromiohumeral distance. In patients with rotator cuff disease, there may be superior subluxation of the humeral head with an associated decrease in the acromiohumeral distance. However, there can be the false appearance of superior humeral head subluxation with posterior subluxation of the humeral head (**Figure 1**).

In the setting of glenoid erosion, there is a relative decrease in the amount of humeral head offset from the lateral border of the acromion. Specifically, the lateral border of the greater tuberosity may be medial to the lateral edge of the acromion in shoulders with significant glenoid erosion.

In addition, AP radiographs are helpful in determining the thickness of the cortices, the size of the humeral canal, and the overall degree of osteopenia. The axillary view allows assessment of glenoid version, glenoid erosion, and humeral head subluxation.

CT scans can be an extremely valuable evaluation tool before shoulder arthroplasty, providing valuable information regarding glenoid version and quantifying

3: Upper Extremity

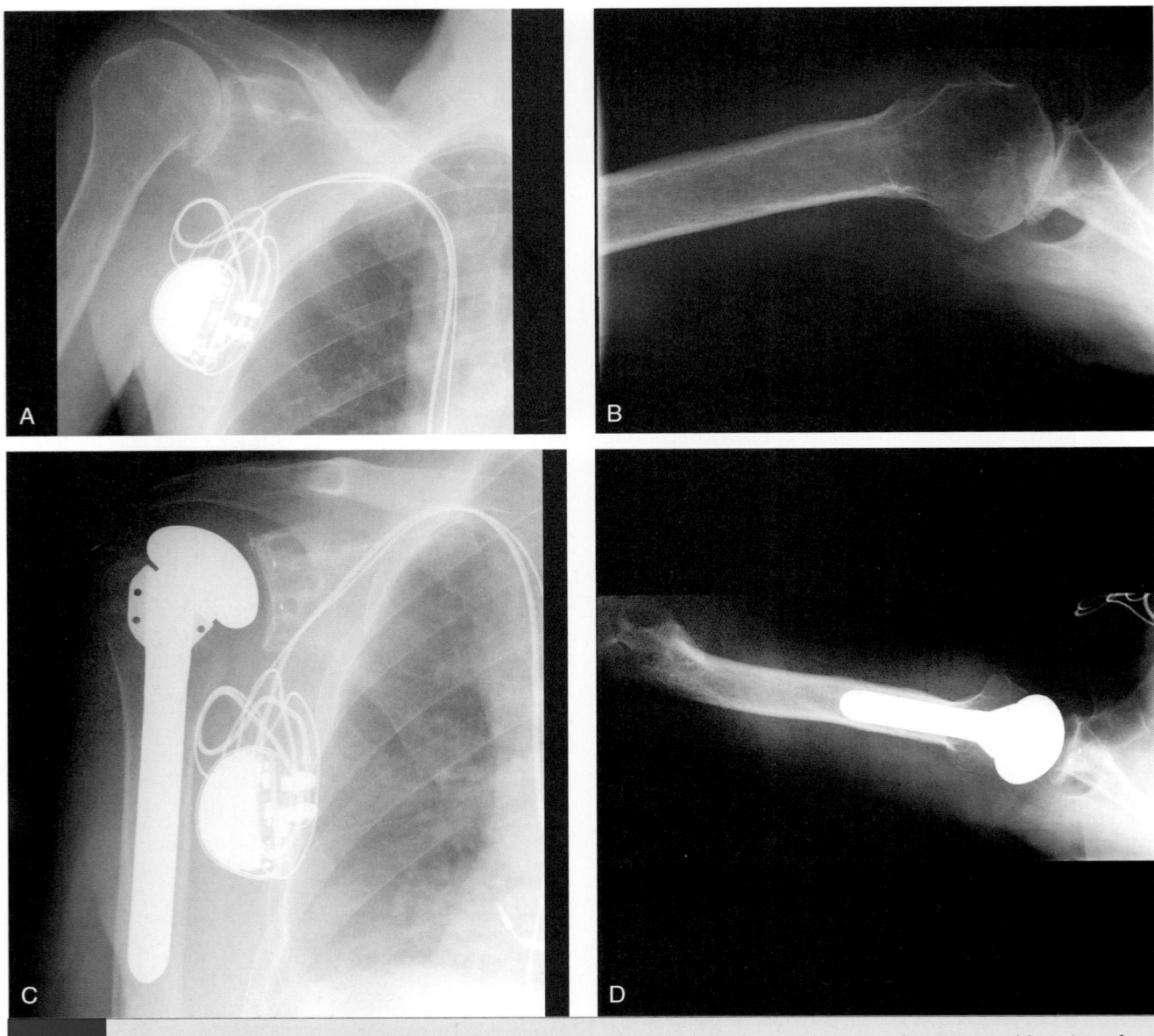

Figure 1 **A** and **B,** The AP radiograph has the false appearance of superior subluxation because of posterior subluxation of the humeral head. **C** and **D,** There is an increased acromiohumeral distance with correction of the posterior subluxation.

the amount of bone loss. A new development is the use of three-dimensional CT, which can further assist in evaluating the humerus and glenoid. Some surgeons prefer to perform an MRI to determine the integrity of the rotator cuff as well as to confirm the presence of associated muscle atrophy.

Treatment

The early stages of shoulder arthritis can be treated nonsurgically. Treatment modalities may include nonsteroidal anti-inflammatory agents and intra-articular steroid and/or hyaluronic acid injections. A physical ther-

apy program can be instituted that focuses on maintaining range of motion and strengthening exercises. Local pain-relieving modalities include heat and cold therapy; ultrasound may reduce the inflammatory response and provide pain relief. Patients with more advanced disease may require surgical intervention. It is critical to clearly understand the patient's goals to determine the most appropriate treatment. The patient must be amenable to postoperative rehabilitation and restrictions.

Arthroscopic Treatment
In a young, active patient with isolated Outerbridge grade I, II, or III chondral lesions, arthroscopic débridement may be a potential treatment option. Several stud-

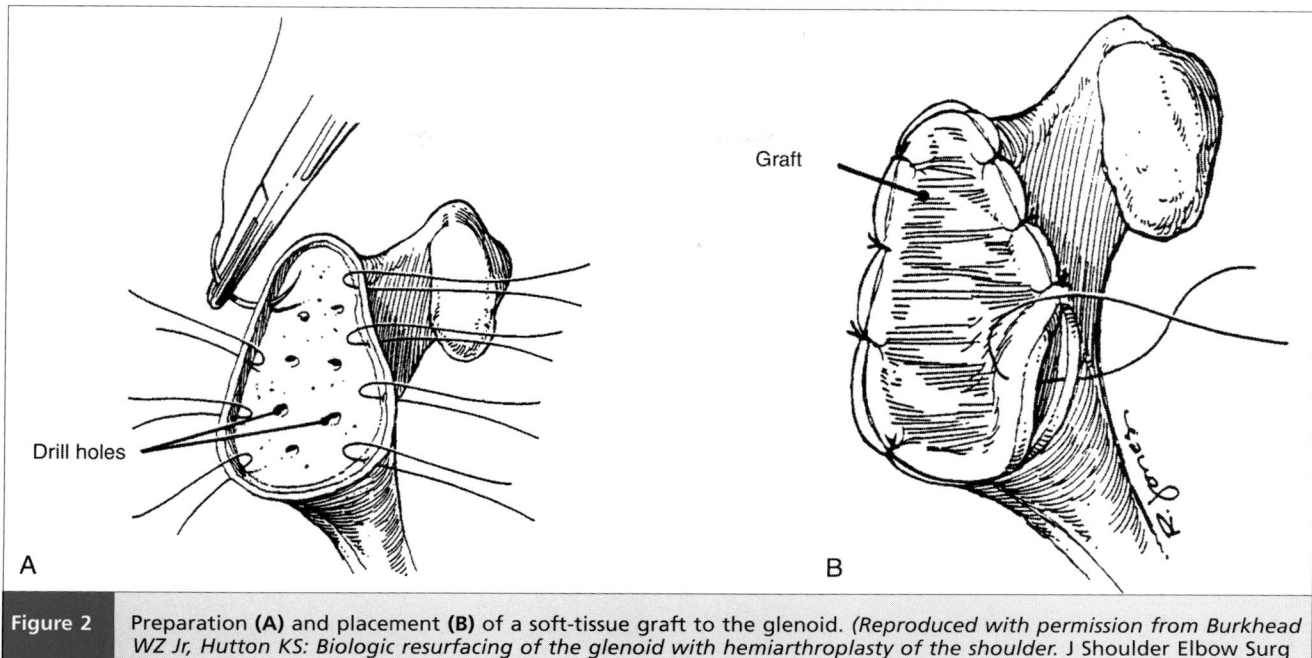

Drill holes

A

Graft

B

Figure 2 | Preparation **(A)** and placement **(B)** of a soft-tissue graft to the glenoid. *(Reproduced with permission from Burkhead WZ Jr, Hutton KS: Biologic resurfacing of the glenoid with hemiarthroplasty of the shoulder. J Shoulder Elbow Surg 1995;4:263:270.)*

ies have noted that the severity of the arthritis and the congruity of the joint are related to the outcome with débridement.[1-3] Arthroscopic lavage is believed to help remove inflammatory enzymes and proteins from the joint fluid. Débridement of chondral flaps and labral tears with removal of loose bodies may alleviate mechanical symptoms. Release of capsular contracture may also be performed to help restore motion.

A few studies have been published on the outcome of arthroscopic treatment of shoulder arthritis. According to one early study, approximately 60% of patients with mild disease had improvement; however, only 30% of patients with moderate to severe disease had pain relief.[1] The extent and duration of pain relief after arthroscopic débridement for glenohumeral arthritis was evaluated in another study.[2] Among the 25 patients with a mean follow-up of 34 months, 2 excellent, 18 good, and 5 unsatisfactory results were reported. There was a trend toward worse results with increasing severity of cartilage changes. Ten of 12 patients with marked preoperative stiffness had significant improvement of motion. Patients who had large osteophytes and/or nonconcentric joints had worse results.

Arthroscopic débridement and capsular release was studied among patients with Outerbridge grade IV lesions.[3] Forty-five patients in the study had a minimum 2-year follow-up. There was significant improvement in patient satisfaction scores, with 87% of patients reporting that they would have the surgery again.

Biologic Resurfacing
There has been some recent enthusiasm about the use of biologic resurfacing of the glenoid alone or in combination with hemiarthroplasty. In the past, these pa-

tients (especially heavy laborers) had been considered candidates for shoulder fusion. Although the reported results for fusion are satisfactory in 80% of patients, continued scapulothoracic muscle pain as well as significant loss of motion make this treatment an unattractive option for many patients.[4]

Prior biologic techniques have usually involved an open approach; however, an all-arthroscopic resurfacing technique has been described.[5] The central goals of performing an interposition arthroplasty or hybrid interposition arthroplasty are to provide pain relief and restoration of function while preserving bone stock for future procedures. There have been a variety of different materials described for interposition arthroplasty, including anterior capsule, fascia lata autograft, and allografts of Achilles tendon, lateral meniscus, dura mater, and purified porcine submucosa.

In 1995, biologic resurfacing of the glenoid and placement of a hemiarthroplasty was first described[6] (**Figure 2**). A recent review of long-term results (2 to 15 years) of 36 shoulders (34 patients) that underwent biologic glenoid resurfacing and humeral head replacement revealed that results were excellent in 18 shoulders, satisfactory in 13, and unsatisfactory in 5 using Neer's criteria.[7]

Total Shoulder Arthroplasty Versus Hemiarthroplasty
There continues to be significant debate in the literature comparing the outcome of total shoulder arthroplasty to hemiarthroplasty for osteoarthritis. Two recent prospective studies comparing total shoulder arthroplasty to hemiarthroplasty for osteoarthritis have been published. Fifty-one shoulders with osteoarthritis,

3: Upper Extremity

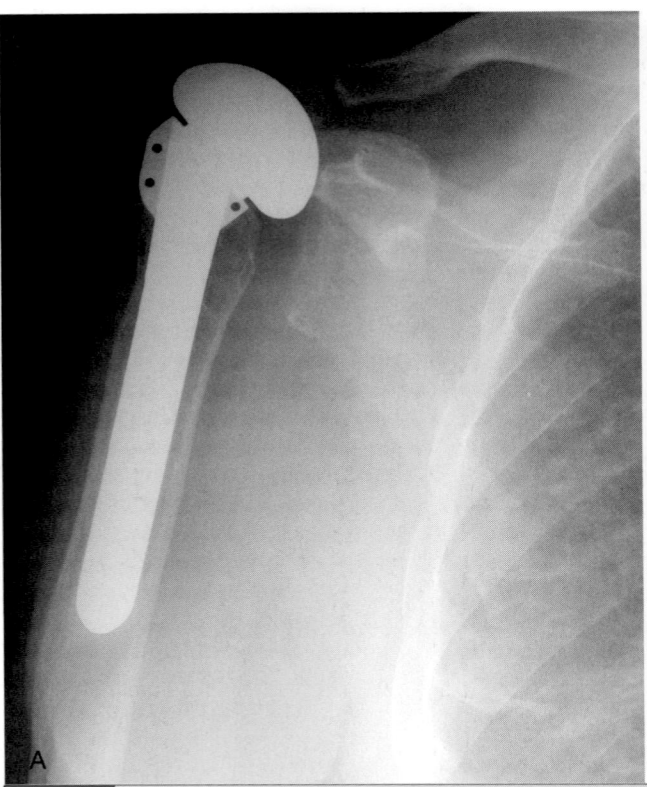
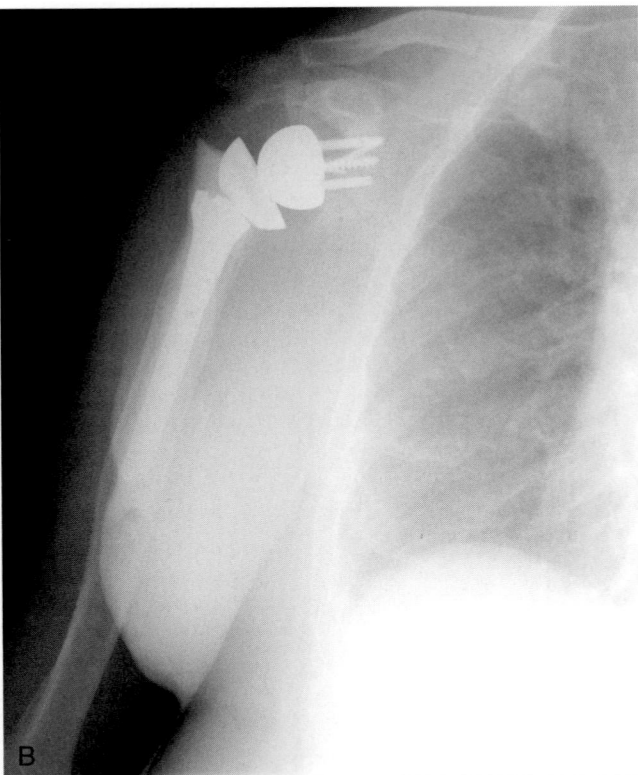

Figure 3   **A,** Radiograph of an unstable hemiarthroplasty that was originally placed for a proximal humerus fracture. **B,** The patient underwent revision to a reverse prosthesis.

a concentric glenoid, and an intact rotator cuff were randomly assigned to hemiarthroplasty or total shoulder arthroplasty.[8] Results of the study demonstrated that patients who received total shoulder arthroplasty had significantly better pain relief. There were no revisions in the total shoulder arthroplasty group, whereas there were three revisions for painful glenoid arthritis in the hemiarthroplasty group.

In another study, 42 patients with osteoarthritis were randomized to receive either a hemiarthroplasty or a total shoulder arthroplasty.[9] At a minimum 2-year follow-up, there were no significant differences between the two procedures in regard to quality of life scores. Two patients in the hemiarthroplasty group did require revision to total shoulder arthroplasty because of painful glenoid arthritis.

Reverse Prosthesis
Originally described in 1993, the reverse prosthesis, which involves a convex glenoid and a concave humerus, is being used more often[10] (Figure 3). The original design was based on the concept of placing the center of rotation in the scapular neck, thereby increasing the lever arm of the deltoid.

The results of 60 patients with rotator cuff deficiency and glenohumeral arthritis who underwent surgery with a reverse shoulder prosthesis have been reported.[11] The mean patient age was 71 years, and

minimum follow-up was 2 years. The authors noted significant improvement in the American Shoulder and Elbow Surgeons (ASES) score as well as the visual analog pain score. Complications were reported in 13 patients; 7 required revision surgery.

The use of a reverse shoulder prosthesis for the treatment of painful pseudoparesis caused by irreparable rotator cuff dysfunction was examined in a recent study.[12] The study included 58 consecutive patients with shoulder pain and less than 90° of active elevation. The mean duration of follow-up was 38 months. There was significant improvement in outcome measures such as the Constant score, and active elevation. The revision rate was 18% for those patients with a primary reverse prosthesis and 39% for those who had undergone prior surgery. The authors noted that complications were common but rarely affected the final outcome.

The outcome of reverse shoulder arthroplasty was assessed at a minimum 5-year follow-up.[13] Sixty shoulders were available for review. There were two breaks observed in regard to the survival curves. The first break occurred approximately 3 years after surgery, reflecting early loosening of the prosthesis. The curve was then seen to be stable. The second break began approximately 6 years after surgery and was believed to be caused by progressive deterioration of the functional result. The authors concluded that the reverse prosthesis should be reserved for patients with a disabling shoulder arthropathy and massive rotator cuff rupture.

In addition, they noted that the reverse prosthesis should be used exclusively in patients older than 70 years with low functional demands.

Rotator Cuff Surgery

Arthroscopic Rotator Cuff Repair

Several recent studies have shed new light on the outcome of arthroscopic rotator cuff repair. In one study, the outcome of all arthroscopic versus mini-open rotator cuff repair with a minimum 2-year follow-up were retrospectively reviewed.[14] There were 33 patients in the mini-open repair group and 38 in the all-arthroscopic repair group. The authors noted no difference in ASES scores when comparing patients in the two groups. Ultrasound revealed that there were recurrent defects in 24% of the arthroscopic repairs and 27% of the mini-open repairs. In addition, the authors reported that patients who had an original tear that was larger than 3 cm were seven times more likely to have a recurrent tear. Patients with a recurrent tear did have significant strength deficits in external rotation and elevation. However, there was no difference in pain or outcome scores in those with a recurrent tear compared with those with an intact rotator cuff.

One of the first prospective studies on the integrity of arthroscopic rotator cuff repair reported on the outcome of 18 patients with a minimum 1-year follow-up.[15] Recurrent tears were seen in 17 of 18 patients. Despite these recurrent tears, 16 patients had improved functional outcome scores at 1 year. Thirteen patients had an ASES score greater than 90. However, at 2 years the results deteriorated, with 12 patients having an ASES score greater than 80.

In another prospective study, the results of 40 patients who underwent arthroscopic rotator cuff repair were compared with those of 32 patients who underwent open repair.[16] At a minimum 1-year follow-up, 69% of repairs in the open group were intact compared with 53% in the arthroscopic group. MRI revealed that among tears smaller than 3 cm, 74% of the repairs in the open group and 84% of those in the arthroscopic group were intact. However, in tears larger than 3 cm, 24% in the arthroscopic group were intact compared with 62% in the open group. The authors noted that the integrity of the rotator cuff was comparable for small tears; however, larger tears had twice the retear rate when done arthroscopically. Continued evolution of techniques to perform arthroscopic rotator cuff repair and additional research will be necessary to determine the long-term outcome of this procedure.

Tissue Transfer for Massive Rotator Cuff Tears

In a recent study, the outcome of 67 patients with 69 irreparable rotator cuff tears treated with a latissimus dorsi transfer was reported.[17] The patients were reviewed at a mean follow-up of 53 months. The subjective shoulder value was significantly improved, from 28% to 66%. The authors concluded that a latissimus dorsi transfer significantly improves painful shoulders with loss of function in the setting of an irreparable rotator cuff tear, particularly if the subscapularis is intact. In another recent study, specific factors were examined that may affect the outcome of latissimus dorsi tendon transfer for irreparable posterosuperior rotator cuff tears.[18] The authors reviewed the results of 14 patients with a minimum follow-up of 24 months. Female patients with generalized muscle weakness and poor shoulder function preoperatively were more likely to have a poor result.

Annotated References

1. Ogilvie-Harris DJ, Wiley AM: Arthroscopic surgery of the shoulder: A general appraisal. *J Bone Joint Surg Br* 1986;68:201-207.

2. Weinstein DM, Bucchieri JS, Pollock RG, Flatow EL, Bigliani LU: Arthroscopic debridement of the shoulder for osteoarthritis. *Arthroscopy* 2000;16:471-476.

3. Cameron BD, Galatz LM, Ramsey ML, Williams GR, Iannotti JP: Non-prosthetic management of grade IV osteochondral lesions of the glenohumeral joint. *J Shoulder Elbow Surg* 2002;11:25-32.

4. Cofield RH: Shoulder arthrodesis and resection arthroplasty of the shoulder. *Instr Course Lect* 1985;34:268-277.

5. Brislin KJ, Savoie FH III, Field LD, Ramsey JR: Surgical treatment for glenohumeral arthritis in the young patient. *Tech Shoulder Elbow Surg* 2004;5:165-169.

   The authors describe an all-arthroscopic resurfacing technique for treating glenohumeral arthritis.

6. Burkhead WZ, Hutton KS: Biologic resurfacing of the glenoid with hemiarthroplasty of the shoulder. *J Shoulder Elbow Surg* 1995;4:263-270.

7. Krishnan SG, Nowinski RJ, Harrison D, Burkhead WZ: Humeral head hemiarthroplasty with biologic resurfacing of the glenoid for glenohumeral arthritis: Two to fifteen-year outcomes. *J Bone Joint Surg Am* 2007;89:727-734.

   According to the results from this study, biologic glenoid resurfacing is a good alternative to total shoulder arthroplasty. Of 36 shoulders studied, 31 had excellent or satisfactory results. Level of evidence: IV.

8. Gartsman GM, Roddey TS, Hammerman SM: Shoulder arthroplasty with or without resurfacing of the glenoid in patients who have osteoarthritis. *J Bone Joint Surg Am* 2000;82:26-34.

9. Lo IK, Litchfield RB, Griffen S, Faber K, Patterson SD, Kirkley A: Quality of life outcome following hemiarthroplasty or total shoulder arthroplasty in patients with osteoarthritis: A prospective, randomized trial. *J Bone Joint Surg Am* 2005;87:2178-2185.

3: Upper Extremity

In a prospective study of 42 patients randomly assigned to receive either a hemiarthroplasty or a total shoulder arthroplasty, there were no significant differences between the two procedures in regard to quality of life scores at a minimum 2-year follow-up. Level of evidence: I.

10. Grammont PM, Baulot E: Delta shoulder prosthesis for rotator cuff rupture. *Orthopedics* 1993;16:65-68.

11. Frankle M, Siegal S, Pupello D, Saleem A, Mighell M, Vasey M: The reverse shoulder prosthesis for glenohumeral arthritis associated with severe rotator cuff deficiency: A minimum two-year follow-up study of sixty patients. *J Bone Joint Surg Am* 2005;87:1697-1705.

    The authors report on the outcome of 60 patients who underwent a reverse prosthesis. There was significant improvement in ASES scores as well as pain relief. The complication rate was 17%.

12. Werner CM, Steinmann PA, Gilbert M, Gerber C: Treatment of painful pseudoparalysis due to irreparable rotator cuff dysfunction with the Delta III reverse-ball-and-socket total shoulder prosthesis. *J Bone Joint Surg Am* 2005;87:1476-1486.

    In patients treated with reverse shoulder arthroplasty for painful pseudoparalysis caused by an irreparable rotator cuff tear, there was significant improvement in function. The revision rate was 18% for patients who received a primary reverse prosthesis and 39% for those who had undergone prior surgery. Although complications were common, they rarely affected final outcome.

13. Guery J, Favard L, Sirveaux F, Oudet D, Mole D, Walch G: Reverse total shoulder arthroplasty: Survivorship analysis of eighty replacements followed for five to ten years. *J Bone Joint Surg Am* 2006;88:1742-1747.

    The authors report the outcome of 60 shoulders treated with a reverse prosthesis at a minimum follow-up of 5 years. The authors concluded that the procedure should be reserved for patients with disabling shoulder arthropathy and a massive rotator cuff rupture and exclusively in patients older than 70 years with low functional demands.

14. Verma NN, Dunn W, Adler RS, et al: All arthroscopic versus mini-open rotator cuff repair: A retrospective review with minimum 2 year follow-up. *Arthroscopy* 2006;22:587-594.

    The authors retrospectively reviewed the outcome of all-arthroscopic versus mini-open rotator cuff repairs with a minimum 2-year follow-up. The authors noted no difference in ASES scores when comparing patients in the two groups. Ultrasound revealed that there were recurrent defects in 24% of the arthroscopic repairs and 27% of the mini-open repairs.

15. Galatz LM, Ball CM, Teefey SA, Middleton WD, Yamaguchi K: The outcome and repair integrity of completely arthroscopically repaired large and massive rotator cuff tears. *J Bone Joint Surg Am* 2004;86:219-224.

    The authors reported on the outcome of 18 patients with a minimum 1-year follow-up after arthroscopic rotator cuff repair. Recurrent tears were seen in 17 of 18 patients. Despite the recurrent tears, 16 patients had improved functional outcome scores at 1 year.

16. Bishop J, Klepps S, Lo IK, Bird J, Gladstone JN, Flatow EL: Cuff integrity after arthroscopic versus open rotator cuff repair: A prospective study. *J Shoulder Elbow Surg* 2006;15:290-299.

    In this prospective study, the results of 40 patients who underwent arthroscopic rotator cuff repair were compared with those of 32 patients who underwent open repair. The integrity of the rotator cuff was comparable for small tears; however, larger tears had twice the retear rate when done arthroscopically.

17. Gerber C, Maquieira G, Espinosa N: Latissimus dorsi transfer for the treatment of irreparable rotator cuff tears. *J Bone Joint Surg Am* 2006;88:113-120.

    The authors report on the outcome of 67 patients with 69 irreparable rotator cuff tears treated with a latissimus dorsi transfer. A latissimus dorsi transfer significantly improved pain and function; however, the procedure is of questionable benefit if the subscapularis is deficient.

18. Iannotti JP, Hennigan S, Herzog R, et al: Latissimus dorsi tendon transfer for irreparable posterosuperior rotator cuff tears: Factors affecting outcome. *J Bone Joint Surg Am* 2006;88:342-348.

    According to this study, preoperative shoulder function influences the outcome of the tissue transfer. In addition, female patients with preoperative generalized muscle weakness were more likely to have a poor clinical outcome.

Chapter 26

Elbow and Forearm Trauma

Julie E. Adams, MD   Scott P. Steinmann, MD

Introduction

Trauma to the elbow and forearm is common. Cadaver studies suggest that fracture patterns vary depending on the flexion angle of the elbow, with radial head and coronoid fractures occurring at flexion less than 80°, olecranon fractures occurring when the elbow is at a right angle, and distal humerus fractures occurring when the angle of flexion exceeds 110°.[1] Diagnosis is usually straightforward; treatment of complicated elbow injuries, however, requires anatomic reduction and stable fixation allowing for early motion to prevent complications of malunion, nonunion, and stiffness.

Radial Head Fractures

Fractures of the radial head may occur in isolation or as a part of more extensive elbow trauma, such as the terrible triad injury (elbow dislocation, radial head fracture, and coronoid fracture). Typically, radial head fractures are caused by a fall on the outstretched and pronated forearm as a result of axial, valgus, and external rotatory loads. Patients with radial head fractures, such as those with an Essex-Lopresti lesion, should be examined for associated injuries, such as medial collateral ligament disruption or interossei ligament and distal radial ulnar joint injury. The most commonly used classification system is the modified Mason classification (Figure 1). This classification system is useful in defining treatment algorithms.

In patients with acute injury, true AP and lateral radiographs should be obtained; oblique radiographs are helpful. A therapeutic aspiration of the hemarthrosis and injection of local anesthetic can help ameliorate pain and allow for evaluation of range of motion and identification of any mechanical block to motion that may require surgical treatment. Type I fractures are treated with sling immobilization for comfort, with early active motion encouraged to begin within days. Weekly radiographs are obtained to evaluate for displacement.

Type II fractures may be treated nonsurgically if stability of the elbow is maintained and no mechanical block to motion is apparent. If there is a mechanical block to motion or the stability of the joint is compromised, surgical therapy is indicated. Most type II fractures do not involve joint instability or a mechanical block to motion. If instability or a block to motion is suspected, then an evaluation with the patient under anesthesia can be performed in the operating room. If instability of the joint is found during this evaluation, then open surgical repair can be performed. Established protocols for determining which type II fractures require fixation (based on displacement) are being revised. Recently, a report from Sweden documented successful nonsurgical treatment of moderately displaced (2 to 5 mm) radial head fractures in a long-term study.[2] Examination with the patient under anesthesia is recommended for assessment of displaced type II fractures

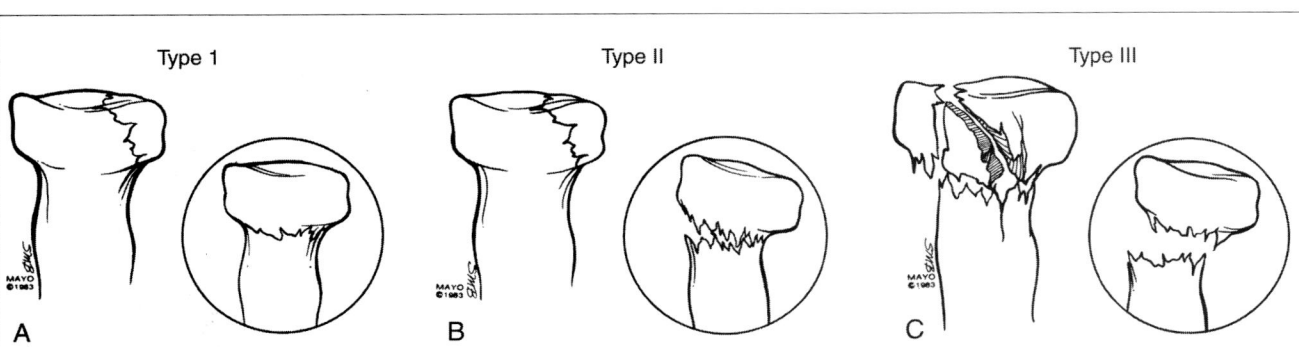

| Figure 1 | Mason classification of radial head fractures. **A,** Type I fractures are minimally or nondisplaced fractures. **B,** Type II fractures have greater than 2 mm of displacement. **C,** Type III fractures are severely comminuted fractures. Type IV fractures (*not shown*) are those associated with dislocation of the elbow joint. *(Reproduced with permission from Mayo, ©1983.)* |

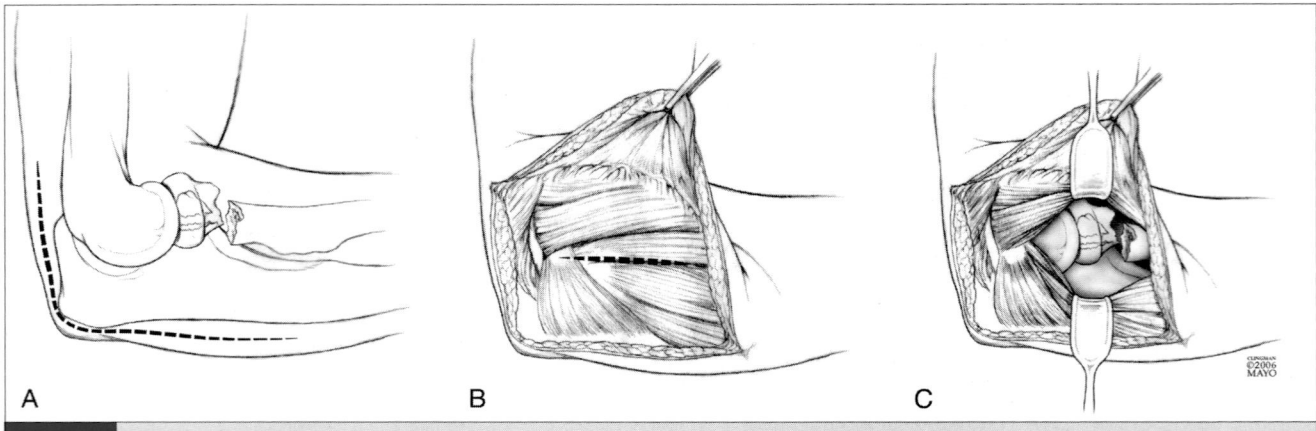

Figure 2 Illustrations showing the skin incision **(A)**, the incision in common extensor tendon **(B)**, and the exposure of a radial head fracture **(C)** during a direct approach for fixation or replacement of the radial head. *(Reproduced with permission from Mayo, ©2006.)*

or those with possible instability. If instability is absent, most patients will undergo arthroscopic débridement of fragments or reduction and screw fixation if the displacement is greater than 3 to 5 mm. Displacement of less than 3 mm seems to be well tolerated in most individuals.

In fractures that require fixation, attention is given to hardware placement to avoid impingement on the ulna. The safe zone for hardware placement has been defined in the literature; it is recommended that imaginary lines be drawn in direct supination, pronation, and neutral placement.[3] Implants may be placed up to the halfway point between the middle and posterior lines and a few millimeters beyond the midpoint between the anterior and middle lines. Likewise, it was determined that the nonarticulating region of the radial head was always found within a 90° angle bounded by the radial styloid and Lister's tubercle distally.[4]

Treatment for type III fractures is open reduction and internal fixation for minimally comminuted fractures (less than three articular fragments) or radial head excision or replacement. Excision alone may be performed for fractures without instability. Previously, excision alone was rarely recommended except in patients with low functional or physical demands or elderly patients without ligamentous instability because of the potential for pain or early ulnohumeral arthritis as a result of altered loads across the elbow joint. However, the findings of a recent study with an average 18-year follow-up suggest that primary or delayed excision of the radial head in the setting of radial head fractures leads to satisfactory results in most patients.[5] Replacement is usually preferred in the setting of young, active patients or patients with associated elbow instability.

The Essex-Lopresti lesion is a longitudinal disruption of the interosseous ligament, distal radial ulnar joint injury, and radial head fracture or dislocation. Treatment involves restoring stability of the elbow and wrist; repair or replacement of the radial head instead of excision is critical to prevent proximal migration of the radius.

Regardless of the procedure selected, all surgical techniques should allow for early active motion by removing mechanical blocks to motion, achieving rigid fixation of fracture fragments, and restoring the stability of the elbow. The patient is best placed supine for open procedures or in the lateral position for arthroscopic treatments. An examination with the patient under anesthesia using fluoroscopy before prepping and draping is critical to evaluate elbow and forearm stability and motion. A direct, muscle-splitting approach through the extensor digitorum communis is recommended, rather than approaching via Kocher's interval (between the anconeus and the extensor carpi ulnaris), which may put the dissection too posterior for unrestricted fixation of fractures and may also result in iatrogenic injury to the lateral ulnar collateral ligament, particularly in the setting of abandoning fixation in favor of radial head replacement (Figure 2).

Complications following radial head fracture include contracture (most commonly, patients will lack full extension), wrist pain secondary to an unrecognized interossei ligament injury, a distal radial ulnar joint or triangular fibrocartilaginous cartilage injury, posttraumatic arthritis, or instability resulting from an unrecognized ligamentous injury. However, longitudinal studies demonstrate that most fractures of the radial head heal well. Two recent reports on outcomes following nonsurgical treatment of type I and II radial head fractures demonstrated satisfactory results in most patients.[2,5] Type II fractures that remained symptomatic were successfully treated at a later date with resection.

Elbow Dislocation

Elbow dislocations may be classified by the position of the ulna relative to the humerus. Simple dislocations occur without fractures, whereas complex dislocations occur in conjunction with radial head or coronoid fractures. Most commonly, dislocations occur posteriorly and typically as a result of a fall on the outstretched hand in association with posterolateral rotatory instability. It is believed that posterior dislocations involve a force transmitted through the extended elbow, which levers out the joint. The valgus moment applied to the forearm with concomitant forearm supination causes the radial head and coronoid to rotate under the capitellum and dislocate. The progression of injury typically proceeds from lateral to medial in three stages (Figure 3). In the first stage, the lateral ulnar collateral ligament is disrupted, leading to posterolateral rotatory instability. In the second stage, with continued anterior and posterior disruption of the capsule, instability increases, and the elbow can subluxate to a perched position. In the first part of the third stage, all the ligamentous structures except the anterior band of the medial collateral ligament are torn, and the elbow hinges about the intact anterior band of the medial collateral ligament. With further disruption, the anterior band of the medial collateral ligament is torn and gross instability is noted. Varus posterolateral rotatory instability occurs in the setting of axial loading of the elbow with extension and with a varus and internal rotation moment of the forearm. This results in dislocation and an anteromedial coronoid fracture.

Initial evaluation in the emergency department includes standard radiographs and clinical examination to document neurovascular status before manipulation. The brachial artery and median and ulnar nerves may be injured. Volar forearm fasciotomy may be necessary if treatment delay is significant. Nerve injuries most commonly represent neurapraxias, and they may be treated with observation. If spontaneous recovery is not evident within 3 to 6 months, surgical exploration may be considered. Closed reduction may proceed with sedation. Longitudinal traction with the forearm in supination and with gentle guiding of the olecranon forward is usually successful.

Simple dislocations are usually stable and may be treated with immobilization for comfort followed by early range of motion, as demonstrated by a series of patients treated successfully at the US Naval Academy with early active motion and no immobilization.[6] If a fracture is present in conjunction with the ligamentous injury, however, treatment requires addressing potential instability by addressing the fracture and/or ligamentous injury. The progression of injury usually proceeds from lateral to medial. Treatment of dislocations resulting in persistent instability after relocation frequently involves focusing on the lateral ulnar collateral ligament. The essential lesion in recurrent or persistent instability following simple dislocation of the elbow typically involves lateral ulnar collateral ligament injury. The medial collateral ligament is repaired only if treatment of associated fractures and lateral collateral ligament injury does not restore stability.

Outcomes generally depend on the nature of the injury. Simple dislocations without significant ligamentous injury generally heal well following closed reduction. Outcomes for more significant injuries depend on repair and reconstruction to restore stability. Contrac-

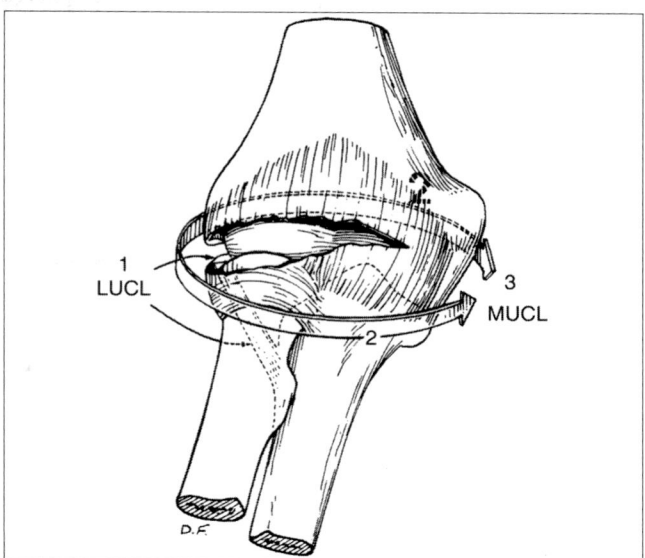

| Figure 3 | Illustration of the spectrum of instability to dislocation of the elbow. In stage 1, the lateral ulnar collateral ligament (LUCL) is disrupted. In stage 2, the other lateral ligamentous structures and the anterior and posterior capsule are disrupted. In stage 3, disruption of the medial ulnar collateral ligament (MUCL) can be partial with disruption of the posterior MUCL only (stage 3A) or complete (stage 3B). *(Reproduced with permission from O'Driscoll SW, Morrey BF, Korinek S, An KH: Elbow subluxation and dislocation: A spectrum of instability.* Clin Orthop Relat Res *1992;280:186-197.)* |

ture, particularly a small loss of terminal extension, is a common complication that appears to be related to the duration of immobilization.[7]

Coronoid Fractures

Coronoid fractures, which are rarely found in isolation, often occur in the setting of elbow trauma, such as radial head fractures and/or elbow dislocation. The optimal treatment of these fractures, therefore, relates intimately to the degree and nature of the other injuries to the elbow.

Classification systems of coronoid fractures include the Regan-Morrey classification, which is based on lateral plain film radiographs (Figure 4); a seven-part classification described by O'Driscoll (Figure 5); and a five-part classification proposed by Steinmann (Figure 6).

The simplicity of the Regan-Morrey classification is both an advantage and a limitation. This classification is commonly used because it allows physicians to easily define fracture type based on an easily and readily obtained single study (lateral plain film radiograph); however, it does not provide guidelines for surgical intervention. In the original description of this classification, only 4 of the 37 patients with coronoid fractures underwent surgical treatment. CT has become more readily

3: Upper Extremity

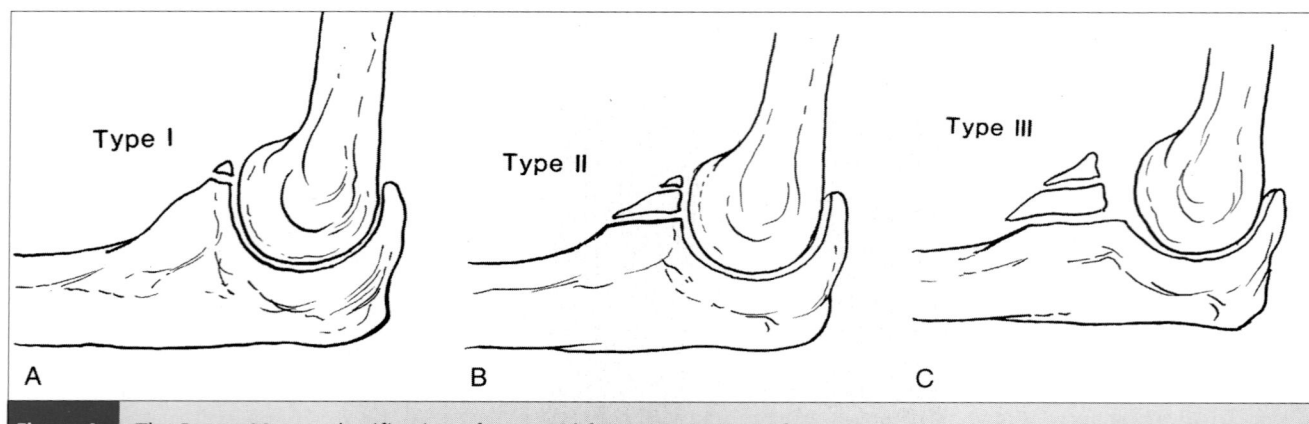

Figure 4 The Regan-Morrey classification of coronoid fractures. **A,** Type I fractures are described as avulsion fractures of the tip of the coronoid, and usually do not require surgical treatment. **B,** Type II fractures involve 50% or less of the height of the coronoid, and frequently do not require treatment. **C,** Type III fractures involve more than 50% of the height of the coronoid. *(Reproduced with permission from Regan WD, Morrey BF: Coronoid process and Monteggia fractures, in Morrey BF (ed):* The Elbow and Its Disorders, *ed 3. Philadelphia, PA, WB Saunders, 2000, pp 396-408.)*

available in recent years and enables physicians to further define the fracture fragments and determine whether surgical fixation is indicated.

The classification described by O'Driscoll includes three parts with seven subtypes, and this system attempts to correlate the presumed mechanism of injury with the fracture type. The classification system proposed by Steinmann is based on three-dimensional CT evaluation of a large number of coronoid fractures and attempts to consolidate five main fracture types, including the three types of Regan-Morrey fractures plus two oblique fracture types.

Small tip fractures typically occur in patients with a terrible triad injury as a result of a valgus and supination moment of the forearm at the time of injury. This is the most common pattern of elbow dislocation, and it has been termed posterolateral rotatory instability. In this setting, the coronoid fracture is of secondary concern; treatment of the radial head fracture and the associated lateral instability is paramount. A small tip fracture can be ignored as long as stable fixation or replacement of the radial head has been performed. With this injury pattern, the lateral collateral ligament is typically torn off the humerus and will require suture fixation at the lateral epicondyle. Cadaver studies have shown that if fixation or replacement of the radial head is performed in the setting of intact ligaments, then stability will be achieved unless greater than 50% of the coronoid is fractured.[8] Therefore, emphasis should be placed on restoring the radial head and lateral ligament stability in patients with less than 50% involvement of the coronoid.

A slightly larger coronoid fracture fragment typically occurs with an anteromedial coronoid fracture. This results from a varus internal rotation moment to the forearm and typically does not involve injury to the radial head. Radiographs are often deceptively benign appearing for patients with this type of injury, with a small bony fragment that may not be recognized initially as a coronoid fracture. On the AP radiograph, subtle incongruity of the joint line may be present. Normally, the joint line between the medial trochlea and the ulna is of equal width. The lateral trochlea and ulnar distance is a bit wider than on the medial side, but, most importantly, the joint space should be symmetric. If a "river delta" sign or narrowing of the joint space from lateral to medial is present, then there is a high likelihood of a coronoid fracture or significant ligamentous instability. If a coronoid fracture is suspected from the standard radiographs, then a CT scan should be obtained and will usually be diagnostic. It is important to diagnose and treat a coronoid fracture in association with joint subluxation or incongruity because, if left untreated, progression to ulnohumeral arthritis will occur because of altered stresses at the ulnohumeral joint. This fracture pattern is distinct from a standard tip fracture associated with a posterolateral elbow dislocation. The elbow instability associated with a tip fracture is based on the lateral collateral ligament injury and the fracture of the radial head. In an anteromedial fracture, the instability is directly related to the fracture of the coronoid. Recently, outcomes on a series of 18 patients with this injury were described.[8] Patients who had inadequate treatment had poor or fair results with malalignment and varus subluxation of the elbow.

Biomechanical studies suggest that a competent lateral collateral ligament is more important to stability in anteromedial fractures, typically those involving less than 25% of the coronoid.[8] Therefore, in patients with small anteromedial fractures, attention should be focused on restoration of ligamentous stability rather than fracture fixation.

Cadaver studies indicate that in larger transverse fractures comprising greater than 50% of the height of the coronoid, fixation of the coronoid is required to restore stability.[9] It is assumed also that large anteromedial coronoid fractures will require surgical fixation. Although biomechanical studies do not replicate in vivo

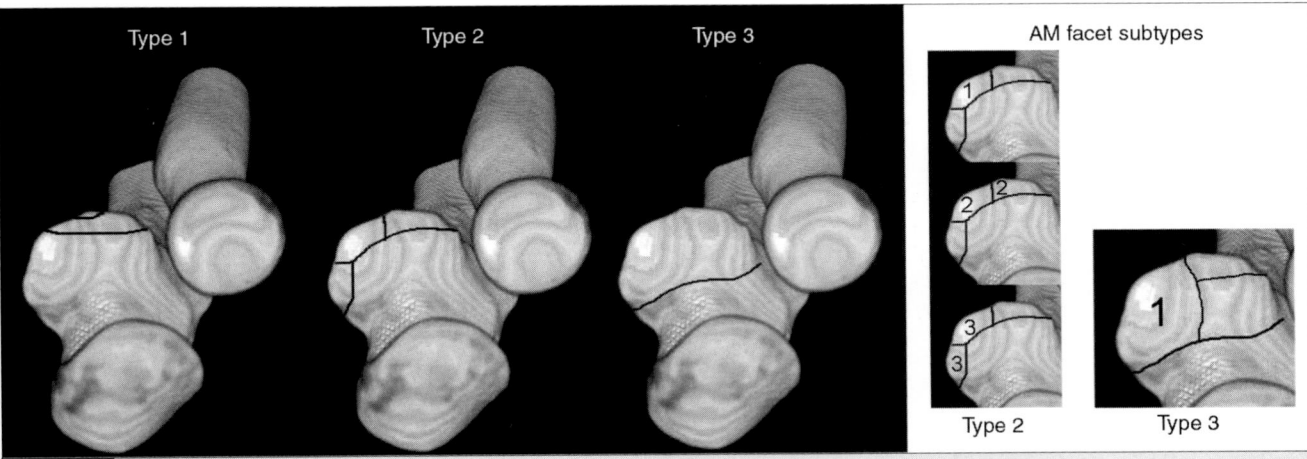

Figure 5 Classification of coronoid fractures by anatomic type according to O'Driscoll. Fracture types include tip fractures, anteromedial (AM) coronoid fragments, and basal fragments with multiple subtypes. *(Reproduced with permission from David Ring, MD.)*

fracture patterns and associated injuries, it appears that a fracture of less than 25% of the coronoid may not require fixation if the radial head and ligamentous structures are repaired or replaced.

In coronoid fractures associated with instability, surgical fixation can be achieved using several methods. As mentioned, a tip fracture associated with a posterolateral rotatory instability injury (terrible triad injury) usually does not require fixation. However, if this fracture is of significant size, fixation can be achieved from the lateral side through the temporary defect in the radial head when the radial head is replaced or retracted during internal fixation (Figure 7). Cannulated screw fixation can be placed from the posterior ulna up into the coronoid fragment. This can be simplified by the use of an anterior cruciate ligament guide to help reduce the coronoid fracture and also guide the cannulated pin to the best position on the coronoid tip. As an alternative, suture fixation of small coronoid tip fractures has been advocated in the past, but this technique results in less stability, and it should not be used for large coronoid fractures. Stable fixation or replacement of the radial head and lateral ligamentous repair is paramount in addressing a terrible triad fracture.

An anteromedial coronoid fracture will often need to be approached from the medial side because the radial head is often intact as a result of the varus rotational moment at the time of injury. Through either a direct medial approach or a posterior incision, the coronoid fracture can be exposed through the "floor" of the ulnar nerve with anterior elevation (not release) of the flexor pronator group (Figure 8). This exposure allows for application of an anterior plate that can buttress and maintain the reduction. In most anteromedial fractures, the lateral collateral ligament has been avulsed off of the humerus and will need to be repaired. It is for this reason that a posterior skin incision, which allows access to both sides of the joint, is favored. The injury to the lateral collateral ligament is usually iden-

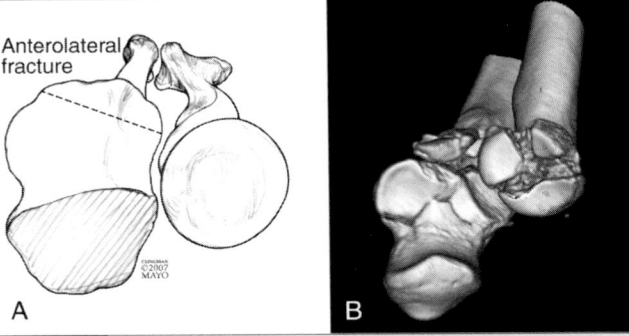

Figure 6 Classification of coronoid fracture type, according to visualization using three-dimensional CT scans as proposed by Steinmann. **A,** Illustration of the pattern of an anterolateral coronoid fracture. This type of fracture often results in a radial head fracture. **B,** Three-dimensional CT scan of an anterolateral coronoid fracture with an associated radial head fracture. *(Reproduced with permission from Mayo, ©2007.)*

tified by the development of a surgical plane between the anconeus and the extensor carpi ulnaris. The ligament can then be repaired back to the lateral epicondyle with multiple suture anchors. In anteromedial fractures involving less than 25% of the coronoid without involvement of the sublime tubercle, secure fixation of the lateral collateral ligament is most important.

Distal Humerus Fractures

Classification systems of fractures of the distal humerus include that of Mehne and Matta, which classifies fractures according to columns involved and level of the fracture into the metaphyseal region (high versus low). The AO/OTA classification system is straightforward: type A

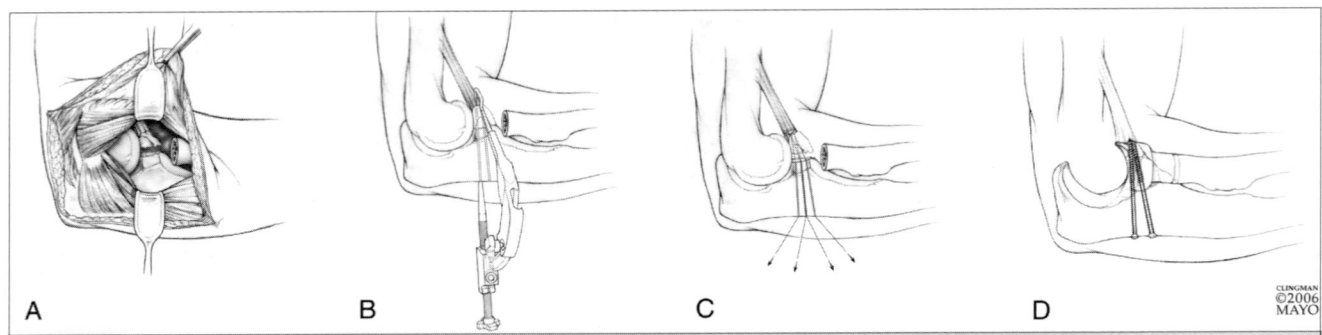

Figure 7 Fixation of small coronoid fractures through a temporary defect in the radial head. **A,** The radial head is resected and the coronoid fracture is exposed. **B,** The large coronoid fracture is reduced with an anterior cruciate ligament guide, which is useful for drilling holes for suture or screw fixation. **C,** Suture is passed over the coronoid fragment and through the ulna drill holes (*arrows*). **D,** Screw placement with large coronoid fracture. *(Reproduced with permission from Mayo, ©2006.)*

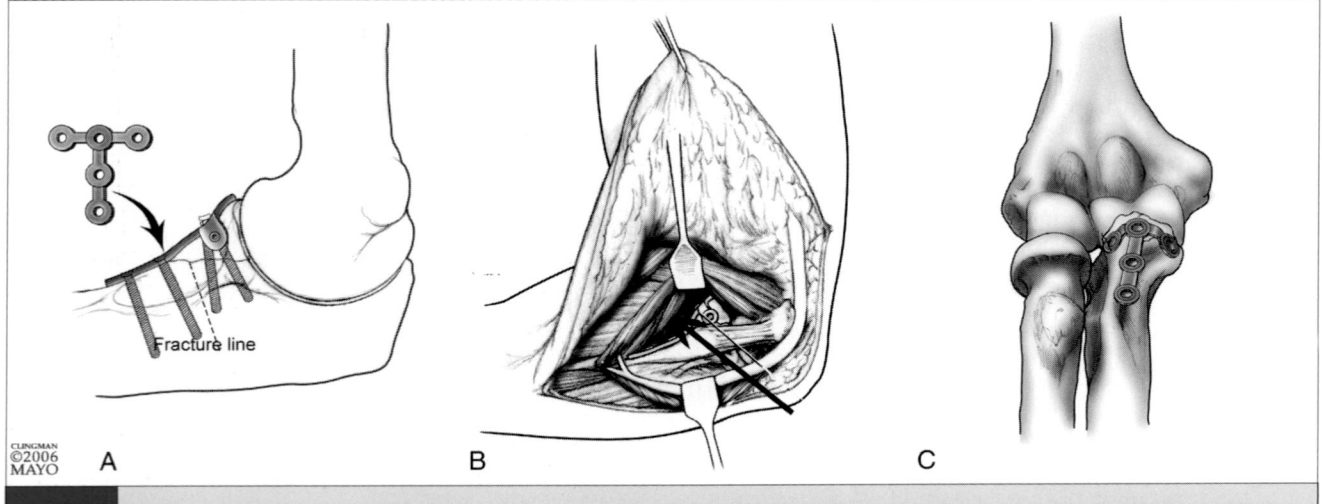

Figure 8 Fixation of an anteromedial coronoid fracture through a medial approach. **A,** Lateral view of plate fixation. **B,** Plate reduction of the coronoid fracture. **C,** Anterior view of the plate fixation. *(Reproduced with permission from Mayo, ©2006.)*

fractures are extra-articular, type B fractures have partial involvement of the articular surface, and type C fractures have complete articular involvement (Figure 9).

Standard radiographic studies should be obtained for the diagnosis of distal humerus fractures. In most patients, a CT scan with three-dimensional reconstructions and joint subtraction views is helpful for preoperative planning. Basic considerations involve an evaluation of the articular surface involvement.

Patients with distal humerus fractures are usually best served by treatment with open reduction and internal fixation of their fracture. Rarely, in selected patients (those with low physical demands, elderly patients, or those with preexisting inflammatory arthritis) other options may be selected. Total elbow arthroplasty may be used in frail patients with extremely low physical demands. It should be avoided in young or active patients because the durability of this procedure is limited in this patient population. The "bag of bones" technique involves the use of a cast or splint immobilization to allow healing, and it is useful in a limited number of patients. A growing body of literature suggests that open reduction and internal fixation of distal humerus fractures is a reliable treatment even in elderly and low-demand patients. Open reduction and internal fixation was compared with nonsurgical treatment of distal humerus fractures in a study of patients older than 75 years (mean age, 85 years).[10] Surgically treated patients had improved Orthopaedic Trauma Association ratings, improved range of motion, improved pain relief, and radiographic evidence of maintained reduction; complication rates were not higher than those reported in the literature for younger patients. Similarly, a recent study found that age was not predictive of results or frequency of complications in treatment of distal humerus fractures with open reduction and internal fixation.[11] In addition, 19 patients (average age, 72 years) who had displaced intra-articular fractures of the distal humerus were studied.[12] During the 10-year study period, only one patient was treated nonsurgically because of health concerns that precluded surgery. All patients were satisfied with their outcomes. Mayo Elbow Performance scores were excellent for 79% of patients and good for 21%, with no fair or poor results. Range of motion measured 17° to 128°, and 79% of patients reported no pain. Studies such as this and others suggest that the role of open reduction and internal fixation may be expanded.

One study reported on the use of total elbow arthroplasty for treating acute distal humerus fractures with good results at an average 2.8-year follow-up; however, nearly one half of the patients in that series had rheumatoid arthritis.[13] In patients without preexisting rheumatoid arthritis, the authors reported a 30% rate of persistent pain and a 30% rate of nerve injury. Mechanical failures of total elbow arthroplasty in patients with posttraumatic arthritis at 2-year follow-up were noted.[9] It appears, therefore, that total elbow arthroplasty in patients with acute trauma should be reserved for those who are elderly, those with inflammatory arthritis, and/or those who have extremely low functional demands.

Surgical approaches include olecranon osteotomy, triceps elevating (Bryan-Morrey approach), triceps splitting, the triceps-reflecting anconeus pedicle approach, and the anconeus flap transolecranon approach (Figure 10).

If open reduction and internal fixation is used to treat a fracture with a significant intra-articular component, a triceps-reflecting anconeus pedicle approach or an olecranon osteotomy approach (such as the anconeus flap transolecranon approach) can then be used. The osteotomy is made with the use of a saw to cut partially through, followed by the use of an osteotome to complete the osteotomy and create fragments that interdigitate and thereby facilitate reduction and stability. The triceps-reflecting anconeus pedicle approach allows for visualization without olecranon osteotomy. Transolecranon approaches provide the best visualization of the distal humerus articular surface. However, an olecranon osteotomy should not be performed if there is a chance that open reduction and internal fixation may be abandoned and the patient treated with total elbow arthroplasty. The anconeus flap transolecranon approach is a modification of transolecranon approaches and it incorporates advantages of the triceps-reflecting anconeus pedicle approach and the use of olecranon osteotomy. The anconeus flap transolecranon approach is designed to preserve the neurovascular supply to the anconeus muscle, which facilitates a vascularized bed over the osteotomy site and preserves the anconeus, allowing it to contribute to stability of the elbow. The anconeus is raised on a flap by incising Kocher's interval and freeing the muscle from the extensor carpi ulnaris laterally and elevation subperiosteally from the ulna. The standard osteotomy is performed, and the anconeus and olecranon are elevated in continuity with the triceps. Fixation of the osteotomy can be done with tension

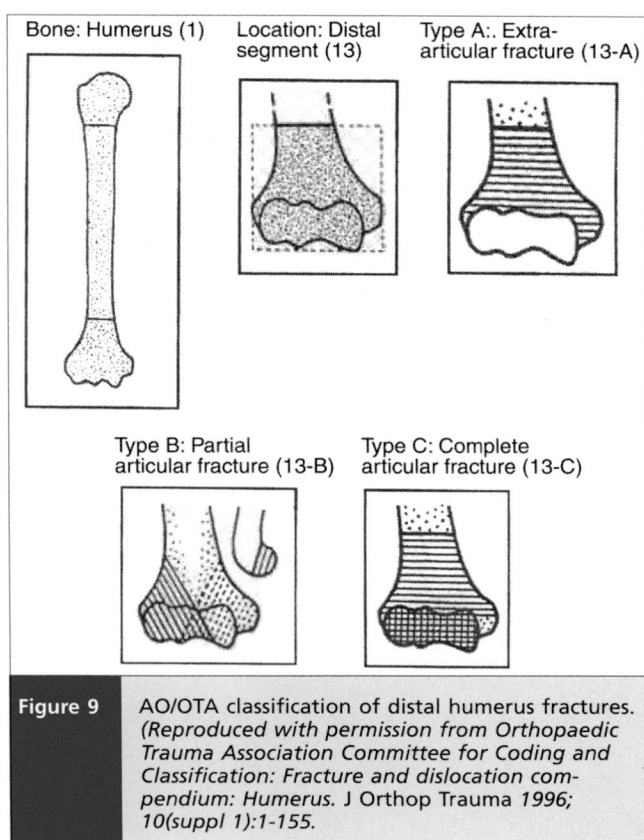

Figure 9 AO/OTA classification of distal humerus fractures. *(Reproduced with permission from Orthopaedic Trauma Association Committee for Coding and Classification: Fracture and dislocation compendium: Humerus. J Orthop Trauma 1996; 10(suppl 1):1-155.*

band wiring, intramedullary screw fixation, or plate and screw fixation according to the preference of the surgeon. In vitro studies indicate that intramedullary screw fixation with tension band wiring results in improved strength, which provides additional rotational stability; however, low-profile plates make hardware prominence with plate and screw constructs less problematic.

The goals of surgical fixation include restoration of the articular surface and achieving adequate stability to allow for early motion to prevent stiffness. Although 90-90 perpendicular plate configurations, as advocated by the AO/ASIF, have been considered the standard of care, recent studies have suggested that parallel plating is at least as mechanically stable as perpendicularly oriented plates and may result in a stronger construct when interdigitating screws are applied.[14]

Technical objectives have been outlined for the treatment of distal humeral fractures with parallel plating systems. Two strong parallel plates should apply compression at the supracondylar level, and screws should be arranged such that they interdigitate with one another and engage and buttress as much of the distal articular portion as possible. Such constructs allow for stable fixation and facilitate early motion protocols, resulting in improved outcomes and less stiffness (Figure 11).

Factors that have been found to adversely affect outcome include multiple trauma, more comminution of the joint surface (AO type C3), and open fractures. Non-

3: Upper Extremity

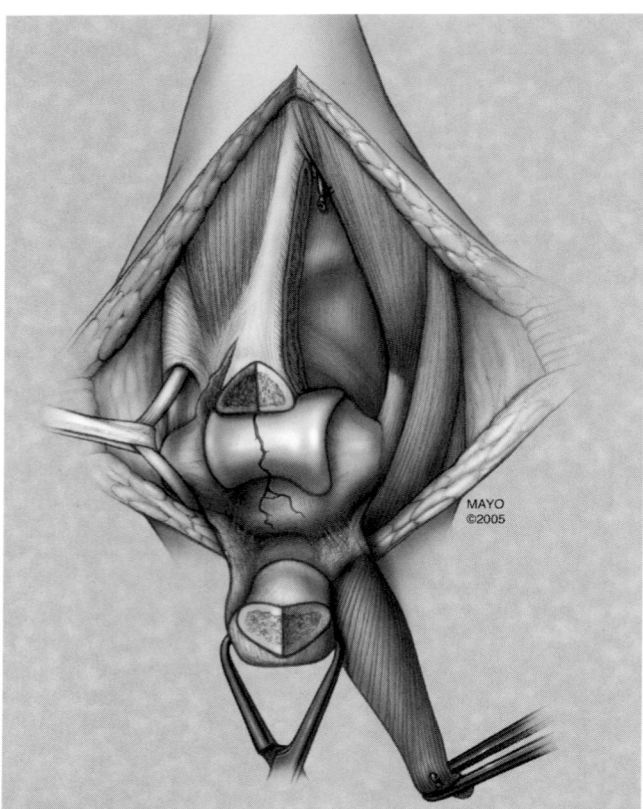

Figure 10 Illustration showing that the anconeus flap transolecranon approach preserves the anconeus and allows for an osteotomy of the ulna. *(Reproduced with permission from Mayo, ©2005.)*

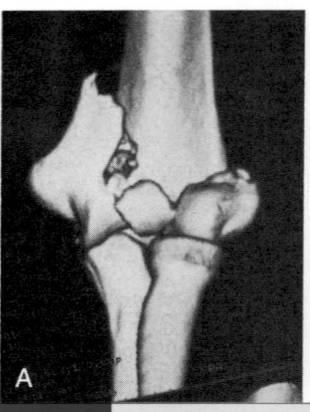 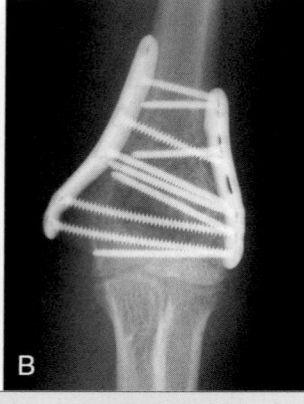

Figure 11 Preoperative **(A)** and postoperative **(B)** imaging studies of a distal humerus fracture. The postoperative radiograph shows that the fracture was treated using parallel plating. *(Reproduced with permission from Scott Steinmann, MD.)*

union is usually the result of inadequate fixation. Elbow stiffness is a common complication, but if adequate stability at the time of fixation is achieved, early motion protocols may be initiated, limiting the amount of residual stiffness. Ulnar neuropathy is also a common com-

plication; use of anterior subcutaneous transposition of the nerve may lessen the frequency of this complication.

Capitellar Fractures

Capitellar fractures do not commonly occur as isolated injuries. When they do occur, they present most often in adults, in women, and in association with a posterior elbow dislocation and/or radial head fracture. The pattern is one of a shear fracture in the coronal plane. This fracture type is more common in women, possibly because of the ability to hyperextend the elbow, allowing the radial head to forcefully shear off the capitellum. Type I capitellar fractures, Hahn-Steinthal fractures, involve shearing of the capitellum from the humerus and are usually treated with open reduction and internal fixation. Type II capitellar fractures, Kocher-Lorenz fractures, are less substantial shear fractures of the cartilage and a thin layer of subchondral bone. Type III capitellar fractures involve comminution or compression of the articular surface. Type II and III capitellar fractures are generally treated with excision of the fracture fragments.

Condylar Fractures

Condylar fractures are uncommon and usually involve the lateral rather than medial condyle. These fractures, unlike capitellar fractures, present with the fracture line in the sagittal plane, typically involving the epicondyle and soft-tissue attachments. Milch type I lateral condyle fractures leave the lateral wall of the trochlea attached to the humerus. In Milch type II fractures, the lateral wall of the trochlea is attached to the fracture fragment. Practically speaking, most fractures are treated with open reduction and internal fixation, particularly displaced Milch type I fractures and all Milch type II fractures (**Figure 12**). A posterior incision with elevation of a lateral flap provides excellent exposure. The articular fracture can often be exposed through distal retraction of the common extensors, which are attached to the fractured lateral epicondyle. In patients with more complex injuries, an olecranon osteotomy can provide access to the fracture.

Olecranon Fractures

The subcutaneous location of the olecranon makes it vulnerable to injury, and olecranon fractures commonly occur as a result of low-energy trauma. Fractures of the olecranon are generally amenable to treatment and usually have a favorable prognosis.

The Mayo classification of olecranon fractures divides olecranon fractures into three types according to criteria regarding stability, comminution, and displacement (**Figure 13**). The Mayo classification thus provides a basis for a rational treatment algorithm by fracture type and subtype and conveys prognostic value.

Complex olecranon fracture-dislocations are associated with injury to the radial head or coronoid process and are typically multifragmentary, complex injuries that may not be adequately described by the Mayo

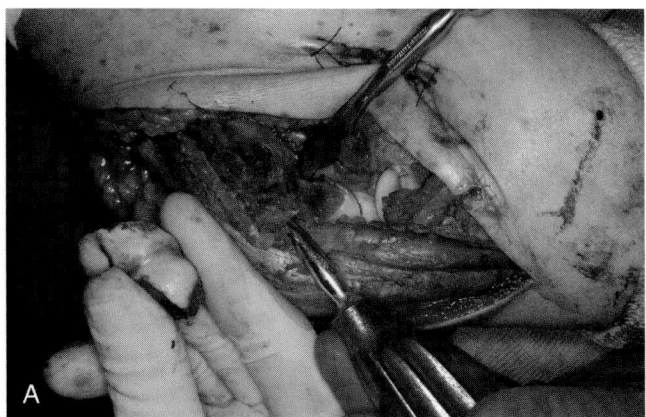

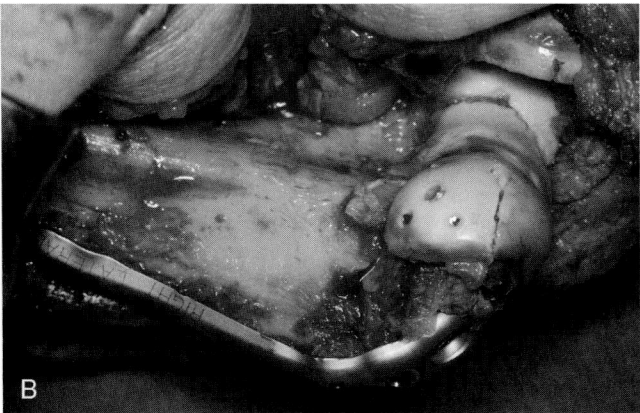

Figure 12 **A,** Intraoperative photograph showing the typical shear fracture pattern that occurs with capitella and trochlea fractures. **B,** This fracture was fixed using a plate and screw construct and headless screws under the articular cartilage. *(Reproduced with permission from Scott Steinmann, MD.)*

classification scheme. Anterior fracture-dislocations are often referred to as transolecranon fracture-dislocations because the mechanism of injury appears to involve anterior displacement of the forearm, resulting in the trochlea being driven through the olecranon process and the radial head being displaced anteriorly. This injury is characterized by instability of the ulnohumeral joint with a preserved radioulnar relationship. Posterior fracture-dislocations of the olecranon involve posterior dislocation of the radial head with an apex posterior fracture of the ulna. These fractures may be considered a variant of the posterior Monteggia lesion. Both posterior and anterior variants are commonly associated with basal fractures of the coronoid.

For Mayo type I olecranon fractures, nonsurgical treatment typically involves sling immobilization for comfort followed by early gentle range of motion initiated within days of injury. Weekly follow-up with radiographs is essential to monitor for displacement; restrictions on active-resisted elbow extension and weight bearing should be maintained for 6 to 8 weeks, with gradual increases in these activities as tolerated. Rarely,

in selected patients, Mayo type I fractures may benefit from open reduction and internal fixation to allow immediate motion and stability; alternatively, some Mayo type I fractures may be treated with immobilization in a long arm cast at 90° of flexion for 3 to 4 weeks. Range-of-motion exercises may be commenced at an earlier point in selected patients, such as the elderly, in whom stiffness occurs more frequently.

Displaced olecranon fractures (Mayo type II and type III) are best treated surgically, with either excision or open reduction and internal fixation. Goals of surgical management include restoring the articular congruity and stability of the elbow, maintaining extension power, and providing stable anatomic fixation such that early range of motion is possible, thereby lessening the risk of postoperative stiffness. Options include tension band wiring, intramedullary screw placement, plate and screw constructs (Figure 14), bioabsorbable pins, or excision. Tension band wiring using standard AO technique is generally accepted and widely used as a treatment for most olecranon fracture patterns amenable to this fixation technique. Tension band wiring converts tensile forces across the fracture to compressive forces that, with motion, exert compression across the fracture site. Prominent pins or wires may be problematic, however; one series reported hardware-related pain (in 24% of patients) and functional difficulties (in 32% of patients) were relieved by hardware removal.[15-17] Hardware removal rates are up to 81% in some series.[15-17] Nevertheless, up to 97% good to excellent results have been widely reported with tension band wiring using proper technique. However, for fractures with fragments distal to the coronoid, plate and screw osteosynthesis is preferred because these more distal fragments are usually not adequately fixed using tension band wiring. Likewise, more comminuted fractures or oblique patterns are best treated with plate and screw osteosynthesis to optimize stability.

Mayo type IIA olecranon fractures are usually adequately treated with tension band wiring or plate fixation. Mayo type IIB olecranon fractures are treated according to the age and activity level of the patient. In patients younger than 60 years, anatomic reduction of fracture fragments followed by plate and screw fixation is the treatment of choice. Care should be taken to avoid shortening the articular groove of the ulna between the olecranon process and the coronoid process because doing so may lead to early arthritis. In older patients, or in those in whom comminution is severe, excision of proximal fragments with advancement and reinsertion of the triceps tendon may be preferred.

Mayo type III olecranon fractures (displaced, unstable fractures) represent the most difficult treatment challenge of all olecranon fractures and are associated with high complication rates and low rates of satisfactory outcomes. Mayo type III fractures are associated with a high incidence of concomitant pathology, such as ligamentous trauma or bony injuries of the radial head or coronoid or distal humerus; these should be addressed at the time of olecranon fixation. Mayo type

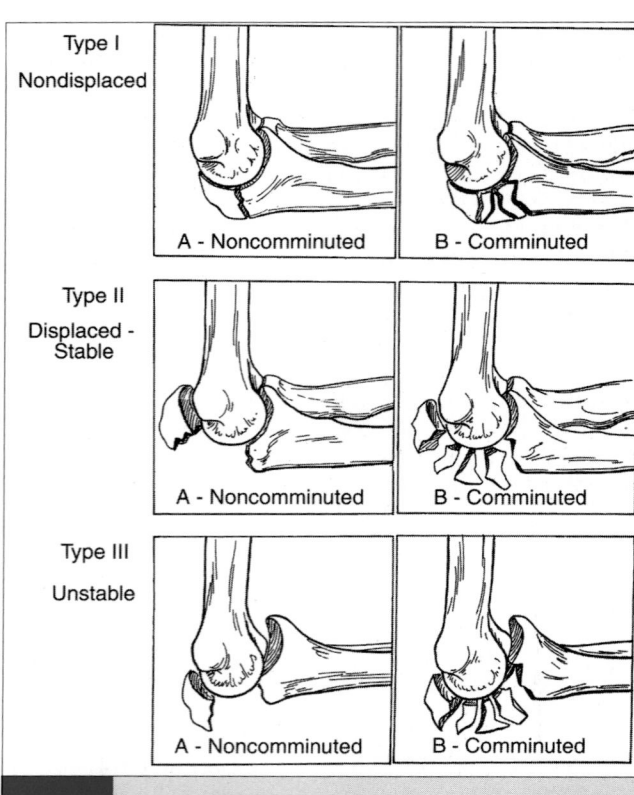

Type I
Nondisplaced

A - Noncomminuted   B - Comminuted

Type II
Displaced -
Stable

A - Noncomminuted   B - Comminuted

Type III
Unstable

A - Noncomminuted   B - Comminuted

Figure 13 Olecranon fractures according to the Mayo classification system. This classification system is useful in treatment algorithms. Mayo type I fractures are nondisplaced (< 2 mm) with no comminution (IA) or with comminution (IB). Mayo type IIA fractures are stable fractures with more than 3 mm of displacement and no comminution. Mayo type IIB fractures are stable with less than 3 mm of displacement and comminution. Mayo type IIIA fractures are unstable, displaced fracture-dislocations without comminution. Mayo type IIIB fractures are unstable, displaced fracture-dislocations with comminution. *(Reproduced with permission from Cabanela ME, Morrey BF: Fractures of the olecranon, in Morrey BF (ed): The Elbow and Its Disorders, ed 3. Philadelphia, PA, WB Saunders, 2000, pp 365-379.)*

ceps weakness, instability, stiffness, and a theoretic risk of increased arthrosis. Biomechanical studies suggest loss of extension strength may be minimized by reattaching the triceps at a more posterior site.[18] Up to 80% of the olecranon may be excised without sacrificing stability if the coronoid and anterior soft tissues are intact.[18] If anterior damage is present or if comminution extends as far distally as the coronoid process, instability results if too much proximal ulna is excised. An increase in instability of the elbow with olecranon excision was noted.[19] Satisfactory clinical outcomes have been described, however, for the treatment of olecranon fracture by excision when used in appropriate patient populations.

After surgical intervention, the arm should be elevated overnight and the initial dressing changed on the second day. Active and passive motion is then initiated. Protected use of the extremity is maintained with minimal weight bearing and no resistance greater than that of gravity for 6 weeks or until radiographic evidence of healing is seen.

Outcomes following surgical treatment are generally good to excellent, with most studies noting satisfactory outcomes and restoration of normal or near-normal function in more than 95% of patients.[15-17]

Complications include nonunion or malunion, infection, loss of motion, ulnar nerve symptoms, arthrosis, and need for additional procedures such as hardware removal. Loss of motion may be problematic, particularly a 10° to 15° extension lag, which appears to be related to immobilization. Radiographic evidence of degenerative changes in the ulnohumeral joint has been documented in 20% to 50% of patients up to 15 to 25 years following olecranon fracture, but it is generally asymptomatic.[15-17] Symptomatic hardware is the most common complication, requiring removal in 11.4% to 81% of patients.[16] Hardware prominence is more common in tension band wiring relative to other fixation techniques, such as figure-of-8 wiring or plate and screw constructs. The risk of problematic hardware with tension band wiring is decreased if attention to proper AO technique is observed and wires are bent 180° and impacted into bone with the triceps securely sutured over wires. Overall, however, decreased range of motion, radiographic evidence of degenerative changes, and requirement for hardware removal are common, but these complications generally are not devastating and may be obviated by attention to proper technique, anatomic reduction, and proper postoperative management.

III olecranon fractures typically require plate fixation and ligamentous reconstruction.

Noncomminuted (Mayo type IIIA) olecranon fractures may be treated with a plate and screw construct and anatomic reduction. Comminuted (Mayo type IIIB) fractures may likewise be treated with plate osteosynthesis or, in rare instances, with excision of fracture fragments, although instability is a possible complication.

Excision of fracture fragments with advancement and reinsertion of the triceps is preferred for elderly, low-demand patients and for patients with nonunions, poor soft-tissue viability, avulsion-type extra-articular fractures, severe comminution (as in Mayo type IIB fractures), or, rarely, Mayo type IIIB fractures. The disadvantages of excision include subsequent risks of tri-

Distal Biceps Ruptures

Ruptures of the distal biceps tendon are readily diagnosed by history in most patients. The patient with a distal biceps rupture is typically a middle-aged man who relates a history of lifting an object or a forced extension of a flexed and loaded forearm.

On clinical examination, the patient exhibits pain and weakness in flexion and supination and may have ecchymoses in the antecubital fossa or an abnormal muscle contour of the biceps. Additionally, with the elbow at 90° of flexion and the pronated forearm rotated to supination, the examiner can, in uninjured patients, hook the tip of his or her thumb about the biceps tendon in the cubital fossa; however, in patients with distal avulsion of the tendon, this feature is lost. Occasionally, some fibers or a fascial sleeve may remain intact, giving an appearance of intact tendon. The examiner must discriminate between the normal lacertus fibrosus, which remains intact even with biceps rupture and the biceps tendon. MRI may show evidence of a distal biceps rupture, but it is not necessary for diagnosis in most patients and occasionally may be read as falsely negative.

Treatment of a distal biceps rupture may be nonsurgical; however, an estimated 40% loss of supination power and a 30% loss of flexion power can be anticipated. If surgical treatment is elected, it should ideally proceed within several days of injury before tissue can become retracted and scarred. In addition, complications of early repairs are less likely. Risks include rerupture and injury to neurovascular structures (especially the lateral antebrachial cutaneous nerve), persistent anterior elbow pain, and heterotopic ossification. Rerupture is uncommon, with most series reporting a 0% to 4.3% reruptured rate.[20-22] Heterotopic ossification is uncommon, and it is likely dependent on patient- and injury-related factors rather than surgical technique. Two-incision techniques offer the ability to limit the size of the anterior exposure (Figure 15) and decrease risk of neurovascular injury; if a muscle-splitting approach is used, there is no higher risk of radioulnar synostoses. Complications with a single-incision technique and a modified Boyd-Anderson two-incision technique were compared.[20] Complication rates were higher (44%) in the single-incision technique group than in the two-incision technique group (10%). In addition, patients who underwent the two-incision technique repair had a slightly more rapid recovery of flexion strength.

The technique of repair to bone is also variable. Options include direct repair to bone through bony tunnels and the use of interference screws, suture anchors, or other devices. Clinical studies have documented that tendon repair to bone through bony tunnels in the bicipital tuberosity appears to be sufficient to withstand forces in vivo, even with early motion protocols, and biologically provides a bone-to-tendon interface for robust healing.[23]

Diaphyseal Forearm Fractures

The use of plate and screw osteosynthesis to treat diaphyseal forearm fractures results in a high union rate, ranging from 95% to 98% in most series.[24-26] Although pediatric fractures may be treated with intramedullary fixation or casting, most adult fractures are best treated with open reduction and internal fixation with plate and screws. Important considerations at the time of surgery include restoration of the radial bow and

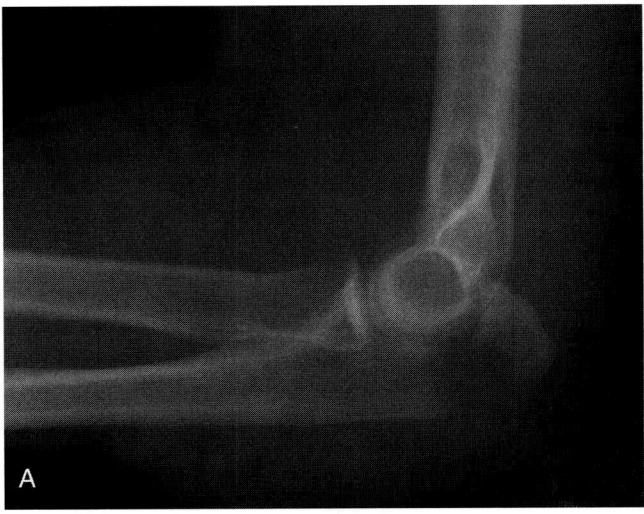
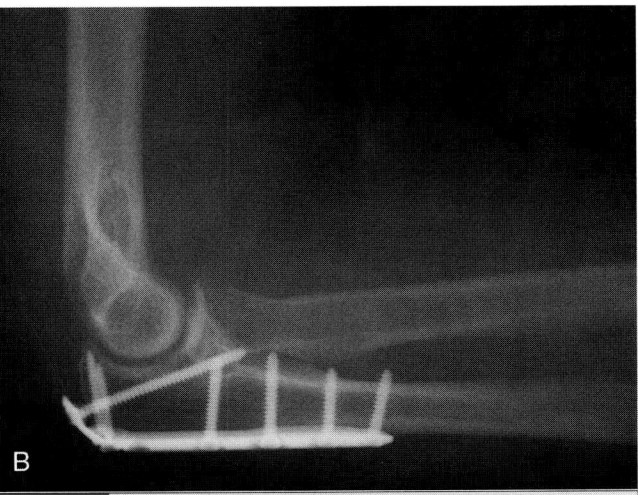

Figure 14 Preoperative **(A)** and postoperative **(B)** radiographs demonstrate open reduction and internal fixation of an olecranon fracture with a plate and screw construct. *(Reproduced with permission from Scott Steinmann, MD.)*

avoiding fixation in malrotation to preserve forearm rotation. Malunion without restoration of the radial bow is related to poor outcomes. It has been demonstrated that restoration of the normal radial bow resulted in a better functional outcome with improved range of motion and grip strength.[27] Some authors recommend primary bone grafting at the time of fixation if comminution exceeds one third of the bone diameter. In a 2004 study, the authors reviewed 319 diaphyseal forearm fractures with variable comminution treated with open reduction and internal fixation without bone grafting.[26] Although fractures with more than two thirds diaphyseal width comminution had a prolonged time to union, no difference in the union rate was noted. Therefore, it appears that primary bone grafting may not be necessary for treatment of diaphyseal forearm fractures. The authors noted that fractures with

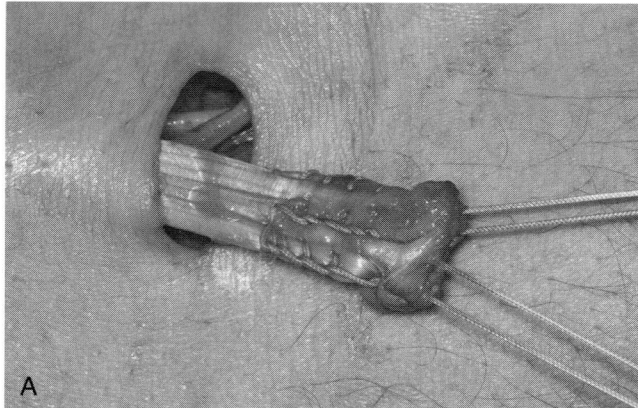

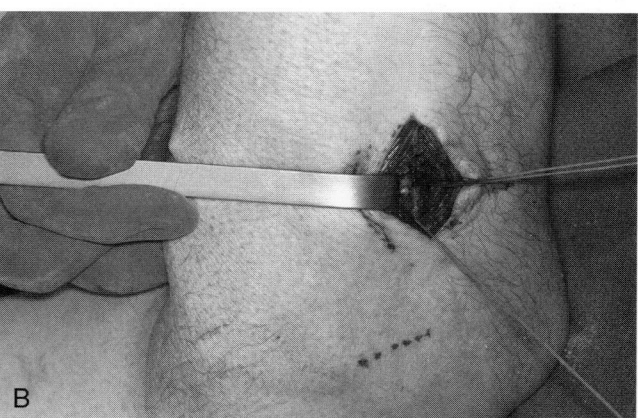

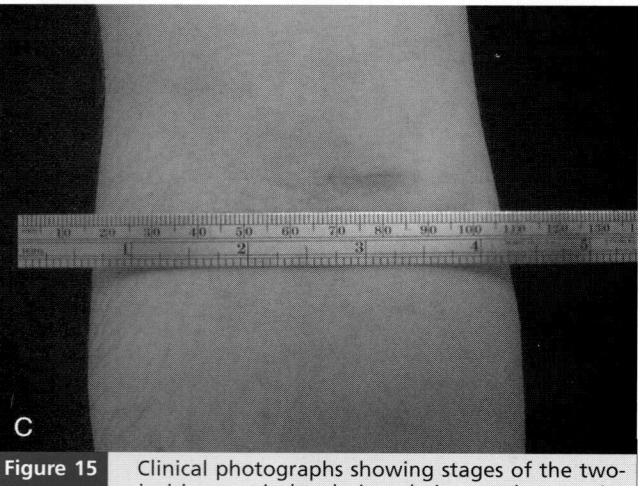

Figure 15 Clinical photographs showing stages of the two-incision surgical technique being used to repair a distal biceps rupture. **A,** The distal biceps is prepared for reinsertion using a Krackow stitch. **B,** The bicipital tuberosity is approached and prepared to accept the tendon. **C,** The healed antecubital fossa incision is highly cosmetic. (*Reproduced with permission from Scott Steinmann, MD.*)

greater than two thirds diaphyseal width comminution were rare, constituting 5% of the fractures in their series. In a study conducted to determine which comminuted fractures are more likely to go on to nonunion,

41 patients with comminuted diaphyseal forearm fractures were treated with dynamic compression plates.[28] Factors including multiple trauma, open fracture, and use of cancellous bone graft at time of surgery did not have a statistically significant association with the development of a nonunion, which occurred in 12% of the patients.

Annotated References

1. Amis AA, Miller JH: The mechanisms of elbow fractures: An investigation using impact tests in vitro. *Injury* 1995;26:163-168.

2. Akesson T, Herbertsson P, Josefsson PO, Hasserius R, Besjakov J, Karlsson MK: Primary nonoperative treatment of moderately displaced two-part fractures of the radial head. *J Bone Joint Surg Am* 2006;88:1909-1914.

   This recent report documented good outcomes in patients with Mason type II radial head fractures treated nonsurgically at an average follow-up of 19 years. On average, small differences in the range of motion in the injured/normal arm were observed (flexion, 137°/139°; extension, 3°/1°; supination, 86°/88°; pronation, 87°/87°); 82% of patients had no continued symptoms. For patients with continued symptoms, delayed radial head excision provided satisfactory treatment.

3. Smith GR, Hotchkiss RN: Radial head and neck fractures: Anatomic guidelines for proper placement of internal fixation. *J Shoulder Elbow Surg* 1996;5:113-117.

4. Caputo AE, Mazzocca AD, Santoro VM: The nonarticulating portion of the radial head: Anatomic and clinical correlations for internal fixation. *J Hand Surg [Am]* 1998;23:1082-1090.

5. Herbertsson P, Josefsson PO, Hasserius R, Besjakov J, Nyqvist F, Karlsson MK: Fractures of the radial head and neck treated with radial head excision. *J Bone Joint Surg Am* 2004;86-A:1925-1930.

   This study demonstrated fair or good results in most patients with radial head fractures that were treated with primary or delayed radial head excision (average follow-up, 18 years). No difference was noted between patients treated with primary or delayed excisions.

6. Ross G, McDevitt ER, Chronister R, Ove PN: Treatment of simple elbow dislocation using an immediate motion protocol. *Am J Sports Med* 1999;27:308-311.

7. Mehlhoff TL, Noble PC, Bennett JB, Tullos HS: Simple dislocation of the elbow in the adult: Results after closed treatment. *J Bone Joint Surg Am* 1988;70:244-249.

8. Doornberg JN, Ring DC: Fracture of the anteromedial facet of the coronoid process. *J Bone Joint Surg Am* 2006;88:2216-2224.

   The authors document the injury, management, and outcomes in a study of 18 patients with anteromedial coronoid fractures. All but three fractures were associated with lateral ulnar collateral ligament injury (two patients had concomitant olecranon fractures and one had a basal coronoid fracture). Patients who were identified retrospectively to have received inadequate treatment had poorer results than those treated with adequate fixation.

9. Schneeberger AG, Sadowski MM, Jacob HA: Coronoid process and radial head as posterolateral rotatory stabilizers of the elbow. *J Bone Joint Surg Am* 2004;86-A: 975-982.

The authors evaluated the role of the radial head and coronoid process in posterolateral rotatory instability of the elbow in this cadaveric study. Posterolateral rotatory displacement of the ulna was measured in intact elbows, after radial head excision or sequential resection of the coronoid, and again after radial head replacement and open reduction and internal fixation of the coronoid. In elbows with greater than a 50% loss of the coronoid, stability could not be restored by radial head replacement alone; stability required additional coronoid reconstruction.

10. Srinivasan K, Agarwal M, Matthews SJ, Giannoudis PV: Fractures of the distal humerus in the elderly: Is internal fixation the treatment of choice? *Clin Orthop Relat Res* 2005;434:222-230.

The authors conducted a retrospective comparison of open reduction and internal fixation and nonsurgical treatment of distal humerus fractures in patients older than 75 years (mean age, 85 years). Surgically treated patients had improved Orthopaedic Trauma Association ratings, improved range of motion, improved pain relief, and radiographic evidence of maintained reduction; complication rates were not higher than those reported in the literature for younger patients. Studies such as this suggest that the role of open reduction and internal fixation may be expanded to include patients who traditionally have been treated with total elbow arthroplasty or nonsurgically. Importantly, the outcomes of patients treated with earlier plating technologies are good; the use of technologically advanced plating systems may result in even better outcomes.

11. Kundel K, Braun W, Wieberneit J, Rüter A: Intra-articular distal humerus fractures: Factors affecting functional outcome. *Clin Orthop Relat Res* 1996;332: 200-208.

12. Huang TL, Chiu FY, Chuang TY, Chen TH: The results of open reduction and internal fixation in elderly patients with severe fractures of the distal humerus: A critical analysis of the results. *J Trauma* 2005;58:62-69.

The authors describe their experience with 19 patients following open reduction and internal fixation of the distal humerus in patients older than 65 years (average age, 72 years). During the 10-year study period, only one patient was treated nonsurgically because of health concerns that precluded surgery. Outcomes were highly satisfactory with minimal complications. Range of motion was 17° to 128° on average; 84% of patients had good or very good motion according to the classification system of Cassebaum, 79% had excellent Mayo El-

bow Performance scores, and 79% reported no pain at final follow-up.

13. Cobb TK, Morrey BF: Total elbow arthroplasty as primary treatment for distal humeral fractures in elderly patients. *J Bone Joint Surg Am* 1997;79:826-832.

14. O'Driscoll SW: Optimizing stability in distal humeral fracture fixation. *J Shoulder Elbow Surg* 2005;14(suppl S):186S-194S.

This principle-based article provides an algorithm and rationale to fixation of distal humerus fractures.

15. Morrey BF: Current concepts in the treatment of fractures of the radial head, the olecranon, and the coronoid. *Instr Course Lect* 1995;44:175-185.

16. Horne JG, Tanzer TL: Olecranon fractures: A review of 100 cases. *J Trauma* 1981;21:469-472.

17. Karlsson MK, Hasserius R, Karlsson C, Besjakov J, Josefsson PO: Fractures of the olecranon: A 15- to 25-year followup of 73 patients.*Clin Orthop Relat Res* 2002; 403:205-212.

18. Didonna ML, Fernandez JJ, Lim TH, Hastings H II, Cohen MS: Partial olecranon excision: The relationship between triceps insertion site and extension strength of the elbow. *J Hand Surg Am* 2003;28:117-122.

19. McKeever FM, Buck RM: Fracture of the olecranon process of the ulna: Treatment by excision of fragment and repair of triceps tendon. *JAMA* 1947;125:1-5.

20. Ider CS, Montgomery WH III, Lindsey DP, Badua PA, Wynne GF, Yerby SA: Distal biceps tendon repair: A biomechanical comparison of intact tendon and two repair techniques. *Am J Sports Med* 2006;34:968-974.

This biomechanical study investigated differences between mean failure strength, maximum strength and stiffness of intact biceps tendon, repaired tendon with bony tunnels and transosseous sutures, and repaired tendon with suture anchors. There was no statistically significant difference in mean maximal strength between the intact tendon and the two repair techniques, although the stiffness and failure strength of the interference screw fixation technique was higher than that of the bony tunnel technique.

21. Kelly EW, Morrey BF, O'Driscoll SW Complications of repair of the distal biceps tendon with the modified two-incision technique. *J Bone Joint Surg Am* 2000; 82A:1575-1581.

22. Morrey BF, Askew LJ, An KN, Dobyns JH: Rupture of the distal tendon of the biceps brachii: A biomechanical study. *J Bone Joint Surg Am* 1985;67:418-421.

23. Hartman MW, Merten SM, Steinmann SP: Mini-open 2-incision technique for repair of distal biceps tendon ruptures. *J Shoulder Elbow Surg* 2007;16:616-620.

A series of distal biceps tendon ruptures were treated

with a two-incision mini-open repair to bony tunnels followed by an immediate active range-of-motion protocol. All patients were satisfied with the surgical outcome. Heterotopic ossification, which was functionally insignificant, developed in one patient. No ruptures were observed.

24. Dumont CE, Thalmann ER, Macy JC: The effect of rotational malunion of the radius and the ulna on supination and pronation. *J Bone Joint Surg Br* 2002;84:1070-1074.

25. Hertel R, Pisan M, Lambert S, Ballmer FT: Plate osteosynthesis of diaphyseal fractures of the radius and ulna. *Injury* 1996;27:545-548.

26. Mikek M, Vidmar G, Tonin M, Pavlovcic V: Fracture-related and implant-specific factors influencing treatment results of comminuted diaphyseal forearm fractures without bone grafting. *Arch Orthop Trauma Surg* 2004;124:393-400.

    The authors reviewed 319 diaphyseal forearm fractures with variable comminution that were treated with open reduction and internal fixation without bone grafting. Although fractures with greater than two thirds diaphyseal width comminution had a prolonged time to union, no difference in the union rate was noted; therefore, it appears that primary bone grafting may not be necessary for treating diaphyseal forearm fractures. The authors noted that fractures with greater than two thirds diaphyseal comminution were rare, constituting 5% of this study.

27. Schemitsch EH, Richards RR: The effect of malunion on functional outcome after plate fixation of fractures of both bones of the forearm in adults. *J Bone Joint Surg Am* 1992;74:1068-1078.

28. Ring D, Rhim R, Carpenter C, Jupiter JB: Comminuted diaphyseal fractures of the radius and ulna: Does bone grafting affect nonunion rate? *J Trauma* 2005;59:438-441.

    Forty-one patients with comminuted diaphyseal forearm fractures were treated with dynamic compression plates. Factors including polytrauma, open fracture, and use of cancellous bone graft at the time of surgery did not have a statistically significant association with development of a nonunion, which occurred in 12% of patients.

Chapter 27
Elbow Reconstruction

George S. Athwal, MD, FRCSC   Kenneth J. Faber, MD, MHPE, FRCSC
*Graham J.W. King, MD, MSc, FRCSC

Instability

Posterolateral Rotatory Instability

The understanding of posterolateral rotatory instability has improved in recent years. Although it was initially believed that the condition was caused by a deficiency of the lateral ulnar collateral ligament, it has become increasingly clear that there are secondary ligamentous, muscular, and osseous stabilizers that may also be involved. Isolated sectioning of the lateral ulnar collateral ligament from the lateral epicondyle does not cause posterolateral rotatory instability in the setting of intact radial collateral and annular ligaments.[1] A recent study showed that arthroscopic sectioning of both the lateral ulnar collateral ligament and radial collateral ligament were needed to cause posterolateral rotatory instability.[2] Sectioning of the overlying muscles and muscular fascia caused an increase in instability. It would therefore seem that patients presenting with this condition likely have deficiency of more than just the lateral ulnar collateral ligament; most have some attenuation of the radial collateral ligament and the overlying muscular fascia. Osseous contributors to development of posterolateral rotatory instability include the presence of chronic cubitus varus and radial head excision.[3] Cubitus varus has been shown to cause an increase in strain in the lateral collateral ligament experimentally, which presumably is the cause of a gradual attrition of this structure over time as has been reported clinically.[4] Other contributing factors to the development of posterolateral rotatory instability would appear to be partial or complete resection of the radial head, which causes a reduction in the intrinsic constraint of the radiocapitellar joint, and a decrease in the tensioning of the lateral collateral ligament. Posterolateral rotatory instability has also been reported to occur in association with lateral epicondylitis.[5] It is not clear whether the steroid injections used to manage this condition caused an attrition of the lateral ligament stabilizers of the elbow or whether the instability occurred primarily. Further

investigations are required to better understand this relationship.

The diagnosis of posterolateral rotatory instability is typically clinical, based on a history of instability or posterolateral elbow pain. Confirmatory tests include the posterolateral rotatory drawer test, as well as the lateral pivot-shift test. The posterolateral rotatory drawer test is performed with the elbow at 90° of flexion. External rotation and posterior forces are applied to the forearm to translate the radius posterior to the capitellum (Figure 1). The lateral pivot-shift test is performed with the patient supine; the shoulder is abducted and externally rotated. Valgus and axial loads are applied to the extended and supinated forearm while the elbow is gradually flexed (Figure 2). The presence of apprehension in an awake patient when performing this maneuver is suggestive of posterolateral rotatory instability. The development of a posterolateral dimple and then a clunk as the elbow relocates with greater flexion is diagnostic of posterolateral rotatory instability; however, this test usually is only positive when the patient is under a general anesthetic. In a recent prospective evaluation of apprehension signs for

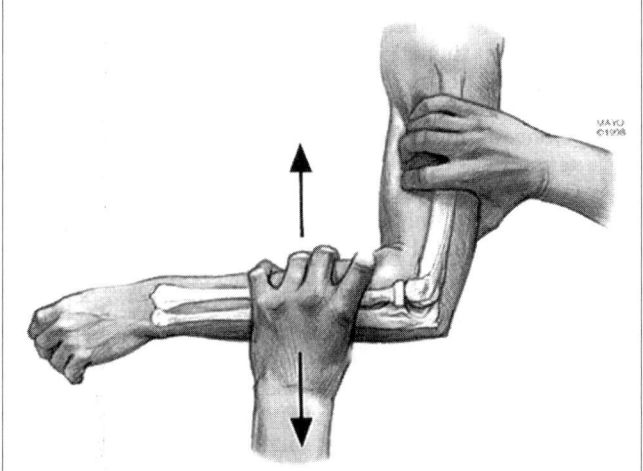

Figure 1 Posterolateral rotatory drawer test. This test is performed with the elbow at 90° of flexion and full supination. A positive test is posterolateral translation of the radial head on the capitellum with a posterior-directed force. *(Reproduced with permission from Mayo, ©1998.*

Graham J.W. King, MD, MSc, FRCSC or the department with which he is affiliated has received research or institutional support from Wright Medical Technology and royalties from Tornier.

3: Upper Extremity

posterolateral rotatory instability, the chair test (**Figure 3**) as well as the push-up sign (**Figure 4**) both were more sensitive than the pivot-shift test in the awake patient and were easily performed in the office environment.[6] MRI, while often demonstrating an abnormality in patients with suspected posterolateral rotatory instability, is not diagnostic of this condition. In a recent

study of normal asymptomatic elbows, the lateral ulnar collateral ligament was not routinely visualized, suggesting that imaging is not reliable in the diagnosis of this condition.[7]

The management of posterolateral rotatory instability continues to be clarified. Lateral collateral ligament repair is effective in managing posterolateral rotatory instability caused by an acute ligament injury. Active flexion and extension of the elbow with the forearm maintained in pronation protects the ligament repair or reconstruction. Extension of the elbow with the forearm supinated and varus forces should be avoided during ligament healing.[8] Reconstruction of the lateral ulnar collateral ligament with a palmaris longus tendon graft combined with plication of the lateral capsuloligamentous structures is effective in treating chronic posterolateral rotatory instability.[9] Isolated plication of the lateral capsule and ligaments without tendon augmentation appears to be less reliable. A recent study demonstrated the effectiveness of arthroscopic electrothermal shrinkage to manage patients with posterolateral rotatory instability.[10] Further investigations will be necessary to clarify the role of arthroscopic shrinkage versus more conventional open ligament reconstruction in the management of this condition.

Medial Collateral Ligament Insufficiency

Attritional rupture of the medial collateral ligament of the elbow is a common condition in male pitchers and javelin throwers. Reconstruction of the ulnar collateral ligament using autogenous tendon grafts continues to be the cornerstone of management for this condition. A recent study of medial collateral ligament insufficiency in women reported that most athletes were not pitchers

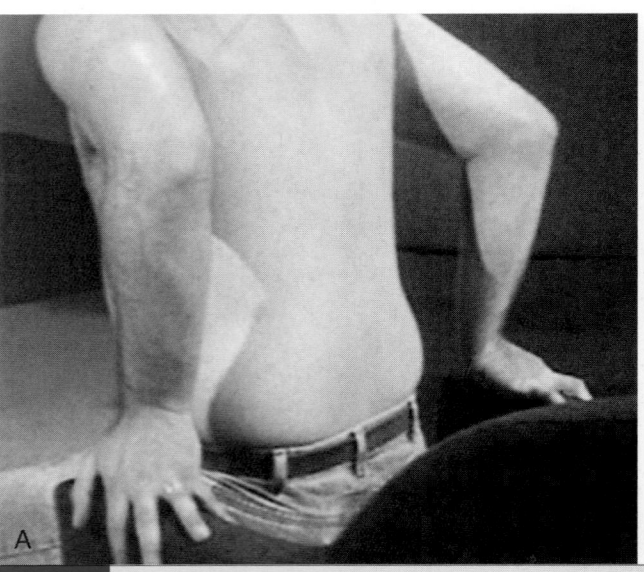

Figure 2	Posterolateral rotatory instability test (lateral pivot-shift test of the elbow). This test is performed with the patient supine and the shoulder abducted and externally rotated. Valgus and axial load is applied to the extended and supinated forearm causing elbow subluxation. While the elbow is gradually flexed, a reduction occurs with a palpable, audible clunk. (*Reproduced with permission from Morrey BF. The Elbow and Its Disorders. Philadelphia, PA, WB Saunders, 2000.*)

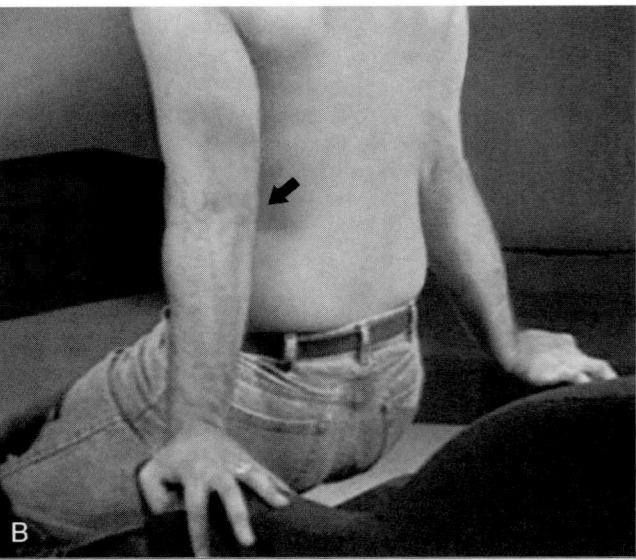

Figure 3	**A** and **B**, The chair test. A positive chair test is characterized by apprehension or dislocation on terminal extension of the arm when rising from a seated position. The apprehension sign occurs with axial load and valgus supination of the forearm. Note the reluctance to fully extend the elbow (*arrow*). (*Reproduced with permission from Regan W, Lapner PC: Prospective evaluation of two diagnostic apprehension signs for posterolateral instability of the elbow. J Shoulder Elbow Surg 2006;15:344-6.*)

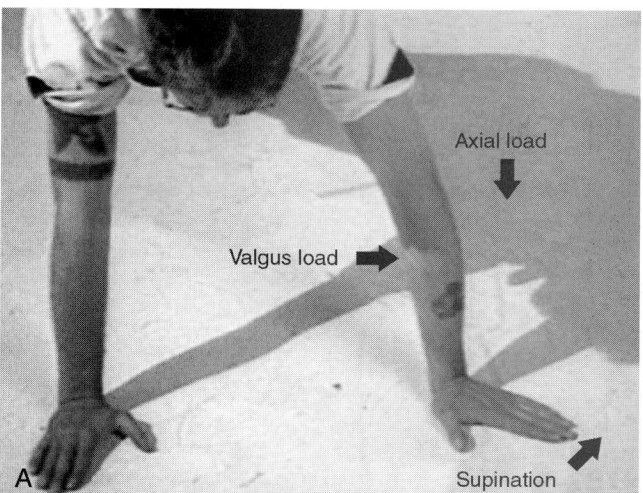
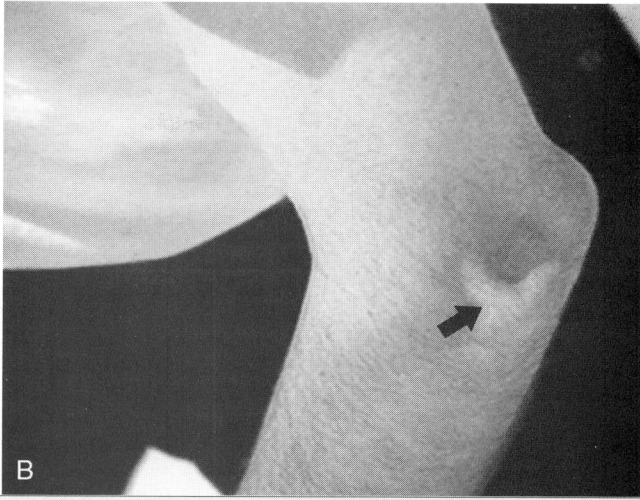

Figure 4　**A** and **B,** Push-up sign. The arm is positioned in full flexion and supination. A positive test is when apprehension or dislocation occurs as the arm goes in to extension as the patient pushes up. Active posterolateral rotatory instability is indicated in **B** (*arrow*). (*Reproduced with permission from Regan W, Lapner PC: Prospective evaluation of two diagnostic apprehension signs for posterolateral instability of the elbow. J Shoulder Elbow Surg 2006;15:344-346.*)

but played other sports such as softball, gymnastics, and tennis.[11] These authors reported that unlike similar studies in men, plication or repair of the medial collateral ligament was typically successful. Only one of their patients, a pitcher, required medial collateral ligament reconstruction. This study suggests that management of medial collateral ligament insufficiency of the elbow in nonthrowing athletes may be successful without ligament reconstruction.

The diagnosis of medial collateral ligament insufficiency of the elbow in throwing athletes is typically based on a history of a decrease in throwing velocity and medial elbow pain in the late cocking and early acceleration phases of the pitch. Tenderness over the medial side of the elbow combined with pain on valgus stress testing in 30° of flexion has typically been the most useful indicator. A recent study demonstrated the superiority of the moving valgus stress test to diagnose this condition[12] (**Figure 5**). In this test, a valgus load is applied to the elbow during flexion and extension. Patients with medial collateral ligament insufficiency have pain in the mid arc of flexion where the ligament provides the most stability to the elbow. Fluoroscopic examination, MRI, and more recently, ultrasound may be helpful to confirm the clinical diagnosis of this condition.

The dynamic contribution of the flexor pronator mass to valgus elbow stability is important. The forces applied to the medial collateral ligament in pitching exceed its tensile strength. This suggests that muscular activation is extremely important to protect the medial collateral ligament from injury. A recent cadaver-based study demonstrated that flexor carpi ulnaris and the flexor digitorum superficialis were the primary and secondary dynamic stabilizers.[13] Forearm supination is helpful to stabilize the elbow during flexion and extension motions following medial collateral ligament injuries and reconstruction.

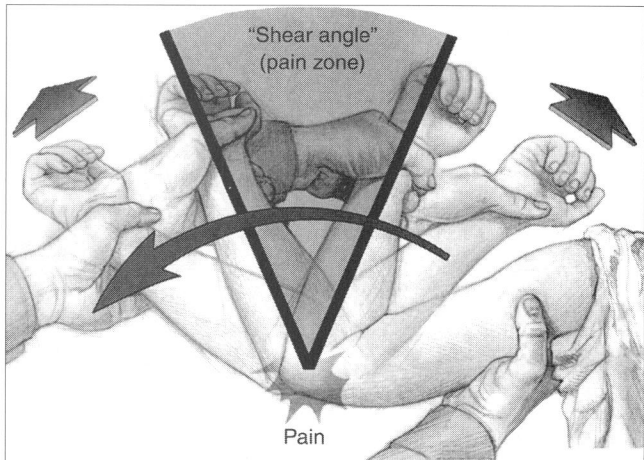

Figure 5　Moving valgus stress test. The shoulder is locked in external rotation and the flexed elbow is extended while applying a valgus stress. Patients with medial collateral ligament injury will experience pain in the mid arc of flexion— the shear angle. (*Reproduced with permission from O'Driscoll SW, Lawton RL, Smith AM: The "moving valgus stress test" for medial collateral ligament tears of the elbow. Am J Sports Med 2005;33:231-239.*)

Reconstruction of the medial collateral ligament has typically been performed with a palmaris longus tendon graft. Docking the graft in the medial epicondyle has superior initial strength and is easier to tension than a figure-of-8 reconstruction (**Figure 6**). Both methods have excellent clinical outcome in reported clinical series. Other modifications that have shown promise are single strand reconstructions and the use of interference screws to secure the grafts. Ulnar nerve transposi-

3: Upper Extremity

tion is no longer recommended except if the patient has motor weakness; sensory symptoms usually resolve following reconstruction.

Arthritis

Osteoarthritis

The treatment of elbow arthritis continues to evolve and the role of arthroscopy is being further defined. Two recent studies have documented the outcome of arthroscopy for the treatment of elbow osteoarthritis with an associated contracture.[14,15] Both reports noted improved patient symptoms and increased range of motion following joint débridement and capsulectomy at a mean of 12 and 25 months, respectively. The procedure remains technically demanding but is safe when performed following established principles. Whether capsulectomy is superior to capsulotomy remains unresolved and the indications for concomitant ulnar nerve decompression require further investigation. Although the long-term durability of arthroscopic débridement remains unknown, the early results are promising and similar to open joint débridement. Arthroscopy may function as an interim treatment of young patients with elbow arthrosis.

Inflammatory Arthritis

Arthroscopy continues to play a role in the management of inflammatory arthritis. When nonsurgical management fails, the most favorable results were achieved in Larsen stage I and II disease where the joint architecture remains relatively normal (**Figure 7**). Poor results were noted in patients with stage III and IV disease. A slight deterioration in outcome was noted during the follow-up period, particularly in more advanced disease stages.[16]

The outcome of linked semiconstrained total elbow arthroplasty following previous resection of the radial head and synovectomy was compared with that of a control group of patients who had elbow arthroplasty with an implant of the same design.[17] Although clinical outcomes and implant survivorship were similar in both groups, a higher rate of complications was observed in the study group.

Arthroplasty

Malpositioning of prosthetic elbow implants has been reported as a possible cause of early implant failure.[18] A cadaveric study has shown that conventional alignment instrumentation fails to recreate normal elbow kinematics following arthroplasty. Newer implant designs attempt to address this concern with improved instrumentation, greater modularity that allows for a more anatomic reconstruction, and convertibility from unlinked (**Figure 8**) to linked components (**Figure 9**)

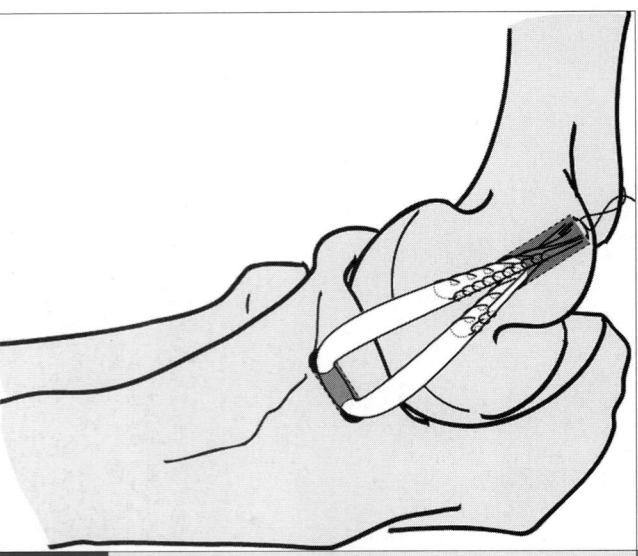

Figure 6 | Medial collateral ligament reconstruction via the docking technique. *(Reproduced with permission from Armstrong AD, Dunning CE, Ferreira LM et al: A biomechanical comparison of four reconstruction techniques for the medial collateral ligament-deficient elbow. J Shoulder Elbow Surg 2005;14:207-215.)*

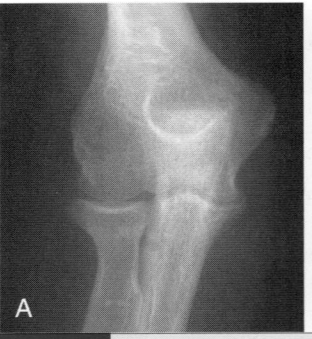 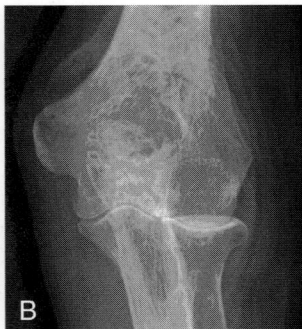 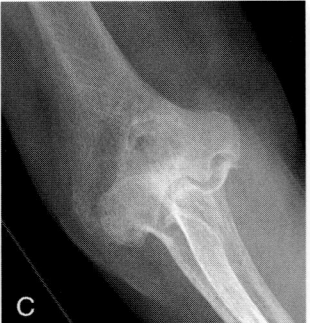 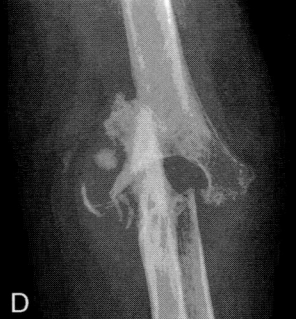

Figure 7 | Classification of inflammatory arthritis. **A**, Stage I; normal architecture, osteoporosis. Synovitis is present. **B**, Stage II; joint space narrowing, intact joint architecture. Synovitis is present. **C**, Stage III; alteration of joint architecture, variable synovitis. **D**, Stage IV; gross joint destruction, minimal synovitis.

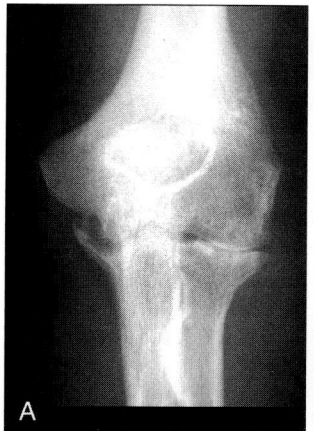
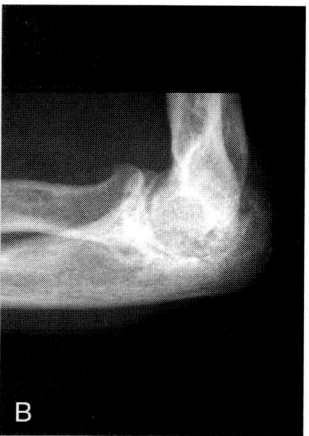
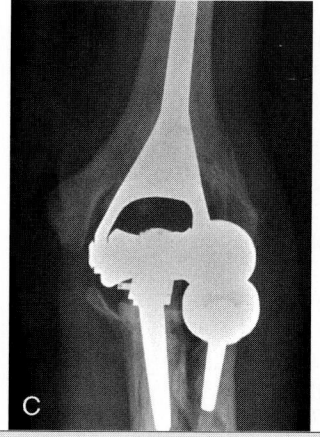
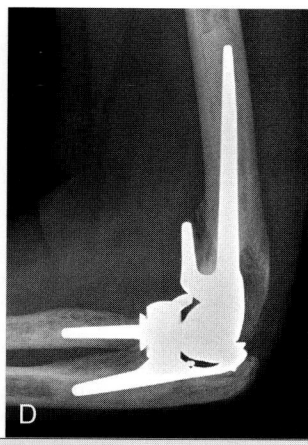

Figure 8   **A** and **B,** Unlinked total elbow arthroplasty. AP and lateral radiographs of a 58-year-old woman with long-standing rheumatoid arthritis. **C** and **D,** AP and lateral radiographs 2 years following an unlinked total elbow arthroplasty. The patient experienced excellent pain relief, had a stable elbow, and a functional range of motion.

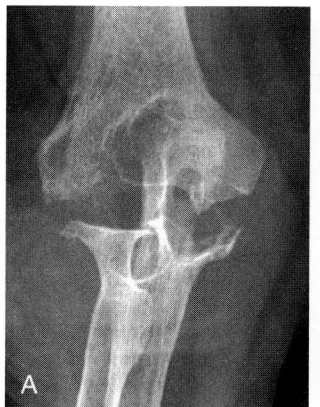
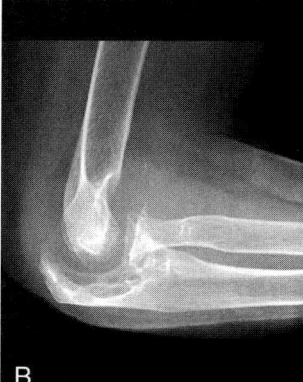
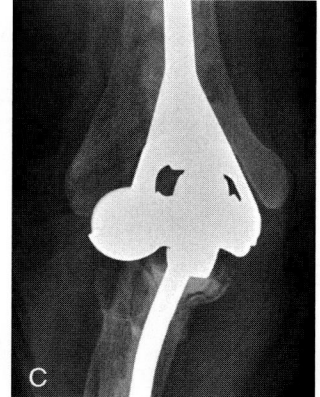
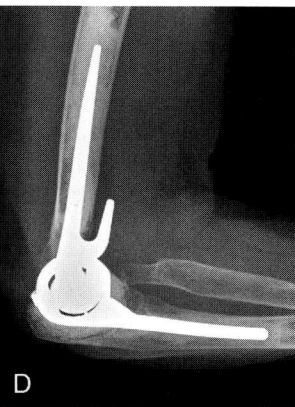

Figure 9   Linked total elbow arthroplasty. **A** and **B,** AP and lateral radiographs of a 76-year-old woman with a painful unstable elbow due to rheumatoid arthritis. **C** and **D,** AP and lateral radiographs 2 years following a linked total elbow arthroplasty. The patient had a stable, pain-free elbow, and a functional range of motion.

but at present, there are no reports of clinical outcomes with new prostheses or comparative studies with more widely used implants.

Elbow Stiffness

Joint contracture is a well-recognized complication of elbow trauma. The etiology of the elbow joint's propensity for contracture is still largely unknown. It is theorized that stiffness and contracture stem from changes in the joint capsule activated by trauma. Immunohistochemistry studies of posttraumatic elbow contracture capsular tissue have demonstrated elevated numbers of myofibroblast cells.[19] An inverse relationship has been described between the myofibroblast numbers in the joint capsule and total arc of flexion-extension motion of the elbow. Regional differences in myofibroblast numbers also exist, as patients with contracture have seven times greater cell numbers in the anterior capsule than in the posterior capsule.

Primary prevention should be used by all surgeons to limit posttraumatic elbow stiffness. For treatment of elbow stiffness, initial management should be nonsurgical with physiotherapy, splints, and braces. Static progressive splinting under the direction of a physiotherapist has been reported as beneficial in gaining additional elbow range of motion.[20] Static progressive splinting involves using a splint to apply torque to a joint statically positioned near its maximal tolerable end range of motion. As the joint tissues lengthen to accommodate the torque, the wearer adjusts the splint to increase torque to a new maximal tolerable end range of motion. A turnbuckle splint is a type of static progressive splint.

When nonsurgical measures fail to obtain functional range of motion, the elbow may be treated using either open or arthroscopic surgical techniques. The application of arthroscopy for the treatment of the stiff elbow has been a major advance. Improvement in range of motion and functional outcome has been reported with arthroscopic techniques, which are comparable to open surgical releases.[14] Open surgical release may be done via an anterior approach, a medial over-the-top exposure, a lateral column procedure, or a combined approach.[21,22] Preoperative assessment of the patient should include identification of previous surgical incisions, careful examination of the ulnar nerve and the adjacent soft-tissue envelope, and clear localization of the pathology to determine the most appropriate surgical approach. The anterior approach is predominantly designed to address lack of extension by excising an anterior tether. The anterior approach does not allow access to the posterior joint to deal with an extension block, such as osteophytes, or a tether to flexion, such as a contracted posterior capsule or a scarred triceps tendon. The medial over-the-top approach is ideal for addressing ulnar nerve pathology or limited flexion by dividing the posterior band of the medial collateral ligament. The key landmarks for the medial approach are the ulnar nerve and the medial epicondyle. After mobilizing the ulnar nerve, the pronator teres is elevated off the anterior capsule to allow access to the capsule and anterior elbow joint. Elevation of the medial triceps allows access to the posteromedial and posterior joint. The lateral column approach is best used when disorders of the radiocapitellar joint coexist with stiffness. The brachioradialis and the extensor carpi radialis brevis and longus are elevated off the anterior capsule to allow access to the capsule, radiocapitellar joint, and anterior ulnohumeral joint. Elevation of the lateral triceps allows access to the posterolateral and posterior joint.

In a recent series of 52 patients who underwent open surgical release for posttraumatic contracture, the authors most often used the combined medial and lateral approach.[22] At 18.7 months' follow-up, the average flexion-extension arc improved from 57° to 116° and the average prosupination arc improved from 119° to 145°. Interestingly, 27% of patients required a closed manipulation under an anesthetic for failure to progress at a mean of 3.5 weeks postoperatively, and 10% required a second surgical release. Excision of heterotopic ossification that is contributing to posttraumatic elbow stiffness is associated with significantly better gains in range of motion than release of soft-tissue contractures.[23]

Tendon Injuries

Lateral Epicondylitis

Lateral epicondylitis is a common condition associated with societal issues such as lost productivity or an increase in the need for health care. The literature, including a randomized clinical trial, has shown no long-term benefit with splinting or forearm straps.[24] Recently, a dynamic extensor brace has shown some promise. A randomized controlled trial comparing a dynamic extensor brace with no brace treatment resulted in a statistically significant reduction in pain, improved arm function, and an improvement in grip strength.[25] The authors also reported that the beneficial results of the brace were sustained over short-term follow-up.

The use of extracorporeal shock wave therapy (ESWT) for the management of lateral epicondylitis is controversial, with variable results reported in the literature. The Cochrane Collaboration recently conducted a systematic review of nine placebo-controlled trials on the effectiveness and safety of ESWT for the management of lateral elbow pain.[26] The authors concluded, based on the nine trials involving 1,006 participants, that there is high-level evidence that ESWT provides little or no benefit in terms of pain and function in lateral epicondylitis.

Lateral epicondylitis that is recalcitrant to nonsurgical treatment may be managed surgically. Surgical options include open release and débridement, extensor carpi radialis brevis lengthening, percutaneous techniques, and arthroscopic débridement. A recent prospective randomized controlled trial compared traditional open release to percutaneous tenotomy.[27] The authors reported at 12-month follow-up that the percutaneous tenotomy group had significantly better patient satisfaction, a quicker return to return to work, and better Disabilities of the Arm, Shoulder and Hand (DASH) scores. The percutaneous technique involves a 1-cm incision over the midportion of the lateral epicondyle with division of the common extensor origin. The patient's wrist is then flexed to complete the division and to create a gap in the extensor origin. The percutaneous procedure is quicker and may be conducted under local anesthesia.

One cause of failure in the nonsurgical management of lateral epicondylitis has been impingement of a posterolateral plica in the radiocapitellar joint.[28] Synovial plicae have been associated with symptoms, such as diffuse lateral elbow pain, that may mimic lateral epicondylitis. Along with lateral pain, patients with a posterolateral plica may present with painful joint snapping occurring maximally in terminal extension and supination. Treatment, when symptoms dictate, involves arthroscopic resection of the plica. The plica is visualized in the posterolateral aspect of the elbow joint as a large enfolded synovial mass covering a portion of the radial head.[29]

An association between lateral epicondylitis and posterolateral rotatory instability has been identified.[5] Posterolateral rotatory instability of the elbow occurring after nonsurgical management of lateral epicondylitis has been reported. It is theorized that repeated corticosteroid injections into the common extensor and lateral collateral ligament origins leads to structural weakening and ultimate failure. Posterolateral rotatory instability should be added to the differential diagnosis of failure of nonsurgical management of lateral epicondylitis, especially in patients with mechanical elbow symptoms.

Distal Biceps Tendon Injuries

The biceps squeeze test, which is analogous to the Thompson test for rupture of the Achilles tendon, has been developed for assessment of distal biceps tendon ruptures.[30] The test is performed with the patient seated, the elbow flexed to approximately 60° to 80°, and the forearm resting slightly pronated. The examiner squeezes the biceps with both hands, one hand at the distal musculotendinous junction and the other around the midmuscle belly. The test is considered positive for a distal biceps tendon rupture when the muscle is squeezed and no forearm supination is seen.

Acute distal biceps tendon ruptures are usually managed surgically to regain elbow flexion and supination strength. Several different surgical techniques exist and most are based on either the single anterior incision approach or the Mayo modification of the Boyd and Anderson two-incision approach. The single best technique with the lowest complication rate remains unknown. One study reviewed patient-oriented functional outcome after repair of acute distal biceps tendon ruptures via a single anterior incision technique.[31] At a mean follow-up of 29 months, 81% of patients were very satisfied, 15% were somewhat satisfied, and 4% were dissatisfied. The mean DASH score at final follow-up was 8.2, which is not statistically different from that of the control group. There were no statistically significant differences between the injured and uninjured sides for any range-of-motion measurement. A subgroup of 22 patients underwent strength testing using a work simulator at a mean of 21 months postoperatively. Compared with the uninjured side, the mean flexion strength was 96%, mean supination strength was 93%, mean power was 94%, and mean grip strength was 99%. Complications were encountered in four patients: one superficial infection, two transient lateral antebrachial nerve palsies, and one transient posterior interosseous nerve palsy. The authors concluded that tendon repair via a single anterior incision with suture anchors was effective in returning injured arms to normal with a low complication rate.

Ulnar Neuropathy

A uniform treatment algorithm for symptomatic ulnar neuropathy at the elbow remains unknown and the outcomes of the various surgical treatments have failed to identify a single best intervention. Recent anatomic investigations have attempted to further define potential sites of compression (**Figure 10**), biomechanical studies have examined alterations in ulnar nerve strain, and a clinical trial has compared two commonly accepted treatments.

The occurrence and relevance of the arcade of Struthers as a point of compression of the ulnar nerve at the elbow region remains controversial. A cadaveric anatomic study identified a musculotendinous arcade in only 13.5% of limbs.[32] No evidence of ulnar nerve compression was found in the specimens where an arcade was

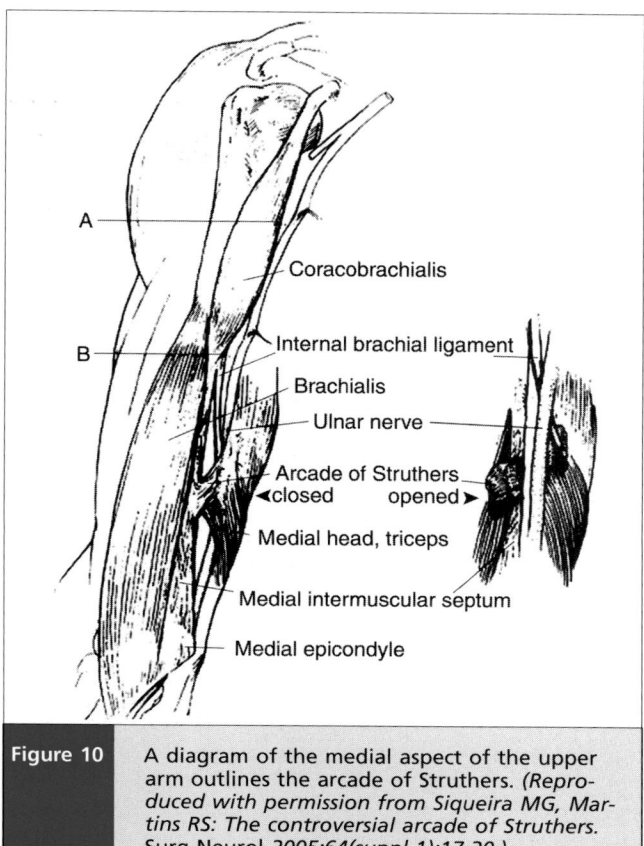

Coracobrachialis

Internal brachial ligament

Brachialis

Ulnar nerve

Arcade of Struthers
◄closed   opened►

Medial head, triceps

Medial intermuscular septum

Medial epicondyle

Figure 10   A diagram of the medial aspect of the upper arm outlines the arcade of Struthers. *(Reproduced with permission from Siqueira MG, Martins RS: The controversial arcade of Struthers. Surg Neurol 2005;64(suppl 1):17-20.)*

identified. In contrast, a second cadaver study identified an arcade of Struthers in 67% of specimens, and Osborne's ligament was present in all specimens.[33] A discrete flexor pronator aponeurosis overlying the ulnar nerve was present in 44% of specimens. Motor branching of the ulnar nerve was highly variable and occurred both proximal and distal to the medial epicondyle.

An anatomic study used radiographic markers to measure ulnar nerve angulation in cadaver upper limbs that underwent ulnar nerve decompression and anterior transposition into subcutaneous and then submuscular positions.[34] A significantly greater angulation was noted after subcutaneous transposition than after submuscular transposition with the elbow held in full flexion. The angulation of the nerve may act as a secondary point of compression that can contribute to the ongoing symptoms after anterior transposition.

Although compression is considered the most frequent cause of ulnar nerve dysfunction, several recent investigations have examined the effect of arm position on ulnar nerve strain. A cadaver study examined the elongation and excursion of the ulnar nerve during passive elbow motion in control conditions, after in situ decompression and after anterior subcutaneous transposition.[35] The authors found that the normal nerve had the greatest elongation (23%) and excursion (14 mm) in the epicondylar groove. In situ decompression reduced nerve elongation within the cubital tunnel, but increased elongation of the nerve was noted proximally, resulting in no overall alteration in the total nerve excursion. After anterior subcutaneous transposition, the nerve elongated during elbow extension to the same extent as occurred with the normal nerve during flexion.

The role of imaging in the diagnosis of ulnar neuropathy remains unknown. In a study to determine the diagnostic value of high-resolution ultrasound, sonographic ulnar nerve diameter measurements were obtained at three levels around the medial epicondyle in a cohort of patients presenting with clinical signs and electrodiagnostic abnormalities associated with ulnar neuropathy and compared with values obtained in healthy volunteer subjects.[36] Patients with ulnar neuropathy had a larger ulnar nerve diameter than control patients. The sensitivity of ultrasound was 80% and the specificity was 91%. The authors concluded that high-resolution ultrasound is a safe, accurate and easily applied test for the diagnosis of ulnar neuropathy. Further studies are required to determine if ultrasound without electrodiagnostic studies is sufficient to establish the severity of ulnar neuropathy and the need for surgical intervention.

A prospective, randomized controlled study compared simple decompression with anterior subcutaneous transposition for idiopathic neuropathy of the ulnar nerve at the elbow.[37] The outcomes of both interventions were equivalent at 1 year; however, a significantly higher complication rate was observed with anterior subcutaneous transposition (31%) than with simple decompression (10%). Simple decompression was recommended for its simplicity, low complication rate, and low cost, even in the presence of nerve subluxation.

Advances in Elbow Reconstruction

Many of the advances in elbow surgery have occurred as a result of an improved understanding of elbow anatomy and function as well as new innovations in implant instrument technology. Arthroscopic surgery has advanced quickly in recent years as equipment has improved and surgical techniques have evolved. The concept of using retractors in the elbow has allowed advanced surgical procedures such as capsulectomy and débridement to be safely and effectively performed. Reliable techniques are now available for medial and lateral collateral ligament reconstruction through more minimally invasive surgical approaches. New designs of total elbow replacements offer thicker polyethylene and some have the option to convert intraoperatively or postoperatively between unlinked and linked configurations. Long-term follow-up studies are required to evaluate these new implants in comparison with conventional devices. The use of hemiarthroplasty for the management of acute distal humeral fractures, nonunions, and osteonecrosis is an exciting development that requires further study.

Annotated References

1. Coonrad RW, Roush TF, Major NM, Basamania CJ: The drop sign: A radiographic warning sign of elbow instability. *J Shoulder Elbow Surg* 2005;14:312-317.

   Following reduction of an elbow dislocation, an increase in the ulnohumeral distance on unstressed postreduction lateral radiographs, the "drop sign" is a common finding that usually resolves as muscle tone returns to the elbow. A persistence of the "drop sign" may be a warning sign of instability.

2. McAdams TR, Masters GW, Srivastava S: The effect of arthroscopic sectioning of the lateral ligament complex of the elbow on posterolateral rotatory stability. *J Shoulder Elbow Surg* 2005;14:298-301.

   Sectioning of both the radial collateral and ulnar collateral ligament were needed to cause significant posterolateral rotatory instability of the elbow in cadaver elbows. Division of the overlying common extensor muscles further increased this instability.

3. Hall JA, McKee MD: Posterolateral rotatory instability of the elbow following radial head resection. *J Bone Joint Surg Am* 2005;87:1571-1579.

   Posterolateral rotatory instability can cause persistent lateral elbow pain and symptoms of instability following radial head resection. Level of evidence: IV.

4. Beuerlein MJ, Reid JT, Schemitsch EH, McKee MD: Effect of distal humeral varus deformity on strain in the lateral ulnar collateral ligament and ulnohumeral joint stability. *J Bone Joint Surg Am* 2004;86-A:2235-2242.

   In a cadaver study, cubitus varus was demonstrated to increase the strain in the lateral ulnar collateral ligament and increase ulnohumeral joint opening consistent with posterolateral rotatory instability. This finding may explain the clinical association of cubitus varus deformity with the development of late posterolateral rotatory instability.

5. Kalainov DM, Cohen MS: Posterolateral rotatory instability of the elbow in association with lateral epicondylitis: A report of three cases. *J Bone Joint Surg Am* 2005;87:1120-1125.

   Posterolateral rotatory instability may occur as a result of repeated steroid injections in patients with lateral epicondylitis.

6. Regan W, Lapner PC: Prospective evaluation of two diagnostic apprehension signs for posterolateral instability of the elbow. *J Shoulder Elbow Surg* 2006;15:344-346.

   The push-up test and chair sign were demonstrated to be more reliable than the pivot-shift sign in the awake patient with suspected posterolateral rotatory instability of the elbow.

7. Terada N, Yamada H, Toyama Y: The appearance of the lateral ulnar collateral ligament on magnetic resonance imaging. *J Shoulder Elbow Surg* 2004;13:214-216.

   The lateral ulnar collateral ligament was not identified

in one half of a group of asymptomatic patients who underwent MRI. The use of this technique is not reliable for the diagnosis of lateral ulnar collateral ligament insufficiency.

8. Wolff AL, Hotchkiss RN: Lateral elbow instability: Nonoperative, operative, and postoperative management. *J Hand Ther* 2006;2:238-243.

Therapeutic approaches for the management of lateral elbow stability are reviewed.

9. Sanchez-Sotelo J, Morrey BF, O'Driscoll SW: Ligamentous repair and reconstruction for posterolateral rotatory instability of the elbow. *J Bone Joint Surg Br* 2005; 87:54-61.

Eighty-six percent of patients had a good outcome with ligamentous repair or reconstruction for posterolateral rotatory instability of the elbow. Better results were noted in patient who had a tendon graft augmentation and those with clinical symptoms of instability.

10. Spahn G, Kirschbaum S, Klinger HM, Wittig R: Arthroscopic electrothermal shrinkage of chronic posterolateral elbow instability: Good or moderate outcome in 21 patients followed for an average of 2.5 years. *Acta Orthop* 2006;77:285-289.

The authors report that arthroscopic electrothermal shrinkage is effective in managing posterolateral rotatory instability of the elbow.

11. Argo D, Trenhaile SW, Savoie FH III, Field LD: Operative treatment of ulnar collateral ligament insufficiency of the elbow in female athletes. *Am J Sports Med* 2006; 34:431-437.

Repair or plication of the medial collateral ligament (without graft augmentation) in female softball players, gymnasts, and tennis players was successful in 18 of 19 patients. Only one patient, who was a pitcher, required a medial collateral ligament reconstruction.

12. O'Driscoll SW, Lawton RL, Smith AM: The "moving valgus stress test" for medial collateral ligament tears of the elbow. *Am J Sports Med* 2005;33:231-239.

The moving valgus stress test was demonstrated to be highly sensitive and specific in the diagnosis of medial collateral ligament insufficiency of the elbow.

13. Park MC, Ahmad CS: Dynamic contributions of the flexor-pronator mass to elbow valgus stability. *J Bone Joint Surg Am* 2004;86:2268-2274.

The flexor pronator mass is an important dynamic stabilizer against valgus elbow loading. The flexor carpi ulnaris is the primary stabilizer whereas the flexor digitorum superficialis and pronator teres provide progressively less dynamic stability.

14. Nguyen D, Proper SI, MacDermid JC, King GJ, Faber KJ: Functional outcomes of arthroscopic capsular release of the elbow. *Arthroscopy* 2006;22:842-849.

Twenty-two patients (14 males, 8 females; mean age, 42 years) undergoing arthroscopic contracture release were retrospectively reviewed at a minimum follow-up of 1 year. Mean arc of motion improved 38° and all patients had improved elbow function.

15. Ball CM, Meunier M, Galatz LM, Calfee R, Yamaguchi K: Arthroscopic treatment of post-traumatic elbow contracture. *J Shoulder Elbow Surg* 2002;11:624-629.

16. Horiuchi K, Momohara S, Tomatsu T, Inoue K, Toyama Y: Arthroscopic synovectomy of the elbow in rheumatoid arthritis. *J Bone Joint Surg Am* 2002;84: 342-347.

17. Whaley A, Morrey BF, Adams R: Total elbow arthroplasty after previous resection of the radial head and synovectomy. *J Bone Joint Surg Br* 2005;87:47-53.

Fifteen elbows with a history of resection and synovectomy were compared with a control group of patients who had elbow arthroplasty with an implant of the same design. Similar functional improvements were noted in both groups; however, complications were more frequent in the study group.

18. Stokdijk M, Nagels J, Garling EH, Rozing PM: The kinematic elbow axis as a parameter to evaluate total elbow replacement: A cadaver study of the iBP elbow system. *J Shoulder Elbow Surg* 2003;12:63-68.

19. Germscheid NM, Hildebrand KA: Regional variation is present in elbow capsules after injury. *Clin Orthop Relat Res* 2006;450:219-224.

Immunohistochemical analysis of posttraumatic elbow capsular tissue showed higher numbers of myofibroblasts with regional variations. Cell numbers are higher in the anterior capsule versus the posterior capsule.

20. Doornberg JN, Ring D, Jupiter JB: Static progressive splinting for posttraumatic elbow stiffness. *J Orthop Trauma* 2006;20:400-404.

Static progressive splinting is described. The authors review their experience with this type of splinting for posttraumatic elbow contractures.

21. Morrey BF: The posttraumatic stiff elbow. *Clin Orthop Relat Res* 2005;431:26-35.

The author thoroughly reviews posttraumatic elbow stiffness, its management, and outcomes.

22. Tan V, Daluiski A, Simic P, Hotchkiss RN: Outcome of open release for post-traumatic elbow stiffness. *J Trauma* 2006;61:673-678.

The authors found that 27% of open contracture release resulted from recurrent stiffness.

23. Park MJ, Kim HG, Lee JY: Surgical treatment of posttraumatic stiffness of the elbow. *J Bone Joint Surg Br* 2004;86:1158-1162.

Open surgical release of posttraumatic elbow contractures in 27 patients are examined. Patients with heterotopic ossification had significantly better postoperative range of motion.

24. Struijs PA, Kerkhoffs GM, Assendelft WJ, Van Dijk CN:

3: Upper Extremity

Conservative treatment of lateral epicondylitis: Brace versus physical therapy or a combination of both: A randomized clinical trial. *Am J Sports Med* 2004;32: 462-469.

A total of 180 patients were randomized into three groups: brace-only treatment, physical therapy, and a combination treatment program. At 26 and 52 weeks follow-up, no significant differences were identified.

25. Faes M, van den Akker B, de Lint JA, Kooloos JG, Hopman MT: Dynamic extensor brace for lateral epicondylitis. *Clin Orthop Relat Res* 2006;442:149-157.

A randomized controlled trial comparing a dynamic extensor brace treatment to no brace treatment of the management of lateral epicondylitis is presented. Level of evidence: I.

26. Buchbinder R, Green SE, Youd JM, Assendelft WJ, Barnsley L, Smidt N: Shock wave therapy for lateral elbow pain. *Cochrane Database Syst Rev* 2005;4: CD003524.

A systematic review of nine placebo-controlled trials involving 1,006 participants to determine the effectiveness and safety of ESWT for lateral epicondylitis is presented. The authors conclude that there is "platinum level" evidence that the use of shock wave therapy provides little to no benefit in the treatment of lateral epicondylitis.

27. Dunkow PD, Jatti M, Muddu BN: A comparison of open and percutaneous techniques in the surgical treatment of tennis elbow. *J Bone Joint Surg Br* 2004;86: 701-704.

A prospective, randomized, controlled trial of 45 patients comparing open release with percutaneous tenotomy for the management of lateral epicondylitis was performed. The percutaneous procedure is described as quicker, simpler, and produces significantly better results.

28. Ruch DS, Papadonikolakis A, Campolattaro RM: The posterolateral plica: A cause of refractory lateral elbow pain. *J Shoulder Elbow Surg* 2006;15:367-370.

Ten patients with symptomatic posterolateral plica who were misdiagnosed with lateral epicondylitis are retrospectively reviewed.

29. Kim DH, Gambardella RA, Elattrache NS, Yocum LA, Jobe FW: Arthroscopic treatment of posterolateral elbow impingement from lateral synovial plicae in throwing athletes and golfers. *Am J Sports Med* 2006;34:438-444.

Twelve patients with symptomatic posterolateral elbow impingement from hypertrophic synovial plicae are reviewed. Arthroscopic resection with focused rehabilitation is reported as highly successful.

30. Ruland RT, Dunbar RP, Bowen JD: The biceps squeeze test for diagnosis of distal biceps tendon ruptures. *Clin Orthop Relat Res* 2005;437:128-131.

A diagnostic study examining the effectiveness of the biceps squeeze test in the diagnosis of distal biceps tendon ruptures. The test is described as simple, reliable, and cost-effective. Level of evidence: II.

31. McKee MD, Hirji R, Schemitsch EH, Wild LM, Waddell JP: Patient-oriented functional outcome after repair of distal biceps tendon ruptures using a single-incision technique. *J Shoulder Elbow Surg* 2005;14:302-306.

The functional outcomes of 53 patients after acute repair of a distal biceps tendon rupture via a single anterior incision with suture anchors are reported.

32. Siqueira MG, Martins RS: The controversial arcade of Struthers. *Surg Neurol* 2005;64:17-20.

This cadaver study identified a musculotendinous arcade of Struthers in 8 (13.5%) limbs. Although no evidence of ulnar nerve compression was found in the specimens where an arcade was identified, the authors suggest that this may be an infrequent site of primary nerve compression and may also become a site of compression after anterior transposition.

33. Gonzalez MH, Lotfi P, Bendre A, Mandelbroyt Y, Lieska N: The ulnar nerve at the elbow and its local branching: An anatomic study. *J Hand Surg Br* 2001;26: 142-144.

34. Grewal R, Varitimidis SE, Vardakas DG, Fu FH, Sotereanos DG: Ulnar nerve elongation and excursion in the cubital tunnel after decompression and anterior transposition. *J Hand Surg Br* 2000;25:457-460.

35. Nikitins MD, Griffin PA, Ch'ng S, Rice NJ: A dynamic anatomical study of ulnar nerve motion after anterior transposition for cubital tunnel syndrome. *Hand Surg* 2002;7:177-182.

36. Beekman R, Schoemaker MC, Van Der Plas JP, et al: Diagnostic value of high-resolution sonography in ulnar neuropathy at the elbow. *Neurology* 2004;62:767-773.

Ultrasonography demonstrated that the diameter of the ulnar nerve was greater in a cohort of patients with clinical signs of ulnar neuropathy than in control patients. The sensitivity of sonography was 80% and the specificity 91%.

37. Bartels RH, Verhagen WI, van der Wilt GJ, Meulstee J, van Rossum LG, Grotenhuis JA: Prospective randomized controlled study comparing simple decompression versus anterior subcutaneous transposition for idiopathic neuropathy of the ulnar nerve at the elbow: Part 1. *Neurosurgery* 2005;56:522-530.

This prospective, randomized controlled study compared simple decompression versus anterior subcutaneous transposition for idiopathic neuropathy of the ulnar nerve at the elbow. Both interventions were equivalent at 1 year; however, a significantly higher complication rate was observed with anterior subcutaneous transposition (31%) than with simple decompression (10%). Simple decompression was recommended for its simplicity, low complication rate, and low cost, even in the presence of nerve subluxation.

Chapter 28

Hand and Wrist Trauma

Seth D. Dodds, MD   Anthony J. Lauder, MD   Thomas E. Trumble, MD

Fractures and Dislocations of the Hand

Bone and joint injuries of the hand are common. They can be classified as stable or unstable: most stable injuries are treated with immobilization, but unstable injuries are best managed with surgical reduction and internal fixation. Some displaced fractures and acute dislocations are stable after closed reduction and amenable to conservative management. After any type of treatment, early mobilization of a stabilized hand fracture leads to improved function. The general principles of hand fracture management are outlined in Table 1.

Phalangeal Fractures

The distal phalanx, especially in the thumb, index, and middle fingers, is susceptible to injury because it extends most distally during hand use. Fractures of the distal tuft or shaft are often associated with soft-tissue injury to the nail bed. Tuft fractures can be immobilized with a clamshell-type splint, and fixation of unstable transverse shaft fractures is with a longitudinal Kirschner wire or screw. Fractures of the base of the distal phalanx are usually associated with a distal flexor or extensor tendon injury. If the joint is incongruent or a significant articular step-off exists, surgical reduction and stabilization of the fracture is indicated. Highly comminuted injuries of the distal interphalangeal (DIP) joint can be treated with delayed or secondary fusion, if necessary. Regardless of the treatment, an associated nail bed injury cannot be ignored. Subungual hematomas should be decompressed, nail bed lacerations should be reapproximated, and pulp lacerations should be débrided and repaired. The proximal nail fold must be kept open. This open injury requires a course of antibiotic therapy, along with débridement of any devitalized tissue.

Mallet fractures are unique, challenging intra-articular avulsion fractures of the terminal extensor tendon. Because of the pull of the extensor tendon, the fracture is typically displaced. If the bony fragment involves a large part of the articular surface, subluxation of the DIP joint occurs. A nondisplaced fracture with a congruent joint can be treated conservatively with the distal phalanx splinted in extension. Displacement of the fracture or joint subluxation is an indication for surgical reduction and internal fixation, although a recent study revealed negligible pain and reasonable patient satisfaction with extension splinting for a dis-

placed mallet fracture.[1] Surgical treatment of these injuries can improve DIP joint function but can lead to complications.[2]

Treatment of extra-articular fractures of the middle and proximal phalanges must take into account the overlying soft tissues, specifically the flexor and extensor tendons. Disregarding the complex anatomy and biomechanics of the flexor tendons, extensor apparatus, and neighboring joints can lead to a stiff and disabled finger.

Fracture stability is less defined by pattern than by the mechanism of injury and displacement at the time of injury. Fractures that cannot be maintained in a splint after a closed reduction are best treated with surgical reduction and fixation. Surgical treatment options range from closed reduction and percutaneous pinning to open reduction and plate fixation. The outcome is typically determined by the accuracy of fracture reduction (maintaining the alignment of the finger to minimize poorly tolerated angular and rotational deformities) and the quality of fixation. A recent prospective, randomized trial found no difference in functional outcome between patients treated with percutaneous Kirschner wires and those treated with lag screw fixation.[3] Results from another study showed adequate fracture healing and no loss of fixation using bicortical screw fixation rather than lag screw fixation.[4] The need for removal of hardware is a limitation of internal fixation; tendon adhesions can form over the hardware or even over the callus at the fracture site. As a consequence, tenolysis to release entrapped extensor or flexor tendons is sometimes necessary after a phalangeal fracture. After the fracture has been reduced and stabilized, early motion of the injured and uninjured fingers leads to improved functional outcomes.

Table 1
Principles of Hand Fracture Management
Immobilization increases hand stiffness
Fracture stability, finger posture, and fracture personality dictate the treatment
Rigid load-bearing fixation is not always required
The preferred method of fixation, if possible, is the use of percutaneously placed pins and screws
The outcome is typically proportional to the injury

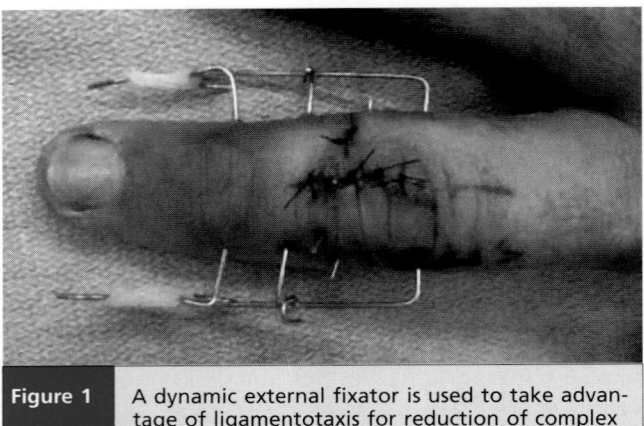

Figure 1   A dynamic external fixator is used to take advantage of ligamentotaxis for reduction of complex fractures involving the base of the middle phalanx, while enabling immediate finger motion.

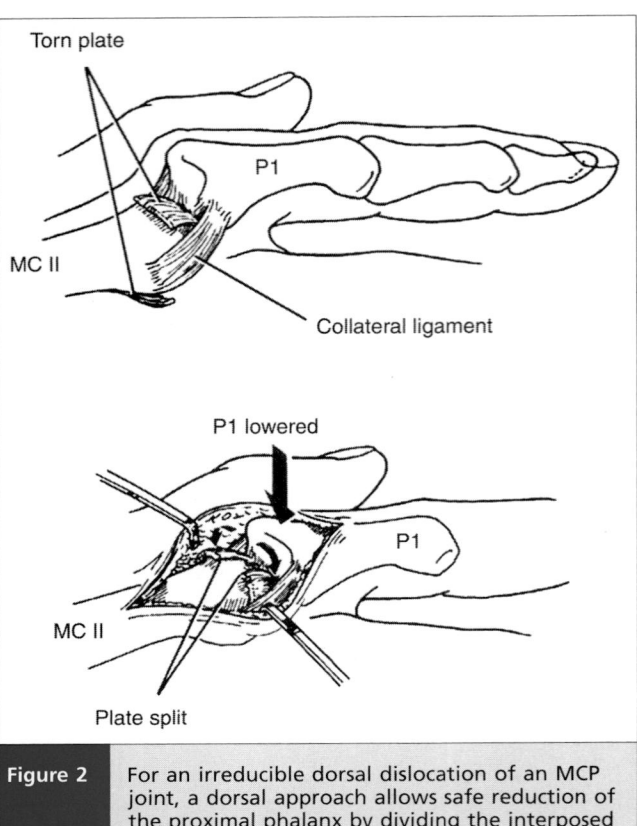

Figure 2   For an irreducible dorsal dislocation of an MCP joint, a dorsal approach allows safe reduction of the proximal phalanx by dividing the interposed volar plate longitudinally. MC = metacarpal, P = proximal phalanx. *(Reproduced with permission from Trumble TE:* Principles of Hand Surgery and Therapy. *Philadelphia, PA, WB Saunders, 1999, p 55.)*

Proximal Interphalangeal Joint Injuries

The proximal interphalangeal (PIP) joint is the cornerstone of digital motion. It is also the most challenging joint in the hand to rehabilitate after an injury. As a result, current treatments of PIP joint injuries all include early motion after stabilization. Straightforward dislocations from hyperextension injuries are reduced under a digital block and tested for stability after reduction. Stable dislocations can be managed by buddy taping to the adjacent finger. If the joint is unstable in extension, it is immobilized with a dorsal blocking splint. Motion can be started immediately within the dorsal blocking splint. Dorsal fracture-dislocations caused by hyperextension with axial loading are managed in the same manner. These injuries most often involve an articular fracture from the base of the middle phalanx. Fracture-dislocations of the PIP joint require surgical reduction and stabilization when concentric reduction of the joint is not possible or cannot be maintained with a splint. Concentric reductions are difficult to achieve and maintain if they involve more than 30% of the joint surface of the base of the middle phalanx. Concentric reductions are especially difficult to achieve with pilon-type axial-loading fractures, which involve both the volar and dorsal articular surface and sometimes the metaphysis of the middle phalanx.

Extension block splinting remains the mainstay of treatment for stable PIP fracture-dislocations that involve a small percentage of the volar joint surface. For extension block splinting to be successful, concentric reduction of the joint must be achieved. Dorsal subluxation of the middle phalanx leads to altered kinematics and poor motion after healing.

If the joint is incongruent after reduction and extension block splinting, surgical reduction is required. A closed reduction in the operating room can frequently be maintained with a Kirschner wire extension block splint or percutaneous fixation of the fracture fragment. Dynamic external fixation is another proven alternative to open reduction and internal fixation.[5] When properly applied, dynamic external fixation allows concentric joint motion and applies traction throughout a full range of motion. Although the fracture reduction may not be perfect, the applied traction stabilizes articular and metaphyseal comminution and should provide a concave containment for the condyles of the proximal phalanx. Immediate joint motion facilitates articular healing and preserves joint flexibility, providing the patient with a functional PIP joint. Dynamic external fixation is particularly useful in pilon-type axial-loading fractures with dorsal and volar comminution. It can be used in conjunction with internal fixation (Figure 1).

Metacarpophalangeal Joint Injuries

Pure dislocations of the metacarpophalangeal (MCP) joint warrant an attempt at closed reduction. However, a dorsal dislocation of the proximal phalanx over the metacarpal is unlikely to be reducible using closed techniques. An interposed volar plate or buttonholing of the metacarpal head between the flexor tendons and radial lumbrical can contribute to an irreducible dorsal dislocation at the MCP joint. Open reduction can be safely performed through a dorsal approach by splitting the extensor tendon and dividing the volar plate longitudinally to allow reduction of the proximal phalanx (Figure 2). An A1 pulley release performed through a volar

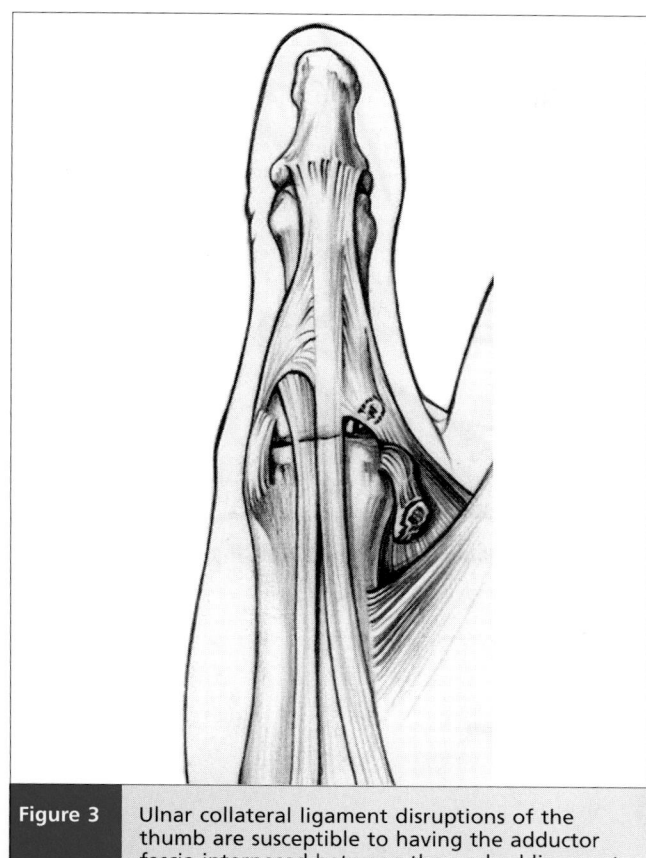

Figure 3 Ulnar collateral ligament disruptions of the thumb are susceptible to having the adductor fascia interposed between the avulsed ligament and the base of the proximal phalanx. *(Reproduced with permission from Trumble TE:* Principles of Hand Surgery and Therapy. *Philadelphia, PA, WB Saunders, 1999, p 49.)*

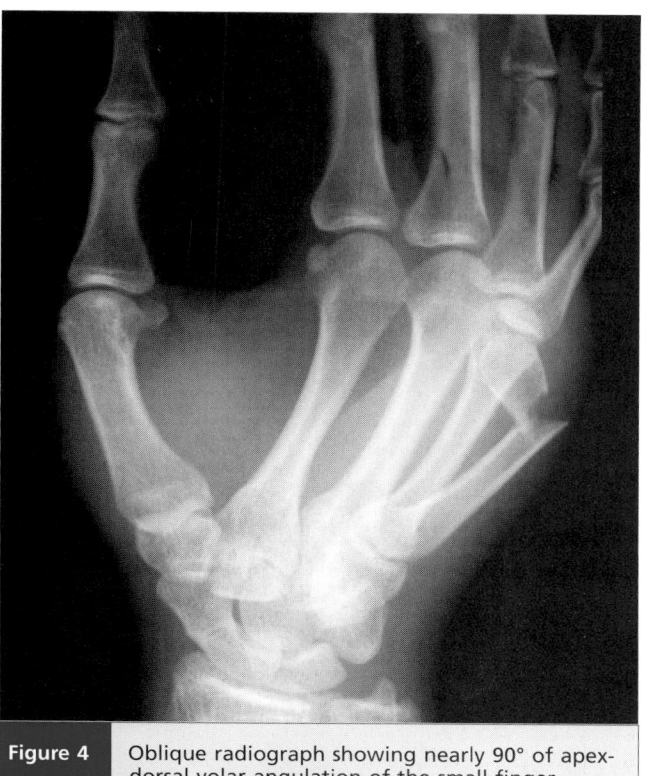

Figure 4 Oblique radiograph showing nearly 90° of apex-dorsal volar angulation of the small finger metacarpal. This view overestimates the actual volar angulation.

approach provides access to the metacarpal head, the lumbrical, and the flexor tendons, but it places the radial digital nerve, which is draped over the protruding metacarpal head, at risk of iatrogenic laceration.

Soft-tissue injury to the radial or ulnar collateral ligaments of the MCP joint is a common occurrence, especially in the thumb. Immobilization alone may be sufficient to treat a partial ligament tear or nondisplaced or minimally displaced avulsion fracture of the collateral ligaments. Surgical repair is indicated if the bulging mass of the torn ligament is palpable and overt instability exists (> 35° of laxity to ulnar stress, with the MCP joint in extension), because of the likelihood of a Stener's lesion[6] (**Figure 3**). Small suture anchors have simplified direct surgical repair of acute ligament disruptions, but traditional pull-out sutures remain an option.

Common pitfalls in collateral ligament surgery include iatrogenic injury to dorsal branches of the radial sensory nerve, overtightening of the repair, and nonanatomic reduction of the ligament insertion. An overly tight repair or reconstruction followed by prolonged immobilization leads to diminished MCP joint range of motion and, perhaps, asymmetric joint loading.

Nonanatomic reduction of the ligament insertion also alters joint kinematics and range of motion.[7] Symptomatic, chronic collateral ligament tears are treated by ligament reconstruction using neighboring autograft tendon or even allograft tendon. Biomechanical testing has demonstrated that a triangular configuration of ligament reconstruction with the apex of the triangle proximal and the base distal (on the base of the proximal phalanx) offers stability without compromising postreconstruction range of motion.[8]

Metacarpal Fractures

Like fractures of the phalanges, stable, minimally displaced fractures of the metacarpals can usually be treated with simple closed reduction and splinting. The intermetacarpal ligaments are stout ligaments that span the metacarpal heads and resist displacement of low-energy fractures involving the metacarpal necks.

The most common hand fracture is the so-called boxer's fracture of the metacarpal neck of the small finger. Metacarpal neck fractures are traditionally managed conservatively, with the apex dorsal angulation determined as follows: small finger, 40° to 50°; ring finger, 30°; middle finger, 15°; index finger, 10°. The degree of apex dorsal or volar angulation at the fracture site is most accurately assessed using a lateral radiograph of the hand; a cadaveric study showed that oblique views often amplify the actual angle of the fracture[9] (**Figure 4**). Apex dorsal angulation, if not reduced, leads to a

3: Upper Extremity

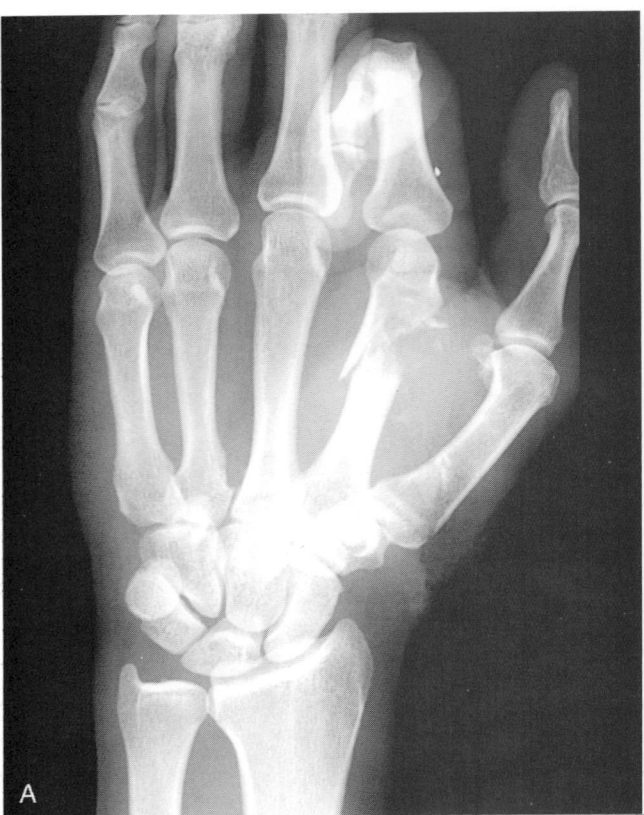
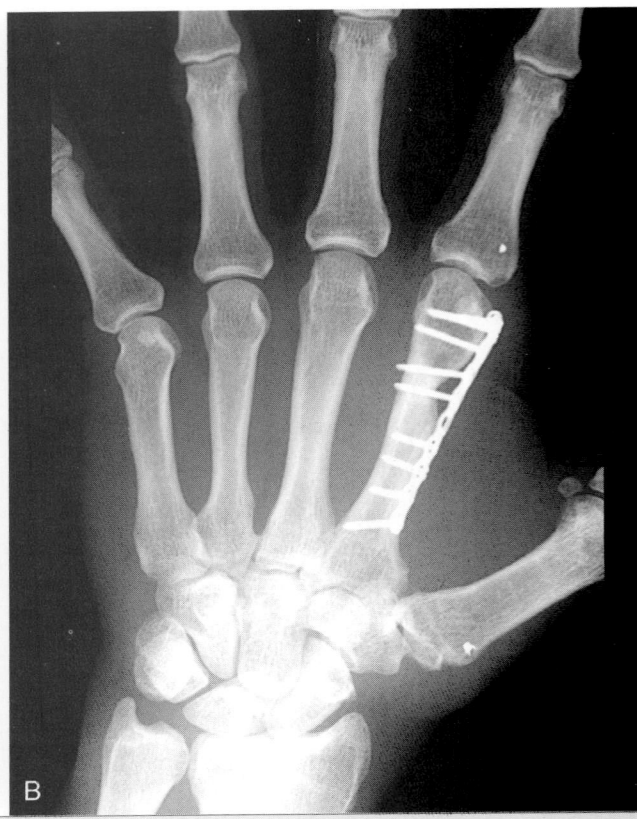

Figure 5 **A,** PA radiograph of a comminuted open fracture shows bone loss involving the index metacarpal. **B,** After surgical débridement and open reduction, internal stabilization of the fracture is done with a plate-and-screw construct to allow early mobilization after soft-tissue healing.

change in the appearance of the cascade of MCP joints on the dorsum of the hand. A retrospective review of three different casting techniques for closed management of extra-articular metacarpal fractures found no differences in the outcomes of the three groups.[10]

These deformities are acceptable only if there is no significant rotational deformity (< 5°). Small finger rotation should be carefully assessed, because fracture site swelling in the fourth web space can exaggerate a perceived rotational deformity.[11] Cadaveric testing has shown that metacarpal shortening of as much as 10 mm can lead to a reduction in grip strength of almost 50%.[12] Adhesions of overlying extensor tendons can be bothersome after treatment of any metacarpal fracture by closed reduction and percutaneous pinning or open reduction and internal fixation. To minimize the impact of extensor tendon adhesions, fixation should be sufficient to permit early digital motion (**Figure 5**).

Carpometacarpal Joint Injuries

Injuries to the base of the hand or carpometacarpal (CMC) joints are uncommon. The metacarpals are well seated onto the distal carpal row with stout volar, dorsal, and intermetacarpal ligament attachments. The CMC joints of the small finger and ring finger act as a fairly mobile hinge, with the convex metacarpal bases articulating on the hamate's two concavities to allow flexion, extension, and some rotation toward the thumb. The inherent mobility of these CMC joints predispose them to injury more than the relatively immobile middle-finger and index-finger CMC joints. Although dislocation of the CMC joints can occur, the typical injury is a dorsal fracture-dislocation. A 30° pronated lateral radiograph of the hand often shows a dorsal dislocation of the ulnar CMC joints that was missed on standard PA and lateral views. CT can confirm a questionable diagnosis. These fracture-dislocations have been referred to as reverse Bennett's fractures, and they should be treated with surgical reduction and internal fixation. Percutaneous Kirschner wire pinning is frequently sufficient, but if avulsion of large fragments of the hamate has occurred, an open reduction can be maintained with screw fixation.

Displaced intra-articular fractures involving the base also should be treated with surgical reduction and internal fixation. A Bennett's fracture is an intra-articular avulsion fracture of the volar oblique ligament of the thumb CMC joint. The adductor pollicis and the abductor pollicis longus act in concert to displace the metacarpal radially and proximally, away from the avulsed bony fragment (**Figure 6**, *A*). A Bennett's fracture should be surgically reduced and internally fixed

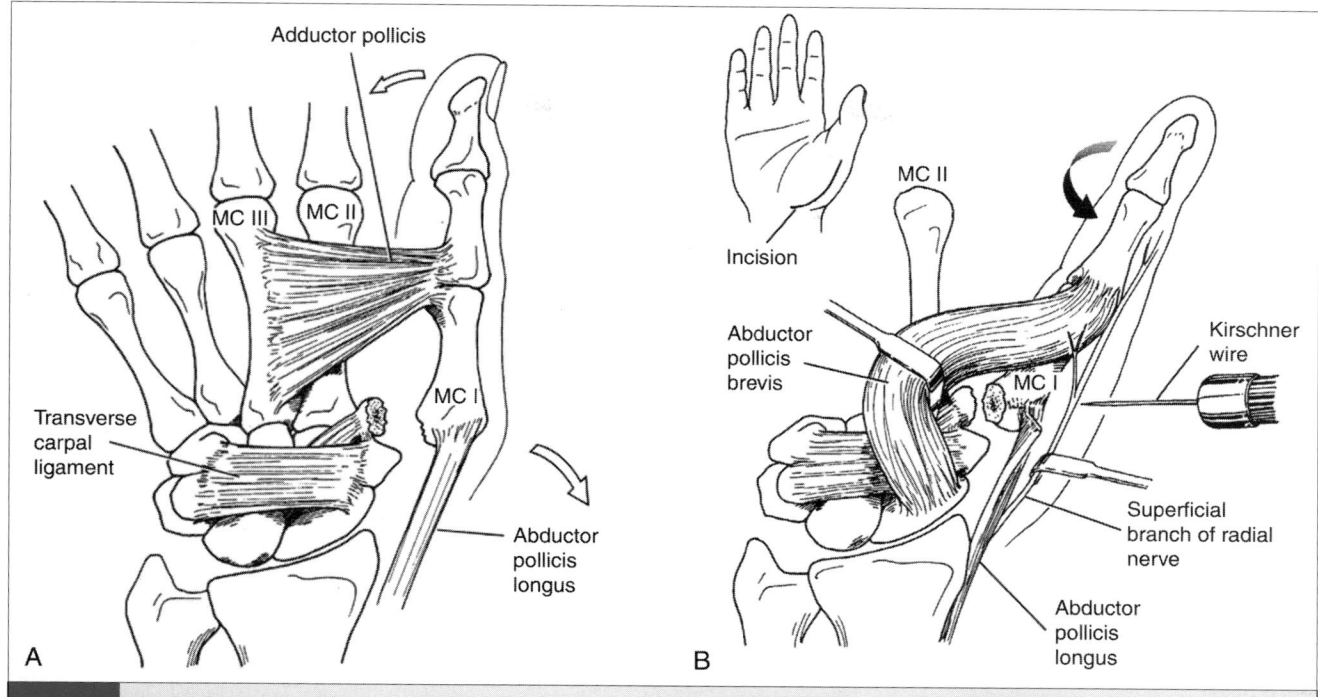

Figure 6 **A,** The adductor pollicis and abductor pollicis longus act in concert to translate the metacarpal base radially and proximally, leading to fracture site displacement and joint subluxation. **B,** Open reduction and internal fixation can be performed through a radial approach, which will avoid branches of the radial sensory nerve and elevate the abductor pollicis brevis from the metacarpal base. MC = metacarpal. *(Reproduced with permission from Trumble TE: Principles of Hand Surgery and Therapy. Philadelphia, PA, WB Saunders, 1999, p 42.)*

to maintain the stability and congruency of the CMC joint (**Figure 6,** *B*). A Rolando's fracture is a pilon-type injury in which the thumb base sustains an axial load, splitting the articular surface into ulnar and radial fragments (**Figure 7**). Occasionally, the forces are sufficient to cause metaphyseal comminution as well as fragmentation of the joint surface. These injuries can be effectively treated by external fixation with gentle axial traction applied through the thumb, using ligamentotaxis to restore the alignment of the metacarpal base.

Fractures and Dislocations of the Wrist

Distal Radius Fractures

Distal radius injuries are exceedingly common and yet problematic to treat, although surgical and implant techniques continue to evolve. The goal continues to be the restoration of a well-aligned, concentric radiocarpal and distal radioulnar joint (**Figure 8**). Most distal radius fractures can be adequately assessed through high-quality PA, oblique, and lateral radiographs.[13] Although technicians often place the forearm flat on the table for the lateral radiograph, elevating the wrist 20° from horizontal places the articular surface on profile. CT can better delineate the fracture pattern or articular disruption, if necessary.

Despite the recent trend toward early surgical intervention for distal radius fractures, it is important to de-

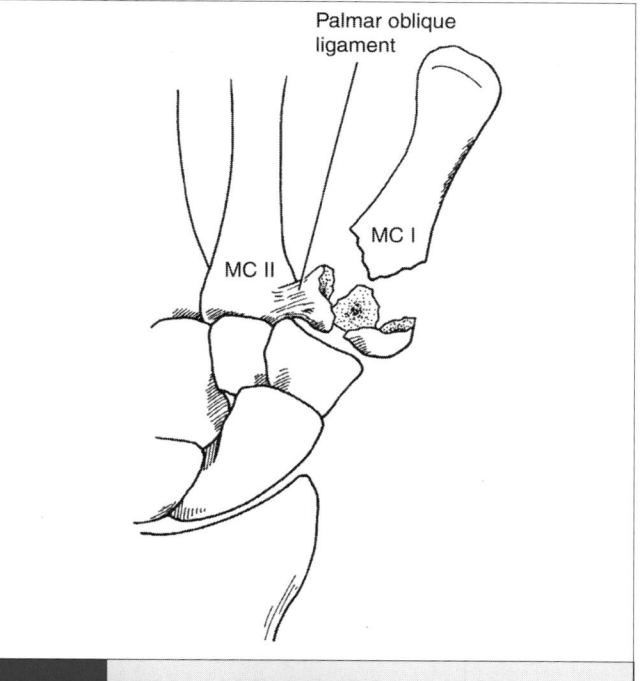

Figure 7 A Rolando's fracture involves an axial load; the articular surface is split into multiple fracture fragments, often in a Y- or T-shaped pattern. MC = metacarpal. *(Reproduced with permission from Trumble TE: Principles of Hand Surgery and Therapy. Philadelphia, PA, WB Saunders, 1999, p 43.)*

3: Upper Extremity

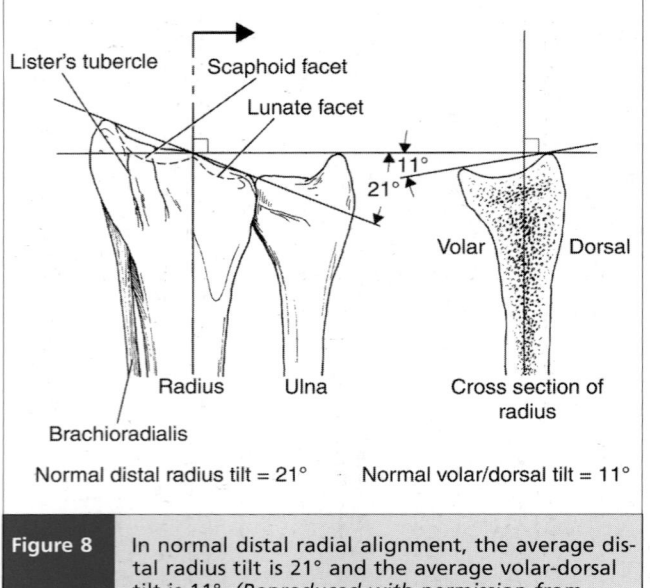

Normal distal radius tilt = 21°   Normal volar/dorsal tilt = 11°

Figure 8	In normal distal radial alignment, the average distal radius tilt is 21° and the average volar-dorsal tilt is 11°. *(Reproduced with permission from Trumble TE:* Principles of Hand Surgery and Therapy. *Philadelphia, PA, WB Saunders, 1999, p 147.)*

sign the treatment plan on a case-by-case basis. In general, closed reduction and conservative management with immobilization should be attempted for fractures of the distal radius, with some exceptions: open fractures, vertical shear injuries (which are inherently unstable), and multiple trauma injuries. The patient's activity level, but not the patient's age, and any comorbid conditions must be taken into account. Fractures with articular displacement of more than 2 mm, metaphyseal instability, or radial shortening, as well as fractures that fail to maintain a reduction, typically benefit from surgical intervention.[14]

Recent data on 4,000 wrist fractures revealed that patient age (older than 80 years), metaphyseal comminution, and radial shortening at presentation consistently predicted radiographically assessed instability; dorsal angulation did not.[15] An earlier study suggested that instability could be predicted if three of the following five factors were present: age older than 60 years, associated ulnar fracture, initial dorsal angulation of more than 20°, comminution of the dorsal metaphysis, and intra-articular extension of the fracture.[16] The surgical treatment options for unstable, significantly displaced, or intra-articular fractures include percutaneous pinning, external fixation with or without supplemental Kirschner wire fixation, open reduction and internal fixation, arthroscopically assisted fixation, and distal radius bridge plating (internal distraction plating).

Percutaneous pinning is generally combined with some form of immobilization (casting, external fixation, or distraction plating). It is an excellent technique for treatment of simple extra-articular fractures or intra-articular fractures with fragments that are amenable to reduction by closed or minimally invasive methods. Percutaneous pinning is intrafocal or interfragmentary. In intrafocal pinning, Kirschner wires are inserted into the fracture site and used to lever displaced fragments into position. Interfragmentary Kirschner wires pass through the fractured distal fragments into the intact proximal fragment. Arthroscopy is a useful tool for assessing the articular reduction.

External fixation with reduction achieved by ligamentotaxis can be a useful method of treating distal radius fractures, especially those associated with a significant soft-tissue injury. Augmenting an external fixation with percutaneously placed pins enhances fracture stability and helps maintain articular congruity. If early wrist motion is desired and the fracture fragments are large and sturdy enough, a nonspanning external fixator can be applied to maintain fracture stabilization without crossing the radiocarpal joint. A recent meta-analysis did not find evidence to support the use of internal fixation rather than external fixation for unstable distal radius fractures, despite the frequent occurrence of pin site infection.[17]

Several new techniques and implant designs have been developed in recent years for internal fixation of distal radius fractures, including dorsal plating, volar plating, and fragment-specific fixation. The dorsal approach to the distal radius is technically simple, and articular exposure is facilitated by the volar location of most radiocarpal stabilizers. Dorsal plating has been associated with extensor tendon irritation and postoperative stiffness; however, a recent study of dorsal implants with relatively low profiles and beveled edges found that only one plate had to be removed because of dorsal wrist pain and extensor tendon rupture had not occurred 1 year or more after surgery.[18]

Most distal radius fractures involve dorsal displacement. Volar plating relies on fixed-angled, locking screw technology for effective stabilization of the distal fragments.[19] The fracture typically can be reduced in a line-to-line fashion from a volar approach, despite dorsal comminution. In contrast to dorsal plating, overlying tendons are protected in volar plating by a repaired pronator quadratus, unless the plate is left prominent. The use of long screws must be avoided in volar plating, because a long screw can cause extensor tendon rupture.

Fragment-specific fixation compels the surgeon to divide distal radius injuries into individual fracture fragments. Typical fracture components include a radial column, dorsal ulnar corner, volar rim, and dorsal wall, as well as intra-articular fragments. A specific implant can be used to stabilize each reduced fragment. Although these implants are surprisingly small, they can provide significant rigidity, especially when applied in orthogonal planes.[20]

Spanning or distraction plating can be an excellent means of treating fractures of the distal radius when the comminution extends into the metaphyseal-diaphyseal region. This method is useful for treating fractures where substantial intra-articular comminution or severe osteoporosis is present and forces across the radiocarpal joint must be neutralized to prevent frac-

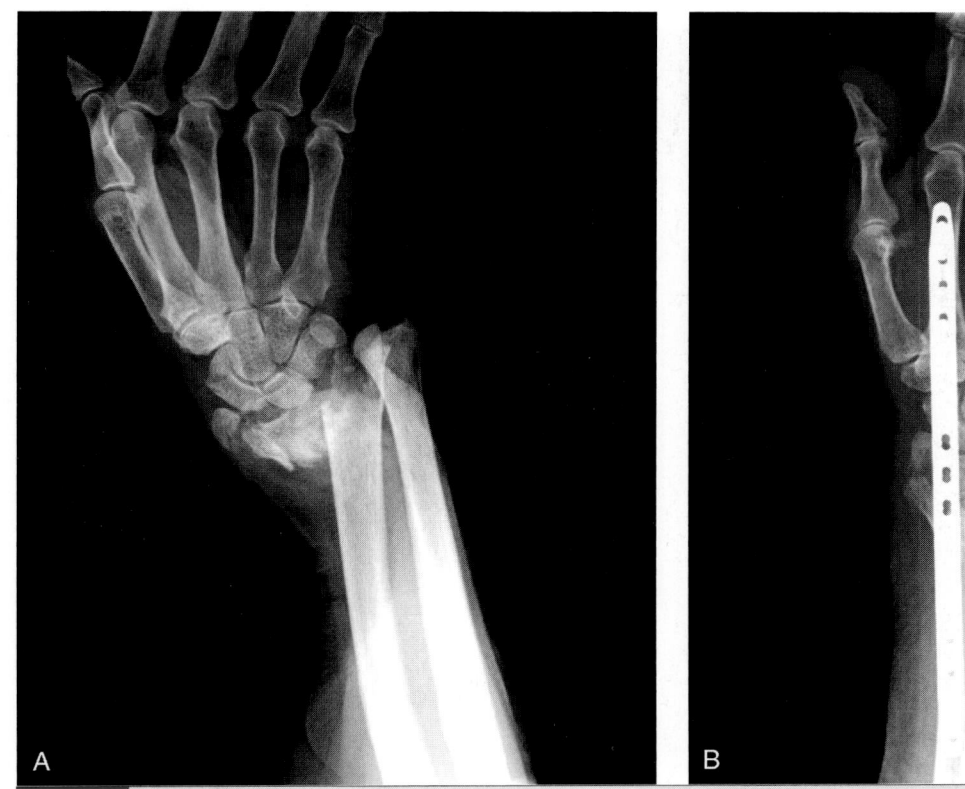
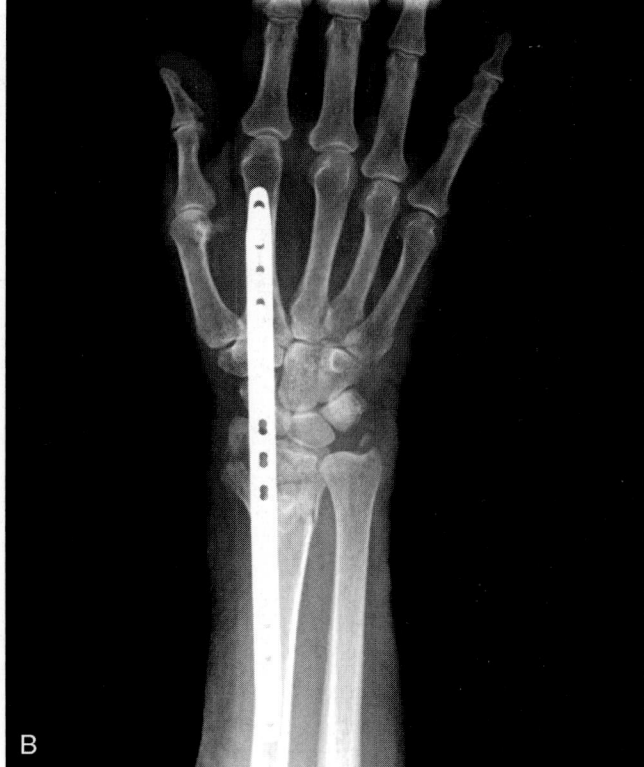

Figure 9   **A,** Preoperative PA radiograph of the wrist shows a significantly displaced open fracture of the distal radius with metaphyseal and articular comminution. **B,** After surgical débridement and reduction, the distal radial alignment is maintained by spanning internal fixation.

ture fragment migration (**Figure 9**). Because these devices are essentially internal external fixators, they are ideal for use in multiple trauma patients, who may require early upper extremity weight bearing for transfers. Maintenance of fracture alignment and a functional range of motion can be expected at 1-year follow-up of a fracture treated with a spanning plate.[21]

Distal Radial Ulnar Joint and Triangular Fibrocartilage Complex Injuries

Distal radial ulnar joint (DRUJ) instability is most commonly the result of a fracture of the distal radius, although it can occur in isolation. When DRUJ dislocation is a purely ligamentous injury, it usually can be reduced under conscious sedation in the emergency department. After a successful reduction, a stable arc of motion should be tested. Volar dislocations are normally stable in pronation, and the more common dorsal dislocations are stable in supination. Most injuries can be splinted in a position of stability for 4 weeks in a long arm cast. However, when the DRUJ is stable only at the extremes of motion, open repair of the distal radioulnar ligament complex or radioulnar pinning with large Kirschner wires should be considered.

In a distal radius fracture, the distal radioulnar ligaments and triangular fibrocartilage complex (TFCC) can only tolerate 5 mm to 7 mm of radial shortening before tearing. Thus, the ability to recreate a concentric sigmoid notch while maintaining radial length and alignment is one of the most important factors in determining DRUJ stability after a wrist fracture. After fractures of the distal radius, associated fractures of the ulnar styloid can lead to instability of the DRUJ. Generally, small or fleck fractures at the tip of the ulnar styloid do not lead to instability, because the tip of the ulnar styloid lacks ligamentous attachments. The volar and dorsal distal radioulnar ligaments of the TFCC are inserted into the fovea at the base of the ulnar styloid (**Figure 10**). Thus, fractures of the distal ulna that occur at the base of the styloid are potentially unstable, and repair of these fractures should be considered.

A traumatic injury of the TFCC is classified as a central perforation, ulnar avulsion (with or without a styloid fracture), distal avulsion (from the carpus), or radial-side avulsion (with or without a sigmoid notch fracture). For a patient who has DRUJ instability or fails to improve after immobilization, an MRI arthrogram can lead to a diagnosis of TFCC tear. Central and radial-side lesions are amenable to arthroscopic débridement. Radial- and ulnar-side TFCC tears can be repaired by arthroscopy or the traditional open approach. Ulnar-side lesions have greater healing potential after repair because of the increased blood flow at the periphery of the TFCC. The dorsal sensory branch

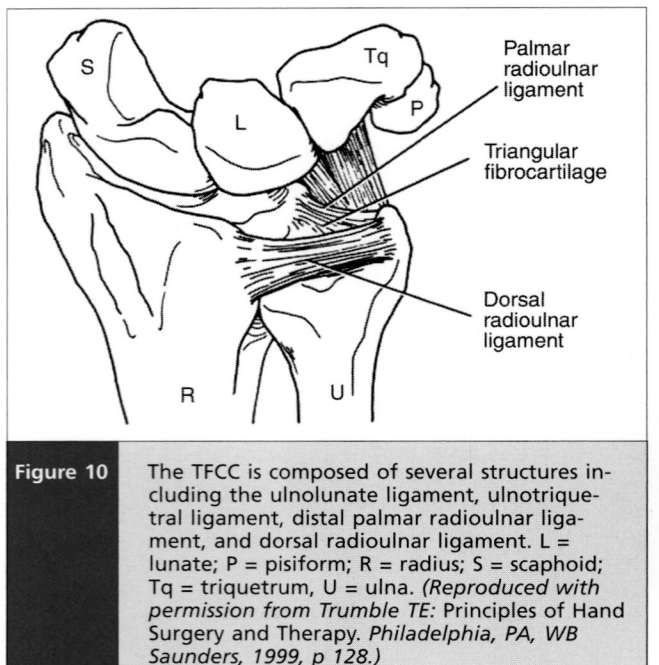

Figure 10 The TFCC is composed of several structures including the ulnolunate ligament, ulnotriquetral ligament, distal palmar radioulnar ligament, and dorsal radioulnar ligament. L = lunate; P = pisiform; R = radius; S = scaphoid; Tq = triquetrum, U = ulna. *(Reproduced with permission from Trumble TE:* Principles of Hand Surgery and Therapy. *Philadelphia, PA, WB Saunders, 1999, p 128.)*

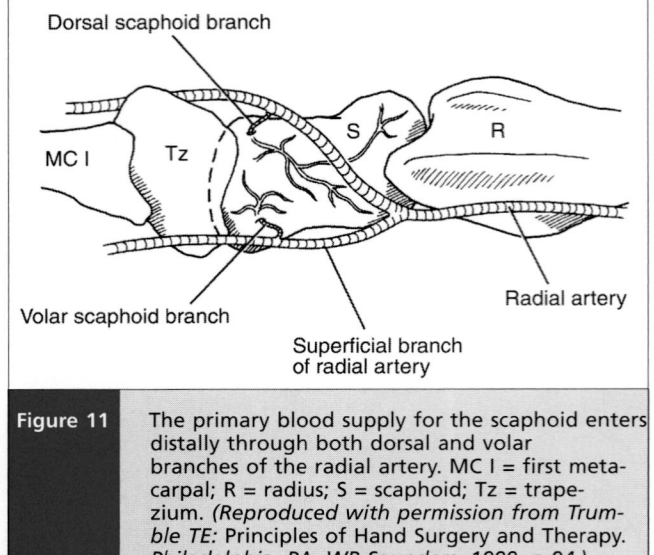

Figure 11 The primary blood supply for the scaphoid enters distally through both dorsal and volar branches of the radial artery. MC I = first metacarpal; R = radius; S = scaphoid; Tz = trapezium. *(Reproduced with permission from Trumble TE:* Principles of Hand Surgery and Therapy. *Philadelphia, PA, WB Saunders, 1999, p 94.)*

of the ulnar nerve must be protected during a TFCC repair.

Carpal Fractures and Nonunions

Most carpal fractures occur in young, active patients who have fallen onto an outstretched hand. These injuries are difficult to diagnose using plain radiography. CT is used to confirm the diagnosis in the emergency department. Occasionally, patients with persistent pain have fractures that are visible only with MRI. Carpal bone fractures, excluding those of the scaphoid, can usually be treated with immobilization for as long as 6 weeks. Most fractures of the lunate and triquetrum are avulsion injuries; they are the bony equivalent of a wrist sprain. Fractures of the hamate generally occur through the hook as the result of a direct blow to the palm. Nondisplaced fractures of the hook of the hamate can be treated with immobilization. Displaced fractures can be treated with internal fixation or excision. Excision of the hook of the hamate can reduce flexor strength to the small finger.

The scaphoid is by far the most commonly fractured bone in the wrist. Scaphoid fractures account for almost 80% of all of fractures of the carpus. A scaphoid fracture typically occurs at the waist, commonly as the result of a fall onto a hyperextended, ulnarly deviated wrist. Because the entire proximal half of the scaphoid is covered with articular cartilage, only the most distal segment and the dorsal ridge carry entering blood vessels. This vascular anatomy means that 70% to 80% of the bone receives its blood supply in a retrograde fashion (**Figure 11**) and is the reason that proximal pole fractures can lead to osteonecrosis or require prolonged healing time.

In general, fractures that are stable (nondisplaced

and not comminuted) can be treated with a thumb spica cast. Fractures that are unstable (displaced > 1 mm and/or comminuted) require surgical management. CT should be used liberally to assess the displacement and comminution of a scaphoid fracture. A prospective, randomized study that compared long arm and short arm-thumb spica casting found a 9% nonunion rate in patients with a short arm cast and no nonunions in patients with a long arm cast.[22] These differences were not statistically significant, and healing was not confirmed by CT. Nonetheless, many surgeons have used the study as the basis for placing patients, at least initially, in long arm casts. A more recent study comparing surgical treatment to casting for nondisplaced scaphoid fractures found that the surgically treated group had better wrist motion at 16 weeks; however, no significant differences were noted at 1 year.[23]

Displaced fractures (≥ 1.0 mm), proximal pole fractures, comminuted fractures, fractures in which the intrascaphoid angle is greater than 35°, and fractures associated with perilunate dislocations or distal radius fractures all warrant surgical fixation to prevent nonunion. Displaced fractures can have nonunion rates as high as 50%. The surgical fixation should take place within 2 to 3 weeks of the injury to prevent difficulty in manipulating the fragments. Variable pitch, headless screw fixation provides compression at the fracture site and therefore is ideal for scaphoid fractures.

The scaphoid is almost entirely intra-articular and, as a result, achieves union by primary bone healing rather than by bony callus formation. For primary bone healing to occur, viable osteocytes, a blood supply, and rigid stability are required. A reduced, viable scaphoid with rigid internal fixation and fracture site compression are the goals of surgery. Studies have found that the longest possible screw should be placed in the center position of the proximal pole, as seen on both AP and lateral radiographs.[24,25] A headless cannulated screw system enables the surgeon to avoid articular prominence of the screw and ensure central placement with a guide pin before screw insertion.

The volar and dorsal approaches are most commonly used for open fixation of unstable scaphoid fractures. The volar approach exposes the scaphoid through the floor of the flexor carpi radialis and is excellent for distal pole and waist fractures because it helps the surgeon avoid inadvertent injury to the vessels entering through the dorsal ridge. The dorsal approach is preferred for proximal pole injuries, although it places the dorsal blood supply at risk if dissection is overly aggressive. Indirect reduction and percutaneous screw placement from the dorsal or volar side of the wrist has been shown to be a satisfactory technique that avoids disruption of the tenuous blood supply.[26]

Many factors can lead to scaphoid nonunion, including the location of the fracture (proximal pole fractures are more prone to nonunion and osteonecrosis), a delay in the fracture diagnosis, inadequate treatment of the fracture, patient noncompliance, and fracture comminution or displacement. Regardless of the etiology, scaphoid nonunions are a significant cause of patient morbidity and surgeon frustration. Often a patient is not aware of a traumatic event leading to a fracture and presents with pain only after wrist arthrosis has set in. MRI with intravenous contrast is effective in evaluating proximal pole viability and the location and extent of arthritis. CT is useful in assessing any scaphoid collapse or humpback deformity.

The treatment algorithms for scaphoid nonunion are based on the location of the fracture, the presence of proximal pole osteonecrosis, the degree of scaphoid collapse or flexion, and the presence of wrist arthrosis. Delayed treatment affects the healing rate. Selected scaphoid nonunions, delayed unions, and fibrous unions that are free of collapse or displacement have been successfully treated by percutaneous fixation.[27] Although this approach can be used to perform cancellous endosteal bone grafting though a dorsally placed drill hole, it does not allow for structural bone grafting to correct a humpback deformity. If proximal pole osteonecrosis is not present, a humpback deformity can be treated volarly with structural autologous bone grafting and rigid internal fixation. If proximal pole osteonecrosis is present, vascularized bone grafting and rigid internal fixation should be considered (**Figure 12**).

Carpal Instability

The proximal carpal row, made up of the scaphoid, lunate, and triquetrum, acts as an intercalated segment coordinating the movements of the distal radius and ulna and the distal carpal row (the trapezium, trapezoid, capitate, and hamate). As the wrist is brought into radial deviation the scaphoid flexes, causing the entire proximal row to flex. In ulnar deviation the reverse is true, and the scaphoid's vertical orientation leads to extension of the lunate and triquetrum.

The most common form of carpal instability stems from injury to the scapholunate interosseous ligament

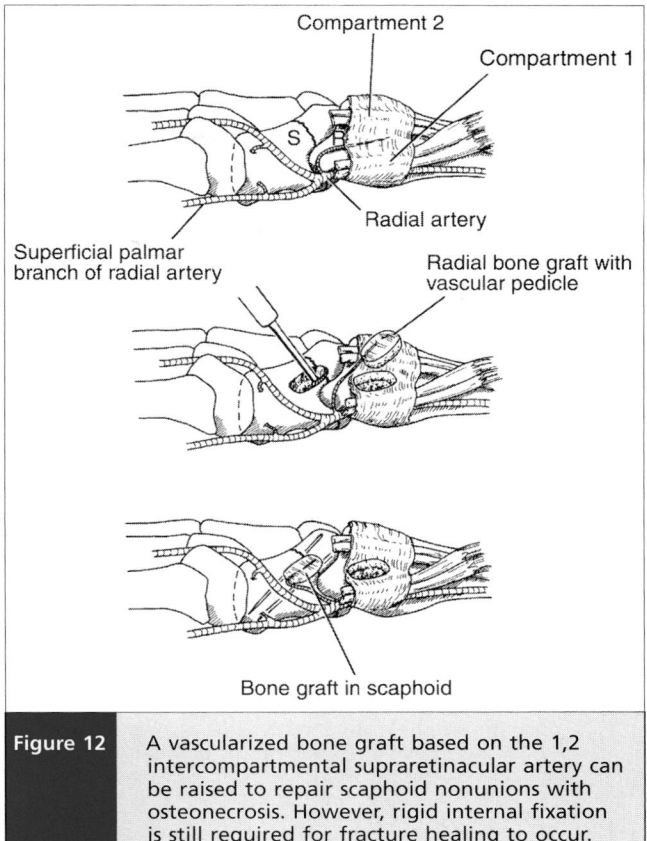

Figure 12   A vascularized bone graft based on the 1,2 intercompartmental supraretinacular artery can be raised to repair scaphoid nonunions with osteonecrosis. However, rigid internal fixation is still required for fracture healing to occur. *(Reproduced with permission from Trumble TE: Fractures and dislocations of the carpus, in* Principles of Hand Surgery and Therapy. *Philadelphia, PA, WB Saunders, 1999, p 102.)*

(SLIL). This U-shaped ligament has three distinct portions: dorsal, volar, and proximal. The dorsal aspect is particularly stout and provides most of the scapholunate joint's stability; the volar and proximal portions are less substantial. The SLIL is the critical link between the scaphoid and lunate. It plays a crucial role in normal carpal kinematics, in which the entire proximal row is required to function as an intercalated segment. Injury to the SLIL disrupts this intricate interplay of carpal motion and leads to an increasingly flexed posture of the scaphoid while the lunate drifts into a dorsiflexed position (termed dorsal intercalated instability). Left untreated, a chronic scapholunate dissociation progresses to carpal collapse and arthritis (termed scapholunate advanced collapse).

Patients with acute SLIL injury generally have dorsoradial wrist pain after falling onto an outstretched hand. If the tear is complete, some patients feel a clunking sensation or have increased motion of the scaphoid as their wrist is taken through a range of motion. Pain can normally be elicited by palpating the scapholunate interval or performing the scaphoid shift test (**Figure 13**). The initial radiographs of a suspected SLIL injury should include a lateral view as well as neutral, bilateral clenched fist, and ulnar deviation (scaphoid) PA views.

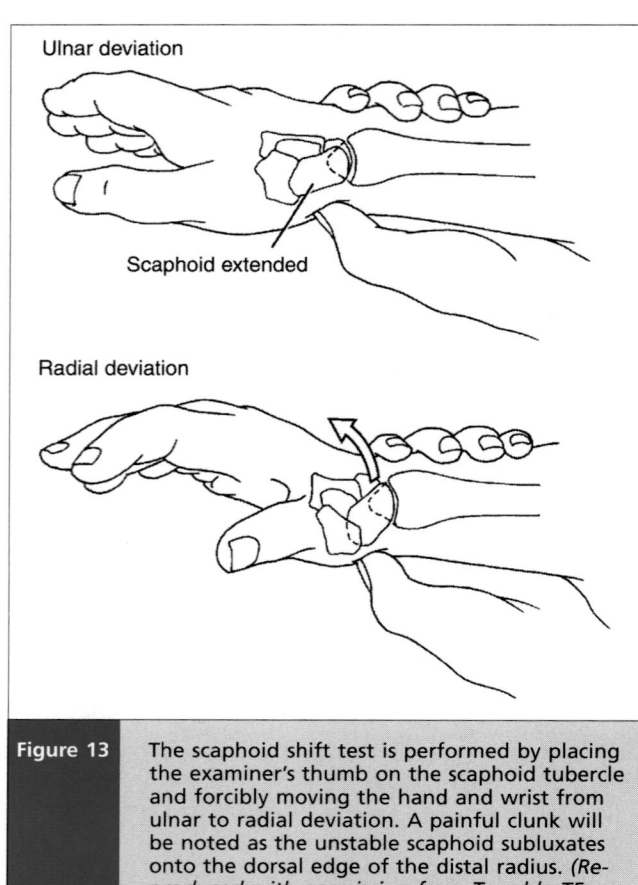

Ulnar deviation

Scaphoid extended

Radial deviation

Figure 13 The scaphoid shift test is performed by placing the examiner's thumb on the scaphoid tubercle and forcibly moving the hand and wrist from ulnar to radial deviation. A painful clunk will be noted as the unstable scaphoid subluxates onto the dorsal edge of the distal radius. *(Reproduced with permission from Trumble TE: Fractures and dislocations of the carpus, in Principles of Hand Surgery and Therapy. Philadelphia, PA, WB Saunders, 1999, p 107.)*

Bone scintigraphy, arthrography, and MRI can also be used to diagnose ligament injuries. Arthrography can be useful in diagnosing a tear, but the leakage of dye only confirms a tear and does not address its significance. MRI used alone has low sensitivity, but adding arthrography can increase sensitivity. Surgeons are using arthroscopy because it is the best tool for determining both the presence of a tear and its extent or severity.

Stable injuries stem from small, partial tears. Patients show no signs of abnormal carpal alignment or kinematics on examination or radiography. They should be treated with a short course of immobilization and close follow-up, although some surgeons argue that arthroscopic evaluation and débridement of these partial tears can be helpful.

Unstable injuries are from large or complete tears of the SLIL. They are further classified as dynamic or static, depending on the radiographic findings. Static instability with scapholunate interval widening and dorsal intercalated instability deformity is readily seen on PA and lateral plain radiographs. Patients with dynamic instability have abnormal carpal kinematics on physical examination and widening between the scaphoid and lunate on stress radiographs (clenched fist

views). Unstable SLIL injuries require surgical treatment, which can range from arthroscopic débridement, reduction, and percutaneous pinning to open, primary repair augmented with internal fixation or soft-tissue reconstruction.

Lunotriquetral instability generally occurs in association with scapholunate injury, as found in lunate or perilunate dislocation. However, isolated instability can occur at the lunotriquetral interosseous ligament and can lead to abnormal carpal kinematics. In contrast to scapholunate instability, in which the scaphoid flexes and the lunate extends with the triquetrum, lunotriquetral interosseous ligament injury can lead to flexion of the lunate and a scapholunate angle that is less than 30°. This type of injury leads to volar intercalated instability. A disruption of the lunotriquetral interosseous ligament does not lead to a volar intercalated instability deformity unless it is associated with another injury to the secondary carpal stabilizers (extrinsic and intrinsic ligaments). Plain radiography and MRI can be helpful in diagnosing lunotriquetral interosseous ligament pathology, but direct or arthroscopic visualization continues to be the best method of assessing lunotriquetral tears and instability. Treatment can include primary repair for an acute injury and ligament reconstruction or limited fusions for a chronic injury. The goal of any surgical treatment is to correct rotational deformity of the proximal row in an effort to restore normal wrist kinematics.

Lunate and perilunate dislocations are relatively rare injuries that usually stem from high-energy trauma and forceful dorsiflexion of the wrist. Injuries of this nature always require a thorough patient evaluation because concomitant injuries are common. In a lunate dislocation, the lunate has been forced from its fossa to a position volar to the distal radius; the rest of the carpus and distal radius remain relatively well aligned. In a perilunate dislocation, the lunate is in position, but dorsal dislocation of the carpus and hand is evident. As shown in Figure 14, the energy of injury is usually transmitted from radial to ulnar; it can progress as a fracture through the scaphoid or capitate (a greater arc injury) or as an interosseous ligament injury around the lunate (a lesser arc injury).

Patients with acute median nerve symptoms do not require emergency carpal tunnel release if the dislocation can be reduced. However, patients with delayed or worsening median nerve symptoms should undergo carpal tunnel release. Open repair of the SLIL and lunotriquetral interosseous ligament is indicated for an acute injury. Additional stabilization should be performed using Kirschner wires to pin the scapholunate and lunotriquetral intervals. Pinning of the scaphocapitate interval blocks midcarpal motion and minimizes scapholunate stress while the ligament heals. Fractures associated with greater arc injuries are treated with surgical reduction and internal fixation. Poor results can be expected after either a high-energy open dislocation or delayed treatment.

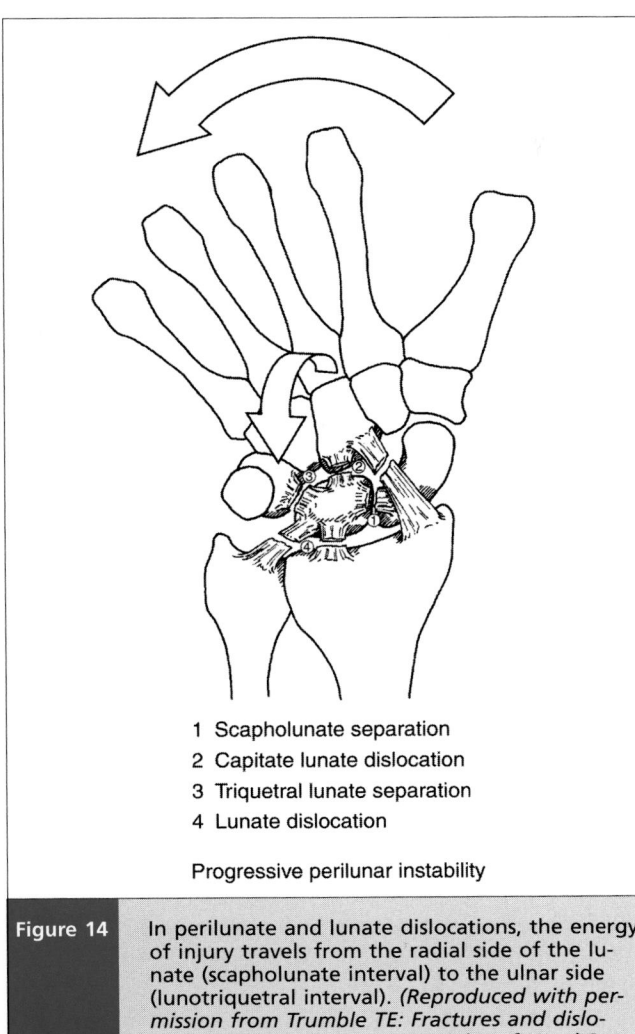

1 Scapholunate separation
2 Capitate lunate dislocation
3 Triquetral lunate separation
4 Lunate dislocation

Progressive perilunar instability

Figure 14	In perilunate and lunate dislocations, the energy of injury travels from the radial side of the lunate (scapholunate interval) to the ulnar side (lunotriquetral interval). *(Reproduced with permission from Trumble TE: Fractures and dislocations of the carpus, in* Principles of Hand Surgery and Therapy. *Philadelphia, PA, WB Saunders, 1999, p 107.)*

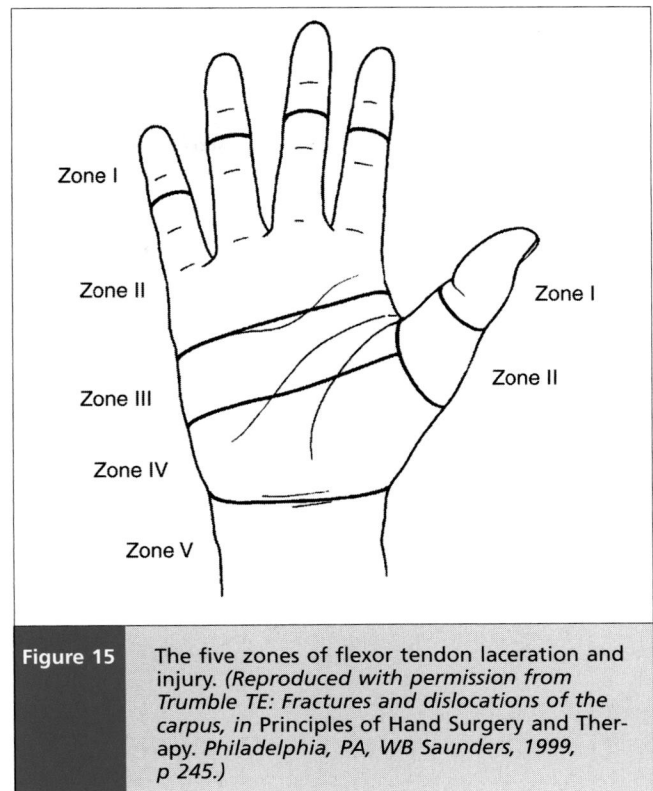

Figure 15	The five zones of flexor tendon laceration and injury. *(Reproduced with permission from Trumble TE: Fractures and dislocations of the carpus, in* Principles of Hand Surgery and Therapy. *Philadelphia, PA, WB Saunders, 1999, p 245.)*

Soft-Tissue Injuries

Flexor Tendon Injuries

Lacerations of the hand and fingers associated with flexor tendon injuries warrant surgical exploration because of the likelihood of digital nerve or artery disruption. A careful examination of the hand must be performed to identify loss of active DIP joint flexion (flexor digitorum profundus injury) or PIP joint flexion (flexor digitorum superficialis injury).

Flexor tendon lacerations can be categorized by anatomic zone of injury (Figure 15). A zone I injury occurs when the flexor digitorum profundus inserts onto the base of the distal phalanx. The tendon either is avulsed from the distal phalanx or lacerated distal to the A4 pulley. If the tendon has been lacerated, great care should be taken to repair it with both a core suture and an epitendinous suture. Tendon avulsions are directly reattached to the insertion site, either with the tradi-

tional pull-out suture method or with small suture anchors. A recent study revealed no significant differences between these two methods.[28] To guard against failure of suture anchors, they should be directed from a distal to a proximal angle in the distal phalanx, rather than from a proximal to a distal angle (Figure 16).

Zone II flexor tendon injuries occur in the flexor tendon sheath between the A1 pulley (over the metacarpal head) and the A4 pulley (over the middle phalanx). The repair frequently requires working around the A1, A2, and A4 pulleys, which if incised can lead to bowstringing of the repaired flexor digitorum profundus. Damage to these pulleys also predisposes the repaired flexor tendons to form scar tissue and adhesions, leading to poor tendon excursion after healing. Increasing the biomechanical strength of the repair allows implementation of an early motion rehabilitation protocol, which can minimize adhesion formation. The ideal balance is being sought between the need for tendon handling and suture passes and the biomechanical strength of the repair. The current thinking is that the surgeon can obtain a biomechanical advantage by increasing the number of core suture strands crossing the repair, locking the core sutures, increasing the strength of the suture material, increasing the length of suture purchase, and implementing an epitendinous repair.[29]

Nerve Injuries

Primary repair of the peripheral nerve should be performed within the first few days after the injury to achieve the best functional results. Care should be

3: Upper Extremity

taken to débride nonviable nerve ends, approximate the nerve ends with minimal tension, and align the fascicles accurately, if possible. The morphology of the peripheral nerves is typically consistent and can aid in the orientation of the repair. An appropriate repair consists of a microneurosurgical epineurial suture using a fine caliber nylon stitch, with minimal joint flexion. Achieving a well-vascularized bed with little or no scarring is im-

portant, as is careful hemostasis. Limited immobilization for as long as 2 weeks is recommended, although early protected motion for tendon rehabilitation has not been shown to jeopardize nerve repair outcomes.[30]

Nerve defects can be caused by the trauma itself, or they can be iatrogenic, as from a tumor or neuroma resection. A direct nerve repair is not always possible. Management of a nerve gap can include reconstruction with a nerve graft or a biologic or synthetic conduit (Figure 17). Recovery of muscle force is reduced if longer nerve graft segments are used or if nerve grafting is delayed. The use of peripheral nerve autografts has been the standard treatment for nerve defects, although autografts have the potential for donor site morbidity resulting from the surgical incision or dissection or from loss of function or sensation at the donor site. The use of biologic or synthetic conduits prevents such complications and allows for a tension-free repair that is likely to be better than a taut primary repair. The most practical form of biologic conduit is a vein graft. A vein graft harvest carries little risk of donor site morbidity and typically can be performed within the surgical site. Synthetic conduits are made from bioabsorbable polyglycolic acid or collagen; a polyglycolic acid conduit has been shown to produce results comparable if not superior to those from autografts in the reconstruction of short nerve gaps (< 4 mm).[31]

Two requirements have guided the development of engineered biologic or synthetic conduits: they must mimic important features of nerve environment, and they must be enriched with elements considered essential for nerve fiber regeneration. Conduits have been enhanced with nerve growth factor, brain-derived neurotrophic factor, glial growth factor, and Schwann cells, but clinical evidence to support these enhancements is limited. Recent research on nerve autograft has demonstrated that the use of sensory cutaneous nerve grafts for bridging motor and mixed nerve gaps can be improved by matching axon and Schwann cell properties.[32]

Tendon transfer can supplement the repair of a major motor nerve. If performed early, a selected tendon

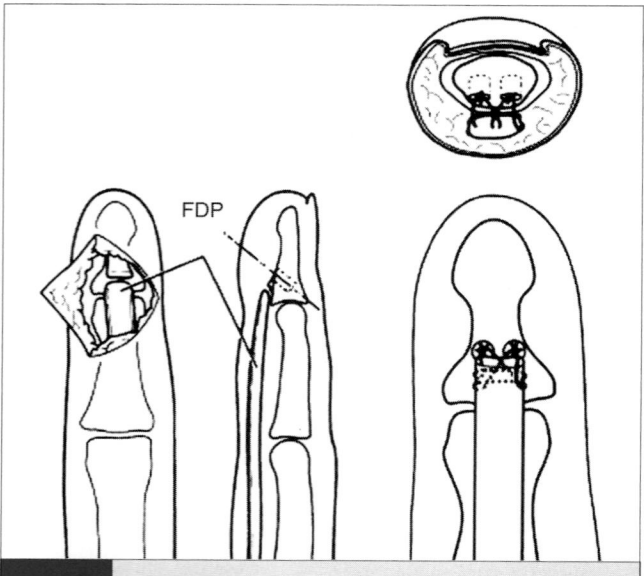

Figure 16 Zone I flexor tendon injuries that involve avulsion of the tendon insertion from the volar base of the distal phalanx can be repaired using a suture anchor technique. A biomechanical advantage against anchor pull-out is gained when the suture anchors are directed from distal to proximal. FDP = Flexor digitorum profundus. *(Reproduced with permission from McCallister WV, Ambrose HC, Katolik LI, Trumble TE: Comparison of pullout button versus suture anchor for zone I flexor tendon repair. J Hand Surg Am 2006;31:246-251.)*

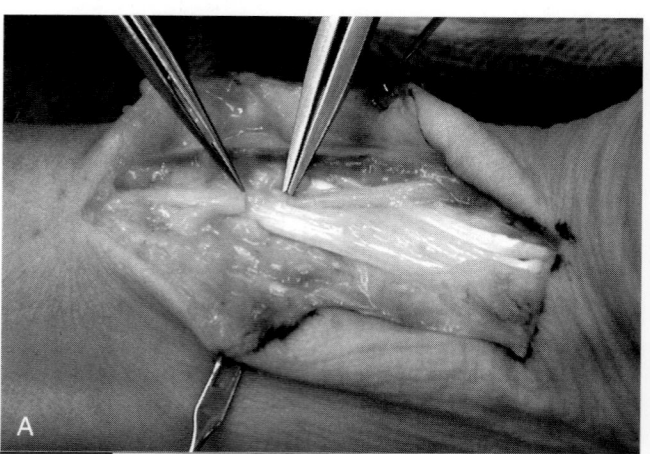
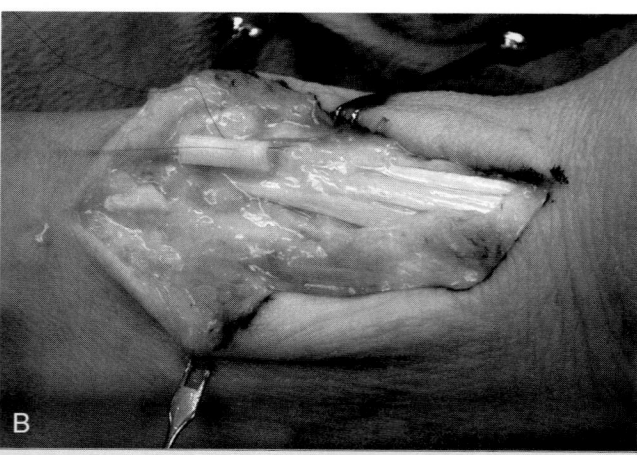

Figure 17 **A,** After resection of a neuroma of the superficial branch of the radial nerve, primary repair is possible only under tension. **B,** As a consequence, to minimize tension, the nerve is repaired using a synthetic conduit.

transfer can act as an internal splint to support function and prevent deformity during nerve recovery. For example, a low median nerve repair can be supplemented by transfer of the ring finger flexor digitorum superficialis tendon to the thumb metacarpal for abduction and opposition.

Annotated References

1. Kalainov DM, Hoepfner PE, Hartigan BJ, Carroll CT, Genuario J: Nonsurgical treatment of closed mallet finger fractures. *J Hand Surg Am* 2005;30:580-586.

2. King HJ, Shin SJ, Kang ES: Complications of operative treatment for mallet fractures of the distal phalanx. *J Hand Surg Br* 2001;26:28-31.

3. Horton TC, Hatton M, Davis TR: A prospective randomized controlled study of fixation of long oblique and spiral shaft fractures of the proximal phalanx: Closed reduction and percutaneous Kirschner wiring versus open reduction and lag screw fixation. *J Hand Surg Br* 2003;28:5-9.

4. Roth JJ, Auerbach DM: Fixation of hand fractures with bicortical screws. *J Hand Surg Am* 2005;30:151-153.

   This retrospective review of 37 assorted hand fractures that were treated with screws using a bicortical fixation technique rather than a lag screw technique found fracture healing in all patients, with no instances of lost fracture reduction or fixation.

5. Slade JF, Baxamusa TH, Wolfe SW: External fixation of proximal interphalangeal joint fracture dislocations. *Atlas Hand Clin* 2000;5:1-29.

6. Heyman P, Gelberman RH, Duncan K, Hipp JA: Injuries of the ulnar collateral ligament of the thumb metacarpophalangeal joint: Biomechanical and prospective clinical studies on the usefulness of valgus stress testing. *Clin Orthop Relat Res* 1993;292:165-171.

7. Bean CH, Tencer AF, Trumble TE: The effect of thumb metacarpophalangeal ulnar collateral ligament attachment site on joint range of motion: An in vitro study. *J Hand Surg Am* 1999;24:283-287.

8. Lee SK, Kubiak EN, Lawler E, Iesaka K, Liporace FA, Green SM: Thumb metacarpophalangeal ulnar collateral ligament injuries: A biomechanical simulation study of four static reconstructions. *J Hand Surg Am* 2005;30:1056-1060.

   Four methods of thumb ulnar collateral ligament reconstruction were tested in a cadaver model. No differences in stability were found, but only a triangular configuration of tendon weave with apex proximal demonstrated a full range of motion at the MCP joint.

9. Lamraski G, Monsaert A, De Maeseneer M, Haentjens P: Reliability and validity of plain radiographs to assess angulation of small finger metacarpal neck fractures: Human cadaveric study. *J Orthop Res* 2006;24:37-45.

   This cadaveric study with a simulated fracture model found substantial validity for angulation measurements on lateral radiographs. Oblique views produced consistently higher readings but not the accuracy and validity of the lateral radiographs.

10. Tavassoli J, Ruland RT, Hogan CJ, Cannon DL: Three cast techniques for the treatment of extra-articular metacarpal fractures: Comparison of short-term outcomes and final fracture alignments. *J Bone Joint Surg Am* 2005;87:2196-2201.

    A retrospective review of three groups of extra-articular metacarpal fractures treated for as long as 5 weeks is presented. The three groups were: MCPs extended, PIPs free; MCPs flexed, PIPs free; and MCPs flexed, PIPs extended. No significant grip strength or range-of-motion differences were found at 9 weeks. Level of evidence: III.

11. Smith NC, Moncrieff NJ, Hartnell N, Ashwell J: Pseudorotation of the little finger metacarpal. *J Hand Surg Br* 2003;28:395-398.

12. Meunier MJ, Hentzen E, Ryan M, Shin AY, Lieber RL: Predicted effects of metacarpal shortening on interosseous muscle function. *J Hand Surg Am* 2004;29:689-693.

    Cadaveric ring metacarpals were translated proximally in an incremental fashion. Proximal translation of 10 mm led to an increased dorsal interosseous sarcomere length of 25%, which was extrapolated to confer an approximately 50% decrease in interosseous muscle force.

13. Medoff RJ: Essential radiographic evaluation for distal radius fractures. *Hand Clin* 2005;21:279-288.

    This review article highlights the key radiographic landmarks and parameters of accurate distal radius fracture assessment.

14. Trumble TE, Schmitt SR, Vedder NB: Factors affecting functional outcome of displaced intra-articular distal radius fractures. *J Hand Surg Am* 1994;19:325-340.

15. Mackenney PJ, McQueen MM, Elton R: Prediction of instability in distal radial fractures. *J Bone Joint Surg Am* 2006;88:1944-1951.

    In a prospectively recorded collection of data on 4,000 wrist fractures, patient age (> 80 years), metaphyseal comminution, and radial shortening at presentation were consistent indicators of instability assessed radiographically; dorsal angulation was not. Level of evidence: Prognostic level I.

16. Lafontaine M, Hardy D, Delince P: Stability assessment of distal radius fractures. *Injury* 1989;20:208-210.

17. Margaliot Z, Haase SC, Kotsis SV, Kim HM, Chung KC: A meta-analysis of outcomes of external fixation versus plate osteosynthesis for unstable distal radius fractures. *J Hand Surg Am* 2005;30:1185-1199.

3: Upper Extremity

This meta-analysis assessed the literature from 1980 to 2004 that compared external fixation and internal fixation for unstable distal radius fractures. Evaluation of clinical outcomes yielded no evidence to support one type of fixation over the other.

18. Simic PM, Robison J, Gardner MJ, Gelberman RH, Weiland AJ, Boyer MI: Treatment of distal radius fractures with a low-profile dorsal plating system: An outcomes assessment. *J Hand Surg Am* 2006;31:382-386.

    This retrospective cohort study of consecutive dorsal implants with lower profiles and beveled edges found that only one plate required removal because of dorsal wrist pain. No extensor tendons had ruptured at a minimum 1-year follow-up. Level of evidence: IV.

19. Orbay JL, Fernandez DL: Volar fixed-angle plate fixation for unstable distal radius fractures in the elderly patient. *J Hand Surg Am* 2004;29:96-102.

    This retrospective review of 24 unstable distal radius fractures with a 63-week follow-up showed that locked volar plating maintained reduction in all but 3 fractures, although all of the patients were older than 75 years of age.

20. Dodds SD, Cornelissen S, Jossan S, Wolfe SW: A biomechanical comparison of fragment-specific fixation and augmented external fixation for intra-articular distal radius fractures. *J Hand Surg Am* 2002;27:953-964.

21. Ruch DS, Ginn TA, Yang CC, Smith BP, Rushing J, Hanel DP: Use of a distraction plate for distal radial fractures with metaphyseal and diaphyseal comminution. *J Bone Joint Surg Am* 2005;87:945-954.

    High-energy fractures of the distal radius were treated using 3.5-mm spanning plates placed in distraction on the dorsum of the wrist from the distal radius to middle finger metacarpal. Joint surfaces were reduced with limited incisions and provisionally fixed with Kirschner wires or screws. Gartland and Werley outcomes were excellent in 14, good in 6, and fair in 2.

22. Gellman H, Caputo RJ, Carter V, Aboulafia A, McKay M: Comparison of short and long thumb-spica casts for non-displaced fractures of the carpal scaphoid. *J Bone Joint Surg Am* 1989;71:354-357.

23. Adolfsson L, Lindau T, Arner M: Acutrak screw fixation versus cast immobilisation for undisplaced scaphoid waist fractures. *J Hand Surg Br* 2001;26:192-195.

24. Dodds SD, Panjabi MM, Slade JF III: Screw fixation of scaphoid fractures: A biomechanical assessment of screw length and screw augmentation. *J Hand Surg Am* 2006;31:405-413.

    Scaphoid fractures maintained within the wrist joint that were repaired with long screws (4 mm less than total scaphoid length) provided significantly more stability than shorter screws. Adding a scaphocapitate Kirschner wire improved stability, although not significantly.

25. McCallister WV, Knight J, Kaliappan R, Trumble TE: Central placement of the screw in simulated fractures of the scaphoid waist: A biomechanical study. *J Bone Joint Surg Am* 2003;85-A:72-77.

26. Slade JF III, Gutow AP, Geissler WB: Percutaneous internal fixation of scaphoid fractures via an arthroscopically assisted dorsal approach. *J Bone Joint Surg Am* 2002;84-A(suppl 2):21-36.

27. Slade JF III, Geissler WB, Gutow AP, Merrell GA: Percutaneous internal fixation of selected scaphoid nonunions with an arthroscopically assisted dorsal approach. *J Bone Joint Surg Am* 2003;85-A(suppl 4):20-32.

28. McCallister WV, Ambrose HC, Katolik LI, Trumble TE: Comparison of pullout button versus suture anchor for zone I flexor tendon repair. *J Hand Surg Am* 2006;31:246-251.

    In retrospectively collected clinical outcomes, no significant differences were found between pull-out sutures and suture anchors used in zone I flexor tendon repairs. However, patients with suture anchor repair returned to work sooner than those with pull-out sutures.

29. Barrie KA, Tomak SL, Cholewicki J, Merrell GA, Wolfe SW: Effect of suture locking and suture caliber on fatigue strength of flexor tendon repairs. *J Hand Surg Am* 2001;26:340-346.

30. Yu RS, Catalano LW III, Barron OA, Johnson C, Glickel SZ: Limited, protected postsurgical motion does not affect the results of digital nerve repair. *J Hand Surg Am* 2004;29:302-306.

    This retrospective review compared cast immobilization for isolated digital nerve repair with early protected motion for combined nerve and tendon repairs. No statistical differences between the two groups were found.

31. Weber RA, Breidenbach WC, Brown RE, Jabaley ME, Mass DP: A randomized prospective study of polyglycolic acid conduits for digital nerve reconstruction in humans. *Plast Reconstr Surg* 2000;106:1036-1045.

32. Hoke A, Redett R, Hameed H, et al: Schwann cells express motor and sensory phenotypes that regulate axon regeneration. *J Neurosci* 2006;26:9646-9655.

    Differences are known to exist between motor and sensory nerves in Schwann cell phenotypes. This study found that a sensory cutaneous nerve graft preferentially supports sensory axon regeneration and a motor ventral root graft preferentially supports motor axon regeneration.

Chapter 29

Hand and Wrist Reconstruction

Marco Rizzo, MD   *William P. Cooney, MD   Hans L. Carlson, MD   *Warren Mays, BS, CPO

Nerve Compression Syndromes, Median Nerve

Carpal Tunnel Syndrome

Compression neuropathy of the median nerve as it travels deep to the transverse carpal ligament results in carpal tunnel syndrome (CTS). It is the most common compression neuropathy of the upper extremity, and it is believed to affect from 0.1% to 10% of the general population. Patients typically report numbness and tingling of the thumb, index, and long fingers, and radial aspect of the ring finger. As the condition worsens, pain is a common symptom. With more severe compression, muscle atrophy and weakness of the thenar muscles will develop. Certain activities such as driving, reading, and prolonged holding of objects will elicit symptoms. Night pain and numbness are commonly reported.

Evaluation of a patient with suspected CTS must include a complete history, review of systems, and a thorough physical examination. Certain risk factors are associated with the development of CTS. Systemic conditions such as diabetes, inflammatory arthritis, obesity, hypothyroidism, amyloidosis, lysosomal storage diseases, renal disease, and pregnancy are associated with CTS. Activities or job-related tasks such as gripping an object (for example, a pen), using a computer keyboard, and exposure to vibration (for example, while driving) have been linked to the pathogenesis of CTS. Aging plays an important role in the development of median neuropathy; nerve cells are diminished as a patient ages and it is believed that the median nerve is less tolerant to pressure shifts and changes within the carpal tunnel. A summary of factors associated with CTS is outlined in **Table 1**.

Physical examination findings consistent with CTS include numbness in the median nerve distribution. Sensory examination can be elicited with Semmes-Weinstein monofilament, vibratory, and two-point discrimination. Semmes-Weinstein monofilament examination is considered to be more sensitive than vibratory and two-point discrimination in detecting early disease. Static and moving two-point discrimination are consid-

ered abnormal when greater than 6 mm and 5 mm, respectively. The use of the Brigham hand diagram, which is performed by the patient marking the areas of numbness/tingling and/or pain, has been shown to be a very sensitive measure of CTS. The Tinel's sign, Phalen's sign, and carpal tunnel compression test are three commonly used provocative tests helpful in confirming the diagnosis. The carpal tunnel compression test is the most sensitive and specific for CTS.

CTS is primarily a clinical diagnosis. It is important to determine and rule out other possible etiologies for numbness, tingling, pain, or weakness of the hand and upper extremity. Conditions such as cervical spine impingement of nerve roots, thoracic outlet syndrome, brachial plexus injuries, or neuropathy such as Parsonage-Turner syndrome, Pancoast's tumor, concomitant peripheral nerve compression syndromes, and vascular pathology or occlusive disease can mimic or coexist with median neuropathy of the wrist. The coexistence of CTS with other compression neuropathies (such as pronator teres syndrome) is called a double-crush phenomenon; electrodiagnostic studies are useful in confirming clinical suspicions. Abnormal nerve conduction sensory latency (> 3.5 ms) is considered most sensitive in detecting early CTS. Motor latencies greater than 4.5 ms are also consistent with CTS. Electromyography typically shows increased insertional activity, positive sharp waves, fibrillations at rest, decreased motor recruitment, and complex repetitive discharges. Unfortunately, the results of electrodiagnostic studies are highly variable and dependent on multiple factors including experience of the technician and the patient's weight, body temperature, and age. In addition, a negative electromyogram does not rule out clinically symptomatic CTS. Up to 20% of patients with clinical CTS and normal electrodiagnostic studies have been reported to improve following carpal tunnel release.

Nonsurgical measures for managing CTS include activity modification, nonsteroidal anti-inflammatory drugs (NSAIDs), and supportive splinting, often at night. The splint holds the wrist where the volume of the carpal tunnel is maximal and helps avoid unconscious flexion and/or extension of the wrist, which can exacerbate symptoms. However, as the severity of median nerve compression worsens, splinting becomes less effective. Another commonly used nonsurgical treatment of CTS is steroid injection into the carpal canal. Both of these measures are very effective, but frequently provide temporary relief. However, it is impor-

*William P. Cooney, MD or the department with which he is affiliated has received research or institutional support and royalties from Small Bone Innovations. Warren Mays, BS, CPO is the President of Artisan Orthotic-Prosthetic Technologies, Inc.

3: Upper Extremity

Table 1

Factors in the Pathogenesis of CTS

Anatomy

Decreased size of carpal tunnel
    Abnormalities of the carpal bones

    Thickened transverse carpal ligament

    Acromegaly

Increased contents of canal
    Neuroma

    Lipoma

    Myeloma

    Abnormal muscle bellies

    Persistent median artery (thrombosed or patent)

    Hypertrophic synovium

    Distal radial fracture callus

    Posttraumatic osteophytes

    Hematoma (hemophilia, anticoagulation therapy)

Physiology

Neuropathic conditions
    Diabetes

    Alcoholism

    Proximal lesion of median nerve (double-crush syndrome)

Inflammatory conditions
    Tenosynovitis

    Rheumatoid arthritis

    Infection

    Gout

Alterations of fluid balance
    Pregnancy

    Eclampsia

    Myxedema

    Long-term hemodialysis

    Horizontal position and muscle relaxation (sleep)

    Raynaud's disease

    Obesity

Congenital
    Mucopolysaccharidosis

    Mucolipidosis

Position and use of the wrist
    Repetitive flexion/extension (manual labor)

    Repetitive forceful squeezing and release of a tool

    Repetitive forceful torsion of a tool

    Finger motion with the wrist extended

        Typing

        Playing many musical instruments

    Vibration exposure

    Weight bearing with the wrist extended

        Paraplegia

        Long-distance bicycling

    Immobilization with the wrist flexed and ulnar deviation

        Casting after Colles' fracture

        Awkward sleep position

Adapted with permission from Szabo RM, Madison M: Carpal tunnel syndrome. Orthop Clin North Am 1992;23:106.

tant to note that patients who fare well with these measures will likely respond favorably to surgery.

The surgical treatment of CTS involves decompression of the nerve by division of the transverse carpal ligament. Both open and endoscopic techniques have been described. Several studies have compared open and endoscopic carpal tunnel release, and other than a shorter return to work with endoscopic release there does not appear to be an appreciable long-term difference in outcomes between methods. Nor is there con-

clusive evidence to suggest one method is safer than the other. Outcomes following surgery are generally favorable with improvement of symptoms in up to 98% of patients. Recent controversy has been noted about outcomes in elderly patients, with debate regarding the benefit of carpal tunnel release in this patient population. Current data suggest patients older than 65 years objectively and subjectively benefit from carpal tunnel release.[1] Another study noted similar improvements in function and symptoms, but less predictable overall patient satisfaction in elderly patients when compared with younger patients.[2] Overall, carpal tunnel release in elderly patients is effective and generally beneficial. Direct carpal release alone is recommended and there is clear clinical evidence that there has been no proven benefit to internal neurolysis of the median nerve or tenosynovectomy of the flexor tendons.[3] Pillar pain, which is caused by a painful palmar scar at the site of release of the transverse carpal ligament, is the most common complication associated with carpal tunnel release. The exact etiology of this condition is unclear. The incidence during the early postoperative period (4 weeks) approaches 50%, and it steadily decreases to less than 10% at 1 year following surgery. In most instances, pillar pain improves by 3 months after surgery with protective splinting and avoidance of forceful use of the hand. No real difference in pillar pain is reported between endoscopic and open techniques.

Recurrence of CTS is related to either a true late redevelopment of compression of the median nerve related to primary pathology such as hypothyroidism or is related to incomplete initial release or decompression of the median nerve. Reasons for early failure following carpal tunnel release include incomplete release of the transverse carpal ligament, double-crush syndrome, peripheral neuropathy, iatrogenic median nerve injury, and a persistent space-occupying lesion in the carpal canal. Repeat clinical examination and electromyographic testing can assist in determining if there is recurrence secondary to incomplete release of the transverse carpal ligament. MRI may also be of benefit. The incidence of late recurrence ranges from 8% to 13%, although repeat surgical intervention is not required in all instances. Late recurrence is most common with systemic illness such as rheumatoid arthritis, diabetes, amyloidosis, and hypothyroidism but can be related to an adverse work environment such as continued use of vibratory instruments or situations such as long haul truck driving.

Pronator Syndrome

Pronator syndrome is proximal compression of the median nerve related to the pronator teres muscle or adjacent anatomic structures. There are multiple potential sites of impingement of the median nerve about the elbow, including the supracondylar process of the medial epicondyle and the ligament of Struthers, the lacertus fibrosus, the deep muscle origin of the pronator teres, and beneath the two muscular heads of the flexor digitorum superficialis. True pronator syndrome is compression of the median nerve as it passes between the two heads of the pronator teres muscle. Statistically it is 100 times less common than CTS. Pronator syndrome is common in patients with well-developed forearm muscles, such as weight lifters. The condition is also associated with repetitive activities, especially forearm pronation with elbow extension.

Symptoms of pronator syndrome are similar to those of CTS with the exception that patients with pronator syndrome commonly have numbness in the palm in the distribution of the palmar cutaneous branch of the median nerve. Night symptoms are less common in patients with pronator syndrome. Provocative tests such as Phalen's sign and Tinel's sign will be negative at the wrist. Rather, the Tinel's sign should be positive at the site of median nerve impingement at the proximal forearm. Pain with forearm pronation and elbow extension will suggest compression between the heads of the pronator. Prominence of a supracondylar process of the humerus and pain with compression along the medial aspect of the distal arm implicates compression proximally between the ligament of Struthers and the bony process. Pain with resisted elbow flexion is consistent with compression of the median nerve beneath the lacertus fibrosus. Finally, pain with resisted interphalangeal long finger flexion will exacerbate the patient's symptoms and will indicate compression of the median nerve deep to the flexor digitorum superficialis.

Electrodiagnostic studies are less reliable in accurately diagnosing nerve compression of the median nerve in the proximal forearm. Local conduction studies with the forearm in a provocative position (stressed pronation) as well as "inching" techniques extending from proximal to distal along the median nerve may be diagnostic. However, it is important to note that CTS can cause "retrograde" median nerve symptoms that simulate pronator teres syndrome. These findings of retrograde axonal atrophy can be seen electrodiagnostically in patients with CTS and normal forearm motor conduction velocities.[4]

Conservative management of pronator syndrome includes activity modification, NSAIDs, and splinting with the elbow at 90°, slight forearm pronation, and wrist flexion. Unlike with CTS, there does not appear to be a role for steroid injections in the treatment of pronator syndrome. Nonsurgical measures can be effective in more than 50% of patients. Surgical treatment of pronator syndrome includes a thorough exploration and release of the nerve at the numerous potential sites of compression, beginning proximal to the elbow in the region of the ligament of Struthers and continued distally releasing the lacertus fibrosus, split heads of the pronator teres, and distally between the arcade of the flexor digitorum superficialis.

Anterior Interosseous Nerve Compression

The anterior interosseous branch of the median nerve innervates the flexor digitorum profundus to the index finger, flexor pollicis longus, and pronator quadratus muscles. It also provides sensation and pain information to the volar aspect of the carpus.

There are several potential sites of compression for the anterior interosseous nerve, including the fibrous bands of the deep or superficial heads of the pronator teres and the fibrous bands of the flexor digitorum superficialis. Additional less common causes of compression include anomalous muscles (such as Gantzer's muscles to the flexor pollicis longus), enlarged or thrombosed vessels, tumors, and enlarged bursae. There is a well documented relationship between

3: Upper Extremity

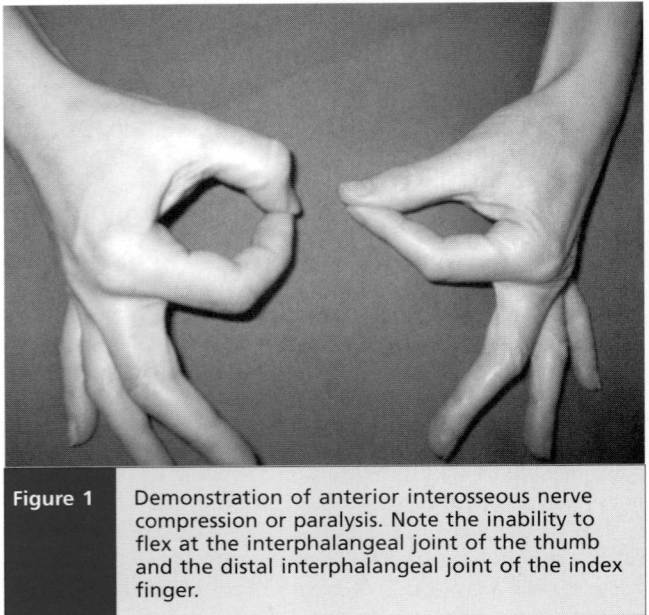

Figure 1 Demonstration of anterior interosseous nerve compression or paralysis. Note the inability to flex at the interphalangeal joint of the thumb and the distal interphalangeal joint of the index finger.

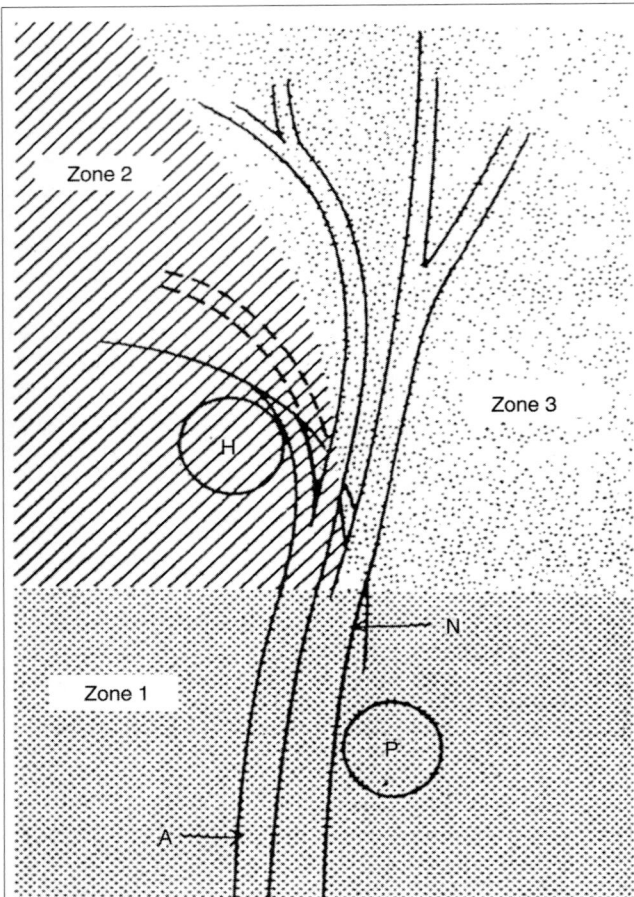

Figure 2 Anatomy of the ulnar nerve as it traverses Guyon's canal. Zone I is before the bifurcation. Zone II represents the distal radial aspect and contains the deep motor branch of the nerve and artery. Zone III is the distal ulnar aspect following the bifurcation. It contains the sensory components of the nerve. H = hamate; P = pisiform; A = artery; N = nerve. *(Reproduced with permission from Gross MS, Gelberman RH: The anatomy of the distal ulnar tunnel. Clin Orthop Relat Res 1985;196:238-247.)*

Parsonage-Turner syndrome (brachial neuritis) and anterior interosseous nerve deficit. It is important to discern these noncompressive conditions from a compressive neuropathy. A history of viral prodrome and/or significant pain may indicate brachial neuritis. Electromyography should include investigation of the shoulder girdle area to rule out the more proximal conditions. Anterior interosseous nerve palsy may also mimic flexor digitorum profundus or flexor pollicis longus tendon ruptures. MRI may be helpful in identifying a specific lesion or compressive process of the anterior interosseous nerve.

Patients with anterior interosseous nerve compression will present with weakness in flexion of the interphalangeal joint of the thumb and weakness of distal interphalangeal joint flexion of the index finger. The physical examination will reveal the inability to formulate a true "OK" sign (**Figure 1**); typically, there will be no sensory loss. The patient may report vague forearm pain. Pinch and grip weakness is predictable.

Nonsurgical treatment of anterior interosseous nerve compression is preferred for a minimum of 3 months. Many cases will resolve spontaneously, especially those related to short-term nerve compression or a viral neuritis. A repeat electromyogram may demonstrate objective improvement of nerve function. Clinical improvement of nerve function has been reported up to 18 months following onset of symptoms with observation, and therefore surgical intervention should be delayed unless there is no evidence of improvement in symptoms or there is clear evidence of a compression neuropathy. If there is no improvement, surgical intervention may be warranted. It is not uncommon to fail to identify an obvious compression site. Unusual causes of anterior interosseous nerve compression include schwannoma and perineurioma as primary tumors of the connective tissue lining of the anterior interosseous

nerve. In such situations, some authors have advocated interfascicular neurolysis and sural nerve grafting of the anterior interosseous nerve.[5,6]

Ulnar Nerve Compression in the Wrist (Ulnar Tunnel Syndrome)

Ulnar nerve compression in Guyon's canal of the wrist (ulnar tunnel syndrome) is significantly less common than compression neuropathy of the elbow or cubital tunnel syndrome. The anatomy of the distal ulnar tunnel is divided into three zones (**Figure 2**). Zone 1 is proximal to the bifurcation of the ulnar nerve and consist of both sensory and motor fibers of the nerve. Zone 2 represents the motor branch of the ulnar nerve distal to the bifurcation. Zone 3 represents the sensory branches of the ulnar nerve beyond its bifurcation. The site or zone of compression will predict the clinical presentation. Zone 1 lesions will have mixed sensory and motor loss. Zone 2 compression will reveal an isolated motor deficit. Patients with a lesion in zone 3 will most likely present with isolated ulnar nerve sensory loss. The most common causes of compression in zones 1 and 2 are ganglions (**Figure 3**) and fractures of the hook of the hamate. In zone 3, the most common cause of isolated sensory nerve branch compression is ulnar artery thrombosis.

In addition to a careful history and physical examination, a complete ulnar nerve motor and sensory evaluation will help to identify the cause and location of the deficit. When there is sensory deficit on the dorsal aspect of the hand (ulnar third) a more proximal ulnar nerve lesion should be suspected. Similarly, the difference in strength between the intrinsic and extrinsic ulna innervated muscle will help to separate a distal from proximal ulnar nerve lesion. To identify ulnar artery thrombosis, Allen's test is critical, along with ancillary studies such as vascular medical examination including ultrasound phlethysmography and flow studies. MRI or ultrasound is useful in identifying ganglia or other space-occupying lesions. CT scans or special radiographic projections (oblique or carpal tunnel views) can help better delineate the bony anatomy to diagnose hook of the hamate fractures. Treatment of ulnar tunnel syndrome is directed at the source of compression but typically involves release of Guyon's canal, resection of any space-occupying lesions, treatment of the hook of the hamate fracture, and revascularization of the ulnar artery if there is distal backflow.

Superficial Branch of the Radial Nerve Compression (Wartenberg's Syndrome)

Compression of the superficial branch of the radial nerve can occur most commonly as the nerve exits from beneath the brachioradialis in the forearm. The nerve can be trapped between the extensor carpi radialis longus and the brachioradialis, especially with pronation of the forearm. Compression can occur as a result of long-standing pressure, repetitive provocative activities or job-related tasks, mass effect, or direct trauma. Patients typically report numbness and/or pain in the dorsal and radial aspects of the hand. Provocative tests include onset of symptoms with forced grip or pinch, and with resisted pronation of the forearm. Differential diagnosis includes de Quervain's tenosynovitis, intersection syndrome, and lateral antebrachial cutaneous nerve compression. Appropriately placed injections can help in the diagnosis. Many patients respond favorably to conservative treatment including steroid injections, NSAIDs, activity modification, splinting, and occupational therapy. Surgical exploration and decompression is warranted for those in whom nonsurgical treatment has failed. Unfortunately, the success with surgery is not significantly better than that with nonsurgical treatment.

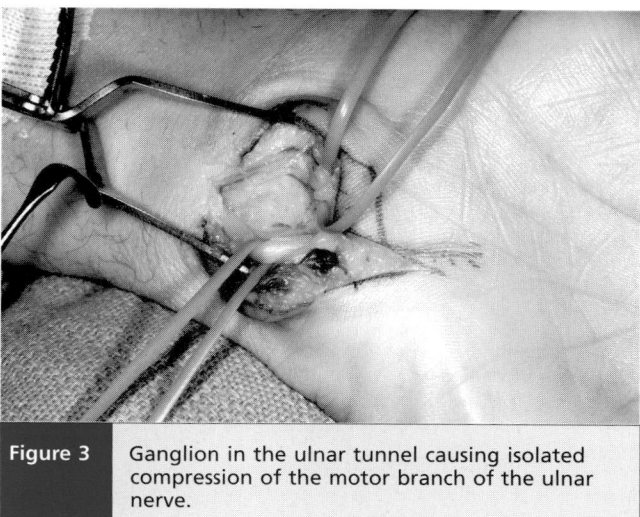

Figure 3   Ganglion in the ulnar tunnel causing isolated compression of the motor branch of the ulnar nerve.

Osteonecrosis of the Carpus

Kienböck's Disease

The lunate is the carpal bone associated with the highest incidence of osteonecrosis. The etiology of Kienböck's disease is most likely multifactorial and includes anatomic, vascular, traumatic, and environmental factors. Anatomically, the vascular supply to the lunate can demonstrate a single nutrient artery and/or poorly organized intraosseous anastomoses. It is believed that lunates with this vascular pattern are predisposed to osteonecrosis. In addition, negative ulnar variance has been associated with Kienböck's disease. The negative variance increases proportional loads across the radiocarpal joint in these patients. There is also a relationship between traumatic injury and Kienböck's disease. However, it is unclear whether injury causes or contributes to the disease process or is the result of lunate fracture and/or fragmentation. The fact that Kienböck's disease is not noticeably associated with perilunate dislocations draws attention from a specific traumatic event as the cause. A loose association between Kienböck's disease and sickle cell anemia, steroid use, gout, and cerebral palsy also has been described.

Kienböck's disease most commonly occurs in the second to fifth decades of life. Men are more often affected than women. The incidence of bilateral disease is rare. Physical examination will vary depending on the stage of the disease. Patients will report pain and difficulty with activities. Symptoms include dorsal wrist pain with direct palpation of the radiolunate joint. Motion is usually limited and grip strength is diminished. Swelling and increased warmth on the dorsal aspect of the wrist may also be present.

Radiographs play an important role in establishing the diagnosis. In early disease, plain films may be normal or show mild sclerosis. MRI is very helpful in assessment of the vascularity of the lunate and diagnosis of early disease. Kienböck's disease is usually characterized by avascular changes throughout the entire lunate.

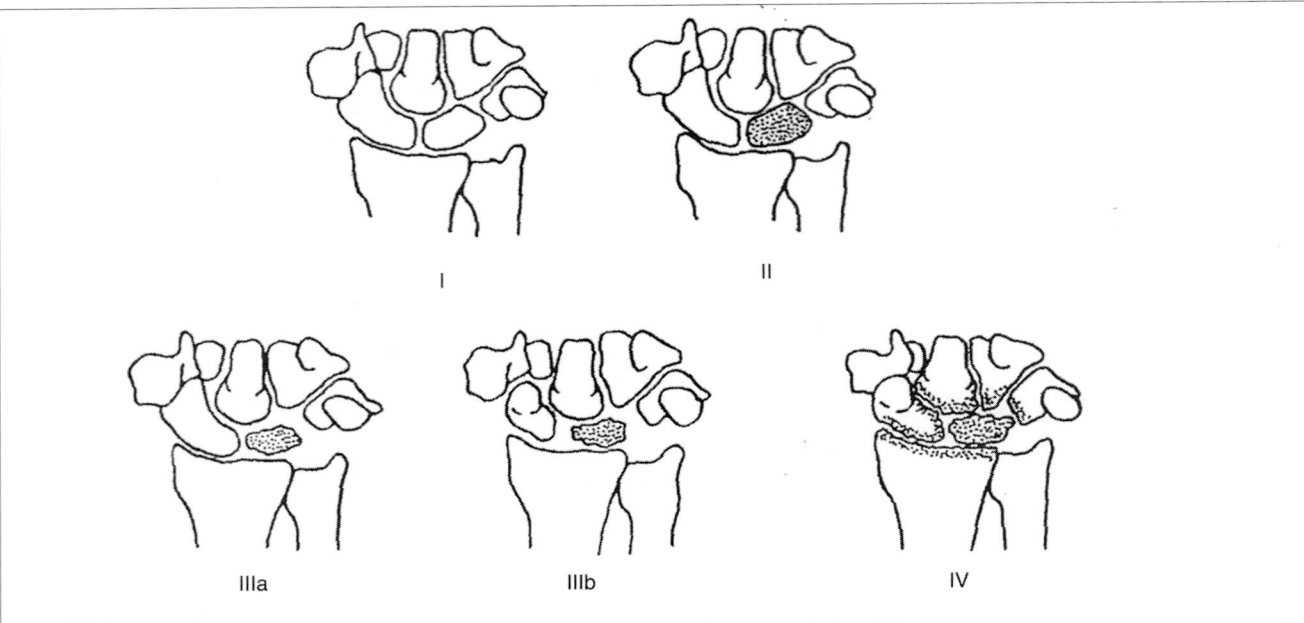

| Figure 4 | The Stahl-Lichtman classification of Kienböck's disease. Stage I: no plain radiographic changes of the lunate; MRI positive. Stage II: sclerosis of the lunate. Stage IIIa: Sclerosis with fragmentation and/or collapse and no rotation of the scaphoid. Stage IIIb: same as IIIA and rotation of the scaphoid. Stage IV: arthritis in the radiocarpal and/or mid-carpal joints. *(Reproduced with permission from Weiss APC, Weiland AJ, Moore JR, Wingis EF: Radial shortening for Kienbock's disease. J Bone Joint Surg Am 1991;73:384-391.)* |

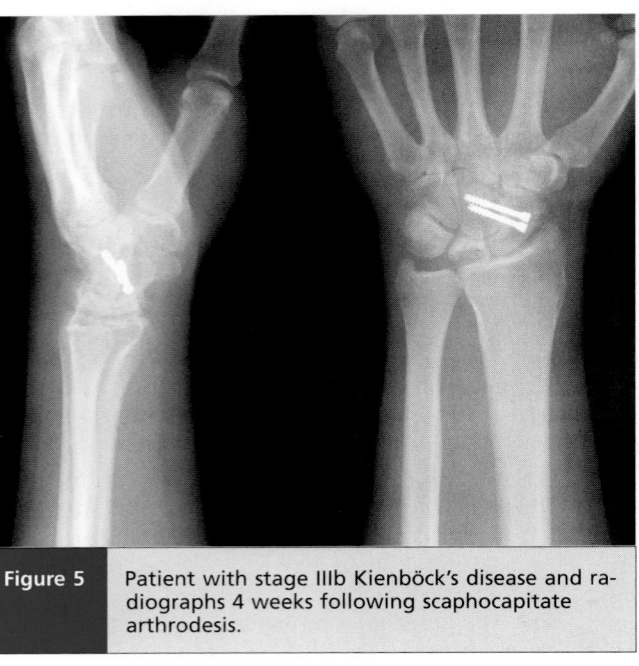

| Figure 5 | Patient with stage IIIb Kienböck's disease and radiographs 4 weeks following scaphocapitate arthrodesis. |

Conditions such as ulnocarpal impaction are typically characterized by cystic changes within the ulnar aspect of the lunate at the site of the ulnocarpal abutment. CT scans are also helpful in showing the degree of fragmentation and collapse.

The Stahl-Lichtman classification for Kienböck's disease has been useful in planning treatment (**Figure 4**). Early-stage disease can be treated symptomatically with splinting, activity modification, and NSAIDs. Precollapse (stages I, II, and IIIa) Kienböck's disease with intact cartilage shell is amenable to pedicled vascularized bone grafting with temporary unloading of the lunate.[7] Additional or alternate treatment options include joint leveling procedures such as ulnar lengthening or radial shortening to balance forces across the wrist in patients with negative ulnar variance. For patients with neutral or ulnar positive variance, wedge osteotomies of the radius, capitate shortening, or capitohamate arthrodesis have been useful. In stage IIIb disease the lunate becomes fragmented and collapsed, and the scaphoid falls into rotatory subluxation. In this stage, intercarpal arthrodeses are commonly used to facilitate and maintain the reduction of the scaphoid and carpal alignment. The two most commonly performed procedures for stage IIIb and stage IV are scaphocapitate (Figure 5) and scaphotrapeziotrapezoid arthrodeses. Proximal row carpectomy has been recommended by some authors for stage IV Kienböck's disease.

Preiser's Disease

Preiser's disease is defined as osteonecrosis of the scaphoid. Its etiology is unclear, and it is much less common than Kienböck's disease. The vascularity to the scaphoid is primarily supplied by the dorsal retrograde vessels from the radial artery and by the volar lateral artery. The blood supply to the scaphoid can be tenuous and susceptible to wrist trauma. Although trauma is believed to contribute to Preiser's disease, there are not enough cases in the literature to confirm

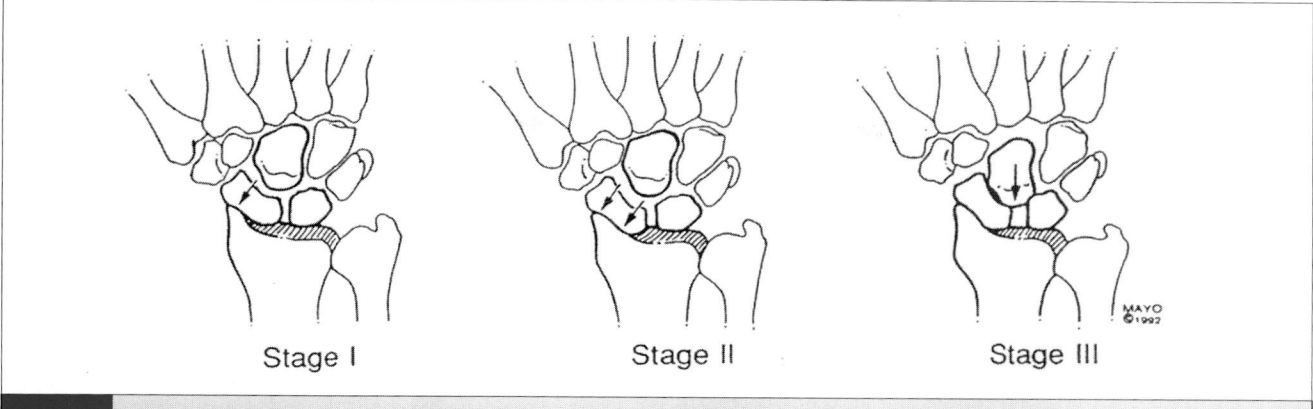

| Figure 6 | Stages of SLAC wrist. Stage I involves the radial styloid. Stage II includes the entire radioscaphoid articulation. Stage III advances to include arthritis at the capitolunate joint. *(Reproduced with permission from Krakauer JD, Bishop AT, Cooney WP: Surgical treatment of scapholunate advanced collapse. J Hand Surg Am 1994;19:751-759.)* |

this speculation. Patients typically present with wrist pain, swelling, and limited motion. Radiographic staging into partial and complete osteonecrosis of the scaphoid has been described for Preiser's disease. In the early stages of the disease, radiographs may be normal. However, as the disease progresses, sclerosis of the scaphoid and subsequent fragmentation with collapse will develop. Ultimately arthritis will occur. As with Kienböck's disease, MRI and CT scans can be very helpful in better assessing the vascularity and degree of fragmentation of the scaphoid. Arthroscopy has been described for inspection of the cartilage shell. The differential diagnosis includes proximal pole osteonecrosis of the scaphoid following fracture.

Treatment of scaphoid osteonecrosis is dependent on the stage of the disease. For precollapse disease, vascularized bone grafting has been shown to improve pain and restore the scaphoid, especially in stage I, partial osteonecrosis. For stage II, complete osteonecrosis vascular grafting is also indicated but the degree of revascularization is less predictable. In some patients a salvage procedure such as intercarpal fusion, scaphoid excision with intercarpal fusion, or proximal row carpectomy may be preferred. Vascularized bone grafting has replaced traditional bone grafting for early disease. A recent review demonstrated that despite incomplete revascularization of the scaphoid following vascularized bone grafting, most patients had good and excellent results.[8] For more advanced scaphoid osteonecrosis with arthritis, alternate treatments include proximal pole excision, complete scaphoid excision and four-corner fusion, proximal row carpectomy, and complete wrist arthrodesis. Unlike Kienböck's disease, surgical outcomes for Preiser's disease are less predictable.

Arthritis of the Wrist and Hand

Scapholunate Advanced Collapse

In many instances, the end result of untreated scapholunate dissociation is a predictable pattern of arthrosis referred to as scapholunate advanced collapse (SLAC) wrist. It is the most common form of wrist arthritis. The stages of SLAC wrist are shown in **Figure 6**. Early SLAC wrist will involve the radioscaphoid articulation. End-stage disease will ultimately include the lunocapitate joint. The radiolunate joint is typically spared. There is some debate about both the length of progression of SLAC wrist following scapholunate disruption.

Patients will present with varying degrees of signs and symptoms consistent with arthritis. Swelling and pain with activity are common. In patients with more severe symptoms, pain at rest is typical. Tenderness over the dorsal radial aspect of the wrist in early arthritis spreads more ulnarly and distally as the disease progresses. Limited range of motion is common. Radiographs will help determine the stage of arthritis. CT scans are more sensitive in detecting early arthritis of either the radioscaphoid joint or the lunocapitate joint.

Nonsurgical treatment options for SLAC wrist include splinting, activity modification, NSAIDs, and steroid injections. When nonsurgical treatment fails to alleviate symptoms, surgery may be warranted. The goal of surgical treatment of stage I SLAC is elimination of the arthritic scaphoid-radial styloid and reduction of the rotatory subluxation of the scaphoid. For very early stage I SLAC wrist, a radial styloidectomy and partial wrist arthrodesis such as scaphocapitate and scaphotrapeziotrapezoid fusion can be effective in eliminating pain. Because of difficulties maintaining carpal alignment, ligament reconstruction and tenodesis are no longer favored. The two main surgical options for stage II disease are scaphoid excision and four-corner arthrodesis and proximal row carpectomy. The decision on which option to use is based in part on patient concerns and needs. Scaphoid excision and four-corner fusion are technically more demanding than proximal row carpectomy, and fusion rates are widely variable. In addition, smokers tend to have higher rates of nonunion. Two recent reports on long-term follow-up of proximal row carpectomy have demonstrated good functional results and good pain relief.[9,10] The ranges of motion and

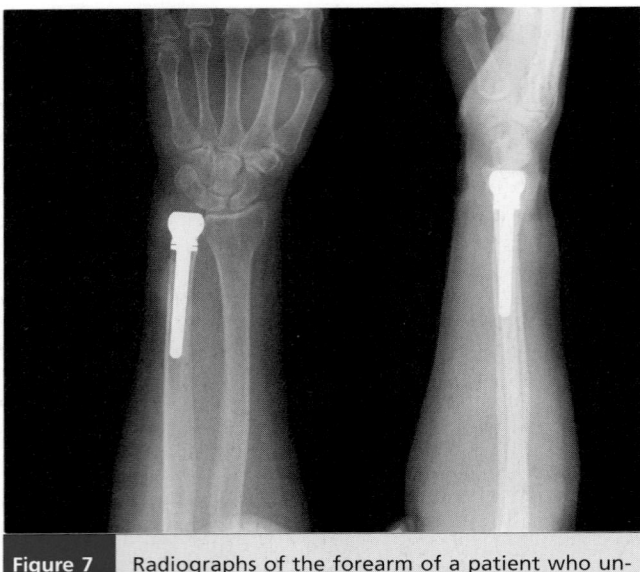

Figure 7 Radiographs of the forearm of a patient who underwent ulnar head arthroplasty for chronic pain, arthritis, and instability following trauma in the remote past.

grip strength are approximately 65% and 85%, respectively, when compared with the contralateral side. Failure rates range from 10% and 20%. The rate of radiographic progression of measurable joint narrowing is variable and has been reported in more than 50% of patients. However, this finding appears to be of little clinical significance. Patients younger than 35 years are more likely to require revision surgery.

Scaphoid excision and four-corner arthrodesis is likely to yield 15° to 20° less flexion-extension arc than proximal row carpectomy, but more grip strength. A recent review compared fixation techniques using circular plate fixation and more traditional fixation methods for helping achieve the four-corner arthrodesis.[11] There was sufficient evidence to suggest improved outcomes with traditional techniques. In patients treated with intercarpal circular fusion plates, higher nonunion and complication rates and increased patient dissatisfaction were reported.

Because of arthritis on the head of the capitate, proximal row carpectomy is not an option for the treatment of stage III SLAC wrist unless it is performed in conjunction with a fascial interposition. Scaphoid excision and four-corner arthrodesis is the favored surgical treatment.

Distal Radioulnar Joint Arthritis

Distal radioulnar joint (DRUJ) arthritis may occur in a variety of clinical settings. Causes include overuse, fracture, ligament injury and instability, or the presence of an inflammatory process or systemic disease. Nonsurgical treatment of DRUJ arthritis is with NSAIDs and a long arm or Munster type splint that restricts or controls forearm rotation. Cortisone injection with bupivacaine hydrochloride or lidocaine can

be helpful to confirm the diagnosis and assist with treatment.

It is important to first determine the stability of the DRUJ in patients with arthritis to facilitate appropriate surgical planning. For patients with positive ulnar variance and early disease, some form of ulnar shortening (distal resection or proximal osteotomy) has been described.[12,13] For patients with arthritis, currently there are four main options for the treatment of the DRUJ: distal ulna resection (Darrach procedure), partial ulna resection and interposition (Bowers or Watson hemiresection procedures), Sauve-Kapandji procedure (radioulnar arthrodesis with more proximal ulna segment resection), and ulnar head replacement. The Darrach procedure (or its variants) is an established treatment of arthritis of the DRUJ. It has been shown to have improved results, more so in patients with rheumatoid arthritis than in those with osteoarthritis or posttraumatic arthritis.[14] Outcomes generally show improved pain, but complications such as joint weakness, ulnar drift of the carpus, and instability of the ulnar stump are well documented. The ulnar hemiresection and tendon interposition procedure is technically demanding and requires adequate bony resection and sufficient soft-tissue interposition. Radioulnar and ulnar styloid-carpal impingement can be difficult complications associated with this procedure. Intact or reconstructible soft-tissue stabilizers to the DRUJ are necessary in improving outcomes. When successful, the hemiresection and interposition procedure can improve pain, strength, and motion. The Sauve-Kapandji procedure has been advocated in younger and more active patients. The procedure involves arthrodesis of the DRUJ while removing a more proximal segment of ulna to allow forearm rotation. Grip strength is better maintained in comparison with the Darrach procedure. However, difficulties with instability of the ulnar stump can be problematic. Varying types of tenodeses have been described to help maintain stability.

Recently, ulnar head replacement has been used in the treatment of both stable and unstable DRUJ arthritis[15] (**Figure 7**). It restores an intact ulnar head, a structure critical for normal function of both the wrist and forearm. Early results of ulnar head replacement have been encouraging; excellent pain improvement, range of motion, and strength have been reported.[15] Adequate soft tissue is needed to ensure stability of the prosthesis. Ulnar head replacement also has been successfully used to treat failed ulnar head resection. Unfortunately, despite promise, long-term follow-up is not yet available for ulnar head arthroplasty.

Basilar Thumb Arthritis

Arthritis of the carpometacarpal (CMC) joint of the thumb is the second most common site of arthritis in the hand, and the most common site for surgical treatment. The incidence is significantly greater in females than males. Because of the shallow articulation between the trapezium and thumb metacarpal, ligamentous support is important in affording stability. Both

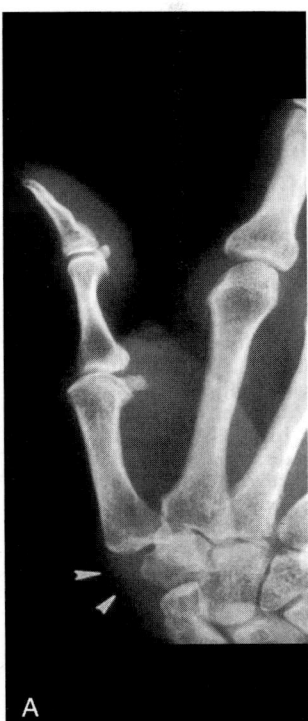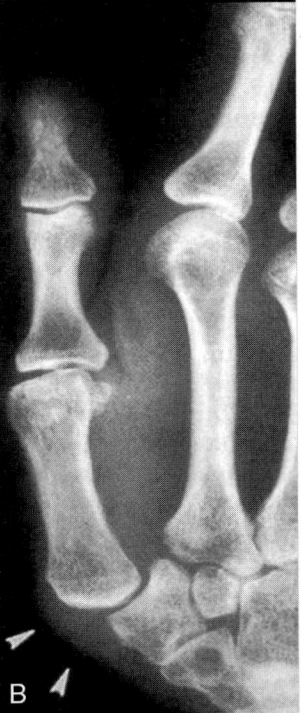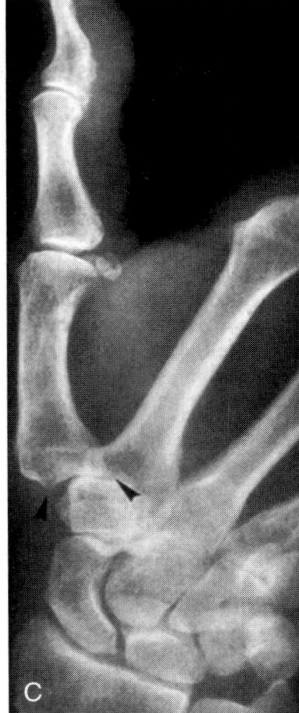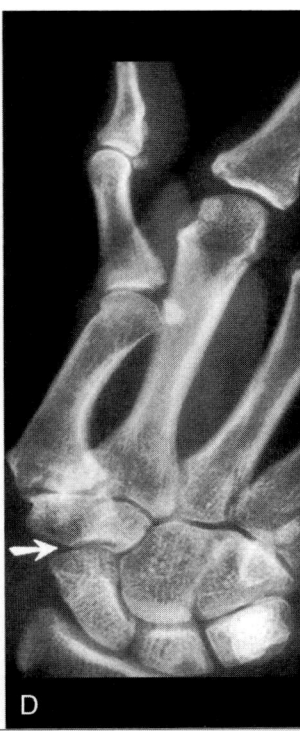

Figure 8 Eaton-Littler classification of basilar thumb arthritis. Stage I: articular contours are normal. There may be slight widening caused by effusion or laxity of the joint. Stage II: mild CMC joint space narrowing. There is minimal sclerosis or cystic changes. If osteophytosis is present, the size is less than 2 mm. Stage III: more extensive arthritic changes. The joint space is markedly narrowed with sclerosis and/or cystic changes. Osteophytes are larger than 2 mm. The scaphotrapezial joint is normal. Stage IV: same as stage III with the inclusion of scaphotrapezial joint arthritis. *(Reproduced with permission from Eaton RG, Glickel SZ: Trapeziometacarpal arthritis: Staging as a rationale for treatment. Hand Clin 1987;3:455-469.)*

the anterior oblique (beak) ligament and dorsal radial ligament are considered major stabilizers of the trapeziometacarpal joint. Disruption of these ligaments leads to abnormal kinematics of the CMC joint, increased shear forces and arthritis.

Patients with trapeziometacarpal arthritis will report pain and weakness with pinch and grip-related activities. Limited radial and palmar abduction of the thumb occurs as the disease progresses. Patients will report pain with direct palpation of the CMC joint. In addition, provocative maneuvers such as grind, compression, and distraction tests should demonstrate pain. Direct palpation over the distal pole of the scaphoid may help discern scaphotrapeziotrapezoid arthritis. Metacarpophalangeal joint hyperextension occurs during attempts to maintain the first web space when opening the hand to grasp objects. Night pain is common in severe disease. The natural history of basilar thumb arthritis can often reveal that, as the disease worsens, motion becomes progressively limited and the pain can subsequently improve. de Quervain's tenosynovitis is important in the differential diagnosis of radial-sided hand pain and it can coexist with basilar thumb arthritis.

A radiographic staging system has been described (**Figure 8**). The radiographs are performed with the

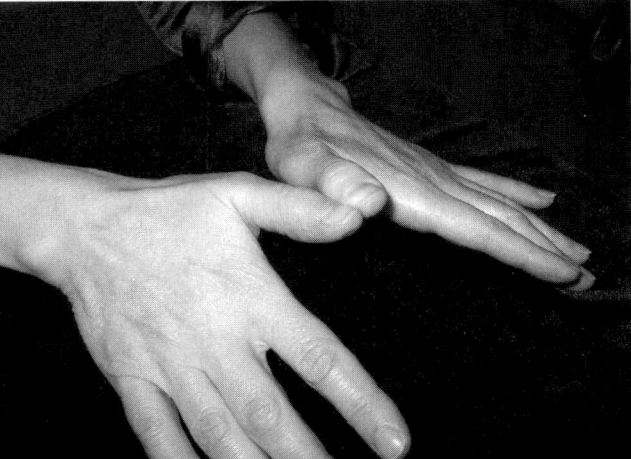

Figure 9 Position of the thumbs when performing Eaton stress views. The thumbs are positioned with the nails parallel to the table and the hands are held obliquely at approximately 30°. The patient is asked to forcibly push the thumbs together while the radiograph is taken centered over the CMC joints.

thumbs pushing against each other with the nails parallel to the table (**Figure 9**). Stage I is considered

3: Upper Extremity

prearthritic with a normal joint with widening suggestive of synovitis. Stages II and III demonstrate progressing arthritis and subluxation of the metacarpal on the trapezium. Stage IV includes scaphotrapezial joint arthritis.

Nonsurgical treatment of CMC arthritis of the thumb includes splinting, NSAIDs, activity modification, and steroid injections. Surgical treatment of stage I disease includes ligament reconstruction. It is important to evaluate the articular cartilage either arthroscopically or by direct visualization at the time of reconstruction to ensure that it appears disease free. The surgeon needs to inform the patient and be prepared to perform an arthroplasty procedure in instances of CMC joint disease. A 30° extension osteotomy of the metacarpal (Wilson-type) is an additional option to treat early disease. Arthroscopic treatments including synovectomy and capsular shrinkage have also been described for early arthritis or prearthritic CMC joints.[16] Surgical options for patients with definitive arthritis include partial or total trapeziectomy. CMC joint arthrodesis is indicated in younger patients and manual laborers. When successful, arthrodesis affords a stable, pain-free, and durable solution. Complications include a significant rate of nonunion. Soft-tissue arthroplasty procedures such as a ligament reconstruction and tendon interposition involving either one half or all of the flexor carpi radialis are common treatments of CMC arthritis (Figure 10). The flexor carpi radialis is harvested from its muscle belly while maintaining its insertion at the base of the index finger metacarpal. The leash of flexor carpi radialis is passed through a drill hole in the base of the thumb metacarpal and secured to itself. This action will effectively recreate the function of the stabilizing ligaments and secure the metacarpal. The remaining leash of flexor carpi radialis is folded into an anchovy and secured into the space created by the trapeziectomy. Suspensionplasty techniques are also commonly used.[17,18] Following trapeziectomy, one half of the flexor carpi radialis or abductor pollicis longus is weaved across the trapeziectomy site and connected or interweaved to create the "suspension." Newer studies evaluating the results of trapeziectomy and ligament reconstruction with and without tendon interposition or suspensionplasty have yielded comparable results.[19] In patients with scaphotrapezial arthritis, a partial trapeziectomy is contraindicated. Patients with significant metacarpophalangeal joint hyperextension require correction with either a volar capsulodesis or arthrodesis at the time of arthroplasty.

Failure of soft-tissue arthroplasty is rare. Recent studies have reported good results with revision ligament reconstruction and/or tendon interposition. Greater than 75% satisfactory outcomes have been reported.[20] There is little evidence that prosthetic replacement of the trapezium or total joint arthroplasty of the CMC joint are effective in the long term, and soft-tissue arthroplasty is currently preferred.

Metacarpophalangeal Joint Arthritis

Etiologies for metacarpophalangeal joint arthritis of the thumb include osteoarthritis, posttraumatic arthritis, and rheumatoid arthritis. Because most of the motion from the thumb arises from the base, arthrodesis of the thumb metacarpophalangeal joint remains the treatment of choice. A successful fusion predictably improves pain, stability, and return to function. The optimal position of fusion is 0° to 15°. Metacarpophalangeal joint arthroplasty in the thumb has attractive features. It maintains length and allows for motion. However, the forces generated at the thumb during pinch may result in early failure or exaggerate the risk of arthritis at the CMC joint, especially in patients with prior ulnar collateral ligament injury.

Metacarpophalangeal joint arthritis of the fingers is more common in patients with rheumatoid arthritis than in those with osteoarthritis. Thus, soft-tissue destruction must be considered when planning reconstruction or arthroplasty. Arthrodesis is not a favorable surgical option in the management of finger metacarpophalangeal arthritis. The mainstay of treatment is the use of a silicone prosthesis. The constrained hinged design is helpful in providing stability, especially in patients with rheumatoid arthritis. However, recent long-term outcome studies of silicone implants reveal that implant fracture rates are significant,[21,22] although not all fractured implants require revision surgery. In addition, early improvements in appearance and range of motion were lost over the long term. Overall patient satisfaction was well below 50%.

Newer unconstrained designs, including metal-plastic and pyrolytic carbon metacarpophalangeal implants (Figure 11) have demonstrated encouraging results.[23] These unconstrained designs are an excellent option for osteoarthritis, where the soft tissues and collateral ligaments are healthier. In patients with rheumatoid arthritis, the results are not as predictable. However, when compared with those of silicone the results in rheumatoid arthritis are comparable, with less bony destruction and implant failure. Although the indications are still being defined, at this time the unconstrained designs are a good option for patients with osteoarthritis or early rheumatoid arthritis.

Proximal Interphalangeal Joint Arthritis

Proximal interphalangeal (PIP) joint arthritis can be caused by inflammatory or noninflammatory conditions. Surgical treatment options include arthrodesis and arthroplasty. A successful arthrodesis can result in a stable and pain-free finger. However, because of the importance of the PIP joint in finger motion, arthrodesis can result in suboptimal function. Fusion currently is recommended for arthritis of the index PIP joint to maintain the pinch strength and stability, and arthroplasty is recommended for the long, ring, and little finger PIP joints. The choices for arthroplasty include the semiconstrained silicone implants and nonconstrained surface replacement implants (Figure 12). Much like treatment of metacarpophalangeal joint arthritis, evalu-

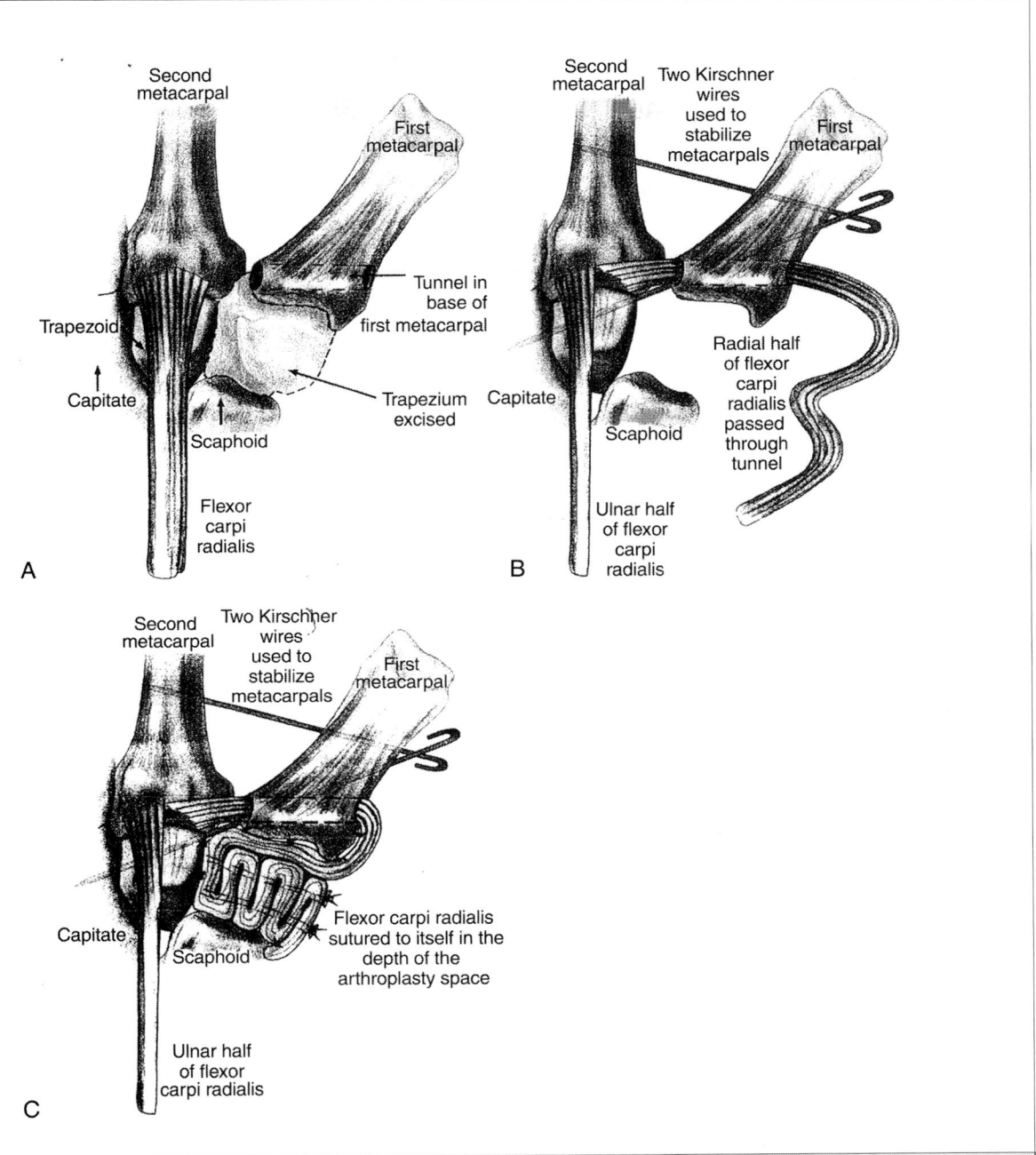

Figure 10   Schematic of ligament reconstruction and tendon interposition. **A,** Upon completion of the trapeziectomy, a drill hole is created in the base of the thumb metacarpal. **B,** One half (or all) of the flexor carpi radialis is passed through the hole and sutured to itself. **C,** The remaining leash of flexor carpi radialis is sewn into an anchovy and secured. Although this schematic demonstrates the use of Kirschner wires, some investigators suggest similar outcomes without their use. *(Reproduced with permission from Bednar MS: Osteoarthritis of the hand: Digits and thumb, in Berger RA, Weiss APC (eds): Hand Surgery. Philadelphia, PA, Lippincott Williams & Wilkins, 2004, vol 2, pp 1279-1288.)*

ation and competence of the soft-tissue stabilizing structures is important in determining the choice of implant. The silicone implants have been used for almost 30 years, and are favored in patients with soft-tissue incompetence or instability. However, durability is a concern with these implants.

Unconstrained PIP implants of both pyrolytic carbon and metal-plastic implants are an alternative to the silicone designs. Early outcome studies with these newer designs are becoming available.[24] With these newer implants, bone cement is not required. Improvement in pain has been predictable, and although motion is im-

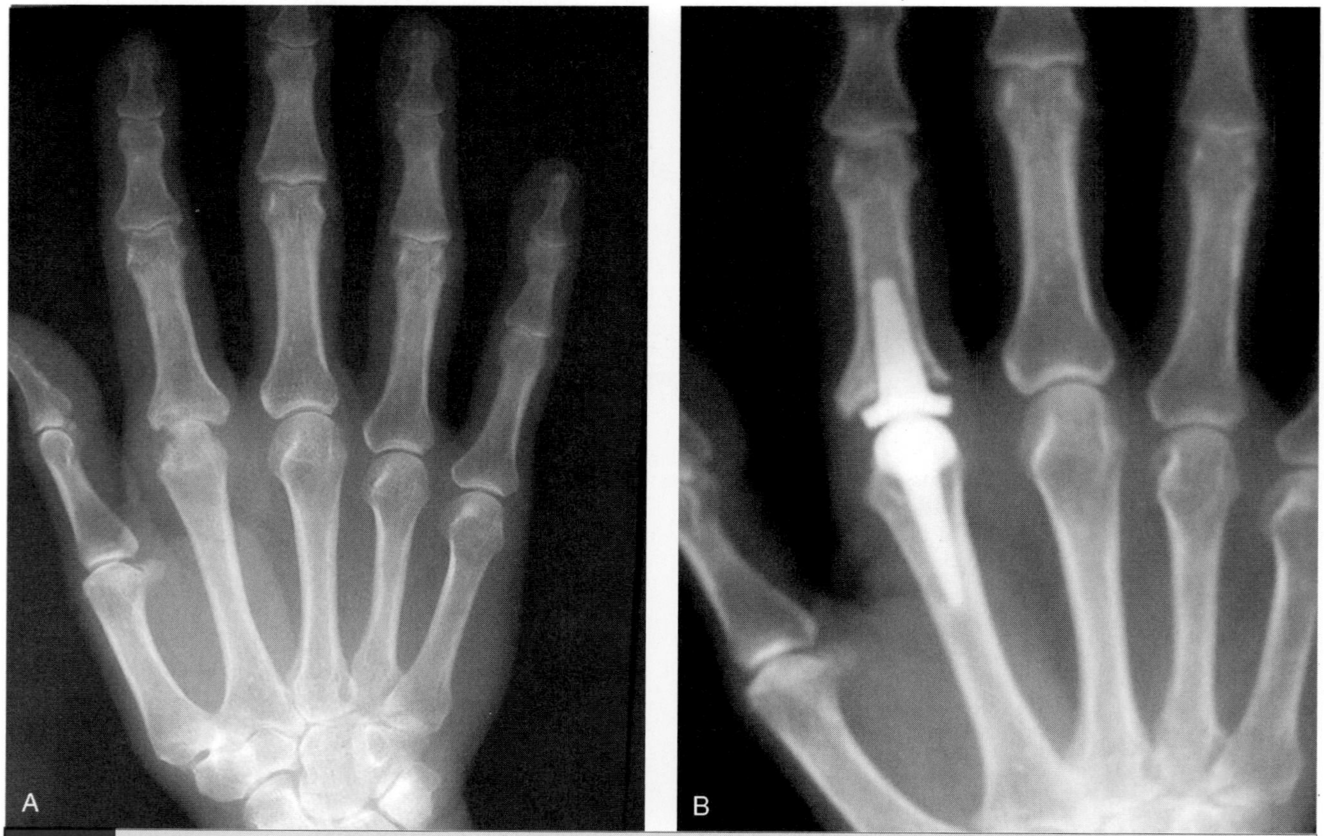

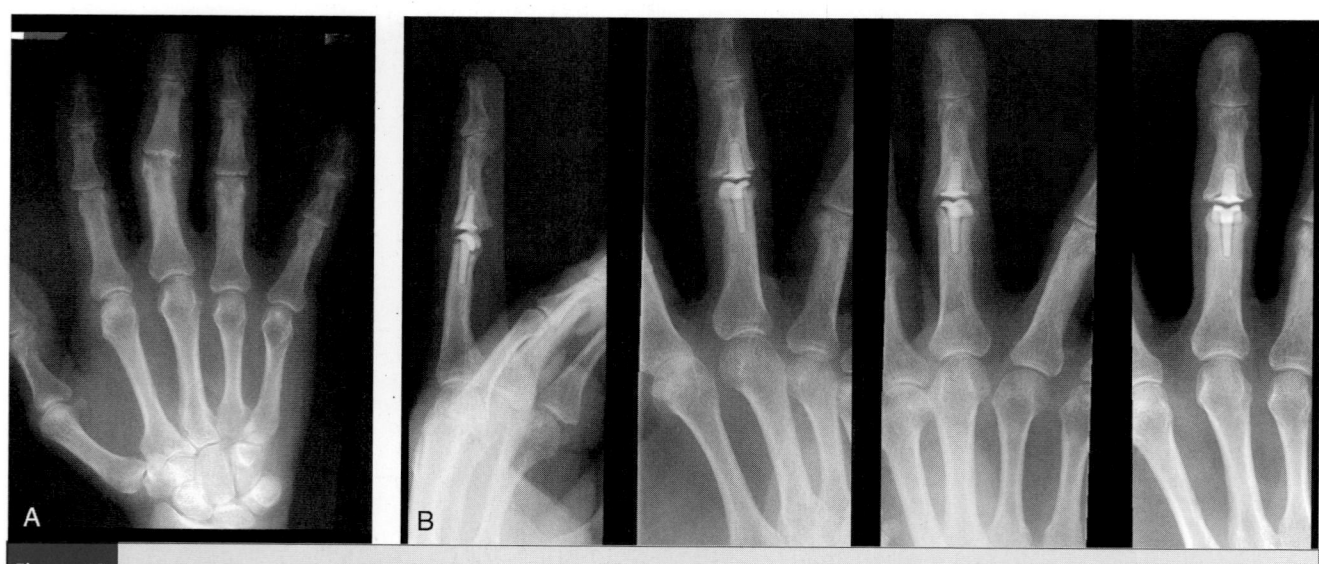

Figure 11 **A,** Preoperative radiograph of the hand of a patient with posttraumatic arthritis of the index finger metacarpopha-langeal joint. **B,** Postoperative radiograph at 17 months following surgery with a pyrolytic carbon nonconstrained metacarpophalangeal implant arthroplasty.

Figure 12 **A,** Preoperative radiograph of the hand of a patient with significant PIP joint arthritis. **B,** Radiographs at 2 years following PIP arthroplasty.

proved (silicone average 47° and metal-plastic 60°) the change in motion is only slightly statistically significant. Complications of resurfacing implants include instability when collateral ligaments are not fully restored, flexion deformity if the extensor tendon is affected, and squeaking in selected pyrolytic carbon joints. Longer follow-up is necessary to determine if these newer unconstrained implants are superior to silicone implants or fusion.

The distal interphalangeal joint is the most common site of arthritis of the hand, but surgery generally is not required. In these small joints, resection of Heberden nodes and mucous cysts is common, and for advanced disease, arthrodesis remains the treatment of choice (Figure 13). A stiff distal interphalangeal joint does little to inhibit function. Successful arthrodesis will result in a stable and pain-free joint with good overall finger function. Complications of arthrodesis include nail bed injury and nail deformity, nonunion, and infection.

Vascular Conditions

Ulnar Artery Thrombosis
Ulnar artery thrombosis is the most common site of upper extremity arterial occlusion. The condition is also known as hypothenar hammer syndrome and is associated with repetitive pounding or pushing, which results in weakness and dilatation of the arterial wall. Thrombi form within the dilatation, leading to emboli and/or complete occlusion of the artery. Anatomic variation will demonstrate 22% of patients will have an incomplete superficial palmar arch and 3% will lack a complete deep palmar arch. The condition most commonly affects males in the second to fifth decades of life, and there is a strong association with smoking. Data suggest that preexisting fibromuscular dysplasia can predispose patients to the development of ulnar artery thrombosis.

The clinical presentation of ulnar artery thrombosis can be subdivided into nerve-related and arterial insufficiency-related symptoms. Nerve-related symptoms typically include numbness, tingling, pain, and weakness. Ischemic symptoms include pain, decreased skin temperature, cold intolerance, pallor, ulceration and gangrene (in more severe cases).

Physical examination will include absent or diminished filling of the ulnar artery on Allen's test. Occasionally a painful or painless pulsatile mass is noted. Differential diagnosis includes autoimmune vasculitides, thoracic outlet syndrome, embolic phenomena, and ulnar nerve compression neuropathy. Additional studies to help confirm the diagnosis include noninvasive vascular studies with cold stress testing, electromyography, and arteriogram.

A variety of nonsurgical treatment options are available in treating ulnar artery thrombosis. Smoking cessation and activity modification are effective measures. Pharmacologic treatment with vasodilators (calcium

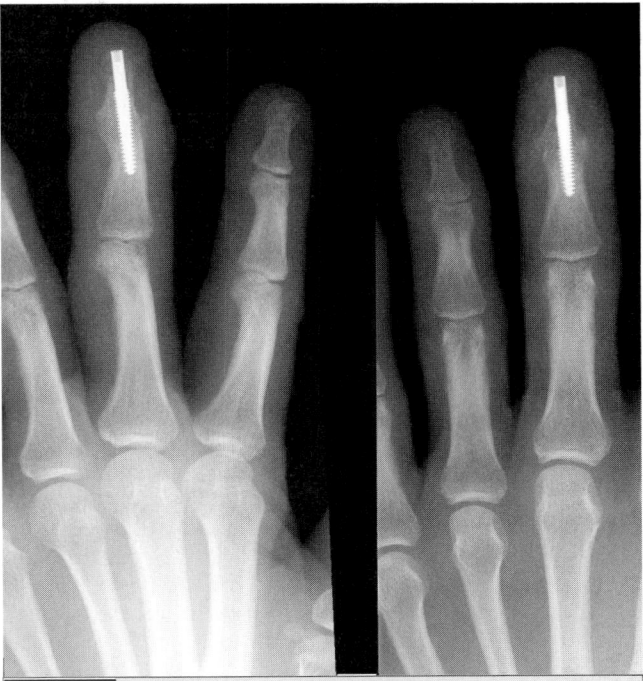

Figure 13 | Distal interphalangeal joint arthrodesis with a small bone screw in a patient treated for gouty arthritis.

channel blockers, α and β blockers), steroids, intravenous prostaglandin, and heparin have been helpful. Urokinase and streptokinase can be used to treat early disease. Stellate ganglion blocks can provide temporary benefit of symptoms.

The goals of surgical treatment are to increase blood flow, remove obstruction, and decrease vasospasm. Treatment options include local or cervical sympathectomy, excision of thrombus and ligation of artery, endarterectomy and excision of thrombus, and ulnar artery reconstruction. Revascularization can be successfully achieved with reverse saphenous vein graft. However, a significant incidence of aneurysm or reocclusion of the anastomosis has been noted in a recent study.[25]

Vasospastic Conditions of the Upper Extremity
Vasospastic conditions can be categorized as primary or secondary. Primary vasospasm is of unknown etiology, and secondary vasospasm is caused by a known agent. Sympathetically mediated occlusion is referred to as Raynaud's phenomenon, whereas Raynaud's disease is defined as vasospasm of unknown causes. Raynaud's disease is typically a diagnosis of exclusion (after 2 years without an underlying etiology).

In patients with suspected occlusive disease, it is important to evaluate for history of smoking, collagen vascular disease, atherosclerosis, renal vascular disease, and trauma. Patients with chronic ischemia may present with cold intolerance, pain, ulceration, or gangrene. A thorough and complete upper extremity exam-

3: Upper Extremity

ination should be performed to evaluate more proximal occlusion. Physical examination should include Allen's test of the digits and wrist. Noninvasive vascular studies with and without cold stress testing help confirm the cause of ischemia. Laboratory measurements demonstrating segmental pressure gradients greater than 20 mm Hg or digital brachial indices less than 0.7 are indicative of occlusion. An arteriogram is helpful in ruling out a specific occlusive lesion. Treatment is based on the presence of underlying vascular disease. In the absence of occlusive disease or vascular abnormalities, patients tend to have good results with nonsurgical treatment. Pharmacologic measures are similar to those used to treat ulnar artery thrombosis. Activity modification, avoidance of cold temperatures, and smoking cessation when applicable are often helpful. Biofeedback and arterial forearm pumps can also improve blood flow and alleviate symptoms. Patients with underlying vascular collagen may respond to the previously mentioned noninvasive options. Depending on the patient's response to noninvasive vascular testing, surgical options such as digital or more extensive sympathectomy have been shown to help improve blood supply to the digits.[26]

Tumors of the Wrist and Hand

Wrist and Hand Ganglions
Ganglions are the most common benign lesions of the wrist and hands. They most often arise from joints or tendon sheaths; the dorsum of the wrist is the most frequent site. Other common locations include the volar wrist, flexor tendon sheath of the fingers, and the distal interphalangeal joint. They are believed to arise from a weakened spot in the capsule or retinaculum, allowing fluid to herniate through the defect. In the distal interphalangeal joint, mucoid cysts are often linked to the presence of arthritis and osteophytosis.

Patients typically present with a painful or painless firm mass of varying size. There appears to be a relationship between size of the mass and symptoms. Because ganglia are filled with clear gelatinous fluid, they usually appear transilluminated. They are prone to rupture when compressed or traumatized. Some ganglia, such as those seen in Guyon's canal, can cause compression of neurovascular structures, leading to functional loss.

Aspiration with and without injection of corticosteroids offers a convenient treatment option and will help confirm the diagnosis. However, recurrence rates are significant following aspiration. Traditional surgical treatment has been open excision of the ganglion. The technique involves dissection of the ganglion and excision after tracing the stalk to its base. Some debate exists regarding reinforcing and closing the defect versus leaving it open. With surgical excision, recurrence rates can be significantly improved. Arthroscopic ganglionectomy is an alternative technique that affords less incision and dissection. Despite inconsistent visualization of the stalk,

outcomes with this technique have been comparable to those of open ganglion resection.[27] Resection of the capsule (1 cm) has been advocated to minimize the risk of recurrence. Care must be taken to avoid overaggressive resection and subsequent tendon injury.

Giant Cell Tumor of the Tendon Sheath
Giant cell tumor of the tendon sheath is the second most common soft-tissue mass in the hand. Peak incidence is in the third through fifth decades of life. The distal interphalangeal joint area is the most common location. Differential diagnosis at the distal interphalangeal joint includes mucous cysts. Giant cell tumor of the tendon sheath, unlike ganglia, do not typically transilluminate.

Physical examination reveals a firm, tender nodule. Larger lesions can elicit greater symptoms because of the mass effect (pain caused by increased pressure on adjacent tissues/nerves). Plain radiographs are usually normal, but can show erosions. MRI can help delineate the mass in better detail and help with preoperative planning. Histologically the lesion resembles pigmented villonodular synovitis. Bony invasion is rare; however, large lesions can infiltrate ligaments and joints, making complete resection extremely challenging.

Marginal surgical excision is the treatment of choice. Tumors that infiltrate the joint or lesions associated with bony erosions carry a higher incidence of recurrence. Multiloculated lesions also carry a higher incidence of recurrence. Reported recurrence rates can be as high as 50%.[28]

Epidermal Inclusion Cyst
Epidermal inclusion cysts are the third most common benign soft-tissue mass of the hand. The lesion is usually the result of penetrating trauma whereby epithelial cells are trapped in the subcutaneous tissues and generate a reaction leading to the mass. Typically they are firm, mobile, and painless. Because they are frequent sites of trauma, the fingertips are the most common site affected. Plain radiographs are essential in evaluation of these cysts. Much like giant cell tumors of the tendon sheath, larger cysts can result in bony erosions. In addition, radiographs may help differentiate foreign body granuloma from epidermal inclusion cyst (although many foreign bodies are not evident with plain radiographs). Treatment includes marginal excision. In patients with significant bony erosions or defects, reconstruction or bone grafting may be necessary.

Glomus Tumor
Glomus tumors are vascular lesions that generally represent only 1% to 4.5% of all hand tumors. However, up to 75% of these masses arise in the hand, and the subungual area of the digits is a common location. They are believed to arise from glomus bodies, which are myoarterial and regulate temperature and blood flow. The typical presentation is that of hypersensitivity to temperature and exquisite pinpoint tenderness with pain that radiates proximally. Subungual lesions have a

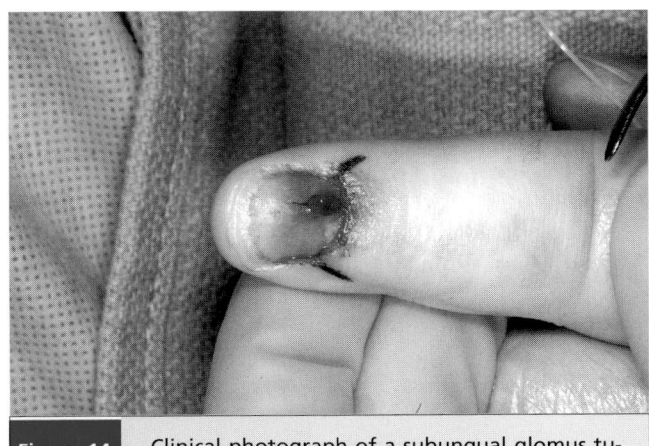

Figure 14 Clinical photograph of a subungual glomus tumor. Tumor is revealed at the time of resection.

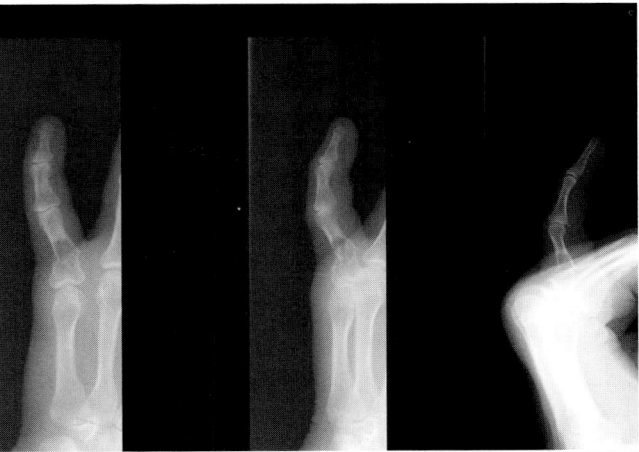

Figure 15 Radiographs of the hand of a patient who presented to the emergency department following a fall onto her hand. Pathologic fracture through an enchondroma in the base of the proximal phalanx is seen, a common presentation for patients with these lesions.

bluish hue. Surgical excision is the treatment of choice (**Figure 14**). Recurrence rates can be significant (as high as 50%).[29]

Hand and Wrist Enchondroma

Enchondroma represents the most common bone tumor in the hand and wrist, accounting for approximately 45% of all primary bone lesions in this area. Although this type of benign tumor is generally asymptomatic, the most common presentation is that of a pathologic fracture (**Figure 15**). The most common sites include the metacarpals, proximal and middle phalanges. Multiple enchondromas can present in conditions such as Ollier's disease. Maffucci's syndrome is a nonhereditary condition also associated with multiple enchondromas. Both Ollier's disease and Maffucci's syndrome carry a significant risk of malignant transformation to chondrosarcoma.

Many enchondromas are diagnosed incidentally. Small lesions generally require no intervention and can be observed. Because of the increased fracture risk, larger lesions that include greater than 50% of the structural integrity of the bone warrant intervention. Pathologic fractures are allowed to heal before formal treatment of the enchondroma. Surgical treatment includes curettage and bone grafting. Fixation may be necessary in some instances.

Giant Cell Tumor of Bone

Giant cell tumor of bone is an aggressive benign lesion that affects the epiphysis of bone, such as the distal radius or metacarpal head. Although generally considered a benign tumor, metastases have been reported in rare instances. The incidence of giant cell tumor is relatively rare in the hand, but when present, recurrence rates are somewhat higher. Only 2% to 5% of all giant cell tumors occur in the small bones of the hand, whereas nearly 15% occur in the distal radius.[30] Radiographically, the lesion is expansile and lytic with indistinct borders. Soft-tissue extension can occur (**Figure 16, A**).

Because of its location and generally aggressive behavior, local recurrence can be an issue. Surgical treatment of tumors retained within bone includes curettage with bone grafting, or polymethylmethacrylate cementation (**Figure 16, B** through D). Cryosurgery and cauterization have been used to minimize recurrence. For larger lesions that extend beyond the bone borders, or recurrent tumors, en bloc resection and allograft with or without wrist fusion may be required.

Hand and Wrist Epithelioid Sarcoma

Epithelioid sarcoma is one of the most common primary soft-tissue malignancies of the hand and wrist. They are often diagnosed late because they resemble a giant cell tumor of tendon sheath or benign fibroma. It usually initially presents as a small painless nodule or mass. They typically occur in young adults. Over time, the lesions ulcerate and can be confused with squamous cell carcinoma or pyogenic granuloma. Treatment should be wide local or radical excision including amputation. Metastases to regional lymph nodes and lungs are common.

Synovial Cell Sarcoma

Synovial cell sarcoma is also one of the most common sarcomas in the hand and wrist. Like epithelioid sarcoma, they notoriously present as a small painless mass, frequently over the dorsum of the hand. It commonly arises from the vicinity of joints or tendons and has been confused with a ganglion cyst. The peak age of occurrence is the second through fourth decades of life. Plain radiographs may demonstrate calcifications within the soft tissues. Treatment includes wide or radical excision with adjuvant radiotherapy. There is a significantly higher incidence of local recurrence with inadequate resection.

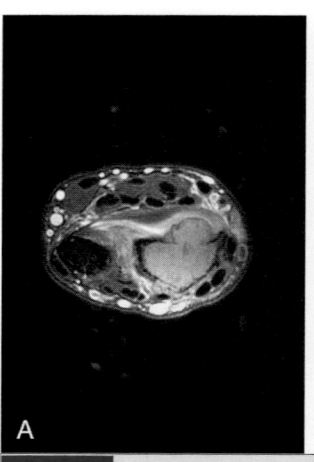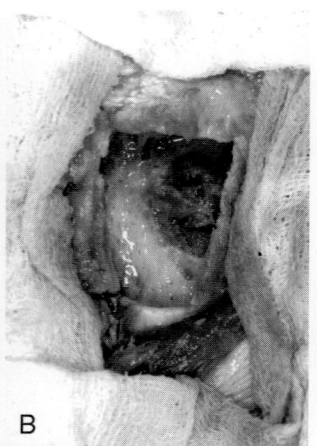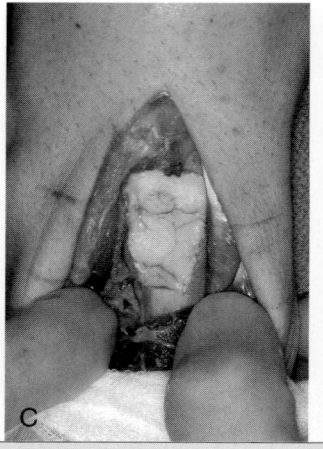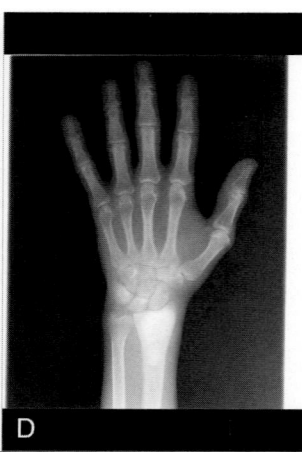

Figure 16 **A,** MRI showing a giant cell tumor of the distal radius. This axial image demonstrated soft-tissue extension of the lesion volarly into the pronator quadratus. **B,** Initial aspect of surgery involved meticulous curettage and cryotherapy. Note the volar defect resulting from tumor invasion into the soft-tissue. **C,** The defect was then filled with polymethylmethacrylate and bone grafting. **D,** Radiograph at 6 weeks following surgery.

Hand and Wrist Chondrosarcoma

Chondrosarcoma is the most common malignant bone tumor of the hand and wrist. It is typically a low-grade malignancy. The peak age of presentation is the sixth decade of life. The proximal phalanx and metacarpals are most often affected. Traditional measures to discern low-grade chondrosarcoma from enchondroma remain difficult. The clinical presentation, radiographs, and histology help to confirm the diagnosis. More expansile lesions with soft-tissue expansion suggest chondrosarcoma. Genetic markers are being investigated to better define malignancy and determine prognosis. Treatment is confined to wide surgical excision.[31]

Osteosarcoma

Osteosarcoma of the hand and wrist is quite uncommon, and represents 0.2% of all osteosarcomas. Unlike other locations where it commonly arises in adolescents and young adults, the peak age of presentation for osteosarcoma in the hand is the fourth through sixth decades of life. Osteosarcoma of the hand is believed to arise secondary to preexisting lesions. It is an aggressive cancer that presents as a rapidly growing, firm, and painful mass. Radiographs demonstrate an expansile mixed lytic and osteoblastic appearance. Tumor grade is important in predicting prognosis, and hand osteosarcomas generally appear to be lower-grade lesions. Treatment includes wide local resection with amputation and chemotherapy.

Metastatic Carcinoma

Despite being exceedingly rare, metastases should always be considered in the differential diagnosis when evaluating bone lesions of the hand. The most common metastasis to the bone of the hand is bronchogenic lung cancer. Other primary cancers that have been noted to metastasize to the hand include renal cell, prostate, colon, esophageal, thyroid, and breast. Treatment is based on pain relief while maintaining function, and can include wide excision or amputation. When amenable, radiation therapy can be helpful.

Hand and Wrist Imaging

When evaluating the hand and wrist radiographically, small changes in the projection and position of the hand can be both helpful and misleading. Developing a consistent method of performing these studies is well worth the effort. Despite growing popularity of newer technologies to evaluate hand and wrist pathology, plain radiographs remain the first step. Standard films should include PA, oblique, and lateral views. In patients with suspected scaphoid injury, a scaphoid view is imperative. When there is concern for ligamentous injury, stress radiographs and motion views (cineradiography with or without contrast) can be helpful.

Over the past 15 years MRI has revolutionized musculoskeletal imaging. It has become an important diagnostic modality in visualizing osteonecrosis, subtle fractures, osteomyelitis, and soft-tissue (ligament triangular fibrocartilage complex, or tendinitis) injuries. MRI remains an important modality in evaluating tumors. T1- and T2-weighted images provide different foci of enhancement. T1-weighted images have high uptake in fat and medullary bone, whereas T2-weighted images enhance edema and fluid with a significant water component. The use of gadolinium is helpful in evaluating the vascularity of conditions such as tumors, infection, and inflammation.

CT scans are helpful in evaluating the bony architecture of fractures. They will identify the degree of bony collapse of scaphoid fractures and the presence of humpback deformities. Complex fractures such as in the distal radius can be better defined and preoperative planning can be based on the CT scan. CT also continues to be helpful in evaluating bone tumors. Healing of scaphoid and other carpal fractures is best confirmed with CT. CT scans are also important in evaluating and detecting early arthritis.

Arthrography is useful in diagnosing ligamentous injuries about the carpus. Following the initial injection, extravasation of dye confirms a ligament injury and presumed instability. This procedure can be performed for virtually any closed compartment of the wrist and hand including the radiocarpal, midcarpal, distal radioulnar, and CMC joints.

Bone scintigraphy has a role in localizing potential sites of pain in patients with diffuse hand or wrist pain. The sensitivity of identifying bone pain is much greater than that of plain radiographs. However, bone scans are not specific. The source of pain can be anything from early arthritis, occult fracture, infection, or osteonecrosis. Bone scintigraphy also maintains a role in helping diagnose early complex regional pain syndrome. Indium-labeled white blood cell scintigraphy remains a valuable tool in evaluating infection.

Ultrasound is helpful in evaluating the cystic nature of a mass. It is an inexpensive and convenient method of characterizing superficial subcutaneous lesions such as ganglia or vascular tumors. In addition, ultrasound has been used as a guide for biopsy or injection.

Overview of Upper Extremity Amputation

The principles of treating upper extremity amputees are focused on restoring activity within a functional range of motion. For most tasks, upper extremity prostheses are not weight bearing and sockets do not require the same ability to accommodate pressure as the lower extremity sockets. Pressure sores or skin breakdown are uncommon in these patients. Upper extremity prostheses are of limited value if they are not capable of tasks requiring some degree of precision and dexterity such as grasping and releasing. Upper extremity prostheses will often combine suspension with control of the prosthesis. Myoelectric control is commonplace in the upper extremity amputee. The positioning of the limb in space is also more critical in the upper extremity amputee than in the lower extremity amputee and the design of the prosthesis needs to take this into account.

Cosmetic requirements are higher for most upper extremity amputees than lower extremity amputees. New silicone glove technology allows for better patient acceptance by allowing less restricted motion and improved perceived hygiene. Cosmetic restorations, which are usually nonfunctional, are quite realistic, but very expensive. Unfortunately these devices are often not covered by insurance.

Technologic Advances

The field of upper extremity prosthetics is a small component of the already small field of prosthetics and orthotics. Research and development by private companies within the field has not grown at the same pace as that of lower extremity prosthetics simply because of

the relatively low number of upper extremity amputees. The increased number of combat veterans with upper extremity amputations has led to government-funded research in upper extremity prosthetic systems. Current 2- and 4-year studies being conducted by the Defense Advanced Research Projects Agency are focusing on reducing overall weight of upper extremity prosthetic systems, as well as providing direct control of these systems through brain activity.[32] Other projects in progress include osseointegration (see chapter 42) and "target muscle reinnervation." There is a need to standardize the connectors and electronic sources for upper extremity prostheses across manufacturers. This will allow the physician and prosthetist to combine the most appropriate choice of components for each patient, regardless of the manufacturer.[33]

Current technology in upper extremity systems is continuing to evolve. Myoelectric systems currently available allow prosthetic limbs that surpass the conventional and myoelectric systems of the past. Current myoelectric systems should not be viewed as merely cosmetic but both durable and functional. Although conventional (body-powered) systems are still appropriate for a segment of upper extremity amputees, current myoelectric systems afford the user two to three degrees of freedom, that is, the simultaneous movement of two or more aspects of the prosthesis. Terminal device opening and closing, wrist pronation and supination, elbow flexion and extension, and shoulder adduction and abduction are motions now being combined to make prosthesis use more natural and functional. Further, new work on a single terminal device to provide more than one type of grasp is close to being commercially available.[32]

One of the coincidental technologic advances affecting the upper extremity prosthetic user is the use of battery technology. Because the prosthetic community is too small to drive any advances in battery technology, the recent movements to make cell phones and laptop computers lighter and longer lasting also has benefited the prosthetic user. Lithium ion and lithium polymer batteries, now in use in upper extremity systems, are the direct result of computer and cell phone advances. Batteries currently may weigh half as much, or last twice as long, for the same weight.

Socket shapes are also changing. Using some of the same concepts of transfemoral socket shapes, transradial and transhumeral muscle-contoured socket shapes are now common. The advantages offered by these new shapes include increased patient comfort, greater range of motion, and improved overall control over the prosthesis.

Two major concepts in upper extremity care in the amputee population are the importance of a team approach, preoperatively and postoperatively, in addressing the needs and goals of the patient, and the "golden window" of success in training and acceptance of an upper extremity system. Further, the expectations of amputees requiring upper extremity prosthetic services is much higher than ever before. The importance of an occupational therapist in prosthetic training has been greatly undervalued and underutilized. The ideal patient care setting allows for prosthetists and occupational therapists working side by side to prepare and train new amputees for a lifetime of prosthetic use.

Annotated References

1. Weber RA, Rude MJ: Clinical outcomes of carpal tunnel release in patients 65 and older. *J Hand Surg Am* 2005; 30:75-80.

   Clinical outcomes of carpal tunnel release in older patients are examined. Both subjective and objective parameters measured revealed improvement following surgery. Overall, 83% of patients were completely or very satisfied with their outcome. The authors concluded that age alone should not be a contraindication to surgery. Level of evidence: II.

2. Hobby JL, Venkatesh R, Motkur P: The effect of age and gender upon symptoms and surgical outcomes in carpal tunnel syndrome. *J Hand Surg Br* 2005;30:599-604.

   In an effort to clarify the efficacy of carpal tunnel release in the elderly, this prospective study compared outcomes in 97 patients following surgery. There were no gender-specific differences identified in both objective and subjective outcomes. In addition, there were no differences in symptom improvement and function between age groups, but the older patients reported less overall satisfaction. The authors concluded that carpal tunnel release is justified in the elderly, but the outcomes are less predictable than in younger patients.

3. Chappell R, Coates V, Turkelson C: Poor outcome for neural surgery (epineurotomy or neurolysis) for carpal tunnel syndrome compared with carpal tunnel release alone: A meta-analysis of global outcomes. *Plast Recontr Surg* 2003;112:983-990.

4. Chang MH, Liu LH, Wei SJ, Chiang HL, Hseih PF: Does retrograde axonal atrophy really occur in carpal tunnel syndrome patients with normal forearm conduction velocity? *Clin Neurophysiol* 2004;115:2783-2788.

   Patients with CTS were evaluated with electrodiagnostic studies and compared with normal age-matched volunteers. The authors found that patients with CTS can exhibit retrograde axonal atrophy with relatively slowed forearm median nerve motor conduction velocity, while demonstrating clear EMG findings across the wrist. Level of evidence: II.

5. Ritt MJ, Bos KE: A very large neurilemmoma of the anterior interosseous nerve. *J Hand Surg Br* 1991;16:98-100.

6. Nagano A, Shibata K, Tukimura H, Yamamoto S, Tajiri Y: Spontaneous anterior interosseous nerve palsy with hourglass-like fascicular constriction within the main trunk of the median nerve. *J Hand Surg* 1996;21:266-270.

7. Moran SL, Cooney WP, Berger RA, Bishop AT, Shin AY: The use of the 4 + 5 extensor compartmental vascularized bone graft for the treatment of Kienbock's disease. *J Hand Surg Am* 2005;30:50-58.

   Review of outcomes using the 4-5 extracompartmental vascularized bone graft for Kienböck's disease. Twenty-six patients were included in the review. Improvement in pain, grip strength, and range of motion were reported at 3-month follow-up. There was an 85% satisfaction rate. Repeat MRI following surgery was performed in most patients and there was a 65% incidence of revascularization. The investigators concluded that vascularized bone graft is a reliable option for the management of precollapse Kienböck's disease.

8. Moran SL, Cooney WP, Shin AY: The use of vascularized grafts from the distal radius for the treatment of Preiser's disease. *J Hand Surg Am* 2006;31:705-710.

   Eight patients with Preiser's disease were treated with vascularized bone grafting. Postoperative MRI was used to evaluate the degree of revascularization. Despite a reduction of range of motion following surgery, all but one patient reported a reduction of pain. Seven of eight patients described good and excellent results. One patient who was a manual laborer underwent revision to a proximal row carpectomy because of recurrent pain following return to work. The authors concluded that vascularized bone graft is a viable option in early stage Preiser's disease.

9. DiDonna ML, Kiefhaber TR, Stern PJ: Proximal row carpectomy: Study with a minimum of ten years of follow-up. *J Bone Joint Surg Am* 2004;86:2359-2365.

   This is a retrospective evaluation of 22 wrists that underwent proximal row carpectomy with a minimum 10-year follow-up. The authors noted an 18% failure rate. Factors associated with failure included age younger than 35 years. Among the remaining wrists, good ranges of motion and grip strength were reported. Despite radiographic progression of arthritis at the capitate and radius in 14 wrists, this finding was not yet clinically relevant. The authors concluded that proximal row carpectomy should be performed with caution in younger patients.

10. Jebson PJ, Hayes EP, Engber WD: Proximal row carpectomy: A minimum 10-year follow-up study. *J Hand Surg Am* 2003;28:561-569.

11. Vance MC, Hernandez JD, DiDonna ML, Stern PJ: Complications and outcome of four-corner arthrodesis: Circular plate fixation versus traditional techniques. *J Hand Surg Am* 2005;30:1122-1127.

    Twenty-seven patients who underwent four corner arthrodesis with a circular plate were compared with 31 patients who underwent fusion with Kirschner wires, staples, or compression screws. The results demonstrated higher complication rates in the circular plate group. The incidence of nonunion was 26% in the plate group versus 3% in the traditional fixation group. In addition, the overall complication rate was higher in the plate group, 48% versus 6%, than in the traditional fixation group. Overall satisfaction rates were 60% and 100%, respectively, between the plate and traditional fixation groups. The study has forced reevaluation of the efficacy of these newer techniques of performing this procedure.

12. Baek GK, Chung MS, Lee YH, Gong HS, Lee S, Kim HM: Osteotomy in idiopathic ulnar impaction syndrome. *J Bone Joint Surg Am* 2005;87:2645-2654.

    The authors evaluated outcomes of ulnar shortening osteotomy for ulnar impaction. Thirty-one patients were evaluated retrospectively. Radiographic and patient-related outcomes were improved according to radiographic findings and Gartland-Werley scores. Twenty-nine wrists were noted to have good/excellent results.

13. Tomaino MM, Weiser RW: Combined arthroscopic TFCC debridement and wafer resection of the distal ulna in wrists with triangular fibrocartilage complex tears and positive ulnar variance. *J Hand Surg Am* 2001;26:1047-1052.

14. Fraser KE, Diao E, Piemer CA, Sherwin FS: Comparative results of resection of the distal ulna in rheumatoid arthritis and posttraumatic conditions. *J Hand Surg Br* 1999;24:667-670.

15. Berger RA, Cooney WP: Use of an ulnar head endoprosthesis for treatment of an unstable distal ulnar resection: Review of mechanics, indications, and surgical technique. *Hand Clin* 2005;21:603-620.

    This article is a review of the indications, technique, and outcomes of ulnar head replacement arthroplasty for DRUJ pathology. The authors report on its use for failed distal ulna resections and note encouraging early results.

16. Culp RW, Rekant MS: The role of arthroscopy in evaluating and treating trapeziometacarpal disease. *Hand Clin* 2001;17:315-319.

17. Weilby A: Tendon interposition arthroplasty of the first carpometacarpal joint. *J Hand Surg Br* 1988;13:421-425.

18. Thompson JS: Complications and salvage of trapeziometacarpal arthroplasties. *Instr Course Lect* 1989;38:3-13.

19. Kriegs-Au G, Petje G, Fojtl E, Ganger R, Zachs I: Ligament reconstruction with or without tendon interposition to treat primary thumb carpometacarpal osteoarthritis: A prospective randomized study. *J Bone Joint Surg Am* 2004;86:209-218.

    This article presents a prospective evaluation of trapeziectomy and ligament reconstruction with tendon interposition (16 patients) and without tendon interposition (15 patients) in the management of basilar thumb arthritis. The average follow-up was more than 4 years. Appearance and radial and palmar abduction motion were better in the group that underwent ligament reconstruction without interposition. Strength, dexterity, and overall satisfaction were similar between groups. The amount of metacarpal subsidence did not significantly differ between cohorts. The authors concluded that tendon interposition does not appear to influence outcome.

20. Cooney WP III, Leddy TP, Larson DR: Revision of thumb trapeziometacarpal arthroplasty. *J Hand Surg Am* 2006;31:219-227.

    This article reports on outcomes following failed arthroplasty procedures for thumb CMC arthritis. The incidence of failure was 2.6%. The authors had 75% success rates with revision to a ligament reconstruction and tendon interposition surgery.

21. Parkkila T, Belt EA, Hakala M, Kautiainen H, Leppilahti J: Comparison of Swanson and Sutter metacarpophalangeal arthroplasties in patients with rheumatoid arthritis: A prospective and randomized trial. *J Hand Surg Am* 2005;30:1276-1281.

    This study is a prospective comparison of two common types of silicone implant arthroplasties. Seventy-five Swanson and 99 Sutter implants were inserted; follow-up was an average of 58 months. Outcomes were similar with regard to strength and deviation. The ranges of motion were similar in all digits with the exception of the index finger, where the Sutter implants were superior to the Swanson.

22. Goldfarb CA, Stern PJ: Metacarpophalangeal joint arthroplasty in rheumatoid arthritis: A long-term assessment. *J Bone Joint Surg Am* 2003;85:1869-1878.

23. Cook SK, Beckenbaugh RK, Redondo J, Popich LS, Klawitter JJ, Linscheid RL: Long-term follow-up of pyrolytic carbon metacarpophalangeal implants. *J Bone Joint Surg Am* 1999;81:635-648.

24. Tuttle HG, Stern PJ: Pyrolytic carbon proximal interphalangeal joint resurfacing arthroplasty. *J Hand Surg Am* 2006;31:930-939.

    In this study the authors review the outcomes following PIP arthroplasty with the unconstrained pyrolytic carbon implants. A total of 18 joints were evaluated at an average 13-month follow-up. Results revealed overall improvement in pain, but no significant improvement in range of motion. There had been no failures to date. Numerous complications were noted including eight squeaky joints, five joint contractures, and two dislocations. Most patients were satisfied with their results. The authors concluded that these newer implants have potential to achieve pain relief, but the results can be unpredictable.

25. Dethmers RS, Houpt P: Surgical management of hypothenar and thenar hammer syndromes: A retrospective study of 31 instances in 28 patients. *J Hand Surg Br* 2005;30:419-423.

    This is a retrospective review of surgical outcomes for ulnar artery thrombosis in 29 cases. Two cases of thenar hammer syndrome also were evaluated. A variety of treatment options were performed with and without thoracoscopic sympathectomy. The average follow-up was 43 months. Results demonstrate that only 3 patients were symptom-free at most recent follow-up, 14 were improved, 11 were no better, and two deteriorated. A duplex evaluation of reconstructions were performed in 27 patients. Thirteen of 27 revascularizations were patent.

3: Upper Extremity

26. Phillips CS, Murphy MS: Vascular problems of the upper extremity: A primer for the orthopaedic surgeon. *J Am Acad Orthop Surg* 2002;10:401-408.

27. Rizzo M, Berger RA, Steinmann SP, Bishop AT: Arthroscopic resection in the management of dorsal wrist ganglions: Results with a minimum 2-year follow-up period. *J Hand Surg Am* 2004;29:59-62.

    This study is a retrospective review of 41 ganglia resected arthroscopically with a minimum 2-year follow-up. Outcomes revealed excellent range of motion, strength, and patient satisfaction. Despite not visualizing the stalk in every incidence, there were only two recurrences. There were no complications noted. The authors concluded that arthroscopic ganglionectomy has comparable results to the open procedure.

28. Glowacki KA: Giant cell tumors of the tendon sheath. *J Am Soc Surg Hand* 2003;3:100-107.

29. Theumann NH, Goettmann S, LeViet D, et al: Recurrent glomus tumors of fingertips: MR imaging evaluation. *Radiology* 2002;223:143-151.

30. Harness NG, Mankin HJ: Giant cell tumor of the distal forearm. *J Hand Surg Am* 2004;29:188-193.

    The authors review 45 patients treated at their institution for giant cell tumor of the distal forearm.

31. Rizzo M, Ghert MA, Harrelson JM, Scully SP: Chondrosarcoma of bone: Analysis of 108 cases and evaluation of predictors of outcome. *Clin Orthop Relat Res* 2001;224-233.

32. Guinnessy P: DARPA joins industry, academia to build better prosthetic arms. *Phys Today* 2006;24-25.

    This article discusses the Defense Advanced Research Projects Agency's research program to build a more sophisticated prosthetic arm.

33. Pasquina PF, Bryant PR, Huang ME, Roberts TL, Nelson VS, Flood KM: Advances in amputee care. *Arch Phys Med Rehab* 2006;51:34-43.

    Recent advances in amputee care are discussed, along with the components of a successful amputee program and pertinent issues related to limb preservation and amputation levels.

Section 4

Lower
Extremity

SECTION EDITORS:

MICHAEL J. ARCHIBECK, MD
ANDREW H. SCHMIDT, MD

Chapter 30
Biomechanics and Gait

Ajit M. W. Chaudhari, PhD   Thomas P. Andriacchi, PhD

Introduction

The biomechanics of human locomotion provides a unique insight into normal and pathologic function. This chapter will focus on several kinematic (study of motion) and kinetic (study of the relationship between motion and force) parameters that are particularly relevant to the understanding of the pathomechanics of human movement. The importance of these kinematic and kinetic parameters is illustrated with specific clinically relevant examples.

Joint Kinematics

The kinematics of human movement are normally described in terms of relative angles between adjacent limb segments. Human gait is most often described in terms of sagittal plane motion (flexion-extension and dorsiflexion-plantar flexion). This practice has come about as a consequence of the much larger motions in this plane, making them relatively easy to measure and perhaps most relevant to function. In reality, however, the motion can be much more complex, involving all six degrees of freedom (three rotations and three translations). The complexity of the kinematic analysis substantially increases when going from a sagittal plane analysis to a complete three-dimensional analysis. Many different methods for measuring kinematics have recently been developed, each with its own benefits and limitations in terms of fidelity to natural, unhindered movement and in absolute accuracy of estimating bony motion. Some of these methods use either several passive reflective markers placed on the skin over specific landmarks on each limb, or electromagnetic sensors placed over each limb. The motions of these markers/sensors are tracked, and the underlying bony motion is inferred. Techniques with a redundant set of reflective markers[1] have enabled the analysis of secondary motions at the knee joint, such as internal-external rotation and anteroposterior translation during gait, and other dynamic activities such as jogging, squatting, and cutting.[2,3] Although these and other similar methods still have limited absolute accuracy because of skin motion relative to the underlying bone, they maximize the fidelity of the measurement because they allow natural, unhindered movement.

Other techniques for measuring three-dimensional motion using high-speed radiography or fluoroscopy discern the relative motion of the underlying bone without the errors caused by skin movement.[4,5] However, the limitation of these techniques is that they cannot be used to measure many normal activities of daily living because of their small field of view and/or bulky equipment that must stay within close proximity to the subject. Therefore, one must consider that these methods do not allow subjects to perform unencumbered natural movement and thus do not maintain fidelity of the motions to natural movement.

Flexion-Extension Rotation Patterns

Patterns of flexion-extension motion are surprisingly reproducible and consistent among the normal population. It is useful to examine these kinematic parameters in terms of the subdivisions of the gait cycle, because the timing of deviations from normal patterns often indicates specific pathology.

The stance phase of gait is typically described in terms of five events: initial contact, loading response, midstance, terminal stance, and preswing (Figure 1). The swing phase has been described in terms of initial swing, midswing, and terminal swing. At initial contact, the hip joint is in a flexed position (approximately 30°), the knee joint is near full extension, and the ankle is slightly plantar flexed. As the limb moves into the loading response phase, the hip joint extends, the knee joint flexes, and the ankle joint dorsiflexes. At midstance, the hip joint continues to extend from its initially flexed position, the knee joint reaches a relative maximum flexion, and the ankle remains in a dorsiflexed position. As the limb goes into terminal stance, the hip reaches an extended position, the knee extends in preparation for swing phase, and the ankle plantar flexes. During initial swing phase, the hip and knee flex while the ankle moves toward dorsiflexion from an initially plantar flexed position. In the final portion of swing phase, the hip reaches maximum flexion, the knee extends for heel strike, and the ankle plantar flexes.

It is important to note that the narrow band of normal variation around each of the motion curves at the hip, knee, and ankle suggests that the characteristics of these patterns do not vary substantially during normal gait (Figure 1). However, care must be taken in measuring certain peak amplitudes, as it has been shown that these values are strongly related to walking speed (Figure 2). For example, the maximum stance-phase knee flexion during midstance increases linearly with walk-

4: Lower Extremity

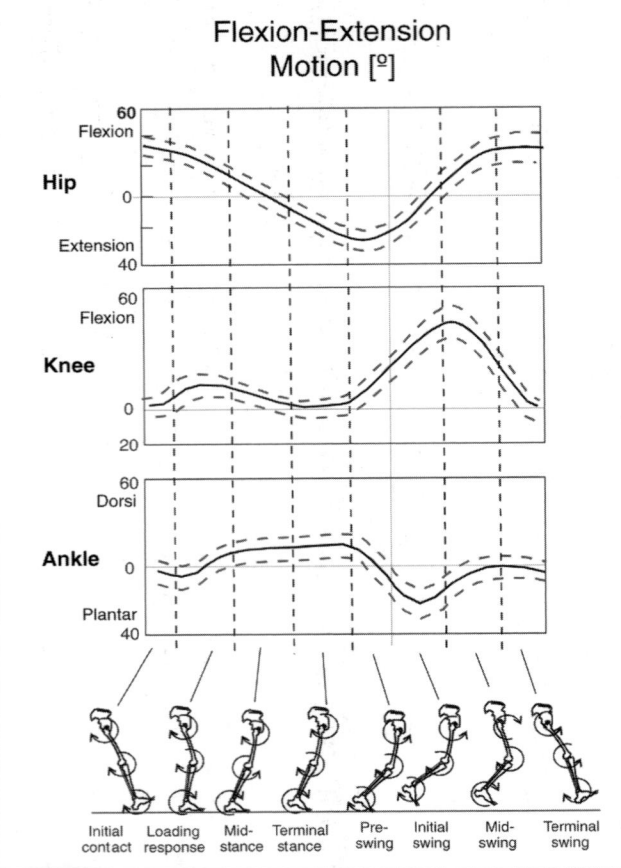

Flexion-Extension Motion [º]

Hip

Knee

Ankle

Initial contact — Loading response — Mid-stance — Terminal stance — Pre-swing — Initial swing — Mid-swing — Terminal swing

Figure 1 The position of the hip, knee, and ankle during gait. The stance phase is divided into five segments, and the swing phase is divided into three segments. The curves represent the normal patterns of motion for the hip, knee, and ankle. The drawings below the curves illustrate the position of the pelvis, thigh, and shank segments as they would be observed during each of these phases of the gait cycle. The normal sequence of events is quite regular and reproducible, as indicated by the relatively narrow bandline segments around the solid bars, which represent the average of the normal motion patterns. *(Reproduced with permission from Andriacchi TP, Johnson TS, Hurwitz DE, Natarajan RN: Musculoskeletal dynamics, locomotion, and clinical applications, in Mow VC, Huiskes R (eds): Basic Orthopaedic Biomechanics and Mechano-Biology, ed 3. Philadelphia, PA, Lippincott Williams & Wilkins, 2005, pp 91-122.)*

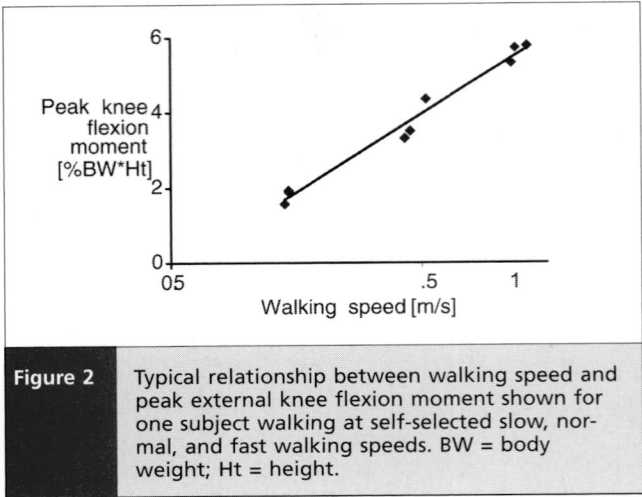

Figure 2 Typical relationship between walking speed and peak external knee flexion moment shown for one subject walking at self-selected slow, normal, and fast walking speeds. BW = body weight; Ht = height.

ing speed. Thus, in attempting to evaluate this parameter between normal subjects and patients with walking pathologies, or even between different normal subjects, controlling for walking speed is critical to making valid, relevant comparisons.

Adduction-Abduction Rotation Patterns

Kinematic patterns in other planes (rotations and translations) also can be quantified to identify gait abnormalities. In the frontal plane, abnormal abduction-adduction motion patterns can be observed at both the hip and ankle when pathologies are present. At the hip, one of the most common of these abnormal kinematic patterns is the Trendelenburg sign, in which the pelvis on the swing side drops, causing increased hip adduction during stance phase. This sign may be indicative of weakened hip abductors. At the ankle, abduction-adduction is also known as eversion-inversion. Excessive eversion of the ankle may be a sign of posterior tibialis tendon dysfunction,[6,7] and it may also be associated with pathologies more proximal in the lower limb, such as knee malalignment or even failures of total knee replacements.[8]

Internal-External Rotation Patterns

Internal-external rotation of the tibiofemoral joint is another biomechanical parameter that has recently received increased attention, because of improvements in marker-based and fluoroscopic techniques. At heel strike, the femur is normally internally rotated relative to the tibia, because of the rotation of the pelvis and the normal "screw home" motion of the knee as it approaches full extension. Throughout the stance phase, the femur rotates externally relative to the tibia as the swing leg is brought forward and the pelvis rotates accordingly, reaching a maximum rotation just after terminal extension. In late stance phase and swing phase, the tibiofemoral joint rotates back to a position of femoral internal rotation in preparation for heel strike. The normal range of internal-external rotation for a healthy subject is approximately 12°.[2] It is important to note the coupling of this motion to flexion-extension, as the knee experiences the external tibial rotation called "screw home" as it extends from approximately 30° to full extension. Abnormal internal-external rotation patterns at the knee have been observed in patients with anterior cruciate ligament (ACL) ruptures as well as in patients with reconstructed ACLs.[3,5,9,10] These abnormal patterns typically involve a rotational offset that remains constant throughout stance phase (Figure 3). During late swing phase in ACL-deficient patients, there appears to be an absence of screw-home motion occurring, leaving the ACL-deficient knee with reduced external tibial rotation at heel strike, which is maintained throughout stance.[3]

Anteroposterior Translation Patterns

Anteroposterior translation of the tibiofemoral joint also has been examined in much greater detail recently because of advances in motion measurement techniques. Anteroposterior translation follows a consistent pattern for most subjects, just as the other motion parameters do. Just before heel strike, the knee extends under quadriceps activation, and the tibia is at its most anterior position relative to the femur. From heel strike to terminal extension, the femur moves anterior relative to the tibia, as the whole upper body passes over the stance limb. During late stance, as the ankle plantar flexes and the knee flexes, the tibia moves in the anterior direction. During early swing phase, relatively little anteroposterior motion occurs, but at late swing, again the tibia moves more anterior as the quadriceps contract and the knee extends. Similar to internal-external rotation, abnormal patterns in anteroposterior translation have been observed in ACL-deficient patients.[3,9,10] These abnormal patterns typically involve an offset toward posterior translation of the tibia relative to the healthy contralateral limb that is maintained through stance phase. This result in particular is very interesting because it appears to represent an adaptation to avoid instability, as the primary function of the ACL is to restrict anterior tibial translation. This adaptation may be accomplished by altering muscle activation patterns to avoid or reduce quadriceps activity,[11,12] or possibly by increasing hamstrings activity as well.[13] To more fully examine this and other interactions between joint loading during gait and the kinematic patterns that are observed, it is necessary to examine the gait measurements known as joint kinetics.

Joint Kinetics

Kinetics is the study of the relationship between force and motion. The motion of the skeletal system is the result of a balance between external forces and internal forces. The external forces on the skeletal system include gravity, inertia, and foot-ground reaction forces during walking. Internal forces are created by muscular contraction, passive soft-tissue stretching, and bony contact at joint articulations. At any instant during walking or any activity of daily living, the external forces and moments must be balanced by internal forces and moments. "Moment" is a short form of "moment of force," and is similar to a rotational torque applied to a joint by a force acting at some distance (the "moment arm") away from the joint.

Interpretation of Joint Moments

External measurements of joint moments can be used to infer and interpret internal forces within the muscles

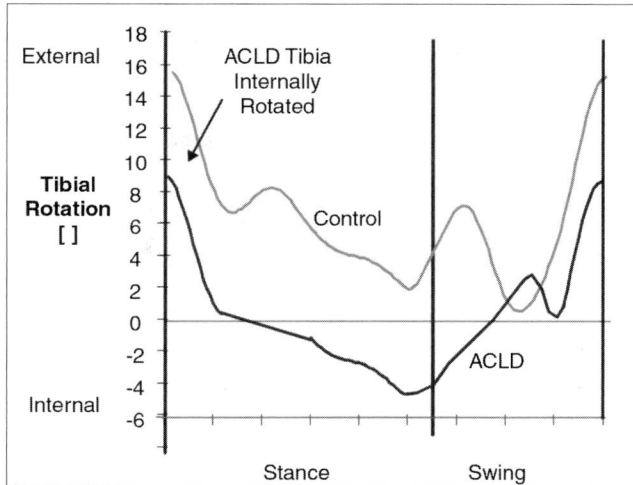

Figure 3   Internal rotational offset observed in ACL-deficient (ACLD) knees (bottom line) relative to uninjured contralateral knees (top line). During late swing, there appears to be a lack of screw-home motion that results in the internal rotational offset that is maintained throughout stance phase. *(Reproduced with permission from Andriacchi TP, Mundermann A, Smith RL, Alexander EJ, Dyrby CO, Koo S: A framework for the in vivo pathomechanics of osteoarthritis at the knee.* Ann Biomed Eng *2004;32:447-457.)*

and on the joint surfaces. However, care must be taken in the interpretation of joint moments. For example, consider an external moment tending to flex the knee (**Figure 4**). This external moment would require a net internal moment tending to extend the knee. The term "net moment" is used because the internal moment is a result of the summation of both antagonistic and synergistic muscle forces in the final equilibrium. If antagonistic muscle activity is present, the net of the balance between the flexors and extensor muscles must still produce a net internal extension moment to balance the external flexion moment. Thus, the moments measured in the gait laboratory (external moments) can be used to infer the net balance between joint flexors and extensor muscles, as these muscles generate most of the internal moment producing flexion or extension at the joint. Similarly, in the frontal plane, the abduction-adduction moments can be directly related to internal forces from the viewpoint of mechanical equilibrium. When appropriate care is exercised in their interpretation, joint moments can be extremely valuable in identifying changes in patterns of muscle activity in joint loading because they are very sensitive to abnormal functional changes.

Factors Influencing Joint Moments

As previously indicated, most gait parameters related to sagittal plane movement are highly sensitive to the speed of walking, including peak magnitudes of the flexion-extension moments at the hip, knee (**Figure 2**), and ankle. The speed dependence of the moment mag-

4: Lower Extremity

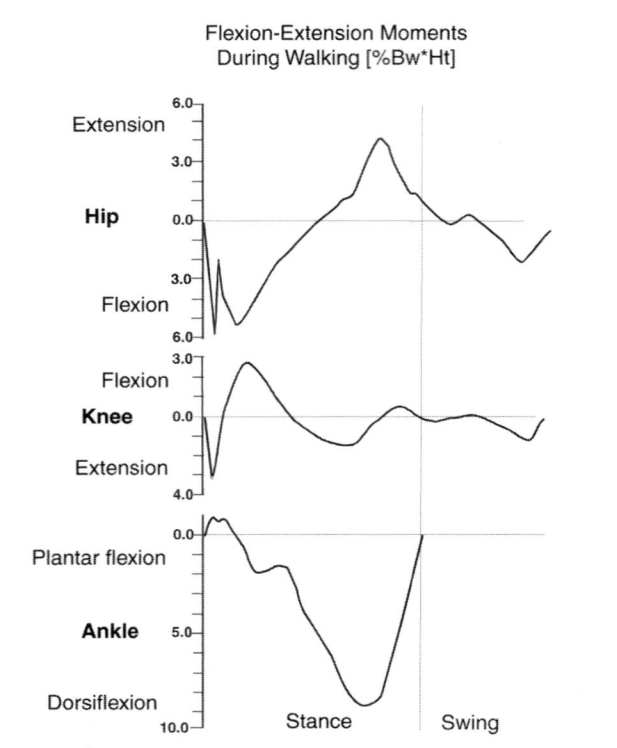

Flexion-Extension Moments
During Walking [%Bw*Ht]

| Figure 4 | Normal patterns of external flexion-extension moments at the hip, knee, and ankle. Bw = body weight; Ht = height. *(Reproduced with permission from Andriacchi TP, Johnson TS, Hurwitz DE, Natarajan RN: Musculoskeletal dynamics, locomotion, and clinical applications, in Mow VC, Huiskes R (eds): Basic Orthopaedic Biomechanics and Mechano-Biology, ed 3. Philadelphia, PA, Lippincott Williams & Wilkins, 2005, pp 91-122.)* |

nitudes is an extremely important consideration when attempting to compare patient populations with normal control groups. One must be able to differentiate the change in moment magnitudes associated with walking speed from a change in the mechanics of walking. Clearly, a normal subject walking at a slower speed will have a lower moment magnitude. Moment magnitudes in the sagittal plane (flexion-extension) should always be compared at nearly the same walking speeds when attempting to identify functional differences. Often, studies report differences in moment magnitudes at different walking speeds, making it impossible to infer whether the difference was associated solely with the change in walking speed or a change in function associated with some type of pathology.

Joint kinetics also are strongly influenced by body size, presenting a challenge when comparing individuals across the normal ranges of body height and weight. The influence of body size can be evaluated and removed from analysis by normalizing moment and force magnitudes to subjects' body dimensions. To account for the influence of body type on moment magnitudes,

moments are often normalized to body mass or the product of height and weight. The normalization to height and weight is quite practical in the sense that it accounts for variations caused by both height and weight. In addition, it normalizes the moment to a non-dimensional quantity and can be expressed as a product of a subject's height and weight. Similarly, joint contact forces can be normalized by body weight, with forces then being expressed in body weights.

Flexion-Extension Moment Patterns

Normal patterns of net flexor and extensor moments at the hip, knee, and ankle are illustrated in **Figure 4**. It is useful to examine the characteristics of the moment curves during the five segments of stance phase. These curves are quite reproducible in a normal population. It should be emphasized that gait analysis measurements provide external measures of moments acting at the limb. The internal net moments described here are inferred from these external measurements. Typically, at initial contact the loads acting on the lower extremity require net internal hip extensor moments, net internal knee flexor moments, and net internal ankle dorsiflexion moments for equilibrium. Moving into the loading response phase, there is still a net internal hip extensor moment, the knee moment reverses to a net internal extensor moment, and the ankle becomes a net internal plantar-flexor moment. In midstance, the net internal hip extensor moment reduces to zero, the knee moment reverses again to a net internal flexor moment, and the ankle moment continues as a net internal plantar-flexor moment. During terminal swing, the hip moment reverses to a net internal flexor moment, the knee moment remains a net internal flexor moment, and the ankle remains a net plantar-flexor moment. During preswing, only the knee moment changes direction from flexor to a net extensor muscle moment. The muscle moments depicted in **Figure 4** are the net balance between the flexors and extensors. Electromyographic activity shows that at heel strike both flexors and extensors are active at both the hip and knee joint. The presence of antagonistic muscle activity at this phase of the gait cycle is probably the result of the need to stabilize the limb for initial contact. Again, these net internal forces and moments are inferred by the measured external forces and moments being applied to the limb as a result of gravity, inertia, and ground contact forces.

The component of the joint moment tending to flex and extend the joint is very important in the analysis of gait. The flexion-extension component is associated with propulsion during walking as well as lowering and raising the body against gravity. Examining the factors that influence the magnitude of the flexion-extension moments is useful, because these parameters can be related to the muscle and joint forces.

One example of the usefulness of flexion-extension moments is in studying patients after ACL rupture. Many of these patients reduce the usage of their knee extensors during gait, and this quadriceps reduction can be identified as a reduced peak external knee flexion moment acting at the knee near midstance.[3,10,12,14] One explanation for this adaptation is that these patients perceive instability in the anteroposterior direction (as mentioned previously) and attempt to avoid any sensation of anterior tibial subluxation by adjusting their gait to reduce the requirements on their knee extensors. This explanation has been further supported by in vivo data showing that lower external knee flexion moments correlate to more normal anteroposterior tibial motion[3] as well as by simulation studies showing increased anterior tibial translation when the ACL is removed.[15] Again, a reduction in external knee flexion moment can be accomplished by increasing hamstrings usage as well as by reducing quadriceps usage; one recent study showed that increased hamstrings usage was more effective at reducing anterior tibial translation than reduced quadriceps usage.[13]

Adduction-Abduction Moment Patterns

At the knee, adduction-abduction moments are also very useful in understanding etiologies of osteoarthritis, because they can be used as a surrogate measure for the load imbalance between the medial and lateral compartments.[16] During the stance phase of gait, the ground reaction force passes medial of the knee joint, creating an adduction moment at the knee. This adduction moment usually has two peaks. The first peak occurs near the peak knee flexion angle at midstance, whereas the second peak occurs during terminal stance. Several studies have shown relationships between the knee adduction moment and the progression of osteoarthritis,[17,18] and between knee adduction moment and symptoms of pain in patients with osteoarthritis.[19]

Relative Magnitudes of Moments During Activities of Daily Living

A comparison of the maximum flexion moments during walking, ascending stairs, descending stairs, rising from a seated position, and jogging shows a substantial variation in the peak flexion moments at each joint (**Figure 5**). It is interesting to note that the largest flexion moment magnitudes during walking occur at the hip and ankle. The magnitude of the flexion moment at the hip and ankle are more than twice the magnitude of the flexion moments that occur at the knee for a walking speed of approximately 1 m/s. Assuming equal muscle lever arms at the hip, knee, and ankle, the difference in moment magnitudes would suggest that the extensor musculature at the hip and the plantar flexor muscles at the ankle would sustain greater forces than the knee extensor muscles for normal walking. The knee joint, which has a relatively small flexion moment during level walking, would sustain substantial increases during several activities, including stair climbing and jogging. The large increases in the flexion moment at the knee joint when jogging are likely associated with the high incidence of patellofemoral conditions in middle- and long-distance runners. Most likely, the relative increase (approximately fivefold) in

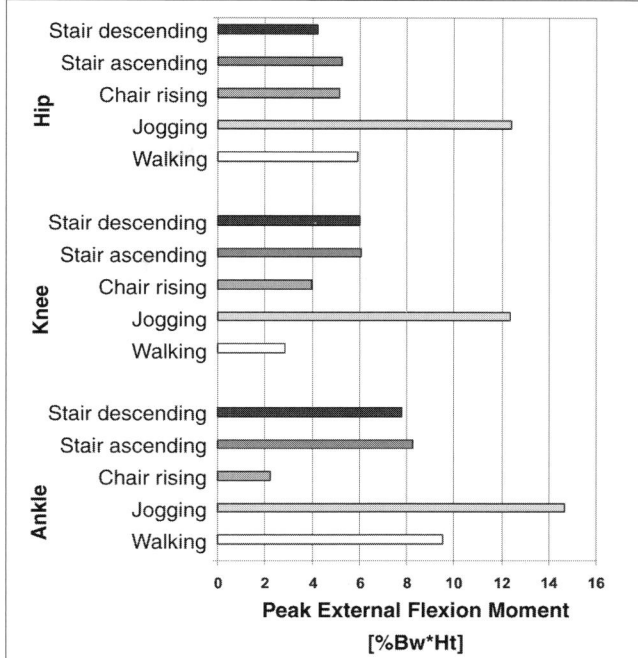

| Figure 5 | Comparison of the magnitudes of peak external flexion moments at the hip, knee, and ankle during various activities of daily living. Bw = body weight; Ht = height. *(Reproduced with permission from Andriacchi TP, Johnson TS, Hurwitz DE, Natarajan RN: Musculoskeletal dynamics, locomotion, and clinical applications, in Mow VC, Huiskes R (eds): Basic Orthopaedic Biomechanics and Mechano-Biology, ed 3. Philadelphia, PA, Lippincott Williams & Wilkins, 2005, pp 91-122.)* |

the flexion moment during jogging over the nominal level of walking is more important on a comparative basis than the absolute magnitudes. For example, the ankle dorsiflexion moment during jogging is higher than the flexion moment at the knee. However, the relative dorsiflexion sustained during jogging, as compared with level walking, is increased by a factor of two as compared with the fivefold increase seen in the knee flexion moment.

Clinical Applications

As previously noted, joint kinematics and moments are excellent indicators of changes from normal function that are quantitative and objective. Abnormal kinematics during functional activities may be an adverse consequence of surgical procedures and may lead to sequelae such as chondral degeneration, meniscal tears, or ligament graft failure. In addition, because the joint moments can be used to infer changes in muscle activity, abnormal moment patterns provide a basis for clinical interpretations of abnormal function. The following examples demonstrate some of these clinical applications of gait analysis that can be used to choose

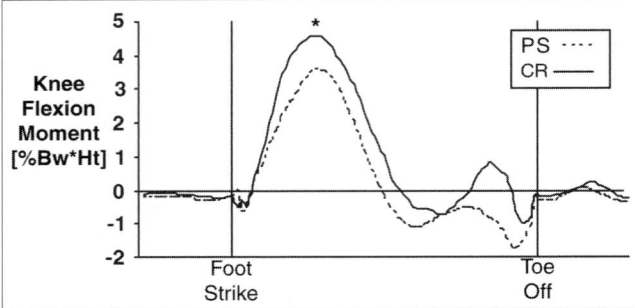

Figure 6 External knee flexion moment during stair climbing for patients after bilateral knee arthroplasty with one PCL-substituting (PS) prosthesis and one PCL-retaining (CR) prosthesis. Knees with CR prostheses showed peak knee flexion moments that were significantly higher and closer to healthy control knees. Bw = body weight; Ht = height. *(Reproduced with permission from Dyrby CO, Tria AJ, Johnson RV, Hartzband M, Andriacchi TP: Bilateral posterior stabilized and cruciate retaining total knee replacements compared during stair climbing. Trans Orthop Res Soc 2004;29:244.)*

between alternative treatments, assess the effectiveness of a treatment, or design new treatments of musculoskeletal conditions.

Total Knee Replacement
A study of patients following bilateral total knee arthroplasty during stair climbing illustrates how differences in function based on the flexion-extension moment during stair climbing can be used to evaluate different designs.[20] Patients received a posterior cruciate ligament (PCL)-substituting knee prosthesis (PS) in one knee and a PCL-retaining knee prosthesis (CR) in the other. A stair-climbing test showed a difference in the knee flexion moment between designs that retained the PCL versus designs that remove the PCL, with the PS design resulting in significantly reduced flexion moments (**Figure 6**). Moreover, the knees that had received the CR prosthesis experienced knee flexion moments similar to height- and weight-matched control subjects. In addition, in these subjects, the peak knee flexion moment occurred near 53° of flexion, below the 70° needed to engage the cam in PS knee prosthesis designs. These results suggest that the PS design may not create femoral rollback at low enough flexion angles to allow the quadriceps to produce a sufficient knee extension moment when climbing stairs, forcing patients to adapt their gait to reduce net quadriceps usage.

Kinematic analysis of knees following knee arthroplasty also can provide insight into the effectiveness of different designs in restoring normal gait. A fluoroscopic study of walking in patients with unicondylar arthroplasties or biunicondylar arthroplasties retaining both cruciate ligaments has shown that these designs maintain more normal range of flexion and more normal patterns of tibiofemoral motion than total knee arthroplasty.[21] A marker-based study has also shown that

PS prosthesis designs result in more anteroposterior sliding in the tibiofemoral joint when compared with CR designs or healthy knees.[22] This additional sliding leads to increased wear in wear-simulation tests,[22] suggesting that a PS design may have a shorter lifetime in the patient than a CR design. However, it should be noted that other investigators have observed different kinematic patterns during gait or stair climbing, with more normal, consistent femoral rollback occurring in PS designs but less consistent femoral rollback in CR designs.[23,24] In fact, in some patients with CR designs, a "paradoxical anterior sliding"[23] of the femur has been reported during gait. It remains unclear whether these variable results are caused by the increased technical challenges of implanting a CR prosthesis[25] or inherent limitations in prosthesis designs, but these results of gait analyses have identified functional deficits after surgery that may better explain the variability in clinical outcomes.

ACL Deficiency and Reconstruction
As mentioned previously, adaptations can be observed in the gait of patients following ACL injury and/or reconstruction. These adaptations allow the patient to resume activities of daily living, but they may be a factor in the long-term consequence of an increased rate of osteoarthritis in this population.[26,27] One of the main adaptations that has been observed is a reduction in quadriceps usage, which may be a subconscious response to proprioception of increased tibiofemoral instability. The adoption of this quadriceps reduction in gait appears to be effective in bringing tibiofemoral motion closer to normal. Patients with a unilateral, isolated ACL rupture in whom knee flexion moments were reduced achieved more normal anteroposterior translation and more normal internal-external rotation in a study of walking 3 months or more after injury.[3] This study showed a more posterior tibial position and more tibial internal rotation in ACL-deficient knees than in contralateral knees (**Figure 3**). Another study showed more lateral translation of the femur during a lunging activity in ACL-deficient patients, resulting in potential impingement of the medial tibial spine.[9] After the ACL is reconstructed, the knee may still retain abnormal kinematics or it may be overcorrected, resulting in different abnormal motion. A study of running in patients following reconstruction of an isolated, unilateral ACL rupture found more external tibial rotation in reconstructed knees than in contralateral knees, but similar anteroposterior translation.[5] These results suggest that ACL reconstructions may properly correct translation, but may not adequately address rotational stability of the tibiofemoral joint. These abnormal motions may lead to altered loading patterns on the articular cartilage. Because cartilage responds to its loading environment, rapid changes in the load seen in different regions of the cartilage may lead to damage and/or catabolic activity that results in the initiation and progression of osteoarthritis.[26,27]

Osteoarthritis Initiation and Progression

Given the evidence that cartilage responds to load and that osteoarthritis seems to be caused at least in part by overloading joints, much research using gait analysis has been devoted to estimating the load in different regions of the joint. As described previously, gait analysis alone can only estimate the net external loading on the joint, so the physician must infer what the true joint load is. Knee adduction moment has widely been used as a surrogate measure for medial compartment load, because it represents the load imbalance between the medial and lateral compartment. Recent studies have shown that the knee adduction moment correlates well with osteoarthritis.[17-19] In addition, direct measurements of medial compartment load using an instrumented tibial prosthesis confirm that peak knee adduction moment is a valid surrogate measure for peak medial compartment load in the knee.[28,29]

Using knee adduction moment as an estimate of medial compartment load, it is possible to estimate the effectiveness of different interventions for knee osteoarthritis, ranging from conservative treatments to surgical ones. One example of the usefulness of gait analysis has been in the study of knee unloader braces. Subjects wearing these braces have been reported to have small but significantly increased medial joint space at heel strike,[30] reduced knee adduction moments, and increased valgus angulation of the knee.[31] These techniques have also demonstrated that different models of braces have different levels of effectiveness in unloading the medial compartment.[30] Other conservative interventions such as shoes and orthotic devices have also shown effectiveness in reducing the knee adduction moment.[32-34] On the opposite end of the spectrum, gait analysis has been able to predict which patients will benefit most from a high tibial osteotomy, which is intended to shift load from the medial to lateral compartment of the knee.[35] Patients with lower adduction moments had more positive clinical outcomes after osteotomies, whereas those with high adduction moments experienced less improvement in their clinical outcomes.

Hip Fracture Risk and Prevention

Hip fracture is one of the most serious injuries that can occur to elderly and weakened populations, and it results in significant morbidity and mortality in these patients. Although it is known that fracture risk is increased when the density of the bone is reduced, gait analysis can provide insight into the mechanical environment that the hip joint experiences. This knowledge may help prevent hip fractures in the future by setting guidelines for how mobile at-risk populations need to be to reduce their fracture risk. Patients left with hemiparetic walking deficiencies after a stroke are a particularly appropriate group that may benefit, because they have an elevated risk of falling and require rehabilitation to restore their walking ability. A recent study of bone density in patients with hemiparesis showed that an index taking into account body weight, number of steps per day, and ground reaction force is a good predictor of bone mineral density in the proximal femur.[36] In the future, such studies may help guide rehabilitation recommendations so that at-risk populations achieve the level of activity needed to avoid hip fractures.

Summary

Biomechanical analysis of human locomotion has been an extremely valuable tool in understanding normal and pathologic function because of its ability to provide quantitative, objective assessments of both the motion and loading on the joints during functional activities. Biomechanical analysis can be a useful complement to clinical examinations that may be subjective in nature, or histologic/biochemical assays that examine the biologic responses to normal or pathologic loading environments rather than the altered loading environments themselves. The examples presented have described just a few of the varied applications for biomechanical analysis. Gait analysis can help improve understanding of etiologies of joint disease, evaluate the effectiveness of conservative and surgical interventions, and develop more appropriate prevention and rehabilitation strategies for patients of all ages.

Annotated References

1. Andriacchi TP, Alexander EJ, Toney MK, Dyrby C, Sum J: A point cluster method for in vivo motion analysis: Applied to a study of knee kinematics. *J Biomech Eng* 1998;120:743-749.

2. Dyrby CO, Andriacchi TP: Secondary motions of the knee during weight bearing and non-weight bearing activities. *J Orthop Res* 2004;22:794-800.

   This study showed that the secondary motions of the knee are coupled to knee flexion, and that this coupling varies with the activity performed, emphasizing the importance of studying activities of daily living directly when attempting to understand the full six degrees of freedom motion of the knee.

3. Andriacchi TP, Dyrby CO: Interactions between kinematics and loading during walking for the normal and ACL deficient knee. *J Biomech* 2005;38:293-298.

   This study showed that kinematic changes associated with ACL deficiency correlate with the net quadriceps moment during weight acceptance, suggesting that adaptations to the patterns of muscle firing during walking may compensate for loss of the ACL.

4. Li G, DeFrate LE, Park SE, Gill TJ, Rubash HE: In vivo articular cartilage contact kinematics of the knee: An investigation using dual-orthogonal fluoroscopy and magnetic resonance image-based computer models. *Am J Sports Med* 2005;33:102-107.

   This study used orthogonal fluoroscopy to demonstrate

that both the medial and lateral tibiofemoral contact points during a lunge activity were located close to the tibial spine, indicating that the tibial spine may play an important role in knee stability.

5. Tashman S, Collon D, Anderson K, Kolowich P, Anderst W: Abnormal rotational knee motion during running after anterior cruciate ligament reconstruction. *Am J Sports Med* 2004;32:975-983.

Using high-speed stereoradiography, this study showed that ACL-reconstructed knees were more externally rotated and more adducted than the uninjured limb during downhill running, while anterior tibial translation was similar. These abnormal motions may contribute to long-term joint degeneration.

6. Pomeroy GC, Pike RH, Beals TC, Manoli A: Acquired flatfoot in adults due to dysfunction of the posterior tibial tendon. *J Bone Joint Surg Am* 1999;81:1173-1182.

7. Guichet JM, Javed A, Russell J, Saleh M: Effect of the foot on the mechanical alignment of the lower limbs. *Clin Orthop Relat Res* 2003;415:193-201.

8. Meding JB, Keating EM, Ritter MA, Faris PM, Berend ME, Malinzak RA: The planovalgus foot: A harbinger of failure of posterior cruciate-retaining total knee replacement. *J Bone Joint Surg Am* 2005;87:59-62.

This retrospective study of revision total knee arthroplasty found that all patients with posterolateral femoral rollback and subluxation also had ipsilateral posterior tibial tendon insufficiency at the time of revision, and that 75% had ipsilateral posterior tibial tendon insufficiency at the time of the index operation. Level of evidence: II.

9. Defrate LE, Papannagari R, Gill TJ, Moses JM, Pathare NP, Li G: The 6 degrees of freedom kinematics of the knee after anterior cruciate ligament deficiency: An in vivo imaging analysis. *Am J Sports Med* 2006;34:1240-1246.

This study used dual-plane fluoroscopy to show abnormal medial translation of the tibia in ACL-deficient patients during a quasistatic lunge, suggesting that future ACL reconstruction techniques should reproduce not only anterior stability but also medial-lateral stability.

10. Georgoulis AD, Papadonikolakis A, Papageorgiou CD, Mitsou A, Stergiou N: Three-dimensional tibiofemoral kinematics of the anterior cruciate ligament-deficient and reconstructed knee during walking. *Am J Sports Med* 2003;31:75-79.

11. Berchuck M, Andriacchi TP, Bach BR, Reider B: Gait adaptations by patients who have a deficient anterior cruciate ligament. *J Bone Joint Surg Am* 1990;72:871-877.

12. Torry MR, Decker MJ, Ellis HB, Shelburne KB, Sterett WI, Steadman JR: Mechanisms of compensating for anterior cruciate ligament deficiency during gait. *Med Sci Sports Exerc* 2004;36:1403-1412.

This study observed several distinct gait compensation patterns that may exist in unilateral ACL-deficient subjects, at least partially accounting for the confounding findings in the literature on the adoption of quadriceps reduction in this population.

13. Shelburne KB, Torry MR, Pandy MG: Effect of muscle compensation on knee instability during ACL-deficient gait. *Med Sci Sports Exerc* 2005;37:642-648.

This study predicted the ability of isolated changes in quadriceps and hamstrings muscle forces to stabilize the ACL-deficient knee during gait using musculoskeletal modeling and computer simulation. The simulations showed that increased hamstring force was sufficient to restore anterior tibial translation to normal levels, whereas reduced quadriceps force was not.

14. Alkjaer T, Simonsen E, Jorgensen U, Dyhre-Poulsen P: Evaluation of the walking pattern in two types of patients with anterior cruciate ligament deficiency: Copers and non-copers. *Eur J Appl Physiol* 2003;89:301-308.

15. Shelburne KB, Pandy MG, Torry MR: Comparison of shear forces and ligament loading in the healthy and ACL-deficient knee during gait. *J Biomech* 2004;37:313-319.

This study predicted shear force and ligament loading in the ACL-deficient knee during walking using musculoskeletal modeling and computer simulation, showing that the medial collateral ligament is the primary restraint to anterior tibial translation after ACL rupture.

16. Schipplein OD, Andriacchi TP: Interaction between active and passive knee stabilizers during level walking. *J Orthop Res* 1991;9:113-119.

17. Sharma L, Hurwitz DE, Thonar E, et al: Knee adduction moment, serum hyaluronan level, and disease severity in medial tibiofemoral osteoarthritis. *Arthritis Rheum* 1998;41:1233-1240.

18. Miyazaki T, Wada M, Kawahara H, Sato M, Baba H, Shimada S: Dynamic load at baseline can predict radiographic disease progression in medial compartment knee osteoarthritis. *Ann Rheum Dis* 2002;61:617-622.

19. Hurwitz DE, Ryals AR, Block JA, Sharma L, Schnitzer TJ, Andriacchi TP: Knee pain and joint loading in subjects with osteoarthritis of the knee. *J Orthop Res* 2000;18:572-579.

20. Dyrby CO, Tria AJ, Johnson RV, Hartzband M, Andriacchi TP: Bilateral posterior stabilized and cruciate retaining total knee replacements compared during stair climbing. *Trans Orthop Res Soc* 2004;29:244.

This study observed more normal kinematics and kinetics during stair climbing in cruciate-retaining knees than in posterior-stabilizing prostheses, with greater peak knee flexion angles and greater peak knee flexion moments, suggesting that cruciate-retaining prostheses may be superior in enabling functional activities.

21. Banks SA, Fregly BJ, Boniforti F, Reinschmidt C, Romagnoli S: Comparing in vivo kinematics of unicondy-

lar and bi-unicondylar knee replacements. *Knee Surg Sports Traumatol Arthrosc* 2005;13:551-556.

This study compared knee kinematics and tibiofemoral contact locations in patients with optimally functioning cruciate-preserving medial unicondylar and biunicondylar arthroplasty using lateral fluoroscopy during activities of daily living. Preserving both cruciate ligaments in knee arthroplasty appeared to maintain more normal knee kinematics.

22. Andriacchi TP, Dyrby CO, Johnson TS: The use of functional analysis in evaluating knee kinematics. *Clin Orthop Relat Res* 2003;410:44-53.

23. Dennis DA, Komistek RD, Mahfouz MR: In vivo fluoroscopic analysis of fixed-bearing total knee replacements. *Clin Orthop Relat Res* 2003;410:114-130.

24. Fantozzi S, Catani F, Ensini A, Leardini A, Giannini S: Femoral rollback of cruciate-retaining and posterior-stabilized total knee replacements: In vivo fluoroscopic analysis during activities of daily living. *J Orthop Res* 2006;24:2222-2229.

    This study observed more consistent, physiologic femoral rollback in patients with posterior stabilized total knee replacements during activities of daily living. In contrast, rollback was inconsistent in patients with cruciate-retaining prostheses; reduced femoral rollback was accompanied by a smaller range of knee flexion.

25. Lampe F, Hille E: Failure in constraint: "Too little", in Bellemans J, Ries MD, Victor J (eds): *Total Knee Arthroplasty: A Guide to Get Better Performance.* Heidelberg, Germany, Springer Medizin Verlag, 2005, pp 74-84.

    This review summarizes the challenges associated with providing too little restraint when performing a total knee arthroplasty and discusses appropriate methodology for choosing between cruciate-retaining and posterior-stabilizing prostheses. It also describes proper surgical techniques when performing an arthroplasty with either prosthesis.

26. Andriacchi TP, Mundermann A, Smith RL, Alexander EJ, Dyrby CO, Koo S: A framework for the in vivo pathomechanics of osteoarthritis at the knee. *Ann Biomed Eng* 2004;32:447-457.

    This article describes a framework for understanding the initiation and progression of idiopathic or posttraumatic osteoarthritis at the knee, based on an analysis of several previous studies describing assays of biomarkers, cartilage morphology, and human function (gait analysis).

27. Andriacchi TP, Briant PL, Bevill SL, Koo S: Rotational changes at the knee after ACL injury cause cartilage thinning. *Clin Orthop Relat Res* 2006;442:39-44.

    This study used an MRI-derived finite-element model to predict accelerated cartilage thinning patterns similar to those observed in osteoarthritis because of an internal rotation offset, as associated with ACL deficiency.

28. D'Lima DD, Patil S, Steklov N, Slamin JE, Colwell

CW Jr: Tibial forces measured in vivo after total knee arthroplasty. *J Arthroplasty* 2006;21:255-262.

This study used an instrumented tibial prosthesis to measure compressive forces in vivo after total tibial arthroplasty during rehabilitation, rising from a chair, standing, walking, and climbing stairs, which should lead to refined surgical techniques and enhanced prosthetic designs.

29. Chaudhari AM, Dyrby CO, D'Lima DD, Colwell CW, Andriacchi TP: A direct test of the relationship between medial compartment load and the knee adduction moment using an instrumented knee. *Trans Orthop Res Soc* 2006;31:608.

    This study used an instrumented total knee replacement to show that the peak knee adduction moment measured during walking correlates well to the peak medial compartment load, suggesting that adduction moment is an appropriate surrogate measure for compressive load.

30. Nadaud MC, Komistek RD, Mahfouz MR, Dennis DA, Anderle MR: In vivo three-dimensional determination of the effectiveness of the osteoarthritic knee brace: A multiple brace analysis. *J Bone Joint Surg Am* 2005;87:114-119.

    Using dynamic fluoroscopy, this study found that five different off-loader braces had varying abilities to create medial joint space during walking.

31. Pollo FE, Otis JC, Backus SI, Warren RF, Wickiewicz TL: Reduction of medial compartment loads with valgus bracing of the osteoarthritic knee. *Am J Sports Med* 2002;30:414-421.

32. Crenshaw SJ, Pollo FE, Calton EF: Effects of lateral-wedged insoles on kinetics at the knee. *Clin Orthop Relat Res* 2000;375:185-192.

33. Kerrigan DC, Lelas JL, Goggins J, Merriman GJ, Kaplan RJ, Felson DT: Effectiveness of a lateral-wedge insole on knee varus torque in patients with knee osteoarthritis. *Arch Phys Med Rehabil* 2002;83:889-893.

34. Fisher D, Andriacchi T, Alexander E, Dyrby C, Morag E: Initial gait characteristics influence the effect of footwear intervention to modify knee loading. *Trans Orthop Res Soc* 2002;27:700.

35. Prodromos CC, Andriacchi TP, Galante JO: A relationship between gait and clinical changes following high tibial osteotomy. *J Bone Joint Surg Am* 1985;67:1188-1194.

36. Worthen LC, Kim CM, Kautz SA, Lew HL, Kiratli BJ, Beaupre GS: Key characteristics of walking correlate with bone density in individuals with chronic stroke. *J Rehabil Res Dev* 2005;42:761-768.

    This study of patients with walking deficits after stroke demonstrated that the bone density index, which incorporates body weight, steps per day, and ground reaction force magnitude, predicted proximal femoral bone mineral density better than other commonly measured demographic and gait parameters. Level of evidence: III.

4: Lower Extremity

Chapter 31
Pelvic and Acetabular Fractures

*David Templeman, MD   *Paul Tornetta III, MD

Introduction

Trauma to the pelvis results in a spectrum of injuries ranging from minimally displaced fractures to complete disruption of the pelvic ring with life-threatening hemorrhage. Injuries to the pelvis can disrupt the pelvic ring, result in fracture of the acetabulum, or both. Either type of injury requires specific diagnostic imaging and careful assessment of the injury mechanism, pattern, and stability to choose an appropriate method of management.

Pelvic Ring Injuries

Most pelvic ring injuries are low-energy injuries that are stable and can be simply treated by limiting weight bearing until healing occurs. In contrast, some pelvic ring injuries occur in hemodynamically unstable patients and are life-threatening emergencies. Although such high-energy pelvic ring injuries comprise just a small percentage of all pelvic fractures seen by orthopaedic surgeons, they require prompt diagnosis and expert management. Despite a multidisciplinary treatment approach, patient survival after such injuries cannot always be assured. Early deaths from pelvic fractures typically result from hemorrhage; late deaths are usually the result of associated injuries or the development of sepsis and multiple organ system failure.[1-4]

The initial assessment of patients with pelvic fractures from high-energy injuries follows Advanced Trauma Life Support protocols. For many patients, the initial assessment and resuscitation are performed simultaneously. The goal of the initial assessment is to identify the source of hemorrhage, pelvic or otherwise, and then control the bleeding. Resuscitation is started at presentation and is directed at correcting hypotension, acidosis, and coagulopathy. Early replacement of clotting factors and es-

tablishment of normal levels of lactate are important in the initial resuscitation and must be monitored. The initial trauma AP pelvis radiograph provides information that identifies the pattern of pelvic ring injury and is often useful in directing early treatment.

Pelvic injuries are defined as being either stable or unstable; however, this definition can apply to the concept of hemodynamic instability as well as mechanical stability. A skeletally stable pelvic ring injury is one that allows load transfer or protected weight bearing without the risk of progressive deformity until complete soft-tissue healing and bony union occur.[5]

Radiographic assessment of the pelvis is an essential part of the initial evaluation of trauma patients. The development of classification systems by Bucholz, Tile, and Young and Burgess has provided consistently reproducible methods for the grouping of various injuries. The Young and Burgess system is particularly useful in the initial evaluation of patients because this classification may be determined with the AP radiograph only and has been correlated with fluid resuscitation requirements, associated skeletal and solid organ injury, energy transmission to the victim, the need for acute stabilization of pelvic ring injuries in hemodynamically unstable patients, and patient survival.[6]

In addition to a plain AP radiograph, 40° inlet and 40° outlet views are obtained. The caudal/inlet view is useful for detecting the integrity of the pelvic ring because it shows the sacroiliac joints and the sacrum, which can help detect either sacroiliac dislocations or sacral fractures and their displacement in the anteroposterior plane. The outlet view detects superior or inferior displacement and sagittal plane flexion or rotation of the pelvis.

CT remains the most sensitive method to determine posterior ring injuries and their degree of displacement. Four anatomic injuries are consistently seen: sacroiliac dislocations, sacral fractures, iliac wing fractures, and sacroiliac fracture-dislocations. Although not routinely obtained, a lateral radiograph of the sacrum identifies transverse fractures of the sacrum and coccyx and the degree of their displacement. A lateral view should be obtained in instances of bilateral sacral fractures and U-shaped sacral fractures in which there are bilateral vertical fractures through the sacral foramina that connect with a transverse fracture line between the second or third sacral segments. Some patients with these fractures have sacral fracture-dislocations with spinopelvic dissociation and a high incidence of neurologic injuries. The

*David Templeman, MD or the department with which he is affilated has received research or institutional support from Smith & Nephew, royalties from Zimmer, holds stock or stock options in Pfizer, and is a consultant or employee for Stryker and Zimmer. Paul Tornetta III, MD or the department with which he is affiliated has received research or institutional support from Smith & Nephew and is a consultant or employee for Smith & Nephew.

4: Lower Extremity

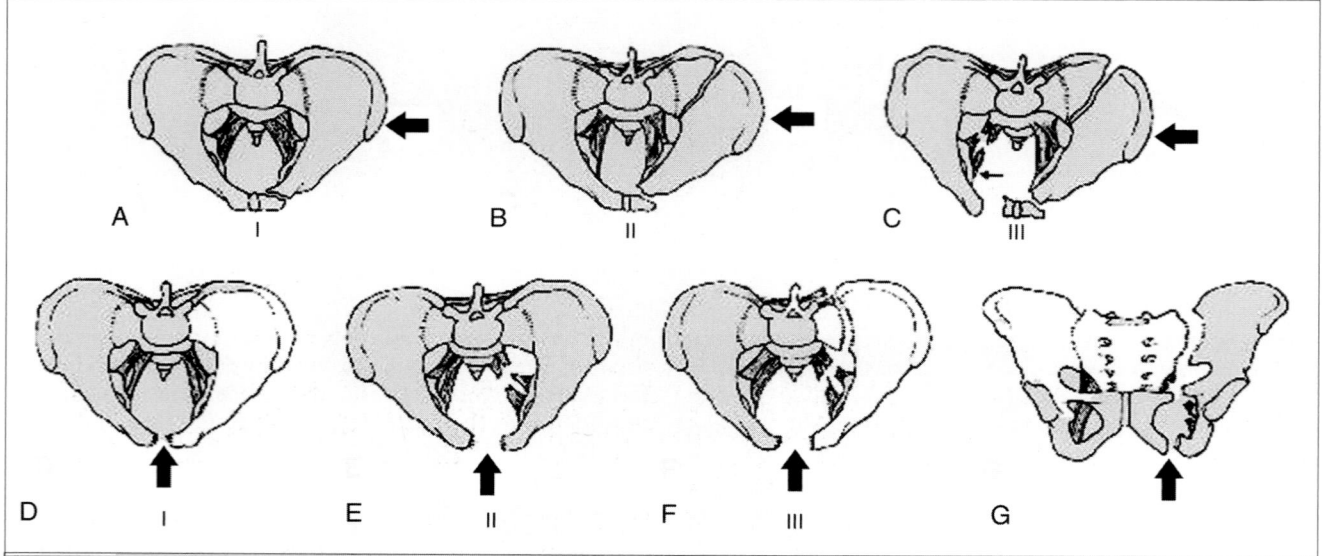

Figure 1 Young-Burgess classification of pelvic injury. The arrows indicate the direction of the force causing the injury. **A**, Lateral compression, grade I. **B**, Lateral compression, grade II. **C**, Lateral compression, grade III. **D**, Anteroposterior compression, grade I. **E**, Anteroposterior compression, grade II. **F**, Anteroposterior compression, grade III. **G**, Vertical shear. *(Reproduced from Tornetta P III: Pelvis and acetabulum: Trauma, in Beaty JH (ed):* Orthopaedic Knowledge Update 6. *Rosemont, IL, American Academy of Orthopaedic Surgeons, 1999, pp 427-439.)*

lateral view will disclose the extent of displacement of the upper sacral segment (usually S2 forward on S3) and the resultant kyphotic deformity. Treatment of these injuries with lumbopelvic fixation has been reported in a small number of patients at tertiary centers, and remains investigational.[7]

The initial examination of the patient requires vigilance to detect open pelvic fractures. Despite advancements in care, a recent study documented a high mortality rate in patients with open pelvic fractures and visceral injuries.[2] Gentle examination of the iliac crests, palpation for instability, and inspection of the perineum and gentle log rolling of the patient to look for open wounds or degloving injuries should be done in all patients. Rectal examination should be performed, and the prostate should be examined. Once the patient has been identified as having an unstable pelvic ring injury, repetitive examinations are contraindicated because they may exacerbate further bleeding.

Urologic injuries are present in 15% of patients with pelvic injuries, and the incidence is higher with greater displacement of the anterior pelvic ring. Urethral injuries occur more often in males because the urethra is longer in males than in females, and a retrograde urethrogram is recommended before passing a Foley catheter when the anterior pelvic ring is disrupted. In females, a Foley catheter can be placed immediately because of the short length of the urethra, and it is followed by careful examination of the perineum and vagina. When the initial urinalysis indicates fewer than 25 red blood cells per highpowered field, an urgent cystogram is not required. The treatment of urethral injuries remains controversial, but studies document that early primary realign-

ment reduces the rates of stricture, incontinence, and impotence. Recent reports continue to document that many patients (both male and female) have sexual dysfunction after pelvic fractures; the causes are multifactorial.[8]

Classification
Several classifications of pelvic ring fractures are used including anatomic descriptions (Letournel and Judet classification of posterior pelvic ring injuries), the mechanistic system of Young and Burgess (**Figure 1**), and systems to predict the stability after injury (Bucholz) (**Figure 2**).[5] All of these classifications are based on the initial radiographic assessment.

Initial Stabilization
Bleeding associated with the pelvic ring fracture is usually from fracture surfaces and from the venous plexus within the pelvis; arterial bleeding is a less frequent cause of significant blood loss.[9]

Skeletal stabilization in the acute setting is most likely to benefit patients with anteroposterior compression injuries that increase the pelvic volume.[3,10] Closure of the anterior pelvic ring is done to decrease pelvic volume and effect tamponade. Pelvic binders, pelvic sheeting with circumferential wraps, military antishock trousers, and external fixation all are effective means to reduce pelvic volume and provide temporary stabilization of the pelvis. Sheeting and pelvic binders can be rapidly applied and are inexpensive.

Pelvic sheeting involves placing a circumferential sheet around the pelvis and then tightening the sheet to reduce its circumference and thereby compress the pel-

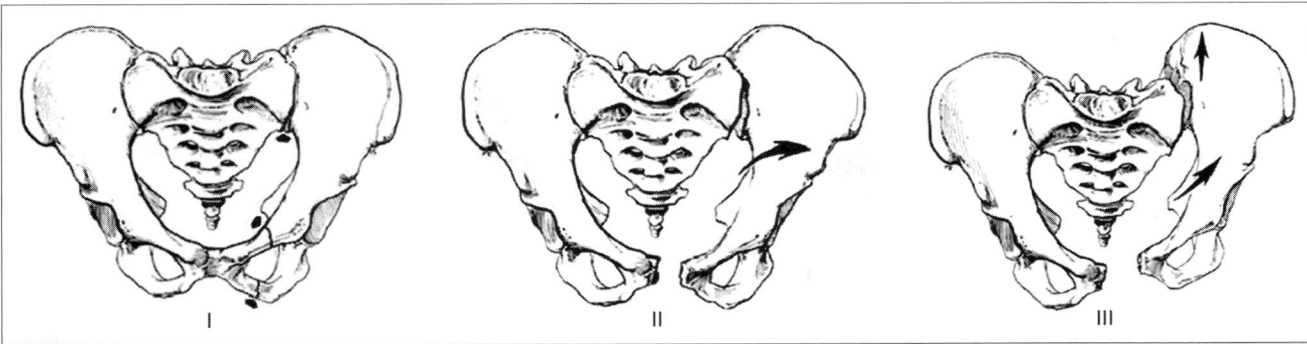

| Figure 2 | Bucholz fracture classification. Type I fractures are stable pelvic ring injuries. Type II fractures have partial or rotational instability and are typically open-book type injuries. Type III fractures have complete instability with disruption at both the anterior and posterior pelvic ring. *(Adapted with permission from Bucholz RW: The pathological anatomy of Malgaigne fracture-dislocations of the pelvis. J Bone Joint Surg Am 1981;63:400-404.)* |

vic ring. Sheeting is indicated in patients with external rotation deformities and is effective in partially reducing the pelvic ring. In contrast, sheeting is of questionable benefit (and may be of potential harm) when applied to patients with lateral compression injuries; however, one study noted no adverse effects in a small number of patients.[3] With cranial displacement of the hemipelvis, skeletal traction achieves further reduction of the pelvic ring. Sheeting should be considered as a temporary treatment because skin ulceration can occur with prolonged use. External fixation applied using a C-clamp with pins inserted into the gluteus medius tubercle and used for patients with anteroposterior compression injuries has been shown to increase systolic blood pressure and improve reduction of the pelvic ring.[10]

In patients with ongoing hemorrhage after initial stabilization, angiography with embolization is effective. The fracture pattern, however, does not always correlate with a vascular injury. Studies have found that arterial bleeding in the pelvis is more common with disruption of the pelvic ring, whereas abdominal bleeding is more common with stable pelvic ring injuries.[11,12] Continued bleeding after arterial embolization mandates that other sources of bleeding be excluded. In one series of patients with persistent hypotension, however, repeated pelvic angiography identified new sources of pelvic bleeding in 68% of patients, recurrent bleeding from a prior site in 18%, and both of these findings in 14%.[9] Institutional resources and their availability play a significant role in determining the timing of these different methods (pelvic sheeting, external fixation, and angiography) to control pelvic bleeding.[5]

Surgical Treatment

Most information available for clinical practice regarding the treatment of pelvic fractures is based on retrospective case studies and a small number of case control studies (level III and level IV evidence-based medicine). Indications for reduction and fixation of pelvic ring injuries include the presence of instability and/or unacceptable deformity of the pelvic ring. These

factors are determined primarily from the radiographic evaluation of pelvic ring injuries and the use of classification systems that predict the stability of the pelvic ring injury; rarely, stress examinations are used to assess vertical stability of the posterior pelvis. Stress examinations should not be used in the setting of zone II (transforaminal) sacral fractures.

A stable pelvic ring injury is defined as one that is able to withstand the physiologic forces incurred with protected weight bearing without resulting in abnormal deformation of the pelvis until bony union or soft-tissue healing occurs. For example, lateral compression can result in injuries to the pelvic ring that are commonly stable. In many patients, lateral compression causes impaction of the anterior part of the sacrum and pubic rami fractures. Nonsurgical treatment is appropriate when there is less than 1 cm of posterior displacement and no neurologic deficit. A series of pelvic radiographs is typically obtained after initial mobilization to confirm that there is no further displacement. Displacement of the innominate bone or sacrum indicates instability, and 1 cm or more of displacement of the posterior pelvic ring is usually considered to be an indication for surgical stabilization.[5]

The approach to the surgical treatment of the pelvic ring requires consideration of both the anterior and posterior ring injuries. Anterior ring injuries are usually pubic ramus fractures or disruptions of the pubic symphysis. Most rami fractures are best managed by nonsurgical treatment because nonunion and symptomatic deformities of the pubic rami are rare. Most authorities emphasize that the initial reduction and fixation of the posterior ring injury usually leads to acceptable position of the pubic rami fractures. In most patients, reduction and fixation of anterior ring fractures is not needed after reduction and fixation of the posterior ring because this restores satisfactory alignment of the pubic rami. When indicated, techniques for stabilization of the anterior ring include anterior pelvic external fixation, open reduction and internal fixation, and intramedullary screw fixation of the superior pubic rami.[5]

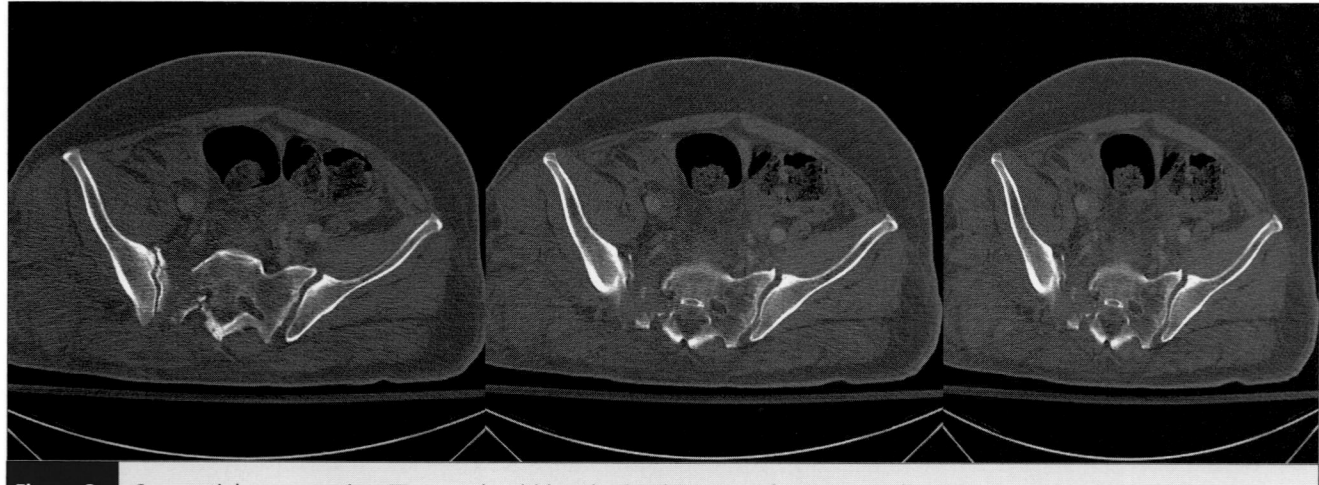

Figure 3 Sequential preoperative CT scans should be obtained to assess for S2 screw fixation; there should be a minimum of 1 cm between the S1 and S2 neural foramina on three sequential preoperative CT 3-mm images.

Closed Versus Open Reduction

The accuracy of the reduction of the pelvic ring has been correlated with good long-term results; loss of reduction and malreductions of 1 cm or greater are associated with inferior results.[13] Whether posterior pelvic ring injuries are best managed by closed reduction and fixation or open reduction and fixation is controversial. Both methods have strong advocates, and no randomized comparative studies have been conducted. The primary issue with the treatment of posterior pelvic ring injuries is the reduction of the deformity rather than the technique of fracture fixation.

For most sacroiliac fracture-dislocations, open reduction and internal fixation are needed to achieve an accurate reduction and appropriate fracture fixation because plate and screw fixation is usually required for this injury pattern. Sacral fractures and sacroiliac dislocations can be stabilized by the percutaneous insertion of iliosacral screws when an accurate reduction is achieved. The success of closed reduction seems to be dependent on early surgical management and accurate intraoperative imaging.

Proponents of closed reduction and percutaneous fixation contend that avoiding open surgical approaches prevents soft-tissue complications, a high incidence of which has been historically reported. A recent multicenter study of open posterior surgical approaches documented a low incidence of complications associated with wound healing (3.9% of patients) and no instances of chronic osteomyelitis.[14] All of these surgical procedures were performed using anatomic dissection of the gluteus maximus as described by Letournel. These data indicate that appropriately performed open reduction is not compromised by soft-tissue complications.

Iliosacral Screw Fixation

Iliosacral screws are used for fixation of sacral fractures, sacroiliac dislocations, and some fracture-dislocations. Mechanical testing indicates that all forms of iliosacral

screw fixation are less stable when compared with mechanical testing of the intact pelvis (with the clinical implication that protected weight bearing is required after fixation). The use of two iliosacral screws is superior to the use of one iliosacral screw with regard to stiffness of the construct and the number of cycles to failure. Iliosacral screw placement is technically demanding, and screw malposition rates of 13% and neurologic complication rates of 8% are documented in different series.[15] The space available for the placement of iliosacral screws is reduced in patients with anatomic variants of sacral formation or in patients in whom the fracture is not accurately reduced. A model of zone II sacral fractures indicated that cranial displacement of greater than 1 cm did not allow for safe placement of an iliosacral screw, underscoring the need for accurate reduction of this fracture pattern.[16]

The safe placement of iliosacral screws into the second sacral segment (S2) has been documented in a clinical series.[17] A minimum distance of 1 cm between the foramina on three sequential preoperative CT slices (thickness, 2 mm) was a prerequisite for this technique (**Figure 3**).

Postoperative loss of reduction and malunion rates as high as 44% have been reported to occur after iliosacral screw fixation.[18] Loss of fixation with this technique has been attributed to the pattern of vertical sacral fractures and osteoporosis.[1]

Outcomes

The meaningful interpretation of much of these data is difficult because multiple injury types were combined when reporting outcomes for groups of patients. It is now known that the injury type (bony or ligamentous), the presence of neurologic or urologic injuries, and the initial displacement play important roles in outcomes.

Outcomes of patients with pelvic injuries correlate with initial displacement and instability. Few outcome data are available for the treatment of stable pelvic in-

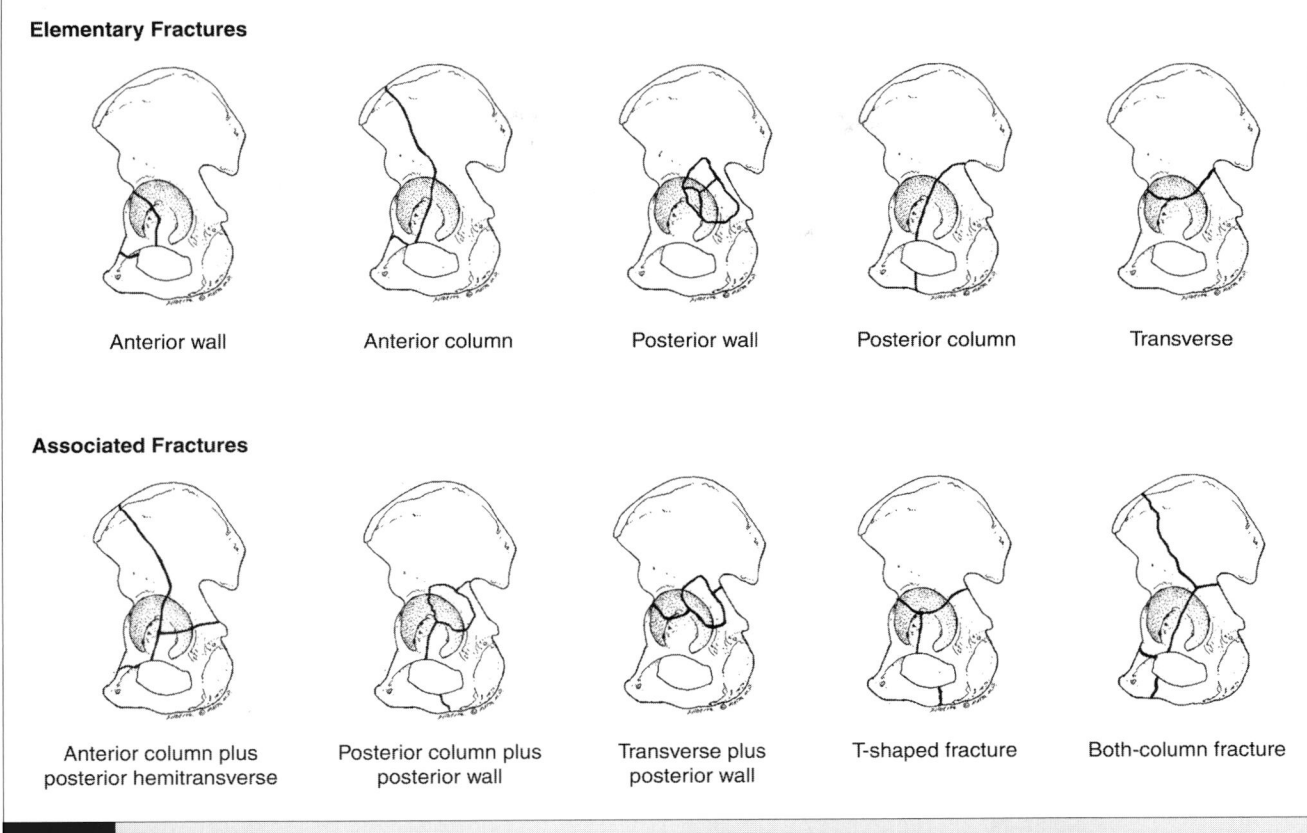

Figure 4 Letournel and Judet classification of acetabular fractures. (Courtesy of Joel M. Matta, MD.)

juries. Rotationally unstable pelvic injuries (Tile type B) tend to have better outcomes than pelvic injuries that are both vertically and rotationally unstable (Tile type C). One series reported 80% good and excellent results in patients with Tile type B injuries compared with only 20% in those with Tile type C injuries.[19] A multicenter study documented a 36% incidence of pain among all patients with pelvic fractures, but a 60% incidence in those with Tile type C injuries.[20] Newer treatment techniques, usually with iliosacral screws for sacroiliac dislocations and sacral fractures and plate and screw fixation for sacroiliac fracture-dislocations, can maintain the reduction to union when the fracture is reduced. Maintenance of reduction reduces the incidence of nonunion, limb-length discrepancy, sitting imbalance, and gait disturbance. The long-term outcome, however, is more likely to be affected by associated injuries than by a properly treated pelvic fracture. It is important to review this information with patients with these injuries.[5]

Acetabular Fractures

Although the incidence of acetabular fractures is relatively low (estimated at 3 per 100,000 patients annually), an increase in the incidence of acetabular fractures caused by simple falls and an increase in the proportion of women with acetabular fractures have been noted; most of these fractures occur in older patients.[21]

Displaced acetabular fractures are best treated with open anatomic reduction and stable internal fixation. The most common long-term complication of this injury is posttraumatic arthrosis. The results of surgical treatment have been highly correlated with the accuracy of reduction, and tertiary centers with trauma specialists report better results than smaller centers with surgery performed by many surgeons.[22,23]

The Letournel classification is widely used to categorize acetabular fractures (**Figure 4**), and high rates of intraobserver and interobserver reliability have been documented using this classification.[24] The radiographic evaluation of acetabular fractures includes an AP pelvic radiograph and the Judet views (45° obturator and iliac oblique projections), which are used to classify the fracture. A CT scan is also obtained to detect posterior pelvic ring injuries, femoral head fractures, intra-articular fragments, and marginal impaction of the articular surfaces.

Treatment

The decision whether nonsurgical or surgical treatment is indicated depends on many factors, including frac-

4: Lower Extremity

ture pattern, fracture displacement, patient comorbidities (including osteoporosis), and the technical ability to anatomically reconstruct the acetabulum. Studies indicate that when fractures involve more than 40% of the posterior wall the hip will be unstable.[25] For fractures with less than 40% involvement or those with marginal impaction, a fluoroscopic stress view of the hip is done. This procedure is performed with the patient under general anesthesia and is considered positive if any widening of the hip occurs with flexion and axial loading of the femur. Both AP and obturator oblique views are used. Instability is reported when 15% or more of the posterior wall is involved.[22]

Posterior Wall Fractures

Posterior wall fractures are the most common type of acetabular fractures, and they also have the highest incidence of poor results. Postoperative CT scans are more sensitive than postoperative plain radiographs in assessing the accuracy of reduction. Reduction as judged by CT scans correlates with long-term results. Factors associated with poor results include delay in the reduction of the dislocation, age older than 55 years, intra-articular comminution, and osteonecrosis. The rate of osteonecrosis after fracture-dislocation is lower than previously believed, approximately 5% of patients.[22]

Associated fracture patterns are more difficult to reduce than simple fracture patterns, and delays to surgical treatment are associated with poor results. Anatomic reduction is more likely to be achieved when associated injury patterns are treated surgically within 5 days of injury, whereas delays of up to 15 days after injury may be acceptable for elementary fractures; therefore, early recognition of posterior wall acetabular fractures and careful evaluation of patients needing surgery for potential transfer are recommended.[23,26]

The quality of reduction for posterior wall fractures is reported with different definitions in published studies. The term "satisfactory reduction" is misleading because it may include displacements that are not consistent with good results. A more precise definition would identify anatomic reduction as within 0 to 1 mm of displacement, imperfect reduction as having 2 to 3 mm of displacement, and poor reduction having more than 3 mm of displacement.

Although the outcome of surgery is most significantly correlated with the quality of reduction, associations with injuries to the femoral head, increasing patient age, and surgical complications are all related to poor results. Surgical complications include neurologic injury, infection, deep venous thrombosis, and heterotopic bone. Body mass index has a significant relationship with estimated blood loss, rate of wound infection, and rate of deep venous thrombosis. Morbidly obese patients (body mass index > 40) are five times more likely to have a wound infection.[27]

Most studies focus on the clinical results after acetabular fractures and have not consistently reported functional outcomes assessments from the patient's point of view. For acetabular fractures, the Merle d'Aubigne scale or one of its modifications is frequently used to assess outcomes, although this evaluation scale has not been validated. Comparison of Musculoskeletal Function Assessment (MFA) and Merle d'Aubigne scale scores indicate a possible ceiling effect of the latter. MFA scores indicate that complete return to normal function is uncommon despite good to excellent Merle d'Aubigne scale scores in the same patients. This finding may limit the usefulness of the Merle d'Aubigne scale in reporting functional outcomes, particularly in young or active patients.[27]

Functional studies have documented that muscle strength after repair of acetabular fractures correlates with MFA scores.[28,29] Decreases in the strength of hip flexion and hip extension have been noted to negatively affect functional outcomes. The ability to detect and improve factors related to the recovery of muscle strength may make it possible to improve the results of future treatment.

Heterotopic ossification is related to the degree of muscle injury and/or surgical approach. The use of an extensile approach is associated with the consistent formation of heterotopic bone, and some form of prophylaxis is recommended with the use of extensile approaches. Treatment with indomethacin, radiation therapy, and combinations of these have been described with conflicting results; however, the use of some form of prophylaxis is recommended when extensile approaches are used.[30]

Deep Venous Thrombosis

Deep venous thrombosis is a cause of morbidity and mortality after pelvic and acetabular fractures, and thrombosis rates as high as 61% have been reported when patients with these injuries do not receive prophylaxis. The mortality rate from pulmonary embolism in the absence of treatment is 2% in this population. There is no recognized gold standard for diagnosing pelvic thrombi. Magnetic resonance venography, contrast CT, and direct cannulation venography can detect pelvic clots, but do so with different rates of false-positive and false-negative results. Duplex ultrasound, although reliable for the detection of extremity thrombosis, is considered inaccurate for the detection of pelvic thrombi. A recent study of surveillance screening with duplex ultrasound found that this strategy was not effective in reducing the rate of pulmonary embolism when compared with a group of patients who did not have screening.[31] Because no gold standard exists to diagnose pelvic thrombi, no widely accepted protocols for the prophylactic treatment of patients with pelvic or acetabular fractures have been established. Forms of mechanical prophylaxis as well as warfarin, heparin, and low-molecular-weight heparin are all used.[31,32]

The use of pulsatile pneumatic compression stockings applied at the time of admission with the addition of low-molecular-weight heparin at a later time was found to be more effective in preventing large or occlusive thrombi than the use of low-molecular-weight heparin alone.

Patients who are older and those with delay to surgery are at increased risk for the development of deep venous thrombosis. Patients with thrombi identified before surgery are often treated with vena caval filters to allow the surgery to proceed. Long-term follow-up of patients with pelvic fractures who received inferior vena caval filters has shown low rates of complications.[33]

Annotated References

1. Griffin DR, Starr AJ, Reinert CM, Jones AL, Whitlock S: Vertically unstable pelvic fractures fixed with percutaneous iliosacral screws: Does posterior injury pattern predict fixation failure? *J Orthop Trauma* 2006; 20(suppl 1):S30-S36.

   This retrospective review was conducted to measure the failure rate of percutaneous iliosacral screw fixation of vertically unstable pelvic fractures and to test the hypothesis that fixations for which the posterior injury is a vertical fracture of the sacrum are more likely to fail than those for dislocations or fracture-dislocations of the sacroiliac joint. The authors found that this increased likelihood of failure did not occur in patients with dislocations or fracture-dislocations of the sacroiliac joint, leading them to conclude that percutaneous iliosacral screw fixation is a useful technique for treating vertically unstable pelvic fractures. For patients with vertical sacral fractures, however, the authors cautioned surgeons to be wary of fixation failure and loss of reduction. Level of evidence: IV.

2. Dente CJ, Feliciano DV, Rozycki GS, et al: The outcome of open pelvic fractures in the modern era. *Am J Surg* 2005;190:830-835.

   In this study, 44 patients were identified as having open pelvic fractures (average injury severity score, 30). The overall mortality rate was 45%, with 11 early deaths and 9 late deaths (average time to death, 17 days). The risk factors for overall mortality included vertical shear pattern of injury, revised trauma score, transfusion requirements, and injury severity score. Level of evidence: IV.

3. Krieg JC, Mohr M, Ellis TJ, Simpson TS, Madey SM, Bottlang M: Emergent stabilization of pelvic ring injuries by controlled circumferential compression: A clinical trial. *J Trauma* 2005;59:659-664.

   This article presents the results of a prospective clinical trial of pelvic circumferential compression using a commercially available device comparable to pelvic sheeting. The authors evaluated 16 patients with pelvic ring injuries. In patients with external rotation injuries, pelvic circumferential compression significantly reduced pelvic width and closely approximated the reduction of pelvic width that was achieved by later definitive stabilization. In patients with internal rotation injuries, pelvic circumferential compression did not cause significant overcompression. Level of evidence: III.

4. Lindahl J, Hirvensalo E: Outcome of operatively treated type-C injuries of the pelvic ring. *Acta Orthop* 2005;76:667-678.

   The reported findings suggested a correlation between an excellent reduction followed by sufficient fixation of the pelvic ring and functional outcome. Unsatisfactory reduction (displacement > 5 mm), failure of fixation, loss of reduction, and a permanent lumbosacral plexus were the most common reasons for an unsatisfactory functional result. Level of evidence: IV.

5. Olson SA, Burgess A: Classification and initial management of patients with unstable pelvic ring injuries. *Instr Course Lect* 2005;54:383-393.

   The authors discuss current methods of evaluating, assessing, and treating unstable pelvic ring injuries in hemodynamically unstable patients. They recommend that surgeons first determine whether patients have hemodynamic instability and identify the source of the hemorrhage. Patients should then be assessed for stabilization of unstable pelvic ring injuries. Level of evidence: IV-V.

6. Dalal SA, Burgess AR, Siegel JH, et al: Pelvic fracture in multiple trauma: Classification by mechanism is key to pattern of organ injury, resuscitative requirements, and outcome. *J Trauma* 1989;29:981-1000.

7. Schildhauer TA, Bellabara C, Nork SE, Barei DP, Routt ML Jr, Chapman JR: Decompression and lumbopelvic fixation for sacral fracture-dislocations with spinopelvic dissociation. *J Orthop Trauma* 2006;20:447-457.

   The authors of this study reported the results of sacral decompression and lumbopelvic fixation of neurologically impaired patients with displaced comminuted sacral fracture-dislocations that resulted in spinopelvic dissociation. The sacral fractures healed in 18 of 19 patients available for 12-month follow-up without loss of reduction. Of these 18 patients, all had been treated with open reduction, sacral decompression, and lumbopelvic fixation. Level of evidence: IV.

8. Ozumba D, Starr AJ, Benedetti GE, Whitlock SN, Frawley WH: Male sexual function after pelvic fracture. *Orthopedics* 2004;27:313-318.

   The authors asked 51 male patients with prior pelvic fracture to complete a Brief Sexual Function Inventory questionnaire 2 years after injury and compared their scores to those of 53 men with ankle fractures. Patients with pelvic fractures were noted to have significantly poorer sexual function than those with ankle fractures. Older patients had significantly poorer sexual function than younger patients. Level of evidence: IV.

9. Gourlay D, Hoffer E, Routt M, Bulger E: Pelvic angiography for recurrent traumatic pelvic arterial hemorrhage. *J Trauma* 2005;59:1168-1173.

   The authors describe a small subset of patients requiring repeat pelvic angiogram for continued arterial bleeding after an initial angiographic embolization. At repeat angiogram, 68% of the patients were identified as having a new bleeding site. The authors concluded that although angiographic control of traumatic pelvic arterial hemorrhage is successful, recurrent pelvic arterial hemorrhage can occur. This small subgroup of patients benefited from repeat angiography and embolization. Level of evidence: IV.

4: Lower Extremity

10. Archdeacon MT, Hiratzka J: The trochanteric C-clamp for provisional pelvic stability. *J Orthop Trauma* 2006; 20:47-51.

    The authors modified the pelvic clamp technique by applying the clamp to the trochanteric region of the femur. They reported that this resulted in a reduction force comparable to that of a pelvic binder or external fixator. Level of evidence: IV.

11. Kryer HM, Miller FB, Evers BM, Rouben LR, Seligson DL: Pelvic fracture classification: Correlation with hemorrhage. *J Trauma* 1988;28:973-980.

12. Poole GV, Ward EF: Causes of mortality in patients with pelvic fractures. *Orthopedics* 1994;17:691-696.

13. Matta JM, Tornetta P III : Internal fixation of unstable pelvic ring injuries. *Clin Orthop Relat Res* 1996;329: 129-140.

14. Stover MD, Sims SH, Templeman DC, Merkle P, Matta JM: Is the posterior approach to pelvic ring injuries associated with a high rate of soft tissue complications? *14th Annual Meeting Proceedings*. Rosemont, IL, Orthopaedic Trauma Association, October 1998.

15. Moed BR, Ahmad BK, Craig JG, et al: Intraoperative monitoring with stimulus-evoked electromyography during placement of iliosacral screws: An initial clinical study. *J Bone Joint Surg Am* 1998;80:537-546.

16. Reilly MC, Bono CM, Litkouhi B, Sirkin M, Behrens FF: The effect of sacral fracture malreduction on the safe placement of iliosacral screws. *J Orthop Trauma* 2003;17:88-94.

17. Moed BR, Geer BL: S2 iliosacral screw fixation for disruptions of the posterior pelvic ring: A report of 49 cases. *J Orthop Trauma* 2006;20:378-383.

    The authors present a retrospective study of 49 patients treated with placement of 53 S2 iliosacral screws. The authors reported no intraoperative iatrogenic nerve injuries. Two patients had postoperative loss of reduction secondary to osteopenia. Satisfactory screw position was documented on postoperative CT scans for all patients. Level of evidence: IV.

18. Keating JF, Werier J, Blachut P, Broekhuyse H, Meek RN, O'Brien PJ: Early fixation of the vertically unstable pelvis: The role of iliosacral screw fixation of the posterior lesion. *J Orthop Trauma* 1999;13:107-113.

19. Pohlemann T, Gänsslen A, Schellwald O, Cullemann U, Tscherne H: Outcome after pelvic ring injuries. *Injury* 1996;27(Suppl 2):B31-B38.

20. Kellam JF, McMurty RY, Paley D, Tile M: The unstable pelvic fracture: Operative treatment. *Orthop Clin North Am* 1987;18:25-41.

21. Laird A, Keating JF: Acetabular fractures: A 16-year prospective epidemiological study. *J Bone Joint Surg Br* 2005;87:969-973.

    The authors present a prospective study of the epidemiology of acetabular fractures at a center in the United Kingdom over a 16-year period (1988 to December 2003). The authors noted a significant decrease in the mortality rate and a reduction in the median injury severity score of patients treated during this period. This was likely the result of an increased number of elderly patients falling and sustaining acetabular fractures during this period. The rate of osteoarthritis during this treatment period was reduced from 31% to 14%, which was believed to be because of increasing subspecialization. Level of evidence: III.

22. Tornetta P III: Displaced acetabular fractures: Indications for operative and nonoperative management. *J Am Acad Orthop Surg* 2001;9:18-28.

23. Giannoudis PV, Grotz MR, Papakostidis C, Dinopoulos H: Operative treatment of displaced fractures of the acetabulum: A meta-analysis. *J Bone Joint Surg Br* 2005; 87:2-9.

    The authors conducted a meta-analysis of 3,670 acetabular fractures reported in the literature and found that osteoarthritis was the most common long-term complication, occurring in approximately 20% of patients. The authors believed that the timing for tertiary referral should be undertaken as early as possible after injury because the timing of surgery was noted to be "of the utmost importance." Level of evidence: IV.

24. Beaule PE, Dorey FJ, Matta JM: Letournel classification for acetabular fractures: Assessment of interobserver and intraobserver reliability. *J Bone Joint Surg Am* 2003;85-A:1704-1709.

25. Tornetta P III: Displaced acetabular fractures: Indications for operative and nonoperative management. *J Am Acad Orthop Surg* 2001;9:18-28.

26. Madhu R, Kotnis R, Al-Mousawi A, et al: Outcome of surgery for reconstruction of fractures of the acetabulum: The time dependent effect of delay. *J Bone Joint Surg Br* 2006;88:1197-1203.

    This retrospective review of 237 patients who were treated for displaced fractures of the acetabulum was conducted to assess the effect of the length of time to surgical reconstruction. For patients with elementary fracture patterns, an increase in the time to surgery of greater than 15 days was associated with poorer results. For those with associated fractures, an excellent and good functional outcome was more likely when surgery was performed within 10 days. The authors concluded that the time to surgery is a significant predictor of radiographic and functional outcome for patients with elementary and associated displaced fractures of the acetabulum, highlighting the importance of early recognition and, if needed, timely transfer of these patients to tertiary care centers. Level of evidence: III.

27. Kreder HJ, Rozen N, Borkhoff CM, et al: Determinants of functional outcomes after simple and complex acetabular fractures involving the posterior wall. *J Bone Joint Surg Br* 2006;88:776-782.

    Marginal impaction and residual displacement of

greater than 2 mm were associated with the development of arthritis, which correlated with poor function and the need for hip replacement. There was a high rate of early conversion to total hip replacement in patients older than 50 years who presented with marginal impaction and comminution of the posterior wall. The authors concluded that this specific subset of patients should be considered for early total hip replacement. Level of evidence: IV.

28. Karunakar MA, Shah SN, Jerabek S: Body mass index as a predictor of complications after operative treatment of acetabular fractures. *J Bone Joint Surg Am* 2005;87: 1498-1502.

   The authors of this study reported that patients who were morbidly obese with a body mass index of greater than 30 were 2.1 times more likely than patients of normal weight to have increased blood loss and 2.6 times more likely to have deep venous thrombosis. Patients with a body mass index of greater than 40 were five times more likely to have a wound infection. The authors concluded that body mass index is predictive of complications after surgical treatment of acetabular fractures. Level of evidence: IV.

29. Borrelli J Jr, Ricci WM, Anglen JO, Gregush R, Engsberg J: Muscle strength recovery and its effect on outcome after open reduction and internal fixation of acetabular fractures. *J Orthop Trauma* 2006;20:388-395.

   The authors compared the hip muscle strength and MFA scores of patients treated for acetabular fractures via an anterior approach to determine the relationship between muscle strength recovery and functional outcome. They reported that hip muscle strength after surgical repair of displaced acetabular fractures directly influenced patient outcome. For all measures of hip muscle strength, the affected side was typically weaker than the unaffected side. Level of evidence: III.

30. Griffin DB, Beaule PE, Matta JM: Safety and efficacy of the extended iliofemoral approach in the treatment of complex fractures of the acetabulum. *J Bone Joint Surg Br* 2005;87:1391-1396.

   The authors reviewed the use of the extended iliofemoral approach as described by Letournel in 106 patients. At a mean 6.3-year follow-up (range, 2 to 17 years), all patients had achieved union of the fractures and reduc-

tion was graded as anatomic in 76 patients (72%), imperfect in 23 (22%), and poor in six (6%). The authors concluded that the extended iliofemoral approach can be safely used in selected patients with complex acetabular fractures and that it results in acceptable clinical outcomes and an acceptable complication rate. The authors strongly advised the use of prophylaxis against heterotopic ossification in this patient population. Level of evidence: IV.

31. Borer DS, Starr AJ, Reinert CM, et al: The effect of screening for deep vein thrombosis on the prevalence of pulmonary embolism in patients with fractures of the pelvis or acetabulum: A review of 973 patients. *J Orthop Trauma* 2005;19:92-95.

   In this study, patients were treated with the same prophylaxis against deep venous thrombosis, and two time periods were compared: one during which a screening protocol for deep venous thrombosis using ultrasound and magnetic resonance venography was used (486 patients) and one during which no screening was used (487 patients). The authors reported no significant difference in the prevalence of pulmonary embolism when comparing the two groups. Level of evidence: IV.

32. Stannard JP, Singhania AK, Lopez-Ben RR, et al: Deep-vein thrombosis in high-energy skeletal trauma despite thromboprophylaxis. *J Bone Joint Surg Br* 2005;87: 965-968.

   The authors of this study reported the incidence and location of deep venous thrombosis in 300 patients who were assessed using magnetic resonance venography and duplex ultrasound. Despite thromboprophylaxis, 11.5% of the patients developed venous thromboembolism disease, with an incidence of 10% in those with nonpelvic trauma and 12.2% in the group with pelvic trauma. When compared with magnetic resonance venography, duplex ultrasound had a false-negative rate of 77% in diagnosing pelvic deep venous thrombosis. As this study notes, there is no gold standard yet available for the diagnosis of pelvic venous thrombosis. Level of evidence: III.

33. Webb LX, Rush PT, Fuller SB, Meredith JW: Greenfield filter prophylaxis of pulmonary embolism in patients undergoing surgery for acetabular fracture. *J Orthop Trauma* 1992;6:139-145.

4: Lower Extremity

Chapter 32
Hip Trauma

Robert V. Cantu, MD   *Kenneth J. Koval, MD

Introduction

As the population continues to age, it is estimated that the number of low-energy hip fractures in elderly individuals will increase exponentially. It is predicted that by the year 2050, 6.3 million hip fractures yearly will occur worldwide.[1] In younger individuals, high-energy trauma can result in hip fractures and dislocations. These injuries can be technically challenging to treat and can result in substantial morbidity.

Hip Dislocations

Hip dislocations, excluding prosthetic dislocations, typically result from high-energy mechanisms such as a motor vehicle collision or a fall from a height. The direction of the dislocation depends on the position of the hip at the time of impact and the direction of the applied force. Most hip dislocations (90%) are posterior.[2] Associated injuries are common and Advanced Trauma Life Support treatment guidelines should be followed. Radiographic evaluation of the pelvis and entire femur may show the most common associated musculoskeletal injuries including fractures of the ipsilateral acetabulum, pelvis, and femoral head, neck, and shaft. Associated injuries to the ipsilateral knee are common. Dashboard impact injuries can result in ligamentous knee injuries, such as posterior cruciate ligament injuries or complete dislocation. Once the hip is reduced, a thorough knee examination should be performed to rule out a ligamentous injury.

The risk of osteonecrosis, with a reported incidence varying from 2% to 40%, is a concern after hip dislocation.[3,4] When reduction is performed within 6 hours of injury, the rate of osteonecrosis seems to be lower with rates from 2% to 10%.[5] Signs of osteonecrosis are most likely to occur within the first year after injury, but have been reported as late as 5 years.[6] Weight bearing is typically limited for 6 weeks after the dislocation and then advanced as tolerated. For patients who remain symptomatic for more than 2 to 3 months after injury, MRI can be useful in detecting osteonecrosis be-

fore structural changes have occurred. Patients whose plain radiographs show changes in the femoral head should also undergo MRI to better evaluate for osteonecrosis.

Posterior Hip Dislocations

Posterior hip dislocations are far more common than anterior dislocations. The hip is typically flexed and adducted at the time of impact, as is the case with knee injuries caused by impact with an automobile dashboard. Patients present with the leg in a flexed, adducted, and internally rotated position. Depending on the position of the leg at time of impact, a posterior wall acetabular fracture may result from the dislocation (**Figure 1**). Sciatic nerve injury can occur, with the risk increasing with delayed reduction or if a patient is transferred between hospitals without hip reduction.[7] Closed reduction of a posterior dislocation involves flexing the hip while applying traction, adduction, and gentle external rotation. To achieve a successful reduction without undue force, muscle relaxation and stabilization of the pelvis are essential. Femoral neck fracture has occurred from repeated, forceful attempts at reduction. If closed reduction is unsuccessful, open reduction is performed through a posterior Kocher-Langenbeck approach. It is important to identify and carefully protect the sciatic nerve when using this approach. Large posterior wall fractures that result in instability should be reduced and stabilized.

After closed reduction, hip stability should be assessed. Cadaveric studies have suggested that most pos-

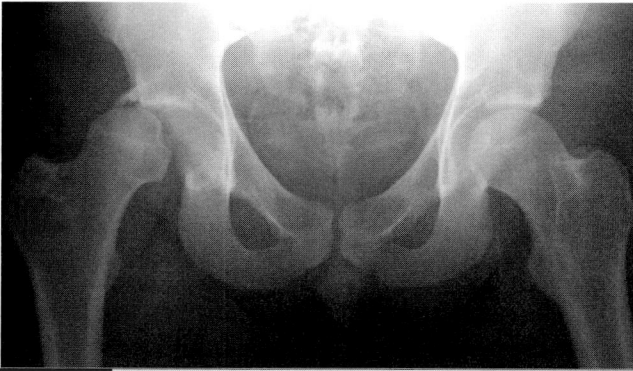

Figure 1   Radiograph of a right hip posterior dislocation with a posterior wall acetabular fracture.

4: Lower Extremity

Kenneth J. Koval, MD or the department with which he is affiliated has received royalties from Biomet and is a consultant or employee of Stryker.

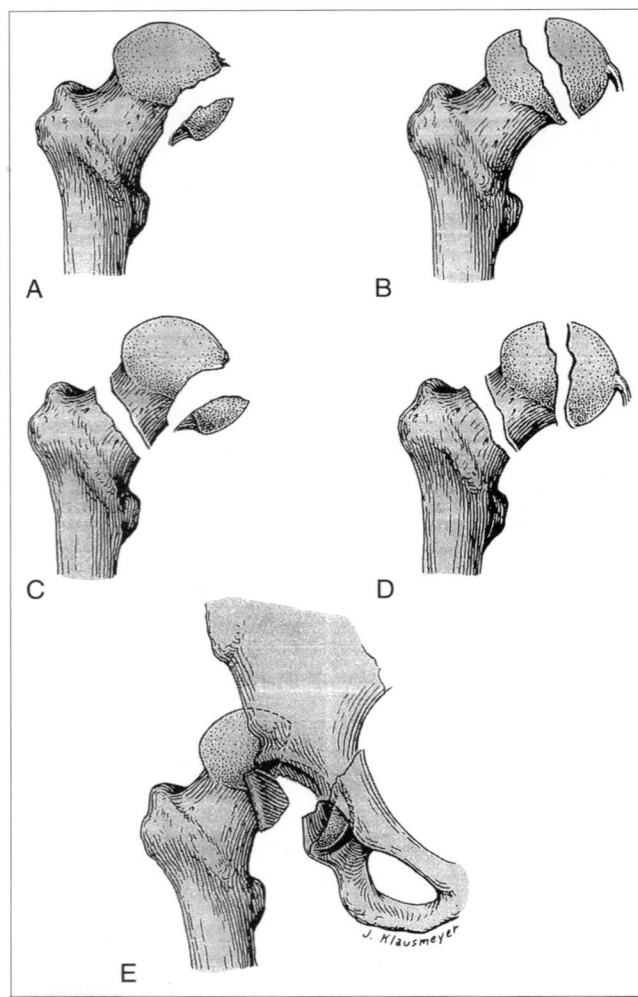

Figure 2 Pipkin classification of femoral head fractures. **A,** Infrafoveal fracture, Pipkin type 1. **B,** Suprafoveal fracture, Pipkin type II. **C** and **D,** Intrafoveal fracture or suprafoveal fracture associated with a femoral neck fracture, Pipkin type III. **E,** Any femoral head fracture configuration associated with an acetabular fracture, Pipkin type IV. *(Reproduced with permission from Swionkowski MF: Intrascapular hip fractures, in Browner BD, Jupiter JB, Levine AM, Trafton PG (eds): Skeletal Trauma: Basic Science, Management, and Reconstruction, ed 2. Philadelphia, PA, WB Saunders, p 1756.)*

to detect associated fractures or loose intra-articular fragments. Some authors have recommended hip arthroscopy to assess for loose fragments and labral and cartilage pathology.[10] Arthroscopy has limitations because only portions of the femoral head and acetabulum can be visualized. The torn hip capsule does not permit the same degree of distention and visualization as in a nontraumatic setting.

Anterior Hip Dislocations

Although anterior hip dislocations are less common (10% incidence) than posterior dislocations, anterior hip dislocations are important to recognize because they have a higher risk of vascular injury (external iliac or femoral vessels).[11] The mechanism producing an anterior dislocation is usually a combination of a forceful hip abduction and external rotation. On initial presentation, the leg is often in a moderately flexed, abducted, and externally rotated position. The reduction maneuver involves applying traction to the extremity while extending and internally rotating the hip. Muscle relaxation is essential to facilitate a gentle reduction. Following reduction, CT is recommended to evaluate the reduction and detect associated fractures or intra-articular loose fragments.

Associated femoral head fractures can occur and are described as either transchondral or indentation fractures. Transchondral fragments preventing concentric reduction require either open reduction and internal fixation (ORIF) or excision, depending on their size and location, whereas indentation fractures are managed with observation. Hip precautions following reduction include avoidance of external rotation until the capsule and soft tissues around the hip have healed. Inability to perform a closed reduction can result from an associated femoral head or acetabular fracture, or entrapment of the hip capsule. In this situation, open reduction is necessary using an anterior approach.

Complications

Anterior hip dislocations can result in major vascular injury requiring emergent surgical treatment. Posterior dislocations are less likely to produce a significant vascular injury, but commonly cause injury to the sciatic nerve (in up to 16% of patients).[7] Delayed complications following dislocation include osteoarthritis and osteonecrosis. MRI is helpful in making the diagnosis of osteonecrosis before structural changes in the femoral head have occurred. When advanced osteonecrosis has occurred, hip arthroplasty may be required to relieve pain and help restore function.

Femoral Head Fractures

Femoral head fractures occur in 6% to 16% of hip dislocations and also can occur without dislocation of the hip.[12] The Pipkin classification system is commonly used to describe femoral head fractures (**Figure 2**). A Pipkin type I injury is a femoral head fracture inferior

terior wall fragments involving less than 25% of the wall are stable, whereas fragments involving more than 50% are unstable.[8] Stability for fragments involving from 25% to 50% of the posterior wall is less predictable. The stability of the hip can be assessed by examining hip range of motion under fluoroscopy.[9] If instability is indicated by any subluxation of the hip with flexion, adduction, and internal rotation, the posterior wall fracture should be fixed. Precautions following closed or open reduction include avoiding hip flexion of more than 90°, avoiding internal rotation, and avoiding adduction. Postreduction CT scanning is used

to the fovea centralis of the femoral head. A type II injury occurs when the fracture extends superior to the fovea. A type III injury is defined as a femoral neck fracture associated with either a type I or II femoral head fracture. A type IV fracture involves an acetabular fracture associated with either a type I or II femoral head fracture.

Treatment of femoral head fractures depends on the location and size of the fracture and the stability of the hip. If the hip is dislocated, it should be reduced as soon as possible. Following reduction, CT is used to assess the location, size, and displacement of the fracture. Pipkin type I fractures with minimal displacement can be treated nonsurgically. Displaced type I fragments can be excised if small, but larger fragments require ORIF to maintain hip stability. Because Pipkin type II fractures involve the weight-bearing portion of the femoral head, anatomic reduction and stable internal fixation is needed. Most type II fractures are best visualized using the anterior Smith-Petersen approach. It has been suggested that using an anterior approach following a posterior hip dislocation may lead to increased rates of osteonecrosis, but this has not been proven.[13] Anatomically, a direct anterior approach does not threaten injury to the vascular supply to the femoral head. An experienced surgeon can consider using a trochanteric flip osteotomy and surgical dislocation of the femoral head; this approach may be especially valuable for Pipkin type IV fractures.

After the fracture is exposed and reduced, either headless screws or countersunk small fragment screws are used to provide fixation. Titanium screws are advantageous if later MRI is needed to assess for osteonecrosis. Type III fractures in young, active patients are treated with ORIF of the femoral neck fracture, followed by internal fixation of the femoral head fracture. In elderly patients with low functional demands, treatment usually involves prosthetic replacement. Treatment of type IV fractures depends on the acetabular fracture size, pattern, and displacement and on the concentricity of the hip. For unstable patterns or nonconcentric reductions, treatment includes ORIF of the acetabular and femoral head fractures.

Long-term complications following femoral head fractures include osteonecrosis and degenerative arthritis. Type I fractures have the best prognosis, with complication rates similar to those of simple dislocations. Type III and IV fractures have a worse prognosis with increased rates of osteonecrosis and decreased functional outcomes.[14]

Hip Fractures

Hip fractures are a significant public health concern. In the United States, the elderly population is the fastest growing segment of society and it is estimated that as many as 1 in 3 women and 1 in 12 men will sustain a hip fracture during their lifetime.[15] Hip fracture is the second leading cause of hospitalization for elderly patients. Approximately 50% of elderly patients are un-

Table 1

Risk Factors for Osteoporosis and Hip Fracture

Nonmodifiable Risk Factors	Modifiable Risk Factors
Older age	Decreased physical activity
Family history	Smoking history
Female gender	Poor nutrition
Medical history	Medication usage
Hyperthyroidism	Glucocorticoids
Hyperparathyroidism	Anticonvulsants
Rheumatoid arthritis	Methotrexate
Hypercalciuria	Cyclosporin
Testosterone/estradiol deficiency	Excessive alcohol intake
Previous fragility fracture	Inadequate calcium/ vitamin D intake

able to walk independently after a hip fracture.[16] Inpatient mortality for elderly patients with a hip fracture ranges from 3% to 10% and the 1-year mortality rate ranges from 14% to 36%.[17] Inpatient survival seems to be improved when surgery is performed within 48 hours of hospital admission.[18] Factors associated with increased mortality include advanced age, male gender, comorbid illnesses, institutionalized living, and psychiatric illness.

Multiple risk factors are associated with osteoporosis and subsequent hip fracture (**Table 1**). Some risk factors cannot be changed, such as the patient's age, gender, family history, and certain medical conditions. Other risk factors can be modified by, for example, improving diet, smoking cessation, avoidance of excessive alcohol intake, and increasing the level of physical activity. In male patients, a low level of either estradiol or both estradiol and testosterone, but not testosterone alone, has been associated with an increased risk for hip fractures.[19] Recent studies have shown that a structured program that includes strength conditioning and exercises to improve balance along with activities such as tai chi can reduce the likelihood of falls in older individuals.[20]

Although most hip fractures in older patients result from low-energy falls, young adults usually sustain hip fractures from high-energy trauma. Motor vehicle crashes and falls from a height are the most common causes of these higher-energy fractures. These patients often have associated injuries that may be life threatening.

Femoral Neck Fractures

Classification
Multiple classification systems exist for femoral neck fractures. Fractures can be classified based on their anatomic location—subcapital, transcervical, or basicervical. The Garden classification system consists of four fracture types based on displacement of the frac-

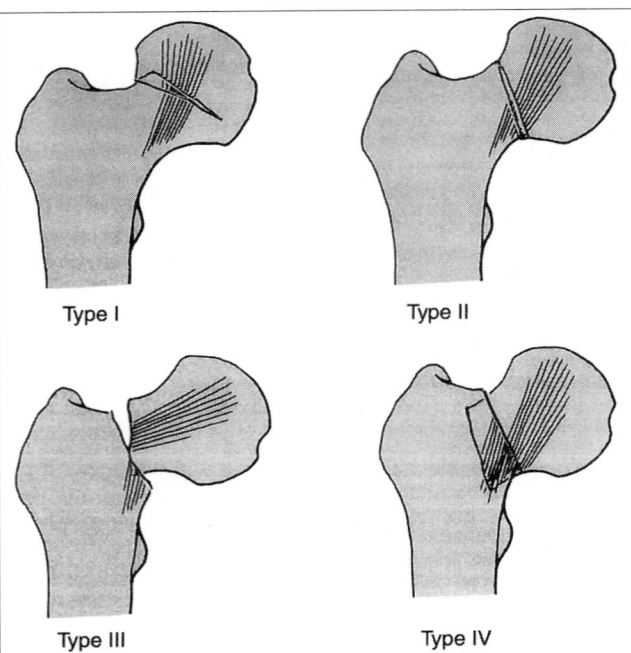

Type I

Type II

Type III

Type IV

Figure 3   The Garden classification of femoral neck fractures. Type I is an incomplete, impacted fracture in valgus malalignment (generally stable). Type II is a nondisplaced fracture. Type III is an incompletely displaced fracture in varus malalignment. Type IV is a completely displaced fracture with no engagement of the two fragments. The compression trabeculae in the femoral head line up with the trabeculae on the acetabular side. *(Reproduced with permission from Swionkowski MF: Intrascapular hip fractures, in Browner BD, Jupiter JB, Levine AM, Trafton PG (eds): Skeletal Trauma: Basic Science, Management, and Reconstruction, ed 2. Philadelphia, PA, WB Saunders, p 1775.)*

ture. Garden type I is an incomplete fracture with valgus impaction; type II is a complete but nondisplaced fracture; type III is a displaced, complete fracture with disruption of the trabecular pattern of the femoral neck. Garden type IV fractures are completely displaced with tearing of the capsule (**Figure 3**). Interobserver agreement of the Garden classifications has been shown to be only fair to moderate, but is improved when fractures are described as either nondisplaced (types I and II) or displaced (types III and IV).[21,22] The Pauwels classification consists of three types based on the verticality of the fracture: type I (< 30°), type II (30° to 50°), and type III (> 50°) (**Figure 4**). As fractures become more vertical, shearing forces increase and the likelihood for loss of reduction also increases. The Orthopaedic Trauma Association classification takes into account both location and verticality of the fracture and is usually used for research purposes.

Treatment
Nondisplaced Fractures
Surgical treatment of nondisplaced femoral neck fractures is often beneficial (even for patients with limited mobility) to help with pain control and to prevent later displacement. Nonsurgical treatment is reserved for patients with severe medical comorbidities who are considered medically unstable for surgery. Preoperative traction has not been shown to improve pain control and is associated with development of sciatic neuropathy in approximately 0.7% of patients.[23] Most nondisplaced femoral neck fractures are treated with internal fixation, commonly performed with parallel cannulated screws (**Figure 5**). Biomechanical studies have shown that three screws are more stable than two screws.[24] If three screws are used, an inverted triangle pattern is recommended with screws placed near the femoral cor-

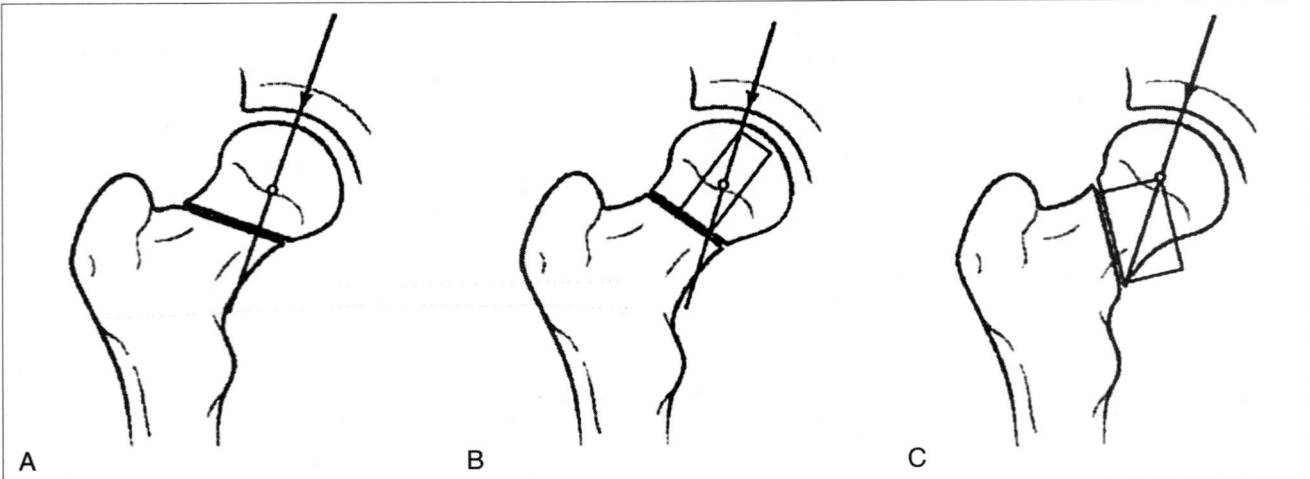

A   B   C

Figure 4   Schematic representation of the Pauwel classification of femoral neck fractures. **A,** In type I patterns, the fracture is relatively horizontal (< 30°) and compressive forces caused by the hip joint reactive force predominate. **B,** In type II patterns, shear forces at the fracture are predicted. **C,** In type III patterns, when the fracture angle is 50° or higher, shear forces predominate. Arrows indicate joint reactive force. *(Adapted with permission from Bartonicek J: Pauwels' classification of femoral neck fractures. J Orthop Trauma 2001;15:358-360.)*

tex to help prevent varus collapse of the fracture. Screws should be placed above the lesser trochanter, and screw threads should not cross the fracture site. With these techniques, nonunion rates of approximately 5% and osteonecrosis rates of 10% have been reported.[25] Postoperatively, most patients are allowed to bear weight as tolerated. Cognitively intact patients will limit weight bearing based on pain levels. Patients who can ambulate within 2 weeks after surgery have a higher likelihood of living at home 1 year after surgery. Patients who have a shorter duration of immobility following a hip fracture have an improved 6-month survival rate and improved functional scores.[26]

Displaced Fractures in Young Adults

Displaced femoral neck fractures in young adults usually arise from high-energy trauma. Treatment is surgical and should be performed as soon as possible. Delaying surgery has been associated with higher rates of osteonecrosis. Theoretically, early fracture reduction preserves stretched or twisted vessels supplying the femoral head that eventually would thrombose. Anatomic reduction and stable fixation is the goal of surgery.

For displaced fractures, surgical treatment begins with fracture reduction in the operating room. An anatomic reduction or a slight valgus deformity (up to 15°) is acceptable. If reduction cannot be obtained closed, then an open reduction is required through an anterior or anterolateral approach to the hip. For most fractures, internal fixation is achieved using parallel cannulated screws. For fractures with high verticality or severe comminution, or for lateral basicervical fractures, fixed-angle devices such as a sliding hip screw (with a derotation screw) should be considered to prevent loss of fixation. Nonunion rates range from 10% to 30% and osteonecrosis rates from 15% to 33%.[25] Nonunions in young patients are typically treated with a valgus osteotomy. Arthroplasty may be considered for either nonunion or osteonecrosis. Capsulotomy appears to improve femoral head blood flow in laboratory studies, but has not been conclusively shown to decrease the risk of osteonecrosis in clinical studies; therefore, the clinical benefits of capsulotomy remain unknown. Because capsulotomy is a simple procedure that does not add significant risk, it should be considered during surgery, although it cannot be definitively recommended.[27] Revision rates are high with approximately 33% of patients with osteonecrosis and 75% of patient with nonunion requiring further surgery. Nonunion of the femoral neck in young patients is treated with valgus osteotomy.

Displaced Fractures in Elderly Patients

Displaced femoral neck fractures in elderly patients are associated with high rates of nonunion and osteonecrosis when treated with ORIF. Loss of fixation rates average 30% to 40%.[28] Even when the fractures unite, shortening and malunion are common. To improve fixation, using four screws instead of three, sliding hip screws instead of multiple cannulated screws, and bone

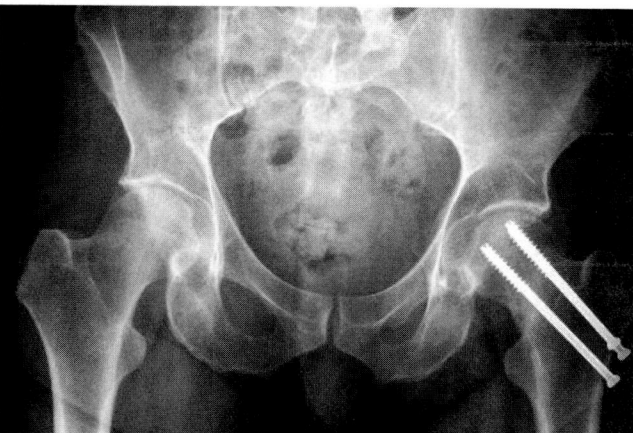

Figure 5 | A nondisplaced femoral neck fracture treated with three cannulated screws in inverted triangle configuration.

augmentation with some form of calcium phosphate cement have all been described with inconsistent results. For these fractures in older patients, hemiarthroplasty (Figure 6) and total hip arthroplasty (THA) have yielded consistently better results than ORIF. Revision surgery rates are much lower with arthroplasty (2% to 10%), and functional outcomes including pain relief and ambulatory status are improved.[29]

Controversy exists regarding the type of arthroplasty that is optimal. Options include hemiarthroplasty, both unipolar or bipolar, and THA. Bipolar hemiarthroplasty is designed to allow two points of articulation: one between the inner and outer heads of the construct and the other between the outer head and the acetabulum. Theoretically, the inner bearing relieves pressure on the acetabular cartilage and results in less articular wear; however, radiographic studies have shown the articulation between the two heads of the prosthesis is often lost, sometimes as early as 3 months after surgery. Acetabular erosion is most strongly correlated with patient activity levels and duration of follow-up. Dislocation rates are low with both unipolar and bipolar prostheses; however, the design of the bipolar prosthesis more often necessitates an open reduction. The bipolar prosthesis, unlike the monopolar design, typically has a metal-on-polyethylene articulation, which can lead to polyethylene debris and osteolysis.

In contrast, THA provides a durable and highly functional result for most patients. The biggest concern about THA is the increased risk of dislocation, which may be especially common (approximately 10% incidence) in elderly patients who have difficulty complying with postoperative precautions. The use of larger femoral heads and techniques incorporating anterior or posterior approaches with capsular repair can lessen the risk of dislocation. In patients with demonstrated recurrent dislocation, revision to a constrained acetabular component may be necessary. Primary use of constrained liners cannot be recommended at this time because of the lack of information about long-term complications.

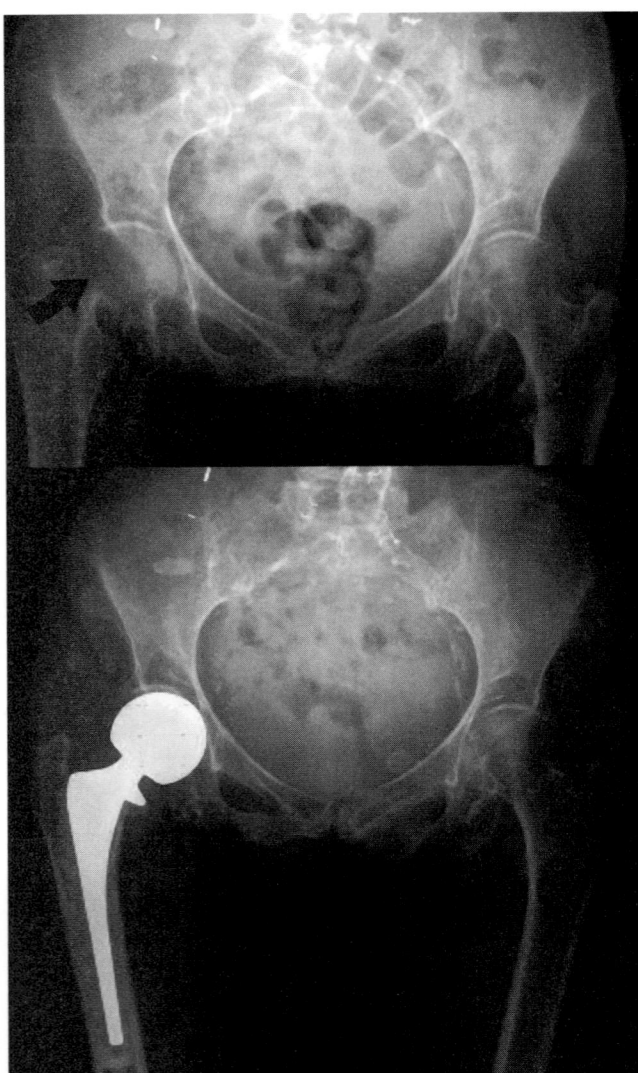

Figure 6 A displaced femoral neck fracture treated with cemented monopolar hemiarthroplasty.

thigh pain.[30] Some patients treated with polymethylmethacrylate experience a reaction to the monomer as it circulates, resulting in intraoperative hypotension and even sudden death. Polymethylmethacrylate should be used cautiously in patients with advanced cardiac or pulmonary disease, and it is important that the patient be well hydrated before surgery.

Intertrochanteric Fractures

Classification
Several classification systems exist for intertrochanteric fractures, including the Evans and Seinsheimer classification proposed more than 50 years ago, and the more recent AO classification (Figure 7). No particular classification system has been universally accepted. Fracture characteristics that should be assessed include the number of fragments, the direction of the fracture, and whether the posteromedial buttress is involved. Reverse obliquity fractures, fractures with subtrochanteric extension, and fractures involving the posteromedial buttress tend to be less stable.

Treatment
Stable Fractures
Stable, two-part intertrochanteric fractures have been treated successfully with a sliding hip screw and sideplate construct (Figure 8). Fractures are reduced using traction on the fracture table, and the lag screw is inserted into the "center-center" position in the femoral head. The tip-apex distance is the sum of the distances from the tip of the lag screw to the apex of the femoral head on AP and lateral radiographs (Figure 9). A tip-apex distance of more than 2.5 cm increases the risk of lag screw cutout and nonunion.[31]

When using a lag screw and a sideplate construct for a stable fracture, various lengths can be used for the sideplate. Biomechanical studies have shown the two-hole sideplate to function similarly to a four-hole plate.[32] When hardware failure occurs, it most commonly results from varus collapse and cutting out of the lag screw from the femoral head. Prospective clinical studies have confirmed the results of the biomechanical studies regarding the two-hole versus four-hole sideplates.[33] These findings presume that both screws in the sideplate have a good purchase; if this is not the case, a four-hole plate should be used.

Unstable Fractures
Unstable fractures include most three- and four-part fractures and reverse obliquity patterns, those with medial comminution, or those with disruption of the lateral cortex. These fractures have substantially higher overall failure rates (up to 32%).[34] For these fractures, a more stable construct such as the cephalomedullary nail, 95° dynamic condylar screw, blade plate, or locked plate should be considered (Figure 10). Although some unstable intertrochanteric fractures may be well treated with a sliding hip screw, this treat-

Comparative studies are ongoing to determine whether THA or hemiarthroplasty provides better overall results for displaced femoral neck fractures in elderly patients. Recent studies have suggested that functional outcomes such as pain and activity level may be better with THA. For the active elderly patient, THA is an option that should be considered. THA also should be considered for patients with preexisting acetabular disease (such as osteoarthritis, rheumatoid arthritis, and Paget's disease). Hemiarthroplasty is the better option for patients at high risk for a dislocation, such as those with advanced Parkinson's disease, patients with neurologic impairment caused by a prior stroke, and patients with advanced dementia.

Controversy also exists on the use of cemented or cementless stems. Cemented stems have shown improved functional outcomes with a decrease in the incidence of

ment choice should be avoided in fractures with a reverse obliquity pattern. The design of the implant may allow continued lateral displacement of the fracture. Intertrochanteric fractures with an associated femoral neck fracture should not be treated with a sliding hip screw because of excessive lag screw sliding and high failure rates (25%). Cephalomedullary nails allow less lag screw sliding than sliding hip screws, because the proximal fragment will eventually contact the nail. Some nails can be locked to prevent sliding, which result in less deformity for unstable fracture patterns. If a cephalomedullary nail is the chosen implant, long nails should be used to prevent a stress riser in the subtrochanteric region. For most intertrochanteric fractures, distal locking of the nail is not necessary; however, if the fracture extends into the subtrochanteric region or is a reverse obliquity pattern where rotational instability is possible, distal locking is necessary. One potential biochemical marker of healing is the patient's alkaline phosphatase level. Alkaline phosphatase levels typically increase for the first 3 weeks postoperatively then gradually decrease back toward normal levels by 8 weeks. Persistently elevated levels at 8 weeks suggest delayed union.[35] Indications for prosthetic replacements include pathologic fractures and fractures in patients with preexisting degenerative joint disease. Patients with unstable fractures and medical conditions associated with difficult healing, such as advanced renal failure or chronic steroid use, also should be considered for prosthetic replacement.

Subtrochanteric Fractures

Classification

Multiple classification systems have been proposed for fractures of the subtrochanteric region, which includes the area from the lesser trochanter to the beginning of the femoral isthmus. The Fielding classification groups fractures based on location: type I, 0 to 2 cm from the

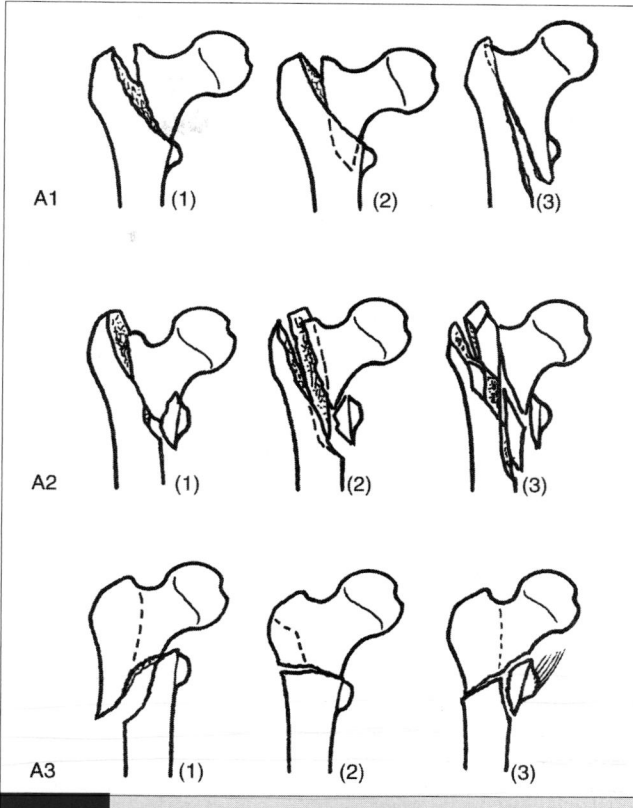

Figure 7 The Müller/AO classification of peritrochanteric femur fractures (incorporated into the Fracture and Dislocation Compendium of the Orthopaedic Trauma Association). Top row, (1) Extraarticular fracture, (2) trochanteric area, (3) peritrochanteric, simple. Middle row, (1) Extraarticular fracture, (2) trochanteric area, (3) peritrochanteric, multifragmentary. Bottom row, (1) Extra-articular fracture, (2) trochanteric area, (3) intertrochanteric. *(Reproduced with permission from Müller ME, Nazarian S, Koch P, Schatzker J (eds): The Comprehensive Classification of Fractures of Long Bones. Berlin, Germany, Springer-Verlag, 1990, p 121.)*

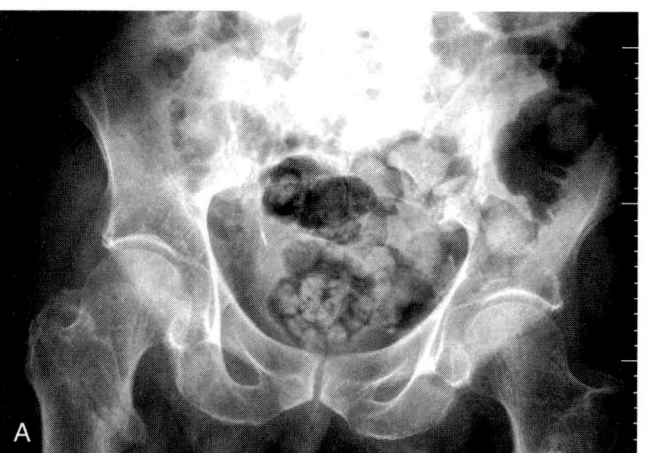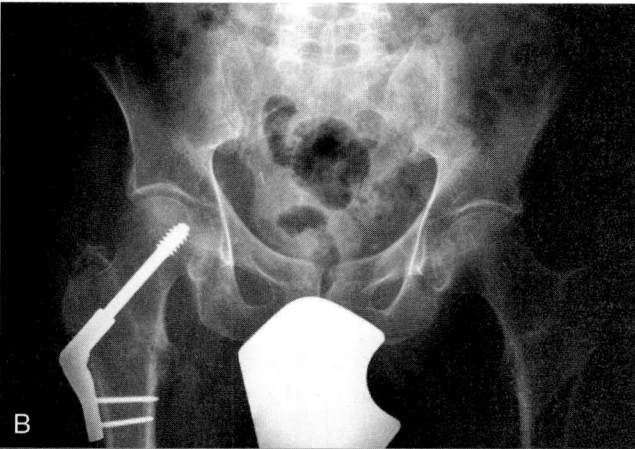

Figure 8 Stable intertrochanteric fracture **(A)** treated with two-hole sideplate and sliding hip screw **(B)**.

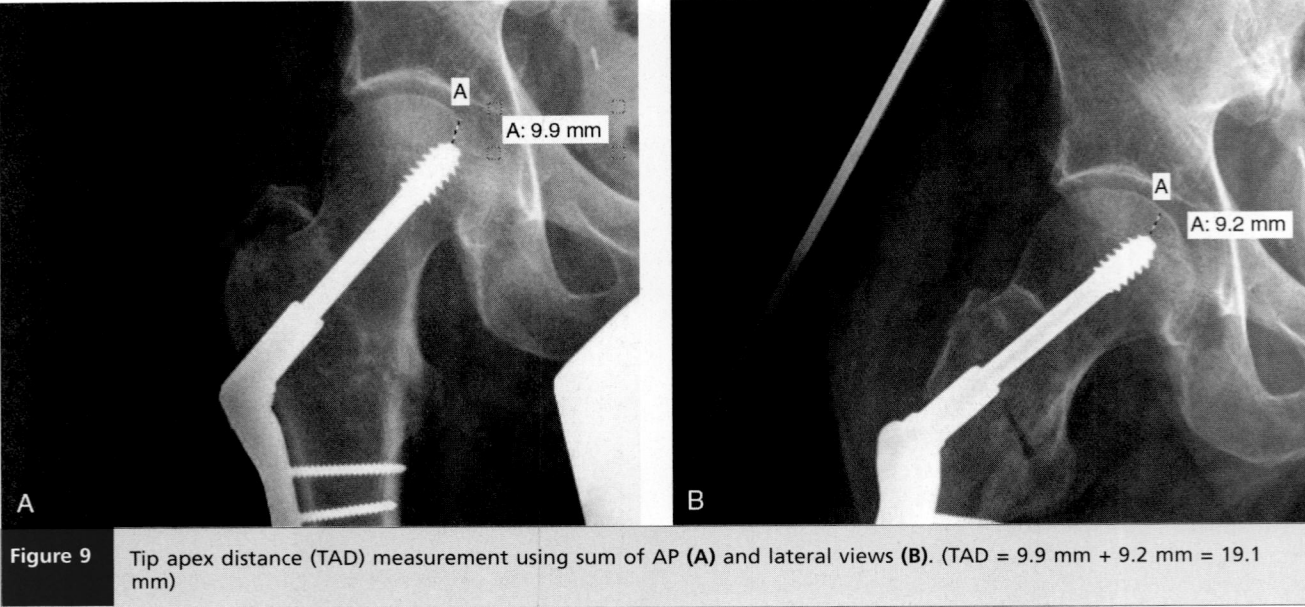

Figure 9   Tip apex distance (TAD) measurement using sum of AP **(A)** and lateral views **(B)**. (TAD = 9.9 mm + 9.2 mm = 19.1 mm)

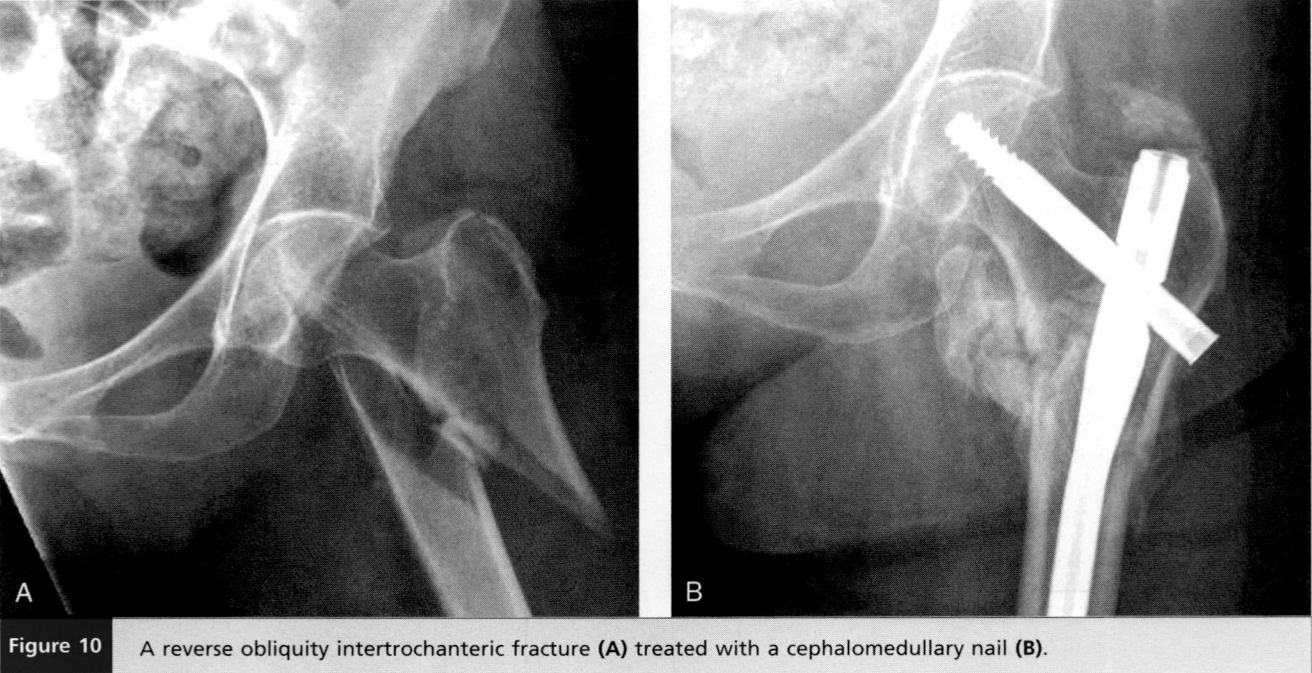

Figure 10   A reverse obliquity intertrochanteric fracture **(A)** treated with a cephalomedullary nail **(B)**.

lesser trochanter; type II, 2 to 5 cm; and type III, more than 5 cm. The Russell-Taylor classification groups fractures based on whether the lesser trochanter is intact and whether the fracture extends into the piriformis fossa. The least stable pattern occurs when both the lesser trochanter and the piriformis fossa are involved in the fracture.

Treatment
In low subtrochanteric fractures in which the piriformis fossa is intact, standard antegrade femoral nails with

traditional proximal locking are appropriate. In fractures that extend above the lesser trochanter, cephalomedullary nails provide a stable construct with the advantages of indirect fracture reduction with minimal soft-tissue disruption. When using a cephalomedullary nail, similar results have been achieved with either a piriformis or a trochanteric starting point. The challenge when using closed techniques is to obtain indirect reduction. The proximal segment typically assumes a flexed, abducted, and externally rotated position. If reduction maneuvers using the fracture table fail to fully

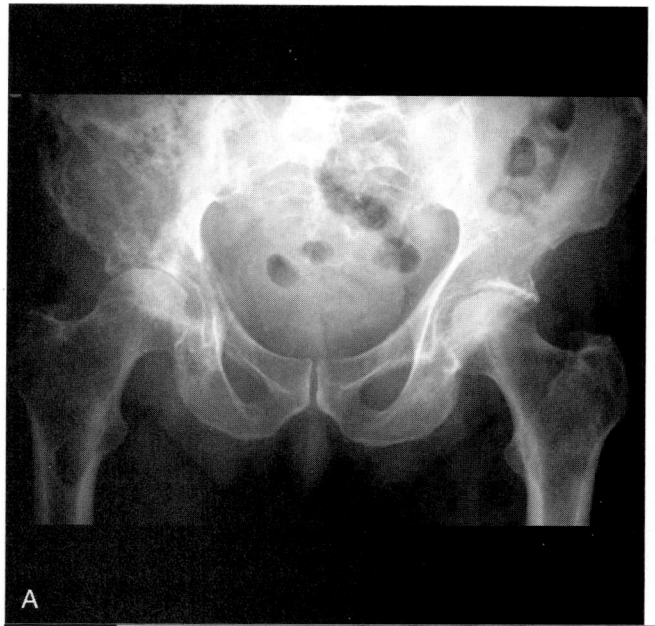
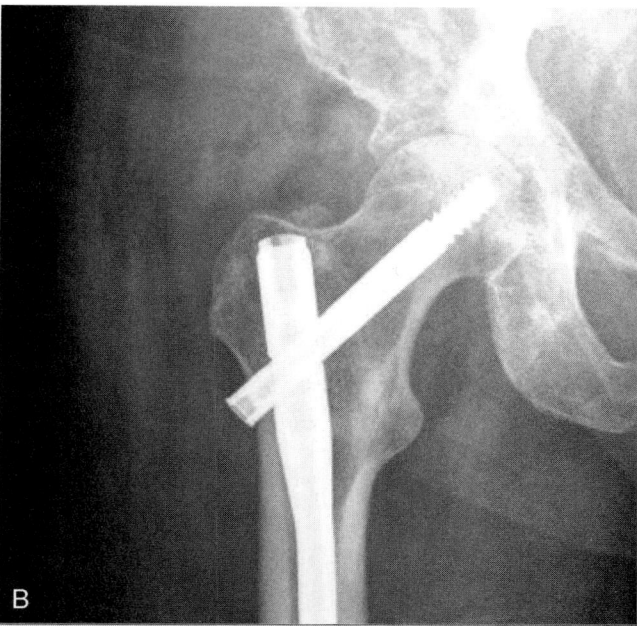

Figure 11 An impending fracture **(A)** caused by a pathologic lesions in the right proximal femur is stabilized with a cephalo-medullary nail **(B)**.

reduce the fracture, percutaneous insertion of a peri-osteal elevator or ball spike instrument can assist in fracture reduction. Alternatively, blocking screws can be inserted to help direct reduction as the intramedul-lary nail is passed, provided the proximal femur is not too comminuted. Varus malreduction is not uncommon when using cephalomedullary nails and attempts should be made to avoid this malposition. Blade plates, 95° dynamic condylar plates, and some newer locked plates also can be used and may facilitate more ana-tomic reduction, but generally at the expense of more soft-tissue disruption. Sliding hip screws should be avoided in these fractures because they may result in loss of fracture reduction as the lag screw slides within the plate barrel.

Pathologic Fractures

The proximal femur is a common site for metastatic le-sions. When treating a pathologic fracture or impend-ing fracture in the proximal femur, the first step is to determine if the lesion is metastatic or represents a pri-mary bone tumor. If there is any question about the ori-gin of the tumor, biopsy and tissue diagnosis should be completed before proceeding. Treatment of primary malignant bone tumors typically involves wide resec-tion and prosthetic replacement.

Metastatic lesions of the proximal femur are often treated surgically. Mirel's classification can be used to help determine the risk of fracture and guide treatment. Mirel's criteria include the location of the lesion, its size, the amount of cortical involvement, and degree of pain. A Mirel's score of 8 or higher generally indicates

the need for surgical treatment. Surgical treatment in-volves either stabilization of the lesion or prosthetic re-placement. When stabilizing a lesion in any part of the proximal femur or femoral shaft, long cephalomedul-lary nails should be used because the tumor can ad-vance into the femoral neck (**Figure 11**). For femoral neck lesions that have already fractured, prosthetic re-placement is the treatment of choice because of the low rate of healing with ORIF. If prosthetic replacement is done, long-stem cemented implants are usually selected.

Osteoporosis Evaluation and Treatment After Hip Fracture

The American Academy of Orthopaedic Surgeons has recommended that osteoporosis should be recognized as a national health priority. Osteoporosis is defined by the World Health Organization as a bone mineral den-sity value of 2.5 standard deviations or more below the young adult mean.[36] The prevalence of osteoporosis continues to rise. It is estimated that 44 million Ameri-cans have osteoporosis, and approximately 30% of postmenopausal women have the disorder. Increasing age is the most sensitive predictor for osteoporosis. Ap-proximately 1.5 million fractures per year in the United States are caused by osteoporosis. About 20% of pa-tients with a fragility fracture (a low-energy fracture caused by osteoporosis) sustain a second fracture within 1 year.[37] The best predictor of a fragility fracture is a history of a previous fragility fracture.

Although it is well known that osteoporosis affects aging woman, it also affects many aging men. It is esti-mated that 2.3 million men in the United States have

4: Lower Extremity

osteoporosis and 11.8 million have low bone density.[38] Despite the fact that 30% of all hip fractures occur in men, osteoporosis remains largely underdiagnosed in males. One study at a tertiary medical center found that following a hip fracture, 27% of women were referred for osteoporosis treatment compared with only 4.5% of men.[39] These numbers are very significant because the rate of mortality for men following a hip fracture is approximately twice that of women.[40]

For patients who have sustained an osteoporotic hip fracture, multiple treatments exist. Dual energy x-ray absorptiometry scanning can be used to measure the results of treatment. The National Osteoporosis Foundation recommends such scanning in all women older than 65 years with any fracture, regardless of other risk factors. Communication between the orthopaedic surgeon and the internist is important to ensure that patients receive proper care after a fragility fracture. Non-pharmacologic treatments include a well-balanced diet and exercise, adequate sunlight exposure, not smoking, vitamin D and calcium supplementation, and selected use of hip protectors. Adequate exercise seems to be an important modifiable factor in the prevention of fragility fractures because exercise not only helps prevent osteopenia and osteoporosis, but also improves balance and aids in fall prevention in elderly individuals. Medical treatments include the antiresorptive bisphosphonates such as alendronate, risedronate, and ibandronate. Nasal calcitonin and raloxifene also have been used to limit bone resorption. Teriparatide is an anabolic agent which improves bone density by increasing osteoblast activity. The Food and Drug Administration has withdrawn approval of hormone replacement with estrogen for osteoporosis prevention, except in selected postmenopausal women.[41]

Annotated References

1. Dennison E, Cole Z, Cooper C: Diagnosis and epidemiology of osteoporosis. *Curr Opin Rheumatol* 2005;17:456-461.

   The authors of this review article discuss the epidemiology of osteoporosis, the associations of disease and medications with osteoporotic fractures, and advancements in treatment.

2. Dreinhofer KE, Schwarzkopf SR, Haas NP, Tscherne H: Isolated traumatic dislocation of the hip: Long-term results in 50 patients. *J Bone Joint Surg Br* 1994;76:6-12.

3. Sahin V, Karakas ES, Aksu S, Atlihan D, Turk CY, Halici M: Traumatic dislocation and fracture-dislocation of the hip: A long term follow-up study. *J Trauma* 2003;54:520-529.

4. Pape HC, Rice J, Wolfram K, Gansslen A, Pohlemann T, Krettek C: Hip dislocation in patients with multiple injuries: A follow-up investigation. *Clin Orthop Relat Res* 2000;377:99-105.

5. Rodriguez-Merchan EC: Osteonecrosis of the femoral head after traumatic hip dislocation in the adult. *Clin Orthop Relat Res* 2000;377:68-77.

6. Hougaard K, Thomsen PB: Traumatic posterior dislocation of the hip: Prognostic factors influencing the incidence of avascular necrosis of the femoral head. *Arch Orthop Trauma Surg* 1986;106:32-35.

7. Hillyard RF, Fox J: Sciatic nerve injuries associated with traumatic posterior hip dislocations. *Am J Emerg Med* 2003;21:545-548.

8. Vailas JC, Hurwitz S, Wiesel SW: Posterior acetabular fracture-dislocations: Fragment size, joint capsule, and stability. *J Trauma* 1989;29:1494-1496.

9. Tornetta P III: Non-operative management of acetabular fractures: The use of dynamic stress views. *J Bone Joint Surg Br* 1999;81:67-70.

10. Mullis BH, Dahners LE: Hip arthroscopy to remove loose bodies after traumatic dislocation. *J Orthop Trauma* 2006;20:22-26.

    The author present a retrospective review of 36 patients with traumatic hip injuries who were treated with hip arthroscopy. Loose bodies were found in 92% of hips including seven of nine in which radiographs did not show the fragments.

11. Holt GE, McCarty EC: Anterior hip dislocation with an associated vascular injury requiring amputation. *J Trauma* 2003;55:135-138.

12. Asghar FA, Karunakar MA: Femoral head fractures: Diagnosis, management, and complications. *Orthop Clin North Am* 2004;35:463-472.

    This review article summarizing the current information regarding diagnosis and treatment of femoral head fractures.

13. Swiontkowski MF, Thorpe M, Seiler JG, Hansen ST: Operative management of displaced femoral head fractures: Case matched comparison of anterior versus posterior approaches for Pipkin I and Pipkin II fractures. *J Orthop Trauma* 1992;6:437-442.

14. Marchetti ME, Steinberg GG, Coumas JM: Intermediate-term experience of Pipkin fracture-dislocations of the hip. *J Orthop Trauma* 1996;10:455-461.

15. Chami G, Jeys L, Freudmann M, Connor L, Siddiqi M: Are osteoporotic fracture being adequately investigated?: A questionnaire of GP and orthopaedic surgeons. *BMC Fam Pract* 2006;7:7.

    This article presents the results of a survey of general practitioners and orthopaedic surgeons on the need to assess patients for osteoporotic care after a fragility fracture. When presented with the case of a 50-year-old woman with a Colles' fracture, only 56% of surgeons recommended osteoporosis investigation; 67% of general practitioners did not recommend investigation unless prompted by the orthopaedic surgeon.

16. Johnell O: The socioeconomic burden of fractures: Today and in the 21st century. *Am J Med* 1997;103:20S-25S.

17. Farahmand BY, Michaelsson K, Ahlbom A, Ljunghall S, Baron JA: Survival after hip fracture. *Osteoporos Int* 2005;16:1583-1590.

    A case control study was done to assess the risk factors for mortality after a hip fracture. Although the highest mortality risk was found in the first 6 months after fracture, a relative increased risk persisted for 6 years in the patients with the hip fracture compared with a control group.

18. Bottle A, Aylin P: Mortality associated with delay in operation after hip fracture: Observational study. *BMJ* 2006;332:947-951.

    A multicenter review of mortality after hip fracture is presented. After adjustment for comorbidities, delay in surgery was associated with increased mortality after a hip fracture.

19. Amin S, Zhang Y, Felson DT, et al: Estradiol, testosterone, and the risk for hip fractures in elderly men from the Framingham study. *Am J Med* 2006;119:426-433.

    A review of the Framingham study regarding the role of estradiol and testosterone levels and risk of hip fracture is presented. Men in the low and middle estradiol groups had a 3.1 higher risk of hip fracture compared with those in the high estradiol group.

20. Faber MJ, Boscher RJ, Chin A, et al: Effects of exercise programs on falls and mobility in frail and pre-frail older adults: A multicenter randomized controlled trial. *Arch Phys Med Rehabil* 2006;87:885-896.

    This multicenter, randomized, controlled trial assessed the effects of two exercise programs on physical performance and the risk of falls in frail and prefrail older adults. Exercise programs reduced falls and improved performance in prefrail patients but not in frail patients.

21. Beimers L, Kreder HJ, Berry GK, et al: Subcapital hip fractures: The Garden classification should be replaced not collapsed. *Can J Surg* 2002;45:411-414.

22. Oakes DA, Jackson KR, Davies MR, et al: The impact of the Garden classification on proposed operative treatment. *Clin Orthop Relat Res* 2003;409:232-240.

23. Kemler MA, de Vries M, van der Tol A: Duration of preoperative traction associated with sciatic neuropathy after hip fracture surgery. *Clin Orthop Relat Res* 2006;445:230-232.

    The authors of this article present the results of a retrospective review of 2,202 patients treated for hip fracture. The duration of preoperative skin traction associated with sciatic nerve palsy had an overall incidence of 0.7%.

24. Maurer SG, Wright KE, Kummer FJ, Zuckerman JD, Koval KJ: Two or three screws for fixation of femoral neck fractures? *Am J Orthop* 2003;32:438-442.

25. Damany DS, Parker MJ, Chojnowski A: Complications after intracapsular hip fractures in young adults: A meta-analysis of 18 published studies involving 564 fractures. *Injury* 2005;36:131-141.

    Meta-analyses on the rates of nonunion and osteonecrosis after hip fracture are presented. The incidence of nonunion is greater after open reduction (11.2%) compared with closed reduction (4.7%).

26. Siu AL, Penrod JD, Boockvar KS, Koval KJ, Strauss E, Morrison RS: Early ambulation after hip fracture: Effects on function and mortality. *Arch Intern Med* 2006;166:766-771.

    A prospective cohort of 532 patients underwent surgery for hip fractures. A delay in mobilizing patients from bed was associated with poor function at 2 months, and a decreased rate of 6-month survival.

27. Rodriguez-Merchan EC: In situ fixation of nondisplaced intracapsular fractures of the proximal femur. *Clin Orthop Relat Res* 2002;399:42-51.

28. Karaeminogullari O, Demirors H, Atabek M, Tuncay C, Tandogan R, Ozalay M: Avascular necrosis and nonunion after osteosynthesis of femoral neck fractures: Effect of fracture displacement and time to surgery. *Adv Ther* 2004;21:335-342.

    The authors present a retrospective analysis of 30 patients who had ORIF of femoral neck fractures. Nonunion and osteonecrosis rates increased from 6% and 18% respectively for nondisplaced fractures to 23% and 38% respectively for displaced fractures.

29. Bjorgul K, Reikeras O: Hemiarthroplasty in worst cases is better than internal fixation in best cases of displaced femoral neck fractures: A prospective study of 683 patients treated with hemiarthroplasty or internal fixation. *Acta Orthop* 2006;77:368-374.

    A prospective cohort of 683 patients with displaced femoral neck fractures was treated with ORIF or hemiarthroplasty. The revision rate was 24% in ORIF group compared with 2% in hemiarthroplasty group.

30. Parker MJ, Gurusamy K: Arthroplasties (with and without bone cement) for proximal femoral fractures in adults. *Cochrane Database Syst Rev* 2006;3:CD001706.

    A review of the results of cemented or cementless arthroplasties for the treatment of hip fractures in 1,920 patients is presented. The authors concluded that a cemented prosthesis may reduce postoperative pain and lead to better mobility.

31. Baumgaertner MR, Solberg BD: Awareness of tip-apex distance reduces failure of fixation of trochanteric fracture of the hip. *J Bone Joint Surg Br* 1997;79:969-971.

32. McLoughlin SW, Wheeler DL, Rider J, Bolhofner B: Biomechanical evaluation of the dynamic hip screw with two- and four-hole side plates. *J Orthop Trauma* 2000;14:318-323.

33. Bolhofner BR, Russo PR, Carmen B: Results of intertrochanteric femur fractures treated with a 135-degree slid-

ing screw with a two-hole side plate. *J Orthop Trauma* 1999;13:5-8.

34. Haidukewych GJ, Israel TA, Berry DJ: Reverse obliquity fractures of the intertrochanteric region of the femur. *J Bone Joint Surg Am* 2001;83:643-650.

35. Nakagawa H, Kamimura M, Takahara K, et al: Changes in total alkaline phosphatase level after hip fracture: Comparison between femoral neck and trochanter fractures. *J Orthop Sci* 2006;11:135-139.

    A prospective cohort of 69 patients with hip fracture received follow-up evaluation for alkaline phosphatase levels at 1, 2, 3, 4, 6, and 8 weeks after surgery. Levels rose to a maximum at 3 weeks postoperatively and decreased from 3 to 6 weeks in all but one patient.

36. Borgstrom E, Johnell O, Kanis JA, et al: At what hip fracture risk is it cost-effective to treat? International intervention thresholds for the treatment of osteoporosis. *Osteoporos Int* 2006;17:1459-1471.

    The Markov cohort model was used to investigate cost effectiveness of interventions for osteoporosis.

37. Reginster JY, Burlet N: Osteoporosis: A still increasing prevalence. *Bone* 2006;38(2 suppl 1):S4-S9.

    A review article on the prevalence of osteoporosis and fragility fractures is presented. It was found that 20% of patients with a fragility fracture will sustain a second fracture within 1 year.

38. National Osteoporosis Foundation: *America's Bone Health: The State of Osteoporosis and Low Bone Mass in Our Nation.* Washington, DC, National Osteoporosis Foundation, 2002.

39. Kiebzak GM, Beinart GA, Perser K, Ambrose CG, Siff SJ, Heggeness MG: Undertreatment of osteoporosis in men with hip fracture. *Arch Intern Med* 2002;162: 2217-2222.

40. Wright VJ: Osteoporosis in men. *J Am Acad Orthop Surg* 2006;14:347-353.

    A review article on the incidence of osteoporosis and fragility fractures in men is presented.

41. Mauck KF, Clarke BL: Diagnosis, screening, prevention, and treatment of osteoporosis. *Mayo Clin Proc* 2006; 81:662-672.

    The authors present a review article on the diagnosis, screening, prevention, and treatment of osteoporosis.

Chapter 33

Hip and Pelvic Reconstruction and Arthroplasty

*Richard L. Illgen II, MD   Matthew Squire, MD   John P. Heiner, MD

Hip Arthritis

Epidemiology

Hip arthritis is a major cause of disability worldwide. In the United States, hip arthritis results in the need for more than 200,000 total hip replacements annually, and this incidence will increase substantially as the population ages. The causes of hip arthritis include childhood disorders (such as developmental dysplasia, Legg-Calvé-Perthes disease, and slipped capital femoral epiphysis), inflammatory arthritis, osteonecrosis, trauma, and infection. In many patients, the cause of hip arthritis is unknown. A growing body of evidence suggests that in many instances more subtle morphologic changes in the hip, such as femoroacetabular impingement and subtle forms of dysplasia, may contribute to hip arthritis.[1]

Clinical Evaluation

Evaluation of the history, physical examination findings, and plain radiographic results leads to a diagnosis of the correct hip pathology in most patients. Intra-articular pathology will usually present with pain localized to the groin that will be exacerbated with internal rotation of the hip. Pain often limits a patient's ability to ambulate, climb stairs, and reach to their shoes. Loss of internal rotation of the hip when compared with the contralateral side is often an early indication of hip pathology. Pain at the level of the greater trochanter is nonspecific and can be caused by either intra-articular or extra-articular processes. Some neuropathies, such as lateral femoral nerve entrapment or diabetic mononeuropathy, may also present as hip pain. A careful examination of the spine, abdomen, and neurovascular structures should always be completed to eliminate the possible presence of spinal stenosis, vascular claudication, or other causes of pain in the region of the hip.

Standard hip assessment should also include documentation of the presence of flexion contractures (Thomas test), asymmetric hip abductor weakness (Trendelenburg sign), and labral impingement signs (pain with flexion, adduction, and internal rotation of the hip). It should be recognized that many clinical signs of hip pain (for example, groin pain and provocative testing with flexion, adduction, and internal hip rotation) are sensitive measures to identify the hip as the cause of pain, but often are nonspecific and fail to identify the exact cause of the hip pathology. Further radiographic testing usually is required. Leg lengths also should be carefully evaluated. The "snapping hip" is usually caused by the iliotibial band snapping across the greater trochanter or the iliopsoas tendon snapping across the iliopectineal prominence. The iliotibial band is tested with the patient standing, and pain is reproduced with adduction and rotation of the hip. The iliopsoas is tested by moving the hip from a flexed and internally rotated position to an extended and externally rotated position while the patient is supine. In equivocal cases, anesthetic injection of the psoas bursa under ultrasound guidance can provide diagnostic utility.[2] In patients with concurrent hip and back arthritis, anesthetic injection into the hip joint (anesthetic arthrogram) can be useful when standard history and physical examination findings fail to provide an accurate diagnosis.[3]

Radiographic Evaluation

Plain radiographs of the hip combined with a thorough history and physical examination provide adequate information to make the correct diagnosis in most patients. Standard radiographic assessment of the hip should include an AP view of the pelvis, AP view of the involved hip, and a frog-lateral view of the involved hip. In patients with pincer-type femoroacetabular impingement, the AP hip view can demonstrate retroversion of the acetabulum as evidenced by a "cross-over" sign[4] (Figures 1 and 2). In patients with developmental dysplasia of the hip, the acetabular deformity includes a shallow socket, decreased lateral and anterior acetabular coverage, and lateral subluxation of the femoral head. Plain radiographs, including an AP pelvis view and a false-profile view (a true lateral view of the acetabulum) can define the degree of acetabular dysplasia[5] (Figure 3). The frog-lateral view will provide improved visualization of the articular surface in patients with

---

*Richard L. Illgen II, MD or the department with which he is affiliated has received research or institutional support from Zimmer and is a consultant or employee for Zimmer.

4: Lower Extremity

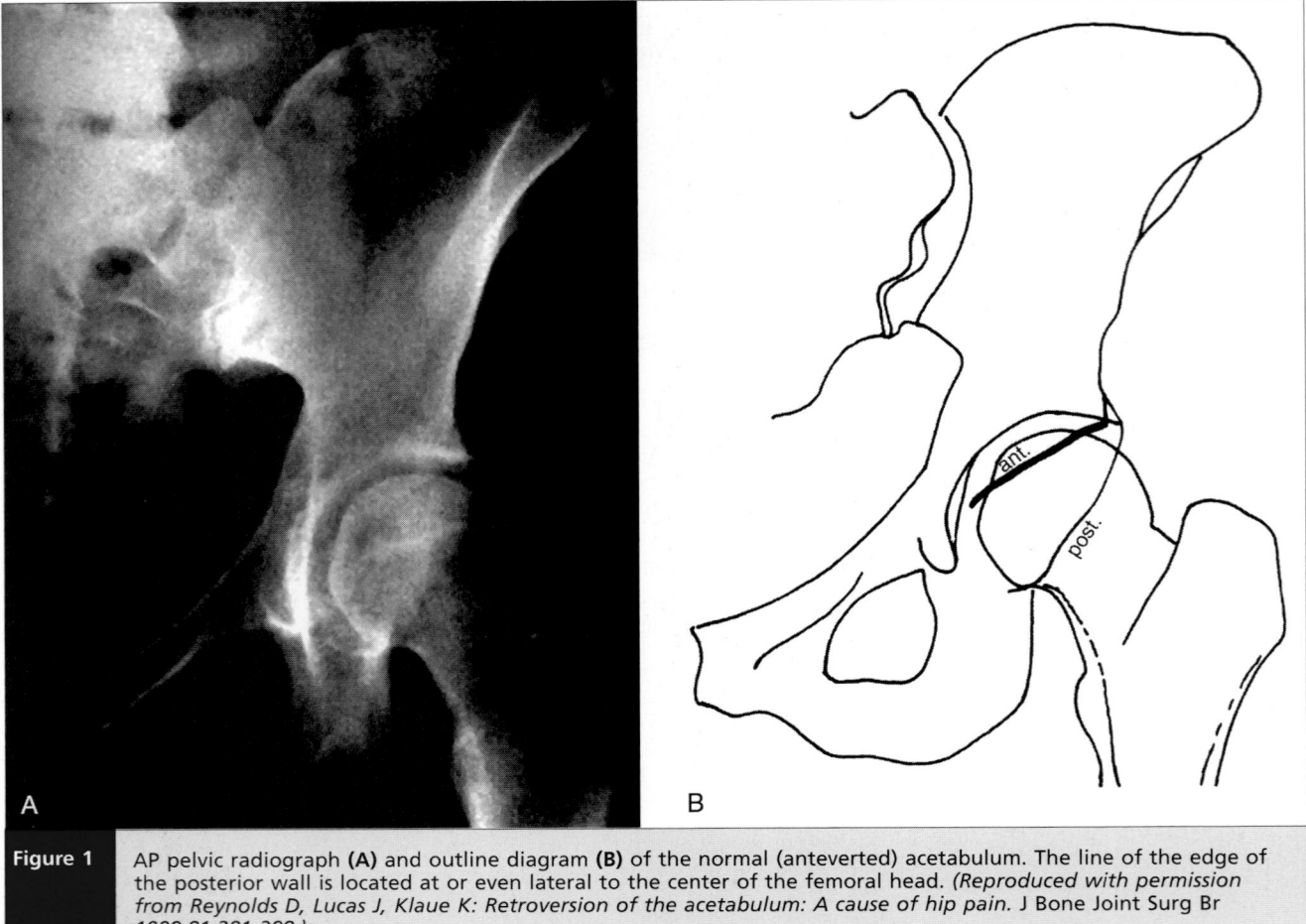

Figure 1 AP pelvic radiograph **(A)** and outline diagram **(B)** of the normal (anteverted) acetabulum. The line of the edge of the posterior wall is located at or even lateral to the center of the femoral head. *(Reproduced with permission from Reynolds D, Lucas J, Klaue K: Retroversion of the acetabulum: A cause of hip pain. J Bone Joint Surg Br 1999;81:281-288.)*

suspected osteonecrosis. The crescent sign, which is evidence of a subchondral femoral fracture, is best seen on the frog-lateral view. A cross-table lateral view will provide additional information about acetabular anteversion and anterior hip coverage.

When plain radiographic assessment fails to provide a diagnosis, additional diagnostic imaging may include MRI, magnetic resonance arthrography, CT, and bone scanning. MRI is the study of choice for the evaluation of osteonecrosis, stress fractures, and neoplasms. MRI can be used to identify patients with an abnormal femoral head-neck junction and to quantify femoroacetabular impingement by measuring the alpha angle[5] (**Figure 4**). MRI is also an important tool for identifying bilateral disease in the asymptomatic contralateral hip of patients with osteonecrosis (in up to 50% of patients), as well as for the staging of osteonecrosis. The role of MRI to quantify osteoarthritic changes remains investigational. Magnetic resonance arthrograms (using intra-articular gadolinium contrast agent) can document labral and perhaps hyaline cartilage pathology, but in some series false-negative rates of 20% to 30% have been reported.[6] CT scans provide fine bone detail and are useful for assessing posttraumatic arthritis. Bone scans can be used to evaluate femoral neck stress

fractures and pathologic lesions, although MRI is more sensitive and may more accurately identify injuries at an early stage.

Osteonecrosis of the Femoral Head

Osteonecrosis of the femoral head is a challenging disorder often occurring in young patients. The pathophysiology of this disease remains poorly understood. Risk factors include steroid use, alcoholism, trauma, marrow-replacing diseases (such as Gaucher's disease), high-dose radiation treatment, and hypercoagulable states (such as sickle cell disease, hypofibrinolysis, thrombophilia, and protein S and C deficiencies). In many patients with osteonecrosis of the femoral head, the cause is unknown. The pathology usually consists of decreased blood flow to the femoral head, resulting in increased intraosseous pressure, osteonecrosis, subchondral fracture, and eventually collapse.

Evaluation and Staging

Plain radiographs should include an AP radiograph of the pelvis, AP radiograph of the involved hip, and a frog-lateral radiograph of the involved hip. The frog-

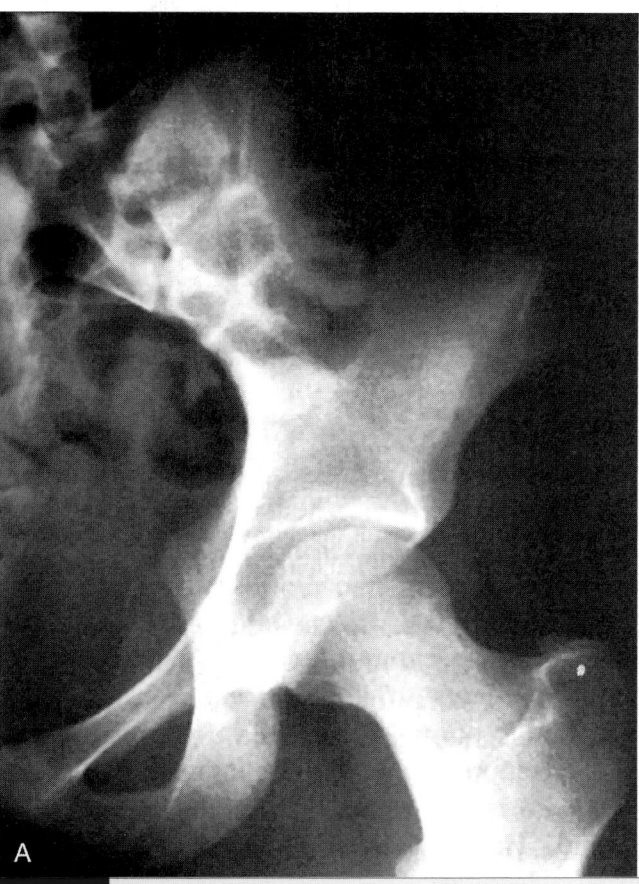
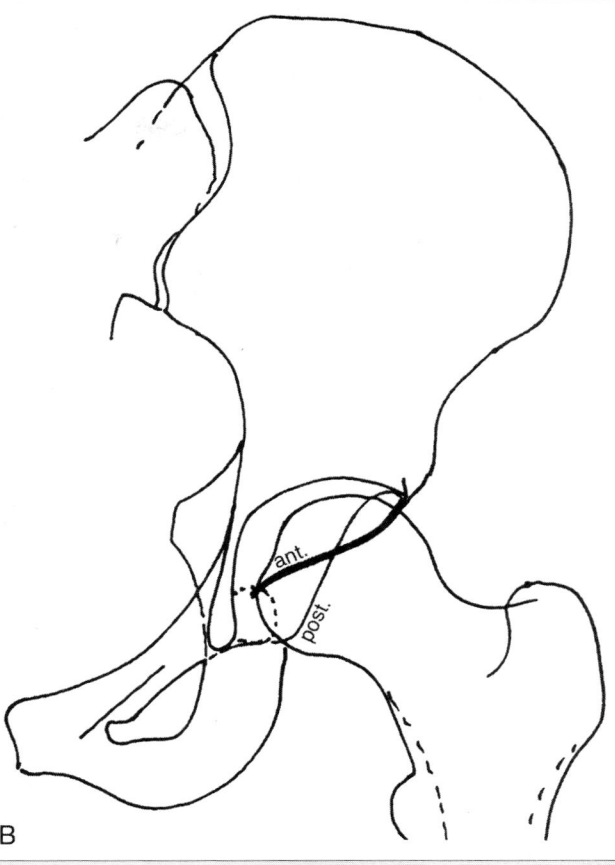

Figure 2 AP pelvic radiograph **(A)** and outline diagram **(B)** showing acetabular retroversion and the "cross-over" sign. *(Reproduced with permission from Reynolds D, Lucas J, Klaue K: Retroversion of the acetabulum: A cause of hip pain. J Bone Joint Surg Br 1999;81:281-288.)*

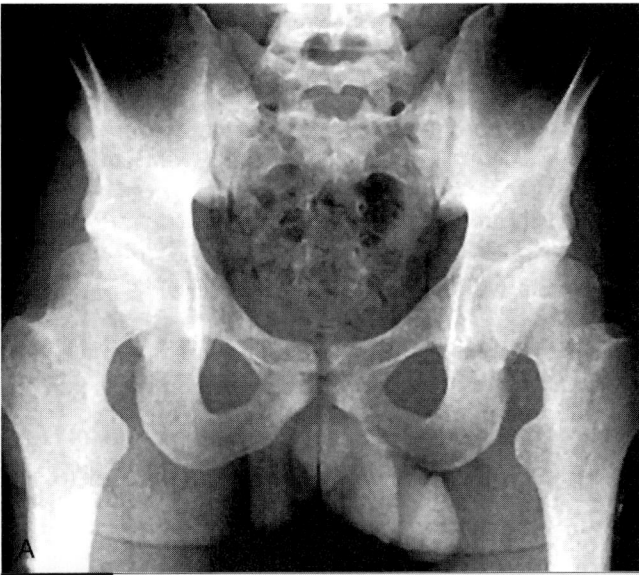
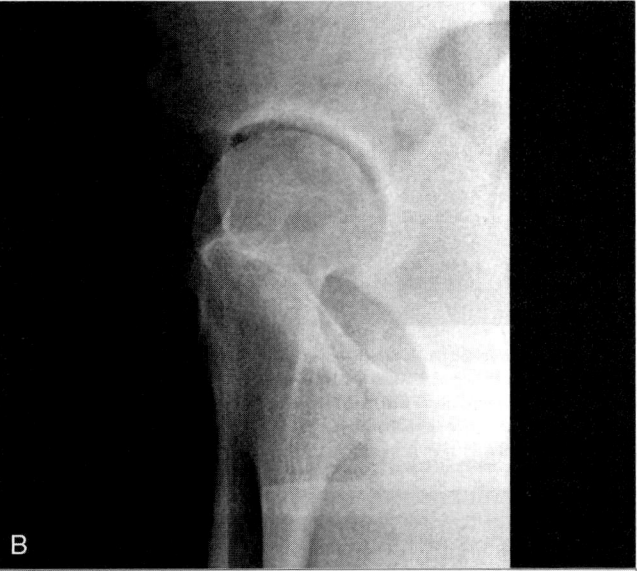

Figure 3 **A,** AP pelvic radiograph demonstrating a shallow acetabulum and lateral subluxation of the femoral head in a patient with bilateral hip dysplasia. **B,** False-profile lateral radiograph demonstrating decreased anterior coverage of the hip. *(Reproduced with permission from Peters CL, Erickson J: The etiology and treatment of hip pain in the young adult. J Bone Joint Surg Am 2006;88-A(suppl 4):20-26.)*

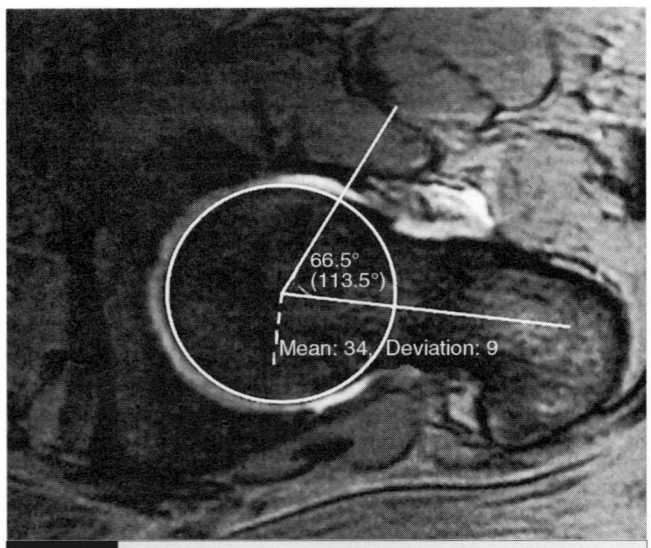

Figure 4 Three-dimensional, gradient-echo magnetic resonance arthrographic image used to quantify femoroacetabular impingement. The alpha angle measures the femoral head-neck offset of 66.5°. The alpha angle in a normal hip is less than 50°. (*Reproduced with permission from Peters CL, Erickson J: The etiology and treatment of hip pain in the young adult. J Bone Joint Surg Am 2006;88-A(suppl 4):20-26.*)

lateral radiograph often demonstrates the subchondral fracture most clearly. MRI is the imaging study of choice for patients with normal radiographs and in whom osteonecrosis is suspected. The most common regions of involvement include the lateral and anterior aspects of the femoral head. The extent and location of the lesion are prognostic factors affecting the treatment options. Several classification systems have been used, including the Ficat and the University of Pennsylvania classification systems. The Ficat system, described in 1960 and modified in 1985, uses plain radiographs and bone scans to classify patients as having precollapse (Ficat stages 0 through II) or postcollapse (Ficat stages III and IV) disease. The University of Pennsylvania system incorporates data from plain radiographs, bone scans, and MRI scans to provide important prognostic information related to the size, location, and extent of the lesion. Large lesions (involving > 30% of the femoral head) and patients with postcollapse disease (University of Pennsylvania stages III through VI) have a poor prognosis compared with patients with small lesions (involving < 15% of the femoral head) and precollapse disease (University of Pennsylvania stages 0 through II).

Treatment
Precollapse Osteonecrosis
Without intervention, progression of disease will occur in most patients, even those with early stage osteonecrosis. However, surgical intervention for asymptomatic patients generally is not recommended and there-fore observation is reasonable for patients with preclinical (asymptomatic) osteonecrosis. Symptomatic precollapse osteonecrosis will likely benefit from intervention. The type of intervention remains controversial. Core decompression, with or without bone graft, remains a common treatment.[7] The role of nonvascularized and vascularized fibula grafting, pedicle grafts, and trap-door procedures for precollapse osteonecrosis remains controversial. Recently, a randomized clinical trial demonstrated that early intervention with oral bisphosphonates (alendronate at a dose of 70 mg weekly for 25 weeks) for nontraumatic, precollapse disease prevented collapse more effectively than placebo at 2-year follow-up (the rate of collapse for the alendronate therapy group was 6.9%; for the placebo group it was 76%; $P < 0.001$).[8] The roles of bone morphogenetic protein and other growth factors is investigational and further study is needed with long-term follow-up to determine the role of such growth factors in the management of patients with osteonecrosis.

Postcollapse Osteonecrosis
Collapse is a poor prognostic sign in patients with osteonecrosis. Failure rates with core decompression are higher in patients with collapse than those without collapse (71% versus 35%, respectively). The role of vascularized fibula grafts for the treatment of postcollapse osteonecrosis remains controversial, with some series demonstrating reasonable results in this challenging group of patients (64% success at 5-year follow-up).[9] Rotational osteotomies have been done for patients with postcollapse osteonecrosis, but this treatment technique has had more success in Japan than in the United States.[10]

For most patients with postcollapse osteonecrosis, arthroplasty represents a more reliable method of pain relief than joint preservation treatment options. Bipolar and unipolar arthroplasty have relatively high rates of conversion to total hip arthroplasty because of the eventual loss of the remaining acetabular cartilage and recurrent pain.[11] Young patients who undergo total hip arthroplasty with conventional polyethylene components have a high rate of osteolysis and revision. Alternative bearing materials demonstrate promising early results in this challenging subgroup of patients.[12] For some patients, surface replacement arthroplasty may be an option, but results are short term and indications are limited to patients with acceptable amounts of femoral head involvement with minimal deformity.[13] Indications for surface replacement arthroplasty in young patients with osteonecrosis are under investigation.

Hip and Pelvic Reconstruction Options

Hip Arthroscopy
Hip arthroscopy has evolved as a method to treat a variety of hip conditions including intra-articular and extra-articular pathology. Intra-articular pathology can

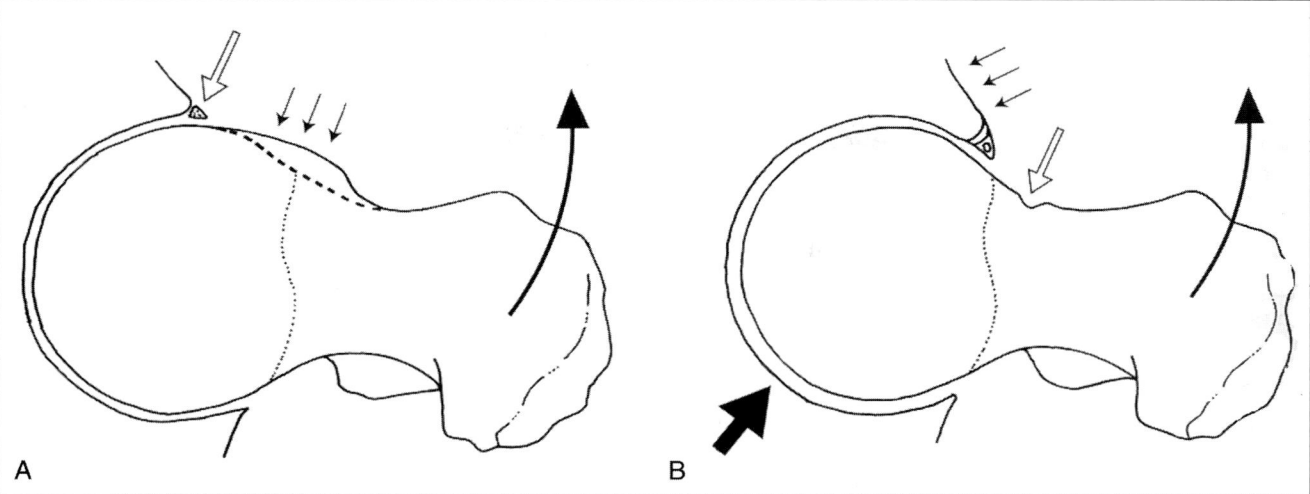

Figure 5 **A,** Line drawing illustrating the pathomechanism of cam-type impingement. The dashed line represents the normal femoral head-neck contour. The small black arrows indicate the abnormal anterior bone that decreases the normal head-neck ratio and causes impingement in flexion, internal rotation, and adduction, leading to damage of the acetabular labrum (*white arrow*). The large curved arrow indicates internal rotation of the hip. **B,** Line drawing illustrating the pathomechanism of pincer-type impingement. The white arrow indicates an indentation on the femoral neck (kissing lesion) that is caused by an acetabular prominence (*small black arrows*). High shearing forces (*large, broad black arrow*) between the posterior aspect of the femoral head and the acetabulum are produced in internal rotation. The large curved arrow indicates internal rotation of the hip. *(Reproduced with permission from Espinosa N, Rothenfluh DA, Beck M, Ganz R, Leunig M: Treatment of femoro-acetabular impingement: Preliminary results of labral refixation. J Bone Joint Surg Am 2006;88-A:925-935.)*

be addressed arthroscopically with the aid of limb traction on a fracture table. Indications include débridement of labral tears, removal of loose bodies (including synovial chondromatosis), débridement of chondral lesions, resection of osteophytes, biopsy, and synovectomy. Resection of the anterior femoral neck and anterior acetabular osteophytes in patients with femoroacetabular impingement can also be performed arthroscopically. More controversial areas of intra-articular arthroscopy include resection or repair of the ligamentum teres and débridement of the femoral head in patients with osteonecrosis. Extra-articular pathology usually can be approached with the hip out of traction. The major indications for extra-articular hip arthroscopy include treatment of the snapping hip by lengthening or releasing of the iliopsoas tendon. Treatment of chronic pain caused by iliopsoas or trochanteric bursitis with arthroscopic release or débridement remains controversial.

Complications of hip arthroscopy, including pudendal and sciatic nerve dysfunction, have decreased because of improved patient positioning, improved surgical technique, the use of fluoroscopy for accurate portal placement, and limiting the duration and amount of hip traction. The most commonly reported complication remains inadvertent damage to the articular surface of the femoral head during introduction of the required cannulas. More long-term studies are needed to assess the effectiveness of hip arthroscopy for the treatment of intra-articular and extra-articular hip pathology.

Osteochondroplasty and Osteotomy

Osteochondroplasty of the hip involves resection of osteophytes and débridement of damaged cartilage. The indication for this procedure is usually femoroacetabular impingement. Femoroacetabular impingement occurs via two known mechanisms: cam-type impingement and pincer-type impingement (**Figure 5**). The cam-type impingement occurs as a result of an abnormal anterior femoral neck impinging on a normal acetabulum and labrum with resulting damage to the acetabular labrum.[1,14] Treatment requires resection of a portion of the anterior femoral neck to improve the femoral head-neck ratio and either débridement or repair of labral pathology. The pincer-type impingement occurs as a result of an abnormal anterior acetabular osteophyte that abuts the anterior femoral neck in hip flexion or retroversion of the acetabulum.[15,16] Treatment involves resecting the anterior acetabular osteophyte, addressing labral abnormalities, correcting acetabular anteversion (periacetabular osteotomy), and in some instances correcting pathology on the anterior femoral neck. Published results demonstrate good outcomes at short-term follow-up for treatment of femoroacetabular impingement with open procedures and surgical dislocation of the hip.[16]

Osteotomy of the adult hip is indicated for treatment of dysplasia, residual deformity from slipped capital femoral epiphyses, cerebral palsy with hip instability, and osteonecrosis. The choice of femoral or acetabular osteotomy is dictated by the type of deformity present. Varus derotational femoral osteotomies are indicated in patients with hip dysplasia and valgus femoral defor-

4: Lower Extremity

mity with persistent femoral anteversion. Valgus femoral osteotomies are indicated for coxa vara in symptomatic patients without significant osteoarthritis and retained hip range of motion. Osteonecrosis with a small area of involvement of the femoral head may benefit from a valgus-flexion osteotomy to decrease the stress on the involved portion of the head. The best results with osteotomies for patients with osteonecrosis of the femoral head occur when the sum of the arcs of the involved osteonecrotic regions on the hip AP and lateral radiographs are less than 200°. Femoral osteotomies can be done to treat severe deformity caused by slipped epiphyses, but the indications for this procedure remain controversial because of the risk of osteonecrosis.

Pelvic osteotomies are most commonly done to correct developmental dysplasia. The most common pelvic osteotomy used to correct adult hip deformity is the periacetabular osteotomy (Ganz osteotomy). Indications for periacetabular osteotomy include deficient lateral and anterior coverage of the femoral head caused by acetabular dysplasia. Prerequisites for pelvic osteotomy include significant deformity (center edge angle < 17°), preservation of joint space on weight-bearing radiographs, and adequate hip motion. New techniques, including gadolinium-enhanced MRI, demonstrate promise to better define which patient subgroups are likely to benefit from corrective pelvic osteotomy.[17]

Resection Arthroplasty
Resection arthroplasty of the hip is a salvage procedure. Indications include severe hip infection (such as infection with antibiotic-resistant organisms and infection in medically debilitated patients), failed total hip arthroplasty with unreconstructible bone defects, previous high-dose pelvic radiation exposure, and inability to tolerate a complex reconstructive procedure. Nonambulatory patients at high risk for dislocation (for example, those with severe cerebral palsy or paraplegia) with osteoarthritis of the hip may benefit from resection arthroplasty for pain control and improved hygiene. All patients who undergo resection arthroplasty will have a significant limb-length discrepancy that requires a shoe lift as well as the use of walking aides.

Arthrodesis
Hip arthrodesis is usually done in young patients with acquired hip abnormalities (such as those caused by posttraumatic arthritis or infection) or developmental hip abnormalities (such as dysplasia). The optimal position for hip arthrodesis is 5° to 10° of external rotation, 20° to 30° of flexion, and neutral adduction. Gait studies have shown that patients with hip fusion increase their lumbar lordosis to accomplish hip extension during gait and decrease coronal plane moments to reduce joint loading on the fused hip.[18] Although pain relief can be excellent and a high level of function can be achieved, patients with hip fusions have energy expenditures during ambulation approximately 30% higher than those of patients without hip fusions. Pain or deformity of the lumbar spine, ipsilateral knee, and contralateral hip in potential candidates for hip arthrodesis should be minimal. Polyarticular arthritis is a relative contraindication to a hip arthrodesis. Nonunion is the most common short-term complication, and osteoarthritis of the lumbar spine and knee are the most frequent late complications.

Primary Total Hip Arthroplasty

Cemented Acetabular Components
Excellent results have been noted with cemented acetabular fixation in elderly patients.[19] In younger patients, cementless designs provide more durable fixation than cemented components. The choice to use cemented acetabular fixation is influenced by surgeon experience. Because of the excellent results with cementless designs in young and old patients, the frequency of cemented acetabular fixation has diminished substantially in the United States over the past decade.

Cementless Acetabular Components
Durable results have been noted with cementless acetabular components using a variety of designs.[19] Stress shielding, polyethylene wear, and osteolysis remain concerns at long-term follow-up intervals. Suboptimal outcomes have been noted with certain cementless acetabular components with inadequate liner locking mechanisms, thin polyethylene, or poor design (for example, threaded acetabular components). Novel porous surfaces have recently been introduced that closely simulate trabecular bone morphology in an effort to improve bone ingrowth and have encouraging results at intermediate follow-up intervals.[20] Longer-term studies are still necessary to determine whether these new bone ingrowth surfaces are superior to previous designs.

Cemented Femoral Components
The optimal choice for femoral fixation in primary total hip arthroplasty remains controversial. Excellent long-term results have been noted with certain cemented femoral component designs.[21] The outcome is influenced by many factors, including the stem geometry, surface finish, stem offset, patient selection, implant material, and surgical technique.[22] Risk factors for failure of cemented stems include young age, male sex, obesity, and high activity level.[21] Modern cement techniques using porosity reduction, pressurization, proximal and distal centralization, and appropriate preparation of the femoral canal to optimize the cancellous bone-cement interface are required to obtain a uniform cement mantle and to maximize the long-term performance of these cemented devices.

Cementless Femoral Components
Excellent long-term results have been noted with proximally and fully porous-coated cementless femoral designs.[21] Many fully porous-coated stems have excellent long-term survival, but thigh pain and proximal stress

shielding have been noted. Many proximally porous-coated femoral designs have documented success at intermediate- and long-term outcome when circumferential coatings are used.[23] The issue of the relative rate of thigh pain in patients with proximally and fully porous-coated femoral components remains controversial. Several hydroxyapatite (HA)-coated cementless femoral designs have demonstrated excellent intermediate-term clinical performance, but they have not been proven superior to non–HA-coated femoral designs to date.[24]

Alternative Bearing Options in Primary Total Hip Arthroplasty

Conventional polyethylene coupled with conventional femoral head sizes (22 to 32 mm) has performed well at long-term follow-up in older patient populations (age 60 years or older).[21] However, dislocation remains a concern, with rates of 1% to 5% with conventional femoral head sizes in patients undergoing primary total hip arthroplasty. In younger, more active patients (younger than age 60 years), polyethylene wear and osteolysis represent the most common cause of long-term failure. Alternative bearing options have been introduced to address the concerns of dislocation and polyethylene wear, including ceramic-on-ceramic, metal-on-highly cross-linked polyethylene, and metal-on-metal designs. These alternative bearing options are discussed in detail in chapter 7.

Large Femoral Heads in Primary Total Hip Arthroplasty

Dislocation remains a challenging complication with primary total hip arthroplasty. Historically, femoral heads were limited to smaller sizes (22 to 32 mm) because of concerns regarding conventional polyethylene wear and failure with the use of larger femoral heads (> 32 mm). The introduction of alternative bearings has provided the opportunity to reevaluate the issue of optimal head size in primary total hip arthroplasty.

Early clinical data suggest that large femoral heads can be used to prevent and treat dislocation after primary total hip arthroplasty.[25,26] Controversy exists regarding the routine use of large femoral heads in patients with no known risk factors for dislocation in primary total hip arthroplasty. It is also unclear whether dislocation precautions are necessary postoperatively with the use of large femoral heads. Further study is needed to determine whether the excellent wear rates noted for these large heads in hip-simulator testing and short-term follow-up intervals[26] will be supported by long-term clinical performance. Issues related to patient selection, optimal bearing material, and cost-effectiveness remain controversial.

Total Hip Resurfacing

Historically, total hip resurfacing has had poor outcomes, but substantial changes have been made to improve the tribology of surface replacement arthroplasty, and these new designs have been used in Europe for ap-

proximately 8 to 10 years.[27,28] The early encouraging results with these new implants[27,28] prompted the US Food and Drug Administration to approve total hip resurfacing (or surface replacement arthroplasty) for use in the United States in May 2006. Although these relatively short-term studies are encouraging, longer-term studies are needed to determine the relative revision rates for surface replacement arthroplasty and total hip arthroplasty with alternative bearings, especially for young, active patients at high risk for implant failure.

The potential advantages of surface replacement arthroplasty compared with traditional total hip arthroplasty include femoral bone preservation, lower dislocation risk, and rapid recovery. However, surface replacement arthroplasty is not less invasive than traditional total hip arthroplasty. Acetabular exposure requires more extensive soft-tissue release than is required with traditional total hip arthroplasty. Accurate placement of the surface replacement arthroplasty femoral component is challenging and heterotopic ossification may occur at a higher rate compared with traditional total hip arthroplasty.

Potential complications with surface replacement arthroplasty include femoral neck fracture (complication rate, 1% to 3%), osteonecrosis, and early loosening of the cemented femoral component. Risk factors for femoral neck fracture include female sex, poor bone quality, varus femoral component positioning, and taller patients.[29] Surgeon experience will likely affect the rate of complications and risk of early failure. The indications and patient selection criteria for surface replacement arthroplasty remain controversial.

Minimally Invasive Total Hip Arthroplasty

There are many minimally invasive surgical approaches available, including the two-incision, mini-posterior, mini-direct lateral, and mini-anterolateral approaches. No single approach has proven superior to any other in published series. Surgeon experience likely influences complication rates, and debate exists regarding the learning curve and potential for complications with these approaches.[30,31]

Benefits from minimally invasive surgical approaches for total hip arthroplasty are likely multifactorial and include modifying surgical techniques, optimizing anesthetic techniques, improving postoperative rehabilitation protocols, and managing patient expectations. Patient selection for minimally invasive total hip arthroplasty and the relative benefit of minimally invasive total hip arthroplasty compared with traditional total hip arthroplasty remain controversial.[30,31]

Revision Total Hip Arthroplasty

Preoperative Assessment

Common indications for revision total hip arthroplasty include periprosthetic osteolysis resulting in aseptic loos-

4: Lower Extremity

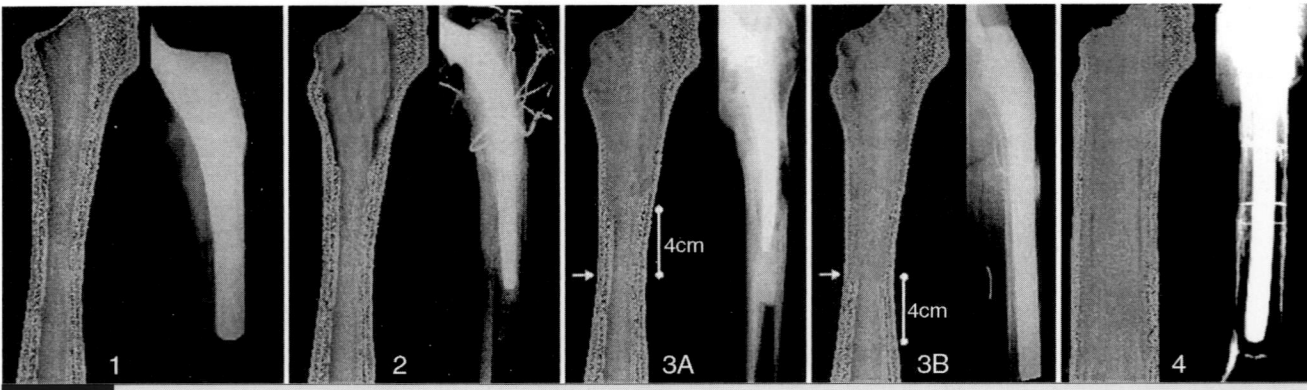

Figure 6 Paprosky femoral defect classification. Type 1 has minimal metaphyseal involvement and adequate cancellous bone. Type 2 has metaphyseal damage with a minimally involved diaphysis. Type 3A has metadiaphyseal damage with 4 cm of reliable cortex proximal to the isthmus. Type 3B has metadiaphyseal damage with 4 cm of reliable cortex distal to the isthmus. Type 4 has extensive metadiaphyseal and thin ballooned cortices with widened canals precluding reliable fixation. *(Reproduced from Berry DJ, Garvin KL, Lee SH, et al: Hip and pelvis: Reconstruction, in Beaty JH (ed):* Orthopaedic Knowledge Update 6. *Rosemont, IL, American Academy of Orthopaedic Surgeons, 1999, pp 455-492.)*

ening, dislocation, and sepsis. Standard preoperative evaluation includes a thorough history, physical examination, and assessment of the erythrocyte sedimentation rate and C-reactive protein level. In patients with suspected infection, a hip aspiration should also be performed. For patients with confirmed infection, a two-stage exchange is often needed to eradicate the infection and provide the highest likelihood of success. In patients with aseptic loosening, the surgeon must assess the degree of acetabular and femoral bone loss to determine the appropriate components needed to perform the reconstruction (the process of preoperative templating). The surgeon must obtain all necessary prior medical records, including the previous surgical notes and the implant stickers listing the manufacturer, the catalog number, and the lot number of the implants currently in place. Extensile surgical techniques, including trochanteric osteotomies, are sometimes needed to provide adequate exposure in complex reconstructive cases.

Osteolysis

Aseptic loosening caused by periprosthetic osteolysis is the most common cause of long-term failure after total hip arthroplasty. The pathology of this process has been reviewed in detail.[32] Briefly, wear of the bearing surface generates particulate debris that stimulates macrophages and other cells to secrete proinflammatory cytokines (such as tumor necrosis factor-α) that ultimately results in activation of the receptor activator of nuclear factor-$\kappa\beta$ (RANK), the receptor activator of nuclear factor-$\kappa\beta$ ligand (RANKL), and the endogenous soluble RANKL inhibitor, osteoprotegerin (OPG)—the RANK/RANKL/OPG system.[33] Osteoclast differentiation and activation via this system can result in periprosthetic bone loss, implant loosening, periprosthetic fracture, and can prompt the need for revision surgery. The degree of femoral and acetabular bone loss dictates the type of reconstruction required.

Femoral Bone Loss

The Paprosky classification system (**Figure 6** and **Table 1**) is useful for categorizing the extent of femoral bone loss and providing guidance regarding treatment options. Type 1 (minimal bone loss) and type 2 (proximal metaphyseal bone loss) defects have no diaphyseal bone loss. Type 3 defects have diaphyseal bone loss. Type 3A defects have at least 4 cm of intact diaphyseal bone proximal to the isthmus. Type 3B defects have less than 4 cm of diaphyseal bone remaining proximal to the isthmus. Type IV defects involve loss of diaphyseal bone distal to the isthmus.

Treatment is dictated by the amount of remaining bone. To achieve stable fixation and reliable bone ingrowth, fully porous-coated stems require approximately 90% canal fill over at least 4 cm of diaphyseal bone. In Paprosky type I and type II defects, adequate stability can generally be achieved with primary fully porous-coated stems (approximately 6 inches in length). In Paprosky type IIIA and IIB defects, adequate stability usually requires the use of revisions stems between 7 and 10 inches in length.[34] Some more extensive type IIIB and most type IV defects require alternative salvage strategies, including impaction grafting, modular tapered stems, allograft prosthetic composites, and megaprosthesis.[34] Treatment strategies that use this femoral revision classification system and fully porous-coated stems have demonstrated excellent results with a 4% mechanical failure rate at a 14-year follow-up interval.[35]

The indications for cemented femoral revisions have diminished because of their inferior long-term survival compared with that for cementless implants.[36] In revision total hip arthroplasty, the suboptimal remaining cancellous bone likely reduces cement interdigitation and reduces the strength of the bone-cement interface, predisposing cemented femoral revisions to early failure. However, specific indications for cemented revision

Table 1

Classification of Acetabulum Defects

Type of Defect	Superior Migration of Hip Center*	Osteolysis of Ischium†	Medial Migration of Hip Center‡	Osteolysis of Teardrops§
I	Minimum	None	None	None
IIA	Minimum	Mild	Grade I	Mild
IIB	Minimum to marked	Mild	Grade II	Mild
IIC	Minimum	Mild	Grade III	Moderate to severe
IIIA	Marked	Moderate	Grade II+ or III	Moderate
IIIB	Marked	Severe	Grade III+	Severe

*Minimum = at least 3 cm proximal to the superior transverse obturator line, and marked = more than 3 cm proximal to the superior transverse obturator line.
†Mild = 0 to 7 mm distal to the superior transverse obturator line, moderate = 8 to 14 mm distal to the obturator line, and severe = 15 mm or more distal to the obturator line.
‡Grade I = lateral to Köhler's line, grade II = migration to Köhler's line, grade II+ = medial expansion of Köhler's line into pelvis, grade III = migration into pelvis with violation of Köhler's line, and grade III+ = marked migration into the pelvis.
§Mild = minimum loss of the lateral border, moderate = complete loss of the lateral border, and severe = loss of the lateral and medial borders.
(Reproduced from Barrack R, Berry D, Burak C, et al: Hip and pelvis reconstruction, in Koval KJ (ed): Orthopaedic Knowledge Update 7. Rosemont, IL, American Academy of Orthopaedic Surgeons, 2002, pp 417-451.)

techniques still exist.[37] Long-stem cemented femoral revisions are most often reserved for older patients with lower physical demands.

Acetabular Bone Loss

To achieve reliable bone ingrowth, cementless acetabular components require adequate initial stability (< 40 μm of micromotion) and at least 50% to 70% contact with host bone. When these criteria are met, excellent results have been noted for cementless hemispherical reconstructions in revision total hip arthroplasty at minimum 10-year follow-up intervals.[38] More sophisticated reconstruction techniques (impaction grafting, antiprotrusio cages, and bulk allografts) are required in challenging patients in whom bone loss is too severe to use hemispherical shells.

The Paprosky classification system uses plain radiographs to determine the degree of acetabular bone loss and provides guidance regarding treatment options (Figure 7 and Table 2). In type 1 defects, the rim and columns are supportive with more than 50% of the cup in contact with host bone. In type 2 defects, the columns are intact, and there is partial loss of the superomedial (type 2A), superolateral (type 2B), or medial wall (type 2C) with intact anterior and posterior columns. Excellent results have been noted for the treatment of type 1 and 2 defects using allograft to fill contained defects and a cementless cup fixed with supplemental screw fixation at 10-year follow-up.[38] In type 3 defects, there is severe bone loss involving the acetabular walls and pelvic columns (type 3A) and pelvic discontinuity (type 3B). Patients with severe (type 3) bone loss require more complex reconstruction, including bulk allograft and antiprotrusio cages. Results with allografts and antiprotrusio cages for these defects have deteriorated over time.[39] These high failure rates have prompted some investigators to use porous tantalum components and metal augments to reconstruct type

3A and 3B defects with promising early (2- to 3-year follow-up) results.[40,41] Contemporary indications for cemented acetabular revision are limited because of the superior performance of cementless acetabular components in most patients. Cemented acetabular revisions are generally reserved for patients in whom a polyethylene liner is cemented into a well-fixed shell or those in whom a polyethylene liner must be cemented into a bulk pelvic allograft or antiprotrusio cage.

Complications

Patients requiring primary and revision total hip arthroplasty often have significant medical comorbidities. The physiologic stress of total hip arthroplasty can result in cardiovascular, pulmonary, renal, and other organ system complications. The incidence of death after primary total hip arthroplasty for osteoarthritis has been estimated to be as high as 6% after total hip arthroplasty for acute hip fracture. Death following total hip arthroplasty is usually the result of cardiac or pulmonary complications.

Neurovascular injury can be a devastating and, in some patients, a life-threatening complication after total hip arthroplasty. Peroneal, sciatic nerve, and femoral nerve palsies have been reported after total hip arthroplasty. Injury to the peroneal portion of the sciatic nerve can result in peroneal nerve palsy and this represents the most common associated neurovascular injury, occurring with an incidence of 0 to 3% after primary total hip arthroplasty and up to 7% after revision total hip arthroplasty. Although the incidence of intraoperative injury to the femoral, iliac, and obturator vessels is low (< 1%), major vessel injury can threaten both life and limb. Major vessel injuries can result from retractor placement, acetabular screw penetration, or femoral cerclage wire placement. If major vessel injury is suspected, immediate notification of the anesthetic team as well as appropriate vascular surgery and/or in-

4: Lower Extremity

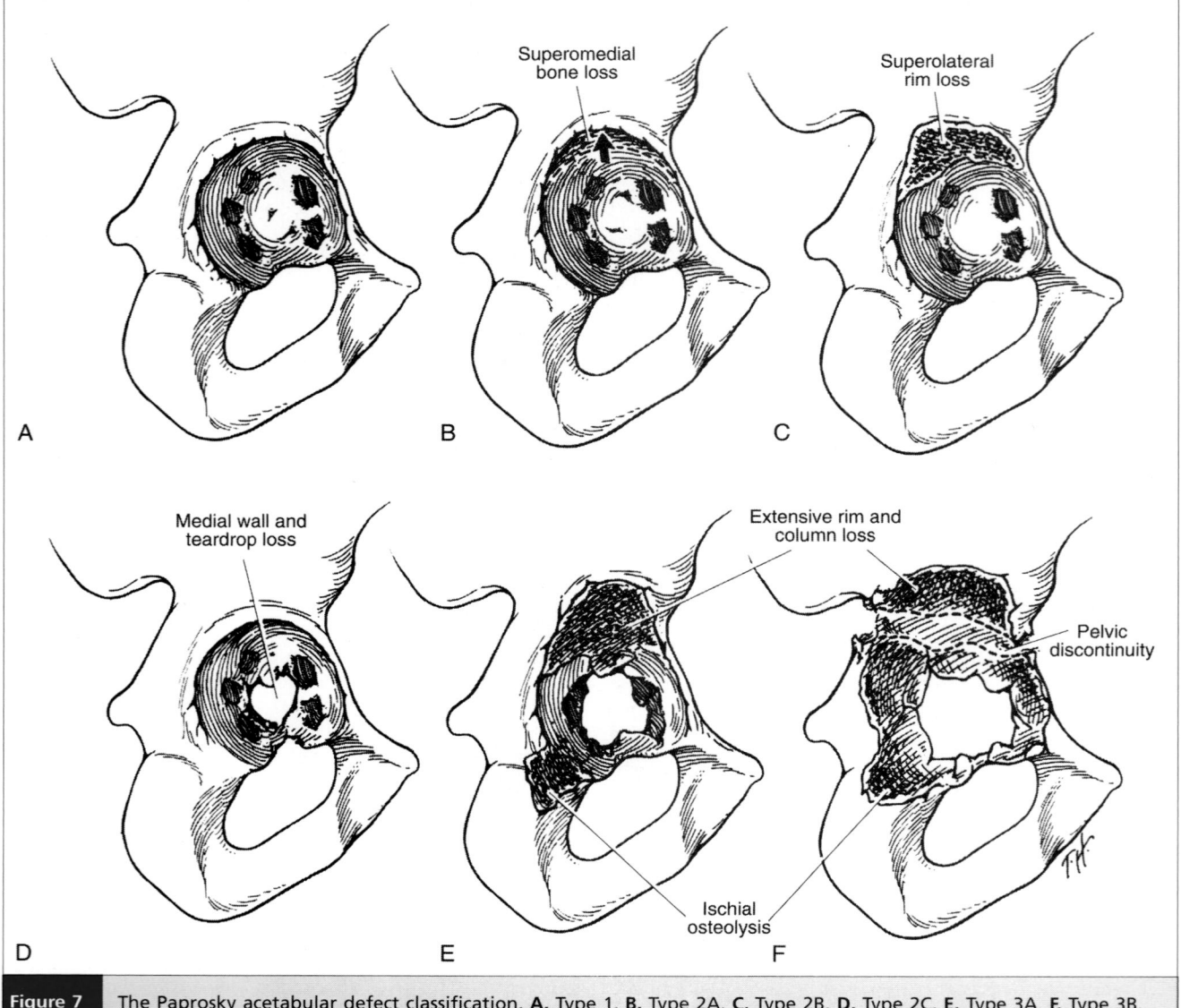

Figure 7 The Paprosky acetabular defect classification. **A,** Type 1. **B,** Type 2A. **C,** Type 2B. **D,** Type 2C. **E,** Type 3A. **F,** Type 3B. *(Reproduced with permission from Buly RL, Nestor BJ: Revision total hip replacement, in Craig EV (ed): Clinical Orthopaedics. Philadelphia, PA, Lippincott Williams & Wilkins, 1999.)*

Table 2

The Paprosky Acetabular Defect Classification

Type 1	Minimal lysis or component migration
Type 2A	Superomedial migration < 2 cm
Type 2B	Superolateral migration < 2 cm
Type 2C	Teardrop lysis, loss of medial wall
Type 3A	Migration > 2 cm, ischial lysis present
Type 3B	Same as 3A plus disruption of Köhler's line, indicative of profound medial loss; pelvic dissociation may be present

(Reproduced with permission from Paprosky WG, Lawrence JM: Acetabular defect classification and surgical reconstruction in revision arthroplasty: A 6-year follow-up evaluation. J Arthroplasty 1994;9:33-44.)

terventional radiology consultation is required.

Despite appropriate prophylactic measures, deep venous thrombosis commonly occurs after total hip arthroplasty. In the absence of appropriate prophylaxis, the incidence of asymptomatic deep venous thrombosis after total hip arthroplasty is approximately 40% to 60%, and the incidence of fatal pulmonary embolism is estimated to be 0.5% to 2.0%.[42] With appropriate prophylactic agents, the incidence of asymptomatic deep venous thrombosis after total hip arthroplasty has been estimated to be 3% to 30%, whereas the incidence of symptomatic pulmonary embolism in some studies has been reported to be less than 0.5%.[42] The optimal perioperative strategy to reduce the incidence of deep venous thrombosis after primary and revision total hip arthroplasty remains controversial. Nevertheless, some form of prophylaxis is recommended. The American College of Chest Physicians suggests warfarin (goal international normalized ratio: 2.0 to 3.0), fondaparinux, or low-molecular-weight heparin for at least 10 days after total hip arthroplasty (all are grade 1A recommendations) with or without the use of graduated compression stockings and/or intermittent pneumatic compression devices (grade 1C+ recommendation). Recommendations from the American College of Chest Physicians are based on deep venous thrombosis prevention as a surrogate for the most clinically relevant end-point symptomatic and fatal pulmonary embolism. The American Academy of Orthopaedic Surgeons (AAOS) will introduce new guidelines in the near future that will be based on preventing symptomatic and fatal pulmonary embolism.

Limb-length discrepancy following total hip arthroplasty can be a source of significant patient dissatisfaction and potential litigation. Patient education concerning limb-length discrepancy should be initiated before total hip arthroplasty, and patients with profound femoral or acetabular deformity, pelvic obliquity, spine deformity, and preexisting limb-length discrepancy should be informed that restoration of equal leg lengths may not be possible. Prevention of significant limb-length discrepancy includes careful preoperative radiographic templating and requires intraoperative assessment of limb-length restoration. The availability of extended offset devices and large femoral heads has diminished the tendency to excessively lengthen the leg to achieve intraoperative stability. Patients with persistent reports of limb-length discrepancy may require a contralateral shoe lift.

The incidence of hip dislocation ranges from 0.5% to 7% for primary total hip arthroplasty and from 10% to 25% for revision total hip arthroplasty. Approximately 66% of dislocations occur within the first 3 months after surgery and most occur posteriorly. Previous investigations have indicated that the dislocation rates for direct lateral (0.5%) and anterolateral (2.2%) approaches are lower when compared with the posterior approach (3.2%).[43] If repair of the posterior capsule and short external rotators is performed, the dislocation rate following the posterior approach is comparable to that for lateral and anterior approaches.[44] Risk factors for dislocation after total hip arthroplasty include previous hip surgery, neuromuscular or spastic disorders (such as Parkinson's disease), acute fracture, developmental dysplasia, cognitive dysfunction, advanced age (80 years or older), female sex, and drug or alcohol abuse. Component malposition and failure to reconstruct appropriate soft-tissue tension are the most common technical factors predisposing patients to dislocation. Fortunately, 60% to 70% of dislocations are isolated events and can be successfully treated with closed reduction and abduction bracing. Patients who experience multiple (three or more) dislocations have a high likelihood of future dislocations, and revision surgery is often indicated. Optimally, the cause of instability is identified and surgically corrected. Options for surgical treatment of recurrent dislocations include removal of well-fixed

malpositioned components, femoral head/liner exchanges, use of captured acetabular components, use of large femoral heads, and trochanteric advancement.

Deep infection is a serious cause of morbidity following total hip arthroplasty. With the use of appropriate surgical theater air-handling and prophylactic antibiotics, the incidence of deep infection ranges from 0.5% to 2%. An increased risk of infection occurs in patients who are malnourished, immunosuppressed (for example, patients who have undergone transplantation or those with rheumatoid arthritis), renal dialysis-dependent, positive for human immunodeficiency virus, morbidly obese, and diabetic. In healthy patients without conditions predisposing them to sepsis resulting from total hip arthroplasty, early infections (< 3 months after total hip arthroplasty) can often be successfully treated with aggressive irrigation and débridement, exchange of modular components, and intravenous antibiotics. In general, two-stage component exchange and intravenous antibiotic treatment remains the gold standard for chronic infections and infections in patients with health issues that compromise the immune system.[45] The rising incidence of antibiotic-resistant infection in patients who have undergone total hip replacements and those with severe bone loss following multiple prior orthopaedic procedures represents a growing challenge of treatment.

Annotated References

1. Ganz R, Parvizi J, Beck M, Leunig M, Notzli H, Siebenrock KA: Femoroacetabular impingement: A cause for osteoarthritis of the hip. *Clin Orthop Relat Res* 2003; 417:112-120.

2. Blankenbaker DG, De Smet AA, Keene JS: Sonography of the iliopsoas tendon and injection of the iliopsoas bursa for diagnosis and management of the painful snapping hip. *Skeletal Radiol* 2006;35:565-571.

   The authors review the technique and results of ultrasound-guided iliopsoas injection for the evaluation of the snapping hip and conclude that patients with groin pain and a clinically suspected snapping iliopsoas tendon can benefit from injection into the iliopsoas bursa even if the snapping tendon is not visualized sonographically. The authors also found that a corticosteroid can provide long-term pain relief, and pain relief after injection is a predictor of good outcome after iliopsoas tendon release. Level of evidence: IV (therapeutic).

3. Illgen RL, Honkamp NJ, Weisman MH, Hagenauer ME, Heiner JP, Anderson PA: The diagnostic and predictive value of hip anesthetic arthrograms in selected patients before total hip arthroplasty. *J Arthroplasty* 2006;21:724-730.

   The authors review the use and diagnostic utility of hip anesthetic arthrograms in the evaluation of patients with concurrent hip and spine osteoarthritis and report that their findings support the selected use of hip anesthetic arthrograms in the preoperative assessment of these patients when associated with nondiagnostic history and physical examinations. Level of evidence: IV (diagnostic).

4. Reynolds D, Lucas J, Klaue K: Retroversion of the acetabulum: A cause of hip pain. *J Bone Joint Surg Br* 1999;81:281-288.

5. Peters CL, Erickson J: The etiology and treatment of hip pain in the young adult. *J Bone Joint Surg Am* 2006;88 (suppl 4):20-26.

    The authors provide a comprehensive review of the concept of femoroacetabular impingement and the causes of hip pain in the young adult. Level of evidence: IV.

6. Byrd JW, Jones KS: Diagnostic accuracy of clinical assessment, magnetic resonance imaging, magnetic resonance arthrography, and intra-articular injection in hip arthroscopy patients. *Am J Sports Med* 2004;32:1668-1674.

    This study was a retrospective review of prospectively collected data. Clinical assessment accurately determined the existence of intra-articular abnormality but was poor at defining its nature. Magnetic resonance arthrography was much more sensitive than MRI at detecting various lesions but had twice as many false-positive interpretations. Response to an intra-articular injection of anesthetic was a 90% reliable indicator of intra-articular abnormality.

7. Mont MA, Marulanda GA, Seyler TM, Plate JF, Delanois RE: Core decompression and nonvascularized bone grafting for the treatment of early stage osteonecrosis of the femoral head. *Instr Course Lect* 2007;56: 213-220.

    More than 40 previous studies of core decompression and nonvascularized bone grafting were reviewed. In general, core decompression is most successful for patients with early stage, small- and medium-sized lesions before collapse of the femoral head. Various methods of nonvascularized bone grafting have been used with varied results. A 60% to 80% success rate has been achieved at 5- to 10-year follow-up.

8. Lai KA, Shen WJ, Yang CY, Shao CJ, Hsu JT, Lin RM: The use of alendronate to prevent early collapse of the femoral head in patients with nontraumatic osteonecrosis: A randomized clinical study. *J Bone Joint Surg Am* 2005;87:2155-2159.

    The authors of this randomized clinical study demonstrated that alendronate can effectively prevent collapse at intermediate follow-up intervals for patients with precollapse (Ficat stage I-II) osteonecrosis. Level of evidence: I (therapeutic).

9. Aldridge JM III, Berend KR, Gunneson EE, Urbaniak JR: Free vascularized fibular grafting for the treatment of postcollapse osteonecrosis of the femoral head: Surgical technique. *J Bone Joint Surg Am* 2004;86-A(suppl 1): 87-101.

    The authors review the use of vascularized free fibular grafting for the treatment of postcollapse osteonecrosis of the femoral head and demonstrate reasonable success rates using this surgical technique. Level of evidence: IV (therapeutic).

10. Miyanishi K, Noguchi Y, Yamamoto T, et al: Prediction of the outcome of transtrochanteric rotational osteotomy for osteonecrosis of the femoral head. *J Bone Joint Surg Br* 2000;82:512-516.

11. Lee SB, Sugano N, Nakata K, Matsui M, Ohzono K: Comparison between bipolar hemiarthroplasty and THA for osteonecrosis of the femoral head. *Clin Orthop Relat Res* 2004;424:161-165.

    The authors of this article illustrate the tradeoffs when considering hemiarthroplasty compared with total hip arthroplasty for treatment of osteonecrosis of the femoral head in young patients. They report that hemiarthroplasty tends to have fewer short-term complications, particularly dislocations, but poses a higher risk for late conversion to total hip arthroplasty because of persistent or progressive hip pain. Level of evidence: IV (therapeutic).

12. Seyler TM, Cui Q, Mihalko WM, Mont MA, Saleh KJ: Advances in hip arthroplasty in the treatment of osteonecrosis. *Instr Course Lect* 2007;56:221-233.

    This review article discusses the multiple approaches to hip arthroplasty in patients with osteonecrosis, a population that historically has shown poor outcomes. More recent studies have shown improved outcomes of these patients by using second- and third-generation designs, especially when incorporating alternative bearing surfaces, in particular, ceramic-on-ceramic and metal-on-metal.

13. Revell MP, McBryde CW, Bhatnagar S, Pynsent PB, Treacy RB: Metal-on-metal hip resurfacing in osteonecrosis of the femoral head. *J Bone Joint Surg Am* 2006; 88(suppl 3):98-103.

    A consecutive series of 73 hip resurfacing procedures performed by a single surgeon between 1994 and 2004, with a mean follow-up of 6.1 years, was reviewed. There were four revision operations and one planned revision of the 73 hips during the follow-up period. Two of these revisions were necessitated by aseptic failure of the femoral component. This represents an overall survival rate of 93.2%. On the basis of this study, metal-on-metal resurfacing of the hip for osteonecrosis can be considered a safe and effective form of surgery for this group of patients.

14. Ito K, Minka MA, Leunig M, Werlen S, Ganz R: Femoroacetabular impingement and the cam-effect: An MRI-based quantitative anatomical study of the femoral head-neck offset. *J Bone Joint Surg Br* 2001;83:171-176.

15. Beck M, Kalhor M, Leunig M, Ganz R: Hip morphology influences the pattern of damage to the acetabular cartilage: Femoroacetabular impingement as a cause of early osteoarthritis of the hip. *J Bone Joint Surg Br* 2005;87:1012-1018.

    This study was conducted to determine whether cam impingement caused by a nonspherical femoral head and pincer impingement caused by excessive acetabular cover each results in different patterns of articular damage. In the 42 hips studied (26 with isolated cam impingement and 16 with isolated pincer impingement), cam impingement was noted to cause damage to the anterosuperior acetabular cartilage with separation between the labrum and cartilage, and pincer impingement was noted to cause cartilage damage circumferentially and included only a narrow strip. The authors discuss femoroacetabular impingement as a cause of osteoarthritis; the senior author (Dr. Ganz) is the originator of this concept. Level of evidence: IV (diagnostic).

16. Beck M, Leunig M, Parvizi J, Boutier V, Wyss D, Ganz R: Anterior femoroacetabular impingement: Part II. Midterm results of surgical treatment. *Clin Orthop Relat Res* 2004;418:67-73.

    The authors treated 19 patients (14 men and 5 women; mean age, 36 years; age range, 21 to 52 years) with surgical dislocation and offset creation of the hip. At an average 4.7-year follow-up (range, 4 to 5.2 years), 13 hips were reported as excellent to good, with pain scores improving from 2.9 to 5.1 at latest follow-up. No osteonecrosis of the femoral head was noted. The authors concluded that surgical dislocation with correction of femoroacetabular impingement yields good results in patients with early degenerative changes that do not exceed grade 1 osteoarthrosis, but that this procedure is not suitable for patients with advanced degenerative changes and extensive articular cartilage damage. Level of evidence: IV (therapeutic).

17. Cunningham T, Jessel R, Zurakowski D, Millis MB, Kim YJ: Delayed gadolinium-enhanced magnetic resonance imaging of cartilage to predict early failure of Bernese periacetabular osteotomy for hip dysplasia. *J Bone Joint Surg Am* 2006;88:1540-1548.

    The authors discuss a cohort study of 47 patients undergoing a Bernese periacetabular osteotomy for the treatment of hip dysplasia. The goal was to identify preoperative radiographic factors, such as the grade of arthritis, joint congruency, and the delayed gadolinium-enhanced magnetic resonance imaging of cartilage (dGEMRIC) index, that are associated with a poor outcome after osteotomy. Hips in which the osteotomy did not fail had a significant decrease in pain compared with their status preoperatively (p < 0.0001). Hips in which the osteotomy did fail had had significantly more arthritis on preoperative radiographs (p = 0.01), more subluxation (p = 0.02), and a lower dGEMRIC index (p < 0.001) than the hips in which the osteotomy did not fail. Multivariate analysis identified the dGEMRIC index as the most important predictor of failure of the osteotomy. Bernese periacetabular osteotomy for the treatment of hip dysplasia can decrease pain and improve unction in symptomatic dysplastic hips. The dGEMRIC index, as an early measure of osteoarthritis, appears to be useful for identifying poor candidates for a pelvic osteotomy.

18. Thambyah A, Hee HT, Das DS, Lee SM: Gait adaptations in patients with longstanding hip fusion. *J Orthop Surg (Hong Kong)* 2003;11:154-158.

19. Illgen R, Rubash HE: The optimal fixation of the cementless acetabular component in primary total hip arthroplasty. *J Am Acad Orthop Surg* 2002;10:43-56.

20. Komarasamy B, Vadivelu R, Bruce A, Kershaw C, Davison J: Clinical and radiological outcome following total hip arthroplasty with an uncemented trabecular metal monoblock acetabular cup. *Acta Orthop Belg* 2006;72: 320-325.

    This study represents one institution's experience with an uncemented trabecular metal monoblock acetabular cup in 113 hips, from 1999-2002. The average age at surgery was 56.8 years. Patient satisfaction was very high (99%), Oxford hip scores improved dramatically, and there were no radiologic signs of cup loosening or wear.

21. Berry DJ, Harmsen WS, Cabanela ME, Morrey BF: Twenty-five-year survivorship of two thousand consecutive primary Charnley total hip replacements: Factors affecting survivorship of acetabular and femoral components. *J Bone Joint Surg Am* 2002;84-A:171-177.

22. Berry DJ: Cemented femoral stems: What matters most. *J Arthroplasty* 2004;19:83-84.

    The author reviews the design features and surgical technique issues that affect survival for cemented femoral stems and reports that most important factors influencing arthroplasty success using a cemented femoral stem include patient selection, intramedullary implant geometry, implant surface finish, implant design above the femoral neck resection level, and surgical technique. Level of evidence: IV (therapeutic).

23. Parvizi J, Keisu KS, Hozack WJ, Sharkey PF, Rothman RH: Primary total hip arthroplasty with an uncemented femoral component: A long-term study of the Taperloc stem. *J Arthroplasty* 2004;19:151-156.

    This is a retrospective case series of 129 hips that underwent primary total hip arthroplasty with the use of a single, proximally and circumferentially porous-coated femoral stem. Average follow-up was 11 years and yielded excellent outcomes, with a low revision rate and high patient satisfaction.

24. Capello WN, D'Antonio JA, Jaffe WL, Geesink RG, Manley MT, Feinberg JR: Hydroxyapatite-coated femoral components: 15-year minimum followup. *Clin Orthop Relat Res* 2006;453:75-80.

    This multicenter study was retrospectively reviewed from a larger prospective cohort. It consisted of 166 hips with a follow-up interval of 15 to 18 years. The femoral aseptic revision and mechanical failure rates were both 0.6% at minimum 15 years follow-up. This demonstrates excellent long-term survivorship of HA-coated femoral components in a relatively young cohort.

25. Amstutz HC, Le Duff MJ, Beaule PE: Prevention and treatment of dislocation after total hip replacement using large diameter balls. *Clin Orthop Relat Res* 2004; 429:108-116.

    The authors of this study demonstrate that femoral heads of 36 mm or larger can reduce the risk of dislocation after primary total hip arthroplasty and in some instances can be used to address recurrent dislocation problems in patients undergoing revision total hip arthroplasty. Level of evidence: IV (prognostic).

4: Lower Extremity

26. Geller JA, Malchau H, Bragdon C, Greene M, Harris WH, Freiberg AA: Large diameter femoral heads on highly cross-linked polyethylene: Minimum 3-year results. *Clin Orthop Relat Res* 2006;447:53-59.

This was a prospective study of 42 patients (45 hips) who underwent total hip replacement using large diameter cobalt-chrome femoral heads articulating with highly cross-linked polyethylene. At a minimum 3 years follow-up (mean, 3.3 years), the authors reported excellent clinical results with a low rate of dislocation. Level of evidence: IV (therapeutic).

27. Treacy RB, McBryde CW, Pynsent PB: Birmingham hip resurfacing arthroplasty: A minimum follow-up of five years. *J Bone Joint Surg Br* 2005;87:167-170.

The authors review early experience with hip surface replacement at one center; 144 consecutive metal-on-metal resurfacings of the hip were studied, and failure was defined as revision of either the acetabular or femoral component for any reason. The survival rate at 5-year follow-up was 98% overall (99% for aseptic revisions only). These data were instrumental in securing US Food and Drug Administration approval of surface replacement arthroplasty in May 2006. Level of evidence: IV (therapeutic).

28. Daniel J, Pynsent PB, McMinn DJ: Metal-on-metal resurfacing of the hip in patients under the age of 55 years with osteoarthritis. *J Bone Joint Surg Br* 2004;86:177-184.

The authors report on a series of 446 hip resurfacings (384 patients) done by a single surgeon using cemented femoral components and HA-coated uncemented acetabular components. Of the 378 patients available for a mean follow-up of 3.3 years, only 1 revision (0.02%) out of 440 hips was reported. Data from this study were also instrumental in securing US Food and Drug Administration approval of surface replacement arthroplasty in May 2006. Level of evidence: IV (therapeutic).

29. Amstutz HC, Beaule PE, Dorey FJ, Le Duff MJ, Campbell PA, Gruen TA: Metal-on-metal hybrid surface arthroplasty: Surgical technique. *J Bone Joint Surg Am* 2006;88 (suppl 1, pt 2):234-249.

The authors review important patient selection and surgical technique factors that influence the risk of femoral neck fractures and affect the long-term survival of the femoral component in surface replacements. Level of evidence: IV (therapeutic).

30. Berger RA, Jacobs JJ, Meneghini RM, Della Valle CJ, Paprosky W, Rosenberg AG: Rapid rehabilitation and recovery with minimally invasive total hip arthroplasty. *Clin Orthop Relat Res* 2004;429:239-247.

A seminal paper on the minimally invasive two-incision hip arthroplasty technique describes with very high successes the rapid rehabilitation of patients receiving this technique. The 100 indexed procedures were performed between 2001 and 2003, with patients an average age of 56 years. Whereas the reported results were outstanding, subsequent reports have noted that such high levels of success are difficult to reproduce by other surgeons. It should also be noted that only 20% of the total hips performed at this institution during this interval were eligible for inclusion. This technique is only appropriate for certain patients meeting defined criteria.

31. Pagnano MW, Leone J, Lewallen DG, Hanssen AD: Two-incision THA had modest outcomes and some substantial complications. *Clin Orthop Relat Res* 2005;441:86-90.

This article reviews the two-incision minimally invasive total hip arthroplasty technique described by Berger in 2004. In this study, the authors performed a randomized trial, including all patients in a series of 80 consecutive hips, average age 70.5. The authors documented longer surgical times, higher complication rates, and less striking early outcomes than reported in the original article by Berger. The authors recommend tempered enthusiasm for this procedure. This report corroborates that the indications for proper patient selection for this procedure are less robust than for a standard posterior approach.

32. Illgen R, Shanbhag AS, Jacobs JJ: Periprosthetic osteolysis: Pathophysiology and medical management. *Semin Arthroplasty* 2002;13:238-255.

33. Granchi D, Pellacani A, Spina M, et al: Serum levels of osteoprotegerin and receptor activator of nuclear factor-kappaβ ligand as markers of periprosthetic osteolysis. *J Bone Joint Surg Am* 2006;88:1501-1509.

The authors report that an increase in osteoprotegerin levels may suggest the presence of a protective mechanism of the skeleton to compensate for the osteolytic activity that occurs in patients with severe osteoarthritis and those with aseptic loosening of total hip arthroplasty components. Level of evidence: III.

34. Sporer SM, Paprosky WG: Revision total hip arthroplasty: The limits of fully coated stems. *Clin Orthop Relat Res* 2003;417:203-209.

35. Weeden SH, Paprosky WG: Minimal 11-year follow-up of extensively porous-coated stems in femoral revision total hip arthroplasty. *J Arthroplasty* 2002;17:134-137.

36. Callaghan JJ, Salvati EA, Pellicci PM, Wilson PD Jr, Ranawat CS: Results of revision for mechanical failure after cemented total hip replacement, 1979 to 1982: A two to five-year follow-up. *J Bone Joint Surg Am* 1985; 67:1074-1085.

37. Lieberman JR: Cemented femoral revision: Lest we forget. *J Arthroplasty* 2005;20:72-74.

The author reviews the patient selection criteria and results for the use of long cemented stems in patients (particularly low-demand individuals) undergoing revision total hip arthroplasty. Level of evidence: IV (therapeutic).

38. Hallstrom BR, Golladay GJ, Vittetoe DA, Harris WH: Cementless acetabular revision with the Harris-Galante porous prosthesis: Results after a minimum of ten years of follow-up. *J Bone Joint Surg Am* 2004;86-A:1007-1011.

The authors report excellent results with the use of a ce-

4: Lower Extremity

mentless acetabular component in patients who underwent revision total hip arthroplasty. Level of evidence: IV.

39. Paprosky W, Sporer S, O'Rourke MR: The treatment of pelvic discontinuity with acetabular cages. *Clin Orthop Relat Res* 2006;453:183-187.

    Acetabular cages in the setting of pelvic discontinuity were associated with a high failure rate at intermediate follow-up. Sixteen acetabular cage reconstructions in 15 patients were studied for an average of 5 years (range, 2 to 8 years).

40. Sporer SM, Paprosky WG: The use of a trabecular metal acetabular component and trabecular metal augment for severe acetabular defects. *J Arthroplasty* 2006; 21:83-86.

    The authors review the use of trabecular metal acetabular components with augments in 28 patients (28 hips) with challenging Paprosky type 3A defects. At an average 3.1-year follow-up, only 1 patient required re-revision for recurrent instability, and the remaining 27 hips remain radiographically stable. Level of evidence: IV (prognostic).

41. Sporer SM, Paprosky WG: Acetabular revision using a trabecular metal acetabular component for severe acetabular bone loss associated with a pelvic discontinuity. *J Arthroplasty* 2006;21:87-90.

    The authors review the use of trabecular metal acetabular components with augments in 13 patients (13 hips)

with challenging Paprosky type 3B defects. At an average follow-up of 2.6 years, only 1 patient demonstrated radiographic evidence of loosening, and the remaining 12 patients had radiographically stable hips. Level of evidence: IV (prognostic).

42. Lieberman JR, Hsu WK: Prevention of venous thromboembolic disease after total hip and knee arthroplasty. *J Bone Joint Surg Am* 2005;87:2097-2112.

    The authors of this article review the use of modern prophylaxis for deep venous thrombosis in patients who have undergone total hip arthroplasty and total knee arthroplasty. These issues will gain further importance as the federal government introduces pay for performance measures requiring the appropriate use of deep venous thrombosis prophylaxis to improve patient safety. Level of evidence: I (therapeutic).

43. Masonis JL, Bourne RB: Surgical approach, abductor function, and total hip arthroplasty dislocation. *Clin Orthop Relat Res* 2002;405:46-53.

44. Weeden SH, Paprosky WG, Bowling JW: The early dislocation rate in primary total hip arthroplasty following the posterior approach with posterior soft-tissue repair. *J Arthroplasty* 2003;18:709-713.

45. Masterson EL, Masri BA, Duncan CP: Treatment of infection at the site of total hip replacement. *Instr Course Lect* 1998;47:297-306.

4: Lower Extremity

Chapter 34

Femoral Fractures

Lisa K. Cannada, MD   Michael T. Charlton, MD

Femoral Shaft Fractures

Femoral shaft fractures are defined as fractures of the femoral diaphysis occurring from 5 cm distal to the lesser trochanter and proximal to the adductor tubercle. A common orthopaedic injury involving high-energy trauma, these fractures are routinely seen in patients with multiple injuries. Associated orthopaedic injuries may occur in up to 94% of patients and include pelvic disruptions, hip dislocations, and fractures of the acetabulum, spine, femoral head, distal femur, patella, and tibial plateau. Associated internal derangement of the knee is also possible, especially when the mechanism of injury is a motor vehicle crash in which the knee is driven into the dashboard. Ipsilateral femoral neck fractures may occur in up to 6% of patients and have historically been associated with high rates of missed fractures.

Evaluation

Clinical evaluation includes assessment of the entire patient in accordance with Advanced Trauma Life Support principles. A complete musculoskeletal examination during the secondary survey often reveals obvious deformity of the thigh with limb shortening. Open fractures and associated soft-tissue injuries should be noted. A well-documented neurovascular examination is imperative. The patient should be evaluated for additional areas of injury, and any evidence of ecchymosis, crepitus, soft-tissue injuries, and other areas of deformity should be noted. Factors that may impact surgical decision making, including concomitant chest and abdominal injures necessitating supine versus lateral positioning, or the practicality of fracture table use (in patients for whom additional procedures are necessary) should be considered. Additionally, the body habitus of the patient and the degree and location of soft-tissue injuries that could impact the placement of surgical incisions should be noted.

Radiographic assessment includes standard AP and lateral views of the entire femoral shaft to adequately assess the diaphyseal fracture, and the location, degree of comminution, fracture pattern, and amount of bone loss should be noted. Patients must always be assessed for an associated femoral neck fracture, which requires specific diagnostic imaging of the femoral neck. Although it is standard protocol to obtain the AP pelvis radiograph in the initial trauma series, and recommended that this radiograph be carefully evaluated for the presence of a femoral neck fracture, it is often not sufficient to assess the femoral neck because of overlying splints or external rotation of the proximal femur. Nondisplaced fractures can easily be missed on the pelvis radiograph alone. These nondisplaced fractures are at risk for displacement during or after femoral fixation with intramedullary nailing. Many femoral neck fractures that occur with an ipsilateral shaft fracture are vertically oriented, making radiographic detection even more difficult.

It has been reported in a recent study that between 20% and 50% of associated femoral neck fractures are missed initially, and protocols that include fine-cut CT evaluation of the femoral neck to further aid in the diagnosis of these fractures have been advocated.[1] According to this study, an established protocol decreased the rate of missed femoral neck fractures from 57% to 5%. The protocol includes an internal rotation AP pelvis radiograph, a fine-cut CT scan through the femoral neck, a preoperative lateral fluoroscopic radiograph, a postoperative AP pelvis radiograph, and a lateral radiograph.

Classification

Fracture classification systems are only valuable if they are able to suggest a prognosis and guide treatment options. Unfortunately, interobserver reliability in most fracture classification systems has repeatedly been shown to be quite poor, especially when relying on detailed systems that are often used for research purposes, calling into question the validity of recommendations based on classification systems alone. As a result, most orthopaedic surgeons describe femoral diaphyseal fractures by the location of the fracture (proximal, middle, or distal third), fracture pattern (transverse, short oblique, or spiral), and degree of comminution (including the presence or absence of large butterfly fragments).

Historically, two main classification systems for femoral shaft fractures have been well described, and a working knowledge of these systems may still be of some benefit. The Winquist and Hansen classification of comminuted femoral shaft fractures is based on the amount of comminution in relation to the diameter of the femoral shaft (**Figure 1**). Type 0 fractures have no comminution. Type I fractures have minimal comminution with greater than 75% of diameter of bone in continuity. Type II fractures have comminution that is less than 50% of the cortical circumference. Type III frac-

4: Lower Extremity

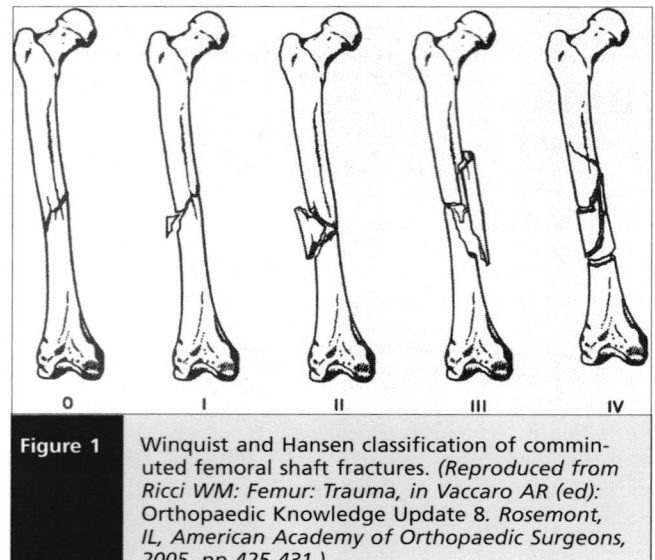

Figure 1 Winquist and Hansen classification of comminuted femoral shaft fractures. *(Reproduced from Ricci WM: Femur: Trauma, in Vaccaro AR (ed): Orthopaedic Knowledge Update 8. Rosemont, IL, American Academy of Orthopaedic Surgeons, 2005, pp 425-431.)*

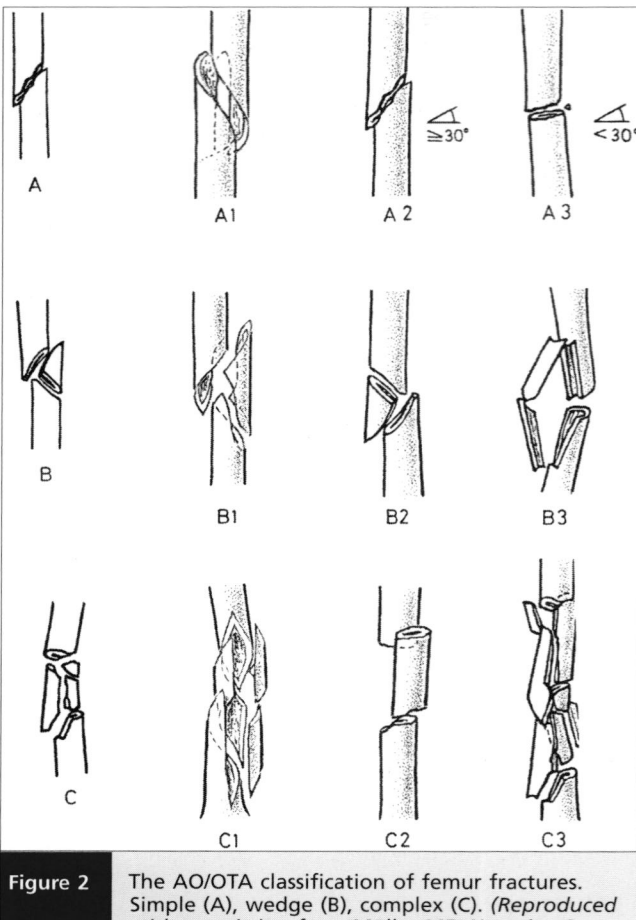

Figure 2 The AO/OTA classification of femur fractures. Simple (A), wedge (B), complex (C). *(Reproduced with permission from Müller ME, Nazarian S, Koch P, Schatzker J (eds): The Comprehensive Classification of Fractures of Long Bones. Berlin, Germany, Springer-Verlag, 1990.)*

tures have comminution and less than 50% cortical contact. Type IV fractures have no cortical contact at the fracture site.

The AO/Orthopaedic Trauma Association (OTA) fracture classification is a universal classification system that, although currently used commonly, is limited in its ability to help guide treatment options (**Figure 2**).

Treatment

Intramedullary nailing has become the universal standard for the treatment of femoral shaft fractures in patients whose overall medical condition is amenable to primary definitive fracture fixation. Union rates in excess of 98% are readily achievable, and rates of infection, even in most patients with open fractures, are extremely low. The low risk of infection is likely attributable to the robust soft-tissue envelope and generous blood supply that places these fractures in stark contrast to those involving the tibial shaft. Nevertheless, the high degree of energy required to fracture the strongest bone in the appendicular skeleton often leads to significant injuries involving vital organ systems. The extension of damage control surgery to the field of orthopaedic trauma, and specifically to the initial management of femoral shaft fractures, has led to the emergence of staged procedures in which the most minimally invasive and expedient methods of fracture stabilization are used. Damage control orthopaedics (DCO) is practiced to avoid the so-called second hit involved in extensive surgical procedures following significant trauma in the multiply injured patient. This concept has impacted the management of femoral shaft fractures in the unstable patient, where primary external fixation is used acutely followed by secondary intramedullary nail stabilization after the patient has been appropriately resuscitated. Recent retrospective studies comparing the changes in the systemic inflammatory response syndrome following immediate intramedullary nailing versus DCO

techniques point to smaller, shorter periods of postoperative systemic inflammatory response syndrome without significantly more pronounced organ system failure in the DCO group.[2] Unfortunately, these studies fail to consider other significant factors, including total surgical time, transfusion requirements, and the stratification of patients into separate subsets of those with thoracic trauma, abdominal trauma, and neurotrauma. Furthermore, the wide disparity in the capabilities of hospitals and surgeons that treat these injuries, or even differences of opinion among surgeons within the same hospital, often dictate how these fractures are initially managed, irrespective of the patient's overall medical status.[3] This reality makes broad comparisons regarding DCO to primary intramedullary nailing difficult at best, and further studies are clearly indicated before the universal adoption of DCO methodologies can be advocated. Nevertheless, immediate external fixation of the femur should be considered in the unstable or stable patient who has persistent hypotension or hypoperfusion as manifested by an elevated lactate level or base deficit, significant pulmonary injury, or a severe traumatic brain injury.

Nonsurgical Treatment

Nonsurgical treatment of femoral shaft fractures is rarely considered for definitive fracture management in the adult patient. In those instances in which the patient may be too sick for surgical treatment in the operating room, skeletal traction may be used for definitive treatment. The long period of bed rest to treat these fractures in traction, however, can often exceed 12 weeks and may be detrimental to the patient. Several studies have shown that the pulmonary status of patients is significantly improved with femoral stabilization that allows patient mobilization, even if only into an upright position in bed. In certain circumstances, external fixators can be applied in the intensive care unit. If nonsurgical management is necessary, the patient must be closely evaluated for pin tract infection, decubiti caused by prolonged immobilization, and the avoidance of fracture site distraction during the course of treatment.

Intramedullary Nailing

Reamed locked antegrade intramedullary nailing through the piriformis fossa has long been held to be the gold standard in the surgical fixation of femoral shaft fractures. Over the past decade, alternative methods have gained greater attention, including antegrade nailing through a trochanteric portal or retrograde nailing.

Antegrade Versus Retrograde Approach

Although antegrade intramedullary nailing has long been considered the gold standard in femoral shaft fracture care, the ease of retrograde nailing and the advantages it provides in certain circumstances has led to numerous comparative studies of these techniques over the past decade. Current indications for retrograde nailing include multiply injured trauma patients, ipsilateral extremity trauma (most commonly floating knee injuries), ipsilateral acetabular trauma, pelvic trauma, bilateral femur fractures, spine trauma, pregnancy, and morbid obesity. Potential advantages of retrograde nailing include ease of insertion, avoidance of a fracture table, and possibly decreased surgical times. Numerous studies have compared antegrade and retrograde intramedullary nailing, with most noting comparably high union rates in both techniques. Early concerns regarding decreased knee motion and septic knee arthritis following retrograde nailing of the femur have not been substantiated in randomized prospective trials. Limited evidence suggests that increased numbers of secondary procedures, including nail dynamization and exchange nailing, may be required to achieve union in fractures treated with small-diameter, unreamed retrograde nails in which significant canal-to-nail diameter mismatch exists or for fractures involving the junction of the middle and distal thirds of the femoral shaft.[4] A higher incidence of thigh pain and abductor lurch is seen in patients with antegrade placed nails, whereas knee pain is more common in patients who undergo the retrograde approach.[5] Fractures in the proximal third of the femur

may be more prone to malalignment with retrograde nailing, presumably because of increased difficulty maintaining fracture reduction during the stabilization process. With retrograde nails, it is important that the upper end of the nail be above the lesser trochanter to avoid a stress riser that could lead to refracture above the tip of the nail. Insertion of anteroposterior proximal interlocking screws is also safer around the lesser trochanter because of the lack of arterial perforators in this region.

Piriformis Versus Trochanteric Starting Approach

Antegrade nailing through the piriformis fossa has been the traditional management of femoral shaft fractures because it offers access to the intramedullary canal in line with the axis of the femoral shaft. If the piriformis starting point is too anterior, however, femoral neck fracture is possible because of increased hoop stresses. The piriformis entry site is also contraindicated in pediatric patients because of differences in the blood supply to the femoral head. The trochanteric starting point has recently gained popularity because of its ease of use, reduced potential for vascular damage, reduced fluoroscopic time, and reduced surgical time. Initial issues with a trochanteric starting point centered around nail design—namely, the exceptionally large entry hole in early designs and the absence of a lateral curve in the proximal portion of the nail. These issues have largely been eliminated with newer nail designs that have smaller proximal nail diameters and a lateral proximal bend that facilitates nail insertion. Future prospective randomized studies evaluating optimal nail design and comparing both antegrade methods, especially with regard to fracture location and type, are necessary.

Reamed Versus Nonreamed Nailing

In the past, femoral reaming was associated with adult respiratory distress syndrome (ARDS) and other pulmonary complications of fractures treated in patients with a concomitant lung injury. The bulk of the current evidence, however, indicates that there is no increased incidence of lung complications in patients managed with reamed femoral nails.[6] A recent study comparing patients with a pulmonary contusion who underwent early (< 24 hours after injury) intramedullary nailing of either femoral or tibial fractures and similarly injured patients without a fracture found no difference in the length of ventilator treatment, oxygenation ratio (PaO_2/FiO_2), or the incidence of ARDS, pneumonia, multiorgan failure, or mortality.[7] Open fractures with extensive soft-tissue damage and periosteal stripping, however, may be a contraindication to reamed nailing. Reamed intramedullary nailing, which allows for the use of larger diameter, stronger implants and reduces the amount of canal-to-nail diameter mismatch, has been shown repeatedly to decrease the rate of nonunion, improve rotational control, and restore femoral length. As a result, reamed intramedullary nailing is still recommended as the treatment of choice for most femoral shaft fractures.[8]

Flat Table Versus Fracture Table

Antegrade femoral nailing can be performed on a fracture table or standard radiolucent table. Considerations include the fracture pattern, patient body habitus, the number of available assistants, associated injuries, and surgeon preference. In one study comparing use of a fracture table versus no fracture table, no difference was reported in fracture alignment, fluoroscopic time, or surgical time.[9]

Plate Fixation

Plate fixation of femoral shaft fractures is not commonly used in adults and has few indications. When performed, efforts to reduce the amount of periosteal stripping and soft-tissue dissection, usually through the use of percutaneous, submuscular techniques, are paramount.

External Fixation

External fixation of femur fractures has been described as the initial treatment of choice when performing DCO. External fixation is useful for the unstable trauma patient or in patients whose skin or soft tissue does not permit definitive intramedullary nailing initially. Additionally, immediate intramedullary nailing is contraindicated in some high-grade open fractures with significant contamination of the intramedullary canal, and external fixation may be used as a temporizing measure in these instances. Primary concerns regarding external fixation include pin tract infection and the timing of external fixation removal and conversion to intramedullary nailing. The literature supports safe conversion to intramedullary nailing within the first 2 weeks after application of the external fixator.[10]

Special Considerations

Ipsilateral Femoral Neck and Shaft Fractures

A combined femoral neck and shaft fracture is challenging to treat. The treatment is dependent on the timing of discovery of the femoral neck fracture. When the fracture is identified preoperatively, priority is given to reduction (if necessary) and stabilization of the femoral neck before treatment of the femoral shaft. A nondisplaced fracture is at risk for displacement during or after femoral fixation with intramedullary nailing.[11,12] Difficulty arises when the identification of a femoral neck fracture intraoperatively (iatrogenic or not) or postoperatively can lead to difficulty with fracture reduction, suboptimal selection of fixation constructs, and may contribute to higher rates of nonunion or malunion. Although some authors still support the use of antegrade-inserted cephalomedullary nails for the combined fixation of these fractures,[13] a decrease in complications is noted with the use of separate implants to treat each fracture individually.[12] Multiple combinations of retrograde nails, plates, lag screws, and compression hip devices are available, all with varying rates of success. Although ultimately the choice of implant may be dictated by the timing of the discovery of the femoral neck fracture, there is no consensus on the optimal treatment option.

Open Femoral Shaft Fractures

Open femoral shaft fractures should be treated with urgent irrigation and débridement (although timing of surgery for open fractures is somewhat controversial, less than 6 to 8 hours from the time of injury is considered ideal) and immediate intramedullary nailing, unless significant intramedullary contamination exists. Intravenous antibiotics in the form of a first-generation cephalosporin (with additional gram-negative coverage in type III open fractures) should be administered for 48 hours. Penicillin should be added for wounds with heavy soil contamination. Repeat irrigation and débridement should occur within 48 hours for higher-grade open injuries. Wound culture is unnecessary and often clouds the clinical picture. Primary wound closure should be considered in patients without severe contamination or soft-tissue crushing and whose soft tissues allow closure.

Gunshot Fractures

Femoral shaft fractures resulting from low-velocity (handgun) gunshot wounds with small entrance and exit wounds can be treated as closed injuries with local wound care only and the wounds left open. Wounds resulting from high-velocity weapons (shotguns and military assault rifles) typically present with extensive soft-tissue exit wounds and should be treated according to the principles outlined for high-grade open fractures. It is important to note that the cavitation and blast effect from these devastating injuries often leads to soft-tissue damage at the cellular level that is far greater than is clinically apparent initially. Serial débridement and early planning for definitive wound closure or coverage are often required. Furthermore, incomplete neurovascular injuries are common, emphasizing the need for close examination.

Bilateral Femur Fractures

Bilateral femur fractures are associated with significant morbidity and mortality—a 26% mortality rate in one study.[14] In a recent retrospective analysis from a large trauma registry at a level 1 trauma center, the authors found a 3.8 times increased risk of mortality in patients with bilateral femur fractures versus those with unilateral femur fractures when injury severity was controlled and both groups were treated with reamed intramedullary nails.[15] In patients who survive the initial injury, bilateral femur fractures are associated with an increased incidence of pulmonary dysfunction, ARDS, compartment syndrome, peroneal nerve palsy, and delayed union.[16] In multiply injured patients, initial external fixation in accordance with DCO principles should be considered, with conversion to an intramedullary nail once the patient has been adequately resuscitated. Bilateral reamed retrograde nailing is commonly used for these injuries.

Complications

Perioperative Complications

Fat Embolism Syndrome

Fat embolism syndrome occurs between 24 and 72 hours after trauma in a small percentage of patients with long-bone fractures. Often associated with multiple long-bone fractures, this condition can be fatal in up to 15% of patients. Classic symptoms include tachypnea, tachycardia, hypoxemia, mental status changes, and petechiae (Table 1). Treatment includes mechanical ventilation with high positive end-expiratory pressure levels. Risk is decreased with early (< 24 hours after injury) stabilization of long-bone fractures.

Thromboembolism

Deep venous thrombosis (DVT) is a serious concern in trauma patients, especially those with long-bone fractures, pelvic and acetabular trauma, and spine injuries. Proximal thrombi are more significant than distal thrombi in that they lead to higher rates of fatal pulmonary embolism. A duplex ultrasound can be used to diagnose a DVT involving the extremities; spiral CT scan, ventilation-perfusion scan, or pulmonary angiography can be used to diagnose pulmonary emboli. The diagnosis of a pulmonary embolism should be suspected in patients with acute-onset tachypnea, tachycardia, low-grade fever, hypoxia, mental status changes, and possible chest pain. Preventive measures for DVT include mechanical compression with sequential compression devices or foot pumps and chemical pharmacoprophylaxis with low-molecular-weight heparin (LMWH) administered twice daily. LMWH has been shown to be superior to unfractionated heparin (UH) in several studies evaluating DVT prophylaxis in trauma patients.[17,18] For acute DVT, treatment recommendations from the Seventh American College of Chest Physicians Conference on Antithrombotic and Thrombolytic Therapy are at least 5 days of treatment with LMWH or UH, with initiation of a vitamin K antagonist (warfarin) on the first treatment day, and discontinuation of the LMWH or UH when the international normalized ratio is stable and greater than 2.0. The international normalized ratio should be maintained between 2.0 and 3.0, and warfarin treatment should be continued for 3 months.[19] Early surgical stabilization and subsequent mobilization are important additional preventive measures.

Adult Respiratory Distress Syndrome

ARDS is acute respiratory failure with pulmonary edema. Often seen in multiply injured trauma patients secondary to multiple etiologies, ARDS is commonly associated with concomitant thoracic injury and hypovolemic shock. Mechanical ventilation may be difficult because of decreased lung compliance. Other signs and symptoms include tachypnea, tachycardia, and hypoxemia. Treatment involves supportive ventilatory management; mortality can be as high as 50% for patients with ARDS. Several studies have shown that early stabiliza-

Table 1	
The Major and Minor Criteria for Diagnosis of Fat Embolism Syndrome*	
Major Criteria	**Minor Criteria**
Hypoxemia (PaO_2 < 60 mm Hg)	Tachycardia (heart rate > 110 bpm)
Central nervous system depression	Pyrexia (temperature > 38.3°C)
Petechial rash	Retinal emboli on fundoscopy
Pulmonary edema	Fat in urine
	Fat in sputum
	Thrombocytopenia
	Decreased hematocrit level

*A positive diagnosis requires at least one major and four minor signs. (Reproduced with permission from Roberts CS, Gleis GE, Seligson D: Diagnosis and treatment of complications, in Browner BD, Jupiter J, Levine AM, Trafton PG (eds): Skeletal Trauma: Basic Science, Management, and Reconstruction, ed 3. Philadelphia, PA, WB Saunders, 2003, pp 437-482.)

tion of long-bone fractures can decrease the incidence of ARDS.

Compartment Syndrome

Compartment syndrome after femur fractures is rare; when it occurs, it is usually associated with a crush injury. Patients with prolonged extrication times following motor vehicle crashes should be thoroughly evaluated for compartment syndrome secondary to extended thigh compression from an impacted dashboard console. Compartment syndrome also has been reported in rare circumstances following intramedullary nailing on the fracture table. Symptoms of thigh compartment syndrome may be easily missed because of the associated trauma and include severe pain with knee motion, pain at rest, and tense swelling of the thigh. Compartment pressure measurements can assist in the diagnosis. Immediate surgical decompression of the quadriceps, adductor, and posterior hamstring compartments is necessary when thigh compartment syndrome occurs.

Nerve Palsy

In femur fractures fixed on a fracture table, a pudendal nerve palsy may occur because of excessive traction and/or improper positioning with the perineal post. A peroneal nerve neurapraxia also may occur if excessive traction is used.

Late Complications

Nonunion/Malunion

The risk of nonunion in the treatment of femoral shaft fractures is relatively low in comparison with that of other major long bones. In patients with hypertrophic nonunions, simple reamed exchange nailing is the treatment of choice. Compression plating with bone grafting is a viable alternative, especially in the setting of failed exchange nailing or angular deformity requiring

4: Lower Extremity

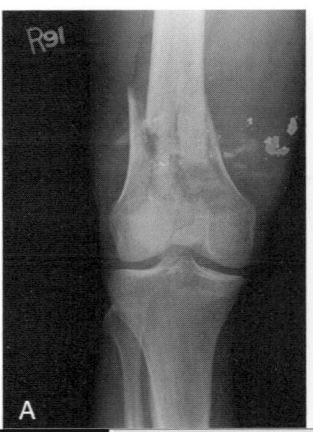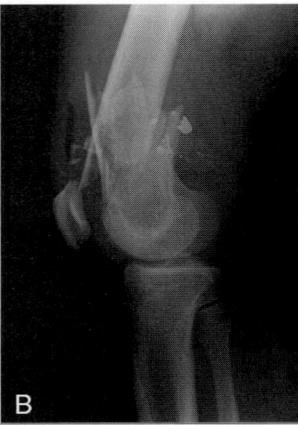

Figure 3 — AP **(A)** and lateral **(B)** radiographs of a distal femur fracture.

correction. A recent study reported 100% union rates at an average of 7.2 months using this technique and leaving the nail in situ.[20] Additionally, the availability of recombinant bone morphogenetic protein (BMP) as a bone-stimulating agent has drawn attention in the recent literature. One such study reported eight femur nonunions healed after treatment with recombinant BMP-7 in patients who had failed other standard treatment protocols for nonunion, including the use of autologous bone graft and marrow injection.[21] Six of the eight patients healed with a single application, and the other two patients required a repeat application of BMP-7 to achieve union. With an infected nonunion, the use of chronic suppressive antibiotics until healing is recommended, followed by implant removal. Antibiotic-impregnated methylmethacrylate beads or similarly fashioned antibiotic rods are additional treatment options. Delayed unions may result from technical issues, and dynamization by removal of the interlocking screw may allow compression across the fracture site and allow union to occur. Rotational deformities have been reported in up to 20% of patients, although internal rotation deformities up to 20° are generally well tolerated.[22]

Heterotopic Ossification
The insertion site for a piriformis antegrade nail involves soft-tissue dissection of the abductors. As a result, heterotopic ossification about the hip may develop in up to 26% of patients, although it is usually of little clinical significance.[23] The occurrence rate and clinical significance with nails placed through a trochanteric starting point not been thoroughly evaluated.

Distal Femur Fractures

Although fractures involving the supracondylar region of the femur are often caused by the same high-energy mechanisms seen in fractures of the femoral shaft, they also occur in older patients as fragility fractures after a minor fall. Furthermore, they increasingly occur as periprosthetic fractures of the distal femur in patients with previous total knee arthroplasty. These fractures generally have severe metaphyseal comminution with varying degrees of intra-articular involvement. As a result, these injuries pose substantial challenges to the orthopaedic surgeon; meticulous attention to preoperative planning with full consideration of all patient factors (condition of the soft tissue, concomitant injuries, comorbidities, and functional level before injury) is paramount.

Although the basic indications for surgery and the general surgical techniques for treating supracondylar femur fractures have not changed significantly, the surgical treatment of distal femoral fractures (with or without intra-articular involvement) continues to evolve. Recent changes in surgical techniques primarily relate to available implants, as well as to an increasing emphasis on minimally invasive plating techniques. The current revolution in locked plating of periarticular fractures in general began several years ago with the introduction of the Less Invasive Stabilization System (LISS) (Synthes, Paoli, PA) for the distal femur. With the increasing popularity of locked plating for the treatment of distal femur fractures, there seems to be less enthusiasm for intramedullary nailing techniques.

Classification
To accurately assess a fracture of the distal femur, good quality AP and lateral radiographs are essential (**Figure 3**). Traction views can be helpful in assessing fractures with significant axial and/or translational displacement. A CT scan with both coronal and sagittal reconstructions is helpful in characterizing complex articular injuries (**Figure 4**).

The AO/OTA classification is the universally accepted system for characterizing distal femur fractures (**Figure 5**). Type A fractures are extra-articular injuries. Type B fractures are intra-articular injuries and involve a single condyle. Type C fractures are intercondylar or bicondylar intra-articular injuries with varying degrees of comminution. Type C fractures are subcategorized depending on the degree of comminution into C1 (no comminution), C2 (metaphyseal comminution only with a simple articular split), and C3 (both metaphyseal and intra-articular comminution).

The surgical approach and the specific implant chosen to treat distal femur fractures are determined to a large degree by the fracture pattern. When reviewing radiographs and deciding on a treatment plan, many specific fracture characteristics should be considered. It should be determined whether the fracture is intra-articular. If so, it should be determined whether there is comminution within the intercondylar notch and an associated coronal (frontal) plane fracture (often referred to as a Hoffa fragment) (**Figure 4**). Such coronal fragments are present in more than one third of type C fractures. Making these determinations allows the surgeon to choose the appropriate implant and surgical

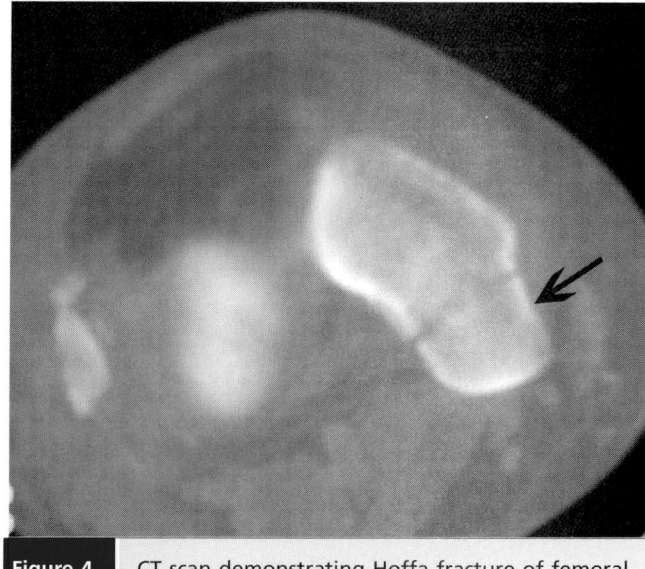

Figure 4 CT scan demonstrating Hoffa fracture of femoral condyle (*arrow*).

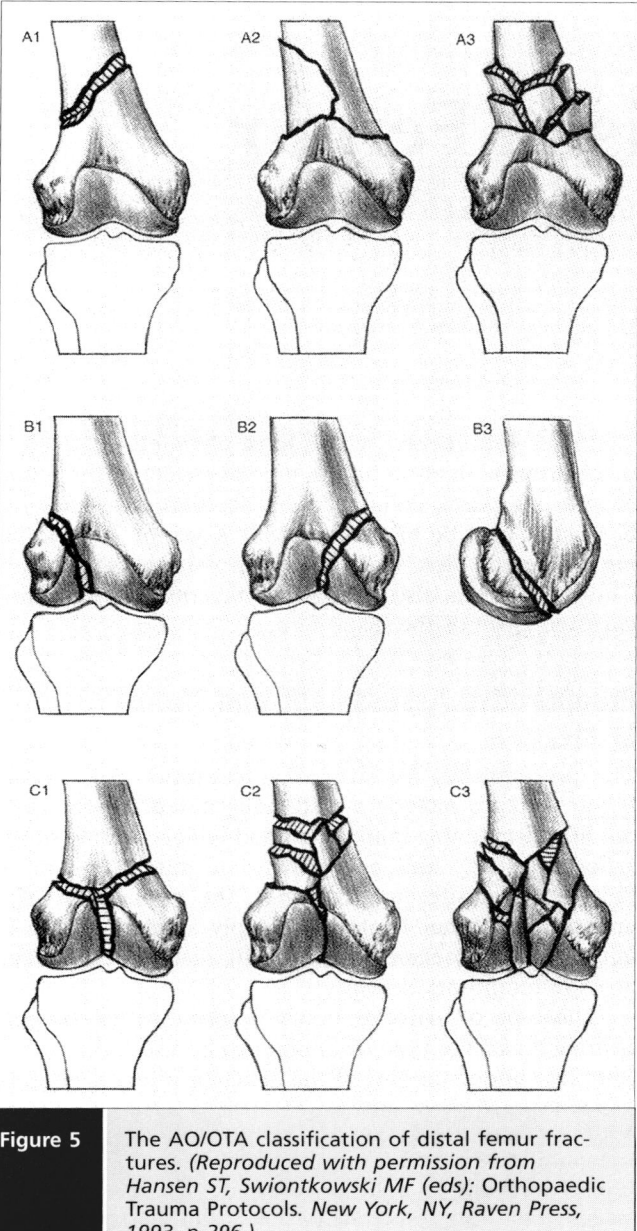

Figure 5 The AO/OTA classification of distal femur fractures. (*Reproduced with permission from Hansen ST, Swiontkowski MF (eds): Orthopaedic Trauma Protocols. New York, NY, Raven Press, 1993, p 296.*)

approach. If there is a Hoffa fragment or significant articular comminution, use of an extensile lateral peripatellar approach is best. For simpler fracture patterns, a standard anterolateral approach is sufficient.

Treatment

Fractures of the distal femur can have several characteristics that make them challenging to manage, including a small, often osteoporotic distal femoral segment in which to insert fixation, comminution with articular injury in multiple planes, associated soft-tissue wounds, and possible extensor mechanism disruption. In patients with a supracondylar or intercondylar distal femur fracture, the goals of treatment are restoration of normal alignment of the limb, anatomic reconstruction of the normal articular surface (when disrupted), rapid fracture healing, and ultimately returning patients to prior activity levels.

Surgical repair is the gold standard for all such fractures, whether open or closed, intra-articular or extra-articular. Nonsurgical management of these injuries should only be used in exceptional circumstances or for absolutely nondisplaced injuries.

Nonsurgical Treatment

Nonsurgical treatment of supracondylar femur fractures is generally associated with poor results and should be reserved for patients for whom surgery poses unacceptable risks. A brief period of traction may prove beneficial, followed by a well-fitting hinged knee brace locked in 20° to 30° of flexion. These braces are often better tolerated by patients than a long leg cast. Range of motion in the brace can then be initiated with evidence of radiographic healing, although motion through the fracture site is a well-described complication. Overall knee function following nonsurgical treatment has historically been quite poor. The origin of the gastrocnemius muscle characteristically pulls the distal fragment into extension.

Surgical Treatment

Surgical treatment of supracondylar femur fractures has consistently been associated with superior results when compared with nonsurgical treatment. Contemporary surgical options for fractures of the distal femur include intramedullary nailing or open reduction and internal fixation. With regard to intramedullary nailing, retrograde nails are typically used because they allow more distal fixation and better control of the condylar fragment. Union rates as high as 95% with low complication rates have been reported using this technique.[24] The use of antegrade nails should be limited to treating fractures at or above the metaphyseal flare of the distal femur. Retrograde nails can be used for fractures with simple intra-articular extension in the sagittal plane, but they are inappropriate for fractures associated with a Hoffa fragment. Conventional open reduction and internal fixation for intra-articular fractures with a variety of implants (usually a combination of plate and screw constructs) is widely accepted as the standard treatment of these injuries. A variety of plates are available, including traditional condylar buttress plates, condylar blade plates, dynamic condylar screw, locking blade plates, locked internal fixator (LISS), and locking periarticular plates. Limited open reduction with percutaneously performed plating techniques have also been used in the treatment of extra-articular fractures with good results.[25]

Positioning

For either plating or nailing, patients should be positioned supine on a radiolucent table with an optional bump under the hip of the affected limb. Open fractures should be treated in accordance with established principles, and temporizing knee-spanning external fixators should be used until the soft tissue is amenable to internal fixation. Once the soft tissues have been stabilized, the surgical approach and tactic are dictated by the degree of articular comminution. In type A fractures in which the joint is spared, intramedullary nailing and plate fixation both are viable options for treatment and have been associated with good results.[26] Plating of simple fractures can be performed through an isolated lateral approach to the distal femur, exposing only the portion of the lateral condyle necessary to facilitate placement of the implant. Type B fractures are generally amenable to lag screw fixation, often through percutaneous techniques. Type C fractures, or those involving more extensive articular involvement, are generally best treated with open reduction and internal fixation using a variety of plate implants via a lateral parapatellar arthrotomy or modification.[27] This exposure, which can include eversion of the patella as required, provides direct visualization of the entire joint and is necessary to facilitate the anatomic reduction of the articular surface.

Plating

Surgical plate fixation historically involved anatomic reduction of all fragments. Condylar plating systems were used with nonlocked screws and required the placement of medial fixation and the liberal use of autogenous bone graft to promote union and prevent varus collapse. These techniques often required large open exposures leading to unacceptably high rates of infection—up to 10% of patients in one recently reported series.[28]

Submuscular locked plating has generally replaced open plating in the treatment of distal femur fractures. With the recognition of the importance of biologic plating techniques and indirect fracture reduction, there is no need to expose and repair the typically comminuted metaphyseal region. Direct exposure of the articular surface is easily accomplished with an anterolateral arthrotomy with medial subluxation of the patella; this approach allows a plate to be easily passed proximally beneath the vastus lateralis muscle. Proximal fixation can be performed through a second incision or percutaneously. Submuscular plating of distal femur fractures has been shown to result in a low incidence of nonunion and infection, less need for autogenous graft, and a substantial decrease in the rate of infections and other soft-tissue complications.[29]

Although most orthopaedic surgeons agree that these fractures usually benefit from surgical intervention, the debate in recent years has now shifted to the optimal application of a host of newer implants, including locked precontoured plating systems and retrograde femoral nails with distal locking holes specifically designed for the treatment of supracondylar fractures. The main advantages to these newer plating systems include the ability to insert them percutaneously with the use of targeting jigs and the need for less periosteal stripping. In addition, the stability with the use of the locking plate screws is provided without bone-plate friction (**Figure 6**). Locking plates have been shown to be biomechanically superior to the 95° blade plate and femoral nails in mechanical studies.[30] Several recently published clinical studies evaluating locked plates have shown consistently excellent to good results with low rates of failure.[25,29] These newer implants are not a panacea, however, and several disadvantages exist, including the increased complexity and cost of these implants, as well as an increased risk of malreduction. A recent case series demonstrated six failures of the locking condylar plate in patients with either poor bone stock or substantial bone loss associated with an open fracture.[31] Selective use of autogenous bone graft, methylmethacrylate cement, and/or the cautious advancement of weight-bearing status based on clinical and radiographic signs of union are critical in the treatment of these complex fractures.

Intramedullary Nailing

Retrograde intramedullary nailing and less commonly antegrade intramedullary nailing remain viable treatment options for many distal femur fractures. Femoral shaft fractures with associated unicondylar (type B) fractures may be stabilized with percutaneous lag screws and are not a contraindication to nailing. The ideal indication for a retrograde intramedullary nail is an extra-articular or simple articular fracture with metaphyseal comminution for which the distal articular block can be easily reconstructed with two or three interfragmentary lag screws.

Retrograde intramedullary nailing is generally performed with the patient supine and with the knee flexed 40° with the use of supportive bumps under the knee. The ideal starting portal for the nail is just above the roof of the intercondylar notch and slightly medial. With less knee flexion, the proximal tibia blocks the desired entry site; with more knee flexion, damage to the

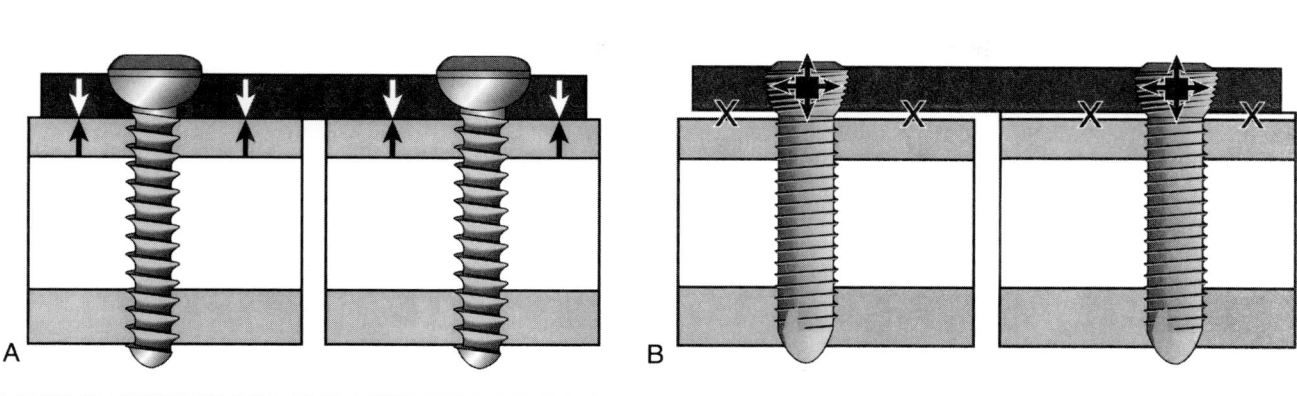

Figure 6	A, Method of stability (by friction of plate against bone) with use of conventional screws and plate. B, Method of stability provided with locking screws and plate (without plate-bone friction). *(Adapted with permission from AO North America Archives.)*

patella is possible. Intraoperative fluoroscopy is used to ensure proper position and trajectory of the guide pin.

As with the newer plating systems, recent advances have been made in the implants used for retrograde femoral nailing. The latest generation of nails enables the placement of multiple orthogonally directed distal locking screws. A recent biomechanical study using osteoporotic cadaver bone found that there was a modest improvement in fixation with locked distal screws, which had less fracture collapse, less anterior and medial translation of the nail at the fracture site, and less varus angulation after cyclic loading when compared with traditional nonlocking interlocking screw fixation.[32]

The clinical results of intramedullary nailing seem to be similar to those of plating. A recent systematic review found one prospective cohort study that compared the LISS with retrograde nails. The rates of nonunion (10%), fixation failure (0%), and revision (10%) were the same at 1-year follow-up, whereas infection was more common after retrograde nailing (6% versus 0%).[33]

Periprosthetic Fractures

The incidence of distal femur fractures adjacent to a total knee arthroplasty or distal to a long-stem total hip arthroplasty is increasing. Although both retrograde nails and locked plating can be used for these fractures, locked plating is the method of choice (Figure 7). Retrograde nailing of periprosthetic distal femur fractures risks damage to the prosthetic patella or tibial tray and may introduce particulate debris into the joint. The geometry of some total knee implants may preclude introduction of a nail, and at the least, the starting point must be more posterior than normal so that an extension deformity may be produced. Occasionally, the nail may shift anteriorly within the distal femur after insertion, making later removal impossible. Additionally, ar-

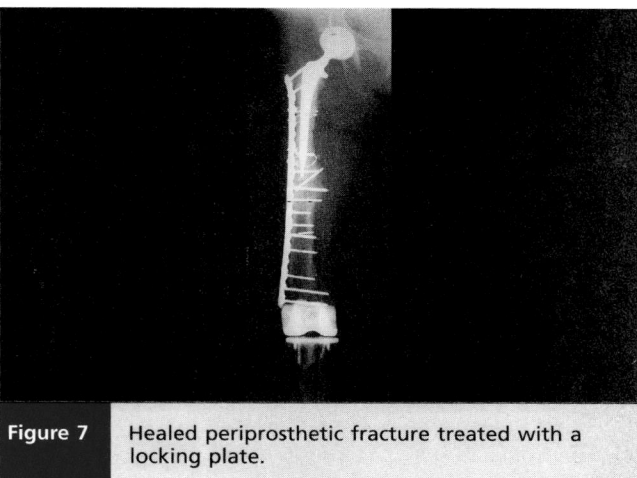

Figure 7	Healed periprosthetic fracture treated with a locking plate.

throtomy may increase the risk of later sepsis. In contrast, locked plating provides acceptable fixation, can be performed with less invasive approaches, and does not interfere with the existing implants.

The clinical results of locked plating of periprosthetic distal femur fractures with less invasive plating techniques have been good. Even without bone grafting, union rates are high and complications are rare.[34]

Annotated References

1. Tornetta P III, Kain MS, Creevy WR: Diagnosis of femoral neck fractures in patients with a femoral shaft fracture: Improvement with a standard protocol. *J Bone Joint Surg Am* 2007;89:39-43.

    The authors reported that an established protocol reduced the rate of missed femoral neck fractures from 57% (4 of 7) to 5% (1 of 19). The protocol included an internal rotation radiograph, a fine-cut CT scan through the femoral neck, a preoperative lateral fluoroscopic radiograph, and postoperative AP and lateral radiographs.

4: Lower Extremity

The authors reported that the fine-cut CT scan was the most sensitive of these studies. Level of evidence: II.

2. Harwood PJ, Giannoudis PV, Griensven MV, Krettek C, Pape HC: Alterations in the systemic inflammatory response after early total care and damage control procedures for femoral shaft fracture in severely injured patients. *J Trauma* 2005;58:446-454.

    The authors of this retrospective review found that multiply injured patients whose femur fractures were treated with DCO had a lesser systemic inflammatory response than those who were treated with early intramedullary nailing. Level of evidence: III.

3. Rixen D, Grass G, Sauerland S, et al: Evaluation of criteria for temporary external fixation in risk-adapted damage control orthopaedic surgery of femur shaft fractures in multiple trauma patients: "Evidence-based medicine" versus "reality" in the trauma registry of the German trauma society. *J Trauma* 2005;59:1375-1395.

    The authors conducted a literature review of 63 trials to evaluate femoral shaft fracture treatment and found that injury severity appears to influence the choice of initial treatment. Level of evidence: II.

4. Ostrum RF, Agarwal A, Lakatos R, Poka A: Prospective comparison of retrograde and antegrade femoral intramedullary nailing. *J Orthop Trauma* 2000;14:496-501.

5. Ricci WM, Bellabarba C, Evanoff B, Herscovici D, Dipasquale T, Sanders R: Retrograde versus antegrade nailing of femoral shaft fractures. *J Orthop Trauma* 2001;15:161-169.

6. Anwar IA, Battistella FD, Neiman R, Olson SA, Chapman M, Moehring HD: Femur fractures and lung complications: A prospective randomized study of reaming. *Clin Orthop Relat Res* 2004;422:71-76.

    The authors conducted a prospective, randomized trial comparing reamed and unreamed intramedullary nailing; however, the study was underpowered to reach conclusions regarding pulmonary or clinical outcomes. Level of evidence: II.

7. Handolin L, Pajarinen JT, Lassus JES, Tulikoura I: Early intramedullary nailing of lower extremity fracture and respiratory function in polytraumatized patients with a chest injury. *Acta Orthop Scand* 2004;75:477-480.

    The authors of this retrospective review of early intramedullary nailing in patients with chest injury and long-bone fractures reported that pulmonary function or outcome was not compromised with intramedullary nailing within the first 24 hours. Level of evidence: III.

8. Bhandari M, Guyatt GH, Tong D, Adili A, Shaughnessy SG: Reamed versus nonreamed intramedullary nailing of lower extremity long bone fractures: A systematic overview and meta-analysis. *J Orthop Trauma* 2000;14:2-9.

9. Stephen DJ, Kreder HJ, Schemitsch EH, Conlan LB, Wild L, McKee MD: Femoral intramedullary nailing: A comparison of fracture table and manual traction. A prospective, randomized study. *J Bone Joint Surg Am* 2002;84:1514-1521.

10. Nowotarski PJ, Turen CH, Brumback RJ, Scarboro JM: Conversion of external fixation to intramedullary nailing for fractures of the shaft of the femur in multiply injured patients. *J Bone Joint Surg Am* 2000;82:781-788.

11. Miller SD, Burkart B, Damson E, Shrive N, Bray RC: The effect of the entry hole for an intramedullary nail on the strength of the proximal femur. *J Bone Joint Surg Br* 1993;75:202-206.

12. Watson JT, Moed BR: Ipsilateral femoral neck and shaft fractures: Complications and their treatment. *Clin Orthop Relat Res* 2002;399:78-86.

13. Okcu G, Aktuglu K: Antegrade nailing of femoral shaft fractures combined with neck or distal femur fractures. *Arch Orthop Trauma Surg* 2003;123:544-550.

14. Copeland CE, Mitchell KA, Brumback RJ, Gens DR, Burgess AR: Mortality in patients with bilateral femur fractures. *J Orthop Trauma* 1998;12:315-319.

15. Nork SE, Agel J, Russell GV, Mills WJ, Holt S, Routt ML Jr: Mortality after reamed intramedullary nailing of bilateral femur fractures. *Clin Orthop Relat Res* 2003;415:272-278.

16. Giannoudis PV, Cohen A, Hinsche A, Stratford T, Matthews SJ, Smith RM: Simultaneous bilateral femoral fractures: Systemic complications in 14 cases. *Int Orthop* 2000;24:246-267.

17. Geerts WH, Jay RM, Code KI, et al: A comparison of low-dose heparin with low molecular weight heparin against venous thromboembolism after major trauma. *N Engl J Med* 1996;335:701-707.

18. Knudson MM, Morabito D, Paiement GD, et al: Use of low molecular weight heparin in preventing thromboembolism is trauma patients. *J Trauma* 1996;41:446-459.

19. Buller HR, Agnelli G, Hull RD, et al: Antithrombotic therapy for venous thromboembolic disease: The Seventh ACCP Conference on Antithrombotic and Thrombolytic Therapy. *Chest* 2004;126(suppl 3):401S-428S.

    The authors report the recommendations of the Seventh American College of Chest Physicians Conference on Antithrombotic and Thrombolytic Therapy. The recommendations cover those patients with DVT diagnosed, high clinical suspicion of DVT, prevention of post-thrombotic syndrome, and treatment of pulmonary emboli. The medication for treatment and duration of therapy are discussed.

20. Choi YS, Kim KS: Plate augmentation leaving the nail in situ and bone grafting for non-union of femoral shaft fractures. *Int Orthop* 2005;29:287-290.

    The authors of this small study reviewed 15 patients

with oligotrophic nonunion after interlocking intramedullary nailing treated with plate augmentation and bone grafting with the nail in situ. At an average 7.2-month follow-up, all patients healed. Level of evidence: IV.

21. Dimitriou R, Dahabreh Z, Katsoulis E, Matthews SJ, Branfoot T, Giannoudis PV: Application of recombinant BMP-7 on persistent upper and lower limb nonunions. *Injury* 2005;36:S51-S59.

    This study was conducted to evaluate the efficacy and safety of recombinant BMP-7 (rhBMP-7 or OP-1) as a bone-stimulating agent in the treatment of persistent fracture nonunions. Twenty-five consecutive patients (19 men, mean age, 39.4 years; age range, 18 to 79 years) with 26 fracture nonunions were treated with rhBMP-7. There were eight recalcitrant femoral nonunions in the study group, six of which achieved union with a single application of rhBMP-7. The remaining two achieved union after a second application of rhBMP-7. Level of evidence: III.

22. Jaarsma RL, Pakvis DF, Verdonschot N, Biert J, van Kampen A: Rotational malalignment after intramedullary nailing of femoral fractures. *J Orthop Trauma* 2004;18:403-409.

    This cohort study of 76 patients found rotational malalignment in 28% of patients. The patients with external rotational malalignment had more difficulty with more demanding activities than those with internal rotational malalignment. Level of evidence: III.

23. Brumback RJ, Wells JD, Lakatos R, Poka A, Bathon GH, Burgess AR: Heterotopic ossification about the hip after intramedullary nailing for fractures of the femur. *J Bone Joint Surg Am* 1990;72:1067-1073.

24. Handolin L, Pajarinen J, Lindahl J, Hirvensalo E: Retrograde intramedullary nailing in distal femoral fractures: Results in a series of 46 consecutive operations. *Injury* 2004;35:517-522.

    The authors used a distal femoral nail to treat 44 patients with 46 distal femur fractures and reported good results, including a 95% union rate with a low rate of complications. Level of evidence: II.

25. Kregor PJ, Stannard JA, Zlowodzki M, Cole PA: Treatment of distal femur fractures using the less invasive stabilization system. *J Orthop Trauma* 2004;18:509-520.

    This retrospective review of early results of the LISS to treat 119 consecutive patients with 123 distal femur fractures found favorable results with minimal complications, even in elderly patients. High union rates without autogenous bone grafting were reported in 93% of patients. The authors also reported a low incidence of infection (3% of patients), maintenance of distal femoral fixation (100% of patients), and no loss of fixation in the distal femoral condyles even though 30 patients were older than 65 years. Level of evidence: III.

26. Markmiller M, Konrad G, Sudkamp N: Femur-LISS and distal femoral nail for fixation of distal femoral fractures. *Clin Orthop Relat Res* 2004;426:252-257.

    This study prospectively followed two groups of pa-

tients with distal femoral fractures that were treated with either the LISS or distal femoral nailing. At 1-year follow-up, there were no significant differences in outcomes and complication rates when comparing the two minimally invasive systems. Level of evidence: III.

27. Starr AJ, Jones AL, Reinert CM: The "Swashbuckler": A modified anterior approach for fractures of the distal femur. *J Orthop Trauma* 1999;13:138-140.

28. Rademakers MV, Kerkhoffs GMMJ, Sierevelt IN, Raaymakers EL, Marti RK: Intra-articular fractures of the distal femur: A long term follow-up study of surgically treated patients. *J Orthop Trauma* 2004;18:213-219.

    The authors reported good long-term results after open reduction and internal fixation of intra-articular distal femur fractures and found that although knee function improved over time, range of motion did not improve after 1 year. The authors also concluded that secondary osteoarthritis did not necessarily adversely affect outcome. Level of evidence: III.

29. Weight M, Collinge C: Early results of the less invasive stabilization system for mechanically unstable fractures of the distal femur (AO/OTA types A2, A3, C2, and C3). *J Orthop Trauma* 2004;18:503-508.

    This retrospective study found good results using the LISS to treat patients with unstable distal femur fractures. The authors concluded that this treatment allows for early initiation of postoperative range-of-motion exercise. Level of evidence: III.

30. Zlowodzki M, Williamson S, Cole PA, Zardiackas LD, Kregor PJ: Biomechanical evaluation of the less invasive stabilization system, angled blade plate, and retrograde intramedullary nail for the internal fixation of distal femur fractures. *J Orthop Trauma* 2004;18:494-502.

    This study was conducted to biomechanically evaluate three types of internal fixation for distal femur fractures: the LISS, the angled blade plate, and the retrograde intramedullary nail. All three devices were able to withstand axial load without failure. The LISS provided better fixation distally in osteoporotic bone, but it resulted in more fracture site displacement.

31. Vallier HA, Hennessey TA, Sontich JK, Patterson BM: Failure of LCP condylar plate fixation in the distal part of the femur: A report of six cases. *J Bone Joint Surg Am* 2006;88:846-853.

    The authors of this article describes six cases of Locking Compression Plate (Synthes, West Chester, PA) failure. Four of the patients had open fractures, and the average patient age was 62 years. The authors concluded that additional procedures should be considered to promote union rather than just relying on newer fixation plates. Level of evidence: IV.

32. Tejwani NC, Park S, Iesaka K, Kummer F: The effect of locked distal screws in retrograde nailing of osteoporotic distal femur fractures: A laboratory study using cadaver femurs. *J Orthop Trauma* 2005;19:380-383.

    In a biomechanical study using matched pairs of cadaveric femora with supracondylar gaps, the authors re-

4: Lower Extremity

ported slightly improved fixation with retrograde nails that used locked distal screws when compared with traditional nonlocking interlocking screw fixation. The authors also noted a significant risk of fracture with proximal locking screws placed distal to the lesser trochanter (proximal femur failure occurred at the level of the proximal screw hole in the nail at the subtrochanteric level in 7 of the 14 samples).

33.   Zlowodzki M, Bhandari M, Marek DJ, Cole PA, Kregor PJ: Operative treatment of acute distal femur fractures: Systematic review of two comparative studies and 45 case series (1989-2005). *J Orthop Trauma* 2006;20: 366-371.

The authors conducted a systematic analysis of the literature regarding fresh distal femoral fractures and found grade B evidence suggesting that surgical fixation reduces the risk of poor results by 32% when compared with nonsurgical management. In terms of surgical techniques, they found grade C evidence that does not favor any implant over another; however, it was noted that submuscular locked plates may be associated with lower infection risk but higher risk of fixation failure. Level of evidence: II.

34.   Ricci WM, Loftus T, Cox C, Borrelli J: Locked plates combined with minimally invasive insertion technique for the treatment of periprosthetic supracondylar femur fractures above a total knee arthroplasty. *J Orthop Trauma* 2006;20:190-196.

The authors treated 24 consecutive patients with periprosthetic fractures about a well-fixed total knee arthroplasty with a locking condylar buttress plate. Nineteen fractures (86%) healed. The three nonunions were all in diabetic patients. A few instances of proximal screw failure occurred with later change in alignment. The authors recommend this technique for nondiabetic patients, but note there may not be any technique that is without a high risk of complications in diabetic patients. Level of evidence: IV.

Chapter 35

Fractures About the Knee

Thomas J. Ellis, MD

Patella Fractures

The patella is a sesamoid bone embedded within the extensor mechanism of the knee; its position defines the quadriceps tendon and the patellar ligament. Collagen fibers of the quadriceps tendon and patellar ligament are in continuity over the dorsal aspect of the patella, and the medial and lateral expansions of the quadriceps tendon insert into the medial and lateral retinacula. Complete injuries of the knee extensor mechanism disrupt both the patella and the lateral retinacular expansions. A rare exception occurs when a direct blow, while the knee is extended, fractures the patella. In such injuries, a stellate fracture of the patella can occur without injury to the retinacula, and the overall extensor mechanism can remain intact.

Diagnosis

A patella fracture is usually diagnosed by the presence of a combination of symptoms including pain, knee effusion, and inability to actively extend the knee, and with the use of simple AP, lateral, and tangential (Merchant or sunrise) radiographs of the knee (**Figure 1**). MRI may be considered to evaluate possible associated soft-tissue injuries (such as retinacular tears) or occult osteochondral injury.

Classification

Patella fractures are classified by the orientation of fracture line(s) as seen on plain radiographs. Displaced transverse fractures are the most common type and result from either direct or indirect mechanisms that cause the patella to fail in tension. Vertical or stellate fractures more commonly occur from direct trauma to the anterior knee. Vertical fractures do not necessarily tear the retinacula, and may not result in disruption of the extensor mechanism. Vertical tears may involve the main body of the patella or only the patellar margins. Simple fractures are distinguished from comminuted fractures because of the implications that fracture comminution has on methods of surgical treatment. Osteochondral fragments are best seen on tangential radiographs or MRI scans. Bipartite patella exists in 1% to 2% of patients and should not be confused with an acute fracture.

Treatment Options

Nonsurgical Treatment

Nondisplaced patella fractures with an intact knee extensor mechanism can be treated successfully in a cast or brace. Because it may be difficult to assess a patient's ability to actively extend the knee because of pain, the intra-articular injection of local anesthetic will allow better assessment of motor function. If nonsurgical treatment is considered, it is important to recognize that transverse fractures are likely to have associated retinacular tears. Minimally displaced vertical patellar fractures are more appropriate for nonsurgical treatment because the retinacula are more likely to be intact. If the fracture is extra-articular and the extensor mech-

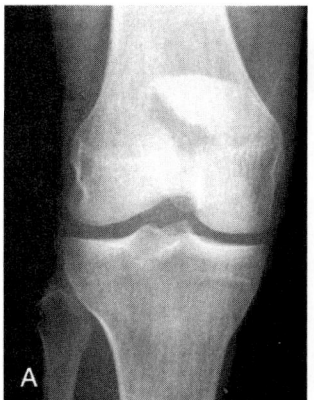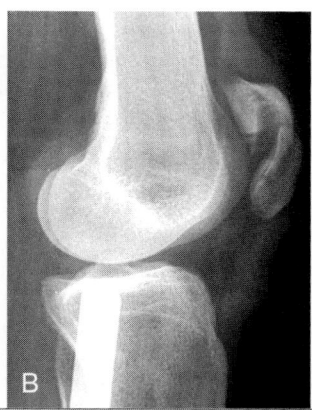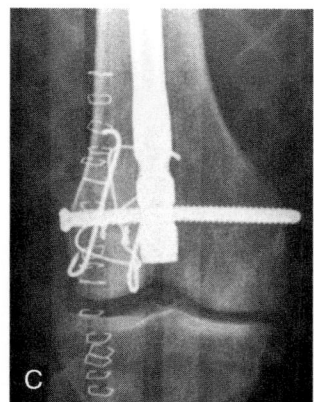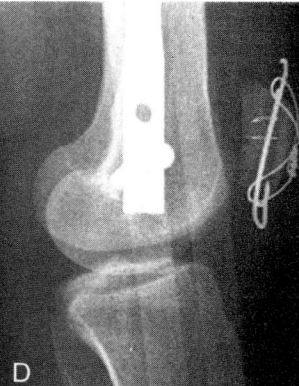

Figure 1 Preoperative AP (**A**) and lateral (**B**) views of a patella fracture. Postoperative AP (**C**) and lateral (**D**) views after open reduction and internal fixation with a tension band construct.

4: Lower Extremity

anism is intact, the fracture can be safely treated nonsurgically with early, unrestricted range-of-motion exercises.

Surgical Treatment

For displaced intra-articular fractures or those with an extensor lag, surgical treatment is recommended. Surgery also should be considered for fractures with articular step-offs or gaps greater than 2 mm. Patella fractures associated with other fractures about the knee should be surgically treated to allow early knee rehabilitation.

The three general methods of repair for patella fractures are partial patellectomy with patellar tendon reconstruction, open reduction and internal fixation of the patella, and total patellectomy. Partial patellectomy is usually chosen when the distal pole (which is mostly extra-articular) is comminuted. In such instances, secure repair can be achieved by reattaching the patellar tendon to the proximal fragment after débriding the comminuted distal pole. This approach obviates the need for internal fixation and its complications, and the patient can be rapidly rehabilitated without concern for loss of fixation or nonunion. Displaced transverse fractures are treated with open reduction and internal fixation with wires or screws and an anterior tension band. Total patellectomy is rarely performed for the primary treatment of patella fractures.

Surgery is performed with the patient supine on a radiolucent table and through a vertical midline incision. The medial and lateral retinacula are exposed to the extent that they are disrupted. Patella fractures are usually repaired with a combination of a tension-band wire, cerclage wire, and/or interfragmentary screws. For successful repair with a tension band, the primary fracture line must be transverse and fracture fragments must withstand compressive forces. In fractures with severe comminution, tension-band fixation is not appropriate, and simple cerclage fixation or partial patellectomy should be considered. Single out-of-plane fragments are first repaired to the main fragment with screws, and then the two primary fragments are reduced to each other. If free osteochondral fragments are present, they should be stabilized or excised. The two main fragments of the superior and inferior patella are reduced to one fragment and held with one or two pointed reduction clamps. Using the anterior cortex of the patella as a reduction guide can be misleading; some assessment of the articular reduction should be done by digital palpation, direct visualization of the articular surface, and/or fluoroscopy. After reduction, standard anterior tension-band wiring is used. It has recently been shown that a braided polyester suture tied with a modified Wagoner's hitch knot showed less gaping at the fracture site compared with other methods of tension-band fixation.[1]

An elegant option is to use cannulated screws instead of wires, and to insert the tension band through the screws and then over the anterior patella. This technique may allow better compression of the two fragments in patients with good bone stock. If this technique is used, it is important to ensure that the tip of the screw is buried in the bone so that the wire will not be cut as it exits the screw. Biomechanical studies have reported increased strength when screws are used, most noticeably in terminal extension.[2,3]

Recently, percutaneous methods of repair of displaced patella fractures have been advocated.[4] In one study comparing open with percutaneous repair in 53 patients followed for 2 years, percutaneous repair of displaced patella fractures was associated with less pain, shorter surgical time, improved functional outcome, and fewer complications than open surgery.[4]

Partial patellectomy is useful for comminuted inferior pole patella fractures. There appears to be no correlation between outcome and the size of the remaining patella.[5] The tendon is repaired through parallel drill holes to the site where the distal patella was resected. It is important to maintain the appropriate length of the patellar tendon as measured by the Insall-Salvati criteria.[5] Using this criteria, the patellar tendon to patellar length ratio, or index, should be 1.0. An index of greater than 1.2 indicates patella alta and less than 0.8 indicates patella baja.

Postoperative Treatment

Supervised active knee range-of-motion exercises are usually started immediately, allowing up to 90° of flexion depending on the stability of fixation and the status of the surgical incision. Intraoperative assessment of fracture stability after fixation helps determine the initial degree of flexion that can be allowed. For severely comminuted fractures, it is prudent to immobilize the knee in extension and gradually increase flexion. A knee brace with adjustable hinges is useful for this purpose. A continuous passive motion machine also may be used. Patients are allowed to walk with full weight bearing with the knee locked in extension.

The postoperative protocol should be modified for fractures with severe comminution, tenuous fixation, and/or wounds at risk for dehiscence. Generally, these knees are immobilized in extension for some period of time. Delayed flexion is accepted as a reasonable alternative to avoid wound dehiscence or fixation failure.

Tibial Plateau Fractures

Displaced fractures of the tibial plateau are challenging injuries that are difficult to treat. Just as with distal femoral fractures, tibial plateau fractures generally occur in two groups of patients—geriatric patients with osteopenic bone injured in low-energy falls and younger patients injured in high-energy traumatic events. The former group typically has good outcomes, whereas outcomes for those with high-energy injuries are dictated by the fracture pattern and severity of the soft-tissue injuries. It is important to assess the condition of the soft-tissue envelope when determining the treatment plan for these high-energy fractures. It is also important to remember that compartment syndrome is as common

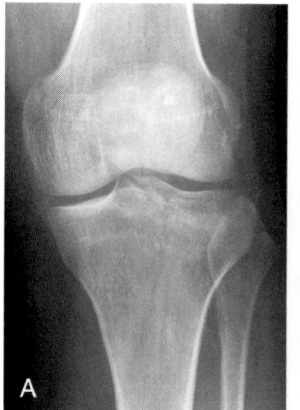 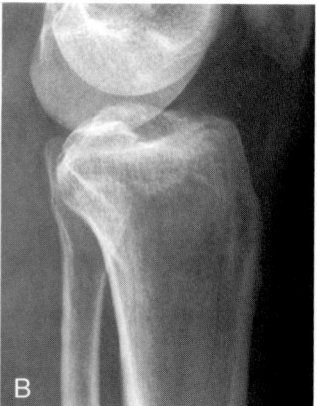 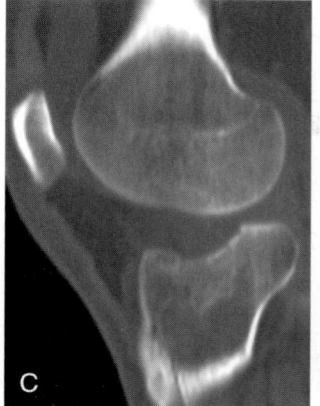 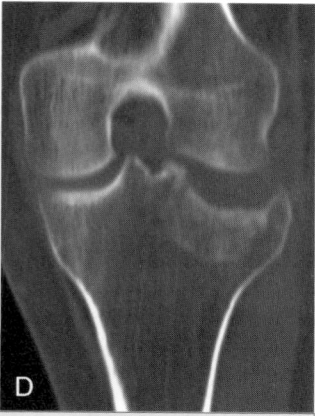

Figure 2 Example of a tibial plateau fracture. AP (**A**) and lateral (**B**) views of the knee. Sagittal (**C**) and coronal (**D**) CT scans are shown.

in patient with tibial plateau fractures as in those with tibial shaft fractures.[6]

Traditional AO techniques of open reduction and internal fixation, when applied to high-energy tibial plateau fractures, often require significant stripping of the soft tissues of the proximal metaphysis of the tibia, resulting in poor outcomes and frequent complications.[7] Recognition of the need for preservation of the biologic environment for fracture healing and advances (in the early 1990s) in external fixation resulted in a dramatic trend away from standard internal fixation techniques in favor of limited internal fixation and hybrid or circular external fixation.[8] However, dissatisfaction with complications of external fixation, including pyarthrosis, combined with increasing experience with staged reconstruction techniques has resulted in the continued evolution of treatment protocols for these complex injuries. The use of temporary knee-spanning external fixation combined with delayed surgical approaches using techniques of indirect reduction have resulted in remarkable decreases in complication rates and improved outcomes.[6,9,10]

Classification

Tibial plateau fractures are first grouped into high- and low-energy patterns, which alone dictates the initial surgical tactic (immediate versus delayed repair), influences the type of fixation used, and affects the likelihood of complications. There are two well-known classification systems based on fracture pattern—the system developed by Schatzker and associates[11] (Table 1) and the system developed by the AO group and adopted by the Orthopaedic Trauma Association.[12]

Radiographic Evaluation

Initial radiographs to evaluate tibial plateau fractures should include AP and lateral views of the knee and tibia (**Figure 2, *A* and *B***). Right and left oblique views and a 10° caudal radiograph also may be needed. Traction radiographs are helpful, but may require the patient to be anesthetized. CT scans with sagittal, coro-

Table 1

Schatzker Classification System

Type I   Split fracture of the lateral tibial plateau

Type II   Split depression fracture of the lateral tibial plateau

Type III Depression fracture of the lateral tibial plateau

Type IV   Fracture of the medial tibial plateau

Type V   Bicondylar fracture that involves a split of the lateral and medial plateau

Type VI   Bicondylar plateau fracture with diaphyseal extension

nal, and three-dimensional reconstruction can be used to detail any articular depression and allow study of the detailed anatomy of the fracture (**Figure 2, *C* and *D*)**. Recently, MRI has been recommended for patients with tibial plateau fractures.[13] Clinical studies of patients with tibial plateau fractures evaluated by MRI show a high incidence of associated soft-tissue injuries of the knee, including meniscal tears, anterior and posterior cruciate ligament tears, posteromedial corner or medial collateral ligament tears, and posterolateral corner tears. Many of these injuries are difficult to reliably detect with physical examination alone. Results from MRI scans frequently lead to a change in the treatment plan for patients with tibial plateau fractures.[13]

Treatment Options

Many factors should be considered when choosing between surgical and nonsurgical treatment of a patient with a tibial plateau fracture, including knee stability, condition of the surrounding soft tissues, the presence of other injuries, the fracture pattern, and the patient's overall health and expectations.

Nonsurgical Treatment

Nonsurgical treatment with a hinged cast or brace is appropriate for some fractures of the tibial plateau. In-

4: Lower Extremity

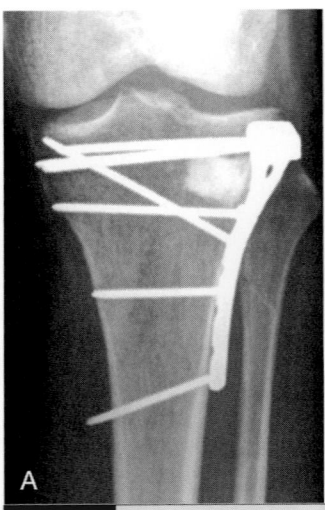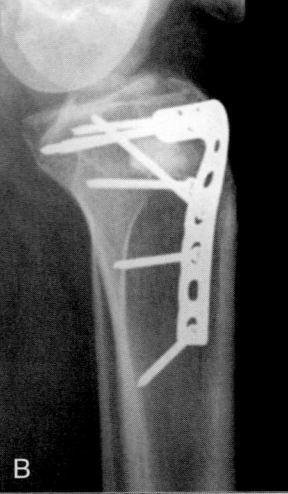

Figure 3 Example of a tibial plateau fracture. AP (**A**) and lateral (**B**) radiographs with calcium phosphate cement maintaining elevation of the depressed segment.

dications for closed management include fractures with less than 3 mm of articular depression, those that are stable to varus and valgus stress, peripheral rim fractures, low-energy fractures with minimal comminution, and fractures in patients with low activity demands or those with medical contraindications to surgery.

Surgical Treatment
Fractures with significant articular impaction and/or disruption, instability, and soft-tissue injury are best treated with surgery, although the timing of surgery must be carefully considered. Surgical options include standard open reduction and internal fixation, arthroscopically-assisted reduction and percutaneous fixation, and external fixation. Some of these techniques can be overlapped.

High-energy, displaced tibial plateau fractures should be considered to represent an impending compartment syndrome until proved otherwise. Careful, frequent neurovascular evaluation must be performed and documented. If there is any joint subluxation or significant shortening, consideration should be given to application of a knee-spanning external fixator. In these instances, it may be necessary to defer definitive surgery for several weeks until soft-tissue swelling and fracture blisters resolve.

Low-energy, lateral split-depression injuries are treated by standard techniques of open reduction, bone grafting, and fixation with a nonlocking buttress plate. Locked plates are not indicated for isolated lateral plateau fractures (**Figure 3**). Use of calcium phosphate cement may result in less late collapse than cancellous autograft or allograft.[14]

Split and split-depression fractures of the lateral plateau that are minimally displaced are treated with arthroscopic reduction and percutaneous screw fixation. An anterior cruciate ligament drill guide can be used to drill a tunnel beneath any depressed fragments to allow percutaneous elevation and bone grafting. Fixation with a "raft" of small-fragment screws placed beneath the articular surface completes the fixation.

The treatment of bicondylar injuries depends on the status of the soft tissues and the morphology of the medial fracture. Surgery (except for fasciotomy or temporary external fixation) is deferred until the soft-tissue injuries stabilize. If the medial fracture is in the sagittal plane, repair with a lateral locking plate is sufficient. If the medial fracture is in the coronal plane, a posteromedial tibial buttress plate should be used first, followed by repair of the lateral plateau fragment with a locking plate. Direct posterior approaches rarely may be necessary.[15] In bicondylar plateau fractures with articular comminution, reduction and stabilization of the medial and lateral plateau using a rim plate and nonlocking screws and buried, small-diameter wires is performed first. Once the joint is reconstructed, a lateral locking plate is used to connect the articular block to the tibial diaphysis. Locking plates help prevent varus collapse in the presence of medial plateau bony instability. However, the use of locking plates alone to treat these fractures may make it difficult to maintain joint reduction in the presence of articular comminution.

External fixation is used as an emergency temporizing measure in patients with unstable high-energy fractures, and occasionally as definitive treatment. In the first scenario, the fixator is applied as a uniplanar frame over the anterior knee with the knee extended. In most situations, such frames are not left in place for more than 4 weeks. When applying a knee-spanning external fixator, care must be taken to place the pins away from the zone of injury and away from potential incisions or hardware; therefore, pins are typically inserted into the distal tibia. When used for definitive fixation, a circular wire frame (Ilizarov type) or a hybrid ring external fixator is used. It should be realized that all wires placed in the proximal tibial metaphysis are potentially intra-articular, and pin tract sepsis should be treated to avoid pyarthrosis. These devices are used to stabilize the metadiaphyseal junction, and patients can begin knee movement and weight bearing. External fixation can be combined with limited or arthroscopic reduction of the articular surface.

Compartment Syndrome
Compartment syndrome complicates up to 15% of high-energy tibial plateau fractures; the placement of knee-spanning external fixation may increase the risk, although this has not been well quantified. Careful monitoring is mandatory. Fasciotomy should be performed when indicated by typical clinical findings or by perfusion pressure criteria (diastolic blood pressure minus intramuscular pressure > 30 mm Hg). Fasciotomy incisions should be placed with consideration of later surgical approaches, but should not compromise fascial decompression.

Medial Tibial Plateau Fractures

Medial tibial plateau fractures warrant special consideration because they commonly represent a variant of a knee fracture-dislocation and may be especially prone to neurovascular complications and compartment syndrome. Ankle-brachial indices should be obtained by computing a Doppler-derived pulse pressure at the foot in both the injured and contralateral legs. If the injured leg has an ankle-brachial index of less than 90% of that of the uninjured leg, vascular consultation is needed. Most medial tibial plateau fractures warrant internal plate fixation. Unstable vertical split fractures of the medial plateau require plate fixation.

Tibial Spine Fractures

Fractures of the tibial spine occur in adults and are often considered to be the bony equivalent of an anterior cruciate ligament tear. The diagnosis is made on the basis of plain radiographs. In adults, treatment usually depends on whether the patient has a block to motion. When pain, intercondylar impingement, and/or instability exist, arthroscopically assisted repair is usually considered, often with associated anterior cruciate ligament reconstruction, because of concerns about ligament elongation before the avulsion occurred. Reduction and fixation of displaced, malunited tibial spine fractures in symptomatic adults with loss of knee extension can result in clinical improvement.

A unique characteristic of tibial spine fractures in adults is the likelihood of other intra-articular damage and/or associated ligament injury. In a review of MRI findings in 10 children and 15 adults with tibial spine fractures in the setting of acute injury, none of the pediatric patients had ligament or meniscal injury.[16] In contrast, both medial and lateral meniscal tears occurred in several of the adult patients. Based on these findings, MRI is recommended in adults because tibial spine fractures may be accompanied by concomitant injuries that require surgical treatment.

Annotated References

1. Hughes SC, Stott PM, Hearnden AJ, Ripley LG: A new and effective tension-band braided polyester suture technique for transverse patellar fracture fixation. *Injury* 2007;38:212-222.

    In a biomechanical model, despite less rigid fixation, the use of braided polyester suture secured with a modified Wagoner's hitch knot led to less fracture gaping than other tension-band techniques. More clinical evaluation is needed before this technique should be widely adopted in the clinical setting.

2. Carpenter JE, Kasman R, Matthews LS: Fractures of the patella. *Instr Course Lect* 1994;43:97-108.

3. Burvant JG, Thomas KA, Alexander R, Harris MB: Evaluation of methods of internal fixation of transverse patella fractures: A biomechanical study. *J Orthop Trauma* 1994;8:147-153.

4. Luna-Pizarro D, Amato D, Arellano F, Hernandez A, Lopez-Rojas P: Comparison of a technique using a new percutaneous osteosynthesis device with conventional open surgery for displaced patella fractures in a randomized controlled trial. *J Orthop Trauma* 2006;20:529-535.

    In a randomized controlled trial, 53 patients with displaced patellar fractures were treated with traditional open reduction and internal fixation or a percutaneous patellar osteosynthesis system technique developed by the authors. The patients in the percutaneous group had fewer complications and better functional outcome scores at 2 years compared with the group treated with open reduction and internal fixation. These results should be considered preliminary until validated in other larger studies with longer follow-up.

5. Saltzman CL, Goulet JA, McClellan RT, Schneider LA, Matthews LS: Results of treatment of displaced patellar fractures by partial patellectomy. *J Bone Joint Surg Am* 1990;72:1279-1285.

6. Mills WJ, Nork SE: Open reduction and internal fixation of high-energy tibial plateau fractures. *Orthop Clin North Am* 2002;33:177-198.

7. Young MJ, Barrack RL: Complications of internal fixation of tibial plateau fractures. *Orthop Rev* 1994;23:149-154.

8. Weiner LS, Kelley M, Yang E, et al: The use of combination internal fixation and hybrid external fixation in severe proximal tibia fractures. *J Orthop Trauma* 1995;9:244-250.

9. Stannard JP, Wilson TC, Volgas DA, Alonso JE: The less invasive stabilization system in the treatment of complex fractures of the tibial plateau: Short-term results. *J Orthop Trauma* 2004;18:552-558.

    The authors report a consecutive series of 39 patients with complex tibial plateau fractures who were treated with the LISS plate (Synthes USA, Paoli, PA). At more than 1 year follow-up, 34 fractures had healed; only two superficial infections occurred.

10. Weigel DP, Marsh JL: High-energy fractures of the tibial plateau: Knee function after longer follow-up. *J Bone Joint Surg Am* 2002;84-A:1541-1551.

11. Schatzker J, Lambert DC: Supracondylar fractures of the femur. *Clin Orthop Relat Res* 1979;138:77-83.

12. Muller ME, Nazarian S, Koch P, Schatzker J: *The Comprehensive Classification of Fractures of Long Bones.* New York, NY, Springer-Verlag, 1990, pp 453-458.

13. Yacoubian SV, Nevins RT, Sallis JG, Potter HG, Lorich DG: Impact of MRI on treatment plan and fracture clas-

sification of tibial plateau fractures. *J Orthop Trauma* 2002;16:632-637.

14. Trenholm A, Landry S, McLaughlin K, et al: Comparative fixation of tibial plateau fractures using alpha-BSM, a calcium phosphate cement, versus cancellous bone graft. *J Orthop Trauma* 2005;19:698-702.

    The authors of this study performed biomechanical testing on 10 matched pairs of cadaveric tibiae, and used either calcium phosphate cement or cancellous bone to fill a simulated lateral split-depression fracture with a metaphyseal defect. The bones repaired with the bone substitute had greater stiffness and less collapse during subsequent loading.

15. Carlson DA: Posterior bicondylar tibial plateau fractures. *J Orthop Trauma* 2005;19:73-78.

    The author describes a study of eight patients with comminuted bicondylar posterior tibial plateau fractures treated with separate posteromedial and posterolateral approaches. A detailed description of the surgical approaches is provided.

16. Ishibashi Y, Tsuda E, Sasaki T, Toh S: Magnetic resonance imaging aids in detecting concomitant injuries in patients with tibial spine fractures. *Clin Orthop Relat Res* 2005;434:207-212.

    MRI scanning was done in 25 patients (10 children and 15 adults) with tibial spine fractures. No associated lesions were seen in the pediatric patients, except for one meniscus tear in a patient with a chronic injury. In contrast, in the 15 adult patients there were medial meniscus lesions in 2 patients with chronic injuries and in 1 patient with an acute injury, as well as 4 lateral meniscus tears (1 patient had a chronic injury and 3 patients had acute injuries). Based on these findings, MRI is recommended in adults because tibial spine fractures may be accompanied by concomitant injuries that require surgical treatment.

4: Lower Extremity

Chapter 36

Soft-Tissue Injuries About the Knee

*Dennis Crawford, MD, PhD

Knee Dislocations

Dislocation can occur in the patellofemoral, proximal tibiofibular, and tibiofemoral joints of the knee. Tibiofemoral dislocations are typically characterized by purely ligamentous injuries, although the pathology can include associated periarticular femoral and/or tibial fractures and fractures of the proximal fibula. Conversely, the spectrum of injury in periarticular knee fractures is now recognized to include significant soft-tissue injury. MRI shows associated soft-tissue injury in most surgical tibial plateau fractures.[1] The clinical consequence of such combined injuries is not fully known. Regardless of the presence of a fracture, initial evaluation of all tibiofemoral dislocations mandates prompt assessment of the neurovascular status because vascular injury requires immediate treatment to avoid the devastating sequelae of prolonged ischemia.

Multiple ligaments must be disrupted for a knee dislocation to occur. Patterns of injury can be considered either complex or simple, based on associated nerve and vascular function. Complex injuries include those with popliteal artery disruption, significant motor nerve dysfunction, and open injuries. Each component requires an urgent and thorough evaluation to avoid prolonged ischemia, to allow decompression of nerves, and to reduce the risk of septic arthritis. Physical examination including ankle-brachial index for evaluation of arterial injury in reduced knee dislocations is highly predictive of the need for surgical arterial repair. Noninvasive systolic blood pressure recordings taken distal to the injury can be compared with those of an uninjured upper extremity to standardize the measurement of potential vascular injury in normotensive patients after reduction of the knee joint. When the ankle-brachial index ratio is less than 0.9, close observation is required, and consideration of angiographic evaluation or surgical exploration is recommended.[2] When arterial repair is done, concomitant fasciotomies of the lower extremity are often done, either prophylactically or therapeutically. External fixation is recommended in this situation to maintain reduction and to allow access to the soft tissue. External fixation also is indicated if residual subluxation of the knee remains after reduction, usually with the tibia posterior to the femur, or in patients in whom orthotic management is precluded (such as in obese patients).

For cruciate ligament tears after a knee dislocation, surgical treatment is generally favored over nonsurgical treatment. Subacute repairs are recommended and should be done within the first 3 weeks after injury to allow primary repair of collateral ligaments and posterolateral structures when possible.[3] Outcome studies consistently indicate that despite successful surgical reconstruction, return to preinjury high-level athletic participation and vigorous labor generally is compromised.

Posterior Cruciate Ligament Injury

Posterior cruciate ligament (PCL) injury typically occurs when a flexed knee sustains a direct blow to the tibia tubercle. This injury is classified from grade 1 (partial) to grade 3 (complete). Combined injury patterns that can include PCL rupture are associated with hyperextension, hyperflexion, and severe rotational force mechanisms. Physical examination allows characterization of this injury based on the position of the tibia tubercle relative to the anterior aspect of the medial femoral condyle, with the contralateral knee used for comparison. In the presence of a posteriorly subluxated tibia, this test will help to avoid the mistake of interpreting anterior laxity as a positive Lachman's test. Assessment of the collateral ligaments and lateral corner integrity using a dial test along with varus and valgus stress testing at both 0° and 30° of knee flexion will provide a complete examination. A dial test involves external rotation of the tibia at 30° and 90° of knee flexion. When increased rotation (> 10°) occurs in comparison with the uninjured knee it is considered indicative of lateral corner injury (30°) or posterior cruciate injury (90°). Initial radiographic evaluation should include AP, lateral, and Merchant views to identify fractures and potential subluxation. MRI is the gold standard for assessment of ligamentous and chondral injuries and nondisplaced fractures.

Long-term outcome studies consistently identify arthrosis of the patellofemoral joint. Surgical intervention using an algorithmic approach is based on the chronicity of the injury and associated pathology. **Figure 1** outlines a systematic approach to the treatment of the various ligament injury patterns associated with PCL

*Dennis Crawford, MD, PhD or the department with which he is affiliated holds stock or stock options in Histogenics.

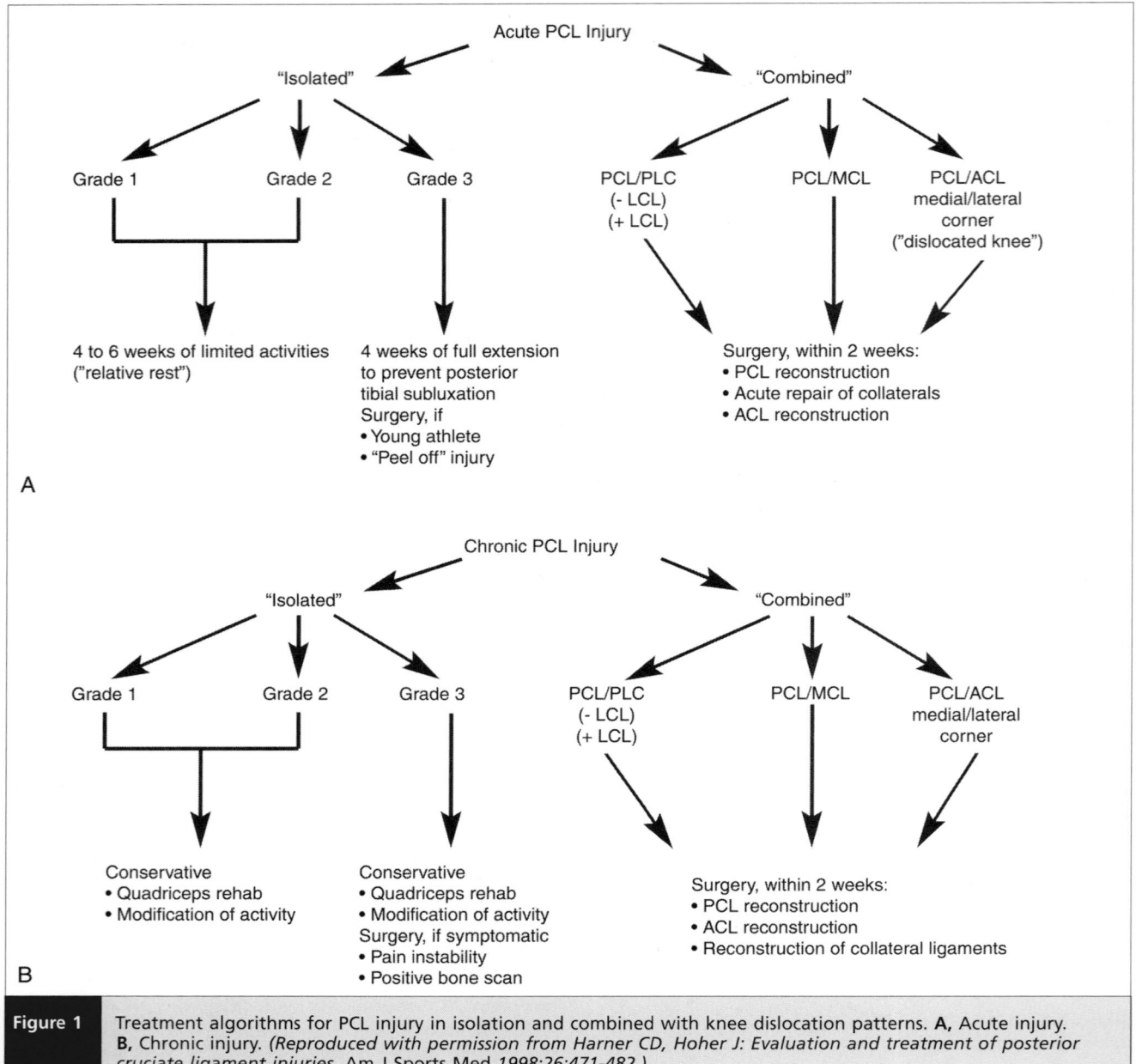

Figure 1 Treatment algorithms for PCL injury in isolation and combined with knee dislocation patterns. **A,** Acute injury. **B,** Chronic injury. *(Reproduced with permission from Harner CD, Hoher J: Evaluation and treatment of posterior cruciate ligament injuries. Am J Sports Med 1998;26:471-482.)*

injury. Repair of chronic injuries with symptomatic instability is generally recommended because improved function can be expected, although some degree of persistent laxity is common.[4,5]

The current trend in PCL reconstruction is to reestablish the anatomic character of the anteromedial and posterolateral bundles. Primary repair is recommended in the acute setting for avulsions involving periosteum (femur) or associated fractures (tibia). Reconstruction with a variety of graft sources and techniques is generally recommended for midsubstance and chronic tears. Transtibial approaches are typified by a single-bundle reconstruction that recapitulates more of the anterolateral fibers and is thus fixed with the knee

in 90° of flexion while applying an anteriorly directed load. Clinical data indicate generally satisfactory outcomes and return to activity with this approach. Tibia inlay techniques have the theoretic advantage of avoiding graft fraying, but clinically no difference appears to exist between the inlay and transtibial technique.[6,7]

Double-bundle techniques provide increased stability through the full range of knee motion in laboratory biomechanical testing. These techniques include a variation of the arthroscopic transtibial approach using two femoral tunnels and fixing the second posteromedial bundle in 30° of knee flexion, or the open "onlay" (inlay) approach.[8] The relative risk of morbidity, particularly vascular injury to the popliteal artery, and post-

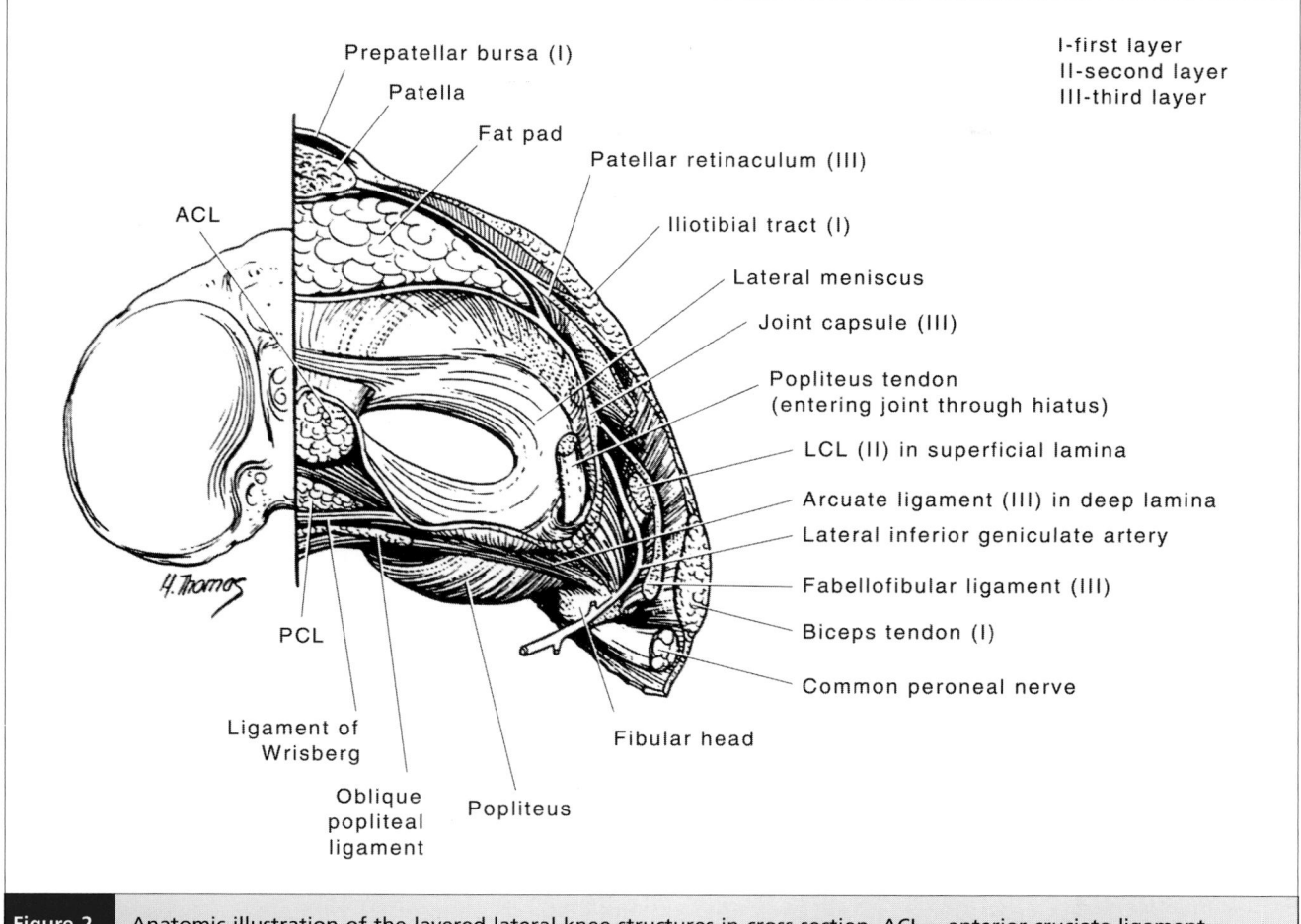

I-first layer
II-second layer
III-third layer

Prepatellar bursa (I)
Patella
Fat pad
Patellar retinaculum (III)
ACL
Iliotibial tract (I)
Lateral meniscus
Joint capsule (III)
Popliteus tendon
(entering joint through hiatus)
LCL (II) in superficial lamina
Arcuate ligament (III) in deep lamina
Lateral inferior geniculate artery
Fabellofibular ligament (III)
Biceps tendon (I)
Common peroneal nerve
PCL
Fibular head
Ligament of
Wrisberg
Oblique
popliteal   Popliteus
ligament

| Figure 2 | Anatomic illustration of the layered lateral knee structures in cross section. ACL = anterior cruciate ligament. *(Reproduced with permission from Seebacher JR, Inglis AE, Marshall JL, Warren RF: The structure of the posterolateral aspect of the knee. J Bone Joint Surg Am 1982;64:536-541.)* |

4: Lower Extremity

operative motion loss should be considered when choosing from these technically demanding procedures.

Injury to Posterolateral Structures

The lateral collateral ligament (LCL), popliteus myotendinous complex, popliteofibular ligament, popliteomeniscal attachment, iliotibial band, and arcuate ligament complex are commonly referred to as the posterolateral corner of the knee. These structures are organized in several layers (**Figure 2**). The LCL inserts posterior (4.6 mm) and proximal (1.3 mm) to the lateral epicondyle of the femur and posterior (8.1 mm) to the anterior point of the head of the fibula. On the femur, the popliteus tendon inserts distal (11 mm) and either anterior or posterior (mean, 0.84 mm anterior) to the LCL. The popliteofibular ligament inserts distal (1.3 mm) and anterior (0.5 mm) to the tip of the fibula styloid process.[9]

Isolated injury to the LCL is uncommon and the diagnostic maneuvers to assess the integrity of the lateral ligament complex typically involve the varus stress and

the dial tests. In the absence of posterolateral corner injury, the knee will be stable in full extension with a varus stress test; if lateral knee joint opening occurs at full extension, a posterolateral corner injury is suspected. An assessment of tibial external rotation (dial test) is then done to determine the potential for concurrent PCL injury as the leg is taken from 30° to 90° of knee flexion. Addition of a valgus stress test at both full extension and 30° of flexion can assess the integrity of the medial collateral ligament (MCL), which can confound the dial test result (a false positive dial test occurs when the MCL is injured).[10]

Selecting the proper surgical treatment for a posterolateral corner injury is based on the degree of symptomatic joint laxity and the presence of associated injuries. Various surgical techniques have been described and generally involve either primary repair or reconstruction with graft supplementation. In chronic injuries, reconstruction (with either allograft or autograft) is recommended over anatomic repair. Anatomic reconstruction is focused on the key structures of the posterolateral corner; principally the LCL, the popliteofibular ligament, and the popliteus tendon (**Figure 3**). In dis-

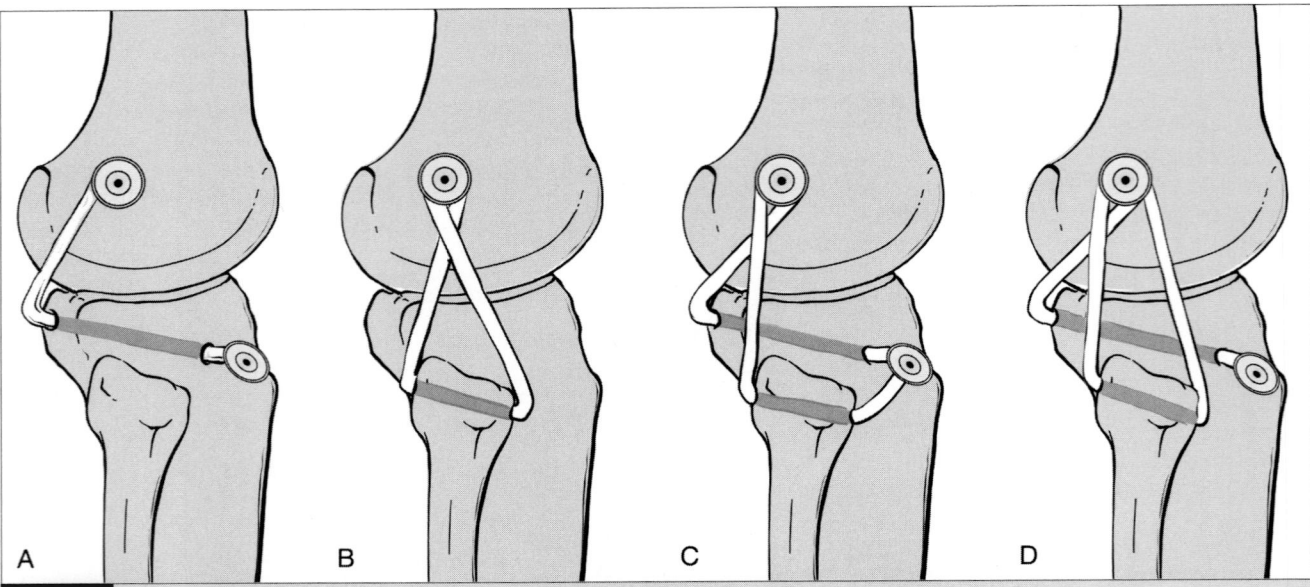

Figure 3 Various techniques for posterolateral complex reconstruction are illustrated. **A,** The popliteal bypass. **B,** The figure-of-8 technique is intended to favor isometry. The two-tailed technique **(C)** and the modified two-tailed technique **(D)** are designed to reconstruct both the LCL and popliteus. *(Reproduced from Bush-Joseph C, Carter TR, Miller MD, Rokito AS, Stuart MJ: Knee and leg: Soft-tissue trauma, in Koval KJ (ed):* Orthopaedic Knowledge Update 7. *Rosemont, IL, American Academy of Orthopaedic Surgeons, 2002, p 495.)*

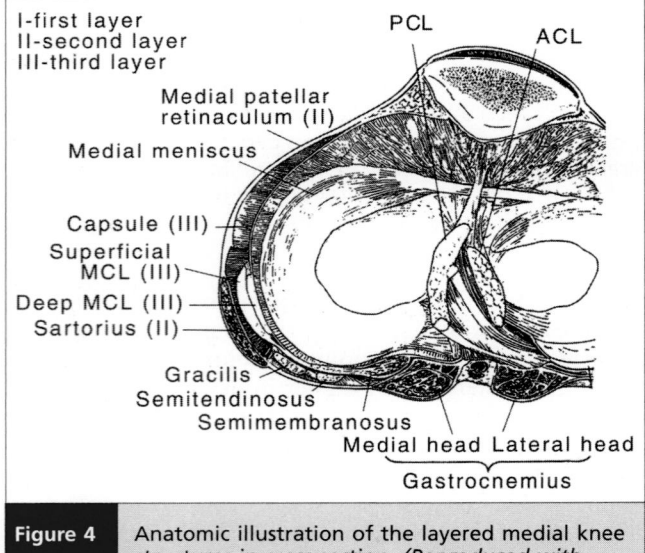

I-first layer
II-second layer
III-third layer

PCL   ACL

Medial patellar retinaculum (II)
Medial meniscus
Capsule (III)
Superficial MCL (III)
Deep MCL (III)
Sartorius (II)
Gracilis
Semitendinosus
Semimembranosus
Medial head   Lateral head
Gastrocnemius

Figure 4 Anatomic illustration of the layered medial knee structures in cross section. *(Reproduced with permission from Warren RF, Arnoczky SP, Wickiewicz TL: Anatomy of the knee, in Nicholas JA, Hershman E (eds):* The Lower Extremity and Spine in Sports Medicine, *ed 2. St. Louis, MO, Mosby-Year Book, 1995, pp 657-693.)*

placed fibula fractures, the functional integrity of the LCL, biceps tendon, and popliteofibular ligament is compromised; therefore, fracture repair should be considered when possible. Reconstruction of a posterolateral corner injury in isolation appears to have a better outcome than in the setting of a multiligament injury.[11] Factors associated with the failure of posterolateral cor-

ner injury repair include nonanatomic graft reconstruction, untreated varus malalignment, and failure to repair all ruptured ligaments.[12]

Injury to Medial Structures

The anatomy of the MCL complex consists of three identifiable passive restraining structures: the superficial MCL, the deep MCL, and the posteromedial capsule (Figure 4). These ligament bundles are described as sustaining maximum loads of 534 N (superficial MCL), 194 N (deep MCL), and 425 N (posteromedial capsule); the bundles fail at 10.2, 7.1, and 12.0 mm mean extension, respectively, in human cadaver testing.[13] MCL and medial capsule integrity have implications for treatment of anterior cruciate ligament (ACL) injuries, because various components make different contributions to rotational and anteroposterior translational integrity.[14] The posteromedial capsule controls valgus, internal rotation, and posterior drawer in extension. The superficial collateral ligament resists valgus loads at all angles and is dominant from 30° to 90° of flexion, and also controls internal rotation in flexion. The deep collateral ligament controls anterior tibial drawer of the flexed and externally rotated knee and is a secondary restraint to valgus stress. Recent data suggest that prophylactic bracing in athletes who participate in contact sports may offer protection for the MCL from valgus injury while sacrificing performance and increasing fatigue and cramping.[15]

Generally, isolated midsubstance tears of the MCL complex can be treated with brace application to prevent recurrent valgus overload. In a rat model, low intensity pulsed ultrasound therapy resulted in accelerated healing, and a nonsteroidal anti-inflammatory drug (celecoxib) delayed knee ligament healing in early injury (after 2 weeks); however, those modalities resulted in no difference in outcomes when used in combination at 2 weeks, or individually after 4 or 12 weeks of healing compared with control groups.[16] The identification and treatment of combined ACL and MCL injuries is more complex. Identifying an MCL injury in the presence of an ACL tear requires a valgus stress test. Cadaver testing indicates that ACL deficiency causes an increase in MCL insertion site and contact forces in response to anterior tibia loading, but not in response to valgus loading. Increased valgus laxity in the ACL-deficient knee indicates a compromised MCL.[17] Treatment of grade III MCL injury in the context of ACL injury remains controversial. One recent study found no clinically significant difference between nonsurgically or surgically treated MCL injuries 2 years after early ACL reconstruction.[18]

Anterior Cruciate Ligament Injury

Advances in the treatment of ACL injuries include extensive investigation of injury susceptibility, effects of different training modalities in preventing ACL injury, outcomes following reconstruction and revision surgery, technical improvements providing more anatomic reconstructions, and consideration of the relative success of the variety of options for graft selection.

Continued study of gender disparity in rates of ACL injury (female athletes sustain a twofold to fourfold increased incidence of ACL rupture in identical sports in comparison with males) has focused on the factors influencing risks and the success of exercise training programs for reducing the prevalence of frequently occurring injury. The multifactorial nature of susceptibility to noncontact ACL injury was reported in a prospective study of military cadets. Data from the study support previous data identifying small femoral notch width, generalized ligamentous laxity, higher body mass index, and female gender as risk factors for ACL injury.[19] Specific neuromuscular training techniques that emphasize balance and plyometrics appear to be an important factor in reducing the positional susceptibility of the knee joint to forces associated with ACL injury.[20] Although controversy exists as to the exact nature, intensity, and type of training program needed, a favorable effect with a reduction in the rate of ACL injury during the training period is usually reported.[21,22]

The standard technique of ACL reconstruction continues to evolve. A long-term study (13 years) of patients treated with endoscopic autogenous patella tendon ACL reconstruction found significant radiographic osteoarthrosis associated with meniscectomy, loss of extension, and greater residual laxity on Lachman testing after reconstruction. In this study, 97% of patients reported normal or near-normal knee function despite radiographic evidence of arthrosis in 79% of the patients.[23] Recent attempts to improve the results of surgical reconstruction of the ACL have focused on recapitulating the anterolateral and posteromedial bundles using a variety of double bundle techniques. Several authors have described the biomechanical effects that suggest the potential for improved clinical results.[24] Outcomes data from clinical trials are limited, but appear to indicate no significant clinical differences despite improvements in stability test measures after early follow-up.[25-27] Others have suggested that results of the pivot-shift test better correlate to outcomes compared with results from the Lachman test or instrumented testing.[28] Independent predictors of poor outcome after ACL reconstruction were recently shown to include smoking, recollection of hearing a pop at the time of ACL injury, a weight gain of more than 15 lb (6.8 kg), and no change in educational level since the surgery.[29,30] Bracing for 1 year after ACL reconstruction does not appear to influence outcomes for isolated ligament injuries.[31] One large prospective study found an equal rate of ACL rupture in knees with previously reconstructed ACL ligaments compared with uninjured contralateral knees.[32]

There is no consensus on a single optimal graft choice for ACL reconstruction. Allograft tissue from various sources is being used in both primary, and more consistently, in revision ACL reconstruction techniques. Arguments in favor of allograft tissue application include the persistent histologic abnormality of both the patella and hamstring tendons after harvesting, the potential for cost reduction, minimized early postoperative pain, and improved early function. It is not recommended that previously harvested patella tendon be considered as a viable graft source for any subsequent procedure, although ipsilateral normal tissue use as a graft source is an acceptable choice in revision surgery. Arguments against the use of allograft tissue include concern for disease transmission and potentially inferior biologic incorporation.[32] Clinical outcome studies generally have found no significant difference in knee function scores after allograft patella tendon reconstruction compared with historic cohorts (autograft patellar tendon).[33] One prospective study consistent with this trend found patients treated with allograft had less perioperative pain and more rapid return to function; however, there was no significant difference in outcome at 5-year follow-up.[34]

Rerupture or failure of ACL reconstruction presents several clinical challenges. Failed ACL reconstruction may be either traumatic or atraumatic. Atraumatic failures may be attributable to technical errors, diagnostic errors, or failure of graft incorporation. Successful revision ACL reconstruction depends on identifying and treating concurrent pathology such as articular cartilage damage, a prior meniscectomy or new tear, malalignment, or additional ligament injuries. An analysis of the spectrum of technical reasons for graft failure such as poor tunnel placement, bone loss or tunnel widening, and hardware interference shows the need for thorough preoperative planning. Published outcomes of revision ACL reconstruction consistently indicate worse outcomes than those achieved for primary ACL reconstruction; however, all results indicate significantly improved function. One technical consideration involves the choice of graft material. Several studies show significantly improved knee function regardless of the graft material applied (such as previously unharvested ipsilateral autografts, quadriceps patella autograft, or allograft irradiated patella tendon).[35,36]

The care of skeletally immature athletes with ACL instability continues to remain controversial. Previous studies have shown that failure of reconstruction results in a high rate of premature degeneration, and a delay in surgical treatment is associated with a higher prevalence of meniscal tears. Other studies have indicated no increase in the rate of additional knee injuries with surgical delay and absolute activity restriction. Among authors who advocate surgical repair, no consensus exists on the technique to be used; however, physeal-sparing techniques are generally favored for patients who have substantial remaining growth. The use of a quadrupled soft-tissue graft for tunnels traversing the tibia and femoral physis has been shown to produce no significant limb-length discrepancy, and in one study was advocated as an effective technique to restore function and maintain isometric graft placement in children from 11 to 14 years of age (mean, 12.5 years).[37] In younger patients (Tanner stage 1 or 2; mean age, 10.3 years) a recent study evaluated the results of a physeal-sparing, combined intra-articular and extra-articular reconstruction using autogenous iliotibial band.[38] No limb-length discrepancy was reported and significant improvement in functional measures occurred across the group at an average of 5 years after surgery. Lachman and pivot-shift test results were normal in 55% of the children age 11 to 14 years and 75% of the younger patients.

Meniscal Cartilage Tears

There are two general types of meniscal tears—acute tears, which usually occur in younger patients after significant trauma; and degenerative tears, which typically occur in older patients after minimal or no trauma. Acute tears are often associated with other intra-articular knee abnormalities and are often amenable to repair. Degenerative tears can be treated nonsurgically or with partial meniscectomy if associated mechanical symptoms are present. Tear patterns have been shown to predict etiology. Radial, longitudinal, and complex meniscal tears shown on MRI scans are strongly related to trauma. Horizontal meniscal tears are more likely preexistent conditions and are more often unrelated to trauma. Similarly, extruded menisci are more commonly associated with degenerative cartilage loss and progression of symptomatic osteoarthritis. Clinical diagnosis of meniscal tears may be improved by adding Ege's weight-bearing test to a panel of physical examination maneuvers. Ege's test is done by placing the feet 8 to 10 inches apart and turned outward (medial meniscal) or inward (lateral meniscal test). The patient squats down while keeping the feet flat. Pain or a click when the knee is bent approximately 90° is considered a positive result.[39]

Surgical treatment of knees with meniscal injury continues to involve a variety of arthroscopic techniques. Simple arthroscopic débridement of knee joints (including subtotal meniscectomy) in knees with minimal evidence of radiographic osteoarthritis (Kellgren-Lawrence grades 0 and 1), normal alignment, and preserved joint space (≥ 3 mm) provides good symptomatic relief. An inverse correlation between the degree of cartilage damage found at arthroscopy and pain relief was described.[40] Multiple devices and techniques have been described to allow preservation of maximal normal tissue during débridement procedures and simplify repair techniques. Although mechanical instruments remain the standard of care, development of new approaches continues. For example, one laboratory study using radiofrequency ablation in a porcine knee (ex vivo) produced no more cell injury within the meniscus or surrounding cartilage during débridement than simple mechanical débridement with a basket punch.[41]

The potential for successful meniscal repair is dependent on several factors including acuity of injury, presence of associated ACL rupture and reconstruction, morphology of the tear, and proximity to the vascular red zone (**Figure 5**). The open suture technique is the gold standard for meniscal repair. Recent technologic advancements with all-inside arthroscopic devices provide opportunity for compression across the zone of injury with a variety of techniques. Use of several of these devices has shown comparable results to open methods. One recent case study identified similar outcomes (90% healing) with an all-inside device compared with a control group treated with the historic inside-out methods.[42] However, it should be noted that this study reflects the limited nature of statistical data in evaluating these repair techniques. Evidence-based review of the outcomes of all-inside meniscus repair devices found that 77% of identified studies were case studies, 10% were retrospective comparative studies, 6.5% were prospective comparative studies, and 6.5% were prospective randomized studies. The failure rates ranged from 0% to 43.5%.[43]

Meniscal transplantation is indicated for young patients who have substantial compromise of the existing meniscus or those who have had a total meniscectomy. Techniques for transplanting the medial and lateral meniscus are shown in **Figures 6 and 7**, respectively. Several recent studies showed that this procedure was associated with encouraging intermediate-term results in terms of reduction of knee pain and improvement of function. In a retrospective review of patients treated with lateral meniscal transplants (fresh-frozen), follow-up at more than 3 years showed preservation of radiographic joint space in comparison with the normal contralateral knee.[44] Longer-term data on patients with medial and lateral meniscal transplants (fresh-frozen) followed for an average of 10 years provide evidence that results are improved with simultaneous valgus-

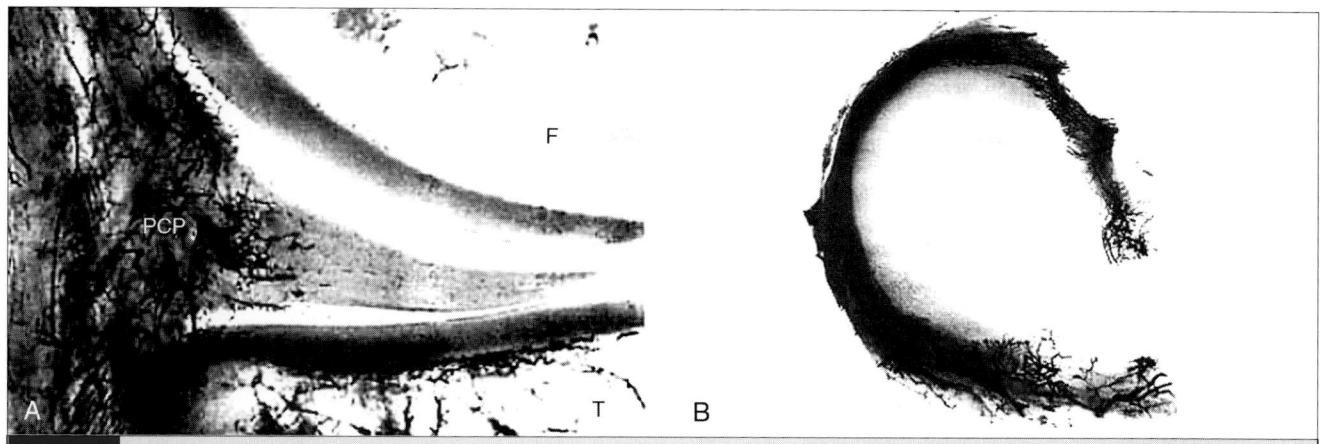

Figure 5 Sagittal **(A)** and axial **(B)** sections of the medial meniscus showing the peripheral vasculature. Branching radial vessels from the perimeniscal capillary plexus (PCP) can be seen penetrating the peripheral border of the medial meniscus. The central portion of the meniscus is avascular. F = femur, T = tibia. *(Reproduced with permission from Arnoczky SP, Warren RF: Microvasculature of the human meniscus. Am J Sports Med 1982:10:90-95.)*

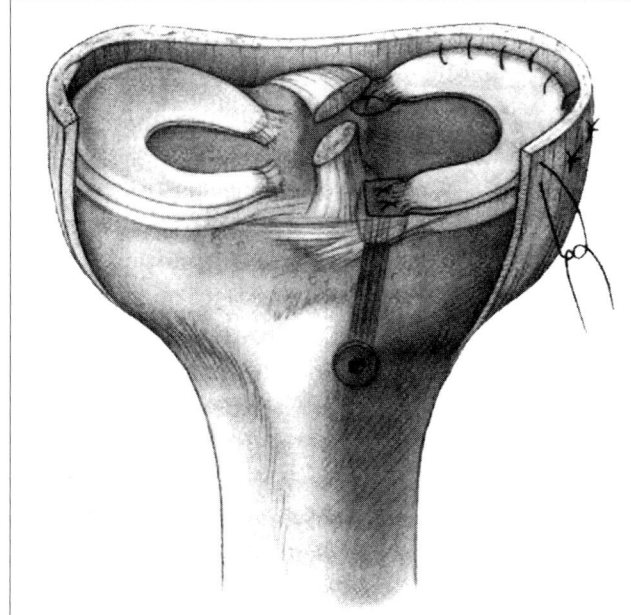

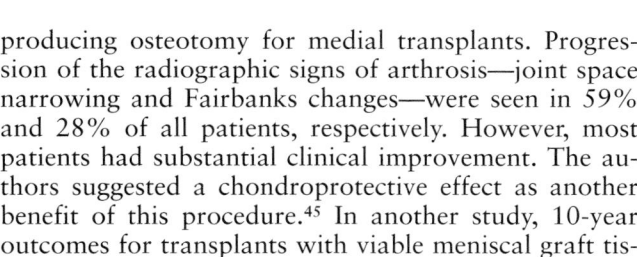

Figure 6 Illustration of the in situ medial meniscal transplant using the two-tunnel technique and vertically oriented peripheral sutures. *(Reproduced with permission from Noyes FR, Barber-Westin SD, Rankin M: Meniscal transplantation in symptomatic patients less than fifty years old. J Bone Joint Surg Am 2005;87(suppl 1):149-165.)*

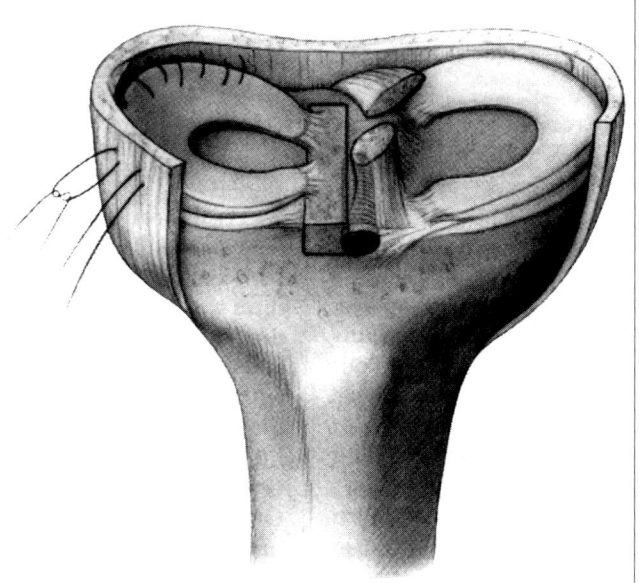

Figure 7 Illustration of the in situ lateral meniscal transplant using a bone-bridge technique (anterior maintained to posterior horn) with vertically oriented peripheral sutures. *(Reproduced with permission from Noyes FR, Barber-Westin SD, Rankin M: Meniscal transplantation in symptomatic patients less than fifty years old. J Bone Joint Surg Am 2005;87(suppl 1):149-165.)*

producing osteotomy for medial transplants. Progression of the radiographic signs of arthrosis—joint space narrowing and Fairbanks changes—were seen in 59% and 28% of all patients, respectively. However, most patients had substantial clinical improvement. The authors suggested a chondroprotective effect as another benefit of this procedure.[45] In another study, 10-year outcomes for transplants with viable meniscal graft tis-

sue showed a 70% to 83% transplant survival rate with a trend toward improved longevity when concurrent unloading osteotomy is performed.[46] Fresh-frozen meniscal transplantation also appears to provide acceptable short-term results with respect to pain relief and functional improvement, even in younger patients treated with concomitant osteochondral autograft transfer and knee ligament reconstruction. Complications reported for this procedure included graft shrinkage, displacement, and tearing.[47]

Articular Cartilage Injury

The treatment of articular cartilage damage includes a spectrum of disorders from focal isolated injury sustained in association with trauma to that associated with degenerative arthritides. Surgical options include simple débridement of small partial-thickness injuries, microfracture, osteochondral transfer (autogenous or allograft), or autologous chondrocyte transplantation. Evolution of these techniques, especially options for chondrocyte-based treatments and structural matrix designed to induce chondrogenesis, continues at a rapid pace. Autologous chondrocyte implantation (ACI) includes the use of porcine-derived type I/type III collagen as a cover, and matrix-induced ACI uses a collagen bilayer seeded with chondrocytes. Important considerations for selecting treatment options involve the degree, extent, and location of cartilage damage, the absence of arthritic degeneration, and relative joint contact forces in the area of injury (limb alignment, joint stability, and body mass index).

Microfracture is reported to provide functional improvement in select patients after short-term follow-up. Best results are achieved in association with increased fill of the defect (radiographic evidence of "replacement" tissue, not necessarily cartilage), low body mass index, and a short duration of preoperative symptoms. Conversely, high body mass index adversely affects short-term outcome, and a poor fill grade is associated with limited short-term durability.[48] Similar early results were reported in a larger study where deterioration of these clinical benefits occurred after 18 months. Specific predictors of higher fill grade (which correlated positively with International Cartilage Repair Society scores) were associated with femoral condyle lesions.[48] The biologic nature of this repair tissue was not identified in either study. One laboratory evaluation considered early histologic changes in primates after microfracture for experimentally created full-thickness defects. Data included evidence of substantial maturation of the fibrocartilage repair tissue from the 6th to 12th postoperative week, with complete fill by the 12th week.[49] The authors suggested maintaining protection of the repair tissue for extended periods. Early activity restrictions and the use of continuous passive motion are considered essential to fibrocartilage formation and clinical improvement. One retrospective review, however, found no significant clinical difference between short-term improvement (up to 5 years) after microfracture with traditional (non–weight-bearing protocols and continuous passive motion for 6 weeks) and accelerated (weight bearing and no continuous passive motion) rehabilitation protocols.[50]

Several studies have focused on the relative efficacy between different treatments of chondral injury. An analysis of the methodology of such studies (63 studies of 3,987 patients) casts doubt on their general validity because deficiencies were consistently found with respect to five criteria: the type of study, description of the rehabilitation protocol, outcome criteria, outcome assessment, and the patient selection process.[51] Similarly, evaluation of autologous chondrocyte transplantation clinical trials by the Cochrane Database of Systematic Reviews allowed inclusion of only four randomized controlled trials including a total of 266 participants. One trial of ACI versus mosaicplasty (osteochondral autograft treatment) reported statistically significant results for ACI at 1 year, but only in a post hoc subgroup analysis of participants with medial condylar defects; 88% had excellent or good results with ACI compared with 69% with mosaicplasty. A second trial of ACI versus mosaicplasty found no statistically significant difference in clinical outcomes at 2-year follow-up. There was no statistically significant difference in outcomes at 2-year follow-up in a trial comparing ACI with microfracture. In addition, one trial of matrix-guided ACI versus microfracture did not contain enough long-term results to reach definitive conclusions.[52] ACI, mosaicplasty, and microfracture are also discussed in chapter 3.

Allograft tissue has application for osteoarticular replacement in the setting of bone compromise with associated cartilage loss of more than 2 cm or in selected patients with premature unicompartmental arthritic degeneration. Transplantation of frozen allograft, although reported by some as successful, is believed to induce significant chondrocyte damage associated with subsequent premature graft degeneration. Use of fresh allograft, which provides improved preservation of chondrocyte viability, remains a significant challenge with respect to procurement, safety testing, and distribution in a timely manner. Use of hypothermic technique has been advocated as a method for preserving the chondrocyte and surrounding matrix. Recent advances are directed to improving preservation and storage; however, the length of time that these grafts maintain clinically significant viability is controversial. One recent study of the time-dependent changes to chondrocyte viability indicated significant change after 20 days.[53] A significant increase in degenerative changes to the allograft following implantation into nonhuman primates was observed following implantation of graft stored for more than 20 days. However, clinical data consistently indicate that the application of this technique throughout the knee (including selected patellofemoral joints) is effective, with success rates of up to 90% at 5 years and 70% at 10 years. Radiographic evidence of bone incorporation favors improved longer-term outcomes. Patients with underlying posttraumatic injury and osteochondritis dissecans typically find more success than those with bipolar lesions (kissing lesions) or lesions caused by osteonecrosis.

Annotated References

1. Gardner MJ, Yacoubian S, Geller D, et al: The incidence of soft tissue injury in operative tibial plateau fractures:

A magnetic resonance imaging analysis of 103 patients. *J Orthop Trauma* 2005;19:79-84.

The authors of this prospective cohort evaluation of acute tibial plateau fractures before surgical repair found that 99% of patients had injury to soft tissue on MRI evaluation. Level of evidence: IV.

2. Mills WJ, Barei DP, McNair P: The value of the ankle-brachial index for diagnosing arterial injury after knee dislocation: A prospective study. *J Trauma* 2004;56: 1261-1265.

This prospective study of the use of the ankle-brachial index to predict vascular injury after knee dislocation found that the sensitivity, specificity, and positive predictive value of an ankle-brachial index of less than 0.90 was 100%. The negative predictive value of an ankle brachial index of 0.90 or higher was 100%. Level of evidence: III.

3. Harner CD, Waltrip RL, Bennett CH, Francis KA, Cole B, Irrgang JJ: Surgical management of knee dislocations. *J Bone Joint Surg Am* 2004;86:262-273.

The authors present the results of a case study comparing acute (< 3 weeks duration) versus chronic simple knee dislocations treated with fresh-frozen allograft tissue. Level of evidence: IV.

4. Khanduja V, Somayaji HS, Harnett P, Utukuri M, Dowd GS: Combined reconstruction of chronic posterior cruciate ligament and posterolateral corner deficiency: A two- to nine-year follow-up study. *J Bone Joint Surg Br* 2006;88:1169-1172.

The authors of this retrospective case study examined chronic grade III PCL and posterolateral corner injuries after combined reconstruction. Level of evidence: IV.

5. Strobel MJ, Schulz MS, Petersen WJ, Eichhorn HJ: Combined anterior cruciate ligament, posterior cruciate ligament, and posterolateral corner reconstruction with autogenous hamstring grafts in chronic instabilities. *Arthroscopy* 2006;22:182-192.

In this prospective case study, outcomes of patients with chronic multiligament knee injuries treated with simultaneous ACL, PCL, and posterolateral corner reconstructions are presented. Level of evidence: IV.

6. Seon JK, Song EK: Reconstruction of isolated posterior cruciate ligament injuries: A clinical comparison of the transtibial and tibial inlay techniques. *Arthroscopy* 2006;22:27-32.

This retrospective case study of two techniques for PCL reconstruction found significant improvement with the use of both techniques and no difference in outcomes between the groups treated with transtibial or tibial inlay techniques. Level of evidence: III.

7. Jung YB, Jung HJ, Tae SK, Lee YS, Lee KH: Reconstruction of the posterior cruciate ligament with a mid-third patellar tendon graft with use of a modified tibial inlay method. *J Bone Joint Surg Am* 2005;87(suppl 1): 247-263.

A modified tibial inlay technique for PCL reconstruction that eliminates the need to reposition the patient during surgery is described. Level of evidence: IV.

8. Chhabra A, Kline AJ, Harner CD: Single-bundle versus double-bundle posterior cruciate ligament reconstruction: Scientific rationale and surgical technique. *Instr Course Lect* 2006;55:497-507.

The authors present a review of the anatomy, mechanics, and technique for two-bundle PCL reconstruction.

9. Brinkman JM, Schwering PJ, Blankevoort L, Kooloos JG, Luites J, Wymenga AB: The insertion geometry of the posterolateral corner of the knee. *J Bone Joint Surg Br* 2005;87:1364-1368.

The results of a human cadaveric laboratory study of the knee are presented.

10. Pritsch T, Blumberg N, Haim A, Dekel S, Arbel R: The importance of the valgus stress test in the diagnosis of posterolateral instability of the knee. *Injury* 2006;37: 1011-1014.

This cadaveric study indicates the confounding possibility of MCL injury in assessing injury to the posterolateral corner of the knee.

11. Stannard JP, Brown SL, Robinson JT, McGwin G Jr, Volgas DA: Reconstruction of the posterolateral corner of the knee. *Arthroscopy* 2005;21:1051-1059.

This case study of patients with posterolateral corner reconstruction who were treated with allograft found improved motion and a lower incidence of failure in patients with isolated posterolateral corner injuries. Level of evidence: IV.

12. Noyes FR, Barber-Westin SD, Albright JC: An analysis of the cause of failure in 57 consecutive posterolateral operative procedures. *Am J Sports Med* 2006;34:1419-1430.

The authors of this case study present a review of the failure mechanism for 57 procedures in 30 consecutive knees after posterolateral corner reconstruction. Level of evidence: IV.

13. Robinson JR, Bull AM, Amis AA: Structural properties of the medial collateral ligament complex of the human knee. *J Biomech* 2005;38:1067-1074.

This cadaveric study characterizes the biomechanical properties of the posterior medial capsule, the long superficial MCL, and the short, deep MCL.

14. Robinson JR, Bull AM, Thomas RR, Amis AA: The role of the medial collateral ligament and posteromedial capsule in controlling knee laxity. *Am J Sports Med* 2006; 34:1815-1823.

The authors of this cadaveric laboratory study indicate that the functional role of MCL structures in controlling tibiofemoral laxity depends on knee flexion and tibial rotation.

15. Najibi S, Albright JP: The use of knee braces: Part 1. Prophylactic knee braces in contact sports. *Am J Sports Med* 2005;33:602-611.

The authors of this review of prophylactic knee bracing suggest protection for the MCL from a valgus contact injury at the expense of some performance factors.

16. Warden SJ, Avin KG, Beck EM, DeWolf ME, Hagemeier MA, Martin KM: Low-intensity pulsed ultrasound accelerates and a nonsteroidal anti-inflammatory drug delays knee ligament healing. *Am J Sports Med* 2006;34: 1094-1102.

Low-intensity pulsed ultrasound therapy after ligament injury may facilitate earlier return to activity, whereas the use of nonsteroidal anti-inflammatory drugs may increase early reinjury risks.

17. Ellis BJ, Lujan TJ, Dalton MS, Weiss JA: Medial collateral ligament insertion site and contact forces in the ACL-deficient knee. *J Orthop Res* 2006;24:800-810.

A cadaveric biomechanical analysis of the effects of ACL deficiency on MCL insertional and contact force during anterior tibial or valgus loading is presented.

18. Halinen J, Lindahl J, Hirvensalo E, Santavirta S: Operative and nonoperative treatments of medial collateral ligament rupture with early anterior cruciate ligament reconstruction: A prospective randomized study. *Am J Sports Med* 2006;34:1134-1140.

This controlled randomized trial showed that nonsurgical and surgical treatment of grade III MCL ruptures leads to equally good results when concurrent ACL injury is reconstructed in the acute phase. Level of evidence: I.

19. Hewett TE, Myer GD, Ford KR: Decrease in neuromuscular control about the knee with maturation in female athletes. *J Bone Joint Surg Am* 2004;86:1601-1608.

Musculoskeletal changes associated with maturation in girls lead to greater total medial knee motion, greater maximum lower extremity valgus angle, and decreased flexor torque in female athletes. These changes result in poor neuromuscular control of the knee joint in female athletes.

20. Hewett TE, Myer GD, Ford KR, McLean SG: The effects of plyometric versus dynamic stabilization and balance training on lower extremity biomechanics. *Am J Sports Med* 2006;34:445-455.

This controlled laboratory study of female athletes found that both plyometric and balance training independently reduce lower extremity valgus moments. Level of evidence: I.

21. Mandelbaum BR, Silvers HJ, Watanabe DS, et al: Effectiveness of a neuromuscular and proprioceptive training program in preventing anterior cruciate ligament injuries in female athletes: 2-year follow-up. *Am J Sports Med* 2005;33:1003-1010.

This prospective cohort compared female athletes receiving training to matched control patients. The authors suggest that training provides a direct benefit in decreasing ACL injury. Level of evidence: II.

22. Hewett TE, Ford KR, Myer GD: Anterior cruciate ligament injuries in female athletes: Part 2. A meta-analysis of neuromuscular interventions aimed at injury prevention. *Am J Sports Med* 2006;34:490-498.

A review of six interventions designed to reduce ACL injury in female athletes identified four that reduced the incidence of knee injury and three that significantly reduced the incidence of ACL injury. A meta-analysis of these studies showed the significant effect of neuromuscular training programs on reducing the incidence of ACL injury in female athletes ($P < 0.001$). Level of evidence: I.

23. Salmon LJ, Russell VJ, Refshauge K, et al: Long-term outcome of endoscopic anterior cruciate ligament reconstruction with patellar tendon autograft: Minimum 13-year review. *Am J Sports Med* 2006;34:721-732.

The evaluation of consecutive study data for endoscopic ACL reconstruction with patella tendon at 13-year follow-up found significant arthrosis, yet sustained improvement in functional outcomes. Level of evidence: IV.

24. Cha PS, Brucker PU, West RV, et al: Arthroscopic double-bundle anterior cruciate ligament reconstruction: An anatomic approach. *Arthroscopy* 2005; 21:1275.

A technique description for arthroscopic ACL reconstruction that restores both the anteromedial and the posterolateral bundle is presented.

25. Muneta T, Koga H, Morito T, Yagishita K, Sekiya I: A retrospective study of the midterm outcome of two-bundle anterior cruciate ligament reconstruction using quadrupled semitendinosus tendon in comparison with one-bundle reconstruction. *Arthroscopy* 2006;22:252-258.

This retrospective comparison of a two-bundle ACL reconstruction versus a one-bundle technique found no significant outcome differences. Level of evidence: III.

26. Yasuda K, Kondo E, Ichiyama H, Tanabe Y, Tohyama H: Clinical evaluation of anatomic double-bundle anterior cruciate ligament reconstruction procedure using hamstring tendon grafts: Comparisons among 3 different procedures. *Arthroscopy* 2006;3:240-251.

This prospective cohort compared one-bundle, nonanatomic two-bundle, and anatomic two-bundle reconstructions at 2 years and found no clinical differences, except improved laxity in the group treated with anatomic two-bundle reconstruction. Level of evidence: II.

27. Williams RJ, Hyman J, Petrigliano F, Rozental T, Wickiewicz TL: Anterior cruciate ligament reconstruction with a four-strand hamstring tendon autograft: Surgical technique. *J Bone Joint Surg Am* 2005;87:51-66.

The authors of this case study of ACL reconstruction using four-strand autologous graft indicated that the 11% failure rate was not correlated with functional knee scores. Level of evidence: IV.

28. Kocher MS, Steadman JR, Briggs KK, Sterett WI, Hawkins RJ: Relationships between objective assessment of ligament stability and subjective assessment of symptoms and function after anterior cruciate ligament reconstruction. *Am J Sports Med* 2004;32:629-634.

The authors of this case study suggest that the pivot-shift examination is a better measure of functional instability compared with instrumented testing or with the Lachman test. Level of evidence: IV.

29. Karim A, Pandit H, Murray J, Wandless F, Thomas NP: Smoking and reconstruction of the anterior cruciate ligament. *J Bone Joint Surg Br* 2006;88:1027-1031.

This cohort study indicated significantly worse outcomes in smokers compared with nonsmokers 5 years after ACL reconstruction. Level of evidence: III.

30. Spindler KP, Warren TA, Callison JC, Secic M, Fleisch SB, Wright RW: Clinical outcome at a minimum of five years after reconstruction of the anterior cruciate ligament. *J Bone Joint Surg Am* 2005;87:1673-1679.

Arthroscopic primary ACL reconstructions using validated tools indicated independent predictors of worse outcome in this consecutive study. Level of evidence: III.

31. McDevitt ER, Taylor DC, Miller MD, et al: Functional bracing after anterior cruciate ligament reconstruction: Prospective, randomized, multicenter study. *Am J Sports Med* 2004;32:1887-1892.

The authors of this prospective randomized trial found no difference in outcomes for patients with ACL injuries treated by reconstruction with or without the use of a brace. Level of evidence: II.

32. Salmon L, Russel V, Musgrove T, Pinczewski L, Refshauge K: Incidence of risk factors for graft rupture and contralateral rupture after anterior cruciate ligament reconstruction. *Arthroscopy* 2005;21:948-957.

The authors of this case study compared 675 pairs of knees for 5 years after unilateral ACL reconstruction. Reconstructed knees (autograft patella tendon or quadrupled hamstring) ruptured at the same rate (6%) as contralateral native ACL. Level of evidence: IV.

33. Bach BR Jr, Aadalen KJ, Dennis MG, et al: Primary anterior cruciate ligament reconstruction using fresh-frozen, nonirradiated patellar tendon allograft: Minimum 2-year follow-up. *Am J Sports Med* 2005;33:284-292.

This case study showed that nonirradiated patella tendon allograft reconstruction for the ACL is comparable to previously published historic cohorts. Level of evidence: IV.

34. Poehling GG, Curl WW, Lee CA, et al: Analysis of outcomes of anterior cruciate ligament repair with 5-year follow-up: Allograft versus autograft. *Arthroscopy* 2005;21:774-785.

The authors of the prospective cohort compared primary ACL reconstruction using Achilles tendon allograft to autograft bone patellar tendon. Similar long-term outcomes were found; however, those treated with allograft had less early pain and fewer activity limitations. Level of evidence: II.

35. Noyes FR, Barber-Westin SD: Anterior cruciate ligament revision reconstruction: Results using a quadriceps tendon-patellar bone autograft. *Am J Sports Med* 2006;34:553-564.

The authors of this case study concluded that quadriceps tendon is a viable graft source for revision ACL reconstruction. Level of evidence: IV.

36. O'Neill DB: Revision arthroscopically assisted anterior cruciate ligament reconstruction with previously unharvested ipsilateral autografts. *Am J Sports Med* 2004;32:1833-1841.

The results of this consecutive case study indicated that previously unharvested ipsilateral autografts improved function and stability in revision ACL reconstruction; however, outcomes were less favorable than in primary reconstructions. Level of evidence: IV.

37. Anderson AF: Transepiphyseal replacement of the anterior cruciate ligament using quadruple hamstring grafts in skeletally immature patients. *J Bone Joint Surg Am* 2004;86A(suppl 1):201-209.

In this case study, 12 patients with a mean age of 13 years (range, 11.6 to 14.4 years) were treated with transepiphyseal replacement of the ACL using quadruple hamstring grafts. At a mean follow-up period of approximately 4 years, leg length was evaluated. Outcome measures found functional improvement and no significant radiographic evidence of growth disturbance. Level of evidence: IV.

38. Kocher MS, Garg S, Micheli LJ: Physeal sparing reconstruction of the anterior cruciate ligament in skeletally immature prepubescent children and adolescents: Surgical technique. *J Bone Joint Surg Am* 2006;88:283-293.

The authors present the results of a case study of children (Tanner stage 1 or 2) who were treated with physeal-sparing ACL reconstruction with a combined intra-articular and extra-articular autogenous iliotibial band graft method. Excellent functional outcome and minimal risk of growth disturbance was reported after 5 years. Level of evidence: IV.

39. Akseki D, Ozcan O, Boya H, Pinar H: A new weight bearing test and a comparison with McMurray's test and joint line tenderness. *Arthroscopy* 2004;20:951-958.

The authors of this case-control study found higher positive predictive values with Ege's test and McMurray's test compared with joint line tenderness or any test in isolation. All methods had similar negative predictive values. Level of evidence: II.

40. Aaron RK, Skolnik AH, Reinert SE, Ciombor DM: Arthroscopic debridement for osteoarthritis of the knee. *J Bone Joint Surg Am* 2006;88:936-943.

The authors of this cross-sectional cohort study to evaluate arthroscopic débridement for knee osteoarthritis found that minimal radiographic signs of arthritis, normal alignment, and minimal cartilage damage predicted symptomatic relief compared with débridement for patients with advanced osteoarthritis. Level of evidence: III.

41. Allen RT, Tasto JP, Cummings J, Robertson C, Amiel D: Meniscal debridement with an arthroscopic radiofrequency wand versus an arthroscopic shaver: Compara-

4: Lower Extremity

tive effects on menisci and underlying articular cartilage. *Arthroscopy* 2006;22:385-393.

This cadaveric study of the response of bovine meniscal cartilage to débridement with an arthroscopic radiofrequency wand versus mechanical shaving found no injury zone or cell viability difference between methods.

42. Quinby JS, Golish SR, Hart JA, Diduch DR: All-inside meniscal repair using a new flexible, tensionable device. *Am J Sports Med* 2006;34:1281-1286.

    The authors of this case study evaluated one flexible, tensionable meniscal device 34 months after meniscal repair and found a 90% success rate, which was comparable to the success rate in historic control subjects. Level of evidence: IV.

43. Lozano J, Ma CB, Cannon WD: All-inside meniscal repair: A systematic review. *Clin Orthop Relat Res* 2007; 455:134-141.

    This article presents an evidence-based literature review of published studies involving all-inside arthroscopic meniscal repair techniques. Level of evidence: IV.

44. Sekiya JK, West RV, Groff YJ, Irrgang JJ, Fu FH, Harner CD: Clinical outcomes following isolated lateral meniscal allograft transplantation. *Arthroscopy* 2006; 22:771-780.

    The authors of this therapeutic case study used radiographic and quality-of-life measures to assess the intermediate outcomes of patients treated with meniscal transplant. Level of evidence: IV.

45. Verdonk PC, Verstraete KL, Almqvist KF, et al: Meniscal allograft transplantation: Long-term clinical results with radiological and MRI correlation. *Knee Surg Sports Traumatol Arthrosc* 2006;14:694-706.

    The authors used a retrospective analysis of prospectively collected data to evaluate three groups of patients: those with lateral meniscal transplants, medial transplants, and medial meniscal transplants with concurrent high tibial osteotomy. Level of evidence: IV.

46. Verdonk PC, Demurie A, Almqvist KF, Veys EM, Verbruggen G, Verdonk R: Transplantation of viable meniscal allograft: Surgical technique. *J Bone Joint Surg Am* 2006;88(suppl 1):109-118.

    This consecutive study provides survival analysis and clinical outcomes for 100 transplantations of viable medial and lateral meniscal allografts. Level of evidence: IV.

47. Noyes FR, Barber-Westin SD, Rankin M: Meniscal transplantation in symptomatic patients less than fifty years old. *J Bone Joint Surg Am* 2004;86:1392-1404.

    The authors evaluated the clinical outcomes associated with transplantation of fresh frozen meniscal allograft after an average of 40 months follow-up. Level of evidence: IV.

48. Mithoefer K, Williams RJ III, Warren RF, et al: The microfracture technique for the treatment of articular cartilage lesions in the knee: A prospective cohort study. *J Bone Joint Surg Am* 2005;87:1911-1920.

    This article presents the results of a prospective study of 48 patients with isolated, full-thickness articular cartilage lesions at 2 years after microfracture treatment. Level of evidence: IV.

49. Gill TJ, McCulloch PC, Glasson SS, Blanchet T, Morris EA: Chondral defect repair after the microfracture procedure: A nonhuman primate model. *Am J Sports Med* 2005;33:680-685.

    The results of a descriptive laboratory study of macaque knees following microfracture treatment of full-thickness cartilage defects at 6 and 12 weeks are presented.

50. Marder RA, Hopkins G Jr, Timmerman LA: Arthroscopic microfracture of chondral defects of the knee: A comparison of two postoperative treatments. *Arthroscopy* 2005;21:152-158.

    The authors of this case-control study found no difference in long-term results based on a comparison of the two initial rehabilitation protocols used for patients after microfracture treatment of chondral injury. Level of evidence: III.

51. Jakobsen RB, Engebretsen L, Slauterbeck JR: An analysis of the quality of cartilage repair studies. *J Bone Joint Surg Am* 2005;87:2232-2239.

    A literature search and methodologic review of several different cartilage repair techniques are presented in this article. Level of evidence: III.

52. Wasiak J, Villanueva E: Autologous cartilage implantation for full thickness articular cartilage defects of the knee. *Cochrane Database Syst Rev* 2002;4:CD003323.

    A systematic literature review of randomized and quasi-randomized trials comparing ACI with other treatments (including no treatment or placebo) for chondral injuries of knee is presented.

53. Malinin T, Temple HT, Buck BE: Transplantation of osteochondral allografts after cold storage. *J Bone Joint Surg Am* 2006;88:762-770.

Chapter 37

Knee Reconstruction and Replacement

*Christopher L. Peters, MD   Carmen D. Crofoot, MD

Clinical Evaluation

History

The clinical evaluation of a patient who has a painful knee begins with a thorough history and physical examination. Anterior knee pain that is exacerbated by stair climbing or squatting usually suggests patellofemoral pathology. Medial or lateral joint line pain or both may indicate meniscal pathology or osteoarthritis, especially if it is aggravated by weight-bearing activity. One should keep in mind that hip or lumbar spine pathology can present as knee pain, so associated reports about symptoms in these areas should be sought.

The history should include the duration, location, and severity of the pain; its impact on the patient's level of activity; and any history of trauma or surgery. The patient should be asked about positions or activities that exacerbate or relieve the symptoms such as knee locking, popping, or giving way. The use of assistive devices or bracing, medications, therapies, and injections should be noted, with specific information regarding their effectiveness. The patient's occupation, hobbies, and treatment goals and expectations are key components of the history.

Physical Examination

The physical examination begins with an evaluation of the patient's gait and limb alignment. Varus or valgus limb alignment and joint contractures should be documented. The range of motion of both knees should be assessed, noting the presence of a flexion contracture. Patellar crepitus or instability, joint line tenderness, and varus or valgus instability should be noted. The drawer and Lachman tests should be performed. It is important to include a thorough assessment of the hip, including range of motion, because hip pathology can masquerade as knee pain. Tenderness in periartic-

ular structures such as the pes anserinus bursa, iliotibial band, or proximal tibiofibular joint should be noted. A distended popliteal cyst can sometimes be palpated.

Several tools commonly used in research are available to evaluate the effect of arthritis and its treatment on the patient's general health. The Western Ontario and McMaster University Osteoarthritis Index focuses on pain, disability, and joint stiffness. The Knee Injury and Osteoarthritis Outcome Score evaluates pain and other symptoms, function in activities of daily living and sports, and knee-related quality of life. The Medical Outcomes Study Short Form-36 is used as a general health survey instrument and an outcomes measure in clinical practice. It can survey both specific and general populations as well as compare the impact of disease states and differentiate the benefits of interventions and treatments.

Radiographic Evaluation

Plain radiographs of the knee should include a weight-bearing AP view as well as lateral and Merchant (sunrise) views.[1] Non–weight-bearing radiographs can underestimate joint space narrowing. A flexion weight-bearing PA view taken at 45° can demonstrate subtle joint space narrowing (Figure 1). A standing long-cassette AP radiograph of both limbs should be obtained to assess the mechanical and anatomic axes of the limb; this information is used in surgical planning. If symptoms or the physical examination suggests hip pathology, it is important to obtain AP pelvic and lateral radiographs of the hip.

MRI is most commonly used to assess meniscal and ligament integrity. MRI can also be helpful in identifying the severity of osteoarthritis, although this finding is most evident on plain radiographs. Predictors of more rapid progression of osteoarthritis include the presence of severe meniscal extrusion, as defined by extending beyond the tibial margin on midcoronal images, a severe medial meniscus tear, medial or lateral bone edema, a high body mass index, female gender, poor range of motion, and stiffness.[2]

*Christopher L. Peters, MD or the department with which he is affiliated has received research or institutional support and royalties from Biomet and is a consultant or employee for Biomet.

4: Lower Extremity

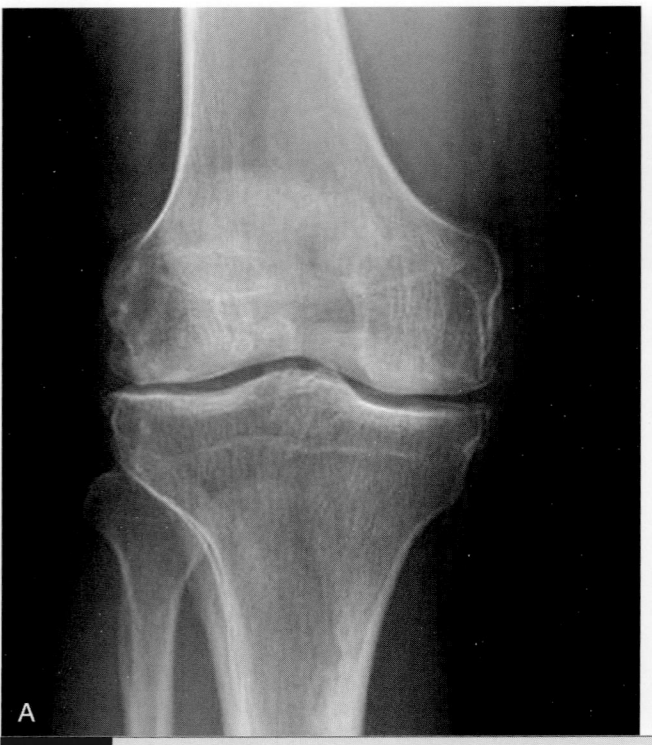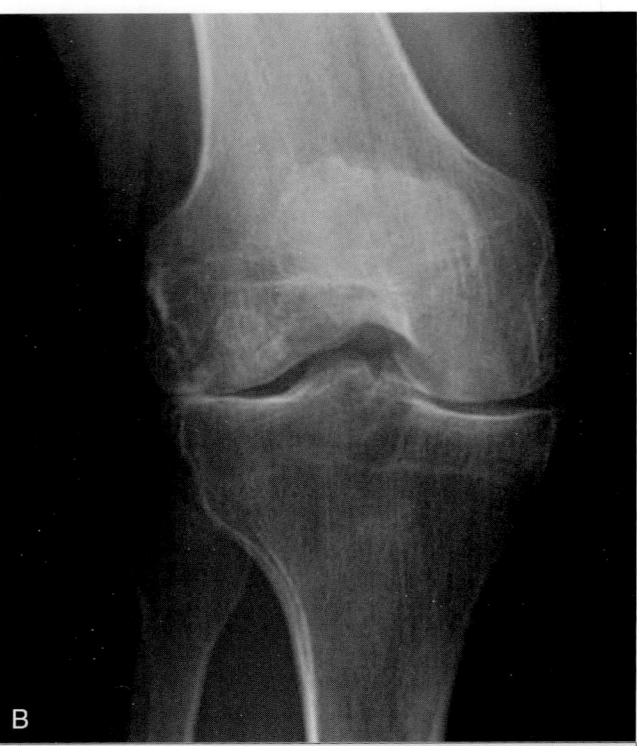

Figure 1 **A,** Weight-bearing AP radiograph showing some narrowing of the joint space. **B,** 45° flexion AP radiograph showing accentuation of joint space narrowing, especially in the lateral compartment.

Nonsurgical Treatment

The initial treatment of knee pain is typically conservative. Activity modification, oral analgesics and anti-inflammatory medications, intra-articular injections, and assisted weight bearing are often beneficial. Pharmacologic options include nonsteroidal anti-inflammatory drugs, acetaminophen, and glucosamine and chondroitin sulfate. Although the efficacy of glucosamine and chondroitin sulfate is debatable, they have minimal adverse effects, and some studies have found reduced joint pain and improved mobility in patients with mild to moderate degenerative joint disease.

Corticosteroid and viscosupplementation injections have been used with varying rates of success; several studies found significant short-term pain relief and functional improvement. Hyaluronic acid was shown to have a slower onset of action when compared with corticosteroids and did not provide superior pain relief with regard to quality and duration.[3] Potential complications of intra-articular injections include infection and local reaction. An unloader brace, which uses a three-point pressure system to decrease the deformity and widen the affected joint space, also may provide relief in the setting of unicompartmental disease. These braces are particularly beneficial in patients either not medically suited for surgical intervention or not wanting to undergo such procedures. Studies have shown that these braces diminish pain, increase walking tolerances, and provide better short-term function.

Joint-Preserving Surgical Procedures

Arthroscopy

Arthroscopic treatment of degenerative joint disease is most appropriate for patients in the early stages of the disease process whose symptoms are predominantly mechanical. Although patients with mild disease may obtain 90% improvement of symptoms, with mild disease defined as joint space greater than 3 mm with normal or varus alignment, those with severe disease may only obtain 25% relief of symptoms.[4] A randomized trial comparing placebo surgery, arthroscopic lavage, and arthroscopic débridement found no significant difference in their outcomes.[5] However, the methodology of this study has been under criticism and the placebo effect of surgery should not be discounted.

Osteotomy

Unicompartmental arthritis in patients younger than 50 years has been treated with tibial or femoral osteotomy to unload the involved compartment and correct malalignment. The results of osteotomy deteriorate over time; multiple studies have found that the rate of survival after 10 years is less than 50% to 70%.[6-8] The recent resurgence in the use of unicompartmental knee arthroplasty (UKA) as a precursor to total knee arthroplasty (TKA) has reduced the number of osteotomies performed.

Valgus-Producing Proximal Tibial Osteotomy

A valgus-producing proximal tibial osteotomy is considered an option in young (≤ 50 years), active patients with isolated medial compartment arthritis and localized symptoms. Contraindications to surgery include degenerative changes in the lateral and patellofemoral compartments, a knee range of motion of less than 90°, flexion contracture greater than 15°, ligamentous instability, and inflammatory arthritis. The goal of correction is 8° to 10° of anatomic valgus. Undercorrection of the deformity is associated with progression of the arthritis.

Technical treatment options include a lateral closing wedge or a medial opening wedge technique. The superiority of one technique over the other has not been identified. Patella baja, alteration of tibial slope, fixation failure, and intra-articular fracture have been reported with both procedures. An opening wedge osteotomy has less potential for peroneal nerve injury and more flexibility in deformity correction, but the disadvantages include medial hardware symptoms and the potential need for plate removal.[9]

Varus-Producing Distal Femoral Osteotomy

Lateral compartment gonarthrosis and valgus deformity can be treated with a varus-producing distal femoral osteotomy. The indications and contraindications are similar to those for high tibial osteotomy. Patellar tracking can improve associated patellofemoral arthritis, and the results of distal femoral osteotomy may not be affected by the severity of patellofemoral disease.[10,11] There is a reported conversion rate to TKA of 13% to 17% over 16 years.[10,11]

Unicompartmental Arthroplasty

There has been a recent renewed interest in UKA with improved published results, the development of less invasive techniques, the potential for a more functional outcome, and a lower complication rate than that reported with osteotomies and TKA.

Indications for UKA include isolated unicompartmental noninflammatory arthritis, deformity of less than 10°, an intact anterior cruciate ligament, and little or no joint subluxation. Young patients weighing more than 90 kg have inferior results. Contraindications include inflammatory arthritis, a fixed deformity of more than 10°, and ligamentous instability, advanced patellofemoral disease, and poorly localizable symptoms.

Early failure has been associated with several factors, including patient weight of more than 90 kg, secondary loosening, and wear and subsidence, as well as errors in surgical technique. Several factors influence the success of UKA, including surgical technique and polyethylene wear. Undercorrection of the mechanical axis by 2° to 3° is the goal. Overcorrection should be avoided because it can result in subluxation or progressive degeneration of the unresurfaced compartments. A posterior tibial slope greater than 7° can lead to degeneration and rupture of the anterior cruciate ligament.[12] Polyethylene components that have been sterilized with gamma irradiation in air and implanted after a long shelf life have been associated with early failure of UKA.

Patellofemoral Arthroplasty

Patellofemoral arthroplasty for treatment of isolated patellofemoral arthritis is controversial, with limited long-term data. The procedure is currently considered for patients who are younger than 60 years and have isolated patellofemoral arthritis and normal patellofemoral alignment. Initial studies of early designs were discouraging, but newer implants have improved short-term outcomes.[13] Failure most commonly occurs because of patellar malalignment, or progression of tibiofemoral compartment arthritis.

TKA generally remains the most common surgical treatment for advanced patellofemoral arthritis. According to several studies, survivorship, function, and pain relief were improved at an average 5.2-year follow-up. Resurfacing of the patella, attention to rotational alignment of the femoral and tibial components, appropriate balancing of the extensor mechanism, and more frequent lateral release are important factors for a successful TKA in these patients.[14,15]

Patellofemoral arthritis can also be treated with tibial tubercle anteriorization or anteromedialization, with or without cartilage transplantation, or patellectomy. Patellectomy should be considered a salvage procedure for pain control because it is associated with residual quadriceps weakness.[16]

Total Knee Arthroplasty

TKA is a highly effective procedure that provides reliable pain relief and improved function in patients with advanced knee arthritis. The principal indication is knee pain from arthritis that is refractory to conservative therapy in medically suitable patients.

Disease Variables Affecting Outcome

Medical Conditions Predisposing the Patient to Infection

Medical comorbidities such as diabetes, obesity, hemophilia, human immunodeficiency virus-positive status, and conditions associated with prolonged steroid use are associated with an increased risk of wound healing complications, deep infection, and aseptic failure. Diabetes has been studied extensively and is associated with a higher infection rate (1.2% for patients with diabetes versus 0.7% in patients without diabetes).[17] Obesity has also been shown to be associated with a higher risk of infection.[18] Patients with hemophilia have an increased risk of infection, although their mechanical survival rate is good.[19]

Inflammatory Arthritis

The long-term results of TKA are excellent for patients with rheumatoid arthritis or juvenile rheumatoid arthritis. TKA can provide substantial pain relief and improvement in function and quality of life for most rheumatoid arthritis patients, although they have a higher rate of complications such as infection, inadequate wound healing, and late instability than patients who do not have rheumatoid arthritis. Most rheumatoid arthritis patients, especially patients younger than 60 years, have required medical management for extended periods of time before undergoing TKA, and they often have poor motion as well as significant deformity and joint contractures. Performing TKA can be more technically demanding in the presence of soft-tissue contractures, bony deformities, and poor bone quality. Attention to soft-tissue balancing, deformity correction, and maintenance of joint stability are therefore essential.[20] Many patients with rheumatoid arthritis and other inflammatory arthropathies take medications such as disease-modifying antirheumatic drugs and tumor necrosis factor-alpha inhibitors. These drugs have the potential to interfere with wound healing and result in dehiscence, delayed healing, impaired collagen synthesis, or infection. Although data are limited, discontinuation of therapy may be required up to 4 weeks before surgery because of the long half-lives of the drugs. In discontinuing therapy, patients may experience an exacerbation or worsening of disease. Several studies do not show a significant increase in infection when medications such as methotrexate, tumor necrosis factor-alpha inhibitors, etanercept, and infliximab are used during the perioperative period for elective orthopaedic procedures, but not specific to TKA.[21-23]

Osteonecrosis

Osteonecrosis of the knee encompasses two separate disorders. One is a spontaneous condition that commonly affects females older than 55 years. It is typically unilateral, affecting one condyle. This condition is referred to as spontaneous osteonecrosis of the knee and is characterized by the sudden onset of severe knee pain. Although treatment consists of UKA and TKA, the results are not as predictable when compared with the results of those procedures performed for osteoarthritis. The second type of osteonecrosis of the knee is related to corticosteroid use, alcohol abuse, sickle cell anemia, or systemic lupus erythematosus. It commonly affects patients who are younger than 45 years of age, is bilateral, and involves more than one compartment. The pain is generally insidious and difficult to localize. In general, survivorship and satisfaction rates after TKA are relatively low for these patients.

Posttraumatic Arthritis

TKA for posttraumatic arthritis is frequently effective in reducing pain and improving function. However, it is associated with a relatively high risk of complications and outcomes are generally inferior to those of TKA for primary osteoarthritis. Prior trauma and surgery frequently compromise soft tissue and bone, making exposure and joint reconstruction more difficult.

Preoperative planning is essential to determine the necessity of hardware removal, bone defect management, and/or compromised soft-tissue management.

Hardware can be removed during the TKA, or removal can be staged. Earlier skin incisions need to be considered to avoid the risk of skin necrosis or wound-healing complications. If the skin bridges are less than approximately 6 cm in width, the earlier incisions should be incorporated into the approach. If multiple incisions are present, the most appropriate lateral incision should be used, as the deep perforating vessels arise from the medial side. Subfascial flaps should be created to avoid compromising the skin. Associated patella baja may render the exposure more difficult and jeopardize the patellar tendon. The use of revision implants, such as stemmed components and metal augmentation, may be necessary to address bone defects or bypass stress risers such as screw holes.

Surgical Technique

Approaches

The median parapatellar approach is the standard, most utilitarian approach for TKA. It is an extensile approach and is familiar to most knee surgeons. This approach can also be used with a smaller skin and quadriceps tendon incision without compromising exposure. This approach facilitates the difficult primary TKA and is generally recommended for revision arthroplasty.

The midvastus approach was developed to minimize violation of the quadriceps tendon. Using a midline skin incision, the vastus medialis oblique is divided in line with its fibers starting at the superomedial border of the patella. The benefits of this approach include preservation of the quadriceps tendon insertion and the vascularity of the patella. Generally, this approach has been shown to reduce the need for lateral retinacular release and potentially provide for more rapid return of quadriceps function.

The subvastus, or southern, approach preserves the extensor mechanism by bluntly dissecting the vastus medialis oblique away from the intermuscular septum. By preserving the medial descending geniculate artery, the subvastus approach preserves the vascularity of the patella. Care must be taken to avoid injury to the inferior intermuscular perforators in the region. The subvastus approach may not be suitable for a patient who is muscular or obese, has marked deformity, is undergoing a revision TKA, or has had prior surgery.[24] Although this exposure is not extensile, it can be performed through a relatively small skin incision in properly selected patients.

All of the above mentioned exposures have been used with so-called minimally invasive techniques. Smaller modified instrumentation has facilitated these minimally invasive surgeries. Limited numbers of outcome studies have shown more rapid recovery and greater range of motion at shorter follow-up intervals; however, the effects of simultaneous modification in pain management has not been well controlled.[25,26] Concerns regarding increased complications such as delayed wound healing, infection, suboptimal implant alignment, or compromised cement technique all are associated with minimally invasive techniques.

Alignment

Preoperative assessment of the anatomic and mechanical axes of the limb is essential to obtain a balanced and long-lasting TKA. The alignment goal of TKA should be a neutral tibiofemoral alignment (approximately 4° to 6° of anatomic valgus).

In most modern TKA systems, the tibial cut is made perpendicular to the long axis of the tibia. For a TKA that will retain the posterior cruciate ligament (PCL), a posterior slope of 6° to 9° may be required; for a PCL-sacrificing TKA, the posterior slope can be 3° or less. The distal femoral cut is made in 4° to 6° of valgus relative to the anatomic axis of the femur to create the final extension alignment of 4° to 6° of anatomic valgus.

Femoral component rotation plays an essential role in flexion space balance and patellofemoral tracking. The femoral component should be aligned rotationally parallel to the epicondylar axis of the femur (**Figure 2**). In general, the epicondylar axis is externally rotated 3° to 5° relative to the posterior condylar axis, which is commonly referenced using posterior referencing instrumentation. The AP axis of the femur (Whiteside's line), which is typically perpendicular to the epicondylar axis, can also be used for femoral component rotational alignment. Proper femoral component rotation facilitates patellar tracking and balancing of an initially asymmetric flexion space created by a perpendicular tibial resection. Release of the PCL causes the flexion space to increase 2 to 3 mm. Therefore, a comparable additional resection of distal femur should be considered in a PCL-sacrificing design to balance the flexion and extension spaces. The joint line should not be altered more than 8 mm in a posterior stabilized design to prevent patellofemoral complications such as patella baja and quadriceps weakness.

Fixation

Polymethylmethacrylate cement fixation has been used in TKA for 30 years with great success. Common technique includes pulsatile lavage of the osseous surfaces, suction drying, and pressurization of cement to provide interdigitation of approximately 3 mm, especially on the tibia. The practice of cementing only the tibial baseplate, avoiding the stem or keel, has been associated with higher failure rates when used with some knee designs. Therefore, full cementation of the tibial component remains the standard for primary TKA.

Cementless fixation has been shown to be a viable alternative to cement in several series. Proponents support its use in active patients age 50 years or younger. Higher failure rates have been reported in comparison with cemented fixation because of failure of ingrowth and osteolysis, primarily of the tibial component. Cementless femoral component fixation has had more predictable ingrowth in many series. Stems, screws, spikes, and bone grafts have been used to improve early fixation and reduce the failure rate. Recently introduced novel ingrowth surfaces may have the potential for increasing the rate of ingrowth, although long-term studies are currently sparse.

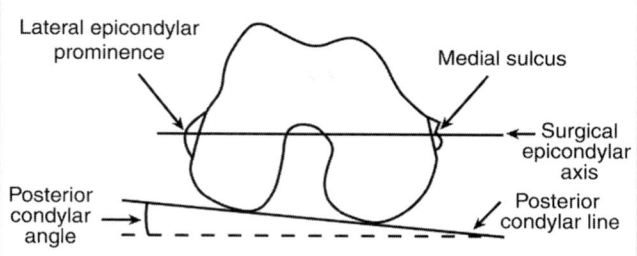

Figure 2	The reference lines for femoral component rotation include the epicondylar axis, posterior condylar axis, and AP axis (Whiteside's line), which is not shown here. In this axial view of the distal femur, with the knee flexed at 90°, the epicondylar axis is externally rotated 3° to 5° relative to the posterior condylar axis. (*Reproduced with permission from Berger RA, Rubash HE, Seel MJ, Thompson WH, Crossett LS: Determining the rotational alignment of the femoral component in total knee arthroplasty using the epicondylar axis. Clin Orthop Relat Res 1993;286:40-47.*)

Soft-Tissue Balancing

Obtaining a well-functioning total knee replacement requires strict attention to soft-tissue balancing. The type and amount of soft-tissue release can be largely anticipated preoperatively based on the magnitude and flexibility of the deformity. In general, the soft tissues become contracted on the concave side of the deformity and attenuated on the convex side of the deformity.

Varus alignment is the most common preoperative deformity in the arthritic knee. It is usually associated with a relatively contracted superficial and deep medial collateral ligament (MCL), PCL, and posterior capsule. This deformity is often accompanied by a variable degree of fixed flexion contracture. For a normally aligned knee with little or no deformity, the initial medial release should be approximately 2 to 3 cm below the tibial joint line. For a severe varus deformity, the release can extend 4 to 6 cm below the joint line to facilitate exposure. Removal of medial tibial osteophytes provides some degree of medial release. The goal of balancing should be laxity equivalent to that of a normal knee, or approximately 2 mm of joint opening in both compartments in flexion and extension. A moderate to severe varus knee that is tight only in flexion usually requires release of the anterior portion of the MCL (**Figure 3, *A***). For extension tightness, release of the posterior oblique fibers of the MCL is usually required (**Figure 3, *B***). Residual flexion contracture requires release of the posterior capsule and removal of posterior osteophytes. Regardless of whether the PCL is retained or sacrificed, collateral ligament balance and flexion contracture management should be accomplished.

In a valgus arthritic knee, the lateral femoral condyle is often hypoplastic and preferentially worn. If the posterior condylar axis is used exclusively to determine femoral component rotation, the component will often be erroneously internally rotated, resulting in subopti-

4: Lower Extremity

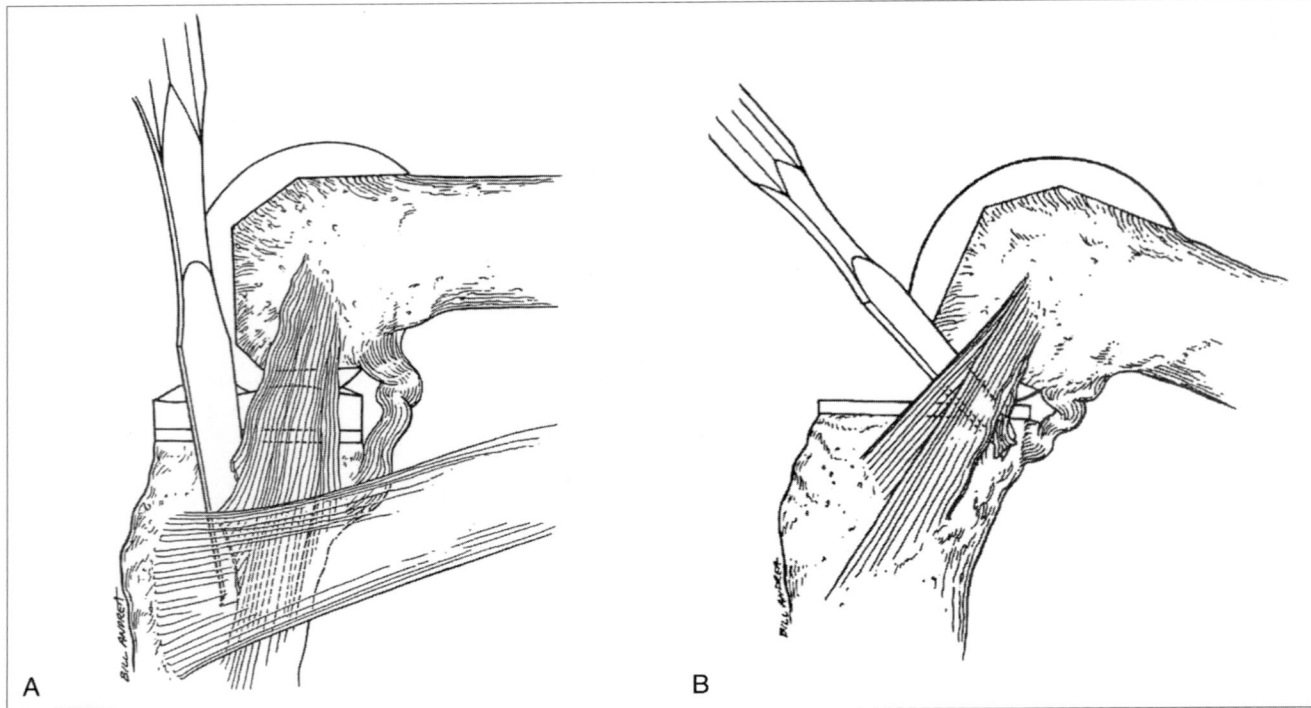

Figure 3 **A,** The medial aspect of the knee in flexion, depicting the release of the anterior portion of the superficial collateral ligament using a curved osteotome. **B,** The medial aspect of the knee in flexion, depicting the release of the posterior oblique portion of the superficial MCL using a curved osteotome. *(Reproduced with permission from Whiteside LA, Saeki K, Mihalko W: Functional medial ligament balancing in total knee arthroplasty.* Clin Orthop Rel Res *2000;380:45-57.)*

mal patellar tracking and an asymmetric flexion gap. More accurate landmarks for determining appropriate rotational alignment include the epicondylar axis and the AP axis of the femur (also known as Whiteside's line). Typically with restoration of a neutral mechanical alignment of the limb, the lateral structures are contracted. For residual tightness in flexion, flexion-influencing structures such as the popliteus and PCL should be released first. The lateral collateral ligament should be released only for the most severe valgus deformities. Residual lateral extension tightness should be addressed by release of the iliotibial band. Recent studies emphasized that results are better when selective release of tight structures is performed, rather than complete release of all structures attached to the lateral epicondyle of the femur. This may result in overstuffing of the joint (inserting a polyethylene liner that is too large to compensate for excessive laxity). For excessive MCL laxity after release of the lateral knee musculotendinous structures, the treatment options include use of a varus-valgus constrained implant to increase the level of prosthetic constraint or advancement or reconstruction of the MCL[27,28] (**Figure 4**).

Constraint

Although debate continues about retention or sacrifice of the PCL, long-term success has been reported with both PCL retention and substitution. PCL substitution can be accomplished using a cam-and-post mechanism or an anterior-lipped, highly conforming tibial bearing. PCL substitution should be considered for patients who have rheumatoid arthritis, prior patellectomy, a prior proximal or tibial osteotomy, or significant preoperative deformity.

Advocates of PCL substitution cite several potential benefits of this design. These factors include simplification of soft-tissue balancing in the absence of the potentially contracted or deficient PCL, its applicability to all patients, its more reproducible kinematics, and excellent long-term results. Although some believe that a better range of motion can be achieved with the cam-and-post mechanism, because of enforced femoral rollback, studies are inconclusive in this regard. Balancing the flexion and extension gaps is crucial to avoid dislocating the post, and cam engagement can lead to polyethylene wear and osteolysis.

Advocates of designs that retain the PCL cite this design as being more bone conserving (lack of femoral box cut); the retained PCL acts as a secondary restraint to varus and valgus forces. Long-term results are excellent. However, late flexion instability can occur if the PCL fails over time. If the PCL is too tight, asymmetric posterior polyethylene wear can result from posterior femoral subluxation, possibly leading to osteolysis.

Generally, it is advisable to use the least amount of constraint needed when performing primary total knee

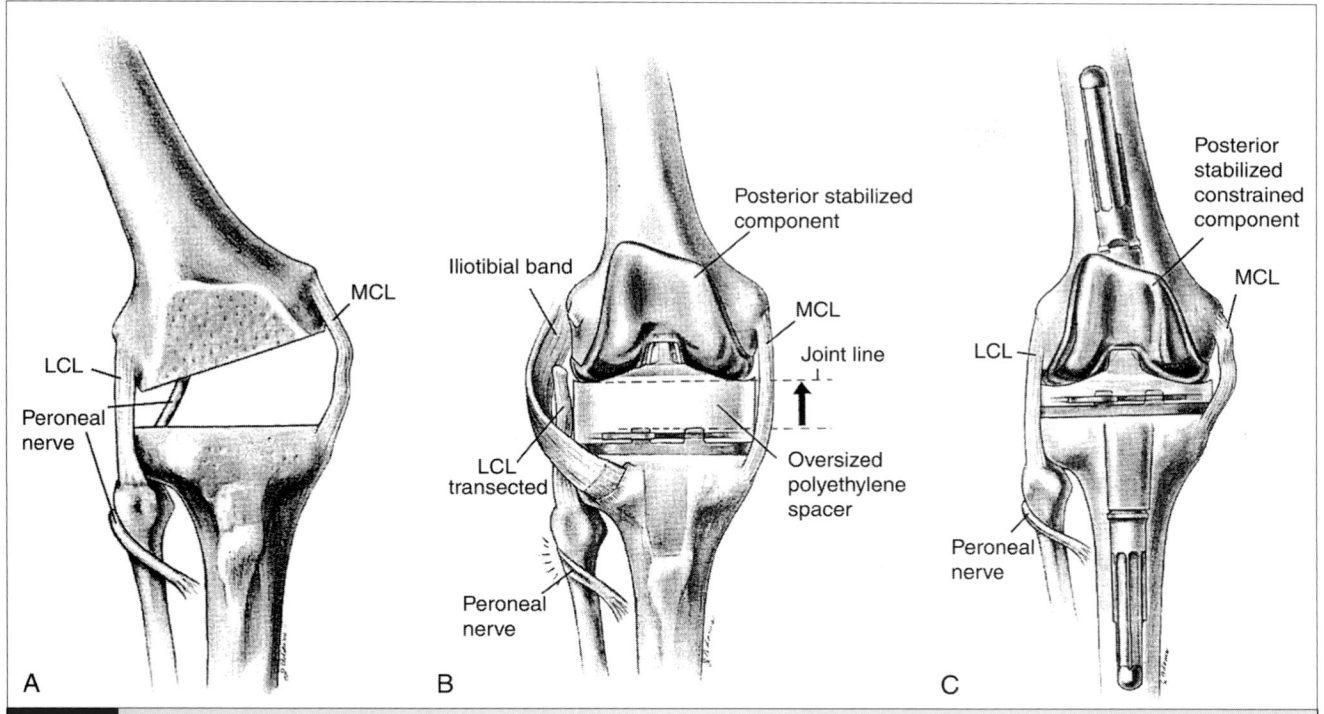

Figure 4 The effect of inserting a polyethylene liner that is too large (overstuffing the joint) after complete release of the lateral knee structures and a lax MCL. **A,** Tight lateral structures and lax MCL. **B,** A posterior stabilized TKA with complete release of the lateral knee structures and overstuffing to tighten the lax MCL. **C,** A varus-valgus constrained TKA to compensate for a lax MCL. LCL = lateral collateral ligament. *(Courtesy of Dobbs KL, Lombardi AV, Berent K, Mallory T, Adams J.)*

replacement. There are situations in which a varus/valgus constrained device is needed in the primary setting. The most common scenario is that of a significantly attenuated MCL in a severe preoperative valgus deformity. This condition can be addressed with more constraint with or without medial soft-tissue reefing or advancement. Rarely, a hinged device may be needed in cases of severe genu recurvatum or global instability. As the level of prosthetic constraint increases, increased force is transmitted to the bone-implant interface, necessitating the use of stems to partially offset the force.

Design Issues

Modularity
TKA using modular tibial components remains commonplace because it provides intraoperative flexibility and allows for subsequent polyethylene exchange if needed. However, modular components have been associated with concerns regarding backside wear and osteolysis. As a result, locking mechanisms have been recently altered and improved. Although monoblock designs have been introduced, modular design remains the most commonly used design.

High-Flexion Designs
Despite careful patient selection, implant design, and surgical technique, most patients cannot flex the knee beyond 125° after TKA. After a conventional TKA, the impingement of the polyethylene on the posterior femoral condyles and bone results in edge loading as flexion increases. High-flexion designs incorporate a thicker posterior femoral condyle to prevent edge loading on the posterior tibial articular surface. The result is an increase in contact areas at high flexion. Although high flexion designs accommodate these higher degrees of flexion, the literature is inconclusive with respect to the clinical benefit of such designs.

Mobile-Bearing Devices
Mobile-bearing tibial articulations have the theoretic advantage of decreasing wear, self-correcting rotational alignment to improve patellar tracking, greater contact area, and greater range of motion compared with fixed-bearing devices. Possible disadvantages associated with such designs include the potential for bearing dislocation, the need for meticulous soft-tissue balancing, and lack of applicability for difficult cases requiring augmentation and increased constraint. However, mobile-bearing knees have generally performed well but have not been clinically demonstrated to be superior to fixed-bearing knees in the areas of longevity, range of motion, and functional results.

Patellar Resurfacing
Debate continues regarding the desirability of resurfacing the patella in TKA. Several studies have reported

4: Lower Extremity

similar knee scores with and without resurfacing. However, reoperation for anterior knee pain is performed in a small percentage (2% to 10%) of patients with unresurfaced patellae. Pain relief after revision to resurface the patella is not as predictable as relief after resurfacing during the index procedure. Patients with a well-tracking extensor mechanism, minimal patellar arthritis, and patellar-friendly femoral components may not be candidates for resurfacing the patella. The proponents of this approach cite the rationale of avoiding the risk of difficult-to-treat patellar complications such as fracture, osteonecrosis, and component loosening.[29,30]

Computer Navigation

Computer navigation is a developing technology that is used to improve the accuracy of component placement. Recent studies found that the use of image guidance systems improved accuracy and decreased the number of outliers but that both cost and surgical time increased. Studies also documented that additional training and practice is needed prior to routine implementation of this new technology.[31-33] Patients with significant femoral deformity that does not allow the insertion of intramedullary instrumentation may be excellent candidates for this new technology. Further information will define the role of this new but costly technology with primary TKA.

Pain Management

Multiple pain control and anesthesia regimens have recently been introduced in an effort to minimize postoperative pain, improve mobility, and minimize side effects of parenteral narcotics. Intraoperative local anesthetic wound infiltration has been shown to reduce narcotic use with minimal adverse effects. A multimodal perioperative protocol combining continuous femoral nerve blocks, oral narcotics, cyclooxygenase-2 inhibitors, and local anesthetic wound infiltration, without intrathecal or patient-controlled analgesia, produced significant improvement in therapy participation rates, with earlier achievement of therapy goals, improvement in pain control and narcotic use, and shorter length of hospital stay.[34] Many multimodal approaches are now being successfully used to reduce pain, narcotic use, and length of hospital stay.

Complications

Infection

Postoperative infection of TKA is a devastating complication. The incidence of infection is increased in patients with diabetes or hemophilia and in obese patients, as well as those who have had prior open knee surgery. The use of antibiotic-impregnated cement has been shown to decrease the incidence of deep infection in these at-risk patients. The presence of persistent pain, wound drainage, or effusion should raise clinical suspicion. Initial workup should begin with clinical examination and radiographic evaluation. Radiographs should be considered suspicious for infection if there is significant change from prior studies with regard to

loosening, osteolysis, or significant progression as well as presence of gas in the soft tissues. The laboratory workup of suspected infection remote to TKA should include a complete blood cell count, erythrocyte sedimentation rate (ESR), and C-reactive protein (CRP). Aspiration of the painful TKA should be performed if sepsis is considered a potential etiology. The synovial fluid should be sent for cell count with differential, Gram stain, crystal analysis, and culture. White blood cell counts greater than 3,000/mm³ with greater than 60% polymorphonuclear leukocytes should raise suspicion of infection. If cultures are negative, repeat aspiration should be considered. If the radiographs are normal and laboratory studies are inconclusive, a leukocyte scan can be helpful. Although interleukin-6 was recently reported to be a marker of periprosthetic infection, the test's lack of sensitivity, limited availability, and cost may limit the application of this finding.[35] Leukocyte gene expression is also being investigated as a potential technique to identify infection. A rising CRP level has been shown to be predictive of septic complications.

Thromboembolic Disease

Patients undergoing TKA are at increased risk of developing venous thromboembolic disease. The need for prophylaxis is well understood, but the choice of agent, duration of treatment, and use of screening are controversial. The most effective chemoprophylactic agents include warfarin, low molecular weight heparin, and fondaparinux. Mechanical devices, such as pneumatic compression boots, have also been shown to be effective. Although the optimum duration of treatment is debated, a minimum of 10 to 14 days is suggested.[36] The current American College of Clinical Pharmacology 1A rated recommendations include fondaparinux, low molecular weight heparin, or adjusted-dose warfarin after TKA.[37]

MCL Injury

Intraoperative disruption of the MCL can be treated by repair, reattachment, or conversion to a varus-valgus constrained prosthesis. For an acute injury, bracing with range-of-motion exercises has been shown to yield acceptable results. For a postoperative disruption of symptomatic attenuation, the treatment options include revision to a more constrained implant or MCL reconstruction. MCL reconstruction has been described using a semitendinosus autograft or an allograft such as Achilles tendon.[38]

Extensor Mechanism Failure

Extensor mechanism failure is a rare complication during TKA. Treatment can be difficult and is directed at the mechanism of failure. Patella fracture can be treated nonsurgically in a cylinder cast if the extensor mechanism is intact; if it is not, patellar revision or patellectomy is usually necessary. Quadriceps tendon rupture requires direct repair and occasional augmentation with local or allogeneic tissue. Acute patella tendon rupture can be treated with direct repair or reconstruction using a semitendinosus autograft or an allograft (Achilles tendon or complete extensor mechanism). A more chronic injury to the extensor mechanism resulting in symptomatic lag is generally treated with extensor mechanism allograft or gastrocnemius transfer. Success of a complete extensor mechanism allograft reconstruction has been shown to depend on being adequately tensioned in full extension.[39] For patients with poor soft-tissue coverage, a history of infection, or a compromised immune system, a medial gastrocnemius rotational flap with an attached portion of the Achilles tendon may be a suitable alternative.[40]

Stiffness and Arthrofibrosis

The most predictive determinant of postoperative range of motion is preoperative range of motion. Appropriate implant selection and proper surgical technique, including exposure, restoration of flexion and extension gaps, and avoidance of raising the joint line excessively can aid in obtaining adequate postoperative range of motion. When significant preoperative stiffness is present, a PCL-substituting design may be desirable.

Stiffness following TKA (less than 90°) occurs in approximately 5% to 10% of patients. Indolent infection, complex regional pain syndrome, component malpositioning, mechanical malalignment, and prosthetic loosening should be ruled out before arthrofibrosis is diagnosed. Knee manipulation is an effective treatment during the first 3 months after the index arthroplasty.[41] Stiffness that is remote to arthroplasty may be relieved with revision arthroplasty, although results are variable.

Periprosthetic Fracture

Supracondylar fracture of the femur is the most common type of periprosthetic fracture associated with TKA. Classification systems have focused on the timing (intraoperative or postoperative) and location of the fracture, as well as the stability of the implant.

A classification system to guide treatment of femur fractures has been proposed. Type I fractures affect patients with adequate bone stock and a stable prosthesis in good position. Type IA fractures are nondisplaced or easily reduced, and they can be treated conservatively; type IB fractures (unstable or displaced) require internal fixation, with intramedullary rod fixation if the femoral component has an open box or locked plates. Type II fractures affect patients with adequate bone stock who have malpositioned or loose components and typically require revision arthroplasty. Type III fractures occur in patients who have poor bone stock and a loose or malpositioned component; they require distal femoral replacement (allograft prosthetic composite or a modular hinged implant).[42]

Tibial fractures are classified in a similar manner. Closed treatment is recommended if the implant is stable and the fracture is nondisplaced. Displaced fractures in the presence of a well-fixed arthroplasty can be treated with fixation. Fractures in the presence of loose components or osteolysis should be treated with revision. Intraoperative fractures should be treated with a longer-stemmed implant.

Patella fractures should be assessed for extensor mechanism integrity, fracture displacement, and loosening of the patellar component. If the extensor mechanism is intact, the fracture should generally be treated nonsurgically because the complication rate of patellar fixation has been shown to be quite high. If, however, the extensor mechanism is disrupted, patellectomy or fixation is recommended. If the patient's bone stock is adequate, open reduction and internal fixation combined with or without component revision should be performed. Partial or complete patellectomy should be considered if the bone stock or vascularity is inadequate.

Revision Total Knee Arthroscopy

Pain Evaluation

The number of revision TKAs performed annually in the United States is projected to increase from 37,000 to 195,000 (522%) between 2005 and 2030.[43] The causes of TKA failure include infection, aseptic loosening or failure of ingrowth, component malalignment, wear, osteolysis, instability, extensor mechanism disruption, and arthrofibrosis resulting in stiffness. Successful revision TKA depends on accurate preoperative determination of the cause of failure. Exploratory surgery for pain about a TKA is generally unsuccessful. If the cause of failure is unknown following a systematic evaluation of the knee, further observation is warranted.

The evaluation of a painful TKA should include a thorough history, physical examination, selective laboratory studies, aspiration, and radiographic evaluation. Extrinsic sources, such as low back pain, thigh pain, or radicular pain, should be separated from intrinsic sources. Failure of the initial arthroplasty to relieve pain can indicate the presence of a second, unrecognized source of pain. A physical examination of the knee, including gait inspection, usually is sufficient to diagnose component malalignment, instability, extensor mechanism malfunction, or arthrofibrosis. Radiographic examination, including a long-standing AP radiograph, can reveal component loosening and malalignment. CT scan has been shown to be of value in evaluation of femoral and tibial component rotational malalignment.

Infection can occasionally be diagnosed clinically, but is facilitated by laboratory studies including blood cell count, ESR, CRP, and knee aspiration. Synovial fluid should be analyzed for cell count with differential, crystal analysis, Gram stain, and culture and sensitivity. A positive culture is highly predictive of infection in a painful knee, but a negative culture does not rule out the possibility of infection. Aspiration of the painful TKA should be performed if sepsis is considered a potential etiology. White blood cell counts greater than 3,000/mm³ with greater than 60% polymorphonuclear leukocytes should raise suspicion of infection. If cultures are negative, repeat aspiration should be considered.

Preoperative Planning

Preoperative planning for revision TKA includes anticipation of approach, the degree of bone loss that will need to be addressed, and the potential need for constraint or ligamentous reconstruction. The surgeon has available a large armamentarium of devices to address ligamentous instability and bone stock deficiency.

An understanding of previous incisions and approaches is important. The standard midline incision is recommended for most patients, although, if multiple incisions are present, the most lateral incision that allows for exposure is recommended. Generally, restoration of the suprapatellar pouch, recreation of the medial and lateral gutters, and excision of the fibrotic patellar fat pad allow adequate exposure. Patellar eversion is not necessary and can increase the risk of tendon avulsion. If these maneuvers do not provide adequate exposure, a quadriceps snip or a tibial tubercle osteotomy are occasionally needed. Patellar turndown is generally avoided secondary to its higher incidence of extensor lag. Component removal is performed in a systematic fashion and typically includes polyethylene removal, femoral component removal, and tibial component removal. The cement or bone-prosthetic interface can be disrupted with thin saws or osteotomes. Meticulous technique is necessary to avoid excessive bone loss with component removal.

Preoperative determination of collateral ligament integrity can help delineate the need for a varus-valgus constrained prosthesis or rotating-hinge implant. Indications for the use of increased constraint can include medial or lateral ligamentous insufficiency, and significant flexion instability despite appropriate component sizing. The use of a constrained hinge-type device is indicated in the setting of MCL instability or global instability in the elderly patient. Typically, with restoration of alignment and appropriate component sizing, increased constraint can be avoided.

The results of revision surgery are improved when the joint line and the flexion-extension gap balance are accurately restored. Anatomic references useful for assessing the position of the joint line include the relationship between the joint line and the tip of the fibular head (usually 1.5 cm) and the relationship between the joint line and the adductor tubercle of the femur (measured from the other knee, if it is intact). In general, it is useful to reestablish the tibial platform with reference to joint line restoration, address the flexion gap by appropriate sizing of the femoral component, and finally, assess the extension gap with distal femoral augmentation if needed.

Flexion-extension gap balancing is critical to successful reconstruction. The surgeon should understand the options available for altering the flexion and extension gaps and their effect on the joint line. The flexion gap is affected by the slope of the tibial resection, the thickness of the polyethylene insert, and the AP dimen-

sion of the femoral component. The extension gap is affected by the height of the tibial surface and the height of the distal femoral augmentation. Because typical landmarks are absent, the epicondylar axis is used as a reference for rotational alignment of the femoral component.

If the host bone is deficient, augmentation may be required to satisfy the dual requirement of joint line restoration and gap balance. The area of implant-bone contact can be maximized by using allograft bone or metallic augmentation blocks or wedges. Metallic augmentation is especially useful for altering the distal and AP position of the femoral implant.

Selective Component Retention

Isolated polyethylene exchange can be considered with polyethylene wear in the presence of appropriate alignment and stability of the knee (this is an unusual occurrence). Single component revision (tibial or femoral component) can be considered but is difficult to accomplish without exposure complications and potential injury to the collateral ligaments.

Fixation

There is general agreement that the femoral metaphyseal regions should be cemented and stem augmentation is needed in the revision setting; however, the optimum method of stem fixation remains controversial. Studies have demonstrated high success rates with fully cemented stems as well as diaphyseal engaging press fit stems with cementation of the components. A cementless stem should engage the femoral or tibial diaphysis and not dangle in the metaphyseal bone. Some studies found slightly higher failure rates after cementless stems were used and prosthetic constraint was increased. This factor should be weighed against the difficulty of removing a fully cemented stem with the adjacent cement[44] (Figure 5).

Bone Loss Management

Bone loss can be the result of osteolysis or can occur during component extraction. Osteolysis is often underappreciated on preoperative radiographs and the surgeon should be prepared for restoration of large bone defects in these instances. Segmental bone loss can be addressed with metal augmentation or bulk bone grafting. Cavitary defects can generally be treated with allogeneic particulate graft.

Patellar Management

A well-fixed patella with minimal wear typically should be retained. Metal-backed components with wear of thin polyethylene edges often require revision. A patella thickness of less than 12 cm is associated with an increased risk of fracture and osteonecrosis. Options for patellar reconstruction in the face of significant bone loss include no resurfacing, bone grafting with the use of a periosteal flap, or augmentation with a trabecular metal device. Patellectomy is rarely needed.

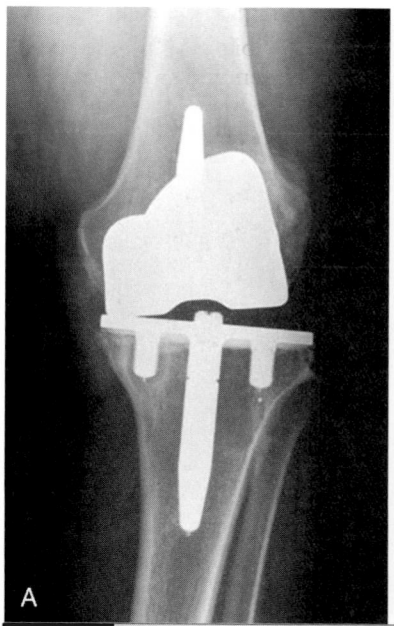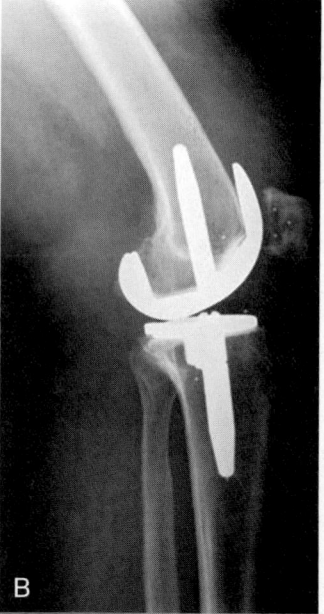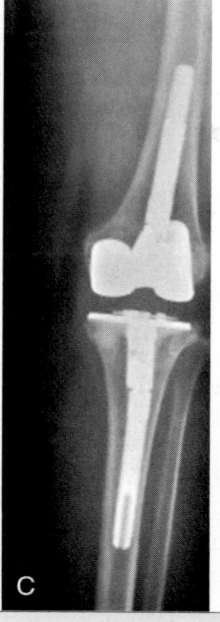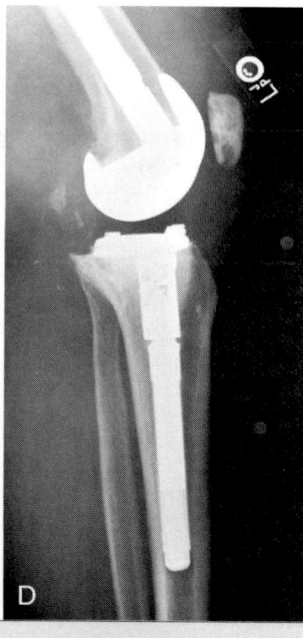

Figure 5 Preoperative AP (**A**) and lateral (**B**) radiographs showing TKA failure caused by extensive eccentric polyethylene wear, with resulting varus malalignment. Tibial and femoral osteolysis is also present. Postoperative AP (**C**) and lateral (**D**) radiograph after revision arthroplasty with hybrid fixation. The femoral and tibial metaphyseal regions are cemented, with the cementless stems engaging the diaphysis of both canals.

Infection Management

Infection is one of the most devastating complications of total joint arthroplasty. An infection can be treated by irrigation and débridement, direct exchange, or two-stage reimplantation. Arthroscopic irrigation and débridement generally are not recommended to treat infection after arthroplasty because it has been shown to have a low success rate.

The choice of treatment depends on the timing of infection onset and the type of bacteria. An acute infection is typically defined as occurring during the immediate postoperative period (within 3 weeks) or subsequently as a hematogenous event without prior symptoms. Urgent irrigation and débridement with polyethylene exchange in the setting of well-fixed implants has been shown to have an acceptable success rate. This process is accompanied by parenteral antibiotics for 6 weeks or longer, under the direction of an infectious disease consultant. Direct exchange has limited application, because it may not eradicate the infection.

Two-Stage Reimplantation

For a chronic infection, which has been present for more than 3 weeks, the treatment of choice is two-stage reimplantation. The first stage includes removal of all components and cement and placement of a static or articulating antibiotic spacer. Several types of articulating spacers are available: a handmade spacer,[45] a spacer created from a mold of the removed components to have similar surface contours,[46] or a spacer that uses the autoclaved explanted femoral component and a new polyethylene insert. None has been shown to be superior to the others. Placement of an articulating spacer allows the patient early range of motion and partial weight bearing, with preservation of the soft-tissue envelope. After placement, the patient is treated with a 6-week course of intravenous antibiotics. Reimplantation can be considered 2 to 6 weeks after the antibiotic course ends, if the patient's health and soft-tissue envelope allow. ESR and CRP should be normalized and repeat aspiration in the absence of antibiotics may be helpful. It is recommended that antibiotic-impregnated cement be used for reimplantation. Two-stage reimplantation has an 80% to 85% success rate. Direct exchange has demonstrated success in some series and may be advantageous in certain instances. Its use in North America is limited.

Salvage

Arthrodesis, resection arthroplasty, and amputation can be considered for salvage of an infected TKA. Arthrodesis, usually performed as a two-stage procedure, can provide a stable, pain-free leg that allows independent ambulation. Successful fusion has been reported using a long intramedullary nail.[47] Other techniques include external fixation and plate fixation. The choice of technique depends on the surgeon's experience, the quality of the patient's bone stock, the availability of the intramedullary canal, and the soft-tissue coverage. Amputation and resection arthroplasty can be life saving but leave little possibility of patient ambulation, especially in a frail, elderly patient.

Annotated References

1. Mason RB, Horne JG: The posteroanterior 45 degrees flexion weight-bearing radiograph of the knee. *J Arthroplasty* 1995;10:790-792.

2. Raynauld JP, Martel-Pelletier J, Berthiaume MJ, et al: Long term evaluation of disease progression through the quantitative magnetic resonance imaging of symptomatic knee osteoarthritis patients: Correlation with clinical symptoms and radiographic changes. *Arthritis Res Ther* 2006;8:R21.

   Three categories of osteoarthritis progression (fast, intermediate, and slow) were identified using MRI, as well as risk factors associated with progression.

3. Leopold SS, Redd BB, Warme WJ, Wehrle PA, Pettis PD, Shott S: Corticosteroid compared with hyaluronic acid injections for the treatment of osteoarthritis of the knee. *J Bone Joint Surg Am* 2003;85:1197-1203.

4. Aaron RK, Skolnick AH, Reinert SE, Ciombor D: Arthroscopic debridement for osteoarthritis of the knee. *J Bone Joint Surg Am* 2006;88:936-943.

   Patients with mild arthritis had a 90% improvement in symptoms after arthroscopic débridement, but patients with severe arthritis had only a 25% improvement. The result is unpredictable for patients with moderate arthritis.

5. Moseley JB, O'Malley K, Petersen NJ, et al: A controlled trial of arthroscopic surgery for osteoarthritis of the knee. *N Engl J Med* 2002;347:81-88.

6. Billings A, Scott DF, Camargo MP, Hofmann AA: High tibial osteotomy with a calibrated osteotomy guide, rigid internal fixation and early motion: Long-term follow-up. *J Bone Joint Surg Am* 2000;82:70-79.

7. Wu LD, Hahne HJ, Hassenpflug T: A long-term follow-up study of high tibial osteotomy for medial compartment osteoarthritis. *Chin J Traumatol* 2004;7:348-353.

   According to results from this study, the survivorship rate for patients receiving high tibial osteotomy to treat medial compartment arthritis is 78.2% after 5 years, with a trend to deterioration.

8. Anglietti P, Buzzi R, Vena LM, Baldini A, Mondaini A: High tibial valgus osteotomy for medial gonarthrosis: A 10- to 21-year study. *J Knee Surg* 2003;16:21-26.

9. Hoell S, Suttmoeller J, Stoll V, Fuchs S, Gosheger G: The high tibial osteotomy, open versus closed wedge, a comparison in 108 patients. *Arch Orthop Trauma Surg* 2005;125:638-643.

   No difference was found between open-wedge osteotomy and closed-wedge osteotomy for treatment of varus gonarthrosis with high tibial osteotomy. Patients should be informed of the need for plate removal.

10. Wang JW, Hsu CC: Distal femoral varus osteotomy for osteoarthritis of the knee: Surgical technique. *J Bone Joint Surg Am* 2006;88:100-108.

    An 83% rate of satisfactory results and an 87% survival rate were found 10 years after distal femoral osteotomy in 30 patients. Severe patellofemoral arthritis did not affect the results, and the surgery improved tracking in seven of eight affected knees.

11. Pach M, Uvizl M, Hulibka R, Zapletalova J: Varus supracondylar osteotomy of femur: Long-term results. *Acta Chir Orthop Traumatol Cech* 2005;72:363-370.

    Results from this study show a conversion rate to TKA of 17% but an overall survivorship of osteotomy of 95% at 16 years.

12. Hernigou P, Deschamps G: Posterior slope of the tibial implant and the outcome of unicompartmental knee arthroplasty. *J Bone Joint Surg Am* 2004;86:506-511.

    The effect of posterior slope on long-term outcome of UKA was studied in patients with intact and deficient anterior cruciate ligaments.

13. Nicol SG, Loveridge JM, Weale AE, Ackroyd CE, Newman JH: Arthritis progressions after patellofemoral joint replacement. *Knee* 2006;13:290-295.

    A prospective evaluation of patellofemoral joint arthroplasty for progressive symptomatic tibiofemoral osteoarthritis found that progression of osteoarthritis was an important cause of failure. It is seen less frequently in patients with femoral trochlear dysplasia.

14. Parvizi J, Stuart MJ, Pagnano MW, Hanssen AD: Total knee arthroplasty in patients with isolated patellofemoral arthritis. *Clin Orthop Relat Res* 2001;392:147-152.

15. Dalury DF: Total knee replacement for patellofemoral disease. *J Knee Surg* 2005;18:274-277.

    At 5-year follow-up, results were satisfactory after TKA for isolated patellofemoral disease.

16. Fulkerson JP: Alternatives to patellofemoral arthroplasty. *Clin Orthop Relat Res* 2005;436:76-80.

    The alternatives to patellofemoral arthroplasty for treatment of patellofemoral arthritis include tubercle realignment, patellectomy, and cartilage transplant.

17. Meding JB, Reddleman K, Keating ME, et al: Total knee replacement in patients with diabetes mellitus. *Clin Orthop Relat Res* 2003;416:208-216.

18. Namba RS, Paxton L, Fithian DC, Stone ML: Obesity and perioperative morbidity in total hip and total knee arthroplasty patients. *J Arthroplasty* 2005;20:46-50.

    Patients with a body mass index of 35 or higher had higher postoperative infection rates; the odds ratio was 6.7 times higher after TKA.

19. Silva M, Luck JV Jr: Long-term results of primary total knee replacement in patients with hemophilia. *J Bone Joint Surg Am* 2005;87:85-91.

    A retrospective review of TKA outcomes in patients

with hemophilia found that 97% had good or excellent functional scores and good mechanical survival rates. The overall infection rate was 16%; the rates were similar for human immunodeficiency virus-positive and human immunodeficiency virus-negative patients.

20. Parvizi J, Lajam CM, Trousdale RT, Shaughnessy WJ, Cabanela ME: Total knee arthroplasty in young patients with juvenile rheumatoid arthritis. *J Bone Joint Surg Am* 2003;85:1090-1094.

21. Busti AJ, Hooper JS, Amaya CT, Kavi S: Effects of perioperative anti-inflammatory and immunomodulating therapy on surgical wound healing. *Pharmacotherapy* 2005;25:1566-1591.

No clear consensus exists on the need and optimum time for withholding therapy before surgery. When data are limited or absent, drugs used for perioperative therapy should be reviewed on an individual basis.

22. Grennan DM, Gray J, Loudon J, Fear S: Methotrexate and early postoperative complications in patients with rheumatoid arthritis undergoing elective orthopaedic surgery. *Ann Rheum Dis* 2002;61:86-87.

23. Bibbo C, Goldberg JW: Infectious and healing complications after elective orthopaedic foot and ankle surgery during tumor necrosis factor-alpha inhibition therapy. *Foot Ankle Int* 2004;25:331-335.

Results indicate that tumor necrosis factor-alpha therapy is safe during the perioperative period and is not associated with an increase in complications related to healing or infection.

24. Kelly MJ, Rumi MN, Kothari M, et al: Comparison of vastus-splitting and median parapatellar approaches for primary total knee arthroplasty: A prospective, randomized study. *J Bone Joint Surg Am* 2006;88:715-720.

No functional differences were found after use of vastus-splitting and median parapatellar approaches for primary TKA, although in the median parapatellar approach the need for lateral retinacular release is greater. Abnormalities seen on electromyography after the midvastus approach, without functional consequences, can be avoided by blunt dissection in the vastus medialis.

25. Tria AJ Jr: Minimally invasive total knee arthroplasty: The importance of instrumentation. *Orthop Clin North Am* 2004;35:227-234.

Issues related to instrumentation during minimally invasive TKA are discussed.

26. Bonutti PM, Seyler TM, Kester M, McMahon M, Mont MA: Minimally invasive revision total knee arthroplasty. *Clin Orthop Relat Res* 2006;446:699-75.

The authors reported on a minimally invasive approach for revision TKA in 17 knees. Initial results were good using improved instrumentation.

27. Peters CL: Soft-tissue balancing in primary total knee arthroplasty. *Instr Course Lect* 2006;55:413-417.

A well-balanced soft-tissue envelope surrounding a well-aligned, well-fixed implant is the goal of a primary TKA. Soft-tissue balancing techniques to address the varus, valgus, and associated flexion contracture deformities commonly encountered in primary TKA are discussed.

28. Elkus M, Ranawat CS, Rasquinha VJ, Babhulkar S, Rossi R, Ranawat AS: Total knee arthroplasty for severe valgus deformity. *J Bone Joint Surg Am* 2004;86:2671-2676.

Long-term results using the inside-out release technique to correct a fixed valgus deformity in patients undergoing primary TKA were excellent. The mean modified Knee Society clinical score improved from 30 points preoperatively to 93 points postoperatively. The mean functional score improved from 34 to 81 points.

29. Burnett RS, Haydon CM, Rorabeck CH, Bourne RB: Patella resurfacing versus nonresurfacing in total knee arthroplasty: Results of a randomized controlled clinical trial at a minimum of 10 years' followup. *Clin Orthop Relat Res* 2004;428:12-25.

The results of resurfacing and nonresurfacing the patella in a randomized controlled, clinical trial at a minimum of 10 years follow-up showed no significant difference between the groups regarding revision rates, Knee Society clinical rating scores, and function, patient satisfaction, anterior knee pain, and patellofemoral and radiographic outcomes.

30. Bourne RB, Burnett RS: The consequences of not resurfacing the patella. *Clin Orthop Relat Res* 2004;428: 166-169.

A meta-analysis revealed that although the evidence seems to support patellar resurfacing, this issue remains inconclusive because of implant issues and the short-term nature of available studies.

31. Haaker RG, Stockheim M, Kamp M, Proff G, Breitenfelder J, Ottersbach A: Computer-assisted navigation increases precision of component placement in total knee arthroplasty. *Clin Orthop Relat Res* 2005;433:152-159.

One hundred navigated knees were compared with 100 conventionally implanted knees after matching the two groups. The radiographic results were significantly better in the computer-assisted group compared with the results in the conventionally treated group when the component positioning in four axes was assessed.

32. Chin PL, Yang KY, Yeo SJ, Lo NN: Randomized control trial comparing radiographic total knee arthroplasty implant placement using computer navigation versus conventional technique. *J Arthroplasty* 2005;20: 618-626.

Computer-navigated TKA helps to increase accuracy and reduce outliers for implant placement. In the coronal view, 93.3% in the computer navigation surgery group had better outcomes compared with those treated with an extramedullary (73.4%) and intramedullary (60.0%) tibia guide. In the sagittal axis, 90% of those in the computer navigation surgery group also has better outcomes compared with the group treated with an extramedullary (63.3%) and intramedullary (76.7%) tibia guide.

4: Lower Extremity

33. Bolognesi M, Hofmann A: Computer navigation verses standard instrumentation for TKA: A single surgeon experience. *Clin Orthop Relat Res* 2005;440:162-169.

    Fifty TKAs performed with an imageless navigation system were compared retrospectively with 50 TKAs using standard instrumentation. Results of the study showed that navigation provides the surgeon with the potential to reduce outliers with regard to component position without an increase in complications.

34. Peters CL, Shirley B, Erickson J: The effect of a new multimodal perioperative anesthetic regimen on postoperative pain, side effects, rehabilitation, and length of hospital stay after total joint arthroplasty. *J Arthroplasty* 2006;21:132-138.

    A multimodal protocol using oral narcotics, cyclooxygenase-2 inhibitors, femoral nerve catheters, and local anesthetic wound infiltration without intrathecal narcotics for TKA improved pain scores and decreased narcotic consumption and length of stay.

35. DiCesare PE, Chang E, Preston CF, Liu C: Serum interleukin-6 as a marker of periprosthetic infection following total hip and knee arthroplasty. *J Bone Joint Surg Am* 2005;87:1921-1927.

    An elevated serum interleukin-6 level was found to be positively correlated with the presence of periprosthetic infection.

36. Lieberman JR, Hsu WK: Prevention of venous thromboembolic disease after total hip and knee arthroplasty. *J Bone Joint Surg Am* 2005;87:2097-2112.

    The ideal agent for prophylaxis against deep venous thrombosis has not been identified. Low molecular weight heparin, warfarin, and fondaparinux are the most effective prophylactic agents after total hip arthroplasty and these agents along with pneumatic compression boots are the most effective against TKA. Duration of prophylaxis remains a controversial topic.

37. Geerts WH, Pineo GF, Heit JA, et al: Prevention of venous thromboembolism: The seventh ACCP Conference on Antithrombotic and Thrombolytic Therapy. *Chest.* 2004;126:338-400.

    This article discusses the prevention of venous thromboembolism. For patients undergoing elective total hip arthroplasty or TKA, low molecular weight heparin, fondaparinux, or adjusted-dose vitamin K agonist is recommended.

38. Peters CL, Dienst M, Erickson J: Reconstruction of medial femoral condyle and medial collateral ligament in total knee arthroplasty using tendinoachilles allograft with calcaneal bone block. *J Arthroplasty* 2004;19:935-940.

    A technique for reconstruction of the medial femoral condyle and MCL using an Achilles tendon allograft with a calcaneal bone block is discussed to restore the deficient medial femoral condylar bar as well as to provide ligamentous stability on the medial side of the knee.

39. Burnett RS, Berger RA, Della Valle CJ, et al: Extensor mechanism allograft reconstruction after total knee arthroplasty. *J Bone Joint Surg Am* 2005;87:175-194.

    The results of reconstruction with an extensor mechanism allograft after TKA depend on the initial tensioning of the allograft. Loosely tensioned allografts result in a persistent extension lag and clinical failure while allografts that are tightly tensioned in full extension can restore active knee extension and result in clinical success.

40. Busfield BT, Huffman GR, Nahai F, Hoffman W, Ries M: Extended medial gastrocnemius rotational flap for treatment of chronic knee extensor mechanism deficiency in patients with or without total knee arthroplasty. *Clin Orthop Relat Res* 2004;428:190-197.

    Medial gastrocnemius flap reconstruction can provide successful salvage of a failed extensor mechanism allograft or an alternative to allograft reconstruction in patients with poor soft-tissue coverage, previous infection, or a compromised immune system.

41. Diduch DR, Scuderi GR, Scott WN, Insall JN, Kelly MA: The efficacy of arthroscopy following total knee replacement. *Arthroscopy* 1997;13:166-171.

42. Kim KI, Egol KA, Hozack WJ, Parvizi J: Periprosthetic fractures after total knee arthroplasties. *Clin Orthop Relat Res* 2006;446:167-175.

    A new classification system for periprosthetic femur fractures is proposed to evaluate prosthesis stability, quality of distal bone stock, and reducibility of the fracture.

43. Archibeck MJ, White RE, Jr: What's new in adult reconstructive knee surgery. *J Bone Joint Surg Am* 2006;88:1677-1686.

    Recent trends in TKA are reviewed in this article.

44. Chon JG, Lombardi AV, Berend KR: Hybrid stem fixation in revision total knee arthroplasty. *Surg Technol Int* 2004;12:214-220.

    The authors present a retrospective clinical and radiographic comparison of a posterior constrained knee system using hybrid fixation versus fully cemented fixation of stems of the same length. A lower but not statistically significant failure rate was observed in the hybrid group in comparison with the cemented group.

45. Villanueva M, Rios A, Pereiro J, Chana F, Fahandez-Saddi H: Hand-made articulating spacers for infected total knee arthroplasty: A technical note. *Acta Orthop* 2006;77:329-332.

    A modified technique for custom-made articulating spacers is described.

46. Ha CW: A technique for intraoperative construction of antibiotic spacers. *Clin Orthop Relat Res* 2006;445:204-209.

    An intraoperative mold can be made from removed components and used to create antibiotic spacers with surface contours similar to those of the original TKA. This allows limited function during the interval before reimplantation of the new TKA. The clinical results of 12 patients are equivalent or better than results reported in previous studies.

47. Bargiotas K, Wohlrab D, Sewecke JJ, Lavinge G, Demeo PJ, Sotereanos NG: Arthrodesis of the knee with a long intramedullary nail following the failure of a total knee arthroplasty as the result of infection. *J Bone Joint Surg Am* 2006;88:553-558.

The outcome of a staged approach for arthrodesis of the knee with a long intramedullary nail after the failure of a TKA as the result of infection was reviewed. There was solid union in 10 of 12 knees. The average time to union was 5.5 months. Obtaining large surfaces of bleeding contact bone during arthrodesis following staged treatment of an infection at the site of a failed TKA contributes to stability and enhances bone healing.

4: Lower Extremity

Chapter 38

Tibial Fractures

John T. Gorczyca, MD

Introduction

Tibial fractures occur fairly commonly in patients of all ages and can be quite debilitating, especially when complications occur. Fracture of the tibia is the most common traumatic long-bone fracture. Because of the subcutaneous nature of the tibia, particularly the medial aspect, soft-tissue wounds are often challenging to manage. Complications such as infection, nonunion, or perceived malalignment make tibial fractures a consistent source of litigation and morbidity. Although nonsurgical methods of managing tibial fractures have long been successfully used, especially for stable, low-energy fractures, surgical intervention is increasingly performed for all tibial fractures because of the benefits of faster recovery time and less residual shortening and/or angulation of the injured limb. Because multiple options are available for successfully treating most tibial fractures, orthopaedic surgeons must balance the benefits and risks of the various treatment options for each patient.

Clinical Examination

Patients with tibial fractures commonly present with leg pain and the inability to bear weight. The leg will have a variable degree of swelling, depending on the energy transmitted by the mechanism of injury and the timing of the examination. The skin may appear intact, it may have contusions, or it may be completely violated by the trauma with associated injuries to the tissues surrounding the bone. The clinical presentation of a tibial fracture varies depending on the mechanism of injury. Patients with high-energy injuries usually present with significant deformity, soft-tissue contusion, and possible vascular or neurologic deficits. Patients with low-energy injuries often present with swelling, pain, and the inability to ambulate. The initial clinical assessment of a patient with a tibial fracture should include determination of the vascular and neurologic status of the limb, the presence or absence of an open fracture, and the determination of possible compartment syndrome.

It is essential to realign the limb, evaluate the circulation to the limb, and identify any neurologic impairment. Evidence of vascular injury, such as decreased pulses, decreased capillary perfusion, or an expanding hematoma, should prompt immediate provisional reduction and splinting of the limb and reassessment of vascular status. Although studies of ankle-brachial indices (ankle-brachial index equals systolic arterial pressure in the limb distal to fracture divided by systolic arterial pressure in the upper extremity) obtained using Doppler ultrasound have not been reported for patients with tibial fractures, studies of vascular injury in patients with knee dislocations have established an ankle-brachial index of less than 0.9 as being highly sensitive and specific for a vascular injury that requires surgical repair. It seems reasonable, therefore, to follow this guideline to rule out limb-threatening vascular injury and to decrease reliance on arteriography to rule out such injury.

Compartment syndrome is a limb-threatening condition caused by swelling within the myofascial compartments of the leg, which decreases perfusion of the tissues below what is necessary to maintain viability. The leg has four compartments encircled by inflexible fascia, and compartment syndrome can occur in any or all of the compartments. The superficial posterior compartment includes the gastrocnemius, soleus, and plantaris muscles. The deep posterior compartment includes the tibialis posterior, flexor hallucis longus, flexor digitorum longus, and popliteus (proximal) muscles, as well as the posterior tibial artery and the tibial nerve. The anterior compartment includes the tibialis anterior, extensor hallucis longus, and extensor digitorum longus muscles, as well as the anterior tibial artery and the deep peroneal nerve. The lateral compartment includes the peroneal muscles, the peroneal artery, and the superficial peroneal nerve. Compartment syndrome in the leg occurs most commonly in the deep posterior and anterior compartments.

Compartment syndrome occurs because the elevated compartment pressure causes an elevated venous pressure as well as reduced venule (but not arteriole) diameter, with a consequent reduction in arteriovenous pressure gradient and decreased tissue perfusion. If the arteriovenous gradient does not allow sufficient perfusion to meet the metabolic demands of the tissue, then tissue necrosis occurs. Early diagnosis and treatment of compartment syndrome are essential to prevent irreversible impairment of the microcirculation and myonecrosis.

Important clinical findings in compartment syndrome include pain out of proportion to the injury, pain on passive muscle stretch, and inability to actively contract muscles in a compartment (which usually occurs late in the course of untreated compartment syndrome). Clinical detection of compartment syndrome may be challenging in a patient with a tibial fracture because the fracture itself may cause substantial pain in the absence or presence of compartment syndrome. Clinical diagnosis is also challenging in obtunded patients, such as those who are intoxicated or have neurologic impairment (such as patients with spinal cord injury or traumatic brain injury). Whenever there is any doubt, intramuscular pressure measurements in all four leg compartments should be made and compared with diastolic blood pressure. Intramuscular pressure measurements should be obtained using the most accurate device available. Arterial line monitors and the Stryker apparatus (Stryker Intra-Compartmental Pressure Monitor System, Kalamazoo, MI) are more accurate than the Whitesides apparatus. Side-port needles and slit catheters are more accurate than straight needles.[1]

In the past, an absolute measurement of greater than 30 mm Hg was considered diagnostic of compartment syndrome. Currently, the diagnosis of compartment syndrome is made when the difference between the compartment pressure and the diastolic blood pressure (ΔP) is less than or equal to 30 mm Hg; if compartment syndrome is not present at that time based on clinical assessment, the patient should continue to be closely monitored for compartment syndrome. Although the precise threshold for fasciotomy is not clear, most surgeons perform four-compartment fasciotomy when any compartment ΔP measures less than 30 mm Hg. Noninvasive methods of measuring compartment syndrome have not yet proven to be clinically useful.

Classification

Tibial fractures are described according to their location, the fracture orientation (transverse, oblique, or spiral), and fracture comminution (wedge, butterfly, comminuted, or bone loss). The AO/Orthopaedic Trauma Association (OTA) classification is the most detailed.[2] This alphanumeric classification grades the bone (tibia = 4), the location (diaphysis = 2), and the fracture type. Type A fractures are simple fractures. Type B fractures are wedge ("butterfly") fractures in which contact between the fragments exists after reduction. Type C fractures are complex fractures without contact between the main fragments after reduction. Classification into subgroups and further qualifications are based on fracture mechanism, fracture orientation, presence and location of fibula fracture, number of fracture fragments, tibia fracture location, and fracture extent. For example, a tibial shaft fracture with extensive shattering (> 4 cm) and extension to the proximal metadiaphyseal region would be classified as 42-C.332. Although the detail and thoroughness of this classification make it ideal for comparing groups of patients from different clinical studies, it is impractical for common use in clinical practice.

Open fractures are classified according to the Gustilo and Anderson classification (discussed later in this chapter). The soft-tissue injury in closed fractures can be classified according to the Oestern and Tscherne classification.[3] Grade 0 injuries have minimal soft-tissue damage, are usually caused by indirect (torsion) force, and have simple fracture patterns. Grade 1 injuries have superficial abrasions or contusions and a mild fracture pattern. Grade 2 injuries have deep abrasion with skin or muscle contusion, are usually caused by direct trauma to the limb, and have a severe fracture pattern. Grade 3 injuries have extensive skin contusion or crush injury, severe damage to underlying muscle, subcutaneous avulsion, or compartment syndrome.

Treatment Options

Indications for Surgery

Many nondisplaced, low-energy tibia fractures can be treated nonsurgically. Strong indications for surgical stabilization include open fractures, fractures with vascular injury, fractures with compartment syndrome, displaced and/or unstable fractures, and fractures in patients with multiple injuries. Stabilization of displaced fractures provides better outcomes than nonsurgical management.[4-6] Therefore, initial radiographs are helpful in determining fracture characteristics that make nonsurgical treatment less likely to be successful. Significant displacement (for example, > 50% of the tibial shaft diameter), fractures with greater than 1 cm of shortening, tibia fractures with fibula fractures at the same level, high-energy fractures, and displaced fractures with intact fibula are more likely to result in nonunion or malunion, and thus are good indications for reduction and stabilization. Irreducible fractures and unstable fractures for which proper alignment cannot be maintained with appropriate nonsurgical treatment will benefit from surgery. Relative indications for surgery include intra-articular extension of the fracture and extensive soft-tissue injury for which frequent monitoring will be necessary. Often, the best treatment is debatable, especially with low-energy fractures that can be reduced to proper alignment. In these circumstances, there is no substitute for discussing the risks and benefits of the treatment options with the patient and involving the patient in the treatment plan.

Nonsurgical Treatment

Nonsurgical treatment of tibial shaft fractures is typically selected for stable, low-energy fractures with acceptable shortening on the initial injury radiograph (because the initial shortening is predictive of the final shortening). Nonsurgical treatment begins with fracture reduction and long leg splints or casts. Although casts are more durable and stronger, they are more likely to restrict acute swelling and cause compartment syndrome for which bivalving the cast and splitting the cast padding will become necessary. Typically, long leg splints/casts are applied with the knee in slight flexion and are used for 2 to 4 weeks, during which time the patient is restricted from bearing weight.

When soft callus forms around the fracture, the patient's comfort level will improve enough to tolerate controlled joint motion. The physician will know that soft callus is present when the patient has minimal tenderness to pressure at the fracture site; this finding may be apparent as soon as 10 days after injury, or it may be delayed for 3 to 4 weeks. At this time, a patellar tendon bearing cast or fracture brace can be applied, and the patient may initiate weight bearing as tolerated. The rate at which soft callus forms is dependent on the patient's age, the severity of the fracture, and the patient's underlying medical condition.

Fracture angulation that occurs during nonsurgical treatment should be treated by cast reapplication with more attention given to three-point molding or with open wedging of the cast. Shortening of more than 1 cm cannot be tolerated in most adults and should be corrected surgically.

Weight bearing is critical to successful functional bracing and should be initiated and progressed as the patient's comfort allows. It is believed that a functional cast or brace results in increased hydrostatic pressure within compartments of the limb, which acts to resist fracture angulation, thereby allowing limited axial motion at the fracture site. This limited axial motion is osteogenic, and stimulates callus formation via endochondral ossification. The cast or brace can be discontinued when evidence of bridging bone appears on radiographs. Discomfort typically persists for more than 1 year, and often for as long as 2 years. Most appropriately chosen tibia fractures treated nonsurgically will heal with acceptable alignment and length. Large case series (albeit with a significant number of lost patients) document a 99% healing rate at an average follow-up of 16.6 weeks.[7] The average shortening at the time of healing was 5 mm, with 94% healing with less than 12 mm of shortening. Ninety percent of the fractures united with less than 8° of angulation in either plane, and 67% united with less than 5° of angulation.

External Fixation

External fixation, a quick, easy, and relatively noninvasive way to achieve fracture reduction and stabilization, has its greatest utility in treating patients who may not tolerate lengthy surgery (such as during damage control surgery on an unstable trauma patient) and those with severe open fractures for which exposure of the fracture ends for a second débridement is indicated. Additionally, external fixation can be used as a temporary stabilizer until the patient's condition or the soft tissues have improved enough to allow definitive surgery. Temporary external fixation will provide improved comfort compared with splinting for patients awaiting definitive fracture stabilization.

External fixator pin sites should be predrilled and inserted manually to prevent cortical cracking and thermal injury that occurs with self-drilled pins. The tips of the pins should not protrude more than 1 to 2 mm beyond the cortex of the bone. Pins should be positioned so that they are not in the joint capsule (which may extend more than 14 mm distal to the tibial plateau) and

so that they are not in the fracture hematoma, if possible. The decision to span the knee or ankle joint is at the discretion of the treating surgeon.

Conversion of an externally fixated tibia to intramedullary nailing carries the risk of disseminating bacteria from the pin site through the intramedullary canal and causing osteomyelitis, whether the pin tract has been infected or not.[8] There is general agreement that short-term use (less than 2 weeks) of an external fixator with clean pin sites is fairly safe. If pin tract infection has occurred, conversion to intramedullary nailing is contraindicated because of the high risk of infection.[8] If no option were available other than intramedullary nailing after pin tract infection, it is probably safest to remove the fixator, débride the infected pin sites, administer antibiotics, and perform delayed nailing.

Definitive treatment of tibial shaft fractures with a standard external fixator can be successful. This method of treatment, however, has been losing popularity in recent years because intramedullary nailing of open tibial fractures has been shown to have a comparable deep infection rate, but results in fewer malunions and nonunions. Definitive treatment of a tibial fracture with external fixation requires attention to detail, including careful pin tract care and consideration of sequential dynamization of the fixator as fracture healing progresses. Nonunions that occur after external fixation of tibial fractures have a high union rate and a low infection rate when treated with plating and bone grafting.[9] Ilizarov and hybrid external fixation are options for treating tibial fractures, and they are sometimes the best options for treating complex fractures with severe soft-tissue wounds. These forms of external fixation are advantageous because they are minimally invasive, allow postoperative adjustment of fracture alignment, and provide stable fixation allowing early weight bearing. These techniques are associated with a high rate of union, but the circular fixators are cumbersome and require pin/wire care that can be dissatisfying to patients, especially when union is delayed.

Open Reduction and Plate Fixation

Plate fixation of a tibial fracture allows anatomic reduction and internal fixation through direct fracture exposure. Simple fractures can be stabilized with techniques that allow interfragmentary compression. Incisions should avoid traumatized soft tissues, which usually are anteromedial. Thus, favored approaches are anterolateral and posteromedial, and the choice of approach requires cautious judgment by the surgeon. Plate fixation using direct fracture exposure is associated with a higher rate of wound healing difficulties than intramedullary nailing, and this technique is not commonly used for acute treatment of tibial fractures. The best indications for plate fixation of tibial fractures are low-energy injuries with intra-articular or periarticular involvement that would complicate intramedullary nailing, or open fractures in which the bone has already been exposed by the traumatic wound.

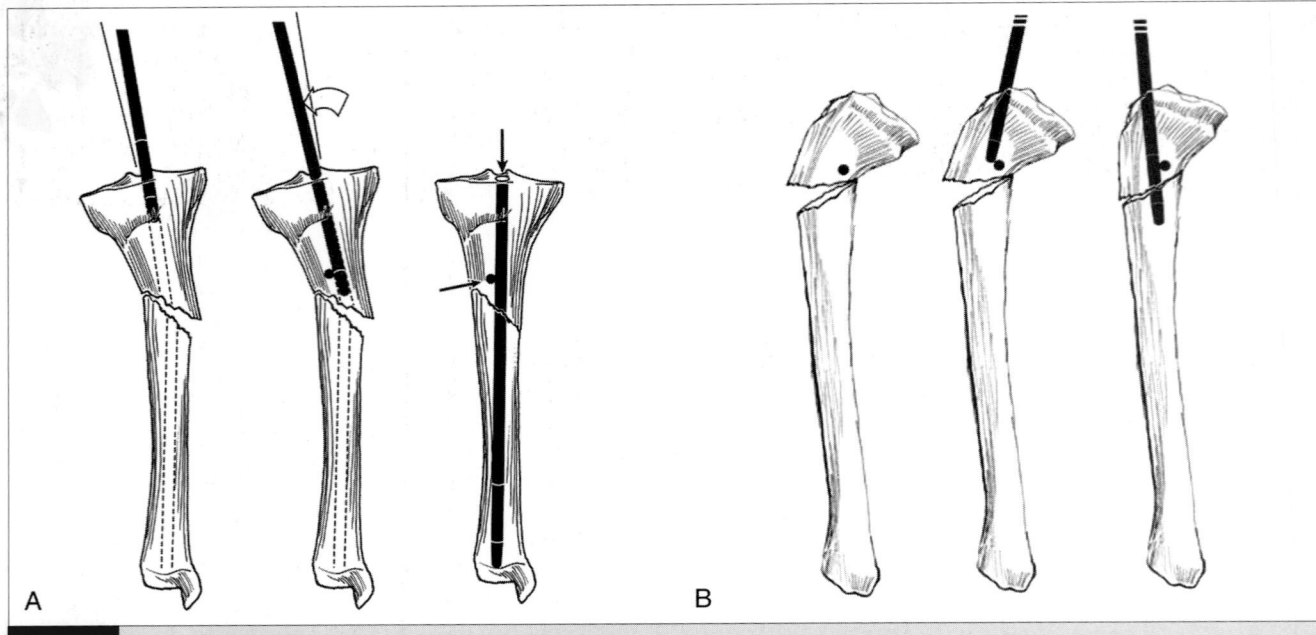

Figure 1 Illustration showing the use of a posterior blocking screw (**A**) and a lateral blocking screw (**B**) to help maintain alignment of the tibia in both coronal and sagittal planes during nailing of a proximal-third tibia fracture. By keeping the nail against the anterior (**A**) and medial (**B**) cortices, deformity is prevented. (*Reproduced with permission from Stannard J, Schmidt A, Kregor P: Surgical Treatment of Orthopaedic Trauma, New York, NY, Thieme Medical Publishers, Inc, 2007.*)

Plate fixation of tibial fractures through minimally invasive or percutaneous techniques is possible and is becoming more popular. The theoretic benefit of percutaneous plating is that the technique preserves the local blood supply and improves healing, although this benefit has not been proven. This technique has been reported mainly for periarticular fractures for which intramedullary nailing is not a good option. Percutaneous plates positioned medially tend to be prominent and may add trauma to the medial soft tissues. Long plates placed laterally carry the risk of damage to the superficial peroneal nerve during percutaneous placement of the distal screws. This risk can be avoided by creating a larger incision and obtaining direct visualization of the bone and tissues.

Intramedullary Nailing

Intramedullary nailing is the standard surgical treatment for displaced tibial shaft fractures. Reamed intramedullary nailing of unstable closed tibial fractures carries a high success rate, with a 96% to 100% union rate at 1-year follow-up.[11,12] The incidence of coronal and sagittal plane malalignment and the incidence of shortening are low after intramedullary nailing of midshaft tibial fractures. Thus, intramedullary nailing has become popular because it has a lower malunion rate than external fixation, and a lower incidence of wound complications than plate fixation.

Nailing of proximal and distal tibial fractures has been associated with higher rates of deformity than midshaft fractures. In particular, proximal tibial frac-tures treated with nails frequently had valgus and flexion deformities of the proximal segment. Techniques such as the use of a lateral starting point, provisional unicortical plating, and the use of blocking screws (**Figure 1**) were developed to prevent this complication. In addition, newer tibial nails incorporate multiple proximal and distal interlocking options as well as instrumentation to facilitate reduction and fixation of fractures in the proximal and distal metaphysis of the tibia. However, whether these specific fractures are best treated with interlocking nails or plates remains a topic of debate and is the subject of studies currently in progress.

The symptom unique to tibial nailing, however, is knee pain. The incidence of knee pain is reported to be between 10% and 86% at 2-year follow-up. The discomfort is probably multifactorial and related to prominent nails and interlocking screws, damage to the infrapatellar fat pad and subcutaneous tissues during reaming, damage to the infrapatellar branch of the saphenous nerve, or damage to the patellar tendon. Every effort should be taken to protect tissues during reaming and during nail insertion, and careful attention to nail length and placement is necessary to avoid prominence. Knee pain is likely to occur, however, even when these steps are taken. It can occur whether a thru-patellar tendon approach is used or not, even when the nail is not prominent, and does not always improve after nail removal. Thus, the risk of postoperative knee pain should be explained to patients before surgery.

Tibial nailing has become the standard treatment for most open tibial shaft fractures. When performed after thorough irrigation and débridement and with limited reaming (that is, reaming until cortical chatter occurs), the infection rates are comparable to those of unreamed tibial nailing and external fixation.[13,14] Contraindications to intramedullary nailing in open tibial fractures include patient medical instability, extremely narrow tibial canal, and profound wound contamination that the surgeon does not believe can be adequately cleaned in one surgical procedure.

Open Tibial Fractures

Open tibial fractures benefit from administration of appropriate intravenous antibiotics in the emergency department, emergent irrigation and débridement, and fracture stabilization. The timing of débridement has been debated, as many trauma centers have orthopaedic trauma surgeons and dedicated operating rooms available each morning, making late night and early morning débridements less necessary. The available literature does not provide definitive support for delaying surgical débridement at this time, and the surgeon should act in his or her best judgment after thorough evaluation of the patient and examination of the wound.

The entire leg should be examined for traumatic wounds that indicate the presence of an open fracture. The wound should be graded according to location, orientation, degree of tissue damage, and amount of contamination. The severity of the wound will influence the antibiotics used, the need for tetanus booster, the timing of surgery, the placement of incisions, and the type of stabilization used.

The Gustilo-Anderson classification of open fractures, which classifies fractures according to wound severity, size, and contamination, is helpful in deciding antibiotic treatment and in quickly communicating the severity of the open tibial fracture.

In general, type I and type II open tibial fractures should be treated with a first-generation cephalosporin. Type III open tibial fractures should have an aminoglycoside added to treat gram-negative bacteria. Farm injuries, mass casualty wounds, and lawn mower injuries should also have penicillin added to cover grampositive anaerobes. Open tibial fractures that have open-water contamination from ponds or streams may benefit from a fourth-generation cephalosporin as prophylaxis against *Aeromonas*. Antibiotic treatment should be initiated as quickly as possible in the emergency department and continued for 48 to 72 hours postoperatively. Antibiotic treatment should resume for each trip to the operating room. Tetanus status should be checked in the emergency department, and a tetanus booster should be administered, if necessary.

Thorough wound débridement remains an essential step in the management of open tibial fractures. Any devitalized tissue or bone should be excised. Badly injured deep tissue may be left in place and examined with a second-look débridement in 48 to 72 hours. Serial débridements are performed until the wound appears clean and healthy enough for closure or coverage.

Recent studies indicate that primary wound closure can be safely performed after the first débridement if the tissues are clean and healthy and the wound edges can be approximated without undue tension. Primary wound closure cannot be routinely recommended at this time; significant experience and skilled judgment are necessary to avoid complications with this method. A deep suction drain should be considered to drain the postoperative hematoma.

If a second débridement is considered necessary, several options for wound treatment should be considered. Vacuum-assisted closure dressings apply sequential negative pressure to a large area of the wound and appear to quickly decrease the postoperative swelling and hematoma. Thus, vacuum-assisted closure dressings seem to be most useful for markedly swollen extremities. Antibiotic-impregnated methylmethacrylate beads can be inserted into traumatic wounds. The antibiotic must be heat stable to tolerate the exothermic reaction of cement curing; therefore, gentamicin and/or vancomycin are commonly used. These beads provide a local concentration of antibiotics that is two orders of magnitude higher than that provided by intravenous antibiotic alone. Thus, these beads seem to be most useful for severely contaminated wounds. Currently, there are no studies that directly compare these two methods of treatment.

If the skin edges cannot be approximated without significant tension, and the swelling seems to have maximally resolved, then coverage of the defect will be necessary. Split-thickness skin grafting is used to cover skin defects over muscle or subcutaneous tissue. Flap coverage is necessary to cover defects over bone, nerves, or vessels. In general, proximal defects are covered with medial gastrocnemius rotational flaps, midleg defects are covered with soleus flaps, and distal defects are covered with free vascularized pedicle flaps. However, traumatized tissue should not be used for flap coverage; thus, free-flap coverage may be the best option for proximal or midleg defects. Recent experience with tunneled sural island pedicle flaps to cover anteromedial defects has been successful.

Proximal and Distal Metadiaphyseal Tibial Fractures

Intramedullary nailing of proximal tibia fractures has been associated with a high rate of valgus and apex anterior malalignment resulting from multiple causes. Use of a small medial plate with unicortical screw, blocking screws (**Figure 1**), use of a lateral tibial starting point, and semiextended positioning of the leg during intramedullary nail insertion all have been reported to address postoperative malalignment.

Many surgeons prefer to treat these injuries with plates. Locking plates, applied either percutaneously or with open techniques, provide a reliable means of achieving proper alignment and may offer a stronger construct to decrease the risk of postoperative displacement of proximal tibia fractures. As stated previously,

4: Lower Extremity

Table 1

LEAP Study Conclusions Regarding Treatment of Patients With Mangled Extremities

Patients with mangled extremities are more extroverted, less agreeable, more likely to drink alcohol, more likely to smoke, and more likely to be blue collar, uninsured, neurotic, and poor.

None of the scoring systems provide useful prognostic information regarding when to amputate.

Patients with mangled extremities treated with thru-the-knee amputations have poorer functional results than patients treated with above-knee amputations.

The presence or absence of protective foot sensation at the time of hospital admission is not predictive of protective foot sensation at 2-year follow-up.

Patients with mangled extremities treated with either amputation or limb salvage have a high rate of poor results at 2-year follow-up.

Patients evaluated at 7-year follow-up have poorer results than at 2-year follow-up.

Patients treated with limb salvage have results comparable with those of patients treated with amputation.

the disadvantage of these plates is their prominence. Comparative studies are underway to assess which of these techniques results in better outcomes; at present both are appropriate.

Obtaining and maintaining alignment of distal metadiaphyseal tibial fractures also can be difficult with intramedullary nailing. Intra-articular extension of the fracture should be reduced and stabilized with lag screws before intramedullary nailing.[15] Prior fracture reduction and stabilization of associated fibula fractures may facilitate reduction and improve stability of intramedullary nailing, resulting in a lower rate of malunion.[16,17]

Plate fixation of distal tibial fractures may provide better fixation than intramedullary nailing, but it carries a higher risk of soft-tissue complications than intramedullary nailing.[18] Use of standard or ring external fixators can be considered, especially for severe wounds. Ring fixators for nonarticular fractures are falling out of favor because the distal wires are not well tolerated by the patient, and fixation strength with intramedullary nailing appears to be adequate with supplemental stabilization of the fibula.

Osseous Defects

Tibial defects usually result from open tibial fractures and can be highly problematic because of (1) traumatized soft-tissue that cannot adequately contribute vascularity to the bony healing response, (2) contamination and risk of infection, and (3) compromised quality of life because of the inability to walk on the leg for

prolonged periods. The use of Ilizarov bone transport for defects greater than 1 to 5 cm has been associated with a high rate of union, but multiple surgeries and use of the fixator for more than 1 year may be required.[19] Numerous bone graft substitutes are commercially available; none has been compared with any other for determination of efficacy. A recent prospective, randomized study of open tibial fractures with a defect of more than 50% of the cortical diameter and measuring 1 to 5 cm in length showed similar results in a group treated with insertion of recombinant human bone morphogenetic protein-2 (rhBMP-2) when compared with a group treated with iliac crest autograft.[20] The rhBMP-2 was inserted on a collagen sponge and with freeze-dried cancellous allograft chips. All traumatic wounds were clean and healed, without evidence of osteomyelitis. This reconstructive surgery was staged between 6 and 12 weeks after initial fracture treatment.

Mangled Extremity

The Lower Extremity Assessment Project (LEAP) is a prospective cohort study of 601 patients with severe lower extremity injuries below the distal part of the femur, admitted to eight level 1 trauma centers over a 42-month period.[21] These injuries include type III open tibial fractures, dysvascular limbs (from knee dislocations, closed fractures, or penetrating wounds with vascular injury), type IIIB open ankle fractures, all type III open tibial pilon fractures, and severe hindfoot or midfoot injuries. Multiple reports from the LEAP group have provided extensive information regarding the treatment of patients with mangled extremities (**Table 1**).

Thus, the mangled extremity with tibial fracture should be treated using the management principles for bone and soft-tissue injuries as described in this chapter. Given the findings of the LEAP group, immediate amputation for trauma does not have long-term support. Clear guidelines for early amputation include widespread necrosis in a medically unstable patient, a rapidly progressive infection in a sick patient, and severe open tibial fracture with a crushed foot. In most other situations, amputation can be postponed until the treatment options, details, and risks can be reviewed with the patient and/or family.

Acceleration of Fracture Healing

Numerous factors contribute to an increased risk of delayed union after fracture of the tibia, including open fracture, tobacco use, diabetes, malnutrition, and increased age. There are two basic means to accelerate healing of tibial fractures believed to be at risk for delayed union: biophysical stimulation and early use of orthobiologic agents such as injection of osteoprogenitor stem cells or application of bone morphogenetic protein.

Although numerous commercially available bone growth stimulators and orthobiologic agents are available, few comparative studies exist that support their use, and existing studies have significant methodological flaws that limit the strength of their conclusions. Comparative studies of ultrasound suggest that fracture healing is improved in fractures treated conservatively, especially in smokers.

With respect to orthobiologics, a large, international, multicenter, prospective, randomized study (that did not involve North American surgeons) reported that rhBMP-2 inserted into open tibial fractures at the time of wound closure leads to a lower infection rate and a higher healing rate. This study also reported that higher concentrations of rhBMP-2 were associated with better results. A second report, which combines the data from the international study with data from a similar North American study, concluded that rhBMP-2 combined with a collagen sponge resulted in a higher healing rate and a lower infection rate in patients with type IIIA and IIIB open fractures.[22] In a subset analysis of reamed tibial nailing procedures, however, the rhBMP-2 did not appear to have clinical benefit. Thus, the benefit of rhBMP-2 in the treatment of open tibial fractures appears to be offset by reaming before nail insertion.

Bone morphogenetic protein-7 (BMP-7) has been compared with iliac crest bone graft for treating tibial nonunions, and comparable results were reported, although the criteria for surgery were not strictly defined in that study.

Tibial Malunion

Tibial malunion is generally defined as angulation of more than 5° in either the coronal or sagittal plane. Angulation, particularly in the coronal plane, will alter the alignment of the knee and ankle and may create symptoms of discomfort in either joint because of malalignment. It is unclear how much malalignment is necessary to cause excessive pressure on the cartilage with consequent degeneration, although it has been reported that as much as 20° of malalignment can be tolerated without significantly increasing the pressure on the cartilage. The location of the deformity is important because proximal fractures will have more of an effect on the knee, and distal fractures will have more of an effect on the ankle. AP weight-bearing alignment radiographs of the entire extremity are the standard for evaluating extremity alignment and assessing the impact of the malunion.

Malunion also can contribute to and exacerbate ligamentous stability. In patients with concomitant tibial malalignment and knee ligament instability, it is generally optimal to correct the tibial malalignment with osteotomy before knee ligament repair. Primary ligament repair is unlikely to have lasting success when malalignment is present. In some patients, correction of the malunion alone will minimize the symptoms of ligament instability, thereby obviating the need for further surgery.

Angular tibial malunions have become increasingly less common now that intramedullary nailing of unstable and open tibial fractures has become the standard of care. Corrective tibial osteotomy with plate fixation, intramedullary nailing, or Ilizarov fixation all have high success rates.[23-26] Preoperative radiographs can reveal that the healed bone at the fracture site may preclude passage of an intramedullary guide wire or reamer, in which instance intramedullary nail stabilization of the osteotomy would be contraindicated. Axial malalignment may be impossible to realign with a single osteotomy and intramedullary nailing, in which instance an alternative means of stabilization would be more favorable. Often, correct alignment cannot be obtained intraoperatively because of fibula malunion; therefore, the surgeon should be prepared to perform fibula osteotomy at the time of corrective tibial surgery. Closing wedge tibial osteotomy or single-cut oblique osteotomy stretches tissue less than opening wedge osteotomy, thereby decreasing the risk of soft-tissue complications and possibly facilitating healing of the osteotomy.[24-26]

Tibial lengthening for excessive shortening after tibial fracture should be considered only if the limb-length discrepancy is greater than 1 inch (2.5 cm). Ilizarov lengthening is the most reliable means of lengthening, but it may require use of the distraction fixator for more than 1 year before the regenerate bone at the distraction site is strong enough to allow removal of the fixator.

Rotational malunion can occur after tibial nailing. CT scan analysis after intramedullary nailing has shown a 22% incidence of rotational tibial malunion of more than 10°.[27] Thus, preoperative measurement of contralateral tibial rotation is necessary, and efforts to match this measurement should be undertaken before placement of final interlocking screws.

Tibial Nonunion

A commonly accepted definition for tibial nonunion does not exist.[28] As a generalization, a tibial fracture that is more than 6 months old and shows no radiographic evidence of progress toward healing for 3 consecutive months can be considered a nonunion. In some instances, this definition is too strict. For instance, tibial fractures with large osseous defects or nonsurgically treated fractures with gross clinical motion more than 1 month after injury are unlikely to heal without surgical intervention, and waiting 6 months to meet this definition of nonunion before performing surgery may not be in the patient's best interest.

After tibial nailing, fractures that are distracted may benefit from removal of interlocking screws to allow fracture compression (dynamization). This procedure offers the theoretic benefit of increased compression across the fracture, but scientific studies have not been performed that show a higher rate of healing when dynamization is performed.

Hypertrophic tibial nonunions require improved stability, which can be achieved with revision to stronger implants (that is, a larger diameter intramedullary nail).

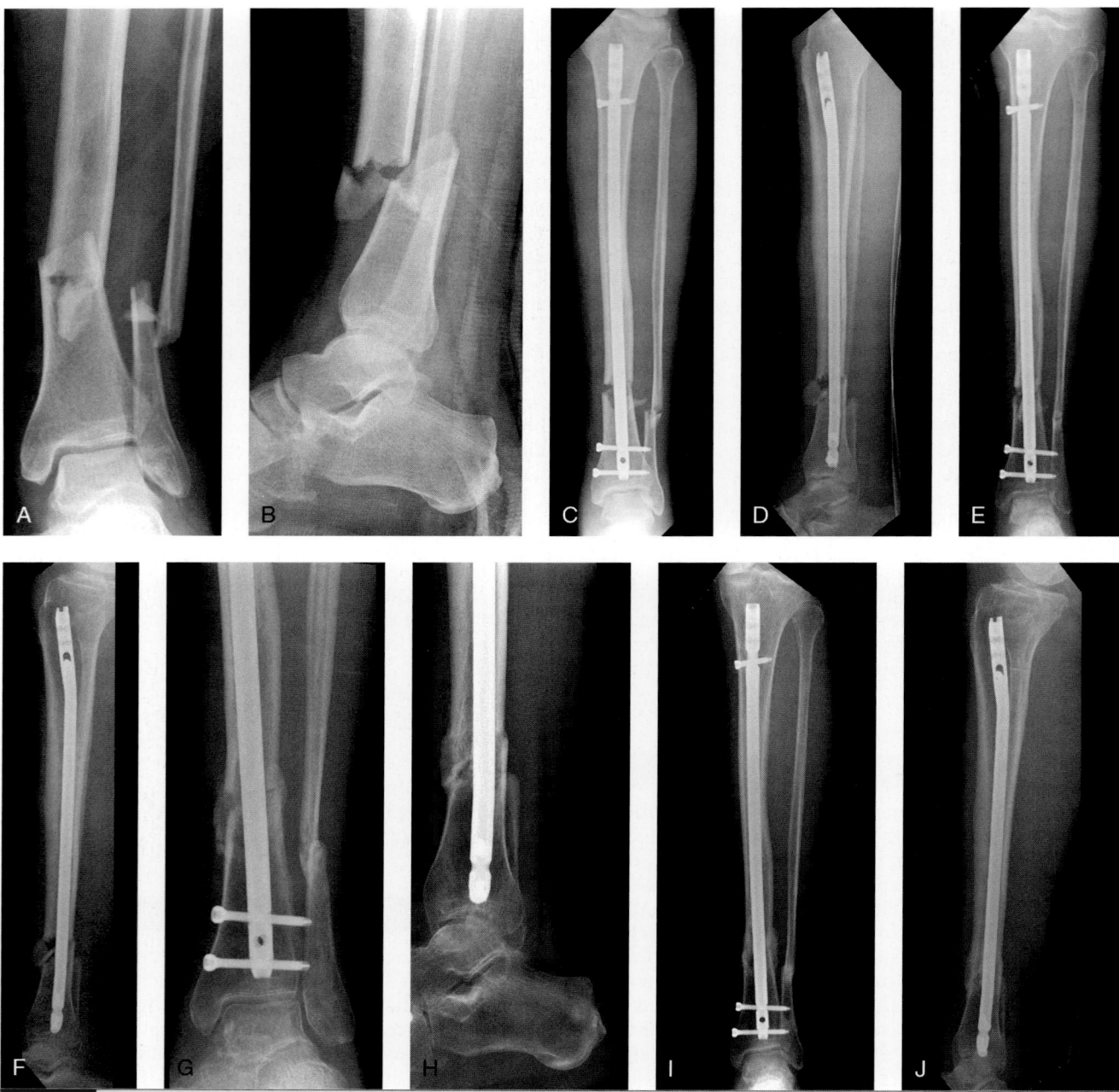

Figure 2 AP (**A**) and lateral (**B**) radiographs of the ankle of a 54-year-old man who was struck by a car while riding a motorcycle. The patient had closed displaced tibial and fibular fractures. Postoperative AP (**C**) and lateral (**D**) radiographs show satisfactory alignment. AP (**E**) and lateral (**F**) radiographs 6 months after surgery show an atrophic tibial nonunion. Laboratory studies were not consistent with infection. As the fracture was in good alignment and the intramedullary nail appeared stable, the nonunion was treated with iliac crest bone grafting through an anterolateral incision. Five months after bone grafting, AP (**G**) and lateral (**H**) radiographs show bridging bone, which matured more completely at 1 year (**I** and **J**).

Atrophic nonunions require both stability and biologic enhancement, which can be achieved with iliac crest bone graft or intramedullary reaming (Figure 2). Reamed tibial nailing for tibial nonunion carries a high success rate, even for atrophic nonunions. This improved success rate is presumably a result of the positive effect of reaming on the healing response.

It is essential to rule out infection preoperatively, using white blood cell count, C-reactive protein level, and erythrocyte sedimentation rate as laboratory guides that are sensitive but not specific. Intraoperative Gram stain and cultures should be obtained. Intraoperative frozen section analysis of tissue has not proven to be helpful in ruling out infected tibial nonunion. Bone

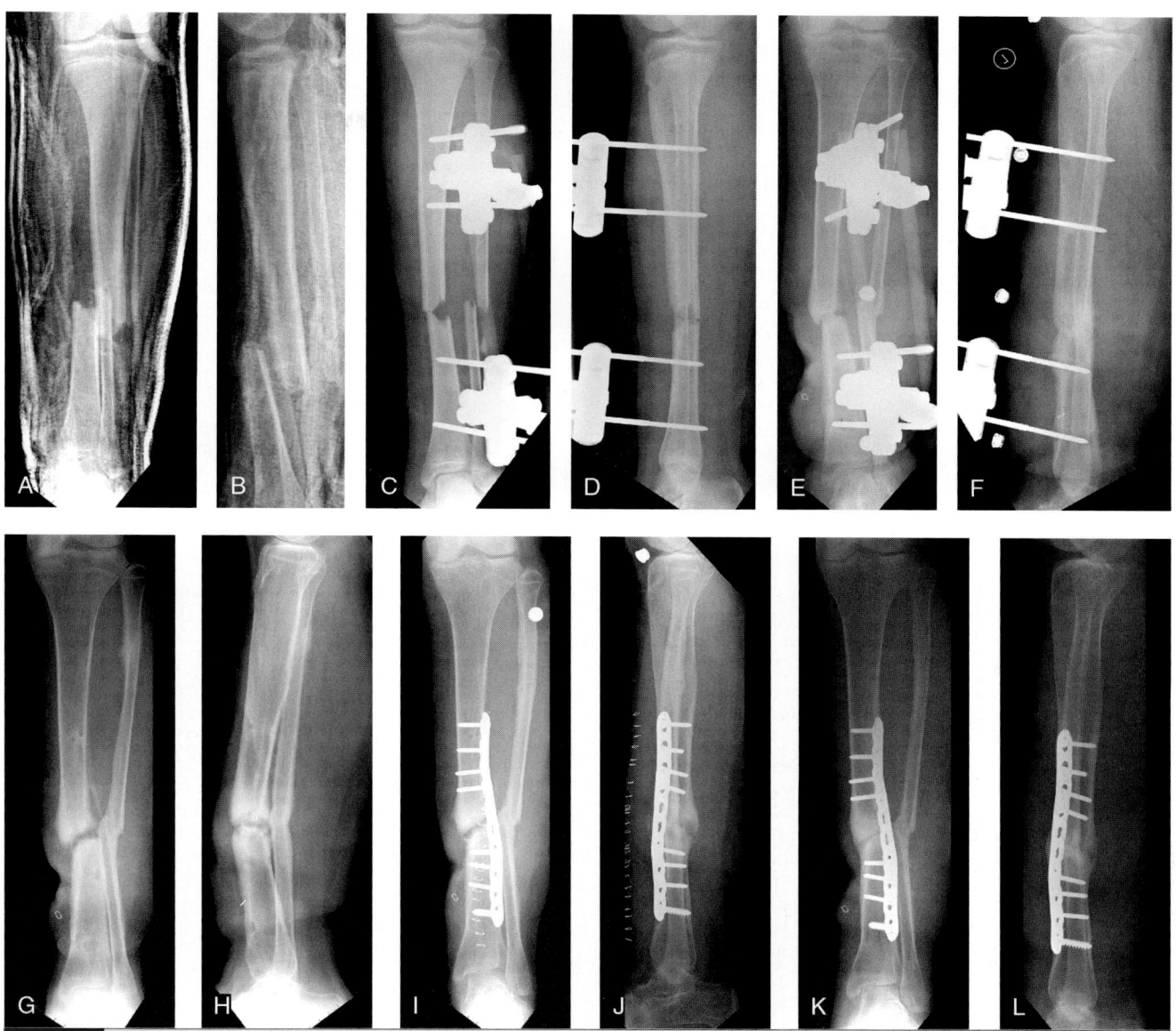

Figure 3 AP (**A**) and lateral (**B**) tibia radiographs of a 14-year-old boy who was struck by a car while riding a bicycle. The patient had a 13 × 15 cm soft-tissue defect of the midleg (Gustilo-Anderson type IIIB) but no neurologic or vascular impairment. AP (**C**) and lateral (**D**) radiographs after irrigation and débridement and external fixator application show satisfactory alignment. The soft-tissue defect was covered with a soleus pedicle flap after the third surgical débridement. The patient's family was reluctant to allow additional surgery. AP (**E**) and lateral (**F**) radiographs 1 year after injury show incomplete fracture healing. The external fixator was loose and the pin tracts were infected, so the external fixator was removed. AP (**G**) and lateral (**H**) radiographs at 15 months show progressive angulation and no further healing. Laboratory studies showed no evidence of infection. AP (**I**) and lateral (**J**) radiographs after open reduction and internal fixation with iliac crest bone grafting are shown. AP (**K**) and lateral (**L**) radiographs 6 months after nonunion surgery and 23 months after injury show complete healing of the tibial nonunion.

graft should not be inserted into a potentially infected nonunion. If it is unclear whether an infection is present, bone grafting should be delayed until definitive cultures can be evaluated.

The best results reported for tibial nonunions after initial external fixation were achieved using plate fixation and iliac crest bone graft[10] (**Figure 3**). Care must be taken to rule out infection preoperatively, to avoid making incisions through badly traumatized tissues, and to clean bone ends without devitalizing them.

Ilizarov treatment of tibial nonunions has been associated with good results, but the fixator is not well tolerated for long periods and has been associated with pin tract infection. However, external fixation can be placed with minimal dissection, provides stable fixation, does not place metal in the region of the non-

4: Lower Extremity

union, and can be adjusted postoperatively, making it ideal for treating infected tibial nonunions with marginal bone quality.

Use of synthetic bone graft and/or BMP avoids donor site morbidity, but neither treatment has convincingly matched the results of iliac crest bone grafting for treating established tibial nonunions. Electrical stimulation and ultrasound therapy have not satisfactorily demonstrated success in treating tibial nonunions and are not a substitute for surgical intervention for established tibial nonunion. Studies of both pulsed electromagnetic field and capacitive-coupling devices are mostly retrospective case series in which the additional contribution of associated treatments is difficult to ascertain. Randomized clinical trials of these devices that have been published to date either show no differences after adjusting for confounding factors, or did not have sufficient follow-up to account for slower healing in the control group. Percutaneous injection of bone marrow aspirate appears promising in treating atrophic tibial nonunions.[29]

Annotated References

1. Boody AR, Wongworawat MD: Accuracy in the measurement of compartment pressures: A comparison of three commonly used devices. *J Bone Joint Surg Am* 2005;87:2415-2422.

   The authors compared tissue pressure measurements of muscle placed in fluid of a known pressure obtained using an arterial line manometer, a Stryker Intracompartmental Monitor System, and a Whitesides manometer apparatus. They found the arterial line manometer to be the most accurate, and the Stryker system also to be accurate. The Whitesides manometer lacked precision. Side-port needles and slit catheters were more accurate than straight needles, regardless of the device used.

2. Orthopaedic Trauma Association: Fracture and dislocation compendium. *J Orthop Trauma* 1996;10(suppl 1): 1-55.

3. Tscherne H, Gotzen L: *Fractures Associated with Soft Tissue Injuries.* New York, NY, Springer-Verlag, 1984.

4. Bone LB, Sucato D, Stegemann PM, Rohrbacher BJ: Displaced isolated fractures of the tibial shaft treated with either a cast or intramedullary nailing: An outcome analysis of matched pairs of patients. *J Bone Joint Surg Am* 1998;80:1084-1085.

5. Hooper GJ, Keddell RG, Penny ID: Conservative management or closed nailing for tibial shaft fractures: A randomised prospective trial. *J Bone Joint Surg Br* 1991;73:83-85.

6. Alho A, Benterud JG, Hogevold HE, Ekeland A, Stromsoe K: Comparison of functional bracing and locked intramedullary nailing in the treatment of displaced tibial shaft fractures. *Clin Orthop Relat Res* 1992;277:243-250.

7. Sarmiento A, Sharpe FE, Ebramzadeh E, Normand P, Shankwiler J: Factors influencing the outcome of closed tibial fractures treated with functional bracing. *Clin Orthop Relat Res* 1995;315:8-24.

8. Bhandari M, Zlowodzki M, Tornetta P III, Schmidt A, Templeman DC: Intramedullary nailing following external fixation in femoral and tibial shaft fractures. *J Orthop Trauma* 2005;19:140-144.

   The authors conducted a meta-analysis of infection and union rates after conversion of external fixation to intramedullary nailing. Weak (grade C) evidence from level IV studies showed a 9% infection rate (95% confidence interval [CI], 7% to 12%) and a 90% union rate (95% CI, 88% to 93%). External fixators converted to intramedullary nailing had higher healing rates than external fixators converted to casts (94% versus 64%, $P = 0.02$). Tibias with external fixators for 28 days or less had an 83% reduced risk of infection compared with those with external fixators for more than 28 days. These findings are limited by the lack of prospective studies.

9. McGraw JM, Lim EV: Treatment of open tibial-shaft fractures: External fixation and secondary intramedullary nailing. *J Bone Joint Surg Am* 1988;70:900-911.

10. Wiss DA, Johnson DL, Miao M: Compression plating for non-union after failed external fixation of open tibial fractures. *J Bone Joint Surg Am* 1992;74:1279-1285.

11. Finkemeier CG, Schmidt AH, Kyle RF, Templeman DC, Varecka TF: A prospective, randomized study of intramedullary nails inserted with and without reaming for the treatment of open and closed fractures of the tibial shaft. *J Orthop Trauma* 2000;14:187-193.

12. Bone LB, Johnson KD: Treatment of tibial fractures by reaming and intramedullary nailing. *J Bone Joint Surg Am* 1986;68:877-887.

13. Karunakar MA, Frankenburg EP, Le TT, Hall J: The thermal effects of intramedullary reaming. *J Orthop Trauma* 2004;18:674-679.

    The authors measured temperature during reaming of five pairs of canine tibia, with and without tourniquet, and reported that the use of a tourniquet did not cause a significant increase in the temperature. Reaming to sizes larger than the intramedullary canal were reported to have produced the highest temperatures. These findings suggest that the risk of thermal necrosis during reaming may be related more to the technique of reaming than to the use of a tourniquet and underscore the importance of limited tibial reaming.

14. Blachut PA, O'Brien PJ, Meek RN, Broekhuyse HM: Interlocking intramedullary nailing with and without reaming for the treatment of closed fractures of the tibial shaft: A prospective, randomized study. *J Bone Joint Surg Am* 1997;79:640-646.

15. Konrath G, Moed BR, Watson JT, Kaneshiro S, Karges DE, Cramer KE: Intramedullary nailing of unstable diaphyseal fractures of the tibia with distal intraarticular

involvement. *J Orthop Trauma* 1997;3:200-205.

16. Egol KA, Weisz R, Hiebert R, Tejwani NC, Koval KJ, Sanders RW: Does fibular plating improve alignment after intramedullary nailing of distal metaphyseal tibia fractures? *J Orthop Trauma* 2006;20:94-103.

This is a retrospective review of 72 distal tibial fractures from three trauma centers; all fractures were treated with intramedullary nailing. Twenty-five patients had fixation of the fibula fracture performed before tibial nailing, and these patients had better maintenance of alignment 12 weeks or more after surgery (*P* = 0.036). The authors recommend plating of the fibula in addition to intramedullary nailing of the tibia for all unstable distal tibial-fibula fractures.

17. Nork SE, Schwartz AK, Agel J, Holt SK, Schrick JL, Winquist RA: Intramedullary nailing of distal metaphyseal tibial fractures. *J Bone Joint Surg Am* 2005;87: 1213-1221.

Thirty-six patients with fractures within 5 cm of the ankle were treated with intramedullary nailing after open reduction and internal fixation of the fibula. Articular extension of the fracture was reduced and stabilized with lag screws before intramedullary nailing. Thirty-three patients (92%) had less than 5% angulation postoperatively. Weight bearing was prohibited for 6 to 12 weeks after surgery. Of the 30 patients who returned for follow-up, all healed at an average of 23.5 weeks. Fracture displacement did not occur in the postoperative period. Dynamization by removal of the proximal interlocking screw(s) was performed in four patients, which allowed up to 1 cm of shortening but prevented angulation at the fracture.

18. Im GI, Tae SK: Distal metaphyseal fractures of tibia: A prospective randomized trial of closed reduction and intramedullary nail versus open reduction and plate and screws fixation. *J Trauma* 2005;59:1219-1223.

The authors prospectively randomized 64 patients with distal metaphyseal fractures of the tibia to either intramedullary nailing or open reduction and internal fixation when the soft tissues appeared ready. The intramedullary angulation group had an average of 2.8° of fracture angulation, whereas the open reduction and internal fixation group had an average angulation of 0.9°. Final ankle dorsiflexion was better in the intramedullary nailing group (14°) than in the open reduction and internal fixation group (7°), but functional ankle scores were similar between the two groups. The intramedullary nailing group had one superficial infection, whereas the open reduction and internal fixation group had six superficial and one deep infection. All three closed fractures with Tscherne grade C2 or higher soft-tissue injury that were treated with open reduction and internal fixation had superficial or deep infection, and the authors recommend intramedullary nailing for these patients.

19. Rozbruch SR, Weitzman AM, Watson JT, Freudigman P, Katz HV, Ilizarov S: Simultaneous treatment of tibial bone and soft-tissue defects with the Ilizarov method. *J Orthop Trauma* 2006;20:197-205.

In this report of 25 patients with large bony (average, 6 cm) and soft-tissue (average, 10 cm) defects who were not candidates for flap coverage, 17 patients (68%) had infection before the procedure, and 11 (44%) had infection involving the bone. Initial treatment was débridement of the devitalized bone and soft tissue and squaring of the bone ends. Gradual bone transport from one, two, or three sites resulted in closure of the soft-tissue defect at an average of 15 weeks and bony healing in 24 patients (96%). The fixator was worn an average of 43 weeks (range, 10 to 82 weeks). There were no amputations. All infections resolved.

20. Jones AL, Bucholz RW, Bosse MJ, et al: Recombinant human BMP-2 and allograft compared with autogenous bone graft for reconstruction of diaphyseal tibial fractures with cortical defects: A randomized, controlled trial. *J Bone Joint Surg Am* 2006;88:1431-1441.

In this randomized, controlled trial of 30 patients with tibial shaft fractures and cortical defects measuring 1 to 5 cm and with 50% or more cortical diameter involvement, the authors compared iliac crest autograft with the use of a combination of rhBMP-2, allograft bone, and collagen sponge. They reported that 10 of 15 autograft patients and 13 of 15 rhBMP/allograft patients healed at 1-year follow-up (*P* = not significant). The Short Musculoskeletal Function Assessment scores were comparable between groups. No patient had antibodies to rhBMP-2. One patient had transient antibodies to the bovine collagen. Six patients were lost to follow-up after fracture healing had occurred. The rhBMP-2 group had one superficial infection and two deep infections, whereas the autograft group had no superficial infections and one deep infection. Larger trials are needed.

21. MacKenzie EJ, Bosse MJ, Pollak AN, et al: Long-term persistence of disability following severe lower-limb trauma: Results of a seven-year follow-up. *J Bone Joint Surg Am* 2005;87:1801-1809.

The LEAP study was a National Institutes of Health investigation to evaluate limb salvage versus amputation in severe lower extremity injuries. An open fracture classification system was clearly defined by the LEAP authors, so that final grading was determined at the time of definitive closure or amputation. This 7-year follow-up of 397 LEAP study patients did not demonstrate a long-term advantage to limb salvage. The authors reported that functional outcome deteriorated between 2- and 7-year follow-up. At 7-year follow-up, half of the patients had substantial disability (Sickness Impact Profile [SIP] score ≥ 10), and only 34.5% had a SIP score typical of the general population, regardless of the treatment. Patients with through-the-knee amputations had worse scores, and patients with severe soft-tissue injuries but no fracture had worse results. Poorer outcomes were associated with older age, female gender, nonwhite race, lower educational level, poverty, history of smoking, low self-efficacy, poor self-reported health status before injury, and involvement with the legal system in an effort to obtain disability payments.

22. Swiontkowski MF, Esterhai JL, Goulet J, et al: Recombinant human bone morphogenetic protein-2 in open tibial fractures: A subgroup analysis of data combined from two prospective randomized studies. *J Bone Joint Surg Am* 2006;88:1258-1265.

4: Lower Extremity

This report combines data from a US study of 60 patients and an international study of 450 patients with open tibial shaft fractures treated with débridement and intramedullary nailing; the patients were randomized to receive rhBMP-2 with collagen sponge at a dosage approved by the US Food and Drug Administration versus no additional treatment. A subgroup analysis of 131 type IIIA or IIIB open tibial fractures demonstrated fewer bone grafting procedures, fewer secondary surgeries, and fewer infections in the rhBMP-2 group. A subgroup analysis of 113 patients treated with reamed intramedullary nailing demonstrated no significant difference between the groups. This treatment is still experimental, and it has not been proven to be of benefit in open tibial fractures treated with reamed intramedullary nailing, which has been the standard treatment in North America. It appears that any implant is most beneficial when unreamed nailing is used to treat open tibia fractures, which was the technique used more commonly outside of North America during this study period (1996-1999). The benefits of the implant appear to be offset by the practice of intramedullary reaming of the tibia before nail insertion.

23. Feldman DS, Sin SS, Madan S, Koval KJ: Correction of tibial malunion and nonunion with six-axis analysis deformity correction using the Taylor Spatial Frame. *J Orthop Trauma* 2003;17:549-554.

24. Sangeorzan BJ, Sangeorzan BP, Hansen ST Jr, Judd RP: Mathematically directed single-cut osteotomy for correction of tibial malunion. *J Orthop Trauma* 1989;3:267-275.

25. Johnson EE: Multiplane correctional osteotomy of the tibia for diaphyseal malunion. *Clin Orthop Relat Res* 1987;215:223-232.

26. Sanders R, Anglen JO, Mark JB: Oblique osteotomy for the correction of tibial malunion. *J Bone Joint Surg Am* 1996;78:151-152.

27. Puloski S, Romano C, Buckley R, Powell J: Rotational malalignment of the tibia following reamed intramedullary nail fixation. *J Orthop Trauma* 2004;18:397-402.

In a consecutive series of 25 tibial fractures treated with intramedullary nailing, CT scans were obtained for 22 bilateral tibiae to evaluate rotational alignment. The fractured tibiae had mean absolute rotational difference of 6.7° (range, 22° internal to 15° external rotation). Five tibiae (22%) were malrotated greater than 10°, and 3 (13%) were rotated 15° or more. Clinical correlation was not reported.

28. Bhattacharyya T, Bouchard KA, Phadke A, Meigs JB, Kassarjian A, Salamipour H: The accuracy of computed tomography for the diagnosis of tibial nonunion. *J Bone Joint Surg Am* 2006;88:692-697.

CT scans were obtained for 35 patients who were suspected of having possible tibial nonunion on clinical examination and after review of plain radiographs. Two radiologists and an orthopaedic surgeon reviewed the CT scans. CT was 100% sensitive for detecting nonunion, but it had a low specificity (62%).

29. Hernigou P, Poignard A, Beaujean F, Rouard H: Percutaneous autologous bone-marrow grafting for nonunions: Influence of the number and concentration of progenitor cells. *J Bone Joint Surg Am* 2005;87:1430-1437.

This European study showed an 88% healing rate in atrophic tibial nonunions treated with injection of centrifuged bone marrow aspirate (53 of 60 patients). The authors reported that the number and concentration of fibroblast colony-forming units correlate with the volume of mineralized callus evident on CT scans at 4-month follow-up. Healing occurred sooner with in this group of patients, with higher concentrations of fibroblast colony-forming units.

Chapter 39
Midfoot and Forefoot Injuries

David P. Barei, MD   Sean E. Nork, MD

Tarsometatarsal Fracture-Dislocations (Lisfranc's Injuries)

Injuries to the tarsometatarsal joint complex are usually referred to as Lisfranc's injuries. These injuries range from high-energy injuries with severe disruption of the midfoot to subtle subluxations or sprains that are easily missed on initial evaluation. Increasing awareness of the potential for long-term disability resulting from even subtle Lisfranc's injuries has resulted in increased vigilance in their diagnosis. It is largely accepted that the best opportunity for a successful functional outcome is provided by anatomic joint reduction and stabilization with internal fixation, and that an open technique is required to reliably achieve these goals. Even when goals are achieved, outcomes are not always good, especially for patients with severe comminution or crush injuries.[1]

Biomechanics

The tarsometatarsal region represents the transition zone between the midfoot and the forefoot. The creation of the transverse and longitudinal arches of the midfoot is a result of the shape of the distal articular surfaces of the cuneiforms and cuboid, their metatarsal attachments proximally, and the weight-bearing metatarsal heads distally. The Lisfranc's joint complex has a relatively rigid medial column (first, second, and third tarsometatarsal joints) and a more mobile lateral column (fourth and fifth tarsometatarsal joints). Within the relatively rigid medial column, the first tarsometatarsal articulation has slightly more mobility than the second and third tarsometatarsal articulations. Lisfranc's joint complex allows a stiff arch that permits the smooth transfer of weight to occur from the ankle-hindfoot region to the forefoot in such a manner that all of the metatarsal heads and sesamoids participate equally in weight bearing. The joint is stabilized by its unique bony structure, as well as by strong capsuloligamentous attachments.

Anatomy

Part of the inherent bony stability of the Lisfranc's joint complex is a result of the dorsally based trapezoidal cross-sectional shape of the medial metatarsal bases and their corresponding cuneiforms. This Roman arch configuration imparts stability by preventing plantar displacement of the metatarsal bases. The second metatarsal base is recessed and dovetailed between the medial and lateral cuneiforms, contributing additional stability to the joint. Because the second metatarsal base is at the apex of osseous stability, it is often fractured at the time of injury. Additional stability of the tarsometatarsal articulation is provided by capsuloligamentous restraints. These restraints can be grouped as dorsal, interosseous, and plantar ligaments. The dorsal ligamentous structures are relatively weak compared with their plantar counterparts. Strong intermetatarsal interosseous ligaments are present between each of the lateral four metatarsals but are absent between the first and second metatarsals. In this region, the base of the second metatarsal is joined to the first tarsometatarsal joint by the medial interosseous ligament (Lisfranc's ligament) and connects the plantar aspect of the second metatarsal base to the medial cuneiform. This represents the largest ligament in the Lisfranc's joint complex and is responsible for the second metatarsal base avulsion that often occurs with Lisfranc's injuries. The absence of a direct ligamentous connection between the base of the first and second metatarsals represents an inherent weakness in the Lisfranc's joint complex. The plantar intertarsal and intermetatarsal ligaments, as is the case with their dorsal equivalents, vary considerably in number and organization. These plantar ligaments are significantly stronger than their corresponding dorsal ligaments.

Mechanism of Injury

Causes of Lisfranc's joint complex injuries are variable. High-energy injuries result in severely displaced fracture-dislocations, whereas less severe twisting injuries may cause more subtle sprains and subluxations. Motor vehicle collisions, crush injuries, falls from ground level or from a height, and sports-related injuries are all common mechanisms of injury.

Impacts to the foot, such as those that occur in crush injuries, apply direct forces to Lisfranc's articulations and often result in severe soft-tissue injury, open wounds, possible vascular compromise, and compartment syndrome.[2] Because the applied force is frequently directed to the dorsum of the foot, plantar displacement of the metatarsal bases is common with this injury mechanism. Indirect injuries are more common and result from a combination of twisting and axial loading of the extremely plantar-flexed foot. Dislocation typically occurs at the site of least resistance, with dorsal dislocation of the metatarsals and secondary me-

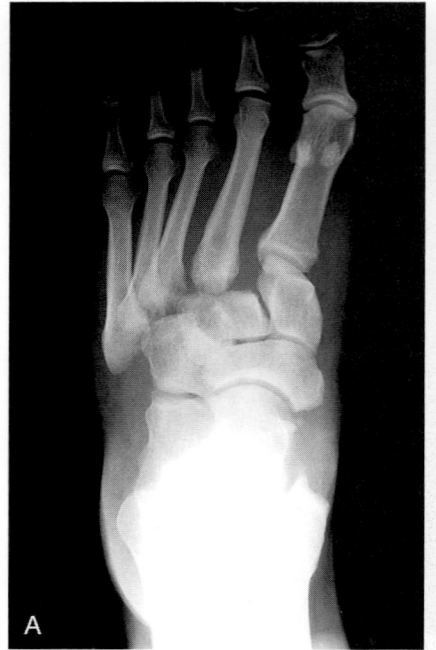
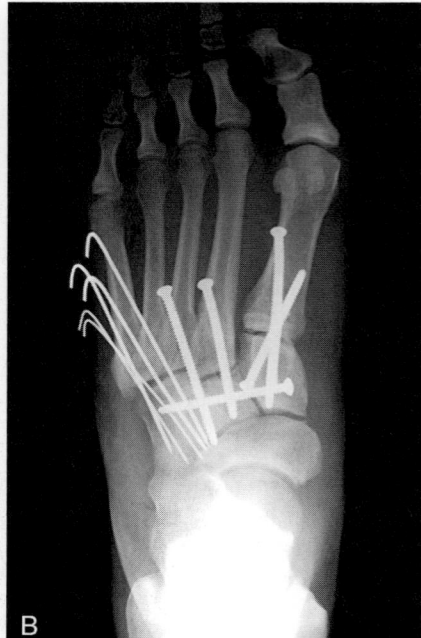
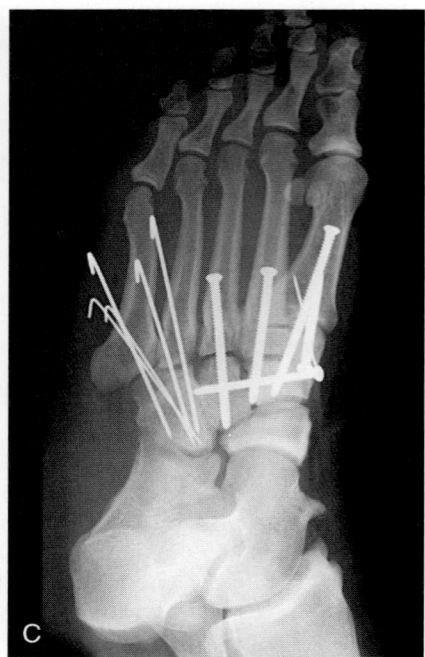
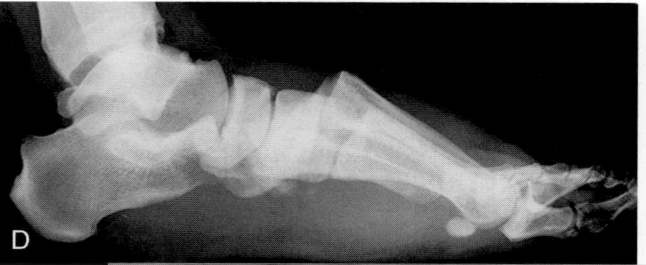
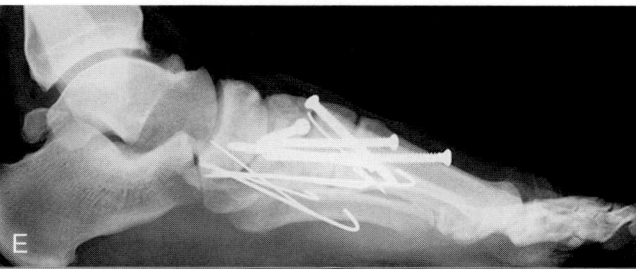

Figure 1 While playing basketball, a 26-year-old man sustained a twisting injury of the left foot that resulted in a Lisfranc's fracture-dislocation. AP **(A)** and lateral **(D)** radiographs show complete ligamentous disruption of all five tarsometatarsal articulations. The patient was treated with open reduction and internal fixation of the medial column and percutaneous temporary Kirschner wire stabilization of the more mobile lateral column. An associated intercuneiform disruption was noted at the time of surgical fixation. The normal radiographic midfoot relationships described by Stein were restored. Postoperative AP **(B)**, internal oblique **(C)**, and lateral views **(E)** are shown.

dial or lateral displacement of the midfoot. These indirect injuries are rarely associated with open wounds or vascular compromise.

Patients usually have pain, swelling, and point tenderness over the Lisfranc's joint after a twisting or axial loading injury to the foot. The plantar ecchymosis sign has been identified as a clinical indicator of a Lisfranc's injury.

Radiographic Evaluation

AP, lateral, and 30° internal (medial) oblique radiographs of the foot are all essential in evaluating the Lisfranc's joint complex (**Figure 1**). The AP view is most useful in assessing the first and second tarsometatarsal joints, whereas the internal oblique radiograph profiles the lateral three tarsometatarsal joints. To facilitate radiographic interpretation of this complex articulation, several consistently normal radiographic parameters have been established. The following guidelines are

provided: on the AP view, the first metatarsal aligns itself with the medial cuneiform both medially and laterally, and the medial border of the second metatarsal aligns itself exactly with the medial edge of the middle cuneiform. On the internal oblique view, the lateral border of the third metatarsal is aligned to the lateral edge of the lateral cuneiform. The medial border of the fourth metatarsal forms a continuous straight line with the medial edge of the cuboid. The relationship of the fifth metatarsal to the cuboid varies, and is not reliable for diagnosing a tarsometatarsal injury. Because the fourth and fifth metatarsals almost always move as a unit, the alignment of the fourth tarsometatarsal joint can be used to identify fifth metatarsal displacement. On the lateral view, the second tarsometatarsal should show an uninterrupted line along the dorsal surface of the tarsal bone proximally and the corresponding metatarsal base distally. Dorsal displacement of the metatarsals is abnormal and indicative of a significant Lisfranc's injury. Slight plantar displacement of 1 mm or less, however, may be a normal radiographic finding. Overlap of bony structures may cause difficulty with interpretation of this view.[3]

Disturbances in the normal relationships described, avulsion fractures around the tarsometatarsal joints, widening of the first intermetatarsal or intertarsal space, and fractures of the second metatarsal base indicate a potentially serious injury to the Lisfranc's joint complex.[4] Fractures of the second metatarsal base occur in approximately 90% of Lisfranc's injuries. Crush injuries to the cuboid or medial cuneiform and avulsion fractures of the navicular tuberosity also should raise suspicion for a Lisfranc's injury. Any disturbance in the normal radiographic alignment on any view confirms a Lisfranc's injury, even if the displacement is not obvious on corresponding views. In some patients, Lisfranc's injury is suspected based on clinical evidence despite the absence of radiographic abnormalities. In these instances, additional options for radiographic evaluation should include stress views to evaluate tarsometatarsal stability, weight-bearing views to evaluate the stability of the longitudinal arch and widening of the first intermetatarsal space, and CT scans for further evaluation of the tarsometatarsal relationships. Recent evidence has suggested that CT scans are more useful for the detection of subtle Lisfranc's injuries when compared with static plain radiographs.[5] Comparison views of the contralateral foot also may be helpful.

Classification

Lisfranc's injuries have been classified according to radiographic findings and mechanism of injury. Despite their obvious value in describing the most common injury patterns, these classifications fail to encompass all injury types and are of little value in classifying crush injuries, which follow an unpredictable pattern. Additionally, there is little evidence to suggest that any of the current classification systems help to determine surgical management or prognosis.

Treatment

The goal of treatment is a painless, stable, plantigrade foot. Treatment of Lisfranc's injuries has evolved from closed reduction and percutaneous pinning to open reduction and rigid internal fixation. Fixation using Kirschner wires (K-wires) is no longer favored, in part because of their mechanical inferiority and their inability to clinically maintain rigidity of the medial column when compared with screw fixation.[6] Current reported studies support the importance of anatomic reduction of the Lisfranc's articulation and maintenance of this reduction as a necessary condition in achieving treatment goals. If anatomic reduction is achieved, 50% to 95% of patients have good or excellent results compared with 17% to 30% of good or excellent results for patients in whom anatomic reduction is not obtained.[7,8] In most situations, open reduction is accomplished through two dorsal longitudinal incisions, one along the interspace between the first and second metatarsals,

and the second along the fourth ray. Reduction typically proceeds from medial to lateral, with provisional fixation obtained using multiple K-wires. Once the adequacy of reduction is ensured with direct visualization and with the use of multiple fluoroscopic views, the tarsometatarsal articulations are definitively secured. Screw fixations are typically performed across the less mobile first through third tarsometatarsal articulations using 3.5-mm cortical screws. The mobile lateral column (fourth and fifth tarsometatarsal joints) is definitively secured with temporary K-wire fixations.

After open reduction and internal fixation (ORIF), a well-padded plaster splint is applied immediately after surgery. Below-knee cast immobilization is used for approximately 6 to 8 weeks. At 8 weeks, the fourth and fifth metatarsal cuboid pins are removed in the clinic. With the use of a removable prefabricated boot, patients begin weight bearing between 8 and 10 weeks after surgery. Weaning out of the boot occurs at approximately the 12th week. After resolution of edema, typically at 6 to 9 months, patients are fitted for a custom-molded semirigid orthotic device to support the arch.

Outcomes

There is almost complete agreement that a satisfactory outcome after a Lisfranc's injury requires anatomic reduction and stable internal fixation.[7,9] Despite this, some patients still develop disabling pain and degenerative changes of the tarsometatarsal articulations.[8] Although selected arthrodesis of the tarsometatarsal articulations has typically been reserved for salvage procedures, it has recently been suggested that there may be a subgroup of patients with purely ligamentous Lisfranc's injuries that are better treated with primary fusion.[9] The rationale for this treatment choice may be related to the relatively poor healing potential of the capsuloligamentous restraints when compared with osseous union, leading to a potentially higher rate of secondary loss of reduction, deformity, and painful degenerative changes.[10] In a 2002 study, a retrospective comparison of tarsometatarsal injuries in patients treated with ORIF, partial arthrodesis (medial column only), and complete arthrodesis was done.[11] The authors found similar results in the group treated with ORIF and the group treated with partial arthrodesis, but poorer results in patients treated with complete arthrodesis. These findings highlight the importance of a mobile lateral column.[9] Although no initial difference was noted between the partial arthrodesis group and the ORIF group, 94% of the ORIF group showed degenerative changes in the tarsometatarsal joints at final follow-up. Despite the similarity in Baltimore Painful Foot scores, it can be postulated that worsening articular degeneration occurs in the ORIF group, with a commensurate worsening in outcome scores over time, compared with the stable partial arthrodesis group.

In a 2006 randomized trial comparing partial (medial column) arthrodesis and ORIF for the treatment of displaced ligamentous tarsometatarsal injuries, results clearly showed that the group treated with primary arthrodesis obtained better short- and medium-term outcomes than patients treated with ORIF.[10] Anatomic open reduction and definitive acute arthrodesis should be strongly considered for the treatment of unstable purely ligamentous medial column tarsometatarsal disruptions.

Complications

The most important early complications of Lisfranc's injuries are compartment syndrome and vascular compromise. Vascular insufficiency is an exceedingly rare complication of a Lisfranc's joint complex fracture-dislocation; however, early reduction of these injuries is important to minimize soft-tissue damage and the risk of circulatory compromise from tented skin. Despite the risk of injury to the dorsalis pedis artery as it courses between the first and second metatarsal bases, vascular compromise rarely occurs and is usually associated with compartment syndrome of the foot. Particularly in direct (crush) Lisfranc's injuries, a high index of suspicion for compartment syndrome and the use of timely fasciotomies are effective in minimizing the potential for vascular compromise and the subsequent need for forefoot amputation.

Posttraumatic deformity (usually planovalgus) and arthritis constitute the major late sequelae of tarsometatarsal joint injury. Patients usually present with gait abnormalities, foot and ankle weakness, chronic pain, and difficulty with footwear. Symptomatic arthritis and late deformity is initially treated with the use of an arch support and a rigid or rocker-bottom shoe, followed by arthrodesis in patients in whom conservative measures fail. Malunion of the second tarsometatarsal joint is most common, resulting in dorsolateral angulation of the metatarsal. Sequelae include arthritis at the tarsometatarsal joint, loss of the midfoot arch, and transfer metatarsalgia at the adjacent metatarsal heads. Treatment involves shoe modifications, selective midfoot fusion, metatarsal osteotomy, and metatarsal head resection as indicated.

Navicular Fractures

The tarsal navicular is a critical component of the medial column of the foot. Its mobile proximal articulation with the talar head is critical for hindfoot function, whereas its rigid distal articulations with the cuneiforms are important for maintaining the longitudinal arch of the foot. Maintaining length of the medial column relative to the lateral column is an important consideration in managing navicular fractures. Relative medial column shortening typically results in cavus deformity whereas relative lengthening results in planus deformity.[12] There are few studies in the recent literature regarding acute traumatic injuries of the tarsal navicular.

Anatomy

Because the navicular is largely covered with articular cartilage, the area available for nutrient blood vessels is limited. Changes resulting from osteonecrosis are more common in the navicular than in the other midfoot bones. Most of the posterior tibial tendon inserts into the navicular tuberosity. The anterior portion of the deltoid ligament attaches to the dorsomedial aspect of the navicular.

Radiographic Evaluation

The initial diagnosis of navicular fractures is made with high-quality AP, internal (medial) oblique, and lateral radiographs of the foot. Fractures of the navicular may occur in isolation, but also may occur as a component of a high-energy, complex, midfoot fracture-dislocation. In the latter situation, radiographic findings may still be subtle. Associated injury patterns may include fractures of the cuboid, talar head, and Lisfranc's joint complex, mandating close examination of these areas. CT scanning is extremely valuable in identifying comminution and/or impaction of the proximal articular surface of the navicular. Bone scans and MRI may be useful for identifying stress fractures.

Injury Patterns

Fractures of the tarsal navicular are relatively rare injuries and can be generally categorized into four main groups: dorsal lip avulsion fractures, tuberosity fractures, body fractures, and stress fractures.

Dorsal Lip Fractures

The mechanism of injury for dorsal lip fractures is typically plantar flexion with inversion, but also may be associated with eversion.[13] Avulsion of the navicular insertion of the dorsal talonavicular ligament and/or the anterior division of the deltoid ligament are responsible for this type of injury. Most injuries can be treated nonsurgically. Large displaced fragments with significant articular involvement should be treated with ORIF, typically with minifragment fixation.

Tuberosity Fractures

Tuberosity fractures represent avulsion fractures of the navicular insertion of the posterior tibial tendon. They typically occur with sudden, acute eversion and/or valgus injury to the foot. Close examination of the cuboid may reveal associated compression injuries signifying a more complex injury of the midfoot. Differentiating an acute fracture from an accessory navicular fracture requires an assessment of the characteristics of the fracture line. Occasionally, the diagnostic dilemma is more problematic because an acute disruption of the accessory navicular synchondrosis may have occurred. Minimally displaced fragments can be treated conservatively. Displaced fragments are treated with ORIF. Small, displaced fragments may require excision with tendon advancement. Treatment is directed at maintaining the integrity of function of the posterior tibial tendon.

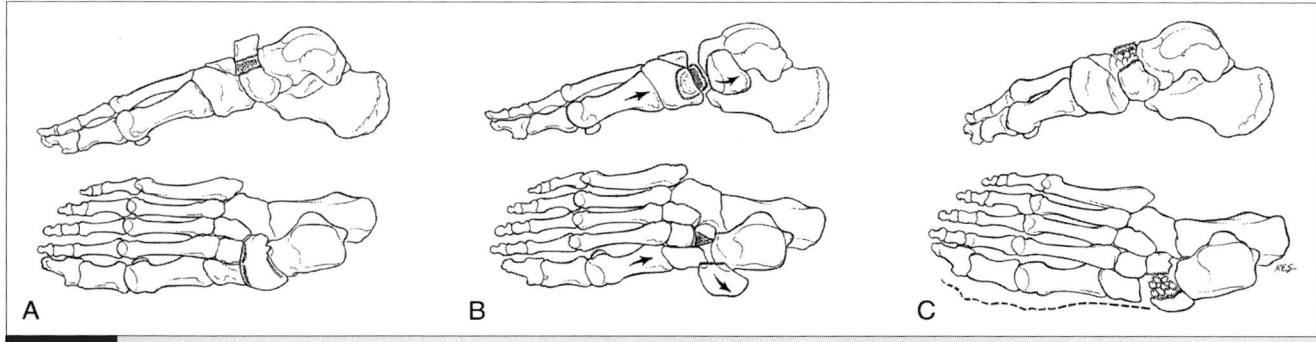

Figure 2 **A,** Diagrammatic representation of a type 1 navicular fracture. The body is split and the dorsal half is displaced dorsally. **B,** A type 2 injury. The navicular is split in the sagittal plane. The body and the medial ray migrate proximally (*arrows*). **C,** The type 3 injury consists of comminution of the navicular in the sagittal plane with displacement of the forefoot laterally.*(Reproduced with permission from Hansen ST, Swiontkowski MF (eds):* Orthopaedic Trauma Protocols. *New York, NY, Raven Press, 1993, p 361.)*

Body Fractures

These injuries have been classified based on the location and orientation of the main fracture line (**Figure 2**).[14] Type 1 fractures are characterized by a coronal plane fracture line and there is no associated forefoot malalignment. Type 2 fractures show a dorsolateral to planar-medial primary fracture line. The major fragment is typically dorsomedial that displaces medially with the forefoot. Type 3 body fractures are comminuted fractures in the sagittal plane with the forefoot displaced laterally. Treatment of these injuries begins with the plain radiographic identification of other subluxations or fractures of the foot, but particularly the midfoot and metatarsals. CT scanning frequently shows the fracture complexity of the articular surface of the navicular and may suggest associated midfoot injuries not identified on plain radiographs. The principles of surgical intervention include anatomic restoration of the proximal articular surface of the navicular to minimize degenerative changes of the talonavicular joint, anatomic realignment of associated midfoot fracture-dislocations, and reestablishment of medial column length.[1-3] Navicular injuries typically require minifragment screws and plates. Fixation should be extended to the cuneiforms if required. In injuries with severe comminution, bridge-type fixation of the medial column may be required, and can be accomplished with transarticular K-wires, temporary external fixation, or temporary bridge plating from the talar neck to the first metatarsal.[12] Bridging fixation is typically removed at 3 months, after union occurs. Postoperatively, the patient usually does not bear weight for 3 months. A semirigid custom-molded orthosis is a reasonable postoperative consideration to facilitate continued support of the arch. Long-term complications of body fractures of the navicular include stiffness, late deformity, and posttraumatic arthritis of the talonavicular joint.

Stress Fractures

Navicular stress fractures are uncommon injuries but tend to occur in young athletes. Pain is located in the midfoot and usually is of insidious onset, worsening with activity. Plain radiographs rarely demonstrate the injury and mandate additional studies to make the diagnosis. CT scanning is currently the diagnostic modality of choice for making the diagnosis and delineating the fracture anatomy. Bone scans and MRI also are helpful modalities but are subject to limited specificity and expense, respectively. Treatment includes cessation of the inciting athletic activity and no weight bearing in a well-molded below-the-knee cast for 6 weeks. Gradual return to sports activity with a supervised physical therapy program is usually successful. Surgical management is indicated for the rare displaced fracture, or when conservative treatment fails.

Cuboid Fractures

The cuboid is an important component of the lateral column of the foot. Its proximal articulation with the calcaneus is relatively rigid compared with the talonavicular articulation. Together, these two joints comprise the transverse tarsal (Chopart's joint). Distally, the cuboid forms mobile articulations with the bases of the fourth and fifth metatarsals. Injuries to the cuboid may result in alterations in the length of the lateral column of the foot relative to the medial column.

Avulsion-Type Injuries

Most cuboid fractures are small avulsion-type injuries secondary to the numerous capsular and ligamentous attachments. These are usually identified on standard AP, oblique, and lateral radiographs of the foot. Treatment is directed at excluding other more extensive midfoot injuries on the basis of the physical examination and radiographs. Additional imaging with CT may show cuboid injuries that may not be readily identifiable with plain radiographs.[15] After other significant associated foot injuries are excluded, symptoms are managed with a brief period of immobilization followed by progressive weight bearing and functional rehabilitation.

Compression Injuries

Conversely, compression injuries of the cuboid are often associated with more significant midfoot injuries to the navicular, cuneiforms, and Lisfranc's joint complex. These compression injuries are typically associated with impaction of the distal cuboid articular surface into the body of the cuboid, leading to two main disorders: incongruence of the fourth and fifth cuboid joints leading to posttraumatic degenerative changes, and relative shortening of the lateral column, leading to planus and abduction deformity of the midfoot. In these situations, treatment is directed at reduction and stabilization of the remainder of the midfoot injury followed by restoration of cuboid length and articular surfaces. Typically surgery is performed with a straight dorsolateral incision over the cuboid with the deep dissection directed between the peroneal tendons and the extensor digitorum brevis musculature.[16] A small distractor or external fixator can be used to regain length to the lateral column. Impacted segments are reduced and the osseous void is filled with bone graft. Fixation is usually achieved with minifragment or periarticular plates and screws.

Metatarsal Fractures

The function of the forefoot is to provide a level platform for standing and a lever for push-off. During the stance phase, weight is borne through the metatarsal heads. The first metatarsal is shorter and wider than the lesser metatarsals, but bears approximately one third of body weight through the tibial and fibular sesamoids. The tibialis anterior tendon generates varus, supination, and elevation moments, whereas the peroneus longus generates valgus, pronation, and depression. The lesser metatarsals are bound to each other by the intermetatarsal ligaments and bear the remaining two thirds of body weight in an equal distribution (one sixth of the body weight each). Recent examination of the cross-sectional geometry of the forefoot determined that the second through fourth metatarsals are the weakest in most cross-sectional geometric properties.[17]

Mechanism of Injury

The second metatarsal experiences high peak pressures that may explain the higher incidence of stress fractures in this metatarsal, and to a lesser extent, the third metatarsal. Injurious forces applied to the forefoot can be direct or indirect. Direct forces, such as those incurred from industrial accidents, motor vehicle collisions, or applied heavy loads are often associated with marked soft-tissue injury.

Radiographic Evaluation

Most acute metatarsal injuries are diagnosed using initial plain radiographic foot trauma imaging studies (AP, oblique, and lateral views). Imaging of the contralateral foot is occasionally useful for comparison. CT scanning is infrequently required.

Treatment

Treatment principles for metatarsal fractures are directed at maintaining even weight distribution. Because of the importance of the metatarsals in weight bearing, most displaced first metatarsal shaft fractures require open reduction and stabilization. Plate and screw constructs are typically used. Nondisplaced fractures can be treated nonsurgically with rigid immobilization and a period of no weight bearing. Displaced fractures of the first metatarsal base are articular injuries that typically require ORIF to maintain integrity of medial column length and alignment, and to decrease posttraumatic arthritic changes. Depending on the degree of comminution, fixation may span the first tarsometatarsal articulation and can be permanent or temporary.

Minimally displaced fractures of the lesser metatarsals (whether affecting single or multiple metatarsals) can usually be treated symptomatically. A recent randomized trial compared cast immobilization with the use of an elastic tubular wrap for these injuries.[18] Both groups were encouraged to weight bear as tolerated. The authors found higher functional outcomes, less pain during treatment, and the absence of complications associated with treatment at 3 months after injury in the group treated with the elastic tubular wrap.

Displaced metatarsal shaft and neck fractures, particularly those with angulation in the sagittal plane, can result in transfer metatarsalgia with dorsal angulation or increased load at the affected metatarsal head with plantar angulation. Treatment options for these injuries include closed manipulation, intramedullary K-wire stabilization, K-wire fixation of the distal segment to an adjacent intact metatarsal, and ORIF with dorsal plating.

Fractures of the Proximal Fifth Metatarsal

Fractures of the proximal aspect of the fifth metatarsal are classified into three zones.[19] Zone 1 fractures occur through the cancellous bone of the tuberosity. The mechanism of injury is inversion causing an avulsion of the peroneus brevis tendon insertion and/or the lateral portion of the plantar aponeurosis. Zone 1 injuries comprise approximately 93% of all proximal fifth metatarsal fractures. Patients are allowed to bear weight as tolerated in a firm or hard-soled shoe. Because of the excellent blood supply to the bone in this area, these fractures heal readily with symptomatic treatment only.[20]

Zone 2 fractures are distal to the tuberosity and extend into the fourth to fifth intermetatarsal articulation. A vascular watershed area has been documented in this region, and is likely responsible for the increased rate of fracture nonunion in this area. Acutely diagnosed fractures are appropriately treated nonsurgically with short leg cast immobilization. Weight bearing is controversial, with reports of increased nonunion associated with early weight bearing.[21] Surgical treatment typically consists of antegrade medullary screw fixation. Surgical treatment can be considered in the acute setting for an elite-level athlete or a worker who requires rapid mobilization, or in instances of delayed union or nonunion of the fracture. In these latter situations, screw fixation is accompanied with open bone grafting. Postoperative weight-bearing restrictions are important for the success of this procedure

Zone 3 fractures occur in the distal metadiaphysis and are usually stress fractures. These injuries often have a delayed presentation and are associated with nonunion. When acutely diagnosed, the patient can be treated nonsurgically with short leg cast immobilization for 6 to 8 weeks, or occasionally longer. Weight bearing is controversial.[22] In situations where the acute presentation shows a previous nonunion, surgical treatment is recommended. Most patients can be treated with medullary screw fixation.

Annotated References

1. Chandran P, Puttaswamaiah R, Dhillon MS, Gill SS: Management of complex open fracture injuries of the midfoot with external fixation. *J Foot Ankle Surg* 2006; 45:308-315.

   The authors report on 11 feet with severe, high-velocity, open injuries to the midfoot treated with external fixation. The mean patient age was 38 years. All patients experienced stiffness at the midfoot and restriction of subtalar and forefoot motion. These results suggest that crush injuries to the midfoot often result in persistent morbidity despite early comprehensive treatment with external fixation. Level of evidence: IV.

2. Myerson MS, McGarvey WC, Henderson MR, Hakim J: Morbidity after crush injuries to the foot. *J Orthop Trauma* 1994;8:343-349.

3. Stein RE: Radiological aspects of the tarsometatarsal joints. *Foot Ankle* 1983;3:286-289.

4. Faciszewski T, Burks RT, Manaster BJ: Subtle injuries of the Lisfranc joint. *J Bone Joint Surg Am* 1990;72: 1519-1522.

5. Haapamaki V, Kiuru M, Koskinen S: Lisfranc fracture-dislocation in patients with multiple trauma: Diagnosis with multidetector computed tomography. *Foot Ankle Int* 2004;25:614-619.

   This study assessed acute phase multidetector CT findings of Lisfranc's fracture-dislocations in multiple trauma patients. The authors concluded that multidetector CT with high-quality multiplanar reconstruction is a complementary examination to plain radiography in multiply injured patients or in patients with equivocal radiographic findings. This imaging modality may reveal Lisfranc's fracture-dislocations, show the extent of the fracture-dislocation, and may show occult fractures in other parts of the foot and ankle. Level of evidence: IV.

6. Lee CA, Birkedal JP, Dickerson EA, Vieta PA Jr, Webb LX, Teasdall RD: Stabilization of Lisfranc joint injuries: A biomechanical study. *Foot Ankle Int* 2004;25:365-370.

   This cadaveric biomechanical study evaluated three fixation techniques: (1) four Kirschner wires; (2) three cortical screws plus two Kirschner wires; and (3) five cortical screws. An unstable tarsometatarsal injury was created, then reduced and stabilized with one of the three methods. The authors demonstrated that cortical screw fixation provided a more rigid and stable method of fixation for Lisfranc injuries compared with Kirschner wire fixation.

7. Arntz CT, Veith RG, Hansen ST Jr: Fractures and fracture-dislocations of the tarsometatarsal joint. *J Bone Joint Surg Am* 1988;70:173-181.

8. Hardcastle PH, Reschauer R, Kutscha-Lissberg E, Schoffmann W: Injuries to the tarsometatarsal joint: Incidence, classification and treatment. *J Bone Joint Surg Br* 1982;64:349-356.

9. Kuo RS, Tejwani NC, Digiovanni CW, et al: Outcome after open reduction and internal fixation of Lisfranc joint injuries. *J Bone Joint Surg Am* 2000;82-A:1609-1618.

10. Ly TV, Coetzee JC: Treatment of primarily ligamentous Lisfranc joint injuries: Primary arthrodesis compared with open reduction and internal fixation. A prospective, randomized study. *J Bone Joint Surg Am* 2006;88: 514-520.

    Using validated functional outcome measures, this randomized controlled trial compared acute medial column arthrodesis with traditional ORIF for purely ligamentous Lisfranc's injuries. The authors concluded that a primary stable arthrodesis of the medial two or three rays appears to have better short- and medium-term outcome than ORIF of ligamentous Lisfranc's joint complex injuries. Level of evidence: I.

11. Mulier T, Reynders P, Dereymaeker G, Broos P: Severe Lisfrancs injuries: Primary arthrodesis or ORIF? *Foot Ankle Int* 2002;23:902-905.

12. Schildhauer TA, Nork SE, Sangeorzan BJ: Temporary bridge plating of the medial column in severe midfoot injuries. *J Orthop Trauma* 2003;17:513-520.

13. Miller CM, Winter WG, Bucknell AL, Jonassen EA: Injuries to the midtarsal joint and lesser tarsal bones. *J Am Acad Orthop Surg* 1998;6:249-258.

14. Sangeorzan BJ, Benirschke SK, Mosca V, Mayo KA, Hansen ST Jr: Displaced intra-articular fractures of the tarsal navicular. *J Bone Joint Surg Am* 1989;71:1504-1510.

15. Miller TT, Pavlov H, Gupta M, Schultz E, Greben C: Isolated injury of the cuboid bone. *Emerg Radiol* 2002; 9:272-277.

16. Sangeorzan BJ, Swiontkowski MF: Displaced fractures of the cuboid. *J Bone Joint Surg Br* 1990;72:376-378.

    The authors report on four cases of fracture of the cuboid treated by ORIF and bone grafting where neces-

4: Lower Extremity

sary. The preliminary results were better than those previously reported for conservative treatment or for later midtarsal fusion. The authors emphasized articular incongruence and lateral column length as surgical indications. Level of evidence: III.

17. Griffin NL, Richmond BG: Cross-sectional geometry of the human forefoot. *Bone* 2005;37:253-260.

This study systematically examined the cross-sectional geometric properties of the human forefoot and their relationship to external loads using CT scans and published plantar pressure data sets recorded during a variety of functional activities. The authors identified that the discrepancy between strength and plantar pressure values in metatarsals 2 and 3 is consistent with the high incidence of stress fractures in these bones and underscores the importance of soft tissues, such as the plantar fascia and flexor musculature, in moderating metatarsal shaft strain.

18. Zenios M, Kim WY, Sampath J, Muddu BN: Functional treatment of acute metatarsal fractures: A prospective randomised comparison of management in a cast versus elasticated support bandage. *Injury* 2005;36:832-835.

A randomized, controlled trial was performed in 50 patients with acute isolated minimally displaced lesser metatarsal fractures to compare plaster immobilization with treatment using an elastic support bandage. Patients treated with an elastic support bandage had significantly higher American Orthopaedic Foot and Ankle Society midfoot scores at 3-month follow-up and reported less pain throughout the treatment period. There was no difference between the two groups in time to independent mobility, midfoot circumference, analgesic requirements, and radiologic union at 3 months. Because plaster casts are associated with serious complications, which occurred during this study, the authors concluded that minimally displaced metatarsal fractures are better treated without a cast. Level of evidence: II.

19. Dameron TB Jr: Fractures of the proximal fifth metatarsal: Selecting the best treatment option. *J Am Acad Orthop Surg* 1995;3:110-114.

20. Dameron TB Jr: Fractures and anatomical variations of the proximal portion of the fifth metatarsal. *J Bone Joint Surg Am* 1975;57:788-792.

21. Torg JS: Fractures of the base of the fifth metatarsal distal to the tuberosity. *Orthopedics* 1990;13:731-737.

22. Larson CM, Almekinders LC, Taft TN, Garrett WE: Intramedullary screw fixation of Jones fractures: Analysis of failure. *Am J Sports Med* 2002;30:55-60.

Chapter 40

Ankle and Hindfoot Trauma

Sean E. Nork, MD   David P. Barei, MD

Ankle Fractures

Evaluation and Classification

Knowledge of both the mechanism of injury and the resultant fracture pattern are important for determining the necessary reduction maneuvers and treatment for ankle fractures. Injuries caused by torsional or bending forces must be distinguished from those caused by axial loading. Ankle instability results from loss of associated osseous and ligamentous supports that constrain the talus in the mortise. Abnormal translation of the talus relative to the tibia results in ankle arthritis and a poor functional result.

The evaluation of the medial soft tissues and radiographic parameters for predicting injury patterns and the need for surgical stabilization have been a focus of several recent studies. Deltoid ligament injury has been assessed with stress radiographs, a gravity stress view, and physical examination of the medial ankle. In cadaver specimens, a medial clear space of 5 mm or more with an external rotation stress test applied to a dorsiflexed ankle was predictive of deep deltoid disruption.[1] However, medial tenderness, ecchymosis, and swelling were poor predictors of deltoid integrity in a study using stress radiographs to confirm lateral talar shift.[2] This finding was confirmed by a study of patients with isolated fibular fractures evaluated clinically and radiographically. Of 65 patients with a positive stress test, 30 patients did not have clinical signs of medial injury. However, the authors found that in patients with a positive stress test but no clinical symptoms of a medial injury, nonsurgical treatment was associated with good results.[3] Despite the superiority of stress radiographs compared with physical examination to confirm medial ligamentous injury and lateral shift of the talus, the indications for surgical stabilization in these patients remain unclear.

Ankle fractures are classified mechanistically and/or radiographically. The well-known Lauge-Hansen classification for ankle fractures specifies four categories of injuries based on foot position and the direction of the applied force (**Figure 1**). Each category describes the pattern of injury and is further divided into several stages based on the theorized sequential disruption of the associated osseous and ligamentous supports of the ankle joint. The most common pattern is the supination-external rotation injury. Despite its name, the actual mechanism and force application is probably reversed when these fractures occur. That is, the foot is firmly planted on the ground, and the tibia internally rotates. The structures that are sequentially injured are the anterior capsule and anterior tibiofibular ligament (stage 1), followed by a spiral (or oblique) fracture of the fibula (stage 2), followed by a disruption of the posterior capsule or posterior malleolus (stage 3), followed by the medial injury, which is either a tear of the deltoid ligament or a transverse medial malleolus fracture (stage 4). The other categories of injury similarly incorporate progressive stages of injury. Although the Lauge-Hansen classification system attempts to categorize and predict injury patterns, its accuracy has been questioned. In one study, MRI was used to analyze the associated soft-tissue injuries in surgically treated ankle fractures and failed to predict the observed ligamentous injury in more than one half of the fractures.[4] Although the Lauge-Hansen system has been used extensively for guidance in the treatment of ankle fractures, reliance on the system and findings from plain radiographs may not be optimal.

Another commonly used and simple anatomic classification system is that of Danis and Weber/AO and is based solely on the location of the fibular fracture (**Figure 2**). Type A fractures occur below the level of the tibial plafond, type B fractures begin at the level of the ankle joint, and type C fractures occur above the level of the plafond. Injuries to the syndesmosis occur with increasing frequency as the level of the fibular fracture occurs more proximally. As a general rule, most Weber/AO type A fractures are not associated with ankle joint instability and can be treated nonsurgically. However, many Weber/AO type B and C fractures are associated with ankle joint instability and require surgical stabilization.

Syndesmosis Injuries

Injuries to the distal tibiofibular syndesmosis are varied and complex. Although certain associated fracture patterns are commonly observed, injury to the syndesmosis should be suspected and specifically evaluated in all ankle fractures, deltoid ligament tears, proximal fibular fractures, proximal tibiofibular disruptions, and ankle sprains. The squeeze test, direct palpation of the syndesmosis, and stress testing have all been recommended and used to evaluate injuries to the syndesmosis. Radiographic parameters commonly used to suggest injury to the syndesmosis include the level of the fibular fracture relative to the joint, and loss of the normal re-

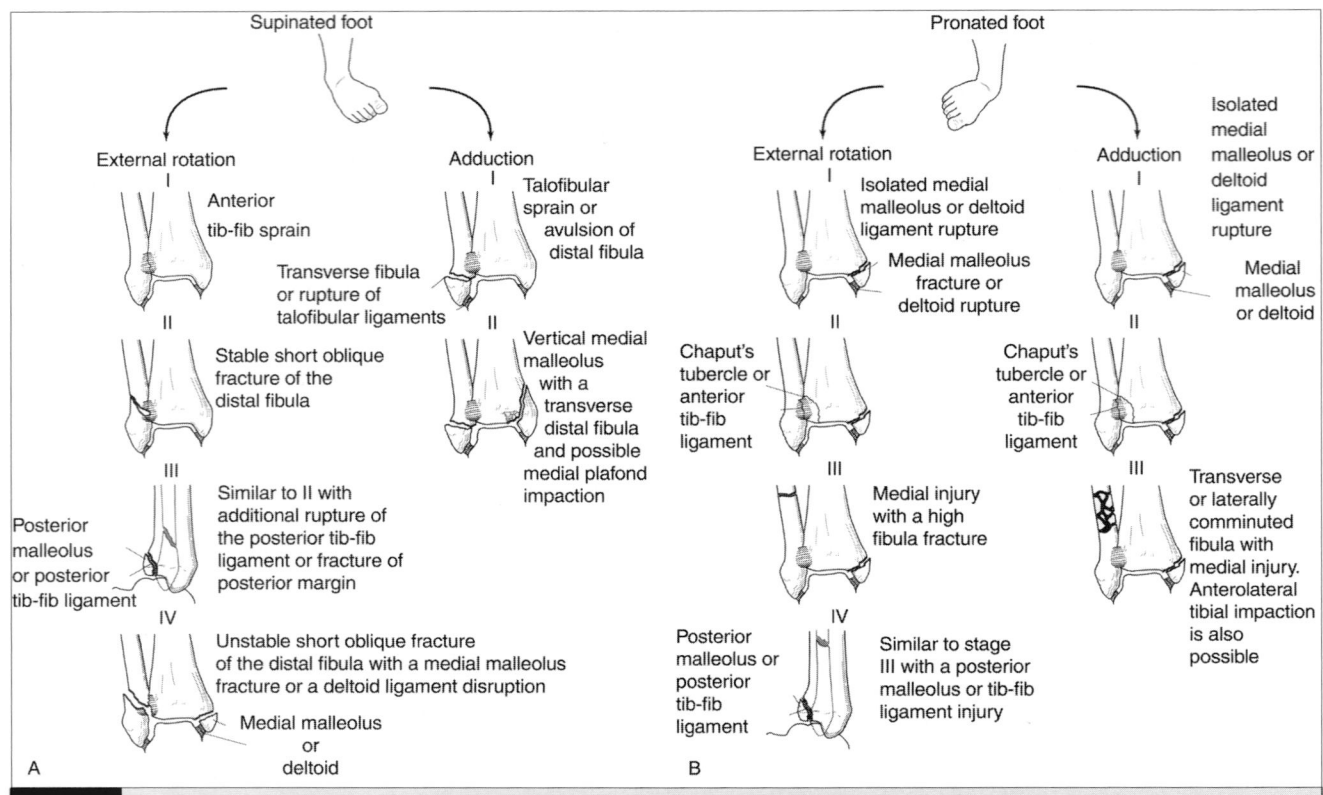

Figure 1 **A,** Schematic diagram and case examples of Lauge-Hansen supination-external rotation and supination-adduction ankle fractures. A supinated foot sustains either an external rotation or adduction force and creates the successive stages of injury shown in the diagram. The supination-external rotation mechanism has four stages of injury, and the supination-adduction mechanism has two stages. tib-fib = tibiofibular. **B,** Schematic diagram and case examples of Lauge-Hansen pronation-external rotation and pronation-abduction ankle fractures. A pronated foot sustains either an external rotation or abduction force and creates the successive stages of injury shown in the diagram. The pronation-external rotation mechanism has four stages of injury, and the pronation-abduction mechanism has three stages. tib-fib = tibiofibular. *(Reproduced with permission from Marsh JL, Saltzman CL: Ankle fractures, in Bucholz RW, Heckman JD (eds): Rockwood and Green's Fractures in Adults, ed 5. Philadelphia, PA, Lippincott William & Wilkins, 2001, pp 2001-2090.)*

lationship between the fibula and the tibia. Fibular fractures above the level of the ankle joint (especially 4.5 cm or more above the joint) are more commonly associated with syndesmotic instability. This is especially true in injury patterns with a deltoid ligament disruption. However, injury to the syndesmosis can occur regardless of the level and location of the fibular fracture. Regardless of the results of the physical examination or the radiographic test used, the syndesmosis should be adequately evaluated because missed or untreated injuries are associated with extremely poor results. CT is valuable if findings from the physical examination and plain radiography are inconclusive. Several recent studies have contributed to a better understanding of these injuries. In a study of 15 patients with pronation-external rotation fracture patterns associated with a posterior malleolar fracture who were evaluated with radiographs and MRI, no posteroinferior talofibular ligament injuries were observed despite widening of the ankle joint and findings of syndesmotic injury.[5] In a study evaluating standard plain radiographic measurements and MRI results, the authors found that a

medial clear space of greater than 4 mm was correlated with disruption of the deltoid and tibiofibular ligaments, but there was no correlation between syndesmotic injury and either tibiofibular clear space or overlap measurements.[6] Other authors have confirmed the usefulness of intraoperative fluoroscopic stress testing to evaluate the syndesmosis.[7]

Treatment of syndesmotic instability includes an accurate reduction of the distal tibiofibular joint and stabilization. The length, translation, and rotation of the fibula must be accurately restored, as well as its relationship with the tibial incisura. Open reduction is necessary if closed reduction is questionable or unsuccessful. Screw placement is directed from posterior to anterior by 20° to 30°, and is ideally located 2 to 4 cm above the ankle joint. Intraoperative stress testing should be performed with forced external rotation of the foot or by grasping the fibula with a towel clip if syndesmotic integrity is questionable. The ideal fixation for syndesmosis injuries has not been determined. There is controversy regarding the implant material (stainless steel versus titanium versus bioabsorbable material), the size of the implant (3.5 mm versus 4.5 mm screws), the number of cortices engaged by the implant (three versus four cortices), the location of the screw(s) relative to the tibial plafond, and the number of screws used (one versus two). Biomechanical studies have shown no difference between stainless and titanium implants, stainless and bioabsorbable implants, and the number of cortices engaged. Although 4.5-mm screws are stronger than 3.5-mm screws placed through four cortices, the minimum strength necessary to maintain the reduction of the syndesmosis is unknown. Because fixation with syndesmosis screws is inadequate to support weight-bearing loads, activity modifications until healing are indicated.[8] In a prospective and randomized study comparing metallic and bioabsorbable screws, the polylevolactic acid implants were associated with an improved return to activities, less swelling, and similar joint motion and ankle reduction compared with metallic implants.[9] Although further study is necessary before bioabsorbable implants can be recommended, some evidence supports their use.

The impact of fixation strategies for combined injuries of the posterior malleolus and the syndesmosis in pronation-external rotation fracture patterns has been studied.[5] Stiffness was restored to 70% of the uninjured ankle after fixation of the posterior malleolus, but to only 40% after syndesmotic fixation. Although this result indicates that attention to the posterior malleolus may be more effective than syndesmotic fixation, intraoperative assessment of the syndesmosis is necessary even after posterior malleolar fixation.

Controversy continues regarding the need for fibula fixation in high fibular fractures associated with syndesmotic disruption. One strategy is to forgo fibular fracture reduction and fixation, and to rely solely on the fixation of the fibula to the tibia using syndesmotic screw fixation. However, achieving proper length and rotation of the fibula may be difficult to accomplish and assess by relying on intraoperative radiographic estimation at the ankle joint. Another strategy is to accurately fix the fibula fracture to restore the proper fibular length and rotation, which is then followed by a more predictable reduction and fixation of the distal tibiofibular joint. The strategy chosen is probably less important than the accuracy of the reduction of the syndesmosis. Outcomes after injury to the syndesmosis are dependent on several factors including maintenance of reduction, accuracy of reduction, and the associated injuries at the ankle joint. In a retrospective study of 51 patients with syndesmotic injuries, the only predictor related to outcome was the reduction of the syndesmosis.[10] Cadaver and radiographic studies have shown that ankle dorsiflexion during fixation of an accurately reduced syndesmosis is unnecessary, and overtightening of the reduced syndesmosis is not possible. Few other factors have an influence on functional outcomes. However, in a prospective, randomized study comparing tricortical and quadricortical syndesmotic fixation in 64 patients fixed with either a 4.5-mm screw placed through four cortices or two 3.5-mm screws placed through three cortices, better function was observed at

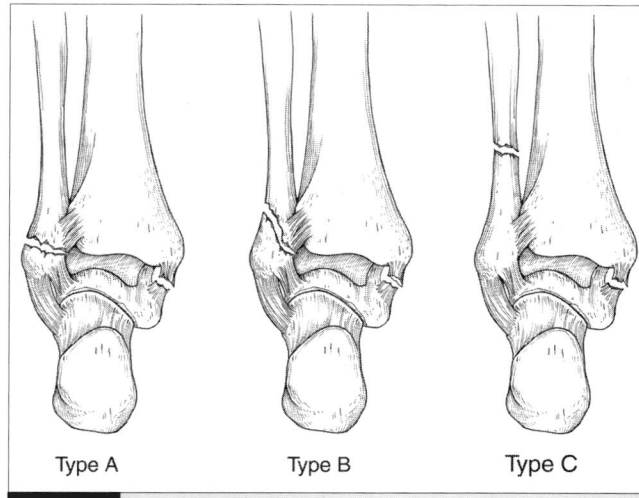

Figure 2 Weber/AO fractures. The staging is completely determined by the level of fibular fracture. Type A occurs below the plafond, type B fractures begin at the level of the ankle joint, and type C starts above the plafond. *(Reproduced from Michelson JD: Ankle fractures resulting from rotational injuries. J Am Acad Orthop Surg 2003;11:403-412.)*

3 months in the group treated with the tricortical screw fixation.[11] No difference in ankle dorsiflexion, loss of fixation, or function at 1 year was observed between the two groups. Given the multiple variables simultaneously evaluated, no recommendation can be made based on these data. The timing and need for syndesmotic screw removal remains controversial. If screw removal is planned, this should be delayed for 8 to 12 weeks to allow for adequate healing of the syndesmotic ligaments. If syndesmotic screws are not removed prior to weight bearing, screw breakage (in screws placed through four cortices) or screw loosening in the tibia (in screws placed through three cortices) is common. The impact of screw loosening or breakage is unknown but is likely of minimal consequence.

Lateral Malleolus Fractures

Fractures of the lateral malleolus below the level of the ankle joint (Weber/AO type A fractures) typically do not result in ankle instability; surgical stabilization of the fibula is not usually indicated. However, the associated medial-sided injury should be independently evaluated and may require treatment. Lateral malleolar fractures at the level of the ankle joint (Weber/AO type B fractures) are the most common type of ankle fracture and treatment is dependent on numerous factors including the presence of medial injury, the integrity of the syndesmosis, and the presence of talar shift relative to the distal tibia. Lateral shift of the talus is associated with altered ankle joint mechanics and is an indication for reduction and fixation. The evaluation of these injuries radiographically and with stress testing has been described. Open reduction and internal fixation of the lat-

4: Lower Extremity

eral malleolus typically consists of plate fixation. This can be accomplished with either a posterior antiglide plate, a lateral neutralization plate combined with a lag screw, or lag screws alone. Lag screw fixation in isolation should be limited to oblique or spiral fracture patterns without comminution that allow multiple screw placements at least 1 cm apart. Plate placement posteriorly is biomechanically superior to lateral plate placement; this technique may minimize hardware irritation.[12] However, to avoid peroneal irritation, extremely distal plate applications and prominent distal screws should be avoided.[13] For fibular fractures above the level of the ankle joint caused by an indirect mechanism (Weber/AO type C fractures), surgical stabilization of the fibular and/or the syndesmosis is usually indicated.

Posterior Malleolar Fractures

Fractures of the posterior malleolus may occur in isolation or, more commonly, in association with bimalleolar and trimalleolar patterns. A recent study showed posterior malleolar fractures in 25% of patients with tibial shaft fractures. Approximately one half of these fractures were initially undiagnosed despite being apparent on later review of the injury radiographs.[14] The posterior malleolus is the attachment for the posterior talofibular ligament and is important for maintaining the stability and reduction of the ankle joint. The decision to treat a fracture of the posterior malleolus has traditionally been determined by the size of the fragment. It is usually recommended that fractures involving less than 25% of the tibial plafond can be treated nonsurgically. However, this recommendation is based on the lateral plain radiographic view that is known to be inaccurate for estimating the size of the fragment as has been determined by CT scans. Several recent studies have provided information for understanding the fracture configuration and size of posterior malleolar fractures associated with ankle injuries. In one study, the posterolateral oblique fracture was the most common pattern (67%), with medial extension fractures (19%) and small-shell fractures (14%) comprising the remaining patterns.[15] The posterolateral oblique fractures were 12% of the total tibial plafond whereas those with medial extension were much larger (30%). Based on these findings, and with the knowledge that lateral radiographs are inaccurate for estimating the size of the posterior malleolar fracture fragments, CT scanning is indicated for many posterior malleolar fractures.[15] Specific information regarding the fracture pattern, the associated impaction, and surgical strategies for use in some trimalleolar fractures were outlined in a study examining trimalleolar ankle fractures with involvement of the posteromedial plafond.[16]

Small posterior malleolar fractures can be treated without surgery assuming that stable fixation of the other components of the ankle can be achieved. Good long-term outcomes have been documented.[17] As the fragment size increases, an accurate restoration of the anatomy is necessary to maintain the stability and con-

gruency of the ankle. The exact size and configuration of the fracture that requires surgical stabilization has not been determined; however, a biomechanical study has shown a shift in the contact stresses anteriorly and medially in a fracture model with a large posterior malleolar fracture.[18] The authors did not identify talar subluxation in their model.

Bimalleolar and Trimalleolar Fractures

In patients without surgical contraindications, most displaced bimalleolar ankle fractures require surgical stabilization of both malleoli. Careful evaluation for associated syndesmotic injury should always follow stabilization. Timing of surgery depends on the associated soft-tissue swelling, but early fixation is preferred. For injuries with a displaced fibular fracture and associated deltoid ligament disruption, deltoid ligament repair is not indicated; only fixation of the lateral injury and syndesmosis are necessary. In some situations, the deltoid ligament may be entrapped in the medial joint and requires attention before fixation of the lateral malleolus. Trimalleolar ankle fractures similarly require surgical fixation of the medial and lateral sides. Supplementary fixation of the posterior malleolus depends on fragment size, the level and fixation of the fibular fracture, and the presence of an associated syndesmotic disruption. Treatment strategies for posterior malleolar reduction and fixation include percutaneous clamp reduction, reduction of large fractures through the medial malleolar fracture, and direct reduction through a posterolateral or posteromedial exposure. The advantage of an open exposure is the ability to accurately reduce the fracture and to place a plate posteriorly, thereby minimizing the risk of late displacement. This technique is preferred in large fractures of the posterior malleolus.

Treatment: Outcomes and Results

In a prospective observational study of patients with unstable Weber/AO type B ankle fractures treated surgically, significant limitations were found even 2 years after treatment. Worse outcomes were associated primarily with patient factors such as smoking, less education, alcohol use, and older age, and with the presence of a medial malleolar fracture.[19] Early weight bearing after open reduction and internal fixation was associated with no negative effects and is recommended for compliant patients.[20] Finally, in a prospective, randomized study of 54 patients to evaluate tourniquet use during surgery, the use of a tourniquet was associated with increased postoperative swelling but no improvement in surgical time.[21]

Distal Tibial Pilon Fractures

Etiology

Distal tibial pilon fractures typically result from high-energy mechanisms such as a motor vehicle crash or fall from a height; however, lower-energy mechanisms can cause torsional injuries with extension into the ankle joint. Articular fractures involve the weight-bearing surface of the distal tibia, thereby distinguishing these injuries from ankle fractures. An important aspect of these injuries is the associated soft-tissue injury in an anatomic region that requires meticulous handling of the tissues.

Evaluation and Classification
Initial management should include careful assessment of the soft tissues, limb realignment, and radiographic confirmation of the position of the foot relative to the tibia. Radiographs include standard ankle views as well as imaging of the entire tibia. Although CT scans are indicated in virtually all articular fractures of the tibial pilon, the timing of the scans should be based on the overall treatment plan for the injury. If a staged protocol with temporary spanning fixation and delayed open reduction is planned, the information obtained from the CT scan is maximized after length is restored. In injuries where immediate or early fixation of some or the entire articular surface is planned, injury CT scans may be helpful.

Classification according to the Ruedi and Allgower system is simplistic and divides fractures based on increasing displacement and comminution.[22] The alphanumeric AO/Orthopaedic Trauma Association classification system is more detailed but studies have failed to show interobserver reliability beyond a moderate level. Of equal importance as the bony injury is appreciation of the associated soft-tissue injury that occurs with each fracture. One recent study noted consistent fracture patterns in the sagittal and coronal planes.[23] Other studies have attempted to gain further understanding of the association between fracture energy absorption and prognosis by quantifying bone comminution.

Treatment
Well-defined principles of treatment according to Ruedi and Allgower[22] include restoration of length by fibular fixation, anatomic reduction of the tibial articular surface, bone grafting of metaphyseal defects, and medial buttress plating to prevent varus.[2-4] Despite poor early results after open reduction, components of these tenets remain valuable for many current treatment strategies for these injuries.

Options for definitive treatment include nonsurgical methods, spanning external fixation, combined limited internal and external fixation, nonspanning external fixation, immediate open reduction and internal fixation, a staged protocol, or a combination of these treatments. Regardless of the option chosen, treatment goals should include accurate restoration of the articular anatomy, restoration of the limb axis in all planes, and minimization of complications. A staged protocol is applicable for most tibial pilon fractures treated by an experienced fracture surgeon. This protocol involves initial fixation of the fibula (if applicable) with temporary ankle spanning external fixation, followed by definitive fixation of the articular surface as allowed by the soft-tissue envelope, typically at 10 to 25 days from injury (**Figure 3**). Good results with acceptable soft-tissue complications have been reported with this technique.[24]

External fixation combined with techniques of internal fixation have been described and advocated for injuries with significant soft-tissue compromise; however, one multicenter, nonrandomized, retrospective study showed that the use of external fixation was the only surgical variable associated with a poorer overall functional outcome.[24] Definitive internal fixation can be performed through anteromedial, anterolateral, posterolateral, and posteromedial surgical exposures or a combination of such exposures. Definitive internal fixation should be of adequate strength to allow unrestricted ankle and subtalar joint range-of-motion exercises. Weight bearing following internal fixation of tibial pilon fractures should be delayed 12 weeks to allow adequate healing.

Complications and Determinants of Outcome
Articular fractures of the distal tibia and associated treatment have numerous potential complications including wound dehiscence, infection, nonunion, malunion, and posttraumatic arthritis. Deep infection has been minimized with the use of a staged protocol consisting of initial spanning external fixation followed by delayed open reduction and internal fixation, with overall rates of infection varying from 0% to 10%. Hybrid external fixation was introduced in an attempt to minimize some of the complications associated with internal fixation of pilon fractures; however, higher rates of complications including nonunions, malunions, and infections have been reported with this method of treatment.[25]

More recently, several studies have evaluated factors associated with outcomes and long-term results following tibial pilon fractures. The posterolateral approach, although potentially useful for some components of reduction and fixation, was shown to have high complication rates and poor reduction results similar to those of a single approach.[26] Another study found that the accuracy of reduction predicted subsequent radiographic arthrosis; however, this finding was not correlated with outcome. Instead, outcome was predicted more accurately by the educational level of the patient and whether the injury was work related.[27] A comprehensive outcomes analysis showed that low income, minimal education, multiple comorbidities, and treatment with external fixation were significantly related to poorer results.[24] A long-term outcomes study (average follow-up of 10 years) after internal fixation of intra-articular and extra-articular pilon fractures found worse outcomes in more severe fracture patterns, those that did not have fibular fixation, open fractures, and fractures with poor reduction.[28] In a study of 56 pilon fractures treated with a combination of ankle spanning external fixation and percutaneous articular fixation, five patients required arthrodesis within 2 years. Most of the remaining patients who were followed for a minimum of 5 years had evidence of ankle arthritis and had limitations in their ability to participate in recreational activities. However, patients perceived improvement for more than 2 years after injury and secondary reconstructive procedures were rare.[29]

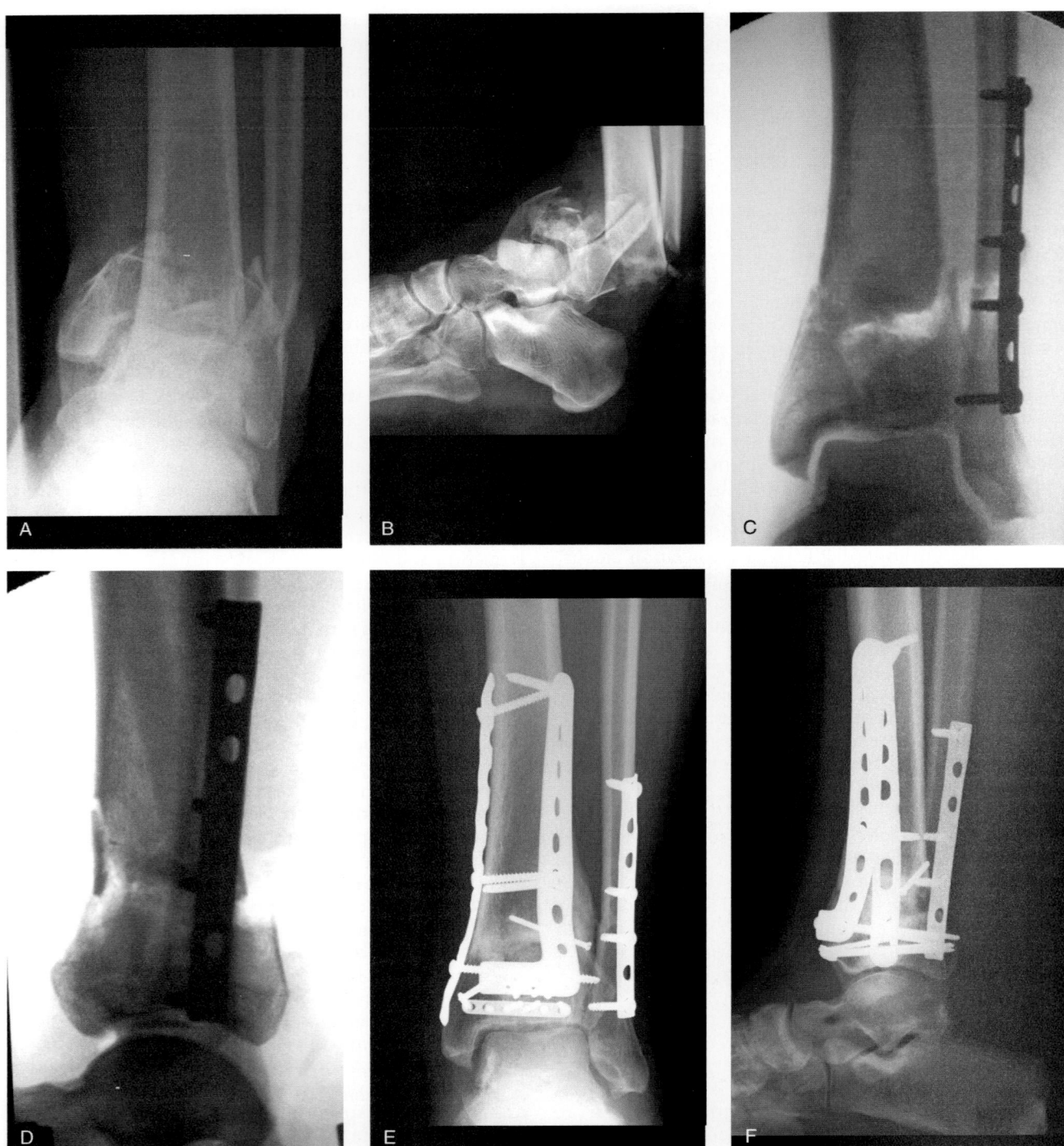

Figure 3   AP **(A)** and lateral **(B)** radiographs show the comminution and foot position in a severe, open pilon fracture. Fibular fixation combined with ankle spanning external fixation allows soft-tissue recovery, centers the talus beneath the articular surface, and allows CT scanning for a better understanding of the fracture. **C**, Mortise view. **D**, Lateral view. Open reduction and internal fixation was delayed for 23 days to allow soft-tissue recovery. AP **(E)** and lateral **(F)** radiographs at 1 year show healing in a reasonable position but with some evidence of joint space narrowing.

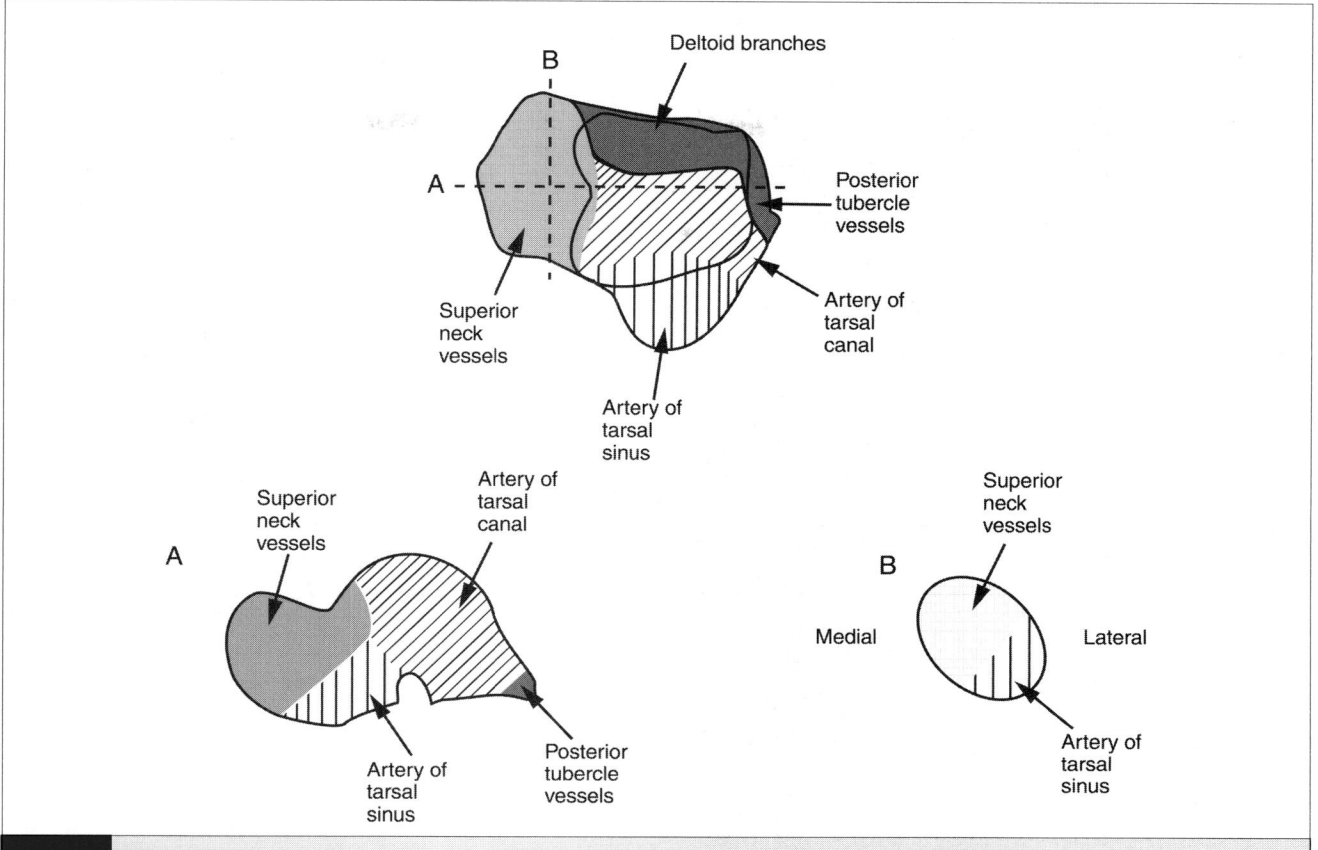

Figure 4 | The locations of the contributions to the talar blood supply from the vessels of the ankle. *(Adapted with permission from Gelberman RH, Morensen WW: The arterial anatomy of the talus.* Foot Ankle *1983;4:64-72.)*

Talus Fractures

Etiology and Classification

Because of its anatomic location and its multiple complex articulations, injuries to the talus and the subtalar joint potentially affect the ankle joint, the hindfoot, and the midfoot. Fractures and dislocations can result in significant functional impairment. An understanding of local anatomy, common injury patterns, and potential treatments can help to optimize long-term outcomes after injury.

The talus has no muscular or tendinous attachments and approximately 60% to 70% of its surface is covered in articular cartilage. Multiple articulations include those with the distal tibia, the distal fibula, the calcaneus, and the navicular. The neck of the talus deviates medially approximately 24°. Even minor varus deformity of the talus limits hindfoot eversion and produces forefoot adduction. The articular body of the talus is wider anteriorly than posteriorly; however, because the axis of rotation is not purely in the sagittal plane, the width of the talus that articulates with the ankle joint is relatively constant with dorsiflexion and plantar flexion. The blood supply to the talus is tenuous and is important when considering the effects of injury patterns and surgical treatment. The intraosseous

blood supply is inconsistent. The extraosseous blood supply comes from the three major vessels of the leg—the posterior tibial, the peroneal, and the dorsalis pedis arteries. The major blood supply is provided by the artery of the tarsal canal with minor contributions from the deltoid vessels, the sinus tarsi vessels, and the leash of vessels along the superior neck (**Figure 4**).

Multiple surgical approaches have been described for reduction and fixation of talar fractures. A dorsomedial approach (centered between the tibialis anterior and tibialis posterior tendons on the dorsomedial aspect of the foot) allows access to the medial talar neck and body. An anterolateral approach (in line with the fourth metatarsal, centered at the ankle joint, and lateral to the anterior compartment musculature and tendons) allows access to the lateral talar neck, the lateral talar body, and the lateral process of the talus. The posterolateral approach (between the peroneal tendons and the Achilles tendon /flexor hallucis longus) allows access to the posterolateral aspect of the talus for hardware placement. The posteromedial approach allows access to the posteromedial talus and the posterior process of the talus. An adjunctive medial malleolar osteotomy expands the potential visualization of the medial talus and may be useful for some talar body fractures.

Fractures to the talus are typically described or clas-

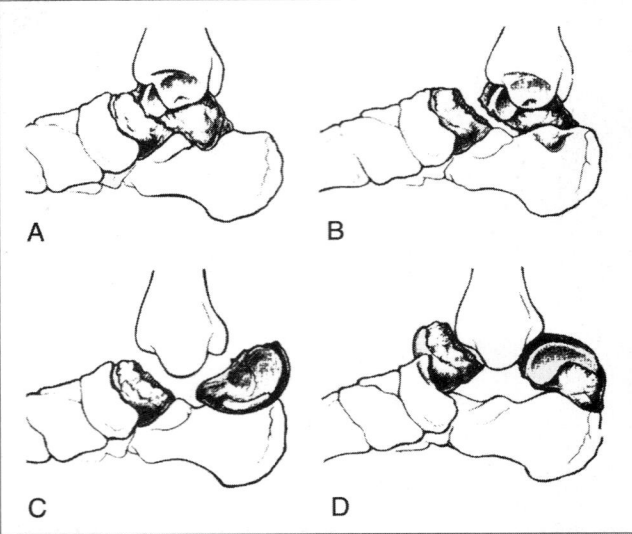

Figure 5 Hawkins classification. **A,** Type I: nondisplaced talar neck fractures. **B,** Type II: displaced talar neck fractures, with subluxation or dislocation of subtalar joint. **C,** Type III: displaced talar neck fractures with associated dislocation of talar body from both subtalar and tibiotalar joints. **D,** Canale and Kelly type IV: displaced talar neck fracture with associated dislocation of talar body from subtalar and tibiotalar joints and dislocation of head/neck fragment from talonavicular joint. *(Reproduced with permission from Sangeorzan BJ: Foot and ankle joint, in Hansen ST Jr, Swiontkowski MF (eds): Orthopaedic Trauma Protocols. New York, NY, Raven Press, 1993, p 350.)*

sified based on anatomic location and include injuries to the body, neck, head, lateral process, and posteromedial talus. Associated foot and ankle fractures commonly occur, especially in displaced neck or body fractures. Radiographic evaluation should include AP, lateral, and oblique views of the foot and three views of the ankle. A modified Canale view of the foot is obtained by internally rotating the foot 15° and angulating the radiographic beam 15° cephalad. This view profiles the neck of the talus and shows subtle subluxations and displacements. A CT scan with multiple reformations can be helpful for further defining fracture displacement, comminution, and articular subluxation.

Talar Neck Fractures

Talar neck fractures are the most common, resulting from forced dorsiflexion. Most talar neck fractures involve some portion of the subtalar joint. The position of the foot at the moment of impact determines the associated injuries, displacements, and comminution, which may include fracture of the medial malleolus, posteromedial displacement of the talar body, and dorsomedial comminution of the talar neck.

Talar neck fractures are classified based on the well-known Hawkins classification system as modified by Canale and Kelly (**Figure 5**). This classification system

may have implications for treatment, and has been shown to predict the incidence of subsequent osteonecrosis.

Treatment of talar neck fractures is dependent on multiple factors including fracture displacement, patient comorbidities, and any associated injuries. The major goal of treatment is to restore the normal anatomy of the talus so that early motion is possible. Subtle deviations and displacements of the talar neck can result in loss of subtalar joint motion and increases in subtalar joint contact pressures, possibly contributing to the development of subtalar joint arthritis. The timing of surgical treatment remains controversial, with multiple underpowered studies failing to establish a relationship between timing and subsequent complications.[30,31] However, associated open wounds, dislocations, and neurovascular compromise remain surgical urgencies or emergencies. An attempted closed reduction of Hawkins type II fracture patterns should be performed to restore the talar relationship to the ankle and the subtalar joint. This reduction is best accomplished with knee flexion (to relax the gastrocnemius), ankle plantar flexion, and manual distraction of the calcaneus.

Nondisplaced (type I) fractures can be managed in a non–weight-bearing, short leg cast for 6 to 12 weeks. Radiographs should be obtained frequently to confirm that subsequent displacement does not occur. Surgical treatment with internal fixation can be considered to avoid subsequent displacement of the talar neck and to allow early range of motion. In displaced type II, III, and IV fracture patterns, an open reduction is required to restore the anatomy of the talus. Simultaneous anterolateral and anteromedial surgical approaches are recommended to allow an accurate reduction. Because of the commonly observed dorsomedial comminution of the talar neck, the lateral and plantar aspects of the talus may show the optimal reduction. The anterolateral approach allows access to the subtalar joint for reduction and débridement of the subtalar joint. Dissection inferiorly and posteriorly on the medial talus should be avoided to limit the surgical insult to the remaining talar blood supply. A medial malleolar osteotomy can be performed to enhance visualization of the medial side, if indicated. Fixation can be accomplished laterally and medially. Typically, screws are countersunk and placed from the head of the talus posteriorly into the talar body. Depending on the location of any associated comminution, these screws may be placed in a static or compressive application. Plates may be added on the nonarticular portion of the lateral talar neck, thereby spanning the fracture (**Figure 6**). Clinically, the use of plates has been shown to be a successful technique. However, in a cadaver study simulating dorsal comminution, improved strength was found with the use of posterior to anterior screws compared with lateral plating combined with a single medial screw. The clinical conclusions of this study are limited because posterior to anterior fixation was accomplished with larger implants compared with those placed laterally and from anterior to posterior.[32]

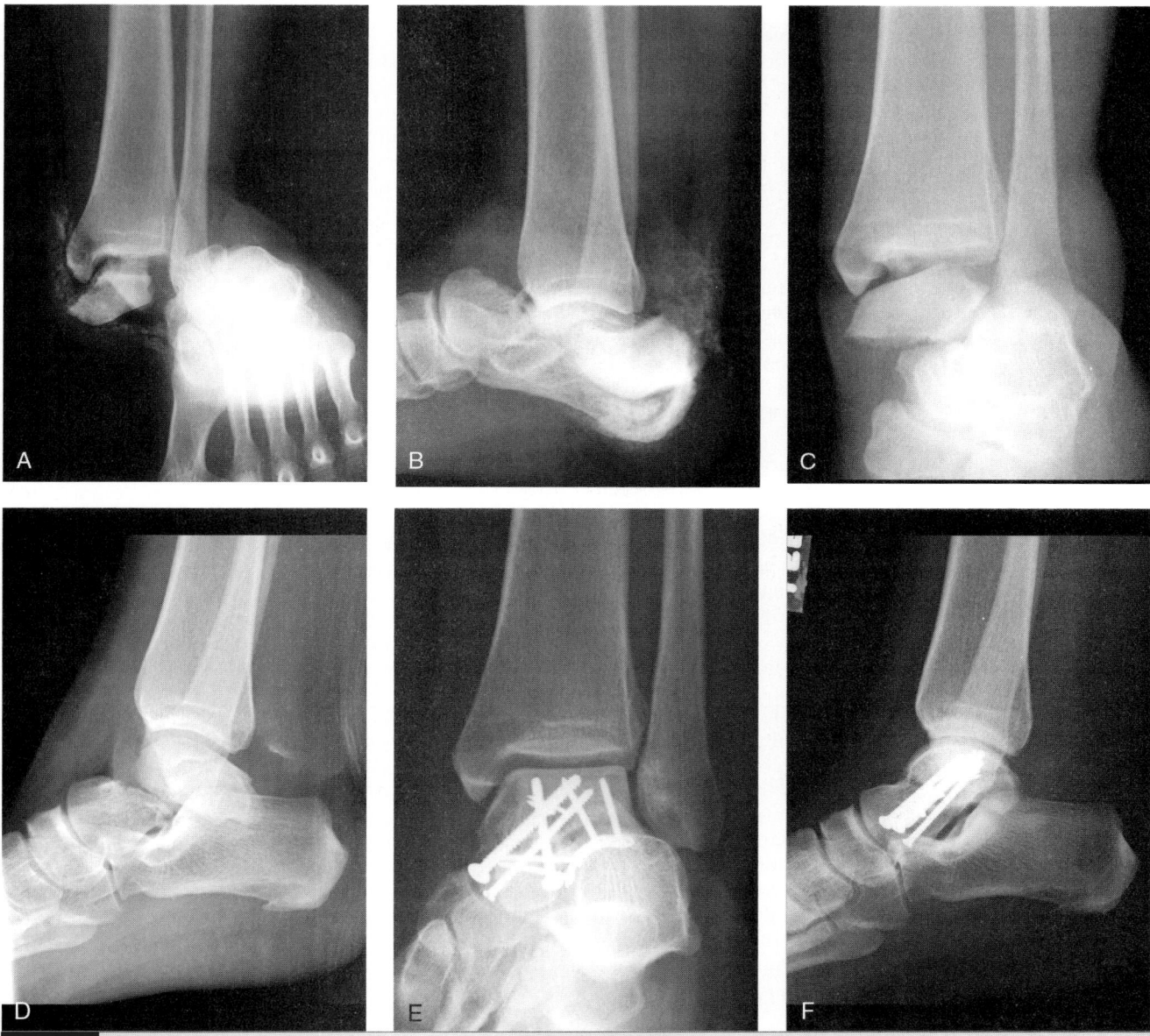

Figure 6 AP (**A**) and lateral (**B**) The injury radiographs show a displaced talar body fracture with rotation of the fragment in the ankle mortise. Mortise (**C**) and lateral (**D**) show that closed reduction was successful, allowing relief of the pressure on the medial soft tissues. Mortise (**E**) and lateral (**F**) radiographs of the ankle show that fixation proceeded uneventfully through two surgical approaches.

Postoperatively, patients should be managed with restricted weight bearing and early motion in fractures that have been adequately stabilized. Radiographic studies should include plain radiographs of the foot and ankle that can be examined to determine fracture healing, maintenance of reduction, and the vascularity of the talus.

Complications associated with both the injury and treatment of talar neck fractures include osteonecrosis, malunion, ankle joint arthritis, and subtalar joint arthritis. The most commonly observed complication following a fracture of the talar neck is subtalar joint ar-

thritis, which has been reported in more than 50% of injuries.[30,31,33] Osteonecrosis is a potentially devastating complication following a fracture of the talar neck; its incidence is related to multiple factors including fracture displacement and the presence of associated open traumatic wounds. Approximate rates of osteonecrosis are 10% to 20% for type I fractures, 20% to 50% for type II, and 60% to 100% for type III patterns. The Hawkins sign is best seen on the AP or mortise radiograph at 6 to 8 weeks following injury and is characterized by subchondral lucency beneath the dome of the talus. This local osteopenia is indicative of talar revascularization and may be incomplete depending on the hazard to the blood supply. However, the absence of early evidence of revascularization does not accurately portend osteonecrosis with collapse. An MRI can be obtained to further evaluate talar revascularization; however, a change in treatment (such as delayed weight bearing, local fusion procedures) of patients with evidence of altered blood flow has not been shown to affect the fate of the talus. MRI before 3 weeks after injury is not indicated. In general, progressive weight bearing is instituted based on timing, healing, and the patient's symptoms and not the presence or absence of talar revascularization. Talar neck malunion is poorly tolerated because of the limitation in subtalar joint motion and the alteration of the mechanics of the hindfoot. Correction with an osteotomy can be considered but should be performed by a surgeon who is familiar with this technique.

The outcomes associated with surgical treatment of talar neck fractures have been shown in several recent studies. One long-term study of 70 displaced talar neck fractures treated over a 10-year period found a low rate of osteonecrosis and better overall function if complications were avoided.[33] Worse functional results occurred in patients with talar malalignment or subtalar joint arthritis; secondary surgical procedures were required in 37% of patients. Another study evaluated a cohort of patients with 26 talar fractures at a minimum follow-up period of 4 years.[30] A high incidence of subtalar joint arthritis and poorer results occurred in patients with open fractures. Osteonecrosis developed in 50% of patients overall and in 86% of patients with open fractures. These findings were confirmed in another retrospective study of 102 talar neck fractures.[31] In the subset of 60 fractures followed for at least 1 year, radiographic evidence of osteonecrosis was seen in 49% of patients but more than one third of these fractures did not progress to collapse of the talar dome. Open injuries and fracture comminution were associated with poorer outcomes.

Talar Body Fractures

Fractures of the talar body typically involve the tibiotalar joint but may be more accurately identified based on the inferior exit point of the fracture. Fractures that extend into the talofibular articulation (including extension into the lateral process of the talus) are probably better classified as talar body fractures. Fractures that involve the dome of the talus can be classified according the major fracture line(s) and include sagittal, coronal, transverse, and comminuted patterns. The radiographic evaluation is similar to that of talar neck fractures, although CT scans are imperative to evaluate most of these injuries. Because of the multiple articulations involved with talar body fractures, a precise understanding of the fracture pattern combined with a precise surgical reduction are necessary to optimize outcomes. Depending on the medial involvement and medial exit point of the fracture, an adjunctive medial malleolar osteotomy may be required to accurately re-

store the anatomy in patients with these injuries. Fixation can be difficult in talar body fractures because of the lack of nonarticular surfaces available for hardware placement. Frequently, countersunk screws are required to secure the multiple fracture components.

Functional outcomes after fixation of talar body fractures are worse in comminuted and open fractures. Most patients (88%) have radiographic evidence of either posttraumatic arthritis or osteonecrosis.[34]

Lateral and Posteromedial Process Fractures

Fractures of the lateral process of the talus frequently present as a lateral ankle sprain and are often missed on plain radiographs. Although these fractures may be viewed optimally on the mortise view of the ankle, they are best delineated by CT. Lateral process fractures may occur in isolation or with other associated foot and ankle fractures. Because these injuries are frequently associated with snowboarding, they should be suspected in that population of patients. Because these fractures involve the talar articulations with both the fibula and the calcaneus at the subtalar joint, an accurate reduction is necessary if allowed by the fracture comminution. In a study of 20 young patients with lateral process fractures secondary to snowboarding, improved outcomes occurred after surgical treatment, although the inherent bias in this retrospective study is unknown.[35]

Fractures of the posteromedial process of the talus, depending on the size of the fracture, typically involve both the tibiotalar and subtalar joints. The mechanism of injury is typically direct and these fractures are associated with medial subtalar dislocations. Because plain radiographs often fail to show the magnitude and comminution of these fractures, CT scans are typically necessary. Because of the involvement of the ankle and subtalar joints, surgical treatment should be considered for patients with displaced fractures. A posteromedial approach with or without an adjunctive medial malleolar osteotomy is usually necessary for reduction and fixation of these difficult patterns.

Subtalar Dislocations

Subtalar dislocations are often the result of high-energy mechanisms, but they also occur during participation in sports and other activities. Classically, both the subtalar joints and talonavicular joints are simultaneously dislocated. The direction of the calcaneus (and the foot) relative to the talus (and the ankle joint) determines nomenclature with medial dislocations occurring much more frequently (incidence, 65% to 80%) than lateral dislocations. Lateral dislocations are typically the result of higher-energy mechanisms, are more frequently open, and are more often associated with a failure of closed reduction.

Closed reduction with intravenous sedation is usually successful and should be urgently attempted. Knee flexion (by an assistant) allows relaxation of the gastrocnemius muscle. The heel and foot are then grasped and distracted in plantar flexion. Slight accentuation of the deformity combined with reversal is combined with pressure on the talar head to simultaneously reduce both dislocations. If reduction is successful, the stability of the subtalar joint is confirmed. A postreduction CT scan is useful to access the congruity of the joint, to evaluate the subtalar joint for small osteochondral fragments, and to identify other associated injuries to the foot and ankle that occur in up to 88% of patients. Irreducible dislocations are usually the result of inadequate sedation, interposed soft tissues, or buttonholing of the osseous structures. Either the posterior tibial tendon or the flexor hallucis longus tendon typically blocks reduction of a lateral subtalar dislocation. Irreducible medial subtalar dislocations are associated with extrusion of the talar head through the extensor digitorum brevis, the inferior retinaculum, or the joint capsule.

Following reduction of the subtalar joint and confirmation with radiographic imaging, patients are immobilized in a short leg cast for 3 to 6 weeks depending on the perceived instability of the subtalar joint. Despite aggressive range-of-motion exercises, subtalar dislocations are associated with pain and with radiographic evidence of subtalar joint arthritis. A study identified radiographic changes of the subtalar joint in 89% of patients; most were symptomatic. Although a similarly high rate of radiographic changes occurred at the midfoot (72%), only 15% of patients were symptomatic.[36]

Calcaneus Fractures

Etiology

Calcaneus fractures account for 1% to 2% of all fractures and approximately 60% of tarsal injuries. Seventy-five percent of calcaneal fractures are intraarticular and are usually the result of an axial-loading mechanism such as a fall from height, or increasingly, secondary to high-speed motor vehicle collisions. Other injuries to the appendicular and axial skeleton, particularly the lumbar spine, frequently occur and should be suspected and sought. Locally, the soft tissues may show substantial swelling, blisters, full-thickness skin necrosis, and open wounds. Despite the relative prevalence of this injury, definitive treatment remains controversial.

Evaluation and Classification

Calcaneal fractures can be identified with standard foot radiographs including dorsoplantar, lateral, and oblique views; the lateral view is best for the initial diagnosis. The dorsoplantar view shows lateral wall displacement and intra-articular involvement of the calcaneocuboid joint. The lateral view allows assessment of the posterior facet, magnitude of calcaneal shortening (Böhler angle), and gives a general impression of overall comminution. The Harris axial view completes the standard plain radiographic investigation when a calcaneal fracture is identified, and shows lat-

eral translation of the calcaneal tuberosity, heel widening, angulation of the tuberosity, lateral wall displacement, and fibular abutment. If desired, multiple oblique hindfoot views (Broden views) may be obtained to further image the posterior facet; however, their use has largely been supplanted by axial CT scanning.

CT is routinely used, although one study found that information on CT scans may not affect decisions about whether surgery is needed compared with information provided by plain radiographs alone.[37] However, in surgically treated patients, CT imaging facilitates preoperative planning and shows previously unrecognized fracture comminution. Reconstructed sagittal and coronal CT images further enhance comprehension of the complex anatomy. Three-dimensional CT reconstructions may further improve conceptualization of the injury but are not routinely obtained. MRI has been used experimentally to evaluate the status of the plantar fat pad after calcaneal fracture, but is rarely used in the acute setting.

Fractures of the calcaneus can be initially classified as intra-articular or extra-articular types. The less common extra-articular fractures are typically the result of avulsion-type mechanisms and often involve the anterior process, the sustentaculum, and the calcaneal tuberosity. Two distinct intra-articular fracture patterns are recognized—the "joint depression" fracture and the "tongue-type" fracture. The main distinguishing characteristic between joint depression and tongue-type fractures is the presence or absence of continuity between the displaced posterior facet fragment and the superior aspect of the calcaneal tuberosity. In a joint depression-type fracture, the posterior facet displaces and is completely separate from the calcaneal tuberosity. In a tongue-type fracture, the posterior facet remains in continuity with the superior aspect of the calcaneal tuberosity, with both osseous structures rotating and displacing as a single unit.

Several CT-based classification systems have been created that focus on the articular injury, particularly to the posterior facet. Sanders' CT classification system is the predominant system currently in use. It is based on the number and location of posterior facet fracture lines relative to the widest portion of the posterior facet of the talus. When assessing intra-articular calcaneal fractures, treatment decisions and prognosis predictions should be based on all the information that is available (patient and injury factors, and full imaging information) rather than simply relying on a fracture classification scheme.

Fracture Anatomy

Calcaneal fractures occur in consistently reproducible patterns. With axial loading, the mid portion of the talus, including the lateral process, impacts the relatively stationary calcaneus and acts as a fulcrum, fracturing the calcaneus. A primary fracture line is common to most intra-articular fractures of the calcaneus and begins in the sinus tarsi near the lateral wall and travels obliquely across the posterior facet to the medial wall.

On the lateral radiograph, the exit point is at the lateral aspect of the Gissane angle, but may extend anteriorly to the calcaneocuboid joint. The posteromedial exit point is posterior to the sustentaculum. This primary fracture line divides the calcaneus into posterolateral and anteromedial fragments. The posterolateral fragment consists of the tuberosity and lateral wall with a variable portion of the posterior facet. The anteromedial segment is composed of the remaining posterior facet, anterior process, and the middle and anterior facets, supported by the sustentaculum tali. The posterolateral tuberosity fragment is typically driven anteriorly and laterally along the primary fracture line, assuming a position beneath the fibula. The anteromedial sustentacular fragment is also known as the "constant" fragment because of its resistance to significant displacement secondary to its strong soft-tissue attachments. Occasionally, this fragment may be rotated downward away from the talus, particularly in high-energy injuries, and requires disimpaction from fragments created by secondary fracture lines.

Additional secondary fracture lines invariably occur. These include a coronal fracture extension that may divide the middle facet from either the posterior facet or the anterior process, and a sagittal anterior fracture extension that divides the anterior process, producing a common anterolateral fragment. Secondary fracture lines in the body of the calcaneus result in posterior facet comminution. During plantar displacement of the posterior facet, the lateral wall of the calcaneus is typically separated and laterally displaced, the entity being commonly described as lateral wall blowout. The final deformity reflects the predictable displacements of the major fracture fragments relative to each other. The calcaneal length and height are diminished. The heel is widened secondary to the displacement of the posterolateral tuberosity fragment and the associated lateral wall blowout. Posterior facet incongruence and the necessarily altered spatial relationship of the three superior facets results in disturbed subtalar mechanics. Anterior process fractures may result in calcaneocuboid incongruity. Loss of the Böhler angle results in a more horizontal attitude of the talus and affects tibiotalar and talonavicular mechanics. Loss of normal talonavicular and calcaneocuboid interaction impacts midtarsal mobility.

Treatment Considerations

Many factors in addition to the fracture pattern influence outcome of calcaneal fractures. A review of the literature suggests that patients with increasing physiologic age, male gender, tobacco use, a pending workers' compensation claim, an occupation requiring heavy labor, bilateral injuries, and increasing comminution of the posterior facet (Sanders classification) do not have significantly improved functional outcomes with surgery compared with outcomes achieved with nonsurgical treatment.[38,39]

Treatment

In patients who are surgical candidates, most displaced intra-articular calcaneus fractures amenable to surgical repair are treated with open reduction and internal fixation. Surgery is usually delayed for 7 to 14 days to allow the swollen soft-tissue envelope to recover and to allow fracture blister reepithelialization. A lateral extensile exposure is used with a vertical limb just posterior to the midpoint between the lateral border of the Achilles tendon and the posterior aspect of the fibula, posterior to the sural nerve. At the transition between the lateral foot skin and the glabrous skin at the plantar-lateral aspect of the foot, the incision curves sharply, paralleling the plantar surface of the calcaneus and extending to the calcaneocuboid joint. The lateral aspect of the calcaneus is exposed by elevating a full thickness flap of skin, subcutaneous tissue, and periosteum. The peroneal tendons, sural nerve, and calcaneofibular ligament are reflected en masse in the flap. The vascularity of the flap is based on the peroneal artery blood supply, which remains protected within the substance of the flap. Reduction typically proceeds from anteromedial to posterolateral, effectively decompressing the central portion of the calcaneus to allow accurate reduction of the posterior facet fragment(s). Anatomic surgical reduction of the posterior facet results in improved outcomes compared with those achieved with reductions with residual steps, gaps, or comminution. The key components of reduction include restoration of calcaneal height (Böhler angle), heel width (identified on the axial view), anatomic restoration of fracture lines traversing chondral surfaces (particularly the posterior facet), and anatomic realignment of the three superior facets to each other and to the corresponding talar facets. Numerous implants are available for definitive fixation including precontoured periarticular multiple-limbed plates and newer locking screw/plate devices. Several areas are available for optimal screw fixation and naturally correspond to those areas subjected to physiologic stress. These include the dense bone in the sustentaculum tali, the thickened bone immediately beneath the posterior facet, the cancellous bone deep to the Achilles tendon insertion, and the bone of the dorsal half of the anterior process near the calcaneocuboid joint. The results of recent biomechanical studies comparing locking with nonlocking screw/plate devices in simulated calcaneal fracture models are conflicting. Without comparative clinical studies, the advantages of locking screw/plate implants in the treatment of calcaneal fractures remain theoretical.

The use of bone graft in the surgical treatment of intra-articular calcaneal fractures remains controversial. The purpose of the graft is to act as an adjunctive supportive structure preventing collapse of the elevated articular segments. However, studies have been unable to show any objective benefits to its use in the treatment of these fractures. Bone graft substitutes can improve the initial compressive strength of the posterior facet reconstruction and may expedite weight bearing.

Other benefits include the ability to combine these products with antibiotics, and the potential for osseous integration.[40] Recent clinical studies using a variety of products appear to show equivalent wound complication rates and reduction maintenance when compared with historic controls.[41] The use of routine bone grafting during the open management of displaced intra-articular calcaneus fractures does not appear to be supported by the current literature. However, supplemental bone graft or bone graft substitutes are reasonable adjuncts for managing large subarticular defects or in situations where mechanical stability of the reduced posterior facet cannot be maintained with fixation techniques.

Closure of the surgical incision is performed in two layers, which has been shown to decrease the incidence of wound dehiscence. The deep interrupted absorbable periosteal suture is followed by a separate nylon modified Allgower-Donati flap stitch with the goal of minimizing tension along the skin incision, particularly at the apex of the exposure. At the conclusion of the procedure, the foot is placed in a well-padded splint. The addition of an immediate postoperative sciatic nerve blockade confers significant analgesic benefit compared with morphine alone, particularly in the first 24 hours after surgery.[42] After surgical wound healing, patients begin a supervised physical therapy program with weight bearing delayed until fracture union, which typically occurs in 10 to 12 weeks. Increasing amounts of subtalar motion appear to be highly correlated with longer-term patient satisfaction.[43]

Approximately 5% to 10% of calcaneal fractures have open wounds. Most of these wounds occur on the medial aspect of the foot and are typically transverse or oblique in orientation. These injuries have a high risk for wound complications, osteomyelitis, poor functional outcomes, and amputation. Gustilo types I and II open fractures with medial wounds can be treated with open reduction and internal fixation with results similar to those of closed fractures.[44] However, with more extensive soft-tissue disruption or type II nonmedial wounds, external fixation and/or percutaneous screw fixation should be considered.

Because there is no strongly convincing evidence that the open treatment of displaced intra-articular calcaneal fractures provides substantial improvement in functional outcomes when compared with nonsurgical methods, and because open surgical treatment carries deep wound complication rates ranging from 2% to 7%, alternate treatment methods continue to be investigated, including percutaneous, limited-incision, arthroscopically-assisted, and ring-fixator techniques.[45-47]

Outcomes

To determine the effect of surgical versus nonsurgical treatment on the rates of union, complications, and functional outcomes after intra-articular calcaneal fractures in adults, the Evidence-Based Orthopaedic Trauma Group performed a recent evaluation.[45] Using the highest quality comparative studies currently avail-

able, the authors concluded that there is no significant difference in pain and functional outcome between surgical and nonsurgical treatment groups, although surgical treatment may demonstrate superiority in the ability to return patients to work and the ability to wear the same shoes as before injury. Hypotheses generated by subgroup analyses include a potential benefit of improved surgical outcomes in females, patients not involved with workers' compensation, younger males, patients with a higher initial Böhler angle, patients with an occupation involving less strenuous labor, and those with simple intra-articular fracture patterns. Similarly, the authors hypothesized a potential benefit from nonsurgical care in patients 50 years of age or older, males, patients receiving workers' compensation, and those patients with an occupation requiring strenuous labor. As noted by the Evidence-Based Orthopaedic Trauma Group, these latter conclusions are considered as hypotheses to emphasize that they be interpreted with caution, because they were obtained using post hoc subgroup analyses and have a higher risk of being obtained by chance. Subsequent subtalar arthrodesis rates, however, were significantly reduced with surgical treatment compared with patients treated nonsurgically. From a societal perspective, surgical treatment is less costly and more effective than nonsurgical care.[48] A potential criticism of all of these studies is that follow-up has been short term, and more significant outcome differences may occur over time. The potential benefits of surgical treatment may not be realized for several years after the initial trauma when the symptoms of posttraumatic subtalar arthrosis become evident.[49] Primary subtalar fusion can be considered in extremely limited circumstances such as open fractures with articular loss and severe articular comminution that cannot be successfully reconstructed.

Annotated References

1. Park SS, Kubiak EN, Egol KA, et al: Stress radiographs after ankle fracture: The effect of ankle position and deltoid ligament status on medial clear space measurements. *J Orthop Trauma* 2006;20:11-18.

   Stress radiographs of cadaver specimens were used to determine how ankle position affects the medial clear space and to determine the predictive value of increased clear space with regard to the integrity of the deep deltoid ligament. The authors found that a medial clear space of 5 mm or more with an external rotation stress applied to a dorsiflexed ankle was most predictive of a deep deltoid ligament injury.

2. McConnell T, Creevy W, Tornetta P III: Stress examination of supination external rotation-type fibular fractures. *J Bone Joint Surg Am* 2004;86-A:2171-2178.

   In a prospective study of patients with supination-external rotation fibular fractures, the authors evaluated the commonly used soft-tissue indicators to determine their relationship with deltoid competence as confirmed

4: Lower Extremity

by intraoperative stress radiographs. Stress radiographs were found to be an effective method for diagnosing deltoid incompetence in patients with fibular fractures and no other osseus injury; however, soft tissue indicators were not found to be predictive of deltoid integrity. Level of evidence: IV.

3. Egol KA, Amirtharajah M, Tejwani NC, et al: Ankle stress test for predicting the need for surgical fixation of isolated fibular fractures. *J Bone Joint Surg Am* 2004; 86-A:2393-2398.

    The authors evaluated 101 patients with isolated fibular fractures using a stress test to evaluate medial widening (defined as ≥ 4 mm) and outcome after treatment. Of the 65 patients with a positive stress test, 36 had clinical signs of a medial injury and 30 did not. Tenderness, swelling, and ecchymosis on the medial side were not sensitive for predicting medial clear space widening on stress radiographs. Nonsurgically treated patients with positive findings on a stress radiograph and no clinical symptoms had a good clinical result. Level of evidence: III.

4. Gardner MJ, Demetrakopoulos D, Briggs SM, et al: The ability of the Lauge-Hansen classification to predict ligament injury and mechanism in ankle fractures: An MRI study. *J Orthop Trauma* 2006;20:267-272.

    In an attempt to determine the accuracy of the Lauge-Hansen classification system to predict associated ligamentous injuries to the ankle, the authors evaluated MRI scans of 59 patients with surgically treated ankle fractures. Most (63%) were supination-external rotation injuries based on findings from plain radiographs, with 17% unclassifiable. In most instances (53%), the predicted patterns of ligamentous injury did not coincide with the Lauge-Hansen system. More than 65% of patients had a complete ligamentous injury combined with a fracture of the malleolus to which the ligament attaches. Level of evidence: IV.

5. Gardner MJ, Brodsky A, Briggs SM, et al: Fixation of posterior malleolar fractures provides greater syndesmotic stability. *Clin Orthop Relat Res* 2006;447:165-171.

    Fifteen patients with pronation-external rotation fracture patterns were evaluated with radiographs and MRI to determine the integrity of the posteroinferior talofibular ligament. A cadaver study was used to better understand the relationship between fixation of the posterior malleolus and the syndesmosis. Stiffness was restored to 70% of ankles after fixation of the posterior malleolus, but to only 40% after syndesmotic fixation. No instances of posteroinferior talofibular ligament injury were observed based on MRI scans. The authors concluded that posterior malleolar fixation may be more effective than syndesmotic fixation in selected patients with this injury pattern.

6. Nielson JH, Gardner MJ, Peterson MG, et al: Radiographic measurements do not predict syndesmotic injury in ankle fractures: An MRI study. *Clin Orthop Relat Res* 2005;436:216-221.

    In a study evaluating standard plain radiographic measurements and MRI results, the authors found that a medial clear space of greater than 4 mm was correlated with disruption of the deltoid and tibiofibular ligaments, but there was no correlation between syndesmotic injury and either tibiofibular clear space or overlap measurements. Level of evidence: II.

7. Jenkinson RJ, Sanders DW, Macleod MD, et al: Intraoperative diagnosis of syndesmosis injuries in external rotation ankle fractures. *J Orthop Trauma* 2005;19: 604-609.

    This prospective study compared intraoperative fluoroscopic stress testing, static radiographs, and published biomechanical criteria to determine the ability of each test to predict injury to the syndesmosis. The authors found, using radiographic clear space measurements as the determinant of syndesmotic injury, that preoperative radiographs and biomechanical criteria were unable to accurately predict the presence or absence of syndesmotic instability. Intraoperative stress fluoroscopy was believed to be a valuable tool for detection. Level of evidence: II.

8. Beumer A, Campo MM, Niesing R, et al: Screw fixation of the syndesmosis: A cadaver model comparing stainless steel and titanium screws and three and four cortical fixation. *Injury* 2005;36:60-64.

    In a biomechanical study to determine syndesmotic fixation strengths, the authors found no difference between stainless and titanium implants, and no difference between those stabilized with three or four cortices. The finding that syndesmotic screw fixation was inadequate to support loads comparable to normal weight bearing supported the need to limit patient activities after fixation.

9. Kaukonen JP, Lamberg T, Korkala O, et al: Fixation of syndesmotic ruptures in 38 patients with a malleolar fracture: A randomized study comparing a metallic and a bioabsorbable screw. *J Orthop Trauma* 2005;19:392-395.

    This prospective and randomized study compared metallic and bioabsorbable screw fixation for syndesmotic injuries. The authors found that polylevolactic screws were associated with a better return to activities, less swelling, and were not detrimental to joint motion or reduction compared with metallic implants. Level of evidence: II.

10. Weening B, Bhandari M: Predictors of functional outcome following transsyndesmotic screw fixation of ankle fractures. *J Orthop Trauma* 2005;19:102-108.

    This retrospective observational study of 51 patients treated with syndesmotic screw fixation showed that the only predictor of outcome was reduction of the syndesmosis. Level of evidence: IV.

11. Hoiness P, Stromsoe K: Tricortical versus quadricortical syndesmosis fixation in ankle fractures: A prospective, randomized study comparing two methods of syndesmosis fixation. *J Orthop Trauma* 2004;18:331-337.

    This prospective randomized study compared tricortical and quadricortical syndesmotic fixation in 64 patients. The authors observed better function at 3 months, but not at 1 year in the tricortical group. There was no difference in ankle dorsiflexion or loss of fixation between the two groups. Level of evidence: II.

12. Lamontagne J, Blachut PA, Broekhuyse HM, et al: Surgical treatment of a displaced lateral malleolus fracture: The antiglide technique versus lateral plate fixation. *J Orthop Trauma* 2002;16:498-502.

13. Weber M, Krause F: Peroneal tendon lesions caused by antiglide plates used for fixation of lateral malleolar fractures: The effect of plate and screw position. *Foot Ankle Int* 2005;26:281-285.

Antiglide plate placement for lateral malleolar fractures was associated with a high rate of hardware removal and peroneal tendinitis. This was correlated with distal plate placement and prominence of the most distal screw. Level of evidence: IV.

14. Kukkonen J, Heikkila JT, Kyyronen T, et al: Posterior malleolar fracture is often associated with spiral tibial diaphyseal fracture: A retrospective study. *J Trauma* 2006;60:1058-1060.

In a study of 72 tibial shaft fractures treated with intramedullary nailing, an associated fracture of the posterior malleolus was identified in 25% of fractures. Although all posterior malleolus fractures were apparent on the original injury plain radiographs when reviewed retrospectively, only 56% of these were initially identified. The authors confirmed the need for dedicated ankle radiographs in all tibial fractures. Level of evidence: IV.

15. Haraguchi N, Haruyama H, Toga H, et al: Pathoanatomy of posterior malleolar fractures of the ankle. *J Bone Joint Surg Am* 2006;88:1085-1092.

The authors used CT to study 57 ankles with a fracture of the posterior malleolus to determine its relative size and location. Most fractures (67%) were posterolateral oblique, with medial extension fractures (19%) and small-shell fractures (14%) comprising the rest. The posterolateral oblique fractures were 12% of the total tibial plafond whereas those with medial extension were much larger (30%). This study supports the use of CT to better understand the fracture and to determine treatment in some posterior malleolar fractures. Level of evidence: IV.

16. Weber M: Trimalleolar fractures with impaction of the posteromedial tibial plafond: Implications for talar stability. *Foot Ankle Int* 2004;25:716-727.

The author of this review expertly describes a variant of the trimalleolar ankle fracture that is characterized by a posterolateral corner fracture combined with a fracture extending into the medial malleolus from the posterior plafond. The radiographic and surgical findings are well described, as is a strategy for surgical treatment. Level of evidence: IV.

17. De Vries JS, Wijgman AJ, Sierevelt IN, et al: Long-term results of ankle fractures with a posterior malleolar fragment. *J Foot Ankle Surg* 2005;44:211-217.

In a long-term outcome study evaluating the size and fixation of posterior malleolar fractures, the authors found good results in patients with small posterior mal-leolar fractures treated nonsurgically. Level of evidence: IV.

18. Fitzpatrick DC, Otto JK, McKinley TO, et al: Kinematic and contact stress analysis of posterior malleolus fractures of the ankle. *J Orthop Trauma* 2004;18:271-278.

In a biomechanical study using dynamic contact stress to determine the effect of a posterior malleolar fracture, no talar subluxation and no increased contact stress was observed near the articular incongruity. However, the center of stress shifted anteriorly and medially with a fracture of the posterior malleolus, resulting in increased loading to cartilage that normally is not subjected to high loads.

19. Bhandari M, Sprague S, Hanson B, et al: Health-related quality of life following operative treatment of unstable ankle fractures: A prospective observational study. *J Orthop Trauma* 2004;18:338-345.

In a prospective observational study evaluating outcomes after Weber/AO type B ankle fractures, the authors found significant improvements over the 24-month study period; however, limitations still existed compared with published normative data even at 2 years. Smoking, less education, alcohol use, increasing age, and the presence of a medial malleolar fracture were associated with worse outcomes. Level of evidence: II.

20. Simanski CJ, Maegele MG, Lefering R, et al: Functional treatment and early weightbearing after an ankle fracture: A prospective study. *J Orthop Trauma* 2006;20:108-114.

In a prospective study examining postoperative weight bearing after open reduction and internal fixation of unstable ankle fractures, the authors compared a group of patients allowed to weight bear early with a historic control group treated with supplementary casting and 6 weeks without weight bearing. The study found no adverse effects of early weight bearing and recommended this protocol in compliant patients judged to have a stable fixation. There was little difference in virtually all outcomes measures with the exception of time to weight bearing. Level of evidence: II.

21. Konrad G, Markmiller M, Lenich A, Mayr E, Ruter A: Tourniquets may increase postoperative swelling and pain after internal fixation of ankle fractures. *Clin Orthop Relat Res* 2005;433:189-194.

The effect of tourniquet use on postoperative swelling, pain; and range of motion after open reduction and internal fuxation was quantified in a prospective, randomized study. Tourniquet use remains controversial. Level of evidence: I.

22. Ruedi TP, Allgower M: The operative treatment of intra-articular fractures of the lower end of the tibia. *Clin Orthop Relat Res* 1979;138:105-110.

23. Topliss CJ, Jackson M, Atkins RM: Anatomy of pilon fractures of the distal tibia *J Bone Joint Surg Br* 2005;87:692-697.

To assist with reduction and fixation techniques, the authors describe the major fracture lines and fracture fragments from a study of 126 consecutive pilon fractures.

24. Pollak AN, McCarthy ML, Bess RS, et al: Outcomes after treatment of high-energy tibial plafond fractures. *J Bone Joint Surg Am* 2003;85-A:1893-1900.

25. Anglen JO: Early outcome of hybrid external fixation for fracture of the distal tibia. *J Orthop Trauma* 1999; 13:92-97.

26. Bhattacharyya T, Crichlow R, Gobezie R, et al: Complications associated with the posterolateral approach for pilon fractures. *J Orthop Trauma* 2006;20:104-107.

    In the authors' experience, a posterolateral approach as an isolated approach was not an effective alternative treatment for tibial pilon fractures. Numerous complications included wound problems, infection, and the need for subsequent fusion. Level of evidence: IV.

27. Williams TM, Nepola JV, DeCoster TA, et al: Factors affecting outcome in tibial plafond fractures. *Clin Orthop Relat Res* 2004;423:93-98.

    The factors associated with outcomes after pilon fractures included level of education and whether the injury was work related. Radiographic arthrosis was predicted by the injury severity and the accuracy of reduction, but this was not related to clinical outcome measures. Level of evidence: IV.

28. Chen SH, Wu PH, Lee YS: Long-term results of pilon fractures. *Arch Orthop Trauma Surg* 2006.

    Fracture pattern, fibular length restoration, quality of reduction, and the severity of the soft-tissue injury were associated with outcome after open reduction and plating for pilon fractures. Level of evidence: IV.

29. Marsh JL, Weigel DP, Dirschl DR: Tibial plafond fractures: How do these ankles function over time? *J Bone Joint Surg Am* 2003;85-A:287-295.

30. Lindvall E, Haidukewych G, Dipasquale T, et al: Open reduction and stable fixation of isolated, displaced talar neck and body fractures. *J Bone Joint Surg Am* 2004; 86-A:2229-2234.

    The authors retrospectively reviewed 26 talar fractures at a minimum of 4 years from injury. Despite good reductions, arthritis was commonly observed. Level of evidence: IV.

31. Vallier HA, Nork SE, Barei DP, et al: Talar neck fractures: Results and outcomes. *J Bone Joint Surg Am* 2004;86-A:1616-1624.

    In a retrospective study of 102 talar neck fractures, osteonecrosis was associated with open injuries and talar neck comminution, confirming that higher-energy injuries have a worse prognosis. Although surgical timing was not found to be related to subsequent complications, the authors recommend urgent reduction of dislocations and open fractures, and definitive fixation when other factors are optimized. Level of evidence: IV.

32. Charlson MD, Parks BG, Weber TG, et al: Comparison of plate and screw fixation and screw fixation alone in a comminuted talar neck fracture model. *Foot Ankle Int* 2006;27:340-343.

    In this biomechanical study using a comminuted talar neck model, plate fixation was compared screw fixations, although different sized implants were used.

33. Sanders DW, Busam M, Hattwick E, et al: Functional outcomes following displaced talar neck fractures. *J Orthop Trauma* 2004;18:265-270.

    In a retrospective review of 70 patients with displaced talar neck fractures, the authors assessed clinical outcome and the need for secondary procedures. The need for secondary procedures was time dependent and was related to complications. Secondary procedures for subtalar arthritis and poor alignment were common. Level of evidence: IV.

34. Vallier HA, Nork SE, Benirschke SK, et al: Surgical treatment of talar body fractures. *J Bone Joint Surg Am* 2003;85-A:1716-1724.

35. Valderrabano V, Perren T, Ryf C, et al: Snowboarder's talus fracture: Treatment outcome of 20 cases after 3.5 years. *Am J Sports Med* 2005;33:871-880.

    The authors present the results of a study of 20 patients with fractures of the lateral process of the talus. Treatment recommendations were made based on fracture type and the injury mechanism was recorded. Level of evidence: IV.

36. Bibbo C, Anderson RB, Davis WH: Injury characteristics and the clinical outcome of subtalar dislocations: A clinical and radiographic analysis of 25 cases. *Foot Ankle Int* 2003;24:158-163.

37. Kumar V, Hameed A, Bhattacharya R, et al: Role of computerised tomography in management of intra-articular fractures of the os calcis. *Int Orthop* 2006;30: 110-112.

    This study examined the role of CT in decision making in the treatment of intra-articular fractures of the calcaneus. The results showed CT should be used when a definite decision is made to operate on a patient, based on plain radiographs. Calcaneal fractures that are selected for nonsurgical treatment based on radiographs do not require routine CT scanning because it provides no valuable additional information affecting the treatment decision.

38. Buckley R, Tough S, McCormack R, et al: Operative compared with nonoperative treatment of displaced intra-articular calcaneal fractures: A prospective, randomized, controlled multicenter trial. *J Bone Joint Surg Am* 2002;84-A:1733-1744.

39. Buckley RE, Tough S: Displaced intra-articular calcaneal fractures. *J Am Acad Orthop Surg* 2004;12:172-178.

    The authors review several parameters necessary to determine a treatment approach. In general, older, sedentary patients and those with no or with minimally displaced fractures may be treated successfully with nonsurgical care. Factors strongly predictive of satisfaction with surgery include age younger than 40 years, simple fracture pattern, and accurate reduction. Smoking, diabetes, and peripheral vascular disease markedly increase the risk of surgical complications. In addition, the quality of surgical reduction affects outcome.

40. Bibbo C, Patel DV: The effect of demineralized bone matrix-calcium sulfate with vancomycin on calcaneal fracture healing and infection rates: A prospective study. *Foot Ankle Int* 2006;27:487-493.

This is the first study to examine human demineralized bone matrix-calcium sulfate bone graft substitute in the treatment of displaced intra-articular calcaneal fractures. Based on initial data, human demineralized bone matrix-calcium sulfate acted as an acceptable and safe autograft alternative in displaced intra-articular calcaneal fractures with moderate (5 mL to 10 mL) central cancellous bone defects. Level of evidence: IV.

41. Thordarson DB, Bollinger M: SRS cancellous bone cement augmentation of calcaneal fracture fixation. *Foot Ankle Int* 2005;26:347-352.

In this small study, patients had no evidence of soft-tissue reaction or loss of reduction with early weight bearing after open reduction and internal fixation augmented with calcium phosphate bone cement.

42. Cooper J, Benirschke S, Sangeorzan B, et al: Sciatic nerve blockade improves early postoperative analgesia after open repair of calcaneus fractures. *J Orthop Trauma* 2004;18:197-201.

This randomized, prospective trial divided 30 patients into three groups of 10 patients, all having open repair of calcaneus fractures. Group 1 used morphine patient-controlled analgesia alone, whereas groups 2 and 3 had morphine patient-controlled analgesia and a one-shot bupivacaine sciatic nerve blockade. This study showed that sciatic nerve blockade confers significant benefit compared with morphine alone for analgesia after open repair of calcaneus fractures. Postsurgical sciatic nerve blockade provides the longest possible postoperative block duration. Level of evidence: II.

43. Kingwell S, Buckley R, Willis N: The association between subtalar joint motion and outcome satisfaction in patients with displaced intraarticular calcaneal fractures. *Foot Ankle Int* 2004;25:666-673.

This study, a retrospective analysis from a randomized, controlled clinical trial, found that the amount of subtalar joint motion at least 12 weeks after a displaced intra-articular calcaneal fracture is significantly related to patient satisfaction at 2 years regardless of the method of treatment. Level of evidence: IV.

44. Heier KA, Infante AF, Walling AK, et al: Open fractures of the calcaneus: Soft-tissue injury determines outcome. *J Bone Joint Surg Am* 2003;85-A:2276-2282.

45. Bajammal S, Tornetta P III, Sanders D, et al: Displaced intra-articular calcaneal fractures. *J Orthop Trauma* 2005;19:360-364.

This evidence-based medicine review summarizes the literature comparing surgical and nonsurgical treatment of displaced intra-articular calcaneus fractures. There was moderate evidence with limitations that surgical treatment may be superior to nonsurgical treatment concerning return to work and the ability to wear the same shoes. Further, surgical treatment was associated with lower costs to society and reduced need for arthrodesis.

46. Carr JB: Surgical treatment of intra-articular calcaneal fractures: A review of small incision approaches. *J Orthop Trauma* 2005;19:109-117.

The specific fracture patterns appropriate for selective small incision approaches are reviewed. A reduction strategy and the commonly observed fracture patterns also are reviewed. Level of evidence: IV.

47. Emara KM, Allam MF: Management of calcaneal fracture using the Ilizarov technique. *Clin Orthop Relat Res* 2005;439:215-220.

The authors reviewed 12 patients with calcaneus fractures with associated poor skin condition treated with open reduction of the articular surface combined with Ilizarov external fixation for reduction of the tuberosity. Outcomes were similar to those of a control group of patients treated with conventional open reduction and internal fixation techniques. Level of evidence: IV.

48. Brauer CA, Manns BJ, Ko M, et al: An economic evaluation of operative compared with nonoperative management of displaced intra-articular calcaneal fractures. *J Bone Joint Surg Am* 2005;87:2741-2749.

Calcaneal fractures are recognized as having relatively poor clinical outcomes and a major socioeconomic impact with regard to time lost from work and recreation. This analysis suggests that surgical treatment of displaced intra-articular fractures is economically attractive. However, further exploration of the impact and valuation of time lost from work and patient outcomes is required. Level of evidence: IV.

49. Allmacher DH, Galles KS, Marsh JL: Intra-articular calcaneal fractures treated nonoperatively and followed sequentially for 2 decades. *J Orthop Trauma* 2006;20:464-469.

This study suggests that after nonsurgical treatment of closed displaced intra-articular calcaneus fractures, clinical results correlate with the presence of subtalar arthrosis on CT scans. Patients with higher grades of arthrosis had increased pain and deterioration in function in the second decade after injury compared with those with minimal arthrosis or those who had spontaneous subtalar fusion. Patients with no arthrosis had good outcomes that remained stable over more than two decades of follow-up. Level of evidence: IV.

Chapter 41

Foot and Ankle Reconstruction

Timothy C. Beals, MD

Ankle Arthritis: Treatment and Reconstruction

Ankle arthritis represents one of the more common pathologic conditions treated by orthopaedic surgeons who perform foot and ankle reconstruction. Although ankle arthritis is less common than hip or knee arthritis, it often represents a significant and complex treatment challenge because the patient population tends to be relatively young and the treatment choices appear to have a significant impact on the adjacent joints. A key component of proper patient care is the identification of the etiology of the arthritis. Most ankle arthritis is posttraumatic (occurring from a fracture or instability); however, it is important not to overlook other causes such as gouty arthrosis, hemochromatosis, or inflammatory arthritides such as psoriatic or rheumatoid arthritis.[1]

It is imperative that treating physicians are aware of the spectrum of options for the nonsurgical treatment of arthritis of the ankle, including over-the-counter medications, nonsteroidal anti-inflammatory drugs, corticosteroid or viscous injections, bracing, physical therapy, and offloading with a cane or other assistive device. Although arthrodesis remains the gold standard for surgical treatment of significant ankle arthritis, there are numerous acceptable treatment options, in contrast to the limited available options for treating most other arthritic joints. In addition to arthrodesis, treatment may include periarticular osteotomy, implant arthroplasty, distraction arthroplasty, osteochondral allograft or autograft surface replacement, or arthroscopic or open débridement with cheilectomy.

Ankle Arthrodesis

The gold standard for treatment of significantly symptomatic ankle arthritis remains arthrodesis. However, the techniques used to achieve fusion continue to evolve, particularly with an emphasis on minimally invasive and arthroscopic techniques.[2] Although there is some disagreement concerning the importance of achieving alignment in the anteroposterior translation of the talus based on gait studies, the goal of achieving a neutral position in the sagittal plane has not been questioned. Irrespective of the method of stabilization, significant pain relief is generally reported in follow-up studies of patients treated with ankle arthrodesis. However, gait is irrecoverably altered by arthrodesis and ipsilateral adjacent joint arthrosis often develops.[3]

Periarticular Osteotomies

Because of the development of adjacent joint arthritis in a significant percentage of patients treated with ankle fusion, and the learning curve for surgeons performing ankle joint arthroplasty, there has been a renewed interest in ankle motion-sparing procedures such as distraction arthroplasty or periarticular osteotomies.[4] Although few data are available describing the outcomes from such treatments, it is important to be familiar with the available options. Osteotomy options include proximal or distal tibial osteotomies or realignment through calcaneal osteotomy. Because only a small translation of force can be achieved through calcaneal osteotomy, such osteotomies may be combined with soft-tissue rebalancing by tendon transfer or ligamentous reconstruction.[5]

Achieving appropriate hindfoot alignment is equally as important in the prevention of arthritis in patients with ankle instability as it is in the treatment of those with established arthrosis. In primary or revision ankle ligament reconstruction, the use of a periarticular osteotomy should be routinely considered.[6] Appropriate alignment should be achieved when malalignment must be corrected (such as hindfoot varus from a cavus foot) to avoid the development of repetitive injury arthrosis (Figure 1). It is important to determine which patients can be helped with periarticular osteotomy. It is interesting to note that the duration of a study of 25 patients treated with distal tibial osteotomy for ankle arthritis was 15 years, which indicates the limited number of appropriate candidates. Patients with less severe disease appeared to have the best outcomes when treated with realignment by tibial osteotomy.[7]

Distraction Arthroplasty of the Ankle

There is only a small body of literature describing distraction arthroplasty of the ankle as a treatment for osteoarthritis; however, successful results can be achieved.[8] The importance of appropriate joint débridement, Achilles mechanism lengthening (if needed), and proper mechanical alignment has been emphasized.[9,10] Because of the young age of many patients with ankle arthrosis, distraction arthroplasty remains an acceptable treatment option. Because weight-bearing radiographs have shown that a joint can maintain an increased joint space after distraction arthroplasty, there is optimism that the technique can be refined and that there will be a better understanding of the response of diseased cartilage to mechanical stress modulation

4: Lower Extremity

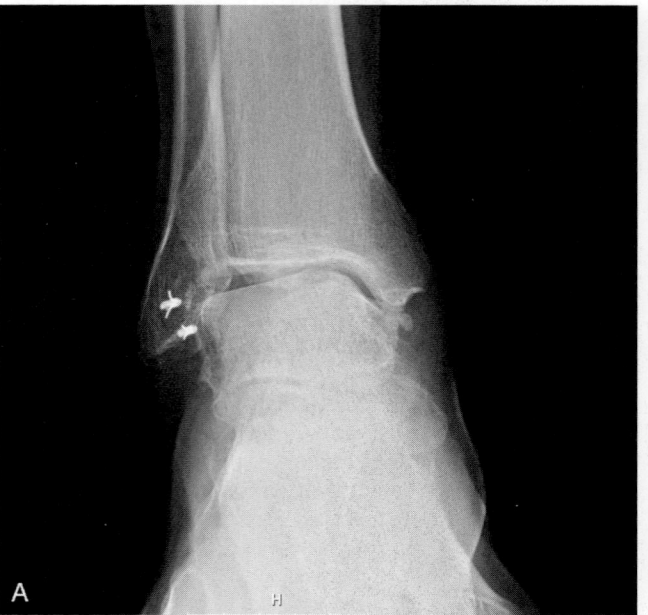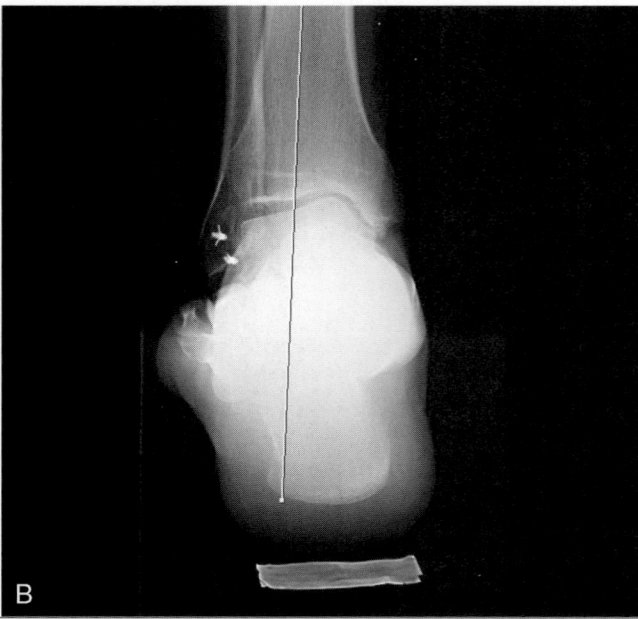

Figure 1 **A,** Radiograph of the ankle of a 31-year-old man 10 years after a lateral ankle instability repair. Cavovarus foot alignment was not initially treated. **B,** Axial hindfoot alignment radiograph shows the varus position of the calcaneus.

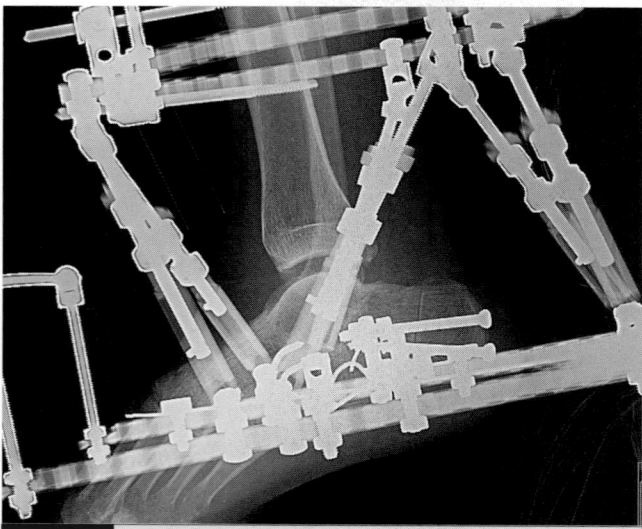

Figure 2 Lateral radiographic view of the ankle of a patient with ankle osteoarthritis treated with prior triple arthrodesis. A translational calcaneal osteotomy and distraction of the ankle was performed.

(**Figure 2**). The technique of distraction involves the use of an external fixator to distract the joint beyond its physiologic norm for approximately 2 to 3 months; motion and weight bearing are resumed after fixator removal.

Osteoarticular Grafting

The use of transplanted articular cartilage to replace defects in the ankle is another treatment method for an-

kle arthrosis. This technique is typically limited in its application to the treatment of relatively small regions of the cartilage, particularly in the setting of an osteochondral defect of the talus. However, in some instances, the entire ankle joint has been replaced with fresh cadaveric tissue, which represents a logical evolution in treatment resulting from a growing understanding of cartilage biology and improved surgical techniques.[11]

Smaller isolated talar or tibial plafond lesions are typically treated with arthroscopic or open débridement of loose fragments of cartilage with either drilling or microfracture applied to the underlying bone. The overall results with such treatments are favorable, but a notable rate of failure has been reported. Although there has been improvement in noninvasive imaging methods such as MRI, the precise locations and size of lesions are not always accurately predicted by preoperative imaging, particularly in instances of delaminated cartilage. This information is important because the size of the lesion is a key determinant in defining the best treatment; however, even patients with large lesions and those with unsuccessful prior surgical treatment can have favorable outcomes after surgery. Primary osteoarticular grafting instead of débridement may be considered for larger lesions, especially those located in the anterior portion of the tibiotalar joint.[12,13]

Total Ankle Arthroplasty

Although ankle arthroplasty has been performed for decades, the use of the procedure has dramatically increased in the past 5 to 10 years because new implant designs have become available and because longer follow-up periods have caused growing concern about adjacent joint arthrosis in patients treated with arthrodesis. Several studies of midrange duration have shown an acceptable level of success with ankle arthroplasty. However, there are also several studies that emphasize the learning curve for surgeons and document the pitfalls associated with implant arthroplasty.[14-16] More recent studies have emphasized the importance of patient selection and strict application to the recommendations concerning the maintenance of appropriate hindfoot alignment and ligamentous stability (**Figure 3**).

Reconstruction After Failed Total Ankle Arthroplasty

Accompanying the increase in the number of total ankle arthroplasties is a commensurate increase in the need to provide treatment for patients in whom arthroplasty has not been successful. Recent studies that have reported on salvage procedures after total ankle arthroplasty have emphasized concern about the longevity of these implants and the implications of removing bone stock during an arthroplasty procedure. Significant loosening of the components, regardless of the arthroplasty design, is clinically challenging to treat. In most patients, however, a failed ankle arthroplasty can be successfully salvaged.[17,18] Such patients may be best cared for by a specialist with experience in complex revision hindfoot surgery.

Causes of Hindfoot Dysfunction

Cavus Foot Deformity

An increased appreciation has occurred over the last few years regarding the implications of the cavus foot shape. Several authors have clarified key elements of the deformities in the cavus foot, which have allowed a better appreciation of the clinically relevant spectrum of disorders.[19] The key to understanding treatment of cavus deformity is recognition of the relative stiffness and deformity in the hindfoot. In 1977, a simple technique in which the patient stands on a block of wood to eliminate the deforming force of the first ray was described to identify whether correction into a valgus alignment will occur in the hindfoot. The importance of that distinction has continued to be emphasized, but an enhanced understanding also has developed regarding the morphologic changes that can be observed in the bones of the hindfoot in long-standing cavus deformities and the relationship of those changes to clinical findings.

Many clinically relevant symptoms are determined by the cavus foot shape. Some patients have simple ankle instability and others present with severe equinocavovarus deformities related to neuromuscular conditions such as Charcot-Marie-Tooth disease, which are some of the most complicated disorders to treat. The orthopaedic surgeon should determine if the foot has a cavus shape, whether it is flexible or rigid, and if the deformity is static or progressive. It is imperative to

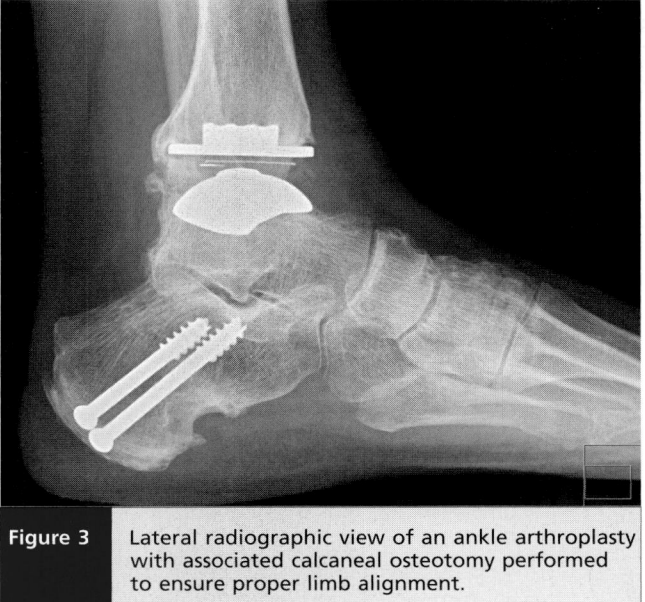

Figure 3 Lateral radiographic view of an ankle arthroplasty with associated calcaneal osteotomy performed to ensure proper limb alignment.

determine whether the cavus shape is representative of a neuromotor abnormality, or if it is characteristic of the individual. It is necessary to appreciate the effect of the foot deformity on the ankle and to incorporate that understanding into a patient-specific treatment plan.[20]

Because of the long-term complications associated with hindfoot or ankle arthrodesis, there is an interest in developing techniques to avoid arthrodesis in the treatment of patients with cavus and cavovarus foot deformities. Disorders that were historically treated with triple arthrodesis are now treated with joint-sparing procedures. Such procedures may involve a lateralizing translational calcaneal osteotomy that is performed with or without a lateral closing wedge osteotomy to augment the degree of deformity correction, or may involve elevation of the medial column of the foot, most commonly through an osteotomy of the first metatarsal. These bony procedures are typically accompanied by soft-tissue reconstruction, which may include transfers of the anterior or posterior tibial tendons depending on the degree of deformity, and transfers of the flexor hallucis longus or peroneal tendons depending on their motor contributions in patients with neuromuscular disease.[21] Midfoot-based procedures also have been described to correct cavus feet with acceptable results.[22]

Adult Acquired Flatfoot Deformity (Posterior Tibial Tendon Insufficiency)

Controversy exists concerning the etiology and most appropriate treatments for adult acquired flatfoot deformity. The development of this condition is most closely associated with degeneration of the posterior tibial tendon; however, other structures also are involved, particularly the degradation of the spring ligament complex that is related to loss of support of hindfoot architecture. The spectrum of severity depends on

4: Lower Extremity

Table 1

The Stages of Posterior Tibial Tendon Insufficiency

Condition	Stage I	Stage II	Stage III	Stage IV
Posterior tibial tendinitis	Present	Present	Present	Present
Forefoot abduction	Absent	Present	Present	Present
Hindfoot valgus	Absent	Flexible	Rigid	Rigid
Ankle valgus	Absent	Absent	Absent	Present

whether the tendon is degenerated or completely ruptured and whether the complete spring ligament complex is dysfunctional or only the superior medial portion of the spring ligament is deficient. In the latest stage of the condition, the deltoid ligament complex becomes incompetent and the ankle may drift into valgus.

Studies have indicated that there may be distinct subpopulations with adult acquired flatfoot. Younger patients are more likely to have inflammatory disorders and enthesopathies in comparison with older patients who are more likely to have isolated dysfunction of the posterior tibial tendon. Obesity has been implicated as a contributing factor in several studies. Posterior tibial dysfunction occurs at an increased rate in patients with rheumatoid arthritis, but there is uncertainty as to the specific mechanism of arch collapse in these patients. Algorithms for treatment have been developed based on the stage of the condition.[23] Table 1 describes the stages of posterior tibial tendon insufficiency and associated clinical findings. Efficacy in the nonsurgical treatment of patients with early stage adult acquired flatfoot was noted in a recent study.[24]

Soft-tissue reconstruction alone for posterior tendon insufficiency with clinically significant deformity is uncommon because there is little evidence in the literature to support such treatment. The primary debate involves whether osteotomies or arthrodesis should accompany soft-tissue treatment. Transfer of the flexor digitorum longus tendon to the navicular, the posterior tibial tendon stump, or the medial cuneiform are the most common soft-tissue transfers to accompany posterior tendon reconstruction. However, the efficacies of these transfers have not been compared nor have they been thoroughly evaluated in comparison with no transfer. Those who support the use of these transfers recognize the importance of achieving a biomechanically aligned foot with the heel beneath the tibia. The spring ligament complex also is repaired. The realignment of the valgus heel is typically accomplished either through a medializing calcaneal osteotomy with or without a lateral column lengthening, or by reduction and fusion of the subtalar joint. Clinical studies of each of these options have shown improved clinical status for most patients (**Figure 4**).

Medial movement of the calcaneal tuberosity achieves an improved static alignment of the foot, and also may improve the ability of the Achilles tendon to function as an inverting muscle. Judiciously performed lateral column-lengthening osteotomies of the calcaneus have not resulted in a high rate of clinically important arthritis at the calcaneocuboid joint, although radiographic changes have been seen. Normal hindfoot motion has not been routinely achieved after any of the osteotomy treatments; however, arthrodesis will eliminate most hindfoot motion in instances of subtalar fusion, and will eliminate all hindfoot motion when either triple arthrodesis or isolated talonavicular fusion is used.[25]

Rheumatoid Arthritis

Methods of both nonsurgical and surgical care continue to evolve for the treatment of inflammatory arthropathies. Although most patients with rheumatoid arthritis are treated with medications such as nonsteroidal anti-inflammatory drugs and methotrexate, orthopaedic surgeons should be aware of newer medications such as those that inhibit tumor necrosis factor-α and other immune system-modulating drugs. Ankle and hindfoot arthrosis or an acquired adult flatfoot deformity often develops in patients with rheumatoid arthritis. The principles of treatment for the general population are applicable to these patients, but the specific limitations of patients with rheumatoid arthritis and the medical complications that often accompany inflammatory disease and medication use (such as osteoporosis) must be recognized. Total ankle arthroplasty is often used in this patient population.[26] Acceptable results have been achieved in the intermediate term, but reconstruction is particularly challenging when arthroplasty fails.

In patients with a rheumatoid forefoot, the gold standard of treatment remains stabilization of the first metatarsophalangeal joint and resectional arthroplasty of the lesser rays, if the degree of articular destruction is severe in subluxated or dislocated joints.[27] Some authors have advocated resectional arthroplasty of the first ray instead of arthrodesis, because greater patient satisfaction is perceived.[28,29] Secondary deformities also can be problematic. Because these deformities often appear after follow-up periods of most studies have ended, longer-term follow-up is needed, especially for younger patients. There is interest in attempts to salvage the subluxated or dislocated metatarsophalangeal joints of the lesser rays, but this salvage must be achieved before significant erosion of the articular surfaces; limited outcome information is available for patients treated with this technique.

Diabetes

The care for diabetic patients with complex deformities resulting from neuropathy, fractures, and/or ulcers remains a challenge for orthopaedic surgeons. The prevalence of such foot disorders continues to increase along with the need for a corresponding increase in treatment expertise. The key to successful care for foot

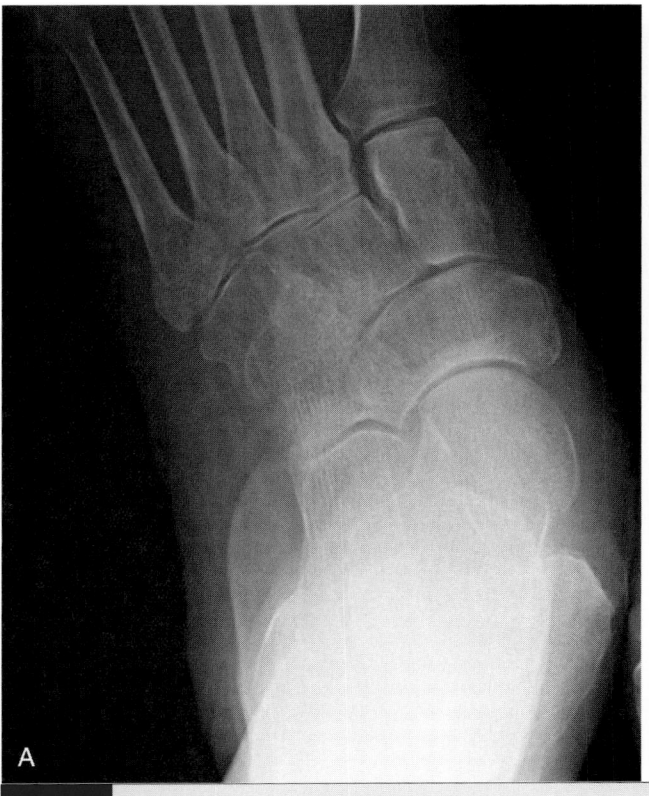 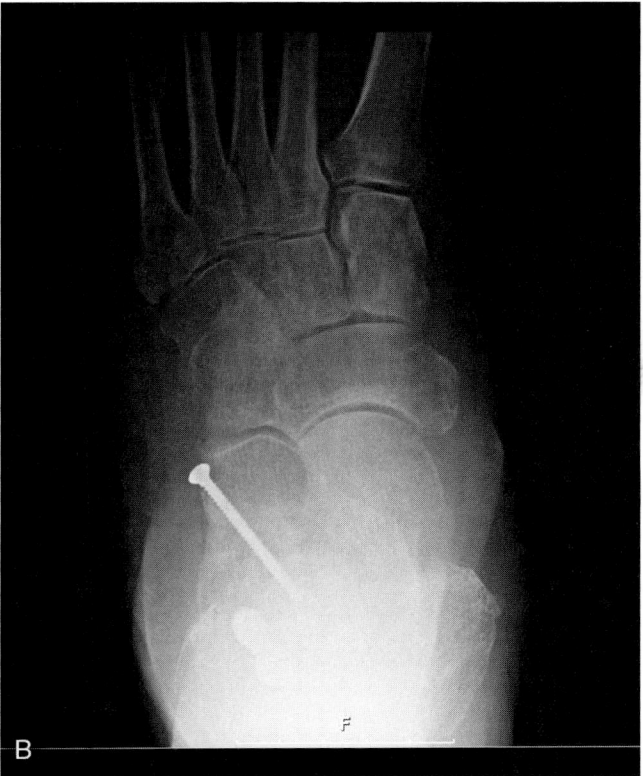

Figure 4 Preoperative **(A)** and postoperative **(B)** AP radiographs showing the correction achieved through extra-articular osteotomy in a patient with posterior tibial tendon insufficiency. The lateral peritalar subluxation is corrected.

and ankle disorders in diabetic patients is an understanding of the mechanical deformities that accompany diabetic neuropathy and a keen appreciation for the physiology that causes these disorders. Although there have been few recent advances in the understanding of joint neuroarthropathy, a 2001 study showed the efficacy of the use of intravenous pamidronate, a bisphosphonate, in the treatment of acute Charcot neuroarthropathy.[30] More recently, a histologic study of neuroarthropathic bone specimens showed a significant increase in the number of osteoclastic cells and a chemical environment of increased bone resorption.[31]

It is important to understand the impact of an equinus contracture of the hindfoot in a diabetic patient with neuropathy. There are several studies showing the effects on forefoot pressures resulting from lengthening of the gastrocnemius or Achilles tendon.[32] Algorithms that use lengthening of the Achilles mechanism to treat and prevent the recurrences of forefoot ulcers have been adopted by some experienced physicians. The importance of Achilles lengthening with partial foot amputations also has been emphasized.

Hallux Valgus Reconstruction

Hallux valgus reconstruction is also challenging to treat and results in a significant percentage of undesirable results. Controversy exists concerning the principle of hypermobility of the first tarsometatarsal joint as a cause or accentuating factor in the development of hallux valgus deformity. The primary clinical determinations that define treatment include the arc of motion of the first metatarsophalangeal joint, the degree of rotation of the toe (pronation), adjacent toe deformities, and the flexibility of the soft tissues. Patients with a significantly limited range of motion of the first metatarsophalangeal joint may be better treated with primary arthrodesis if it is accompanied by radiographic evidence of arthritis. The authors of a few studies have commented on the appearance of the articular surface of the sesamoid bones at the time of hallux valgus reconstruction, but unanticipated articular loss may be a variable that adversely affects the outcome of surgery in these patients (**Figure 5**).

A recent trend is the use of the distal first metatarsal osteotomy (such as a chevron osteotomy) for correcting larger (moderate to severe) deformities. Historically, distal osteotomy was reserved for mild deformities. Some surgeons also are applying limited exposure techniques to treating hallux valgus deformity.[33,34] The surgical options for treatment of symptomatic hallux valgus include distal and proximal metatarsal osteotomies and first tarsometatarsal arthrodesis; each technique is combined with distal soft-tissue procedures. It is recognized that the proximal metatarsal osteotomy, the tar-

4: Lower Extremity

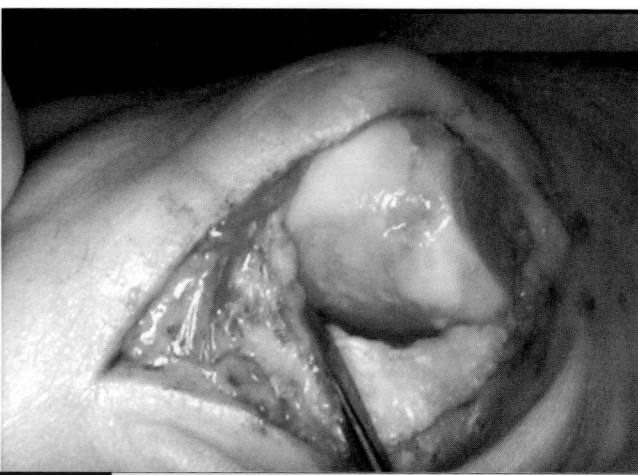

Figure 5 A significant loss of articular cartilage on the plantar aspect of the first metatarsal head is seen in this patient with hallux valgus. No osteoarthritis was apparent on radiographic views.

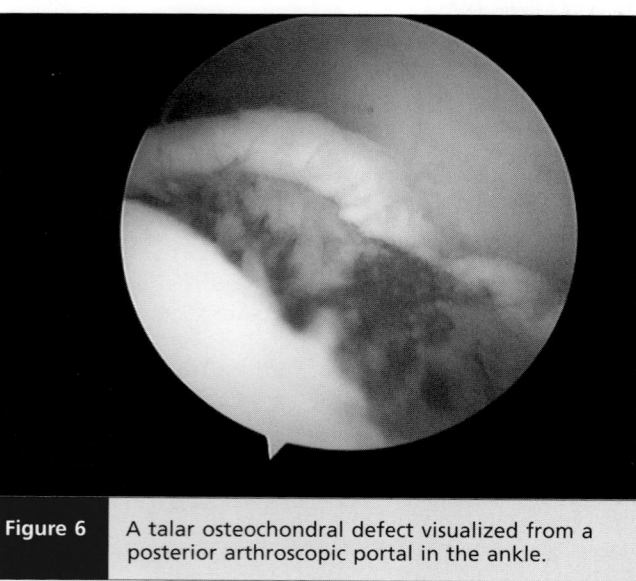

Figure 6 A talar osteochondral defect visualized from a posterior arthroscopic portal in the ankle.

sometatarsal fusion, and the more complicated osteotomies of the midshaft of the first metatarsal (for example, the scarf osteotomy) have a prolonged healing time and are more challenging in terms of technical performance and fixation of the osteotomy.

Arthroscopy of the Foot and Ankle

The role of arthroscopy in the care of foot and ankle disorders continues to expand. Application of arthroscopic techniques in the treatment of hindfoot trauma, arthritis, sports injuries, and chronic conditions are a natural result of improving arthroscopic tools, techniques, and the increasing prevalence of arthroscopy skills in orthopaedic surgeons.[35] Examples of proce-

dures that are more commonly being performed include ankle and subtalar arthrodesis, débridement of loose bodies, treatment of chondral or osteochondral defects, endoscopic calcaneal exostosis excisions (for Haglund's disease) with Achilles tendon insertional débridement, and resection of a symptomatic os trigonum.[36] The ability to safely perform ankle arthroscopy from a posterior approach has improved visualization and treatment options (**Figure 6**). The clinical value of an arthroscopic approach in comparison with more open techniques remains to be proven in many of these procedures, but the goal of limiting soft-tissue injury will likely continue to promote such approaches.

Annotated References

1. Saltzman CL, Salamon ML, Blanchard GM, et al: Epidemiology of ankle arthritis: Report of a consecutive series of 639 patients from a tertiary orthopaedic center. *Iowa Orthop J* 2005;25:44-46.

   At a tertiary medical center, more than 600 consecutive new patients with significant ankle arthritis were assessed to determine the cause of the disorder. Posttraumatic etiology was determined for 70% of patients, 12% were rheumatoid, and 7% were classified as idiopathic. Level of evidence: IV.

2. Winson IG, Robinson DE, Allen PE: Arthroscopic ankle arthrodesis. *J Bone Joint Surg Br* 2005;87:343-347.

   In this study, 116 patients who had been treated with 118 arthroscopic arthrodesis procedures were identified. The patients represented a varied group in terms of diagnoses. At a mean follow-up period of 65 months, 105 ankle fusions were assessed; results showed nonunion in 7.6%. Six patients required subtalar fusions at a mean follow-up of 4 years. Good or excellent results were found in 83 of 105 patients. Level of evidence: IV.

3. Thomas R, Daniels TR, Parker K: Gait analysis and functional outcomes following ankle arthrodesis for isolated ankle arthritis. *J Bone Joint Surg Am* 2006;88: 526-535.

   Twenty-six patients and 27 gender- and age-matched controls were assessed clinically and with gait studies after ankle arthrodesis for isolated ankle arthritis. Twenty patients were completely satisfied (mean follow-up after unilateral arthrodesis, 44 months); however, gait studies showed alterations in gait with a potential for progressive deterioration because of the development of ipsilateral hindfoot arthritis. Level of evidence: III.

4. Coester LM, Saltzman CL, Leupold J, Pontarelli W: Long-term results following ankle arthrodesis for posttraumatic arthritis. *J Bone Joint Surg Am* 2001;83:219-228.

5. Davitt JS, Beals TC, Bachus KN: The effects of medial and lateral displacement calcaneal osteotomies on ankle and subtalar joint pressure distribution. *Foot Ankle Int* 2001;22:885-889.

6. Kuhn MA, Lippert FG: Revision lateral ankle reconstruction. *Foot Ankle Int* 2006;27:77-81.

    The authors present a retrospective review of 15 consecutive patients who had unsuccessful treatment with a revision Gould modification of the Broström procedure for lateral ligament reconstruction. Four patients with hindfoot varus also underwent a lateralizing calcaneal osteotomy. Excellent results were observed in 12 patients at a minimum follow-up of 6 months. Level of evidence: IV.

7. Tanaka Y, Takakura Y, Hayashi K, Taniguchi A, Kumai T, Sugimoto K: Low tibial osteotomy for varus-type osteoarthritis of the ankle. *J Bone Joint Surg Br* 2006; 88:909-913.

    The authors of this retrospective study reviewed 26 ankles treated with an opening wedge valgus-producing tibial osteotomy for arthrosis. All patients were women. Superior results were observed in patients with less severe arthritis. The authors noted the importance of the "Japanese lifestyle" in their study. Level of evidence: IV.

8. van Valburg AA, van Roermund PM, Lammens J, et al: Can Ilizarov joint distraction delay the need for an arthrodesis of the ankle?: A preliminary report. *J Bone Joint Surg Br* 1995;77:720-725.

9. Paley D, Lamm BM: Ankle joint distraction. *Foot Ankle Clin* 2005;10:685-698.

    A review of the principles of ankle joint distraction is presented, with emphasis on technical features and goals of successful distraction and the importance of alignment. Level of evidence: V.

10. Gellman R, Beaman D: External fixation for distraction osteogenesis. *Foot Ankle Clin* 2004;9:489-528.

    This article describes the principles of external fixation distraction for the treatment of symptomatic ankle arthritis. Level of evidence: V.

11. Meehan R, McFarlin S, Bugbee W, Brage M: Fresh ankle osteochondral allograft transplantation for tibiotalar joint arthritis. *Foot Ankle Int* 2005;26:793-802.

    Eleven consecutive patients were treated with fresh osteochondral allografting (bipolar in nine and unipolar in two) and were followed for a minimum of 2 years. A significant improvement occurred in the American Orthopaedic Foot and Ankle Society ankle scores. Three of the five patients who had unsuccessful outcomes were treated with repeat grafting. The authors also present important observations about sizing the grafts and their thickness. Level of evidence: IV.

12. Scranton PE Jr, Frey CC, Feder KS: Outcome of osteochondral autograft transplantation for type-V cystic osteochondral lesions of the talus. *J Bone Joint Surg Br* 2006;88:614-619.

    The authors present a retrospective review of 50 patients surgically treated with talar defects from 8 to 20 mm in diameter (type V lesions). Medial malleolar osteotomies were needed in 26 patients. Autograft was used to fill the defects. At a mean follow-up of 36 months, 90% of patients had good to excellent results. Level of evidence: IV.

13. Kreuz PC, Steinwachs M, Erggelet C, Lahm A, Henle P, Niemeyer P: Mosaicplasty with autogenous talar autograft for osteochondral lesions of the talus after failed primary arthroscopic management: A prospective study with a 4-year follow-up. *Am J Sports Med* 2006;34: 55-63.

    Thirty-four patients who had been surgically treated for osteochondral talar lesions underwent mosaicplasty with an osteochondral graft harvested from the ipsilateral talar articular facet. Two exposure methods for tibial osteotomy were compared. Favorable results were achieved. Level of evidence: IV.

14. Doets HC, Brand R, Nelissen RG: Total ankle arthroplasty in inflammatory joint disease with use of two mobile-bearing designs. *J Bone Joint Surg Am* 2006;88: 1272-1284.

    The authors of this article present a prospective review of 93 ankle replacements at two centers that were treated with two different mobile-bearing designs. At a mean follow-up of 8 years, 15 arthroplasties had been revised. Twenty ankles had malleolar fractures, which were clinically significant only if they occurred with deformity in the frontal plane. Level of evidence: IV.

15. Anderson T, Montgomery F, Carlsson A: Uncemented STAR total ankle prostheses: Three to eight-year follow-up of fifty-one consecutive ankles. *J Bone Joint Surg Am* 2003;85-A:1321-1329.

16. Knecht SI, Estin M, Callaghan JJ, et al: The Agility total ankle arthroplasty: Seven to sixteen-year follow-up. *J Bone Joint Surg Am* 2004;86-A:1161-1171.

    The authors report on 132 ankle arthroplasties in 126 patients who were evaluated at a mean follow-up of 9 years. Of those evaluated at more than 2 years, 76% had some peri-implant lucency, 19% had progressive subtalar arthritis, 15% had progressive talanavicular arthritis, and 8% had a syndesmotic nonunion. Of the 78 surviving patients, more than 90% reported decreased pain and were satisfied with the procedure at 9-year follow-up. Level of evidence: IV.

17. Hopgood P, Kumar R, Wood PL: Ankle arthrodesis for failed total ankle replacement. *J Bone Joint Surg Br* 2006;88:1032-1038.

    The authors describe 23 failed total ankle replacements treated with arthrodesis. Bony union was achieved in 17 ankles. Patients with osteoarthritis were salvaged with tibiotalar arthrodesis with screws, and those with extensive talar destruction (rheumatoid causes) underwent tibiotalocalcaneal arthrodesis. The latter group fared best with treatment using a retrograde nail. Level of evidence: IV.

18. Kotnis R, Pasaula C, Anwar F, Cooke PH, Sharp RJ: The management of failed ankle replacement. *J Bone Joint Surg Br* 2006;88:1039-1047.

    Sixteen patients with failed total ankle replacements were treated over a 5-year period. Two patients had in-

4: Lower Extremity

fections (one was treated with a below-knee amputation). Results showed that 14 patients had aseptic loosening; 5 had revision total ankle replacement, and 9 were treated with arthrodesis. The authors concluded that salvage with fusion was preferable to revision arthroplasty. Level of evidence: IV.

19. Manoli A II, Graham B: The subtle cavus foot, "the underpronator." *Foot Ankle Int* 2005;26:256-263.

This article describes the clinical characteristics of the subtle cavus foot deformity and the clinical presentations that may manifest secondary to the deformity. Level of evidence: V.

20. Fortin PT, Guettler J, Manoli A II: Idiopathic cavovarus and lateral ankle instability: Recognition and treatment implications relating to ankle arthritis. *Foot Ankle Int* 2002;23:1031-1037.

21. Sammarco GJ, Taylor R: Combined calcaneal and metatarsal osteotomies for the treatment of cavus foot. *Foot Ankle Clin* 2001;6:533-543.

22. Giannini S, Ceccarelli F, Benedetti MG, Faldini C, Grandi G: Surgical treatment of adult idiopathic cavus foot with plantar fasciotomy, naviculocuneiform arthrodesis, and cuboid osteotomy. *J Bone Joint Surg Am* 2002;84(supp 2):62-69.

23. Beals TC, Pomeroy GC, Manoli A II : Posterior tibial tendon insufficiency: Diagnosis and treatment. *J Am Acad Orthop Surg* 1999;7:112-118.

24. Alvarez RG, Marini A, Schmitt C, Saltzman CL: Stage I and II posterior tibial tendon dysfunction treated by a structured nonoperative management protocol: An orthosis and exercise program. *Foot Ankle Int* 2006;27:2-8.

Forty-seven consecutive patients with stage I or II posterior tibial tendon insufficiency were treated with a structured protocol involving the use of an orthosis to support the medial arch and with physical therapy. After a median period of 4 months, successful subjective and objective outcomes were reported for 83% of patients. Level of evidence: IV.

25. Myerson MS, Badekas A, Schon LC: Treatment of stage II posterior tibial tendon deficiency with flexor digitorum longus tendon transfer and calcaneal osteotomy. *Foot Ankle Int* 2004;25:445-450.

After surgical treatment for stage II posterior tibial tendon deficiency, 129 patients were evaluated at a mean follow-up of 5.2 years. Most patients were satisfied with the treatment; 97% reported pain relief and 94% noted improved function. Fifty-one percent of patients had slightly decreased subtalar motion and 44% reported normal motion. Significant complications occurred in seven patients. Level of evidence: IV.

26. San Giovanni TP, Keblish DJ, Thomas WH, Wilson MG: Eight-year results of a minimally constrained total ankle arthroplasty. *Foot Ankle Int* 2006;27:418-426.

The authors reviewed 31 ankle arthroplasties in 23 patients at an average follow-up of 8.3 years. Results showed that 89% of patients were satisfied with the outcome and 82% were considered to have stable implants with evidence of bony ingrowth; 32% of patients had intraoperative malleolar fractures (one fracture resulted in a nonunion). The authors stated that these results in low-demand rheumatoid patients were indicative of a predictable procedure over the time period studied. Level of evidence: IV.

27. Mulcahy D, Daniels TR, Lau JT, Boyle E, Bogoch E: Rheumatoid forefoot deformity: A comparison study of 2 functional methods of reconstruction. *J Rheumatol* 2003;30:1440-1450.

28. Thomas S, Kinninmonth AW, Kumar CS: Long-term results of the modified Hoffman procedure in the rheumatoid forefoot. *J Bone Joint Surg Am* 2005;87:748-752.

This consecutive study of 37 feet in 20 patients with an average follow-up of 5.5 years showed that the Hoffman procedure was safe and provided reasonable, if rarely complete, relief of symptoms. Level of evidence: IV.

29. Grondal L, Brostrom E, Wretenberg P, Stark A: Arthrodesis versus Mayo resection: The management of the first metatarsophalangeal joint in reconstruction of the rheumatoid forefoot. *J Bone Joint Surg Br* 2006;88:914-919.

The authors present the results of a randomized prospective study of 31 patients treated with first metatarsophalangeal fusion or with resection arthroplasty with lesser metatarsal head resections. Follow-up at 6 years showed no significant differences in recurrence of the deformity, the need for special shoes, gait velocity, step length, plantar moment, mean pressure, or in the position of the center of force under the forefoot. Level of evidence: II.

30. Jude EB, Selby PL, Burgess J, et al: Bisphosphonates in the treatment of Charcot neuroarthropathy: A double-blind randomized controlled trial. *Diabetologia* 2001;44:2032-2037.

31. Baumhauer JF, O'Keefe RJ, Schon LC, Pinzur MS: Cytokine-induced osteoclastic bone resorption in Charcot arthropathy: An immunohistochemical study. *Foot Ankle Int* 2006;27:797-800.

Results from a histologic review of 20 specimens taken from neuroarthropathic joints showed a significant increase in osteoclastic cells, and was accompanied by an increase in cytokine mediators of bone resorption in comparison with control specimens. Level of evidence: IV.

32. Mueller MJ, Sinacore DR, Hastings MK, Strube MJ, Johnson JE: Effect of Achilles tendon lengthening on neuropathic plantar ulcers: A randomized clinical trial. *J Bone Joint Surg Am* 2003;85-A:1436-1445.

33. Sanhudo JA: Correction of moderate to severe hallux valgus deformity by a modified chevron shaft osteotomy. *Foot Ankle Int* 2006;27:581-585.

The author presents a retrospective review of 50 feet in 34 patients treated with a modified chevron osteotomy for moderate to severe hallux valgus. Based on radiographic studies and limited evaluation of clinical outcomes, the procedure was deemed an appropriate technical treatment option. Level of evidence: IV.

34. Magnan B, Bortolazzi R, Samaila E, Pezze L, Rossi N, Bartolozzi P: Percutaneous distal metatarsal osteotomy for correction of hallux valgus: Surgical technique. *J Bone Joint Surg Am* 2006;88(suppl 1):135-148.

   The authors report that 118 consecutive first metatarsal osteotomies using a percutaneous approach to treat mild to moderate hallux valgus had a 2.5% recurrence rate, and a less than 1% infection rate. Level of evidence: IV.

35. Phisitkul P, Tochigi Y, Saltzman CL, Amendola A: Arthroscopic visualization of the posterior subtalar joint in the prone position: A cadaver study. *Arthroscopy* 2006;22:511-515.

   Working areas of the posterior subtalar joint were defined in cadaveric specimens. A posteromedial portal was determined to increase the working space. Level of evidence: V.

36. van Dijk CN: Hindfoot endoscopy. *Foot Ankle Clin* 2006;11:391-414.

   The author presents a review of hindfoot procedures that can be done arthroscopically or endoscopically.

4: Lower Extremity

Chapter 42
Lower Extremity Amputation

Hans L. Carlson, MD   *Warren Mays, BS, CPO

Introduction

Although the management of amputations is relatively uncommon in a general medical practice, the orthopaedic surgeon will find both the acute and long-term care of lower extremity amputees to be a relatively frequent occurrence.

Current terminology for amputation length is more accurate than in the past. Instead of describing amputation length relative to the nearest joint (for example, below-knee, above-knee), the residual limb is described as being through a specific bone (for example, transtibial or transfemoral). Most limb amputations are of the lower extremity, with the most frequent level being transtibial, followed by the transfemoral level. Lower extremity amputations may be secondary to disease, trauma, tumor, or congenital deformity. Trauma tends to be a common cause of amputation in younger amputees, and peripheral vascular disease is common in older amputees.

The progression from amputation to successful ambulation begins with wound healing. Once the staples or sutures are removed at 3 to 4 weeks after surgery, the patient wears a shrinker sock, a conical elastic sleeve of varying compressive strength and size used in both the transfemoral and transtibial amputee in order to reduce edema and shape the residual limb. Following 1 to 3 weeks of shrinker sock wear, there will be sufficient remodeling of the residual limb to allow casting for fabrication of the socket/prosthesis. The patient generally will receive the prosthesis in 1 to 2 weeks after casting and as therapy visits are often limited, therapy should begin after the amputee is proficient in donning and doffing the prosthesis and able to tolerate standing in the prosthesis for 15 minutes. Four to 8 weeks of therapy should be anticipated for the transtibial/transfemoral amputee, focusing on gait and balance training.

Surgical Management

Preoperative Management

The goals of physical therapy in the preoperative setting include contracture prevention, balance and trans-

*Warren Mays, BS, CPO is the President of Artisan Orthotic-Prosthetic Technologies, Inc.

fer training, and strengthening and endurance exercises. For the patient who is not experiencing complications, this may involve only one or two visits. Early physical therapy also offers the patient the opportunity to have questions and concerns regarding the rehabilitation process addressed before the amputation.

Level of Amputation

The level of amputation (for example, transtibial versus transfemoral) is predicated on many variables, including blood supply, tissue oxygenation, nutritional state, and factors affecting gait efficiency as well as prosthetic fit and available components. Ultimately, the decision on the level of amputation may be based on skin and muscle bleeding at the time of surgery. In general, energy expenditure is increased and gait proficiency is decreased the more proximal the level of amputation (Figures 1 and 2). Patients who have had amputations secondary to vascular disease are less efficient walkers than traumatic amputees.

In choosing a level for amputation, prosthetic management also needs to be considered. For example, the Syme's amputation may leave a long lever and therefore be good for function, but commonly requires adding a lift to the sound-side shoe to provide a level pelvis. If

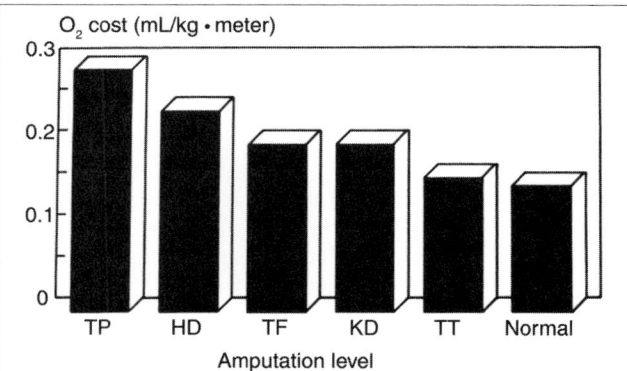

Figure 1 Oxygen cost in unilateral amputees walking with a prosthesis at different amputation levels. TP = transpelvic; HD = hip disarticulation; TF = transfemoral; KD = knee disarticulation; TT = transtibial. *(Reproduced from Bowker JH, Michael JW [eds]: Atlas of Limb Prosthetics: Surgical, Prosthetic, and Rehabilitation Principles. Rosemont, IL, American Academy of Orthopaedic Surgeons, 2001, p 384.)*

4: Lower Extremity

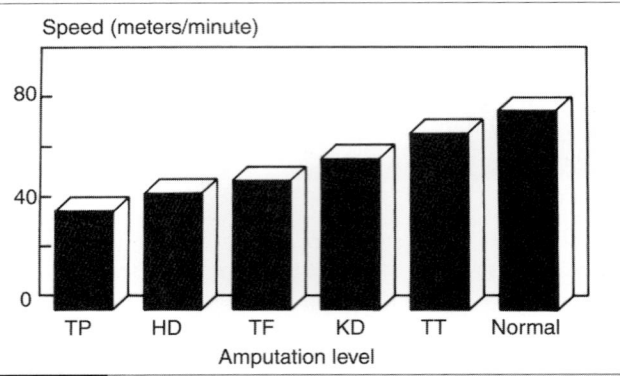

Speed (meters/minute)

Figure 2 Speed in unilateral amputees walking with a prosthesis at different amputation levels. TP = transpelvic; HD = hip disarticulation; TF = transfemoral; KD = knee disarticulation; TT = transtibial. *(Reproduced from Bowker JH, Michael JW [eds]:* Atlas of Limb Prosthetics: Surgical, Prosthetic, and Rehabilitation Principles. *Rosemont, IL, American Academy of Orthopaedic Surgeons, 2001, p 385.*

cosmetic appearance is of greater importance to the patient than power, the patient may be frustrated by the bulky appearance of a Syme's socket and/or the need to have a lift applied to all contralateral shoes. Because the function and comfort afforded by new designs for prosthetic feet and the ability to match height side-to-side are greater in transtibial amputations, it may be advantageous for many patients to proceed with the higher level of amputation.[1] One of the advantages of the Syme's amputation has been that one could walk on the residual limb unsupported by a prosthetic socket. However, the incidence of migration of the distal fatty heel pad is well documented in the Syme's amputation, and this finding may be facilitated by weight bearing without the support of a socket.[2] Furthermore, once the fatty pad has migrated (usually medially and posteriorly), the ability to accept the distal pressures of a prosthetic socket is greatly diminished, often resulting in a limb with no weight-bearing capabilities whatsoever. Therefore, the Syme's amputation should not be considered as a viable weight-bearing option without the support of a rigid socket.

The decision to perform a transfemoral amputation versus a knee disarticulation remains controversial, as there are advantages and disadvantages to each procedure. One potential advantage of the knee disarticulation is that energy expenditure during walking may be less than that for a transfemoral amputee.[3] Another advantage is that the knee disarticulation provides for an end-bearing residual limb. The knee disarticulation also includes complete preservation of the thigh muscles, leading to better muscular balance, and the bulbous shape of the residual limb leads to increased stability of the prosthesis.[4] Disadvantages of knee disarticulation include limitations in knee-joint prosthetic components and concerns regarding the cosmesis of the prosthesis, as well as the asymmetry of the knee

joint with respect to sitting and gait. Because knee disarticulations are relatively uncommon compared with transfemoral amputations, many prosthetists may have less familiarity with the fabrication and fit of this prosthesis. One of the more important issues with respect to knee disarticulation versus transfemoral amputation is the degree of trauma involving the soft tissue around the knee, as increased tissue trauma may lead to painful residual limbs and eventually the need for revision amputation at a higher level.[5] If the residual limb of the knee disarticulation is unable to accommodate the distal-end weight bearing of the socket, then patients with a knee disarticulation may experience decreased levels of function compared with patients undergoing transfemoral amputation.

Length of the Residual Limb
Once the level of amputation has been determined, planning the length of the residual limb is the next step. Important issues to consider include: (1) length of usable lever arm, which also determines the power an amputee will have for ambulation; (2) remaining space for available components; and (3) cosmetic appearance. Patients prioritize these considerations according to their own situation.

The ideal length of a transtibial amputation is at the point where the upper third and middle third of the tibia meet. This length allows the gastrosoleus muscles with a long posterior flap to serve as the padding at the distal end of the tibia. A longer limb is better only to a certain degree. If there is not enough space for inclusion of the technologically advanced feet and shock-reducing pylon systems currently being used, patients may be left with the choice of accepting less responsive and less comfortable components, or adding sizable shoe lifts for every contralateral shoe they own.

The ideal length of a transfemoral amputation preserves 50% to 75% of the femur. A residual limb in the transfemoral amputee that is too short will not only interfere with socket design, but also muscular control of the hip joint. To get the most use out of the more advanced knee systems currently available, the removal of at least 3 inches of bone is necessary to allow for the thickness of the socket, socket adaptor(s), and connection to the knee. Transfemoral amputations leaving less than 2 inches of femur are often fitted as hip disarticulations because of difficulty with socket control. In this instance, the presence of 2 inches of residual femur may further complicate the fitting process in the hip disarticulation socket.

Standard trim lines for a hip disarticulation socket are suprapelvic to stabilize the socket; this configuration is thicker and cosmetically difficult to hide. Some patients may trade off some socket control for a more cosmetic appearance; in these instances, the ipsilateral greater trochanter can assist with suspension and therefore provide a less bulky socket.

Technique: Transtibial Amputation

In general, beveling the bone edges of the distal residual tibia and recessing and beveling the fibula will be helpful in minimizing trauma to the overlying muscle and soft tissue. A variation of this technique is the Ertl procedure, which is usually done as a revision procedure in patients who have experienced continued pain and discomfort long after the initial amputation. The Ertl procedure and variations of this technique create a bony synostosis between the tibia and the fibula, with the advantages of stabilizing the fibula as well as increasing the bony surface area for weight bearing.[6] Proponents of the procedure also espouse the benefits of a closed medullary canal and normal intramedullary pressure gradient with respect to bone nutrition and pain, although this theory is not well established. Currently, there is increased interest in the United States with respect to applying the principles of the Ertl procedure in transtibial and transfemoral amputees.[7]

Immediate Postoperative Care

Postoperative Dressings

Following surgery, many options are available regarding postoperative dressings. Most commonly, simple gauze dressings are used with an elastic wrap. In the transtibial amputation population, other options include rigid plaster dressings with or without an attached prosthesis versus rigid removable dressings. Pneumatic prostheses using air compression within the socket combined with the prosthesis have also been used. The goals of postoperative dressings are to improve wound healing, control pain, protect the residual limb, and speed the process for prosthetic fitting and functional ambulation. Proponents of the rigid dressing with or without attached prostheses support these dressings for the control of edema in the residual limb and protection of the residual limb from inadvertent trauma, as well as prevention of knee contractures with thigh-high rigid dressings. Furthermore, it is thought that early weight bearing may improve early wound healing, although this is not well established.[8] A critical review of the literature regarding postoperative dressings noted that while rigid dressings may lead to a shorter time to initial gait training, the type of dressing management did not affect outcomes of using a prosthesis, time to ambulation, or fitting of the final prosthesis.[8]

Postoperative Rehabilitation Management

The physical therapist can start the rehabilitation process even while the wound is healing. Many of these interventions are progressions of activity that was started before surgery with the goals of preventing hip and/or knee flexion contractures, maintaining conditioning and endurance, and educating the patient regarding wound management and scar tissue mobilization. For successful ambulation, the transtibial amputee should have at least 80% of the strength of the uninjured leg in the involved hip and knee, with full hip and knee extension and up to 70° of knee flexion. Ideally, the transfemoral amputee will have no limitations in hip range of motion but generally can tolerate less than 10° of hip flexion or abduction contractures without significant difficulty in prosthetic fitting. During the healing phase of the residual limb, the superficial scar and soft tissue become adherent to the deep soft tissue and muscle. This creates a residual limb that is less tolerant to pressure or shear forces and may limit the patient's use of the prosthetic limb. The therapist can educate the patient in scar mobilization techniques to minimize this effect; this may also help the patient tolerate phantom pain and/or hypersensitivity of the amputated limb.

Residual limb pain is defined as pain located within the residual limb, whereas phantom limb pain is pain perceived to be coming from the missing portion of the limb. From 46% to 90% of lower extremity amputees will continue to have pain 1 year following their amputation, with 69.2% reporting phantom pain and 41.8% reporting residual limb pain.[9] Almost 40% of these patients rated the residual limb pain as ranging from distressing to more severe. Neuroma development is estimated at 95% to 100% of nerve transactions, but only 40% to 50% may be painful.[10] Some theories of why neuromas may lead to residual nerve pain include traction by scar tissue surrounding the neuroma, chronic inflammation leading to movement of the neuroma, or hypoxia or compression by surrounding tissues. Free nerve fascicles at the location of the painful neuroma are also postulated as an etiology for pain.[11] A technical decision at the time of surgery involves the method of transaction of the peripheral nerve. Techniques to minimize neuroma formation include interosseous nerve transposition,[12] central canal or end-to-side anastomosis of the transected nerve[13,14] as well as transplantation of the nerve stump into veins,[15] and techniques to cap the nerve with the epineural sleeve and/or synthetic tissue adhesive.[11] There are several neuropathic pain medications such as gabapentin or pregabalin that can be effective in treating residual and phantom limb pain.

Prosthetic Management

As the surgical incision heals, the use of elastic wraps or shrinker socks can help to control edema and speed the process of the reshaping of the residual limb. These techniques will allow the new lower extremity amputee to be fit with the prosthesis earlier and, ideally, to ambulate earlier. Generally, amputees do not require the use of the shrinker socks after they have transitioned to using their prostheses. Patients need to be well educated in the proper application of these devices to avoid skin injury.

Rehabilitation/Long-Term Care

Prosthetic Management

The increased number of combat veterans with amputations has forced a rethinking of prosthetic treatment.

4: Lower Extremity

Typically, the time from casting the residual limb to the initial fit is several weeks. With new prosthetic technology and increased efficiency, the design, fabrication, and initial prosthesis fitting on the same day that the surgical staples are removed is now possible. A team approach is required, and these advances may improve a patient's ability to adapt to and use the new prosthesis. This suggests that the "golden window" usually referred to in the treatment of upper extremity amputees may hold true with the treatment of lower extremity amputees as well—the sooner the patient receives the first prosthesis, the better the outcome.[16]

Preparatory Prosthesis Versus Definitive Prosthesis

Socket fit and prosthetic alignment are as critical, if not more critical, than the components of the prosthesis for successful ambulation. If the limb is well healed but significant swelling or edema are present, then the socket fit will be compromised as swelling decreases. Almost all new lower extremity amputees will have continued remodeling of the residual limb when they begin using the new prosthesis; this change in size and shape is accommodated with the use of extra socks or modifications to the socket. When extra socks no longer help with the fit, then a new socket is required. More than one revision of the socket may be necessary during the maturation process. Over time, this shrinking will slow down, but there tends to be some temporal change in shape such that at some point when a prosthesis needs to be replaced secondary to routine wear and tear, a new socket is cast as opposed to relying on the old socket. The "preparatory prosthesis" is defined as an initial prosthesis designed to accommodate radical changes in shape or volume through manipulation of a socket insert. Pin and gel liner systems that do not include the use of a socket insert should be saved for a more stable, mature residual limb; such systems are termed a "definitive prosthesis."

Rehabilitation

Once the new amputee has the prosthesis in place, rehabilitation focusing on gait training begins. The new amputee needs to be advised that there is a breaking-in process for conditioning the limb to accept weight-bearing pressures, as well as for developing a new sense of balance. Slowly increasing the use of the new limb from several 10- to 25-minute sessions to full-time prosthetic wearing may take several weeks.

Prosthetic Prescription

The first step in prescribing a prosthesis is to determine the method of construction and then select the components and accessories. The lower extremity prosthetic prescription has the common elements of the socket, suspension, pylon, and foot. Transfemoral and knee disarticulation amputees will also have a mechanical knee joint. The socket may include the suspension and/or py-

lon (metal tube), depending on the design of the prosthesis.

Construction

Endoskeletal prostheses comprise most of the limbs currently made. Endoskeletal systems depend on a pylon for the structure and strength of the prosthesis. These systems usually can be easily accessed to adjust alignment or to interchange components (feet, sockets, etc). A soft cosmetic cover can be placed over the pylon. Exoskeletal systems are likely to be used for patients who have used them in the past and prefer them over other prostheses. These systems have an anatomically shaped rigid outer shell that provides support and is extremely durable. Exoskeletal systems are often considered to be heavier than endoskeletal systems, and their main drawback is the difficulty in making changes to the alignment of the prosthesis after the prosthesis has been manufactured.

Foot Amputations

Functional goals determine the prosthesis prescription in the partial foot amputee. For phalangeal and distal metatarsal amputations, a "toe filler" is often used. A toe filler is an arch support with a carbon footplate built into it to provide adequate toe lever, as well as to protect the distal end of the amputation. Patients with slightly more proximal amputations can use a silicone boot, with or without zipper closure. Adequate longitudinal foot support requires a carbon plate incorporated into the device or a steel shank placed in the shoe. Lisfranc, Chopart, Pirigoff, Boyd, and Syme's levels all need to be supported by a prosthetic foot and socket, as efficient ambulation is not possible with the short remaining lever from these amputations.[17] The prosthetic foot lever helps to keep the calf musculature from overpowering the lack of anterior musculature, thereby preventing plantar contracture. Surgical technique is important in stabilizing the soft-tissue structures of the partial foot amputee.

Transtibial Amputations

The transtibial amputation is the most common level for lower extremity amputations. Patients who undergo transtibial amputation generally experience good results and are successful ambulators with their prosthetic limbs.

Socket/Suspension

Current options in transtibial sockets include the patellar tendon-bearing (PTB) and total surface-bearing (TSB) designs. The PTB socket is actually a misnomer, as the principal weight-bearing areas are a combination of the medial tibial flare, a popliteal counterpressure, and mild pressure over the patellar tendon. Few patients can tolerate excessive pressure over the patellar tendon. The PTB socket may also be designed with a soft insert (plastic, leather, or foam) that assists with both comfort and suspension. There are many modifications to this socket, including supracondylar and suprapatellar extensions that can add stability to the knee or aid with suspension.

The goal of the TSB socket is to distribute the weight-bearing aspects of the socket over as great an area as possible, thereby reducing overall socket pressures. Typically, this is done with the use of a pin and silicone liner that mechanically engage into a locking mechanism at the bottom of the socket. One TSB socket system can be fabricated directly to the residual limb so that the fabrication time is much quicker. This advance has not translated to any significant difference in gait parameters or socket adjustments and only a minor difference in comfort compared with the PTB socket.[18]

A recent development in TSB socket design and suspension is the suction transtibial socket. There are two different methods of achieving this type of suspension: through the use of a simple one-way valve located in the bottom of the socket, or through the use of the vacuum-assisted suction suspension system, which uses a dynamic vacuum pump that actively removes air and moisture from the socket environment with every step. Suction systems require an additional suspension sleeve, which some patients may object to using.

Pylon

Pylon tubes are usually made of either aircraft-grade aluminum or carbon. An adaptor can be integrated onto one end of the tube to provide an easy connection to other components. These tubes are engineered to different patient weights. A shock absorber and/or transverse rotator mechanism may be incorporated into the pylon design or placed between the pylon and socket or pylon and foot. Transverse rotators are beneficial to those who are involved in activities that require frequent turning (such as golfing or assembly-line work).

Foot Prostheses

There are many options available when selecting the prosthetic foot. The various types include the basic SACH (solid ankle, cushion heel), single axis, multiaxial, energy storing, dynamic, and today's high-energy return carbon feet. A variety of methods of manufacturing combine wood, aluminum, Kevlar, Delrin plastic, carbon, hydraulics, and linkages. The goal of all prosthetic feet is to provide the smoothest rollover possible given a patient's activity level. New patients need stability. "Seasoned" amputees are usually looking for more responsive, active feet. A few foot models have adjustable heel height.

Supplies

The only remaining items to consider are the miscellaneous supplies associated with prosthetic use such as socks, sheaths, and lubricants. If a pin and gel liner system is chosen as the means of suspension, it is customary to provide the patient with two liners because the materials from which the liners are made require 24 hours of nonuse to allow return to the original shape.

Transfemoral Amputations

The transfemoral prosthetic prescription is formulated identically to the transtibial prescription except for the inclusion of a mechanical knee joint.

Socket/Suspension

Socket shapes affect fit and function. Transfemoral socket options include the ischial containment socket and its variants, narrow mediolateral sockets, and quadrilateral sockets. The quadrilateral shapes afford the patient more power, as they are tighter in the anteroposterior dimension. Narrow mediolateral shapes and muscle-contoured shapes tend to be wider in the anteroposterior dimension, sacrificing power for stability in the mediolateral dimension. Suspension options for a transfemoral socket include suction, partial suction, hip joint and pelvic belt, Silesian belt, and gel liner with pin or lanyard. Although suction sockets still comprise most transfemoral fittings, the pin and gel liner systems have become more popular. Suction sockets are prone to fitting complications if there is an increase or decrease in weight. With weight loss, the patient cannot maintain suction. With weight gain, the patient cannot don the socket. With gel liner systems, weight (or volume) is less of an issue because socks can be added or removed as volume fluctuates. Gel liner systems can provide the patient with greater ease in donning and doffing their prosthesis. Residual limbs that have excessive scar tissue or prominent bony anatomy may also benefit from the use of the gel liner system. Usually, to be a candidate for the gel liner system, the patient should have a longer residual limb, with as little redundant tissue as possible, as this will only add to pistoning within the socket. Poor hand strength and lack of hygiene are contraindications for use of liners as the liner must be cleaned after each use.

Knee Prostheses

There are hundreds of prosthetic knee designs, ranging from the single-axis knee to the more technologically advanced microprocessor-controlled knees. Any of these knees may be appropriate based on the component's weight, stability, and cosmetic features as well as the patient's functional goals. Single-axis knees are light and are generally dependent on prosthetic alignment to achieve stability. Some have a stance-phase locking mechanism (safety knee). For the mid- to short-length transfemoral amputation, lightweight hydraulic knees provide greater responsiveness and a smoother gait. For the longer transfemoral and knee disarticulation patients, four-bar knees provide maximum stability, as they have an instantaneous center of rotation posterior to the actual mechanical knee joint. They are also relatively lightweight and are useful cosmetically to help hide the long length of the socket. Pneumatic knees are available in both single and polycentric configurations and generally offer a less expensive alternative to fluid hydraulic knees. Hydraulic knees are typically single-axis knees that may have a stance-phase locking mechanism. They tend to be a heavier but more responsive

4: Lower Extremity

alternative to other knees. There are a few hydraulic knees that are very light, but do not offer stance-phase locking. Microprocessor-controlled knees are quicker to respond than all of the above. Their strength is generally either in stability during stance phase or responsiveness in swing phase. They are heavier than most other knees, and at this point use may be limited secondary to reimbursement issues; however, they are accepted as medically appropriate for the proper patient by the health care community.

Hip Disarticulations

Hip disarticulation prescriptions follow the same criteria as those for transfemoral amputations, with the inclusion of a hip joint. Compared with other components, there are relatively few options for prosthetic hip joints; most are spring-assisted devices.

Technologic Advances in Prosthetics

Plasterless Fittings

Many tools are now available to help expedite prosthetic fittings. One of the new technologies available to the prosthetist is the use of digital scanners to obtain a model of the residual limb. Typically, a digital image of the residual limb is obtained by either running a wand over the surface anatomy, allowing the computer program to record the shape, or by using a ring-type scanner that does not make contact with the residual limb but records the shape by bouncing a laser beam off of it.[19] In either instance, the end result is a digital image that can then be viewed and modified on the computer to improve the weight-bearing aspects of a socket shape or take pressure off of sensitive bony areas. The final shape is then carved out of a foam block for use in the socket fabrication process. Computer-aided socket design is still dependent on input from the prosthetist, and therefore does not represent an improvement in overall socket fit. Digital scanning works well on specific types of devices, such as transfemoral sockets, for which there is more soft tissue relative to bone. The scanner does not have the ability to detect the density of tissue beneath the scanned surface. Heterotopic ossification and other anomalies will be missed if a thorough examination of the underlying anatomy is neglected. Therefore, the advantages of using scanning technology are for producing and fabricating a socket shape quickly, storing the shape digitally for future use, and increasing efficiency with a plasterless facility. Currently, the benefit to the patient may be in time savings only. As technology continues to improve, and the ability to sense density of tissue develops, scanning will become the accepted method of acquiring a socket shape.

Osseointegration

One of the most dramatic changes in the treatment of the amputees is osseointegration. This procedure involves attaching prosthetic limbs directly to titanium implants secured in bone. Osseointegration evolved from experience with dental implants. This use represents an interesting leap in prosthetic philosophy in that the weakest link in the system, the fit of the prosthetic socket, is completely removed. Perceived weight of the prosthesis, lack of prosthetic control, sweating and heat (or cold), socket-induced skin irritation, and weight gain or loss are all common issues associated with the wearing of a prosthetic socket. These issues are eliminated with osseointegration because there is no socket. However, major hurdles face the medical community before osseointegration is accepted in the United States, including the elevated risks of infection around the implant.[20]

Components

Microprocessor-controlled prosthetic knees are becoming more commonplace within the industry. Although the evidence is unclear as to how significantly gait and function are affected by this new technology, patients report improved stability and confidence.[21-23] However, the microprocessor-controlled knees have different advantages relative to one another. The Otto-Bock C-leg (Otto-Bock, Minneapolis, MN), the first microprocessor-controlled knee available in the United States, focuses on providing stance-phase stability. The Rheo knee (Ossur, Aliso Viejo, CA) provides the patient with faster and more predictable swing-phase control, which may be a preference for those wishing to run or participate in other activities requiring the knee to return quickly to the extended position. Many companies have also produced their own versions of these products, providing the rehabilitation team and patient with many choices. New advances are continuing, with one manufacturer (Ossur) introducing microprocessor-controlled "bionic technology" in a line of components that provides powered knee extension and foot dorsiflexion.

Emerging Concepts and Future Directions

Technology is reshaping the care of the amputee. From plasterless laboratories to microprocessor-controlled knees and feet, the care of amputees currently requires electrical and computer engineering skills as opposed to the craftsmanship of the past. The experiences in the military hospitals will be incorporated into the community treatment and rehabilitation of these patients. To improve outcomes, physicians will need to partner with rehabilitation specialists to plan therapy and prosthetic treatment modalities. These advances will allow amputees to be more successful with all types of activities.

Annotated References

1. Pasquina PF, Bryant PR, Huang ME, Roberts TL, Nelson VS, Flood KM: Advances in amputee care. *Arch Phys Med Rehabil* 2006;87(3 suppl 1):S34-S45.

The authors provide a comprehensive review of amputee management including surgical and rehabilitation issues.

2. Gaine WJ, McCreath SW: Syme's amputation revisited: A review of 46 cases. *J Bone Joint Surg Br* 1996;78:461-467.

3. Pinzur MS, Gold J, Schwartz D, Gross N: Energy demands for walking in dysvascular amputees as related to the level of amputation. *Orthopedics* 1992;15:1033-1037.

4. Baumgartner RF: Knee disarticulation versus above-knee amputation. *Prosthet Orthot Int* 1979;3:15-19.

5. MacKenzie EJ, Bosse MJ, Castillo RC, et al: Functional outcomes following trauma-related lower-extremity amputation. *J Bone Joint Surg Am* 2004;86:1636-1645.

This prospective study of 161 lower extremity amputees focuses on functional outcomes and level of amputation.

6. Pinto MA, Harris WW: Fibular segment bone bridging in trans-tibial amputation. *Prosthet Orthot Int* 2004;28:220-224.

This case series reviews an alternative technique to the Ertl procedure for creating a tibia/fibula synostosis.

7. Pinzur MS, Pinto MA, Schon LC, Smith DG: Controversies in amputation surgery. *Instr Course Lect* 2003;52:445-451.

8. Smith DG, McFarland LV, Sangeorzan BJ, Reiber GE, Czerniecki JM: Postoperative dressing and management strategies for transtibial amputations: A critical review. *J Rehabil Res Dev* 2003;40:213-224.

9. Gallagher P, Allen D, Maclachlan M: Phantom limb pain and RLP. *Disabil Rehabil* 2001;23:522-530.

10. Herndon JH: Neuromas, in Green DP (ed): *Operative Hand Surgery*. New York, NY, Churchill Livingstone, 1982, pp 939-955.

11. Martini A, Fromm B: A new operation for the prevention and treatment of amputation neuromas. *J Bone Joint Surg Br* 1989;71:379-382.

12. Goldstein SA, Sturim HS: Intraosseous nerve transposition for treatment of painful neuromas. *J Hand Surg Am* 1985;10:270-274.

13. Barbera J, Albert-Pamplo R: Centrocentral anastomosis of the proximal nerve stump in the treatment of painful amputation neuromas of major nerves. *J Neurosurg* 1993;79:331-334.

14. Low CK, Chew SH, Song IC, Ng TH, Low YP: End-to-side anastomosis of transected nerves to prevent neuroma formation. *Clin Orthop Relat Res* 1999;369:327-332.

15. Koch H, Haas F, Hubmer M, Rappl T, Scharnagl E: Treatment of painful neuroma by resection and nerve stump transplantation into a vein. *Ann Plast Surg* 2003;51:45-50.

16. Sathishkumar S, Manigandan C, Asha T, Charles J, Poonoose PP: A cost-effective, adjustable, femoral socket, temporary prosthesis for immediate rehabilitation of above-knee amputation. *Int J Rehabil Res* 2004;27:71-74.

This article introduces a temporary prosthesis and reviews the benefits of early ambulation.

17. Dillon MP, Barker TM: Can partial foot prostheses effectively restore foot length? *Prosthet Orthot Int* 2006;30:17-23.

This prospective gait analysis of partial foot amputees defines the inability of toe fillers to provide normal gait characteristics.

18. Datta D, Harris I, Heller B, Howitt J, Martin R: Gait, cost and time implications for changing from PTB to ICEX sockets. *Prosthet Orthot Int* 2004;28:115-120.

This randomized trial compared gait, prosthetic visits, and comfort with respect to PTB and TSB socket prostheses.

19. McGarry T, McHugh B: Evaluation of a contemporary CAD/CAM system. *Prosthet Orthot Int* 2005;29:221-229.

This study assesses the accuracy of a digital scanner for measuring dimensions and volumes.

20. Sullivan J, Uden M, Robinson KP, Sooriakumaran S: Rehabilitation of the trans-femoral amputee with an osseointegrated prosthesis: The United Kingdom experience. *Prosthet Orthot Int* 2003;27:114-120.

21. Orendurff MS, Segal AD, Klute GK, McDowell ML, Pecoraro JA, Czerniecki JM: Gait efficiency using the C-leg. *J Rehabil Res Dev* 2006;43:239-246.

This prospective randomized crossover study compared a microprocessor-controlled knee to a more traditional knee and found limited differences with respect to gait efficiency.

22. Klute GK, Berge JS, Orendurff MS, Williams RM, Czerniecki JM: Prosthetic intervention effects on activity of lower-extremity amputees. *Arch Phys Med Rehabil* 2006;87:717-722.

This study compared a microprocessor-controlled knee to a more traditional knee and found no differences with respect to daily activity level or duration of activity.

23. Chin T, Machida K, Sawamura S, et al: Comparison of different microprocessor controlled knee joints on the energy consumption during walking in trans-femoral amputees: Intelligent Knee Prosthesis (IP) versus C-leg. *Prosthet Orthot Int* 2006;30:73-80.

This study compared amputees with microprocessor-controlled knees to able-bodied controls and suggests that these prostheses may provide for a lower energy-consumption gait.

4: Lower Extremity

Section 5

Spine

SECTION EDITORS:

ALAN S. HILIBRAND, MD
JIM A. YOUSSEF, MD

Chapter 43

Intervertebral Disk Degeneration

D. Greg Anderson, MD   Kern Singh, MD   Patrick J. Cahill, MD   Michael J. Lee, MD

Chadi Tannoury, MD   Matthew G. Zmurko, MD

Pathoanatomy of Intervertebral Disk Degeneration

The concept of a cascade of spinal motion segment degeneration invoking progressive wear of the intervertebral disk and facet joints was presented more than 25 years ago.[1] The interdependence of the disk and facet joints for normal spinal function was emphasized and how derangement or injury to either of these articulations leads to abnormal forces and impairment of the other was described. Although insightful, this algorithm was mechanistic and only highlighted biomechanical disturbances associated with degeneration of the motion segment. Over the decades since, research has revealed that spinal degeneration involves a complex interplay of biologic and biomechanical events that are genetically predisposed and modulated by environmental influences.

There are many sources of spinal pain, but the intervertebral disk is the structure that is implicated most often. A host of diagnostics (including diskography) and therapeutic interventions are directed toward the disk. Most treatments of so-called painful disks have, however, met with inconsistent clinical outcomes,[2] probably reflecting a relatively unsophisticated approach to understanding spinal pain. Recent data supporting the idea of facet (zygapophyseal) joint-mediated pain have come from studies of patients sustaining cervical whiplash injuries. Several authors have evaluated cervical zygapophyseal joint pain after whiplash in a diagnostic double-blind study using placebo-controlled local anesthetic blocks. In an evaluation of 68 patients with a predominant report of neck pain and headaches after a whiplash injury, the authors noted that among patients with dominant headache, comparative blocks revealed that the prevalence of C2-3 zygapophyseal joint pain was 50%. Overall, the prevalence of cervical zygapophyseal joint pain was 60% (95% confidence interval, 46% to 73%).[3,4] These studies further support the complex interplay of the intervertebral disk and facet joints in health and disease of the spine.

The understanding of spinal degeneration has advanced as it becomes clear that the degenerative cascade involves interplay of both biologic and biomechanical factors. Biochemical events are important in the pathogenesis of the degenerative process as well as in the pain-signaling pathways responsible for the clinical features of the condition. As the biologic aspects of spinal degeneration are better understood, less invasive, nonablative treatments designed to reverse these biologic processes and restore the disk and facet functioning may become a reality.

Normal Intervertebral Disk and Facet Anatomy

The motion segment of the lumbar spine consists of an anterior intervertebral disk and two posterior facets. This three-joint complex allows for motion and resists the compressive forces across the vertebral column. Although motion occurs at all three joints, the intervertebral disk provides the most resistance to compression, whereas the facets allow for rotation, lateral bending, and extension.

The intervertebral disk acts as a load-bearing structure with two distinct components: the nucleus pulposus and the anulus fibrosus. Each component has very distinct biomechanical properties. The nucleus pulposus, rich in proteoglycan, acts as an internal viscid semifluid mass, whereas the anulus fibrosus, rich in collagen, acts as a laminar fibrous container.[5] The unique combination of biochemical and biomechanical properties of the anulus fibrosus and nucleus pulposus allows the intervertebral disk to absorb and disperse the normal loading forces experienced by the spine.[6,7] The presumption is that when either the anulus fibrosus or nucleus pulposus is structurally compromised, degenerative changes will ensue because of the alteration in mechanical force distribution across the functional spinal unit.

Facet joints are true synovial articulations that undergo degenerative changes similar to those of osteoarthritis seen in other synovial joints. The facet joints are one of the primary stabilizing structures of the spinal motion segment.[8,9] As the degenerative cascade progresses and anterior column support is lost, the facet joints bear more weight and the fulcrum moves dorsally to balance the motion segment. With progressive spinal degeneration, the load-bearing patterns of the facet joints are altered.

Sagittal Subdivisions of the Spinal Canal

The lumbar spinal canal is divided into three regions from midline to lateral—the central zone, the lateral re-

5: Spine

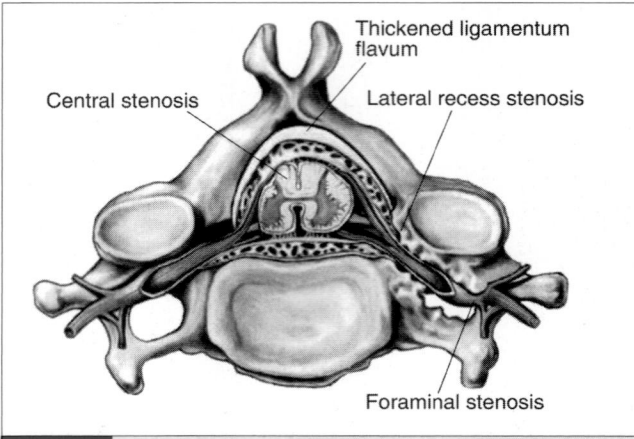

Figure 1   Axial cross-sectional representation of the three zones of spinal stenosis—central, lateral recess, and foraminal. (Reproduced with permission from Gallego J, Schnuerer AP, Manuel C: Basic Anatomy and Pathology of the Spine, ed 2. Memphis, TN, Medtronic Sofamor Danek, 2003, p 106.)

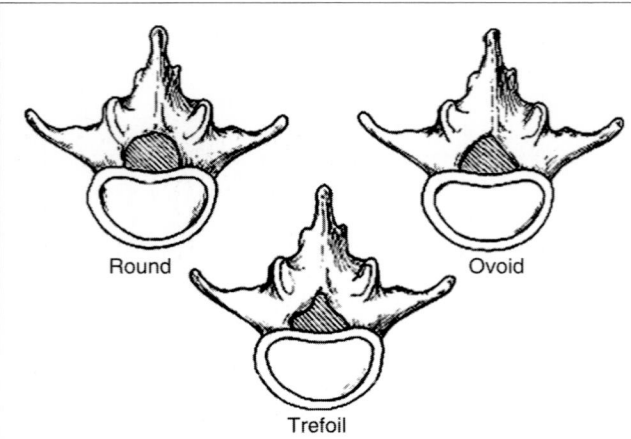

Figure 2   The three typical shapes of the spinal canal. Trefoil canals have the smallest cross-sectional area. (Reproduced from Hilibrand AS, Rand N: Degenerative lumbar stenosis: Diagnosis and management. J Am Acad Orthop Surg 1999;7:239-249.)

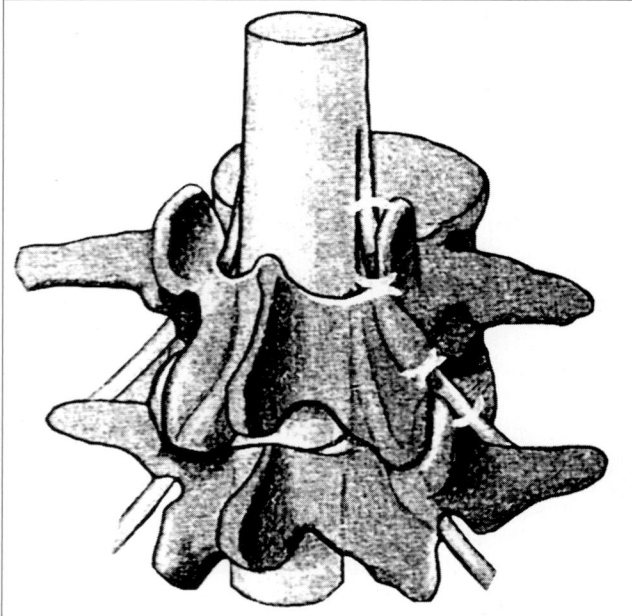

Figure 3   Cross-sectional representation of the zones of the exiting nerve root. (Reproduced with permission from Lee CK, Rauschning W, Glenn W: Lateral lumbar spinal stenosis: Classification, pathologic anatomy and surgical decompression. Spine 1988;13:313-320.)

The lateral recess and foraminal zones have been further defined. The entrance zone is bordered anteriorly by the posterior surface of the disk and posterolaterally by the facet joint. The presence of osteophytes on the superior medial articular process can result in nerve compression in the entrance zone. The midzone is bordered anteriorly by the posterior vertebral wall and posteriorly by the pars interarticularis. Hypertrophy of fibrocartilage from a pars interarticularis defect results in nerve compression in the midzone. The exit zone is the area of the intervertebral foramen bordered posteriorly by the lateral margin of the facet below, and anteriorly by the intervertebral disk of the level below (Figures 2 through 4). Causes for nerve root compression in this zone include a far lateral disk herniation and osteophytic facets.

Pathoanatomy

Intervertebral disk degeneration is a major cause of musculoskeletal disability in humans.[10-12] Degeneration has been linked to low back pain; however, the exact relationship between the two remains uncertain.[13,14] The macroscopic features characterizing disk degeneration include the formation of tears within the anulus fibrosus, and progressive fraying and dehydration of the nucleus pulposus, with eventual loss of the annular-nuclear distinction.[10,12,15] These pathologic alterations result in substantial changes in the functioning of the disk.

Degenerative Disk Biomechanics

Stress distribution across the intervertebral disk and vertebral end plate depends on the degree of disk degeneration.[16] Under pure compressive and eccentric-compressive loading, the healthy lumbar intervertebral disk demonstrated a uniform stress distribution across the entire end plate area. Severely degenerated disks

cess, and the foraminal zone (Figure 1). The central zone is defined as the region between the lateral margins of the dura. Between the lateral margin of dura and the medial border of the pedicle represents an area termed the lateral recess. The foraminal zone lies between the medial and lateral margins of the pedicle and contains the intervertebral foramen.

demonstrated the same uniform shape of stress distribution under compressive loading but a nonuniform stress distribution when loaded eccentrically. The asymmetry of the stress distribution in degenerated disks was found to increase with both angle of inclination and degree of degeneration. The asymmetric stress distribution was presumed to occur because of the relatively solid nature of the degenerated disk and its inability to conform to the eccentric loads.

With advancing degeneration, it appears that the proportion of load transmission shifts to the posterior elements. Several researchers indirectly measured facet forces by using an intervertebral load cell to measure the load transferred through the disk.[14] The model predicted a significant increase in facet load for segments with degenerated disks. The increase was more prominent as the eccentricity of the applied compressive load increased posteriorly. This biomechanical sequence of disk degeneration leading to posterior element load bearing may in fact be what is observed clinically in that disk degeneration typically precedes facet arthrosis.[17]

Clinically, a common observation is that early to midrange disk degeneration creates slight instability of the lumbar spine and, therefore, increases range of motion.[1] The interplay between the intervertebral disk geometric and material properties as well as facet joint competence are important in defining the stability of the involved motion segment.[18] Biomechanical studies suggest that changes in stability with disk degeneration are quite complex. With advancing degeneration the motion segment ultimately becomes less mobile. However, the remaining motion may be painful. The back pain associated with disk degeneration may be related to an increase in pathologic motion despite an overall decrease in motion.

For decades, researchers have attempted to define a relationship between these morphologic and biomechanical intervertebral disk alterations and specific clinical syndromes. More recently, disk dysfunction associated with axial back pain, giving rise to so-called internal disk derangement, has received considerable attention. MRI is a valuable diagnostic tool in assessing the internal architecture of the disk.[19] MRI allows determination of the proton density of the disk indicative of the state of hydration and can also identify the presence of annular tears. The high-intensity zone has been described as a focally increased T2-weighted MRI signal believed to be representative of an annular tear extending to the periphery of the disk.[20] The high-intensity zone can be seen on T2-weighted MRI scans as a high-intensity signal located in the substance of the posterior anulus fibrosus (**Figure 5**). The high-intensity zone has been suggested as, but by no means confirmed to be, associated with discogenic axial back pain.[21,22]

Morphologic Alterations Associated With Intervertebral Disk Degeneration

With degeneration, the intervertebral disk loses proteoglycan and water content. The anatomic result is a de-

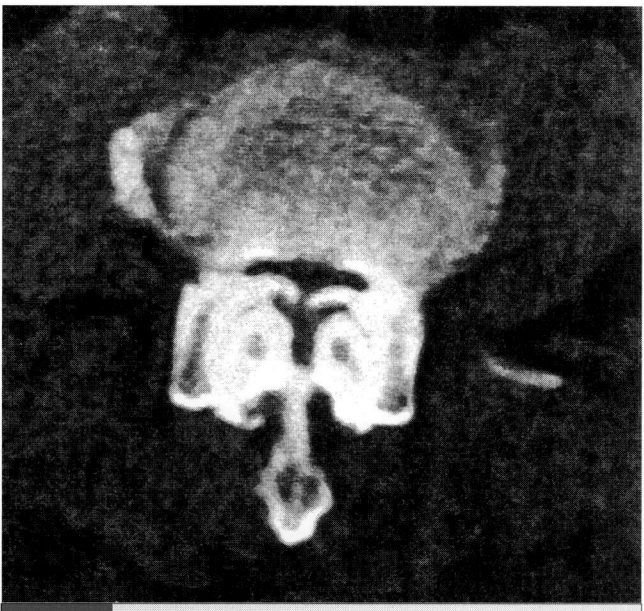

Figure 4 CT scan demonstrating facet osteophytes impinging on the central and lateral recess zones of the spinal canal. *(Reproduced with permission from Kirkaldy-Willis WH, Wedge JH, Yong-King K, Tchang S, de Korompay V, Shannon R: Lumbar spinal nerve lateral entrapment.* Clin Orthop Relat Res *1982;169:171-178.)*

crease in intervertebral disk height, resulting in a decreased cephalad-caudad intervertebral foraminal dimension. One study reported that a posterior disk height less than 4 mm or a foraminal height less than 15 mm correlated with symptomatic nerve root compression.[23] The decrease in disk height also results in tension loss of the ligamentum flavum, causing buckling of the yellow ligament into the canal. A decrease in tension within the posterior anulus fibrosus also contributes to bulging of the disk within the canal.

Further degeneration of the disk can lead to annular fissures and tears. The propagation of these fissures into the periphery has been implicated in the etiology of disk herniations and discogenic back pain. Three types of annular tears have been described. The radial tear is most commonly located in the posterior anulus fibrosus. It has been reported that radial tears are most commonly associated with disk degeneration.[24] Circumferential tears may be secondary to interlaminar shear stresses and are more likely to be observed in older disks. Peripheral rim tears are more commonly located anteriorly and may be associated with trauma. A recent study using both a fluid dynamic model and finite element analysis showed that decreased osmotic pressure may actually enhance the opening of small cracks and fissures in the anulus.[25]

Facet Joint Degeneration

Biomechanical and imaging studies of human cadaveric spinal motion segments have been conducted to deter-

5: Spine

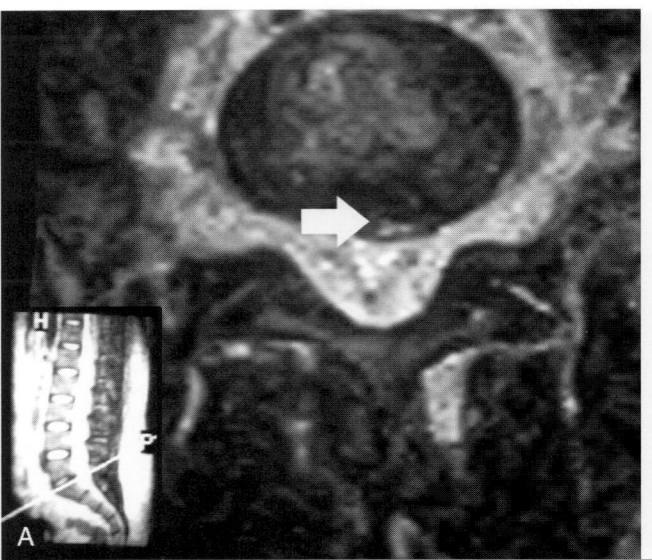
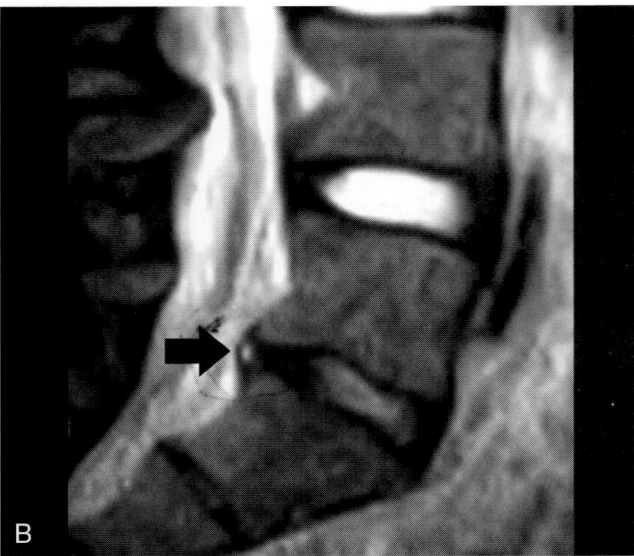

Figure 5   Axial **(A)** and sagittal **(B)** MRI scans demonstrating the high-intensity zone (*arrows*).

mine the effect of disk degeneration and facet joint osteoarthritis on the segmental flexibility of the lumbar spine.[18] The authors noted that axial rotation was most affected by disk degeneration. Facet cartilage degeneration, especially thinning of the cartilage, causes capsular ligament laxity. Capsular laxity may allow abnormal motion or hypermobility of the facet joint. The authors noted a significant linear correlation between facet cartilage thinning and disk degeneration in male cadavers. Cartilage degeneration appeared to further increase the segmental movements already present in the hypermobile, degenerated disk.

Facetectomy studies have been performed in the lumbar spine of immature white rabbits to create a facet-mediated degenerative model.[26] The authors resected the inferior articular process on one side at a selected vertebral level and on the opposite side at the adjacent level. At 9 to 12 months, the disks showed thinning of the posterior anulus fibrosus, circumferential slits in the peripheral anulus fibrosus, and an increased area and decreased organization of the nucleus pulposus. The authors concluded that the facet joint protects the intervertebral disk from rotational stresses.

Unquestionably, the facet joint complex has an important role in stabilizing the segmental spinal unit. As disk disease progresses, increased stress is applied posteriorly, accelerating facet osteoarthrosis. The resultant facet joint osteoarthritis is likely to change the segmental spinal motion, altering the mechanical forces experienced by the intervertebral disk.

Treatment Trends

Over the decades since the degenerative cascade was first presented, it has become apparent that spinal degeneration is the end result of interplay between subtle alterations in mechanical and biochemical properties of the intervertebral disk and facet joint complex. As physicians gain further insight into the degenerative cascade, the treatment of symptomatic spinal degeneration may eventually involve a combination of less ablative reconstructive procedures and biologic manipulations.

Pathophysiology of Intervertebral Disk Degeneration

Intervertebral Disk Development
The spine begins to develop during the third week of gestation with the formation of the ectoderm, mesoderm, and endoderm. As the cells of the primitive streak differentiate, the notochord is formed, and it serves as the basis of axial skeleton formation. The vertebral column develops from a condensation of mesenchymal cells. These cells segment into alternating light and dark bands, which form the vertebral bodies and intervertebral disks, respectively.

The nucleus pulposus develops from an expansion of cells surrounding the primitive cartilage of the notochord itself. The cells of the notochord play a crucial role in the matrix formation of the nucleus pulposus. They are pushed apart into cell clusters, known as chorda reticulum, by the formation of extracellular matrix. Notochordal cells are believed to remain active until the second decade of life, after which they are rarely seen.

Like other connective tissues, the intervertebral disk contains a sparse cell population and abundant extracellular matrix. The outer anulus fibrosus primarily contains type I collagen and fibroblastic cells. In this region, the type I collagen fibrils are oriented in a parallel manner to form concentric lamella; the arrangement resembles the layers of an onion. Each concentric layer in the outer anulus fibrosus contains type I collagen fibers, which are oriented at approximately 30° from the

5: Spine

long axis of the spine. Alternating layers run in opposite directions to provide the tissue with optimal structural integrity and resist torsion and shear stresses. A thin transition zone separates the inner anulus fibrosus and the nucleus pulposus. The nucleus pulposus is the centermost region of the disk. It contains a proteoglycan-rich matrix with randomly oriented collagen fibers (primarily type II collagen). Large, hydrophilic proteoglycan aggregates inside the nucleus pulposus provide stiffness and viscoelasticity to the disk. Within the nucleus pulposus, a small cell population maintains the vast extracellular matrix.

The bony end plates of the vertebral body are made of specialized compact bone. The bone is substantially thicker along the periphery of the disk than in its central region. The thicker peripheral bone provides structural support, whereas the thinner central region allows closer contact between the end plate capillaries and the underlying disk.

The bony vertebral end plates are covered with a hyaline cartilage layer that separates the bone from the nucleus pulposus and acts as a diffusion barrier, allowing only small, uncharged molecules to move into and out of the disk in significant quantity. The vertebral end plates calcify as they age, and the calcification affects disk metabolism by further limiting the delivery of nutrients and removal of waste products. Thus, the cells inside the disk live in a nutritionally challenged environment that worsens with age.

Disk Loading

Unlike most other mammals, humans walk upright and place large compressive loads on their intervertebral disks. The normal nucleus pulposus, which is a hydrated gel, is relatively noncompressible. Compressive loading causes slight deformation of the cartilaginous end plate and vertebral body as well as bulging of the anulus fibrosus. The surrounding tissues must be strong enough to resist the outward tensile stresses transmitted by the nucleus to the surrounding bone and disk. Lateral bending and rotation of the spine places significant tensile stresses on the fibers of the anulus fibrosus and can result in fiber failure if the stresses exceed the tensile strength of the tissue. Fortunately, the healthy anulus fibrosus is strong and capable of withstanding stresses that would fracture the surrounding vertebral bone. In degeneration, the integrity of the anulus fibrosus becomes compromised by the development of fissures. To limit transmission of excessive stresses to the anulus fibrosus, intact facet joints control spinal motion, particularly in lateral bending and torsion. Not surprisingly, when the intact facet complex is lost because of vertebral spondylolysis, pathologic stress applied to the tissues can lead to early degeneration of the intervertebral disk.

To dissipate compressive loads in the spine, the normal disk converts the load into tensile hoop stress in the outer anulus fibrosus while allowing controlled motion of the intervertebral segment. The vertebral end plates transmit the compressive load to the nucleus pul-

Table 1
Factors Associated With Disk Degeneration
Age
Family history
Smoking
Vibration (prolonged driving)
Heavy repetitive loading of the spine
Diabetes

posus, leading to elevated pressure on the hydrated gel of the nucleus pulposus. In a young, healthy disk, the load is transmitted rather evenly outward in all directions to the surrounding tissues of the disk. The result is a viscoelastic deformation of the circumferential fibers of the outer anulus fibrosus, which dissipates some of the stress. The anulus fibrosus has differential stiffness characteristics during loading that lead to a biphasic phenomenon in which the inner anulus fibrosus dampens stress transmission to the outer anulus fibrosus, which is stiffer and resists peak loads.

Significant changes in disk biomechanics occur with aging and disk degeneration. The changes appear to begin in the nucleus pulposus, where loss of the large proteoglycans leads to diminished swelling pressure and results in an uneven transmission of stresses to the surrounding tissues. In the anulus fibrosus, collagen fibers deteriorate, and fissures develop along the inner region and eventually progress outward. As a result, the nuclear material may be expressed outward toward the periphery of the disk. The loss of the normal biomechanical function of the nucleus pulposus and anulus fibrosus leads to overloading of the bony end plates, which become sclerotic and form peripheral osteophytes, as is seen in vertebral spondylosis.

Etiology of Disk Degeneration

The rate and degree of disk degeneration are affected by several factors (**Table 1**). Heavy lifting, vibrational forces, and torsional loads also have been believed to be risk factors. However, studies failed to show a direct correlation between heavy physical loading and degenerative disk disease.[27,28] Tobacco exposure, which was shown to increase degenerative changes in animal models, is under investigation as a cause of disk degeneration in humans.[29]

Genetic predisposition has emerged as perhaps the strongest factor leading to symptomatic degenerative disk disease. Early studies found symptomatic disk degeneration in multiple members of the same family. Disk degeneration was found to be much more likely among family members of patients requiring lumbar surgery than in the general population.[30] Siblings of patients with disk degeneration were found to have a higher prevalence of both disk degeneration and osteoarthritis than the general population.[31] Finally, a study of twins found a strong link between heredity and cervical and lumbar disk degeneration.[32]

5: Spine

Genetic linkage studies have identified links between disk degeneration and a variety of known genes. A link was found between early disk degeneration and certain alleles of the vitamin D receptor.[33] Women who had a lower number of tandem repeats within the aggrecan gene had earlier and more severe disk degeneration.[34] Specific alleles of the matrix metalloproteinase-3 gene were shown to be correlated with disk degeneration in elderly Japanese patients.[35] Single gene abnormalities have also been linked to the process of disk degeneration. A mutation in the type IX collagen α-2 gene was found to result in an amino acid substitution leading to disk degeneration.[36] Another mutation in the α-3 chain of type IX collagen was linked to disk degeneration and shown to act synergistically with obesity. A study of single nucleotide polymorphisms, or variations seen in a single base pair of DNA, found that an allele of cartilage intermediate layer protein produced susceptibility to early disk degeneration.[37] Finally, one allele of the interleukin-6 gene was shown to be correlated with discogenic pain and sciatica. Much remains to be learned about the complex interplay among different genes, disk degeneration, and the presence of back symptoms in humans.

Degenerative Processes

In all tissues, the balance between synthesis and degradation of matrix macromolecules is crucial to tissue homeostasis. Degenerative processes predominate when synthesis of new macromolecules is decreased or the rate of product breakdown increases. Disk degeneration is one of the earliest forms of tissue degeneration seen in the human body; early signs are often present by the second decade of life. However, the onset and rate of degenerative processes vary remarkably among individuals.

One of the earliest changes in the disk is the loss of the large notochordal cells that are abundant in infancy but almost completely absent by adulthood. This change is believed to herald or perhaps initiate some aspects of tissue degeneration. Notochordal cells have been shown to stimulate proteoglycan production in vitro as a result of the release of soluble mediators, and this finding suggests that the disappearance of notochordal cells may remove a necessary stimulus to disk health.[37]

The cell population of the nucleus pulposus changes dramatically over time. Cell necrosis and apoptosis (programmed cell death) both occur. Disk cell apoptosis can be triggered by a number of stimuli, one of which is the Fas/Fas ligand system. Rapid cell death is triggered when a Fas-bearing cell contacts a Fas-ligand–bearing cell.[38,39] The Fas receptor was not found to be expressed by a normal disk in significant amounts but in an experimental model was upregulated after the onset of degeneration.[40] Following a disk herniation, apoptosis and the body's inflammatory process allow the body to break down and resorb a sequestered disk fragment. However, the role of apoptosis in disk degeneration has not been fully defined. Two primary pathways

for Fas-mediated apoptosis have been identified: type I cells carry the Fas receptor on their cell membrane, and type II cells carry the Fas receptor intracellularly at the mitochondrial level. A recent study suggested that type II cells predominate in human disk fragments.[41] Various growth factors may exert a protective effect, decreasing apoptosis within the disk. Some researchers have focused on reducing apoptosis as a method of treating or preventing degenerative changes within the disk.

Inflammatory cytokines and catabolic proteins also play a role in the degenerative process. Catabolic enzymes help turn over macromolecules as a normal part of tissue homeostasis. During disk degeneration, the expression of catabolic factors becomes excessive and leads to tissue breakdown. Disk enzymes including cathepsin, lysozyme, aggrecanase, and several matrix metalloproteinases[42,43] have been found to participate in the disk degeneration process.

Disk metabolism is regulated by a host of cytokines, including interleukins, prostaglandins, and tumor necrosis factor. A complex, poorly understood series of catabolic events seems to be integral to creation of the pain some patients experience during disk degeneration. Interleukin-1, for example, decreases proteoglycan synthesis and upregulates the expression of stromolysin-1 and prostaglandin E_2. Interleukin-8 has been found in patients with sciatic pain. Interleukin-6, tumor necrosis factor-α, and prostaglandin E_2 are believed to play a role in producing discogenic pain.[44,45] These cytokine molecules may be used in the future as targets of therapies to diminish disk-related pain.

Both enzymatic and nonenzymatic processes can cause matrix breakdown. In many patients, the macromolecules of the disk are only partially degraded and contain aggregates of functionless matrix proteins (collagens, proteoglycans, and fibronectins). Some of the partially degraded peptides, such as fibronectin fragments, are biologically active and capable of stimulating the degradative process.[46,47]

The loss of the large, sulfated proteoglycans affects the disk structurally by diminishing its water-binding capacity, leading to loss of disk height. With degeneration, the clear demarcation between the nucleus pulposus and inner anulus fibrosus is lost. The normal lamellar organization of the outer anulus fibrosus becomes disorganized, and gross clefts or fissures appear within the tissue.[48]

Nutrition is believed to play a major role in tissue degeneration within the disk. Because the disk receives virtually all of its nutrients through diffusion, the changes in end plate permeability that occur with aging can greatly affect the vitality of the cells within the disk. The supply of nutrients has been shown to control the density of disk cells.[49] Because the supply of oxygen to the disk is limited, cell metabolism is largely anaerobic, and it produces lactate as a by-product.[50] Lactate increases the acidity of the disk to a pH level between 6.9 and 7.2, although a pH level as low as 6.1 can be observed when the disk is under stress. Cell survival is possible under these harsh conditions, but matrix production declines when the pH is more acidic than is normal for the disk. However, optimal cell metabolism in the disk requires low oxygen tension, elevated levels of carbon dioxide, and a slightly acidic pH in addition to various growth factors.[51]

Degenerative Disk Disease

No consensus exists as to the definition, evaluation, diagnosis, or treatment of degenerative disk disease. Whether disk degeneration should be referred to as a disease is one subject of debate because degeneration is a normal process that usually does not produce significant clinical symptoms. Although the degenerative changes seen on MRI increase with age, they do not closely correspond to the presence or progression of low back pain. Decreased signal intensity on T2-weighted MRI scans, which reflects the loss of hydration of the nucleus pulposus, is the degenerative finding most closely correlated with aging. However, it does not allow symptomatic and asymptomatic degenerative disks to be distinguished from one another.[52] Some have suggested the use of the term symptomatic disk degeneration rather than degenerative disk disease to describe substantial clinical symptoms that appear to stem from degeneration of the intervertebral disks.

Clearly, more than simple dehydration of the disk is necessary to produce discogenic pain. One pathologic finding that may be significant is that an ingrowth of blood vessels and free nerve endings occurs in full-thickness annular fissures.[53] In a normal disk, only the outer 1 mm to 2 mm of the annular surface is innervated, and the inner region of the disk has no nerve supply. In some degenerative disks, nerve fibers with a receptor for nociceptive substances such as substance P and calcitonin gene-related peptide have been found in annular disruptions. These nerve structures may play a role in the production of discogenic symptoms.

Unfortunately, the ability of the clinician to objectively assess a painful disk is limited. Discography, which is widely used to establish a particular disk as a source of pain, has well-documented limitations.[54] Better diagnostic tests are needed to guide both the assessment of patients with symptomatic disk degeneration and the development of new forms of treatment.

Treatment Trends

Although the diagnosis and treatment of spinal disorders have generally focused on biomechanical issues and solutions such as spinal fusion and disk replacement, future treatments are likely to look toward biologic interventions. True biologic therapies are likely to become available as the degenerative process and mechanisms of pain are better understood. Laboratories throughout the world are pursuing strategies such as the use of growth factors, stem cells, and pharmacologic agents to treat the common, vexing problem of the painful degenerative disk.

Annotated References

1. Kirkaldy-Willis WH, Farfan HF: Instability of the lumbar spine. *Clin Orthop Relat Res* 1982;165:110-123.

2. Kompel J, Sobajima S, Clarke C, et al: MRI and histological analysis of a rabbit model of disc degeneration. *Trans Ortho Res Soc* 2003;28:253.

3. Lord SM, Barnsley L, Wallis BJ, McDonald GJ, Bogduk N: Percutaneous radio-frequency neurotomy for chronic cervical zygapophyseal-joint pain. *N Engl J Med* 1996;335:1721-1726.

4. Lord SM, Barnsley L, Wallis BJ, Bogduk N: Chronic cervical zygapophysial joint pain after whiplash: A placebo-controlled prevalence study. *Spine* 1996;21:1737-1744.

5. Gruber HE, Hanley EN Jr: Ultrastructure of the human intervertebral disc during aging and degeneration: Comparison of surgical and control specimens. *Spine* 2002;27:798-805.

6. Lotz JC, Hsieh AH, Walsh AL, Palmer EI, Chin JR: Mechanobiology of the intervertebral disc. *Biochem Soc Trans* 2002;30:853-858.

7. Roughley PJ, Alini M, Antoniou J: The role of proteoglycans in aging, degeneration and repair of the intervertebral disc. *Biochem Soc Trans* 2002;30:869-874.

8. Adams MA, Hutton WC: The mechanical function of the lumbar apophyseal joints. *Spine* 1983;8:327-330.

9. Adams MA, Hutton WC: Cadaver lumbar intervertebral joints. *Spine* 1980;5:483-484.

10. Buckwalter JA: Aging and degeneration of the human intervertebral disc. *Spine* 1995;20:1307-1314.

11. Anderson JA: Epidemiological aspects of back pain. *J Soc Occup Med* 1986;36:90-94.

12. Battie MC, Videman T, Parent E: Lumbar disc degeneration: Epidemiology and genetic influences. *Spine* 2004;29:2679-2690.

    Recent research indicates that heredity has a dominant role in disk degeneration, accounting for 74% of the variance in adult populations studied to date. Level of evidence: III.

13. Vanharanta H, Sachs BL, Spivey MA, et al: The relationship of pain provocation to lumbar disc deterioration as seen by CT/discography. *Spine* 1987;12:295-298.

14. Yang KH, King AI: Mechanism of facet load transmission as a hypothesis for low-back pain. *Spine* 1984;9:557-565.

5: Spine

15. Roughley PJ: Biology of intervertebral disc aging and degeneration: Involvement of the extracellular matrix. *Spine* 2004;29:2691-2699.

    Current research is aimed at trying to restore the integrity of the degenerate disk matrix by biologic means, although at present it is not clear what the structure of the most appropriate repair tissue should be or how it can be achieved.

16. Horst M, Brinckmann P: 1980 Volvo Award in biomechanics: Measurement of the distribution of axial stress on the end-plate of the vertebral body. *Spine* 1981;6: 217-232.

17. Butler D, Trafimow JH, Andersson GB, McNeill TW, Huckman MS: Discs degenerate before facets. *Spine* 1990;15:111-113.

18. Mimura M, Panjabi MM, Oxland TR, Crisco JJ, Yamamoto I, Vasavada A: Disc degeneration affects the multidirectional flexibility of the lumbar spine. *Spine* 1994; 19:1371-1380.

19. Narvani AA, Tsiridis E, Ishaque MA, Wilson LF: "Pig Tail" technique in intradiscal electrothermal therapy. *J Spinal Disord Tech* 2003;16:280-284.

20. Aprill C, Bogduk N: High-intensity zone: A diagnostic sign of painful lumbar disc on magnetic resonance imaging. *Br J Radiol* 1992;65:361-369.

21. Schellhas KP: HIZ lesions. *Spine* 1997;22:1538.

22. Lam KS, Carlin D, Mulholland RC: Lumbar disc high-intensity zone: The value and significance of provocative discography in the determination of the discogenic pain source. *Eur Spine J* 2000;9:36-41.

23. Hasegawa T, An HS, Haughton VM, Nowicki BH: Lumbar foraminal stenosis: Critical heights of the intervertebral disc. *J Bone Joint Surg Am* 1995;77:32-38.

24. Osti OL, Vernon-Roberts B, Fraser RD: 1990 Volvo Award in experimental studies: Anulus tears and intervertebral disc degeneration. An experimental study using an animal model. *Spine* 1990;15:762-767.

25. Wognum S, Huyghe JM, Baaijens FP: Influence of osmotic pressure changes on the opening of existing cracks in two intervertebral disc models. *Spine* 2006;31: 1783-1788.

    An experimental hydrogel model was used to determine the etiology of disk herniations. Experimental simulators demonstrate that a decrease in osmotic pressure results in openings of cracks despite the concomitant decrease in annular stress. Level of evidence: II.

26. Sullivan JD, Farfan HF, Kahn DS: Pathologic changes with intervertebral joint rotational instability in the rabbit. *Can J Surg* 1971;14:71-79.

27. Battie MC, Videman T, Parent E: Lumbar disc degener-

28. Battie MC, Videman T, Gibbons LE, Fisher LD, Manninen H, Gill K: 1995 Volvo Award in clinical sciences: Determinants of lumbar disc degeneration. A study relating lifetime exposures and magnetic resonance imaging findings in identical twins. *Spine* 1995;20:2601-2612.

ation: Epidemiology and genetic influences. *Spine* 2004; 29:2679-2690.

29. Nemoto Y, Matsuzaki H, Tokuhasi Y, et al: Histological changes in the intervertebral disks after smoking and cessation: Experimental study using a rat passive smoking model. *J Orthop Sci* 2006;11:191-197.

    Anulus fibrosus degeneration caused by smoking was partially irreversible after cessation of smoking. The amount of proteoglycan in the nucleus pulposus and anulus fibrosus was increased after smoking cessation. This finding indicates that smoking-induced intervertebral disk degeneration may be repaired to some degree by cessation of smoking.

30. Matsui H, Kanamori M, Ishihara H, Yodoh K, Naruse Y, Tsuji H: Familial predisposition for lumbar degenerative disc disease: A case-controlled study. *Spine* 1998; 23:1029-1034.

31. Bijkerk C, Houwing-Duistermaat JJ, Valkenburg HA, et al: Heritabilities of radiologic arthritis in peripheral joints and of disc degeneration of the spine. *Arthritis Rheum* 1999;42:1729-1735.

32. Sambrook PN, MacGregor AJ, Spector TD: Genetic influences on cervical and lumbar disc degeneration: A magnetic resonance imaging study in twins. *Arthritis Rheum* 1999;42:366-372.

33. Videman T, Leppavuori J, Kaprio J, et al: Intragenic polymorphisms of the vitamin D receptor gene associated with intervertebral disc degeneration. *Spine* 1998; 23:2477-2485.

34. Kawaguchi Y, Osada R, Kanamori M, et al: Association between an aggrecan gene polymorphism and lumbar disc degeneration. *Spine* 1999;24:2456-2460.

35. Takahashi M, Haro H, Wakabayashi Y, Kawa-uchi T, Komori H, Shinomiya K: The association of degeneration of the intervertebral disc with 5a/6a polymorphism in the promoter of the human matrix metalloproteinase-3 gene. *J Bone Joint Surg Br* 2001;83:491-495.

36. Annunen S, Paassilta P, Lohiniva J, et al: An allele of COL9A2 associated with intervertebral disc disease. *Science* 1999;285:409-412.

37. Seki S, Kawaguchi Y, Chiba K, et al: A functional SNP in CILP, encoding cartilage intermediate layer protein, is associated with susceptibility to lumbar disc disease. *Nat Genet* 2005;37:607-612.

    In this case-control study report, the authors identified a

functional genetic polymorphism SNP encoding the cartilage intermediate layer protein that acts as a modulator of lumbar disk disease susceptibility.

38. Park JB, Chang H, Kim KW: Expression of Fas ligand and apoptosis of disc cells in herniated lumbar disc tissue. *Spine* 2001;26:618-621.

39. Park JB, Kim KW, Han CW, Chang H: Expression of Fas receptor on disc cells in herniated lumbar disc tissue. *Spine* 2001;26:142-146.

40. Anderson DG, Izzo MW, Hall DJ, et al: Comparative gene expression profiling of normal and degenerative discs: Analysis of a rabbit annular laceration model. *Spine* 2002;27:1291-1296.

41. Park JB, Lee JK, Park SJ, Kim KW, Riew KD: Mitochondrial involvement in fas-mediated apoptosis of human lumbar disc cells. *J Bone Joint Surg Am* 2005;87: 1338-1342.

    Two principal pathways of Fas-mediated apoptosis have been identified: type I (death-inducing signaling complex) and type II (mitochondrial) pathway. This study suggests that human disk cells are type II cells, which undergo apoptotic cell death through mitochondrial involvement.

42. Crean JK, Roberts S, Jaffray DC, Eisenstein SM, Duance VC: Matrix metalloproteinases in the human intervertebral disc: Role in disc degeneration and scoliosis. *Spine* 1997;22:2877-2884.

43. Kanemoto M, Hukuda S, Komiya Y, Katsuura A, Nishioka J: Immunohistochemical study of matrix metalloproteinase-3 and tissue inhibitor of metalloproteinase-1 human intervertebral discs. *Spine* 1996;21:1-8.

44. Kang JD, Georgescu HI, McIntyre-Larkin L, Stefanovic-Racic M, Donaldson WF III, Evans CH: Herniated lumbar intervertebral discs spontaneously produce matrix metalloproteinases, nitric oxide, interleukin-6, and prostaglandin E2. *Spine* 1996;21:271-277.

45. Onda A, Yabuki S, Kikuchi S: Effects of neutralizing antibodies to tumor necrosis factor-alpha on nucleus pulposus-induced abnormal nociresponses in rat dorsal horn neurons. *Spine* 2003;28:967-972.

46. Oegema TR Jr, Johnson SL, Aguiar DJ, Ogilvie JW: Fibronectin and its fragments increase with degeneration in the human intervertebral disc. *Spine* 2000;25:2742-2747.

47. Anderson DG, Li X, Balian G: A fibronectin fragment alters the metabolism by rabbit intervertebral disc cells

in vitro. *Spine* 2005;30:1242-1246.

    This biochemical and gene expression study in a rabbit model supports a possible detrimental role of the N-terminal fibronectin fragment in the anticipation of intervertebral disk degeneration.

48. Boos N, Weissbach S, Rohrbach H, Weiler C, Spratt KF, Nerlich AG: Classification of age-related changes in lumbar intervertebral discs: 2002 Volvo Award in basic science. *Spine* 2002;27:2631-2644.

49. Horner HA, Urban JP: 2001 Volvo Award Winner in basic science studies: Effect of nutrient supply on the viability of cells from the nucleus pulposus of the intervertebral disc. *Spine* 2001;26:2543-2549.

50. Urban JP, Holm S, Maroudas A, Nachemson A: Nutrition of the intervertebral disc: Effect of fluid flow on solute transport. *Clin Orthop Relat Res* 1982;170:296-302.

51. Risbud MV, Guttapalli A, Stokes DG, et al: Nucleus pulposus cells express HIF-1alpha under normoxic culture conditions: A metabolic adaptation to the intervertebral disc microenvironment. *J Cell Biochem* 2006;98: 152-159.

    Results from this study show that normoxic stabilization of HIF-1alpha is a metabolic adaptation of nucleus pulposus cells to a unique oxygen-limited microenvironment. HIF-1alpha can be used as a phenotypic marker of nucleus pulposus cells.

52. Jensen MC, Brant-Zawadzki MN, Obuchowski N, Modic MT, Malkasian D, Ross JS: Magnetic resonance imaging of the lumbar spine in people without back pain. *N Engl J Med* 1994;331:69-73.

53. Brisby H: Pathology and possible mechanics of nervous system response to disc degeneration. *J Bone Joint Surg Am* 2006;88(suppl 2):68-71.

    The complexity of the nervous system and pain modulation mechanisms, along with psychological aspects, may play a role in the nervous system's response in patients with chronic low back pain as a result of disk degeneration.

54. Carragee EJ, Alamin TF, Carragee JM: Low-pressure positive discography in subjects asymptomatic of significant low back pain illness. *Spine* 2006;31:505-509.

    This study demonstrates that the rate of low-pressure injection in subjects without chronic low back pain is approximately 25%, and correlates with both anatomic and psychosocial factors. This may represent an unacceptable risk of false-positive results.

5: Spine

Chapter 44

Degenerative Disease of the Cervical Spine

*Daniel B. Murrey, MD, MPP

Axial Neck Pain

Axial or mechanical neck pain is a common condition that is typically episodic and short-lived, but can become more chronic. It is characterized by discomfort in the midline or paraspinal muscles of the neck, often extending into the trapezius and periscapular muscle areas. It is often worse at the extremes of a patient's range of motion. It can radiate into the occiput, leading to cervicogenic or tension headaches. Typically, it is not associated with radicular complaints.

Etiology

In most instances, the cause of axial neck pain is multifactorial. Degenerative disks, facet arthropathy, irritation of the greater occipital nerve, root compression, and muscular dysfunction with trigger points all have been implicated as individual causes of neck pain.[1-5] A combination of two or more of these factors can also alter loading patterns in the neck and create less efficient biomechanics, leading to sagittal imbalance and fatigue-related pain.

Disk degeneration is a natural part of the aging process. Most adults will develop radiographically apparent disk degeneration, and yet relatively few will present with persistent painful neck conditions.[6] Still, for some, the tearing of annular fibers and the loss of load-bearing capacity of the nucleus pulposus have been implicated as potential pain generators. The support for this claim is less well delineated in the cervical spine than in the lumbar spine, with few studies of cervical discogenic pain performed. The diagnostic accuracy of cervical diskography is controversial. Because success rates of nonsurgical management for axial neck pain are good, and the risk of esophageal, vascular, infectious, or other complications from cervical diskography are relatively high for a diagnostic test, cervical diskography is infrequently performed and poorly validated.[7]

Daniel B. Murrey, MD, MPP or the department with which he is affiliated has received research or institutional support from Synthes Spine, holds stock or stock options in US Spine, and is a consultant or employee of Stryker Spine, Synthes Spine, and US Spine.

Facet joints, with or without arthropathy, can become painful. They have been implicated as a common source of pain after whiplash injury, but the pain can arise without antecedent trauma. Facet-mediated pain is typically worse with extension and better with flexion.

Chronic axial neck pain often leads to muscular tightness and spasm, which over time can cause shortening or interstitial scarring that creates a locus for recurrent spasm or pain.[8] Often called trigger points, these sites can occur in isolation or as part of a larger syndrome of fibromyalgia.

As multiple disks degenerate and disk height is lost, the anterior column shortens and the natural cervical lordosis is compromised. The occiput gradually shifts forward relative to the base of the neck, increasing the work of the dynamic stabilizers of the posterior cervical spine. In some patients, fatigue-related axial neck pain develops, especially with activities requiring extended periods of cervical flexion.

Atlantoaxial arthrosis can lead to a specific presentation of axial neck pain. Patients with C1-2 arthrosis report suboccipital pain, often associated with a grinding sensation upon lateral rotation of the neck. Flexion and extension typically cause fewer symptoms.

In rare instances, cervical degeneration can lead to atraumatic instability. Most commonly, this would be seen in patients with systemic disease, such as rheumatoid arthritis, or when mechanics have been significantly altered, such as adjacent to a multilevel fusion.

Because much has been written about rheumatoid instability, it will not be covered in detail here. In brief, C1-2 instability is a relatively common finding in patients with rheumatoid conditions and must be ruled out with dynamic lateral radiographs in these patients who present with neck pain.[9,10] Because C1-2 instability is often asymptomatic, radiographic studies should be performed on any patient with rheumatoid arthritis who is preparing for general anesthesia. Subaxial instability can also lead to neck pain and can be similarly evaluated with dynamic films.

Atraumatic listhesis does occur in patients who do not have rheumatoid conditions, particularly above or below multilevel fusions or areas of multilevel spondylosis with minimal residual motion. Although some adjacent segment hypermobility or translation is commonly seen in these scenarios, only rarely does it meet the criteria for instability and/or can be definitively implicated as a source of neck pain. In the presence of axial neck pain without neurologic complaints, such findings would infrequently lead to surgical treatment.

Diagnosis

Physical examination should evaluate range of motion, including flexion, extension, rotation, and lateral bending. A thorough neurologic examination should rule out radiculopathic or myelopathic findings. Because axial neck pain is a clinical syndrome and not easily reducible to a simple pathologic finding, radiographs and more advanced imaging techniques are typically used only to rule out more serious conditions.

Indications for radiographs include a history of trauma, a history of systemic disease such as rheumatoid arthritis or cancer, pain persistent for more than 6 weeks, night pain, or neurologic involvement. Flexion and extension lateral radiographs are used to identify pseudarthrosis or instability, including posterior ligamentous injury. Odontoid views can show atlantoaxial arthrosis. CT scans are useful to evaluate potential fractures, foraminal stenosis, or facet arthropathy. MRI is more helpful to evaluate degenerative disks, neurologic compression, infections, or tumors. Diagnostic injections of the facet joints or medial branch blocks can be useful in confirming a suspicion of facet-mediated pain. Because disk degeneration and facet arthropathy are ubiquitous, even in asymptomatic patients, care must be taken to correlate these findings on imaging studies with symptoms, examination results, and other diagnostic studies before attributing a patient's symptoms to these radiographic findings.

Because the differential diagnosis for axial neck pain includes fracture, dislocation, tumor, infection, and instabilities associated with systemic arthritides, each of these conditions must be reasonably excluded before initiating treatment of degenerative disease. Typically, if a patient presents with no red flags (history of trauma, constitutional symptoms, pain that is constant and unremitting, or physical findings consistent with systemic arthritis or neurologic impairment), then these alternative diagnoses can be excluded and plain radiographs usually are not necessary. However, plain radiographs can provide further confirmation if patient history and physical examination are insufficient to rule out the above conditions.

Nonsurgical Treatment

For most patients with axial neck pain, the treatment is nonsurgical. Physical therapy, traction, chiropractic therapy, heat and other therapeutic modalities, and nonsteroidal anti-inflammatory drugs (NSAIDs) are frequently recommended, although long-term data to justify the use of these treatments is limited. In patients with whiplash-associated disorders, early intervention with physical therapy, analgesics, and NSAIDs can be supported. Bracing is usually not beneficial, and may be detrimental.[11] In patients for whom facet-mediated

pain has been confirmed by facet joint blocks, neuroablation therapy (most commonly with radiofrequency catheters) has met with some success.[2]

Surgical Treatment

In symptomatic patients, if instability is documented on dynamic radiographs, fusion should be considered. In addition, atlantoaxial fusions for patients with arthrosis in whom nonsurgical treatment was unsuccessful have shown good results in small studies.[12]

Fusion for axial neck pain in the subaxial spine without clear evidence of instability is controversial. In controlled studies using diskography and MRI for preoperative selection, satisfactory results have been reported in only 75% to 80% of patients.[13,14] Most authors recommend a conservative approach to this problem.

Radiculopathy

Cervical radiculopathy is characterized by pain in the neck referred into the periscapular area or arm, associated with numbness in the arm or hand in a dermatomal distribution and weakness in a myotomal distribution. Some or all of these symptoms may be present in any given patient, and the distribution can be somewhat variable. Typically, shoulder and arm pain exceed neck pain. The patient may experience relief of pain when the arm is placed overhead (abduction relief sign) and exacerbation of pain when the arm is dropped to the side or with ipsilateral neck rotation and extension (Spurling's maneuver).

The specific area of symptoms depends on the level of pathology. The two most common causes are disk herniation and spondylosis. Both typically produce symptoms in the root exiting at the level of pathology, for example, the C6 root for a C5-6 disk herniation. If invasive treatment is considered, it is obviously imperative that the exact nerve root level of symptomatic pathology be identified. Fortunately, the pain syndromes associated with each level are relatively predictable when pain, numbness, weakness, and reflex changes are all present (Table 1). However, localization can become more challenging in patients with a predominance of pain without significant numbness or weakness, especially when multilevel pathology is present.

Diagnosis

A thorough history and physical examination and correlation with imaging studies are necessary to identify the nerve root level. In addition to sensory, motor, and deep tendon reflexes, the neurologic examination should include testing for long tract signs, such as Babinski's reflex, (upturning and splaying of the toes in response to a plantar stimulus), Hoffman's sign, (flexion of the thumb and index fingers in response to flicking the tip of the outstretched middle finger), Lhermitte's sign, (shooting sensations down the arm with rapid neck flexion), and clonus to rule out myelopathy. Other

Table 1				

Pain Syndromes According to Nerve Root Level

Level	Sensory	Motor	Reflexes	Referred Pain
C4	Top of shoulder			Upper and middle neck
C5	Lateral shoulder	Deltoid	Biceps	Middle and lower neck
C6	Thumb, index finger	Biceps, wrist extensors	Biceps, brachioradialis	Trapezius, elbow
C7	Index, middle, and ring fingers	Triceps, finger extensors	Triceps	Rhomboid, forearm
C8	Ring and small fingers	Finger flexors		Scapula, wrist
T1	Ulnar border of forearm	Intrinsics		

conditions that can mimic cervical radiculopathy include carpal tunnel syndrome, cubital tunnel syndrome, thoracic outlet syndrome, and other peripheral neurologic compression syndromes. The C8 radiculopathy can be particularly difficult to differentiate from other entities, especially if the predominant finding is numbness in the small and ring fingers. Cubital tunnel syndrome, compression in Guyon's canal at the wrist, thoracic outlet syndrome, and myelopathy can all present with ulnar-sided hand numbness. Often electromyography (EMG) is required to delineate the precise source of compression.

Shoulder pathology can create shoulder pain that radiates up to the neck and down to the elbow, often mimicking radiculopathy. To rule out impingement or rotator cuff tear, provocative testing of the neck, such as Spurling's maneuver, and provocative testing of the shoulder should be done. If the diagnosis remains unclear, a diagnostic subacromial and/or acromioclavicular injection will usually confirm the diagnosis.

Lateral radiographs may show loss of disk height, end-plate osteophyte formation, malalignment, or instability. AP radiographs may show uncovertebral degeneration or scoliosis. Open-mouth odontoid views can show degeneration of the C1-2 and occasionally occipitocervical junctions. Oblique radiographs can show foraminal stenosis.

MRI is the most commonly used advanced imaging study, usually demonstrating disk herniations or stenosis with nerve root or spinal cord compression. It can also rule out unexpected pathology such as infections, tumors, demyelinating disorders, or myelomalacia. When a dynamic nerve compression is suspected, CT myelography (or, more recently, dynamic MRI) may be more helpful to confirm the diagnosis. Furthermore, information from a CT myelogram sometimes may complement MRI in surgical planning when multilevel procedures are considered.[15]

Electrodiagnostic studies such as EMG and nerve conduction tests can be helpful to exclude noncervical diagnoses such as neuropathy or peripheral nerve compression syndromes. As previously noted, these tests are particularly helpful when C8 pathology is suspected.

Nonsurgical Treatment

Fortunately, most patients with radiculopathy secondary to disk herniation or spondylosis will resolve their symptoms with conservative care. Initial management typically includes pain and anti-inflammatory medications (either oral steroids or NSAIDs) as well as physical therapy, often with traction. Although some large studies have reported only minor complications, nerve root blocks and epidural steroid injections in the cervical spine have come under increased scrutiny with sporadic reports of quadriparesis and quadriplegia after such procedures. Some theorize that particulate matter in the steroid or its preservative may occlude a spinal cord artery after an inadvertent intravascular injection of steroid, leading to spinal cord infarction. Furthermore, the efficacy of cervical injections in avoiding ultimate surgical treatment has also been questioned. As such, they should probably be used primarily for diagnostic rather than therapeutic purposes.

Most patients with radiculopathy begin noting improvement within the first 4 to 6 weeks and continue to gradually improve over several months. Ongoing use of NSAIDs, muscle relaxants, occasional narcotic use, a home program with stretching and stabilization exercises, and occasionally home traction are often recommended in this subacute phase.

Patients who have a significant and progressive neurologic deficit or who have completed a sufficient trial of conservative treatment and continue to have pain or dysfunction that limit work, exercise, sleep, and other activities of daily living may consider surgical treatment options.

Surgical Treatment

Surgical options traditionally have included laminoforaminotomy and diskectomy with fusion. More recently, experimental techniques that preserve spinal motion are being studied, with most of the focus on total disk replacement.

Laminoforaminotomy is performed through a posterior approach, with a small longitudinal paramedian incision. The lateral edge of the superior and inferior lamina and dorsal aspect of the exiting neuroforamen are removed, exposing the symptomatic nerve root. If

5: Spine

necessary, herniated disk fragments can be removed by gently retracting the exiting root. If less than half of the facet joint is removed, this can be done without destabilizing the spinal motion segment, and as a result no fusion is necessary. If more than 50% of the facet is removed, fusion may be required. Laminoforaminotomy is most appropriate in patients with foraminal stenosis or lateral to foraminal disk herniations without significant neck pain or evidence of instability. Multiple large series have established that under these circumstances, the morbidity of this procedure is low and success rates are good.[16] Recovery time tends to be brief, often only a few weeks. Newer minimally invasive microendoscopic techniques using tube retractors and a muscle-splitting approach have shortened recovery times even further for some patients, while still achieving excellent neurologic outcomes.[17] However, the results of laminoforaminotomy can be inferior to fusion techniques if significant spondylosis is present or can deteriorate over time as disk degeneration progresses.[18]

In patients with generalized spondylosis and/or central or paracentral pathology, anterior cervical diskectomy and fusion (ACDF) is appropriate. Because the pathology is anterior (disk herniations, uncovertebral osteophytes, end-plate osteophytes), this approach allows removal without disturbing the spinal cord or exiting nerve roots. The intervertebral bone graft typically distracts the disk space, enlarging the neuroforamen, and, once incorporated, maintains the foramen's patency. The historical success rates for alleviating radiculopathy with ACDF have been outstanding, with most studies exceeding 90% success rates.[19]

ACDF requires removal of the disk through an anterior approach. Removal of the posterior longitudinal ligament (PLL) is optional, depending on the patient's pathology. Anterior foraminotomy and removal of the medial uncovertebral joint is usually performed.[20] The end plates are decorticated, with care taken to avoid removal of the entire cortical thickness. Some authors recommend no end-plate decortication, favoring multiple cortical perforations with an angled curet to allow contact between the graft and cortical portion of the vertebral body. The autograft (usually iliac crest) or allograft (usually iliac crest, fibula, patella, or composite) is sized and shaped to fit the interspace and placed in position with a tamp. Good results can be achieved with noninstrumented autograft fusions. However, anterior plating is an increasingly popular addition when the environment for healing is challenging, particularly if allograft is used, in multilevel cases, when plating adjacent to previous fusion, in smokers, when maintenance of alignment is important, or when early mobilization without a neck brace is desirable.

Complications include approach-related complications such as recurrent laryngeal nerve palsy (more commonly with right-sided approaches), Horner's syndrome (from neurapraxia of the sympathetic chain on the lateral aspect of the longus colli muscle), and dysphagia or dysphonia, conditions that are often unrecognized and underreported by surgeons. Other complications include neurologic injury and vascular injury,

specifically to the vertebral artery, and pseudarthrosis.

Bone graft harvest-site complications have been largely eliminated with the recent trend favoring the use of allograft and plating over uninstrumented autograft for the fusion. Fusion results for allograft are similar to autograft for short-segment fusions,[21] and fusion rates may be enhanced with plating.[22] Autograft may still be appropriate for patients who have undergone revision, in smokers and other patients at higher risk for pseudarthrosis, and when anterior plating is not performed. Bone morphogenetic protein may also be useful in these challenging cases, but an increased incidence of soft-tissue swelling with concomitant breathing and swallowing dysfunction has been widely reported and is thought to be dose-dependent. Ideal dosing has not been established for this off-label use of the product.

Although plating has reduced the risk of pseudarthrosis, graft collapse, and graft dislodgment, recent evidence has raised the possibility that plating may increase the risk of persistent dysphagia in up to 30% of patients.[23] Further research into this problem is ongoing.

Adjacent-segment degeneration is known to occur after fusion, with an incidence of 2.9% per year after ACDF.[24] The likelihood of developing adjacent-segment disease is further increased when asymptomatic degenerative disk disease exists at adjacent levels before the index procedure. Although some authors speculate that natural history alone may explain this occurrence, biomechanical analyses have shown that fusion increases the loads on adjacent disks and facets.[25]

Mostly because of this concern about adjacent-segment deterioration, motion preservation technology has been developed to allow removal of the offending pathology without requiring fusion. Total disk replacement has been the most widely studied type of motion preservation technology in the cervical spine, with several different implants currently under investigation in US Food and Drug Administration (FDA)-approved trials. Laboratory analyses suggest that disk replacement can maintain normal motion and adjacent-segment disk pressures.[26,27] Two lumbar disk replacements have been approved, and one cervical disk replacement has been granted FDA approval.

Preliminary studies of several of these cervical disk replacements indicate that the short-term results are at least equivalent to ACDF in terms of arm and neck pain relief with fewer complications. However, long-term results are not yet available, and concerns linger regarding durability of the implants, the possibility of recurrent spondylosis, and the procedure's ability to significantly alter the onset of adjacent-segment degeneration.

Myelopathy

Myelopathy is a clinical syndrome caused by compression of the spinal cord. Its manifestations are protean, and the presentation can be subtle. Because of the potentially severe long-term consequences of this clinical syndrome, it is imperative that orthopaedic surgeons seeing patients for spinal symptoms understand the pathology and diagnostic markers, and that they routinely screen for the condition.

Herniated disk material, osteophytes, redundant ligamentum flavum, or ossification of the PLL (OPLL) can all cause spinal cord compression, especially in the presence of a congenitally small spinal canal. OPLL has most often been described in Asian populations, but it certainly can occur in Caucasian or African-American patients.

The clinical syndrome may include any or all of the following symptoms: clumsiness and a loss of coordination, loss of fine motor skills, stiffness of gait and balance disturbance, numbness or burning in the hands or feet (sometimes described as feeling like sandpaper), and urinary retention. Neck or arm pain is usually present but often is not the primary presenting complaint. Incontinence is rare and carries a poor prognosis for recovery.[28]

Diagnosis

A thorough history should include asking whether the patient is capable of buttoning buttons, tying shoes, or performing other fine motor skills. Rapid worsening of handwriting, frequently dropping things, loss of the ability to run, or rapid onset of urinary frequency and retention should raise suspicion. Some patients will describe a reverse Lhermitte's phenomenon, with shooting sensations down the arms and/or legs with neck extension. Patients with myelopathy may not report significant pain and may have difficulty describing their symptoms specifically, but often state that they "can't move well" or "just don't feel right." Because of the sometimes subtle onset of seemingly diverse symptoms without significant neck pain, the diagnosis of cervical myelopathy is often missed. Routinely asking the above questions and examining for long-tract signs can be helpful to avoid missing this important diagnosis.

Physical examination should include a standard sensory and motor examination of all four extremities. Sensation and strength can be normal, but often subjective sensory changes in the hands are present. Deep tendon reflexes typically are increased; however, if radiculopathy or peripheral nerve disease is also present, some levels may be normal or hypotonic. The presence of long-tract signs such as a positive Babinski's sign, a positive Hoffman's sign, sustained clonus, Lhermitte's sign, or an inverted radial reflex (diminished brachioradialis reflex with concomitant flexion of all fingers upon brachioradialis reflex testing) are indications of spinal cord compression.

Imaging studies should show evidence of spinal cord compression and/or instability. MRI may reveal myelomalacia (increased signal intensity indicative of intrinsic cord damage). In some patients, MRI appears to exaggerate the degree of stenosis or spinal cord compression, and interobserver reliability of the decision to treat is greater with CT myelography than with MRI. Still, because of its invasive nature, CT myelography is

usually reserved for patients with multilevel compression requiring complicated decision making.

Nonsurgical Treatment

Historically, myelopathy has been characterized as progressive and leading to spinal cord dysfunction that is not always reversible.[29-31] Although some authors question the benefit of surgery for milder presentations,[32] surgical treatment is recommended for more severe or progressive myelopathy. If the neurologic symptoms are stable, surgery can be scheduled electively. However, if symptoms are progressive, greater urgency is necessary to reduce the risk of long-term functional loss. Although some surgeons attempt to temporize patients' symptoms with steroids while awaiting surgery, no studies validate any long-term benefit in this situation.

The treatment of patients with spinal cord compression but no signs or symptoms of myelopathy is controversial. Because many patients in this situation will never develop myelopathy, surgery is usually not appropriate for these patients. If such patients experience trauma to the neck, such as in a fall or motor vehicle collision, they may be at higher risk for acute spinal cord injury. However, the degree to which the risk of a stenotic patient involved in trauma exceeds that of a normal patient involved in the same type of trauma is ill-defined, as is the comparative known risk of surgical complications versus the unknown risk of spinal cord injury as a result of trauma. This lack of information makes it difficult to advocate definitively for decompressive surgery. Patients must be informed of the treatment options and the potential risks of both surgical and nonsurgical treatment. If observation is elected, patients must be informed of which symptoms to look for and must agree to seek treatment immediately should they occur.

Surgical Treatment

Cervical myelopathy can be successfully managed with several surgical procedures, including both anterior and posterior approaches. The primary goals are to decompress the spinal cord and maintain stability of the cervical spine. Secondary goals are to minimize complications, long-term pain, and motion loss.

Posterior options include laminectomy, laminoplasty, and laminectomy with fusion. Anterior options include multilevel diskectomy with fusion and corpectomy. Both anterior and posterior approaches can produce similar rates of neurologic recovery in appropriately selected patients. As a rule, anterior procedures have less blood loss and a lower infection rate than posterior procedures. Although posterior procedures can result in swallowing dysfunction, it is much more common in anterior procedures. Implant failure and nonunion are also more common with anterior procedures when a fusion is performed.[33]

Laminectomy has been performed for decades with good results. Adequate spinal cord decompression can be achieved, but the success of the procedure is thought to depend on the cord's ability to float posteriorly away from the anterior pathology. The patient must have ade-

5: Spine

quate lordosis for excursion of the spinal cord to occur, and often levels above or below the pathology must also be decompressed to allow sufficient excursion of the cord. The downside to laminectomy has been the incidence of postlaminectomy kyphosis (particularly in patients with multilevel symptoms and in those without adequate lordosis preoperatively), neurapraxic C5 root palsy, and postoperative neck pain, possibly resulting from the removal of the bony attachment site for the posterior neck musculature.

Laminectomy with fusion can achieve the same degree of decompression as laminectomy alone without the risk of postlaminectomy kyphosis. The trade-off is a loss of motion over the fused segments, as well as exposure to fusion-related complications such as nonunion and implant failure.

Laminoplasty was developed in Japan as an alternative to anterior fusions or laminectomy with fusion for the treatment of OPLL.[34,35] Its use has now been expanded to treatment of multilevel stenosis from degenerative causes. Laminoplasty is a canal-expanding procedure in which the laminae are elevated on one side and bent or "greensticked" on the other (Figure 1). As with laminectomy, lordosis allows posterior excursion of the spinal cord to reduce anterior compression. The elevated side of the lamina is held in position by suture, spinous process fashioned as a graft, or any commercially available plates and grafts designed for this purpose.

Laminoplasty may have a lower incidence of postoperative kyphosis than laminectomy, although this has not been definitively proven. As with laminectomy, laminoplasty appears to leave some residual postoperative neck pain, but it is usually not severe enough to require analgesic use.[36] Newer postoperative management protocols with early rehabilitation exercises and little or no bracing have substantially reduced the likelihood of residual postoperative neck pain.[37] Retaining the C7 spinous process may also significantly reduce the incidence of axial neck pain.[38] Although laminoplasty is thought to be a motion-sparing procedure because no fusion is performed, patients can lose 30% to 70% of cervical range of motion. Nerve root palsies also can occur. Laminoplasty can achieve excellent spinal cord decompression in appropriately selected patients. Similar to laminectomy, laminoplasty generally requires a neutral or lordotic alignment, although a recent study suggested that patients with as much as 13° of kyphosis can still achieve good results.[39] Nevertheless, most patients with cervical kyphosis are most reliably treated with anterior approaches.

Anterior approaches must remove the disk herniation, osteophytes, or OPLL that are causing spinal cord compression. Subsequently, the defects created to achieve that decompression must be filled with bone and stabilized. If the pathology is at the level of the disk space, single or multilevel diskectomy and fusion can be performed. However, when pathology behind the vertebral body is involved, such as extruded disk herniations with migration of the fragment or with OPLL, complete corpectomy or multilevel corpectomies are required.

Hybrid techniques with corpectomy and additional diskectomy and fusion above or below are also used. In general, multilevel diskectomy and fusion has greater stability and recreates lordosis better than multilevel corpectomy and fusion, but pseudarthrosis rates may be higher. The treatment approach chosen should be tailored to the pathology of each patient individually.

The diskectomy technique is the same as that described for treatment of radiculopathy. Corpectomy usually requires excision of the disk above and below, followed by removal of the body with a rongeur or burr down to the posterior cortex. The PLL is then incised at one of the disk levels, and dissection is performed in the plane between the PLL and the dura up to the other disk level. From 15 to 18 mm of channel width is usually required to ensure adequate decompression, but the position of the vertebral arteries should be noted using preoperative imaging and taken into account in surgical planning.

OPLL presents a special dilemma in that the dura can become ossified and adherent to the PLL. When this situation occurs, the ossified dura may be removed and a patch can be placed, often in conjunction with a postoperative lumbar subarachnoid drain to reduce cerebrospinal fluid leakage. Alternatively, the ossified PLL and dura can be left intact but detached from the surrounding bone and allowed to float freely away from the spinal cord.

Because most pathology in patients with cervical myelopathy originates from the anterior side and because the anterior procedures stabilize the diseased segments, neurologic recovery from these procedures is typically excellent.[40-42] However, complications are not uncommon. As with any anterior procedure, approach-related complications of dysphagia, dysphonia, esophageal injury, recurrent laryngeal nerve injury, and Horner's syndrome can occur but are typically reversible. Complication rates for corpectomy increase when more levels are removed. Corpectomies of three or more levels have been reported to have up to a 50% incidence of graft dislodgment or subsidence unless accompanied by posterior instrumentation or long-term halo application.

Such reports have further stimulated the ongoing debate over the effectiveness and morbidity of anterior versus posterior approaches. In general, patients with kyphosis should be treated with anterior approaches. Those who have difficulty swallowing or breathing should be treated posteriorly. Patients with multilevel disease requiring corpectomy of greater than two levels should probably have posterior instrumentation to supplement their anterior strut graft fusion. In all other situations, the surgical approach decision should be based on the patient's specific pathology or comorbid conditions that might affect the ability to tolerate potential complications, as well as the surgeon's comfort level with each of the surgical options. As with any surgical procedure, informed consent, including an honest appraisal of the risks and benefits of each option, is of paramount importance.

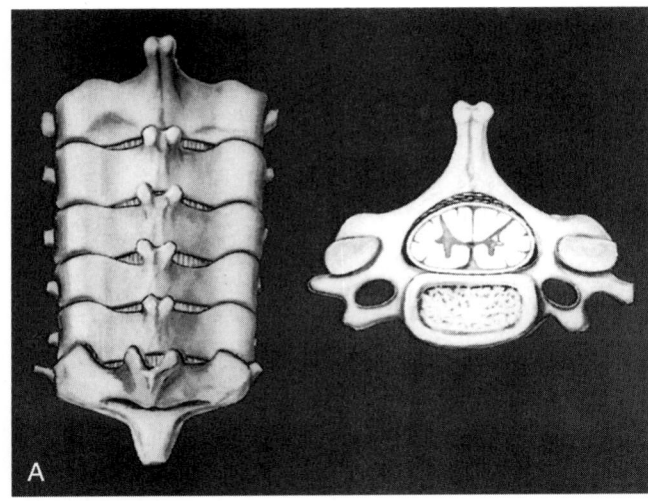
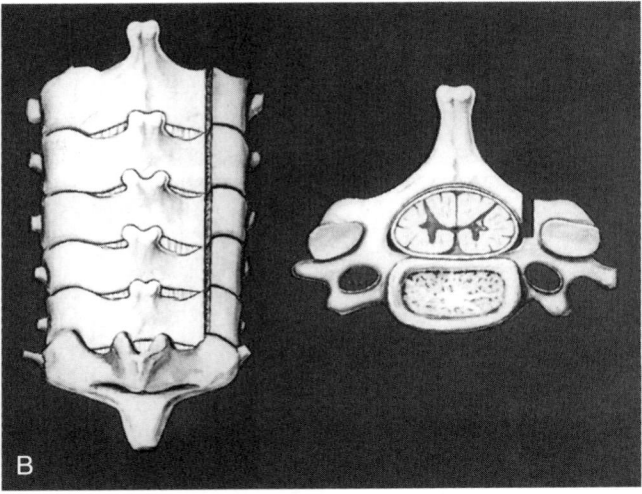
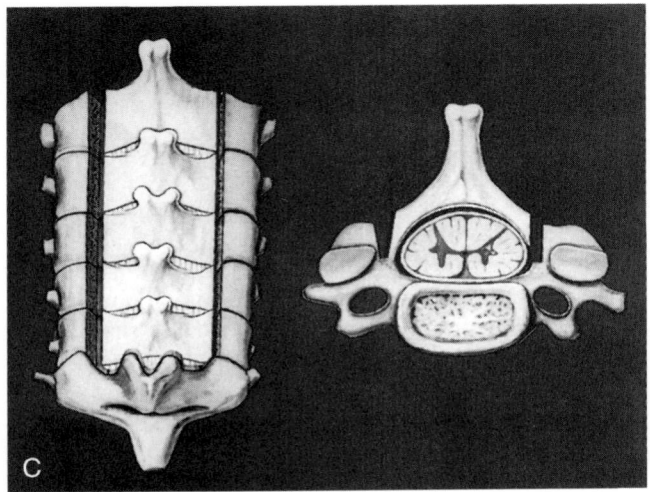
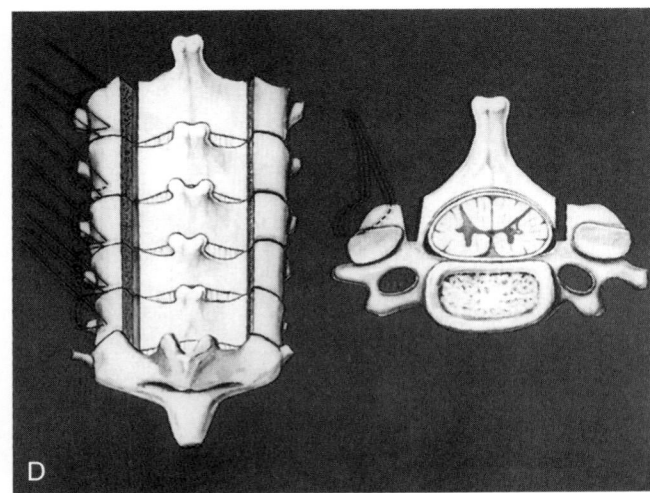
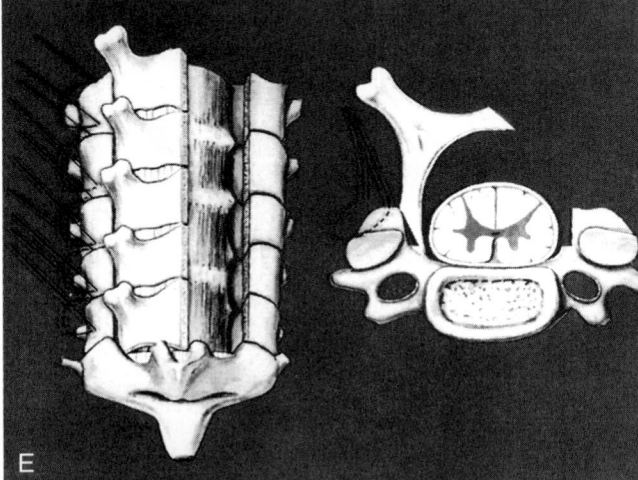
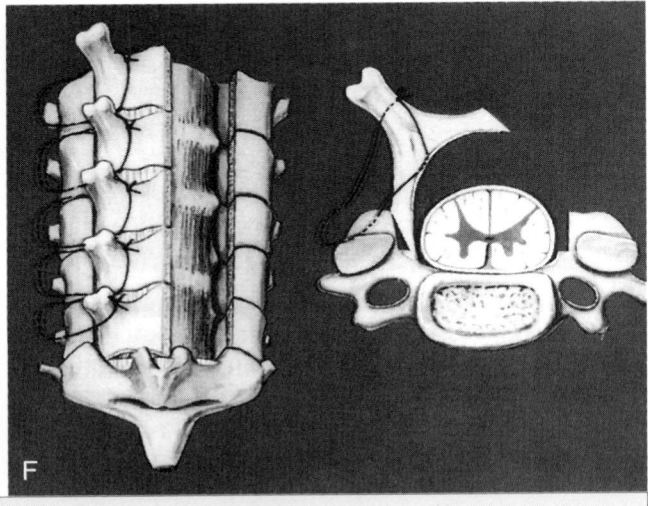

Figure 1 **A,** Posterior elements are exposed without disrupting the facet capsules. **B,** The lamina is incised on the opening side just medial to the facet. **C,** A trough is burred on the hinge side at a depth extending to, but not through, the ventral cortex. **D,** An anchoring device, such as a wire on the hinge side or a plate on the opening side, may be applied. **E,** The laminae are lifted, creating a greenstick fracture of the hinge side. **F,** The hinge is affixed to the anchoring device. *(Reproduced with permission from Denaro V: Surgical techniques, in Denaro V: Stenosis of the Cervical Spine. Heidelberg, Germany, Springer-Verlag, 1991, p 272.)*

5: Spine

Annotated References

1. Aprill C, Dwyer A, Bogduk N: Cervical zygapophyseal joint pain patterns: II. A clinical evaluation. *Spine* 1990; 15:458-461.

2. Lord SM, Barnsley L, Wallis BJ, McDonald GJ, Bogduk N: Percutaneous radio-frequency neurotomy for chronic cervical zygapophyseal-joint pain. *N Engl J Med* 1996; 335:1721-1726.

3. Tanaka Y, Kokobun S, Sato T, Ozawa H: Cervical roots as origin of pain in the neck or scapular regions. *Spine* 2006;31:E568-E573.

   The site of referred axial neck or scapular pain accurately predicted the level of cervical nerve root involvement and was reliably relieved by single nerve root decompression without fusion. Level of evidence: I.

4. Bogduk N, Aprill C: On the nature of neck pain, discography and cervical zygopophyseal joint blocks. *Pain* 1993;54:213-217.

5. Falla D, Bilenkij G, Jull G: Patients with chronic neck pain demonstrate altered patterns of muscle activation during performance of a functional upper limb task. *Spine* 2004;29:1436-1440.

   Patients with greater neck pain and functional disability on National Disability Index scores had increased recruitment of accessory cervical spinal muscles in this cross-sectional study using EMG.

6. Boden SD, McCowin PR, Davis DO, Dina TS, Mark AS, Wiesel S: Abnormal magnetic-resonance scans of the cervical spine in asymptomatic subjects: A prospective investigation. *J Bone Joint Surg Am* 1990;72:1178-1184.

7. Barnsley L, Lord SM, Wallis BJ, Bogduk N: The prevalence of chronic cervical zygapophyseal joint pain after whiplash. *Spine* 1995;20:20-24.

8. Nederhand MJ, Ijzerman MJ, Hermens HJ, Baten CT, Zilvold G: Cervical muscle dysfunction in the chronic whiplash associated disorder grade II (WAD-II). *Spine* 2000;25:1938-1943.

9. Shen FH, Samartzis D, Jenis LG, An HS: Rheumatoid arthritis: Evaluation and surgical management of the cervical spine. *Spine J* 2004;4:689-700.

   A comprehensive literature review of cervical manifestations of rheumatoid disease advocates early diagnosis and treatment. Level of evidence: III.

10. Grauer JN, Tingstad EM, Rand N, Christie MJ, Hilibrand AS: Predictors of paralysis in the rheumatoid cervical spine in patients undergoing total joint arthroplasty. *J Bone Joint Surg Am* 2004;86:1420-1424.

    The prevalence of radiographic signs of instability that predict paralysis in patients with rheumatoid arthritis was studied. Level of evidence: II.

11. Borchgrevink GE, Kaasa A, McDonagh D, Stiles TC, Haraldseth O, Lereim I: Acute treatment of whiplash neck sprain injuries: Randomized trial of treatment during the first 14 days after a car accident. *Spine* 1998;23: 25-31.

12. Ghanayem AJ, Leventhal M, Bohlman HH: Osteoarthritis of the atlanto-axial joints. *J Bone Joint Surg Am* 1996;78:1300-1307.

13. Garvey TA, Transfeldt EE, Malcolm JR, Kos P: Outcome of anterior cervical discectomy and fusion as perceived by patients treated for dominant axial-mechanical cervical spine pain. *Spine* 2002;27:1887-1895.

14. Zheng Y, Liew SM, Simmons ED: Value of magnetic resonance imaging and discography in determining the level of cervical discectomy and fusion. *Spine* 2004;29: 2140-2145.

    A combination of positive cervical diskography and abnormal MRI predicted a satisfactory response to fusion in 76% of patients. Level of evidence: III.

15. Shafaie FF, Wippold FJ II, Gado M, Pilgram TK, Riew KD: Comparison of computed tomography myelography and magnetic resonance imaging in the evaluation of cervical spondylotic myelopathy and radiculopathy. *Spine* 1999;24:1781-1785.

16. Henderson CM, Hennessy RG, Shuey HM Jr, Shackelford EG: Posterior-lateral foraminotomy as an exclusive operative technique for cervical radiculopathy: A review of 846 consecutively operated cases. *Neurosurgery* 1983;13:504-512.

17. Adamson TE: Microendoscopic posterior cervical laminoforaminotomy for unilateral radiculopathy: Results of a new technique in 100 cases. *J Neurosurg* 2001;95 (suppl 1):51-57.

18. Herkowitz HN, Kurz L, Overholt DP: Surgical management of cervical soft disk herniation: A comparison between the anterior and posterior approach. *Spine* 1990; 15:1026-1030.

19. Bohlman HH, Emery SE, Goodfellow DB, Jones PK: Robinson anterior cervical discectomy and arthrodesis for cervical radiculopathy: Long-term follow-up of one hundred and twenty-two patients. *J Bone Joint Surg Am* 1993;75:1298-1307.

20. Smith GW, Robinson RA: The treatment of certain cervical spine disorders by anterior removal of the intervertebral disc and interbody fusion. *J Bone Joint Surg Am* 1958;40:607-624.

21. Zdeblick TA, Ducker TB: The use of freeze-dried allograft bone for anterior cervical fusions. *Spine* 1991; 16:726-729.

22. Wang JC, McDonough PW, Endow K, Kanim LE, Delamarter RB: The effect of cervical plating on single-

level anterior cervical discectomy and fusion. *J Spinal Disord* 1999;12:467-471.

23. Edwards CC, Karpitskaya Y, Cha C, et al: Accurate identification of adverse outcomes after cervical spine surgery. *J Bone Joint Surg Am* 2004;86:251-256.

    Poor correlation was noted between surgeon records and patient surveys in reporting dysphagia and dysphonia after cervical surgery. Dysphagia and dysphonia were underreported or unrecognized in up to 80% of patient records. Level of evidence: III.

24. Hilibrand AS, Carlson GD, Palumbo MA, Jones PK, Bohlman HH: Radiculopathy and myelopathy at segments adjacent to the site of a previous anterior cervical arthrodesis. *J Bone Joint Surg Am* 1999;81:519-528.

25. Schwab JS, Diangelo DJ, Foley KT: Motion compensation associated with single-level cervical fusion: Where does the lost motion go? *Spine* 2006;31:2439-2448.

    Cadaveric biomechanical analysis shows segmental motion increased at levels adjacent to single-level fusion.

26. Eck JC, Humphreys SC, Lim TH, et al: Biomechanical study on the effect of cervical spine fusion on adjacent-level intradiscal pressure and segmental motion. *Spine* 2002;27:2431-2434.

27. Puttlitz CM, Rousseau MA, Xu Z, Hu S, Tay BK, Lotz JC: Intervertebral disc replacement maintains cervical spine kinetics. *Spine* 2004;29:2809-2814.

    Cadaveric biomechanical analysis shows that a ball-and-socket cervical disk replacement can replicate physiologic motion, including coupled motion, at affected and adjacent levels.

28. Nurick S: The natural history and the results of surgical treatment of the spinal cord disorder associated with cervical spondylosis. *Brain* 1972;95:101-108.

29. Brain WR, Northfield D, Wilkinson M: The neurological manifestations of cervical spondylosis. *Brain* 1952;75:187-225.

30. Clarke E, Robinson PK: Cervical myelopathy: A complication of cervical spondylosis. *Brain* 1956;79:483-510.

31. Lees F, Turner JW: Natural history and prognosis of cervical spondylosis. *BMJ* 1963;2:1607-1610.

32. Fouyas IP, Statham PF, Sandercock PA: Cochrane review on the role of surgery in cervical spondylotic radiculomyelopathy. *Spine* 2002;27:736-747.

33. Edwards CC II, Heller JG, Murakami H: Corpectomy versus laminoplasty for multilevel cervical myelopathy: An independent matched-cohort analysis. *Spine* 2002;27:1168-1175.

34. Hirabayashi K, Watanabe K, Wakano K, Suzuki N, Satomi K, Ishii Y: Expansive open-door laminoplasty for cervical spinal stenotic myelopathy. *Spine* 1983;8:693-699.

35. Yonenobu K, Hosano N, Iwasaki M, Asano M, Ono K: Laminoplasty versus subtotal corpectomy: A comparative study of results in multisegmental cervical spondylotic myelopathy. *Spine* 1992;17:1281-1284.

36. Ohnari H, Sasai K, et al: Investigation of axial symptoms after cervical laminoplasty using a questionnaire survey. *Spine J* 2006;6:221-227.

    The percentage of patients undergoing laminoplasty who reported axial neck pain increased from 25% preoperatively to 38% postoperatively, although the pain generally was not severe enough to require analgesic use. Level of evidence: IV.

37. Kawaguchi Y, Kanamori M, Ishiara H, Nobukiyo M, Seki S, Kimura T: Preventive measures for axial symptoms following cervical laminoplasty. *J Spinal Disord Tech* 2003;16:497-501.

38. Hosono N, Sakaura H, Mukai Y, Fujii R, Yoshikawa H: C3-6 laminoplasty takes over C3-7 laminoplasty with significantly lower incidence of axial neck pain. *Eur Spine J* 2006;15:1375-1379.

    Postoperative neck pain was reduced from 29% to 5.4% by limiting cervical laminoplasty to C3-6 rather than the conventional C3-7 levels. Neurologic outcomes were equivalent in both groups. Level of evidence: II.

39. Suda K, Abumi K, Ito M, Shono Y, Kaneda K, Fujiya M: Local kyphosis reduces surgical outcomes of expansive open-door laminoplasty for cervical spondylotic myelopathy. *Spine* 2003;28:1258-1262.

40. Bohlman HH: Cervical spondylosis with moderate to severe myelopathy: A report of 17 cases treated by Robinson anterior cervical discectomy and fusion. *Spine* 1977;2:151-162.

41. Bernard TN Jr, Whitecloud TS III: Cervical spondylotic myelopathy and myeloradiculopathy: Anterior decompression and stabilization with autogenous fibula strut graft. *Clin Orthop Relat Res* 1987;221:149-160.

42. Emery SE, Bohlman HH, Bolesta MJ, Jones PK: Anterior cervical decompression and arthrodesis for the treatment of cervical spondylotic myelopathy: Two- to seventeen-year follow-up. *J Bone Joint Surg Am* 1998;80:941-951.

Chapter 45

Degenerative Disease of the Lumbar Spine

R. Shay Bess, MD   *Darrel S. Brodke, MD

Lumbar Disk Degeneration

Lumbar disk degeneration is noted to some degree in up to 97% of individuals by the fifth decade of life. However, numerous studies have found that degenerative changes to the intervertebral disk do not correlate with patient symptoms nor are these changes predictive of future symptoms. Consequently, the challenge in effectively treating conditions associated with lumbar degenerative disease lies in the ability to correlate patient symptoms with the associated degenerative condition.

Lumbar Disk Herniation

Pathoanatomy
Lumbar disk herniation (LDH) has been defined as a focal displacement of nucleus, anulus, or end-plate material beyond the osseous confines of the vertebral body, resulting in displacement of epidural fat, nerve root, and/or the thecal sac. This is differentiated from a disk bulge, which is a diffuse, nonfocal protrusion of disk material beyond the confines of the normal disk space, with no evidence of neural impingement (Figure 1).

Pathophysiology
The clinical symptoms associated with LDH are likely generated by a combination of mechanical and chemical irritation. Nerve root compression alone has been demonstrated to generate only mild local discomfort in conscious patients who received lumbar diskectomy under local anesthesia. However, when the same patients sustained neural compression following nerve root exposure to nucleus pulposus extract, they reported symptoms consistent with radicular pain. Animal models have also demonstrated that, compared with nerve compression alone, nerve root compression combined

with epidural application of nucleus pulposus extract increases nerve tissue edema, fibrosis, demyelination, and Schwann cell hypertrophy. Tumor necrosis factor-alpha (TNF-α) is produced by the chondrocyte-like cells of the nucleus pulposus, and has been implicated as the key chemical mediator that sensitizes the nerve root to stimulation. The local effects of TNF-α include sodium channel upregulation (predisposing the nerve root to depolarization) and chemotaxis (causing local inflammation), which may then lead to further nerve root irritation. TNF-α may also mediate dorsal root ganglion apoptosis. Consequently, the chemical effects of nerve root exposure to herniated nucleus pulposus likely work in concert with the associated nerve root compression to generate radicular pain.

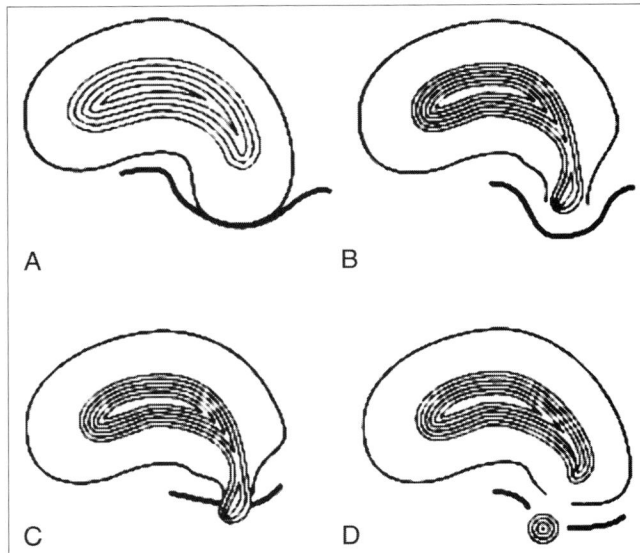

Figure 1 Morphologic types of lumbar disk herniation. **A,** Protruded disk, or contained disk herniation. **B,** Extruded, subligamentous herniation. **C,** Extruded, transligamentous herniation. **D,** Sequestered herniation. *(Reproduced from Rao RJ, David KS: Lumbar Degenerative Disorders, in Vaccaro AR (ed): Orthopaedic Knowledge Update 8. Rosemont, IL, American Academy of Orthopaedic Surgeons, 2005, pp 539-552.)*

Darrel S. Brodke, MD, or the department with which he is affiliated has received research or institutional support from Medtronic, royalties from DePuy, and holds stock or stock options in Amedica.

5: Spine

Clinical Features

Symptoms traditionally associated with LDH are indicative of lower motor neuron pathology causing radiculopathy. Symptoms include pain and/or paresthesias, numbness, and weakness in a dermatomal distribution. Sclerotomal (referred) pain originates from mesodermal tissue (muscle, ligaments, and periosteum). Sclerotomal pain is confined to the low back, buttock, and posterior thigh and does not radiate below the knee.

Findings on physical examination consistent with radiculopathy include dermatomal weakness, sensory loss, atrophy, and hyporeflexia. The straight-leg raise test, defined as production of ipsilateral, concordant leg pain at 35° to 70° of leg elevation in supine or sitting positions, has demonstrated a high sensitivity but low specificity for L4-5 and L5-S1 disk herniations. The contralateral or crossed straight-leg raise test (production of concordant leg pain with contralateral leg elevation) has a lower sensitivity but higher specificity. The straight-leg raise will not produce pain if nerve root pathology is cephalad to the L5 nerve root because the straight-leg raise test maneuver tensions lower nerve roots (L5, S1). Upper lumbar root irritation (L1-4) is reproduced by the femoral stretch test, defined as anterior thigh pain generated by hip extension and knee flexion with the patient in the lateral or prone position.

Cauda equina syndrome (CES), caused by severe compression of lumbar and sacral nerve roots, occurs in approximately 2% of all patients with LDH. Symptoms include severe bilateral leg pain, weakness, saddle anesthesia, bowel/bladder symptoms (urinary retention early, then urine and bowel incontinence as the condition progresses), and impotence. Emergent decompression is traditionally advocated to prevent permanent weakness and loss of bowel/bladder and sexual function. However, a meta-analysis of treatment and outcomes for CES caused by LDH indicated statistically equivalent postoperative outcomes (pain improvement, improved sensory and motor deficits, and resolution of urine and rectal dysfunction) when comparing patients who underwent decompression within 24 hours of symptom onset with those treated 24 to 48 hours after symptom onset. Patients treated later than 48 hours after symptom onset had inferior outcomes for sensory, motor, bladder, and rectal recovery. A subsequent analysis of this study questioned the methodology and conclusions of the meta-analysis.[1] Repeat evaluation of the meta-analysis data demonstrated inconsistent definitions of symptom onset when calculating time to surgery, variable follow-up periods used to report outcomes, lack of inclusion of patients with partial recovery, and too small a sample size for meaningful statistical analysis. The authors emphasized that when evaluating the relationship between the timing of surgery for CES and outcome, the duration of time from symptom onset to treatment should be viewed as a continuous variable instead of definitive blocks of time. As the duration of untreated symptoms increases, the risk for poor outcome also increases. Repeat analysis demonstrated an increased risk for poor outcome for surgery at 24 to 48 hours compared with surgery within 24 hours. The authors concluded that an increased risk for poor outcome in all measures because of delayed surgery cannot be rejected. They also asserted that increased risks for surgery performed at 24 to 48 hours cannot be rejected. These concerns are supported by a 2000 study that reported 44 instances of surgically treated CES caused by LDH.[2] All patients presented with urinary retention or incontinence and saddle anesthesia, and 95% presented with severe bilateral foot weakness. Sudden onset of symptoms (within 24 hours) occurred in 39 patients, 37 of whom sought immediate medical attention. Treatment delay (> 48 hours) was physician-associated in more than 80% of patients, usually occurring during a weekend or holiday admission. Eighteen patients were treated within 24 hours of symptom onset, 2 patients within 24 to 48 hours after onset, and 24 after 48 hours (delayed treatment). Patients treated after 48 hours demonstrated a significantly greater risk for permanent weakness, urologic dysfunction, chronic pain, and sexual dysfunction. All patients treated within 24 hours demonstrated improved motor strength, from 0/5 to 1/5 preoperatively to 4/5 in the early postoperative period. Both patients treated within 24 to 48 hours recovered to 4/5 strength within 2 weeks postoperatively. Of the delayed-treatment patients, 58% had persistent 0/5 to 2/5 weakness at 1-year follow-up. Ninety-five percent of patients treated within 48 hours had recovery of normal bladder function by 6 months, whereas 63% of patients treated with decompression after 48 hours required either an indwelling catheter or self-catheterization at 1-year follow-up.

Diagnostic Imaging

Imaging of the lumbar spine should begin with upright radiographs, including AP, lateral, and flexion/extension views. Although plain radiographs are not often helpful in diagnosing LDH, they provide a global overview of the lumbar spine alignment, help to rule out other potential sources of low back pain and nerve root dysfunction including trauma, tumor, infection, and spondylolisthesis, and aid in surgical planning by defining the regional anatomy.

MRI is the diagnostic imaging modality of choice for LDH. MRI allows localization and classification of the herniated material. T2-weighted images are most commonly used to identify and assess primary LDH. The addition of gadolinium contrast to the T1-weighted images is indicated to differentiate between scar tissue and herniated disk material in patients who have had prior lumbar spine surgery. Herniated disk material has low signal intensity on postcontrast T1-weighted images because it is not vascularized, whereas scar tissue has high signal intensity (Figure 2). CT may be used to visualize bony anatomy in regions of prior surgery or local pathology (for example, in patients with spondylolysis or spina bifida). Myelography and CT myelograms are often poorly tolerated, and are not routinely used to diagnose LDH.

Treatment

When evaluating the efficacy of nonsurgical treatment modalities for LDH, it is important to consider that a large number of studies have focused on low back pain rather than radiculopathy as the primary symptom. One must also consider the favorable prognosis of LDH, as approximately 90% of patients with LDH report improvement of symptoms. Consequently, success of the modalities used to treat LDH may only reflect the ability to make the patient comfortable while the natural history of LDH occurs and symptoms dissipate, rather than truly altering the course of the disease. Physical therapy has been shown to limit the number of missed work days and reduce the severity and duration of symptoms. Nonsteroidal anti-inflammatory drugs (NSAIDs) have been shown to be more effective than placebo when treating acute low back pain associated with LDH. No single NSAID has been shown to be more efficacious than another. The choice of NSAID should be tailored to meet cost, patient tolerance, and efficacy objectives. Muscle relaxants reportedly are more effective than placebo when treating acute low back pain associated with LDH; however, the sedating and habit-forming effects of muscle relaxants must be considered. No single muscle relaxant has demonstrated superiority. The use of systemic (oral or intravenous [IV]) glucocorticoids for acute radiculopathy has demonstrated inconsistent results. Most studies report short-term benefits without lasting benefits. A recent study comparing IV methylprednisolone (500 mg, single bolus) to placebo for acute radiculopathy associated with LDH demonstrated a small, short-term improvement in leg pain (< 3 days), but no effect on functional recovery, clinical findings, or long-term relief.[3] Similarly, infusion of a monoclonal antibody against TNF (anti-TNF; infliximab) for sciatica associated with LDH showed no difference in outcomes at 3 months or 1 year compared with placebo.[4]

Epidural steroid injection (ESI) and selective nerve root injections (SNRIs) have received considerable attention for the treatment of LDH. It was reported in a recent study that at 23-month follow-up, more than 50% of patients treated with SNRIs for lumbar radiculopathy avoided surgery.[5] Injection therapy with corticosteroid (betamethasone) combined with local anesthetic (bupivacaine) was more effective than injections with local anesthetic alone. Minimum 5-year follow-up on the patients who avoided surgery after SNRI therapy in the original study showed that more than 80% of the patients did not later require surgery. Similar results have been reported in the literature, as approximately 50% of patients randomized to receive treatment with ESI for symptomatic LDH avoided surgery at 3-year follow-up.[6] Patients who failed to improve with ESI and progressed to diskectomy demonstrated long-term outcomes similar to those initially randomized to undergo surgery. The author concluded that although surgical treatment of LDH demonstrated better results than ESI, approximately half of the patients treated with ESI avoided surgery, and delayed surgical

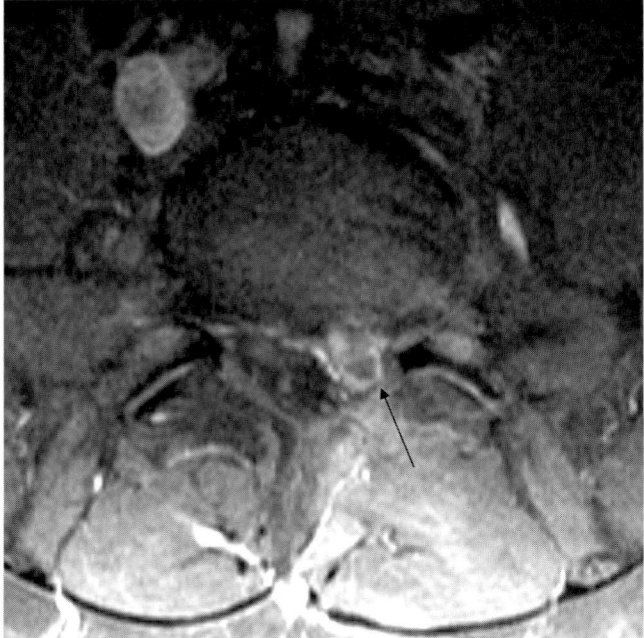

Figure 2 Gadolinium contrast-enhanced images can be used to differentiate scar tissue (high signal on fat-saturated gadolinium-enhanced T1-weighted MRI) from disk material (nonenhancing, low signal) when evaluating for recurrent LDH. Note the enhancing rim of high signal (scar) around the low signal (disk) in the left lateral recess (*arrow*).

treatment because of failed ESI treatment had no effect on surgical outcome. Additionally, the utility of SNRI as a diagnostic and prognostic modality was demonstrated in a recent study, which reported that 91% of patients with symptom relief following SNRI had good surgical outcomes, whereas 60% of patients who had no symptom relief had good surgical outcomes.[7]

The first report on long-term outcomes for surgical versus nonsurgical treatment of LDH was published in 1983. This study indicated that surgery improved short-term outcomes; however, there was no difference in long-term (4- and 10-year) outcomes between the surgical and nonsurgical groups. Criticisms of this study include high crossover rate of patients initially randomized to not undergo surgery and then proceeding to surgery (25%), lack of intent-to-treat analysis, small sample size, and insensitive outcome measures. Despite these criticisms, this study remains the standard against which surgical and nonsurgical treatment of LDH-associated radiculopathy are compared. The Spine Patient Outcomes Research Trial (SPORT) found similar limitations in the 1983 study.[8-10] Intent-to-treat analysis of the SPORT randomized trial for patients with LDH showed small but not statistically significant differences in favor of diskectomy compared with nonsurgical care. The large number of patients who crossed over between assigned groups precluded any conclusions about the comparative effectiveness of surgical

5: Spine

therapy versus nonsurgical care. Subgroup analysis comparing treatment effects of diskectomy versus nonsurgical care found that patients choosing surgical intervention reported greater improvements than patients who elected nonsurgical care. However, the authors reported that these nonrandomized comparisons of self-reported outcomes are subject to potential confounding and must be interpreted cautiously. The Maine Lumbar Spine Study reported results similar to the 1983 study.[11] Ten-year patient follow-up for surgical and nonsurgical LDH treatment demonstrated that 69% of surgically treated patients reported improvement of their predominant symptom, compared with 61% in the nonsurgical group. Both groups had similar work and disability status at 10-year follow-up; however, patients treated surgically reported better functional status, greater satisfaction with treatment, and greater magnitude of improvement than those treated nonsurgically, despite having worse preoperative symptoms and functional status. It has been reported that surgical treatment of LDH that was unresponsive to nonsurgical therapy was more cost-effective and provided an increase in quality-adjusted life in comparison with continued nonsurgical treatment.[12] When comparing selected therapies for various medical conditions, the cost-effectiveness level of diskectomy was superior to medical treatment of moderate hypertension and was superior to coronary artery bypass grafting for single-vessel coronary artery disease, but was inferior to total hip replacement and cervical cancer screening.

Unilateral, limited, open diskectomy (unilateral laminotomy or interlaminar fenestration and removal of free fragments without curetting the disk space and end plates) has demonstrated reduction in postoperative back pain compared with radical or subtotal diskectomy, and reduces the risk of neurologic and vascular injury without significantly increasing the risk of rehernation. Long-term success rates vary between 76% and 93% for open, interlaminar diskectomy. Improved outcomes following surgical treatment are correlated with younger patients without associated degenerative disk changes; large, anteroposterior herniations; sciatica present for less than 6 months; extruded or sequestered fragments with intact or minimal anulus fissure; and no current litigation.

Minimally invasive procedures have been a topic of increased interest. Good results with percutaneous endoscopic lumbar diskectomy have been reported in retrospective studies; however, there is some indication that LDH with canal compromise greater than 50% and herniations that have migrated are at risk for failure with the endoscopic procedure and should be considered for open diskectomy.

Recurrent Herniation and Revision

Recurrent herniation occurs in 5% to 11% of patients following open diskectomy. Recurrent herniation is defined as recurrent radicular pain onset following lumbar diskectomy, with evidence of neural impingement by disk material at the concurrent level. Addition-

ally, patients must report a minimum of 6 weeks of pain relief after the index procedure. Fat-saturated, gadolinium-enhanced T1-weighted MRI is the modality of choice to evaluate recurrent disk herniation and differentiate between disk material (nonenhancing) and scar (enhancing) (Figure 2). CT scans and/or oblique radiographs help rule out iatrogenic pars interarticularis fracture. Surgical treatment options for recurrent disk herniation include repeat diskectomy or fusion. It has been reported that repeat diskectomy was as efficacious as primary diskectomy, with similar outcomes in revision and primary diskectomy groups;[13] however, other studies have reported success rates ranging from 68% to 80%. Patients undergoing surgical treatment of recurrent disk herniation may be at increased risk for further spine surgery. The cumulative risk of needing a third spinal surgery within 10 years following surgery for recurrent disk herniation has been reported to be 25%. Fusion is often recommended to treat symptomatic, recurrent herniations at the involved level.

Lumbar Spinal Stenosis

Pathophysiology
Similar to LDH, the symptoms associated with lumbar spinal stenosis (LSS) are likely a combination of mechanical compression and local inflammation. The rate of compression onset may determine symptomatology, as rapid onset results in more severe symptoms than slow onset. Multilevel compression may also have a greater impact than single-level compression. Symptoms may arise from compression-generated neural ischemia and associated nerve dysfunction. Spinal nerve root blood supply is less than that of peripheral nerves. At least 50% of spinal nerve root nutritional support is dependent on cerebrospinal fluid diffusion. Consequently, mechanical compression may lead to decreased nutrition delivery, reduced neural activity, and ischemic neuritis. It is currently hypothesized that increased neural tension causes local irritation that, combined with mechanical compression and local ischemia, leads to the clinical symptoms associated with LSS.

Clinical Features
Neurogenic claudication refers to the constellation of symptoms ascribed to LSS. Symptoms include buttock and leg pain that worsens with lumbar extension and ambulation and is relieved by lumbar flexion and rest. Patients with LSS most commonly become symptomatic in their 50s and 60s and often have medical comorbidities that may masquerade as neurogenic claudication. Consequently, neurogenic claudication must be differentiated from vascular claudication and degenerative disk disease (Table 1).

Patients with LSS also may have concomitant cervical stenosis causing cervical myelopathy that may mimic or compound the symptoms of neurogenic claudication. The prevalence of combined cervical and lumbar, or tandem spinal stenosis (TSS), is reportedly 5%

Table 1

Clinical Features Differentiating Neurogenic Claudication, Vascular Claudication, and Lumbar Spondylosis

Findings	Neurogenic Claudication	Vascular Claudication	Lumbar Spondylosis
Pain type and location	Lower extremity aching, burning, paresthesias	Calf tightness and cramping	Low back aching
Radiation	Proximal to distal	Distal to proximal	Low back and hips
Exacerbation	Lumbar extension including standing, and upright exercise	All lower extremity exercise	General activity including bending, standing, and lifting
Walking distance	Variable	Constant	Variable
Relief	Lumbar flexion and rest	Cessation of lower extremity exercise	Variable
Back pain	Common	Rare	Common
Bicycle/treadmill test	Bicycle generates minimal symptoms; treadmill generates symptoms	Bicycle and treadmill generate symptoms	Variable
Hill walking	Walking uphill generates minimal symptoms; walking downhill generates symptoms	Walking uphill and walking downhill generate symptoms	Variable
Lower extremity appearance	Normal	Vascular changes including hair loss, toenail atrophy, edema	Normal
Pulses lower extremity	Normal	Diminished	Normal
Lumbar range of motion	Diminished, painful	Normal	Diminished, painful

to 25%. A 10-year review of more than 460,000 hospital admissions was conducted, and a 0.12% TSS incidence (54 patients) or 12 per every 100,000 admissions was reported.[14] Ten patients received lumbar decompression and three underwent lumbar and cervical decompression. No information regarding outcomes was provided. Another study estimated that 5% of patients with either cervical or lumbar spinal stenosis have TSS.[15] Treatment was dictated by the severity of myelopathy, radiculopathy, and canal stenosis. Patients with a cervical spinal canal of 10 mm or less initially received cervical surgery. Patients with predominant lower extremity radiculopathy and a cervical canal of 11 to 13 mm initially received lumbar surgery. Cervical decompression improved myelopathic symptoms; however, neurogenic claudication was not relieved by cervical decompression alone and lower extremity neurogenic claudication symptoms often worsened following cervical surgery, necessitating subsequent lumbar decompression. Good to excellent results were reported in 9 of 19 patients treated with cervical and lumbar decompression for TSS; however, the condition of 5 patients eventually worsened and 1 was unchanged following surgery.[16] Surgical outcome inversely correlated with symptom duration, and surgical sequence and technique was not related to outcome.

Diagnostic Imaging

Initial diagnostic evaluation of patients with LSS should begin with upright AP, lateral, and flexion-extension radiographs to delineate the amount of lumbar degeneration; evaluate for congenital stenosis; evaluate for associated scoliosis and spondylolisthesis; and rule out trauma, infection, or malignancy as a potential source of symptoms. MRI is currently the recommended advanced imaging modality to evaluate LSS. MRI is as accurate as CT myelography and is noninvasive. As previously indicated, one disadvantage of MRI includes high sensitivity to potentially asymptomatic degenerative changes. Patient size, claustrophobia, and the presence of ferromagnetic implants may degrade image quality or preclude MRI.

Electrodiagnostic testing using electromyography has recently been shown to have a high specificity for diagnosing LSS, and may be helpful in differentiating LSS from other neuromuscular disorders including peripheral or diabetic neuropathy, myopathy, and inflammatory neuropathies. Because MRI has a high sensitivity for detecting degenerative changes, electromyography may reduce the high false-positive rate associated with MRI, and may aid in differentiating LSS from symptoms associated with discogenic low back pain.

5: Spine

Despite the various modalities used to evaluate LSS, there is no current gold standard to diagnose LSS. A recent meta-analysis that reviewed the accuracy of different clinical and radiographic tests to diagnose LSS was unable to demonstrate superior accuracy of any imaging modalities (MRI, CT, myelography, and ultrasound).[17] The authors concluded that the overall quality of published information to guide the diagnosis and treatment of LSS is poor, and higher quality research is needed.

Treatment

As previously indicated, patients with lumbar degeneration are often asymptomatic. Studies have also shown inconsistent correlation between the severity of clinical symptoms and/or treatment response and the severity of stenosis, the location of the stenosis (central or lateral), and the number of stenotic levels.

The natural history of LSS is variable. Most patients will not experience severe neurologic deficits or impairment, and paralysis is uncommon. Prior reports indicated that up to 76% of patients with LSS who refused surgery were unchanged or improved at long-term follow-up. Nonsurgical treatment options include activity modification, NSAIDs, physical therapy, and ESI/SNRI. Some studies have indicated that these modalities may be less effective when treating LSS than LDH. However, good outcomes with physical therapy for patients with LSS have been reported, and a greater number of patients randomized to manual therapy combined with exercise indicated symptom improvement at 6-week and 1-year follow-up compared with patients treated with exercise alone.[18] ESI and SNRI have been shown to be effective in relieving pain and can be used as both a therapeutic and diagnostic modality.

The cornerstone of surgical treatment of LSS is decompression of the compressed neural elements. Resection of approximately 50% of the cephalad and caudad lamina and the intervening ligamentum flavum often provides adequate central decompression. Decompression should then extend laterally into the lateral recess to the medial wall of the pedicle and into the foramen. Care must be taken to preserve more than 50% of the bilateral facets because resection of more than 50% of the bilateral facets or complete unilateral facetectomy may result in iatrogenic instability. No guidelines exist as to whether adjacent levels with lesser amounts of stenosis should be included in the decompression. Although decompression of too few levels can result in persistent postoperative symptoms, there is no conclusive evidence that disability for LSS worsens over time; therefore, the goal of decompressive surgery for LSS is to relieve current disability rather than prevent future symptoms.

The Maine Lumbar Spine Study compared short-term (1 year), intermediate-term (4 years) and long-term (8 to 10 years) outcomes for surgical and nonsurgical treatment of LSS.[19] Patients treated surgically (most commonly with decompressive laminectomy) demonstrated greater relief of predominant symptoms, demonstrated greater functional improvement, and reported greater satisfaction with functional status at short- and intermediate-term follow up, despite having worse preoperative symptoms. The differences in postoperative outcome became insignificant at long-term follow-up; however, the surgically treated group continued to report superior relief of leg symptoms, greater improvement in back-related functional status, and retrospectively more often chose the same treatment compared with patients treated nonsurgically. A recent meta-analysis of preoperative predictors for clinical outcome following surgical treatment of LSS showed that improved outcomes were associated with better preoperative health and walking capacity, younger age, higher income, shorter duration of symptoms, and greater central stenosis.[20] Worse outcomes were associated with increased medical comorbidities, depression, back pain, and preoperative scoliosis. Etiology of LSS, spondylolisthesis, obesity, smoking, and marital status had no impact on outcome.

The role of spinal fusion following decompression depends on the presence of associated coronal or sagittal instability. According to results from one study, outcomes were improved following decompression combined with uninstrumented, intertransverse fusion compared to decompression alone for LSS.[21] The same authors then reported greater fusion rates but no improvement in clinical outcome using spinal instrumentation compared with uninstrumented fusion following lumbar decompression. However, long-term follow-up (5 to 14 years) of the uninstrumented patient population demonstrated that patients with a successful spinal arthrodesis had superior clinical outcomes compared with patients with pseudarthrosis. The clinical implication is that lumbar instrumentation itself does not improve outcomes; however, instrumentation was associated with an increased fusion rate, and patients with a solid arthrodesis demonstrated superior clinical outcomes compared with patients with a pseudarthrosis at long-term follow-up. Several studies have since substantiated that patients with pseudarthrosis following attempted lumbar arthrodesis have inferior clinical outcomes in comparison with patients with a solid arthrodesis.

Nonfusion technologies, including interspinous implants and motion-sparing rods, are currently being evaluated to treat LSS. This topic is covered in chapter 53.

Lumbar Spondylosis and Discogenic Back Pain

Pathoanatomy and Pathophysiology

The pathoanatomy and pathophysiology of disk degeneration in covered in detail in chapter 43.

Clinical Features

Despite the large amount of literature pertaining to disk degeneration and degenerative disk disease, there is a lack of consensus on the definition of disk degeneration. It is also unclear how disk degeneration is differentiated from physiologic growth, aging, and remodeling. The process of disk degeneration has been proposed to be an aberrant, cell-mediated response to progressive structural failure of the disk, such that a degenerated disk has evidence of structural failure combined with accelerated or advanced signs of aging. It has also been proposed that, although mechanical loading precipitates degeneration, the most important cause of degeneration is the process that weakens the disk prior to actual disk disruption and the insinuating impaired healing response. Degenerative changes in the lumbar spine occur in most of the population. It is also estimated that 80% of the US population will experience low back pain. However, only 7% of individuals with low back pain have symptoms that last longer than 2 weeks; of these individuals, only 1% will require long-term treatment. Discogenic back pain refers to a pain syndrome that theoretically originates from a lumbar disk, creating low back pain without concomitant radicular symptoms. Discogenic pain syndromes have been divided into two separate categories—internal disk disruption and degenerative disk disease. Internal disk disruption includes conditions in which plain radiographs are normal but disk-space changes, including annular tears and "dark disk disease," are detectable on MRI scans. Symptoms associated with internal disk disruption include deep, midline, low lumbar, aching pain that is exacerbated by bending and rising from sitting and does not resolve with rest, and nonradicular leg pain. Degenerative disk disease includes lumbar spondylosis and isolated disk resorption, with degenerative changes detectable on plain radiographs, including disk-space narrowing, end-plate sclerosis, and osteophyte formation. Symptoms associated with degenerative disk disease are midline back pain and referred pain over the sacroiliac joints and posterior thighs. Buttock and posterior thigh aching with ambulation is common, but this pain does not radiate below the knee and is inconsistent with neurogenic claudication. Disk-space narrowing, radial disk fissures, and disk prolapse are conditions that have been most closely associated with pain. Disk signal intensity on MRI has shown minimal relationship to pain.

Lumbar range of motion is consistently painful for patients with discogenic back pain. The remainder of the physical examination is often nonspecific. A group of physical signs to aid in diagnosing nonorganic low back pain has been developed. Waddell signs are grouped into five types or categories: (1) tenderness—superficial (skin is tender to light touch over the lumbar spine) and nonanatomic (deep tenderness over a wide area in the lumbar spine not confined to an anatomic structure); (2) stimulation tests—axial loading (axial load on the standing patient's skull causes low back pain) and rotation (rotating the patient through the lower extremities while keeping the spine straight causes low back pain); (3) distraction tests—indirect observation (patient can move without pain when not being examined) and the straight-leg raise test (which produces symptoms when the patient is lying supine

Table 2

Modic Classification of Degenerative End-Plate and Vertebral Body MRI Changes

Stage	End Plate	Vertebral Body
Type I	T1 = Decreased signal T2 = Increased signal	T1 = Decreased signal T2 = Increased signal
Type II	T1 = Increased signal T2 = Isointense to mild hyperintense	T1 = Increased signal T2 = Isointense to mild hyperintense
Type III	T1 = Decreased signal T2 = Decreased signal	T1 = Decreased signal T2 = Decreased signal

but not when distracted while sitting); (4) regional disturbances—weakness ("cogwheeling" or multiple muscle group weakness that cannot be explained neuroanatomically) and sensory ("stocking," nonanatomic sensory changes); and (5) overreaction—inappropriate or disproportionate verbalization, facial expression, muscle tension and tremor, collapsing, and sweating. The presence of three or more Waddell signs has been considered clinically significant and has been used to detect malingering and/or nonorganic low back pain. Subsequent research on the prognostic value of Waddell signs has demonstrated variable results. Some reports indicate that the Waddell signs and their correlates might interfere with optimal response to treatment, whereas other studies have indicated that Waddell signs are not predictive for outcomes following intensive, nonsurgical programs such as functional restoration.

Diagnostic Imaging

As previously indicated, plain radiographs may show minimal to no evidence of degeneration or may show variable degrees of spondylosis, including disk-space collapse, end-plate sclerosis, marginal osteophytes, and facet hypertrophy. Segmental instability has been defined as > 4.5 mm or 15° of sagittal displacement on flexion/extension radiographs and is a recognized cause of low back pain. MRI is highly sensitive to degenerative changes; however, the significance of these changes has not been fully clarified. High-intensity zones (HIZs) detected in the anulus fibrosus on T2-weighted MRI scans are thought to represent annular tears consistent with internal disk disruption. Loss of normal disk signal and the presence of dark disks may represent loss of disk hydration and early degeneration; however, the significance of these changes is unclear because similar changes have been shown to be present in up to 57% of asymptomatic volunteers. Degenerative progression of the vertebral body and end plate as seen on MRI scans are now referred to as Modic changes (Table 2). Type I Modic changes are thought to reflect acute vertebral body and end-plate inflammation. Type II Modic changes represent chronic changes, including end-plate disruption and fatty degeneration of the adjacent vertebral body. Type III changes correlate with end-plate

5: Spine

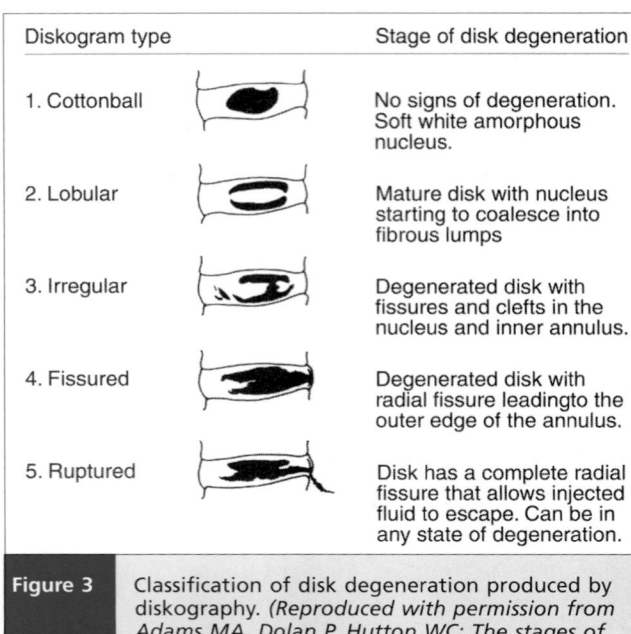

Diskogram type		Stage of disk degeneration
1. Cottonball		No signs of degeneration. Soft white amorphous nucleus.
2. Lobular		Mature disk with nucleus starting to coalesce into fibrous lumps
3. Irregular		Degenerated disk with fissures and clefts in the nucleus and inner annulus.
4. Fissured		Degenerated disk with radial fissure leadingto the outer edge of the annulus.
5. Ruptured		Disk has a complete radial fissure that allows injected fluid to escape. Can be in any state of degeneration.

Figure 3   Classification of disk degeneration produced by diskography. *(Reproduced with permission from Adams MA, Dolan P, Hutton WC: The stages of disc degeneration as revealed by discograms.* J Bone Joint Surg Br *1986;68:36-41.)*

sclerosis and loss of vertebral cancellous bone.

Provocative diskography is often used to evaluate discogenic low back pain. Diskography should only be used as a confirmatory test to evaluate a vertebral level in question and should not be used as a screening tool because of high false-negative test results. Diskography involves injecting radiopaque contrast into the nucleus of the disk suspected of causing symptoms. A minimum of one adjacent control level should also be injected. Results are interpreted according to the disk injection pressure, volume of fluid accepted by the disk, the pattern of contrast distribution in the injected disk, and the subjective pain response to the injection compared with the patient's typical symptoms (**Figure 3**). If the injection demonstrates annular disruption, reproduces the patient's symptoms (concordant pain), and the control levels are negative, it is considered a positive test result.

The clinical implications of Modic changes and HIZ lesions have not been fully elucidated. Additionally, how to interpret the data provided by diskography and the clinical implications remain in question. One study reported no difference in the prevalence of high-intensity annular fissures in patients with low back pain and asymptomatic controls (47% and 31%, respectively).[22] Another study found that patients with low back pain had a higher incidence of HIZ lesions compared with asymptomatic control subjects.[23] Disk segments with HIZ lesions were more consistently positive on provocative diskography in patients with low back pain. Disks with HIZ lesions were also more consistently positive in the asymptomatic control group. Fifty percent of disks with an HIZ lesion were positive on diskography among patients with normal psycho-

metric testing, whereas 100% of disks with an HIZ lesion were diskography-positive in patients with abnormal psychometric testing or chronic pain. The high prevalence of HIZ lesions in asymptomatic individuals (25%) and the similar percentage of asymptomatic and symptomatic patients with a diskography-positive segment with an HIZ lesion led the authors to conclude that the presence of a HIZ lesion does not reliably indicate the presence of symptomatic internal disk disruption. The validity of provocative diskography remains unproven because there is no current gold standard to which diskography can be compared. The clinical results following spinal fusion of diskography-positive levels have been used to verify a true positive test result; however, multiple studies have demonstrated low clinical success of spinal fusion to relieve low back pain. This argument was highlighted in a recent study, which reported a 91% acceptable outcome rate following spinal fusion for patients with segmental instability, compared with a 43% acceptable outcome rate for a matched cohort of patients with discogenic pain confirmed by diskography.[24] The results of diskography also are confounded by multiple factors. It has been reported that asymptomatic patients who have had a prior diskectomy have the same risk of diskography-induced pain at the diskectomy site as are patients with low backpain who undergo diskography at a previous diskectomy site.[25] High injection pressure has been implicated in false-positive diskography results. However, in a select group of asymptomatic patients receiving low-pressure (22 psi) diskography, a 25% incidence of painful injection was reported.[26] Although many argue that positive diskography results and annular tears may herald the future development of low back pain, according to a recent study, painful disk injection did not predict future low back pain 4 years after diskography in asymptomatic volunteers.[23] Annular fissures and HIZ lesions were weakly predictive of low back pain, whereas psychometric profiles strongly and independently predicted the development of low back pain. Consequently, diskography remains controversial and should be used only as an adjunct in the assessment of patients with low back pain.

Treatment
Nonsurgical management remains the cornerstone for the treatment of low back pain. The most effective strategy uses a multidisciplinary approach including education, rehabilitation, medications, and injections. There is no current evidence that "back school" prevents low back pain; however, it may be effective when combined with other rehabilitation modalities. Supervised physical therapy is superior to medical care alone and more effective than chiropractic manipulation for the treatment of chronic low back pain. No single physical therapy modality has demonstrated greater efficacy. A recent study that evaluated therapy for low back pain indicated that exercise therapy appears to be effective for decreasing pain and improving function in adults with chronic low back pain.[27] No benefit was

demonstrated for exercise therapy when treating acute low back pain in comparison with other conservative measures or no treatment. Transcutaneous electrical nerve stimulation and topical magnets have not demonstrated greater efficacy over placebo. Traction has not been shown to be beneficial in treating low back pain. One outcome study indicated greater morbidity associated with traction compared with sham traction.

NSAIDs are the most commonly prescribed medications for low back pain. NSAIDs have demonstrated superiority to placebo in treating acute low back pain; however, chronic NSAID use is associated with hepatic dysfunction, gastric ulceration, and hemorrhage. Although selective cyclooxygenase-2 (COX-2) inhibitors represent a potential group of NSAIDs with limited gastrointestinal and hemorrhagic adverse effects, recent cardiovascular complications associated with COX-2 inhibitors have limited their availability and likely contraindicate chronic use. Narcotics and muscle relaxants should be used judiciously for acute low back pain and rarely for chronic low back pain because of associated addictive and central nervous system adverse effects.

ESIs are more frequently used to treat radiculopathy and neurogenic claudication than low back pain. Facet joint injections and medial branch nerve blocks have also demonstrated short-term relief for chronic low back pain. Facet denervation by radiofrequency dorsal neurotomy has demonstrated variable results, with some studies demonstrating short-term relief of chronic low back pain. Intradiskal electrothermal therapy (IDET) has demonstrated variable results in treating low back pain; however, in a recent prospective, randomized trial there was no benefit of IDET over placebo when treating symptomatic disk degeneration confirmed by CT diskography.[28]

Although several surgical options to treat discogenic low back pain have been proposed, the most common procedures include fusion and, more recently, artificial total disk replacement. Lumbar fusion techniques include posterior spinal fusion, interbody fusion, or combined techniques. Options for lumbar interbody fusion include anterior, posterior, transforaminal, or extreme lateral approaches. Advocates of interbody fusion report more effective removal of discogenic pain generators, greater elimination of painful disk-space motion, and greater fusion rates compared with posterior spinal fusion alone. The advantages of anterior lumbar interbody fusion (ALIF) compared with other interbody fusion options include minimal or no posterior muscle dissection, especially when used as a stand-alone device. Although early experience with stand-alone ALIF indicated good results and minimal complications, one study reported a 30% nonunion rate, 22% revision rate, 22% complication rate, and 70% fair or poor outcome among 33 patients treated with stand-alone anterior Bagby and Kuslich cages at 3- to 6-year follow-up.[29] Other disadvantages of ALIF include vessel damage (2% to 5% incidence), retrograde ejaculation (0.5% to 1% incidence), and difficulty of a repeat anterior approach if revision is necessary.

More recent evaluation of ALIF using cylindrical cages and bone morphogenetic protein (BMP) have shown good results. Posterior interbody fusion devices used for posterior lumbar interbody fusion (PLIF) or transforaminal lumbar interbody fusion (TLIF) obviate the need for an anterior approach. Again, early experience with PLIF indicated good results; however, critics of PLIF cite the increased need for neural element manipulation, high rates of cage subsidence, cage migration and retropulsion, and increased pseudarthrosis rates when PLIF is not supplemented with posterior instrumentation. TLIF has emerged as a viable alternative to ALIF and PLIF. Reported advantages of TLIF include the advantages of a posterior approach, but less neural retraction is required than for PLIF. Several studies have evaluated the biomechanics of PLIF and TLIF constructs with and without posterior instrumentation. All have consistently reported increased stability when PLIF or TLIF is combined with posterior instrumentation. In an effort to improve lumbar fusion rates and reduce donor morbidity, a large body of clinical and basic science research has been devoted to recombinant human BMP (rhBMP) as a substitute for autogenous iliac crest bone graft.

There are two current US Food and Drug Administration–approved applications for rhBMP in the spine: (1) rhBMP-2 carried on a type I collagen sponge in conjunction with a tapered, threaded ALIF cage for the treatment of degenerative lumbar disk disease; and (2) rhBMP-7 as a Humanitarian Device Exemption in the posterolateral lumbar spine for established nonunions or for patients at high risk for nonunion. The pilot Investigational Device Exemption (IDE) for rhBMP-2 enrolled 14 patients in 4 investigational centers.[30] Eleven patients received a stand-alone ALIF lumbar interbody arthrodesis with a tapered cylindrical threaded fusion cage filled with rhBMP-2 (1.5 mg/mL) and three received a similar cage filled with autograft. All 11 rhBMP-2 patients went on to successful fusion by 6 months, while 2 of 3 autograft patients achieved a solid fusion. Serum serology analysis showed no rhBMP-2 patients had increased BMP antibody titers. The pivotal rhBMP-2 IDE trial compared 143 patients treated with stand-alone ALIF filled with rhBMP-2 and 136 autograft patients.[31] Surgical time and blood loss was less in the rhBMP-2 group. At 2-year follow-up, the fusion rates for rhBMP-2 and autograft were 100% and 95.6%, respectively. Success criteria were met by 94.5% of rhBMP-2 patients and 88.7% autograft patients. There was no difference in predetermined criteria for clinical outcome between the two groups. Serology testing indicated that the incidence of a positive antibody response to rhBMP-2 was 0.7% in the rhBMP-2 group and 0.8% in the autograft group. Thirty-two percent of the autograft group reported pain at the harvest site at 2-year follow-up. The pilot IDE trial for rhBMP-7 enrolled 36 patients with degenerative lumbar spondylolisthesis treated with single-level noninstrumented posterior spinal fusion following decompressive laminectomy.[32] Twenty-four patients were randomized to receive rhBMP-7 (osteogenic protein-1; 3.5 mg of rhBMP-7, 1 g of type I collagen, and

5: Spine

200 mg of carboxymethylcellulose carrier), and 12 received autogenous iliac crest bone graft. No local autograft or allograft was used. At 1-year follow-up, 32 patients were available for clinical review and 29 were available for radiographic evaluation. Clinical success was achieved in 86% of rhBMP-7 patients and 73% of autograft patients. Successful posterior spinal fusion was seen in 74% of the rhBMP-7 patients and 60% of the autograft patients. There was no difference in surgical time, hospital stay, or adverse events between the two groups. There were no incidents of systemic side effects or adverse events associated with rhBMP-7.

Despite the ability to achieve a radiographically successful lumbar fusion, clinical outcome following lumbar fusion for discogenic low back pain has been variable. The Swedish Lumbar Spine Study Group demonstrated superior outcomes for pain, disability, depressive symptoms, and return to work among patients treated with lumbar fusion compared with patients randomized to nonsurgical treatment.[33] However, other studies have demonstrated 40% to 70% satisfactory clinical outcomes, despite 60% to 90% radiographically demonstrated solid arthrodesis.

Artificial total disk replacement has received a large amount of attention for the treatment of discogenic back pain. Total disk replacement has been proposed to provide relief of painful motion segments while preserving motion and reducing adjacent-segment degeneration. A review of total disk replacement technology is covered in chapter 53. Biologic repair and/or regeneration of the degenerated disk via local cell or protein delivery, nucleus replacement, or gene therapy has also had a major influence on current research in disk degeneration. This technology is covered in chapter 43.

Summary

The foundation for the diagnosis and treatment of lumbar degenerative disorders rests on accurate correlation of the clinical and radiographic findings with the patient's pathology. Initial nonsurgical treatment modalities are often successful in most patients with lumbar degenerative disorders. In the appropriately selected patient, surgery is often effective when nonsurgical modalities are unsuccessful and the patient's lifestyle is unsatisfactory. Although newer treatment modalities have been developed and may represent a change in treatment paradigm, the long-term benefits of these newer modalities have yet to be demonstrated.

Annotated References

1. Kohles SS, Kohles DA, Karp AP, Erlich VM, Polissar NL: Time-dependent surgical outcomes following cauda equina syndrome diagnosis: Comments on a meta-analysis. *Spine* 2004;29:1281-1287.

   This Journal Club review includes re-evaluation of methodology and data used by Ahn and associates in their meta-analysis evaluating the time dependency of surgical outcomes associated with CES. The authors concluded that a flawed methodology and misinterpretation of results were reported, understating the value of early surgical intervention. Level of evidence: V.

2. Shapiro S: Medical realities of cauda equina syndrome secondary to lumbar disc herniation. *Spine* 2000;25:348-351.

3. Finckh A, Zufferey P, Schurch MA, et al: Short-term efficacy of intravenous pulse glucocorticoids in acute discogenic sciatica: A randomized controlled trial. *Spine* 2006;31:377-381.

   In 60 patients who received an intravenous bolus of glucocorticoids to treat discogenic sciatica, there was short-term improvement in leg pain.

4. Korhonen T, Karppinen J, Paimela L, et al: The treatment of disc herniation-induced sciatica with infliximab: One-year follow-up results of FIRST II, a randomized controlled trial. *Spine* 2006;31:2759-2766.

   This randomized controlled trial evaluated the 1-year efficacy of infliximab, a monoclonal antibody, against TNF-α in patients with acute/subacute sciatica secondary to herniated disk. Sixty-seven percent of patients in the infliximab group reported no pain at 52 weeks compared with 63% in the control group ($P = 0.72$). Similar efficacy was observed between treatment groups for other outcomes. Eight patients in each group required surgery. The response regardless of treatment was significantly better with shorter symptom duration and less straight-leg raise test restriction at baseline. The authors concluded that the 1-year results do not support the use of infliximab compared with placebo for lumbar radicular pain in patients with disk herniation-induced sciatica. Level of evidence: I.

5. Riew KD, Park JB, Cho YS, et al: Nerve root blocks in the treatment of lumbar radicular pain: A minimum five-year follow-up. *J Bone Joint Surg Am* 2006;88:1722-1725.

   A minimum 5-year follow-up of patients who avoided surgery in a previous prospective, randomized, controlled, double-blinded study evaluating the effect of nerve root blocks to prevent surgery for lumbar radicular pain showed that 17 of the 21 patients still had not required surgery. Level of evidence: IV.

6. Buttermann GR: Treatment of lumbar disc herniation: Epidural steroid injection compared with discectomy. A prospective, randomized study. *J Bone Joint Surg Am* 2004;86:670-679.

   In this randomized trial of 169 patients with a large LDH randomized to diskectomy or ESI and followed over a 3-year period, patients who received diskectomy had the most rapid decrease in symptoms, with 92% to 98% of the patients reporting that the treatment had been successful over the various follow-up periods. Forty-two to 56% of patients who received ESI reported that the treatment had been effective. Those who did not obtain relief from the injection had a subsequent diskectomy; however, the outcomes did not appear to have been adversely affected by the delay in surgery resulting from the treatment with ESI. Level of evidence: II.

7. Sasso RC, Macadaeg K, Nordmann D, Smith M: Selective nerve root injections can predict surgical outcome for lumbar and cervical radiculopathy: Comparison to magnetic resonance imaging. *J Spinal Disord Tech* 2005;18:471-478.

   Diagnostic SNRI results were analyzed in 101 patients who underwent lumbar or cervical decompression for radiculopathy and compared with surgical outcome 1 year postoperatively. Ninety-one percent of the patients with a positive result using SNRI had good surgical outcomes, whereas 60% of the patients with a negative result using SNRI had good outcomes. When findings between SNRI and MRI differed, surgery at a level consistent with the SNRI was more strongly associated with a good surgical outcome. Of the patients with a poor surgical outcome, surgery was most often performed at a level inconsistent with the SNRI finding. Level of evidence: IV.

8. Weber H: Lumbar disc herniation: A controlled, prospective study with ten years of observation. *Spine* 1983;8:131-140.

9. Weinstein JN, Lurie JD, Tosteson TD, et al: Surgical vs nonoperative treatment for lumbar disk herniation: The Spine Patient Outcomes Research Trial (SPORT) observational cohort. *JAMA* 2006;296:2451-2459.

   The SPORT randomized intent-to-treat analysis reported that patients with LDH showed small but not statistically significant differences in favor of diskectomy compared with nonsurgical care. The large number of patients who crossed over between assigned groups precluded any conclusions about the comparative effectiveness of surgical therapy versus nonsurgical care. Evaluation of the treatment effects of diskectomy and nonsurgical care at 3 months demonstrated that patients who chose surgery had greater improvement in the primary outcome measures of bodily pain, physical function, and Oswestry Disability Index. These differences narrowed somewhat at 2 years. The authors concluded that although patients with persistent sciatica from LDH improved in both surgical and nonsurgical care groups, patients choosing surgical intervention reported greater improvements than patients who elected nonsurgical care. However, the authors warned that nonrandomized comparisons of self-reported outcomes are subject to potential confounding and must be interpreted cautiously. Level of evidence: I.

10. Weinstein JN, Tosteson TD, Lurie JD, et al: Surgical vs nonoperative treatment for lumbar disk herniation: The Spine Patient Outcomes Research Trial (SPORT). A randomized trial. *JAMA* 2006;296:2441-2450.

    SPORT is a prospective, randomized clinical trial that enrolled patients between March 2000 and November 2004 from 13 multidisciplinary spine clinics to assess the efficacy of surgery for LDH. Adherence to assigned treatment was limited: 50% of patients assigned to undergo surgery received surgery within 3 months of enrollment, whereas 30% of those assigned to undergo nonsurgical treatment received surgery in the same period. Intent-to-treat analyses demonstrated substantial improvements for all primary and secondary outcomes in both treatment groups. Between-group differences in improvements were consistently in favor of surgery for all periods but were small and not statistically significant for the primary outcomes. The authors concluded that patients in both the surgery and nonsurgical treatment groups improved substantially over a 2-year period; however, because of the large number of patients who crossed over in both directions, conclusions about the superiority or equivalence of the treatments are not warranted based on the intent-to-treat analysis. Level of evidence: I.

11. Atlas SJ, Keller RB, Wu YA, Deyo RA, Singer DE: Long-term outcomes of surgical and nonsurgical management of sciatica secondary to a lumbar disc herniation: 10 year results from the Maine Lumbar Spine Study. *Spine* 2005;30:927-935.

    In this 10-year prospective evaluation of patients with sciatica resulting from a lumbar disk herniation treated surgically or nonsurgically, a larger proportion of surgical patients reported that their low back and leg pain were much better or completely gone and were more satisfied with their current status compared with patients treated nonsurgically, despite patients undergoing surgery having worse baseline symptoms and functional status than those initially treated nonsurgically. Improvement in the patients' predominant symptom and work and disability outcomes were similar regardless of treatment received. Level of evidence: II.

12. Malter AD, Larson EB, Urban N, Deyo RA: Cost-effectiveness of lumbar discectomy for the treatment of herniated intervertebral disc. *Spine* 1996;21:1048-1054.

13. Papadopoulos EC, Girardi FP, Sandhu HS, et al: Outcome of revision discectomies following recurrent lumbar disc herniation. *Spine* 2006;31:1473-1476.

    Twenty-seven patients who received revision diskectomies for recurrent LDH were compared with a control group of 30 matched patients who had undergone primary diskectomy. Improvement following the repeat diskectomy was not statistically different from the improvement that occurred in patients who underwent only the primary operation. Level of evidence: IV.

14. LaBan MM, Green ML: Concurrent (tandem) cervical and lumbar spinal stenosis: A 10-yr review of 54 hospitalized patients. *Am J Phys Med Rehabil* 2004;83:187-190.

    A 10-year retrospective review of 460,964 hospital admissions to one hospital identified a base population of 54 patients with TSS. Fifty-one patients were older than 51 years. For all ages, the frequency rate of TSS in this series was 12 per 100,000 admissions. Patients presented with multiple symptoms, including neurogenic claudication, progressive gait disturbances, and neurologic signs of both upper and lower motor neuron dysfunction. The authors found that the symptoms of either the cervical or the lumbar type initially predominated; however, when the primary pathology was treated, the

5: Spine

secondary problem became evident. Level of evidence: IV.

15. Epstein NE, Epstein JA, Carras R, Murthy VS, Hyman RA: Coexisting cervical and lumbar spinal stenosis: Diagnosis and management. *Neurosurgery* 1984;15:489-496.

16. Dagi TF, Tarkington MA, Leech JJ: Tandem lumbar and cervical spinal stenosis: Natural history, prognostic indices, and results after surgical decompression. *J Neurosurg* 1987;66:842-849.

17. de Graaf I, Prak A, Bierma-Zeinstra S, Thomas S, Peul W, Koes B,: Diagnosis of lumbar spinal stenosis: A systematic review of the accuracy of diagnostic tests. *Spine* 2006;31:1168-1176.

    This systematic review of diagnostic studies used to detect LSS showed overall poor quality of studies currently in the literature. Current studies to date showed no superior accuracy for myelography compared with CT or MRI or of any specific clinical test to diagnose LSS. Level of evidence: IV.

18. Whitman JM, Flynn TW, Childs JD, et al: A comparison between two physical therapy treatment programs for patients with lumbar spinal stenosis: A randomized clinical trial. *Spine* 2006;31:2541-2549.

    The multicenter randomized, controlled trial comparing two physical therapy programs for patients with LSS demonstrated a greater proportion of patients in the manual physical therapy, exercise, and walking group reported recovery at 6 weeks compared with the flexion exercise and walking group. At 1 year, 62% and 41% of the manual physical therapy, exercise, and walking group and the flexion exercise and walking group, respectively, still met the threshold for recovery. Improvements in disability, satisfaction, and treadmill walking tests favored the manual physical therapy, exercise, and walking group at all follow-up points. Level of evidence: II.

19. Atlas SJ, Keller RB, Wu YA, Deyo RA, Singer DE: Long-term outcomes of surgical and nonsurgical management of lumbar spinal stenosis: 8 to 10 year results from the Maine lumbar spine study. *Spine* 2005;30:936-943.

    This 10-year prospective observational cohort study evaluating long-term outcomes of patients with LSS treated surgically or nonsurgically demonstrated that patients undergoing surgery had worse baseline symptoms and functional status than those initially treated nonsurgically. Outcomes at 1 and 4 years favored initial surgical treatment. After 8 to 10 years, a similar percentage of surgical and nonsurgical patients reported that their low back pain was improved, their predominant symptom was improved, and were satisfied with their current status. Patients initially treated surgically reported less severe leg pain symptoms and greater improvement in back-specific functional status after 8 to 10 years than nonsurgically treated patients. By 10 years, 23% of surgical patients had undergone at least one additional lumbar spine surgical procedure, and 39% of nonsurgical patients had undergone at least one lumbar spine surgical procedure. Patients undergoing subsequent surgical procedures had worse outcomes than those continuing with their initial treatment. Level of evidence: IV.

20. Aalto TJ, Malmivaara A, Kovacs F, et al: Preoperative predictors for postoperative clinical outcome in lumbar spinal stenosis: Systematic review. *Spine* 2006;31:E648-E663.

    A meta-analysis of randomized controlled or controlled trials or prospective studies dealing with surgically treated LSS was conducted to define preoperative factors predicting clinical outcome after LSS surgery. The authors reported that depression, cardiovascular comorbidity, disorders influencing walking ability, and scoliosis predicted poorer subjective outcome. Better walking ability, self-rated health, higher income, less overall comorbidity, and pronounced central stenosis predicted better subjective outcome. Type of LSS, spondylolisthesis, obesity, smoking, and marital status had no impact on outcome. Male gender and younger age predicted better postoperative walking ability. Level of evidence: I.

21. Herkowitz HN, Kurz LT: Degenerative lumbar spondylolisthesis with spinal stenosis: A prospective study comparing decompression with decompression and intertransverse process arthrodesis. *J Bone Joint Surg Am* 1991;73:802-808.

22. Buirski G, Silberstein M: The symptomatic lumbar disc in patients with low-back pain: Magnetic resonance imaging appearances in both a symptomatic and control population. *Spine* 1993;18:1808-1811.

23. Carragee EJ, Barcohana B, Alamin T, van den Haak E: Prospective controlled study of the development of lower back pain in previously asymptomatic subjects undergoing experimental discography. *Spine* 2004;29:1112-1117.

    A prospective controlled longitudinal study was undertaken to determine if subjects asymptomatic for low back problems who undergo experimental diskography develop low back problems. Results demonstrated a low incidence of low back pain episodes in the experimental and control (no low back pain, no diskography) groups. A painful disk injection, independent of psychological profile, did not predict low back pain or any other functional outcome measure at 4-year follow-up. The presence of an annular fissure seen on diskography was weakly associated with the cumulative incidence of LBP episodes after diskography. The presence of HIZ on MRI in any disk was also weakly associated with the development of low back pain episodes. Psychometric profiles strongly and independently predicted future back pain, medication usage, and work loss. Level of evidence: II.

24. Carragee EJ, Lincoln T, Parmar VS, et al: A gold standard evaluation of the "discogenic pain" diagnosis as determined by provocative discography. *Spine* 2006;31:2115-2123.

    This prospective study evaluated whether provocative diskography accurately identifies low back pain due to primary disk lesion. Patients who underwent spinal fusion for back pain and a positive single-level low-pressure provocative diskogram were compared to patients who received spinal fusion for unstable spondylolisthesis. Seventy-two percent in the spondylolisthesis group met the highly effective success criteria, compared with 27% in the discogenic pain cohort. The proportion of patients who met the "minimal acceptable outcome" was 91% in the spondylolisthesis group and 43% in the presumed discogenic pain group. Adjusting for surgical morbidity and dropout failure, by either criteria of success, the best-case positive predictive value of diskography was calculated to be 50% to 60%. Level of evidence: II.

25. Carragee EJ, Chen Y, Tanner CM, Truong T, Lau E, Brito JL: Provocative discography in patients after limited lumbar discectomy: A controlled, randomized study of pain response in symptomatic and asymptomatic subjects. *Spine* 2000;25:3065-3071.11145818

26. Carragee EJ, Alamin TF, Carragee JM: Low-pressure positive discography in subjects asymptomatic of significant low back pain illness. *Spine* 2006;31:505-509.

    This retrospective review of disk injections at low pressures with positive results among subjects without chronic low back pain illness compared with patients with chronic low back pain undergoing diskography demonstrated that the rate of low-pressure painful injections in subjects without chronic low back pain illness is approximately 25%, and correlates with both anatomic and psychosocial factors and may represent an unacceptable risk of false-positive results. Level of evidence: IV.

27. Hayden JA, van Tulder MW, Malmivaara AV, Koes BW: Meta-analysis: Exercise therapy for nonspecific low back pain. *Ann Intern Med* 2005;142:765-775.

    This meta-analysis of randomized, controlled trials evaluated exercise therapy for adult nonspecific low back pain, measuring pain, function, return to work or absenteeism, and global improvement outcomes. Sixty-one randomized, controlled trials (6,390 participants) met inclusion criteria. Evidence suggested effectiveness of a graded-activity exercise program in subacute low back pain in occupational settings, although the evidence for other types of exercise therapy in other populations was inconsistent. In patients with acute low back pain, exercise therapy and other programs were equally effective. Limitations of the literature included low-quality studies with heterogeneous outcome measures, inconsistent and poor reporting, and possibility of publication bias. Level of evidence: III.

28. Freeman BJ, Fraser RD, Cain CM, Hall DJ, Chapple DC: A randomized, double-blind, controlled trial: Intradiscal electrothermal therapy versus placebo for the treatment of chronic discogenic low back pain. *Spine* 2005;30:2369-2377.

    A prospective, randomized, double-blind, placebo-controlled trial of IDET for the treatment of chronic discogenic low back pain showed that the IDET procedure appeared safe with no permanent complications; however, no subject in either arm met criteria for successful outcome. Further detailed analyses showed no significant change in outcome measures in either group at 6 months, leading the authors to conclude that there is no significant benefit from IDET over placebo. Level of evidence: II.

29. Button G, Gupta M, Barrett C, Cammack P, Benson D: Three- to six-year follow-up of stand-alone BAK cages implanted by a single surgeon. *Spine J* 2005;5:155-160.

    This retrospective review of 3- to 6-year clinical outcomes, including fusion rate, revision rate, complications, and functional status of patients who underwent stand-alone ALIF with Bagby and Kuslich cages by a single surgeon, indicated a 22% revision rate. Ten patients (22%) had 14 total complications not requiring revision surgery. Seventy percent of patients had a fair or poor outcome as assessed by the Prolo rating system, and 58% of patients had at least "severe disability" according to the Oswestry outcome scale. Fifty percent of patients were satisfied with their surgery. The authors concluded that results following stand-alone ALIF with Bagby and Kuslich cages demonstrates significantly worse clinical outcomes than has been previously reported and that the use of stand-alone Bagby and Kuslich cages for degenerative disk disease should be reconsidered. Level of evidence: IV.

30. Boden SD, Zdeblick TA, Sandhu HS, Heim SE: The use of rhBMP-2 in interbody fusion cages: Definitive evidence of osteoinduction in humans. A preliminary report. *Spine* 2000;25:376-381.

31. Burkus JK, Gornet MF, Dickman CA, Zdeblick TA: Anterior lumbar interbody fusion using rhBMP-2 with tapered interbody cages. *J Spinal Disord Tech* 2002;15:337-349.

32. Vaccaro AR, Patel T, Fischgrund J, et al: A pilot study evaluating the safety and efficacy of OP-1 Putty (rhBMP-7) as a replacement for iliac crest autograft in posterolateral lumbar arthrodesis for degenerative spondylolisthesis. *Spine* 2004;29:1885-1892.

    This prospective, randomized, controlled, multicenter clinical study compared the clinical and radiographic outcomes of patients treated with osteogenic protein-1 (BMP-7) Putty with autogenous iliac crest bone graft for single-level uninstrumented posterolateral lumbar fusion following decompressive laminectomy for degenerative spondylolisthesis with spinal stenosis. Clinical success at 1 year was achieved by 86% of the osteogenic protein-1 Putty patients and 73% of the autograft patients. Medical Outcomes Study 36-Item Short Form Health Survey pain index scores showed similar results. Seventy-four percent of the osteogenic protein-1 Putty patients and 60% of the autograft patients achieved successful fusion. No systemic toxicity, ectopic bone formation, recurrent stenosis, or other adverse events related to the osteogenic protein-1 Putty implant were observed. Level of evidence: II.

33. Fritzell P, Hagg O, Wessburg P, Nordwall A: 2001 Volvo Award Winner in clinical studies: Lumbar fusion versus nonsurgical treatment for chronic low back pain: A multicenter randomized controlled trial from the Swedish Lumbar Spine Study Group. *Spine* 2001;26:2521-2532.

5: Spine

Chapter 46

Cervical Spine Trauma

Moe R. Lim, MD   Bikramjit Singh, MD

Evaluation

Clinical Evaluation

The evaluation of a patient suspected to have a cervical spine injury begins with a thorough history of the injury mechanism. After initial resuscitation and primary survey, the patient's entire spinal column should be inspected and palpated for tenderness and step-offs. Care should be taken to preserve spinal stability during the examination by using a log-roll maneuver with an assistant. A complete neurologic evaluation should be performed, including assessment of motor strength, pin-prick sensation, reflexes, cranial nerves, and a rectal examination. A complete neurologic rectal examination includes assessment of perineal pin-prick sensation, sphincter tone, and volitional sphincter control. In patients with spinal cord injury (SCI), a bulbocavernosus reflex should be elicited to determine the presence of spinal shock. In patients with a truly complete SCI determined after the resolution of spinal shock, motor recovery below the zone of injury does not occur.[1] In contrast, initial preservation of sacral or lower extremity pin-prick sensation is associated with improved prognosis for eventual ambulation.[2]

Radiographic Evaluation

Patients with neck pain after trauma should be considered for radiographic evaluation. The Canadian C-spine rule has established a decision-making tool to determine the need for cervical spine imaging in alert and stable trauma patients.[3] Imaging is mandatory in high-risk patients. Indicators for high-risk patients include (1) older than 65 years; (2) paresthesias in the extremities; and (3) dangerous injury mechanism (for example, a fall from more than 3 feet/5 steps, axial load to the head such as a diving injury, rollover or ejection during a high-speed motor vehicle crash, motorized recreational vehicle crash, or bicycle collision). Low-risk patients should undergo a clinical examination to assess cervical range of motion to determine the need for imaging. Low-risk factors that allow for safe assessment of range of motion are (1) simple rear-end motor vehicle crash, (2) the ability to maintain a sitting position in the emergency department, (3) the ability to ambulate, (4) delayed onset of neck pain, or (5) absence of midline cervical spine tenderness. Imaging is not required in low-risk patients who can actively rotate the neck 45° to the left and right. In a study of approximately 9,000 patients, the Canadian C-spine rule was 100% sensitive and 42% specific in detecting clinically significant cervical spine injuries, and also has been shown to be superior to previously established guidelines in terms of sensitivity, specificity, and reduced rates of radiography.[4]

Plain radiography has traditionally been the first imaging modality of choice. A minimum of three views (AP, lateral, and open-mouth) are necessary. The lateral radiograph is the single most important view and is 74% to 86% sensitive and 70% to 97% specific in detecting cervical spine injuries. Flexion-extension views are not useful in the acute emergency department setting but can detect subacute ligamentous instability 1 to 2 weeks after injury. In the presence of a cervical spine fracture and a sufficient injury mechanism, imaging of the entire spine should be done to rule out concomitant noncontiguous spinal injuries.

Screening CT is rapidly replacing plain radiography as the initial imaging study in the evaluation of cervical spine trauma. Proponents of screening CT scans cite greater sensitivity, relative safety, and cost effectiveness in comparison with plain radiographs. The principal advantage of CT is its ability to delineate bony anatomy with superb spatial resolution and detection of bony injuries with close to 100% sensitivity. CT is particularly helpful to identify and characterize fractures in the upper cervical spine and the cervicothoracic junction. The major disadvantage of CT, however, is increased radiation exposure. Despite modern spiral CT technology, radiation exposure from CT is more than six times higher than that of plain radiography.

MRI is indicated in the presence of a neurologic deficit if there is clinical suspicion of ligamentous or disk injury or if the patient requires surgical intervention. MRI can help in the evaluation for causes of neurologic deficit, such as the degree or type of intrinsic SCI, canal stenosis, occult vascular injury, disk disruption, or hematomas. MRI can differentiate between spinal cord transection, contusion, and hemorrhage, and the extent of area involved can be visualized in patients with SCI. Associated soft-tissue injuries, such as injuries to the anterior longitudinal ligament (ALL), posterior longitudinal ligament (PLL), interspinous ligaments, facet capsules, and paraspinal musculature, can be identified using MRI. However, bone cannot be visualized well using MRI, and CT remains the study of choice for the recognition and characterization of bony injuries.

5: Spine

External Immobilization of Cervical Spine Injuries

Stable cervical spine injuries can be successfully treated by external immobilization in a cervical orthosis or halo vest. The choice of orthosis or halo vest depends on the degree of stability of the injury pattern and patient factors such as age, body habitus, and ability to comply with treatment. The soft collar, Philadelphia collar, Miami J collar, cervicothoracic orthosis (CTO), and halo vest offer increasing amounts of cervical immobilization. Hard collars and CTOs, however, may increase motion of the upper cervical spine (occiput-C2). Adequate immobilization of potentially unstable upper cervical spine injuries generally requires the use of a halo vest. Halo vests, however, can be fraught with complications, including pin loosening (36%), pin-site infection (20%), and severe pin discomfort (18%). Less common but more serious complications include dural penetration and subdural abscess. Recent evidence suggests cautious use of halo vests in elderly patients because of unacceptably high rates of complications such as respiratory distress (10%), dysphagia (14%), and death (19% to 40%).[5]

Upper Cervical Injuries and Treatment

Occipital Condyle Fractures

Occipital condyle fractures are the result of high-energy trauma and are associated with head trauma, skull base fractures, lower cranial nerve palsies (most commonly cranial nerve 12), and additional upper cervical spine injuries.[6] Occipital condyle fractures are extremely difficult to diagnose with plain radiography alone and are becoming increasingly recognized with use of cervical screening CT scans. When occipital condyle fractures are identified, associated occipitocervical dissociation must be ruled out. Occipital condyle fractures associated with occipitocervical instability require surgical stabilization. Nondisplaced, impaction, and unilateral injuries can generally be treated with an orthosis for 6 to 12 weeks. Displaced, avulsion, and bilateral injuries tend to require more aggressive immobilization in a halo vest or surgical stabilization.[7]

Occipitocervical Dissociations

Occipitocervical dissociations are caused by high-energy trauma and are frequently associated with other life-threatening injuries such as brainstem injuries, vertebrobasilar arterial injuries, subarachnoid hemorrhages, and posterior pharyngeal wall disruptions. Historically, injuries to the craniocervical junction were considered fatal, with rare case reports of patient survival. With modern emergency services, however, more patients are surviving and these injuries are being more frequently recognized.[8]

Occipitocervical dissociations have been classified based on the direction of displacement of the occiput.[9] The occiput can be displaced anteriorly, posteriorly, vertically, or obliquely. In fatal injuries, the diagnosis is usually obvious. In patients with minimal neurologic deficits, however, symptoms can be subtle and the diagnosis easily missed. Analysis of the imaging studies for the relationship of the occiput to the atlas, small avulsion fractures, bony incongruities, and soft-tissue swelling are the keys to avoiding a delayed diagnosis.

Occipitocervical dissociations are considered universally unstable. These injuries should be immediately reduced and immobilized with a halo vest. Traction should be avoided. Once the associated injuries have been identified and addressed, surgical stabilization with arthrodesis and instrumentation is indicated. Modern occipital plates and upper cervical polyaxial screw instrumentation techniques allow for immediate rigid stability[10] (Figure 1). The caudal extent of the instrumentation can vary from C2 to C4, depending on the injury pattern, bone quality, and fixation methods. Because of the severely unstable nature of these injuries, postoperative halo immobilization is generally recommended.

C1 Ring Fractures

C1 ring fracture patterns include isolated anterior or posterior arch fractures, lateral mass fractures, and Jefferson burst fractures.[11] These fractures (particularly the isolated posterior arch pattern) are commonly associated with C2 fractures, most commonly type II odontoid and hangman's fractures.[12] Neurologic compromise is rare because of the large space available for the spinal cord at this level and the decompressive effect of these fractures. Most isolated anterior or posterior arch fractures and lateral mass fractures can be treated with an orthosis for 6 to 12 weeks. The treatment of combined C1 and C2 fractures is usually dictated by the type and severity of the C2 fracture

Jefferson burst fractures (Figure 2) occur via three or four fracture lines in the C1 ring, leading to radial displacement of the anterior arch, posterior arch, and lateral masses. Displacement of the C1 lateral masses can cause subluxation of the atlanto-occipital and atlanto-axial joints. The key to treatment of Jefferson fractures is determination of the integrity of the transverse ligament. Disruption of the transverse ligament and potential C1-2 instability can be inferred if the combined lateral overhang of the C1 lateral masses (as measured on a magnified open-mouth odontoid radiograph) is greater than 8 mm. With contemporary MRI techniques, disruptions of the transverse ligament and associated craniocervical ligaments can be directly visualized. Patients with an intact transverse ligament or a bony transverse ligament avulsion are treated with an orthosis or halo for 12 weeks, depending on the degree of displacement and estimation of instability. Generally, flexion-extension radiographs are obtained to rule out instability before discontinuing external immobilization. Early surgical treatment is an option in the presence of a midsubstance transverse ligament rupture with C1-2 instability. Surgery involves posterior C1-2 fusion with transarticular Magerl screws or with the Harms technique (C1 lateral mass and C2 pars/pedicle polyaxial screws and rods).

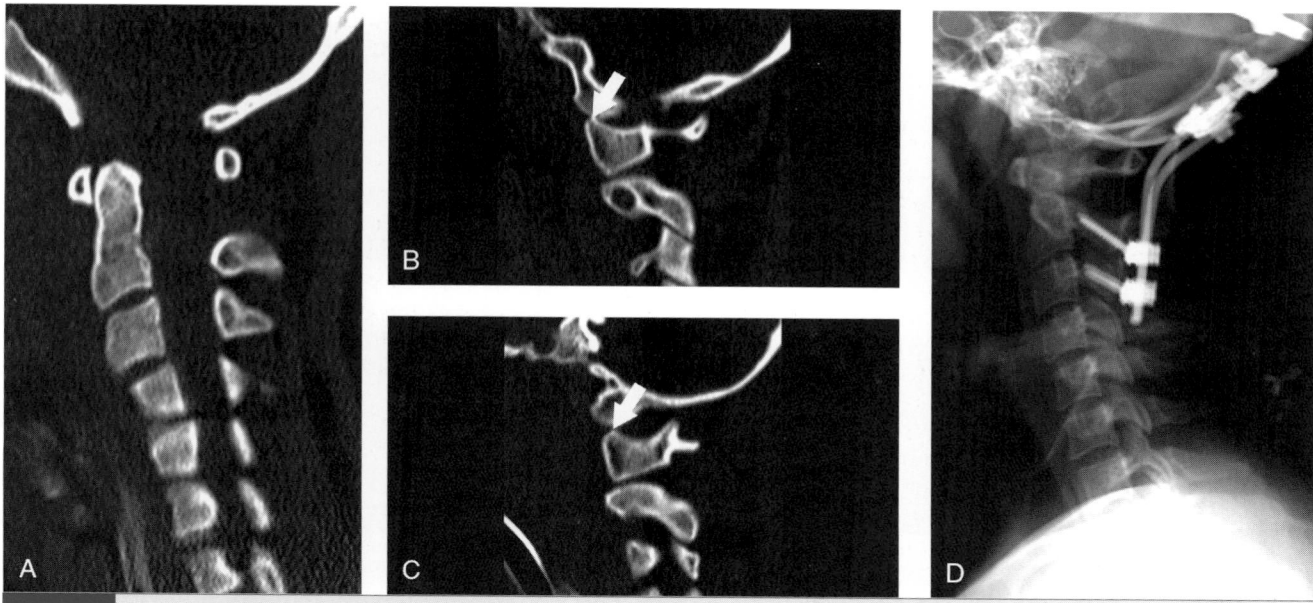

Figure 1   Imaging studies of a 22-year-old woman with craniocervical dissociation that occurred during a high-speed motor vehicle crash. Midsagittal (**A**), left parasagittal (**B**), and right parasagittal (**C**) CT views demonstrate anterior and cephalad displacement of the cranium relative to the cervical spine and subluxation of the O-C1 and C1-C2 joints bilaterally (*arrows*). She underwent O-C3 stabilization with an occipital plate, structural iliac crest bone graft, C2 isthmus screws, and C3 lateral mass screws (**D**).

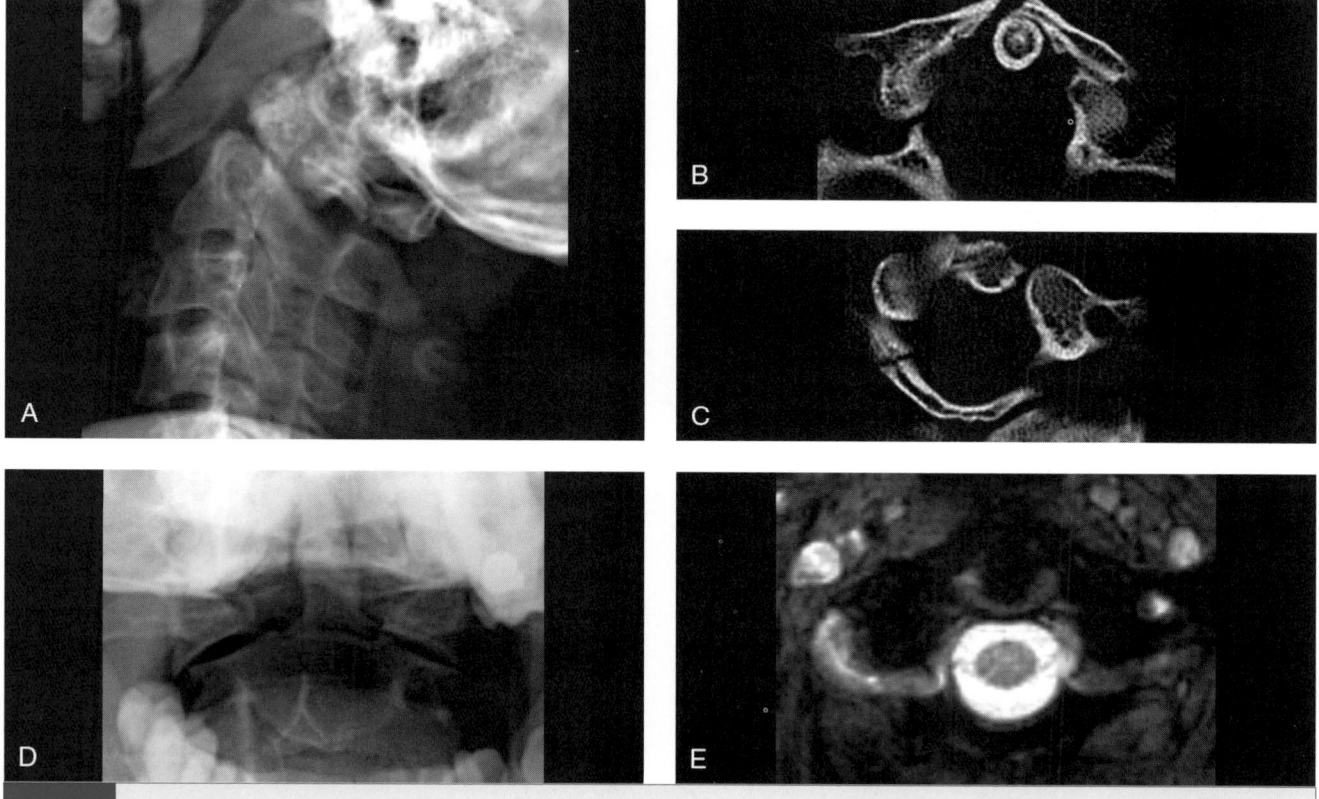

Figure 2   Imaging studies of a 48-year-old man injured during a diving accident. **A,** Three-part Jefferson burst fracture of the atlas with an associated type II odontoid fracture is shown. **B** and **C,** Serial axial CT scans demonstrate one fracture line in the anterior arch and two fracture lines in the posterior arch. **D,** Open-mouth odontoid view and **E,** axial T2-weighted MRI demonstrate an intact transverse ligament. The patient was treated with halo immobilization for the combined C1 and C2 injuries.

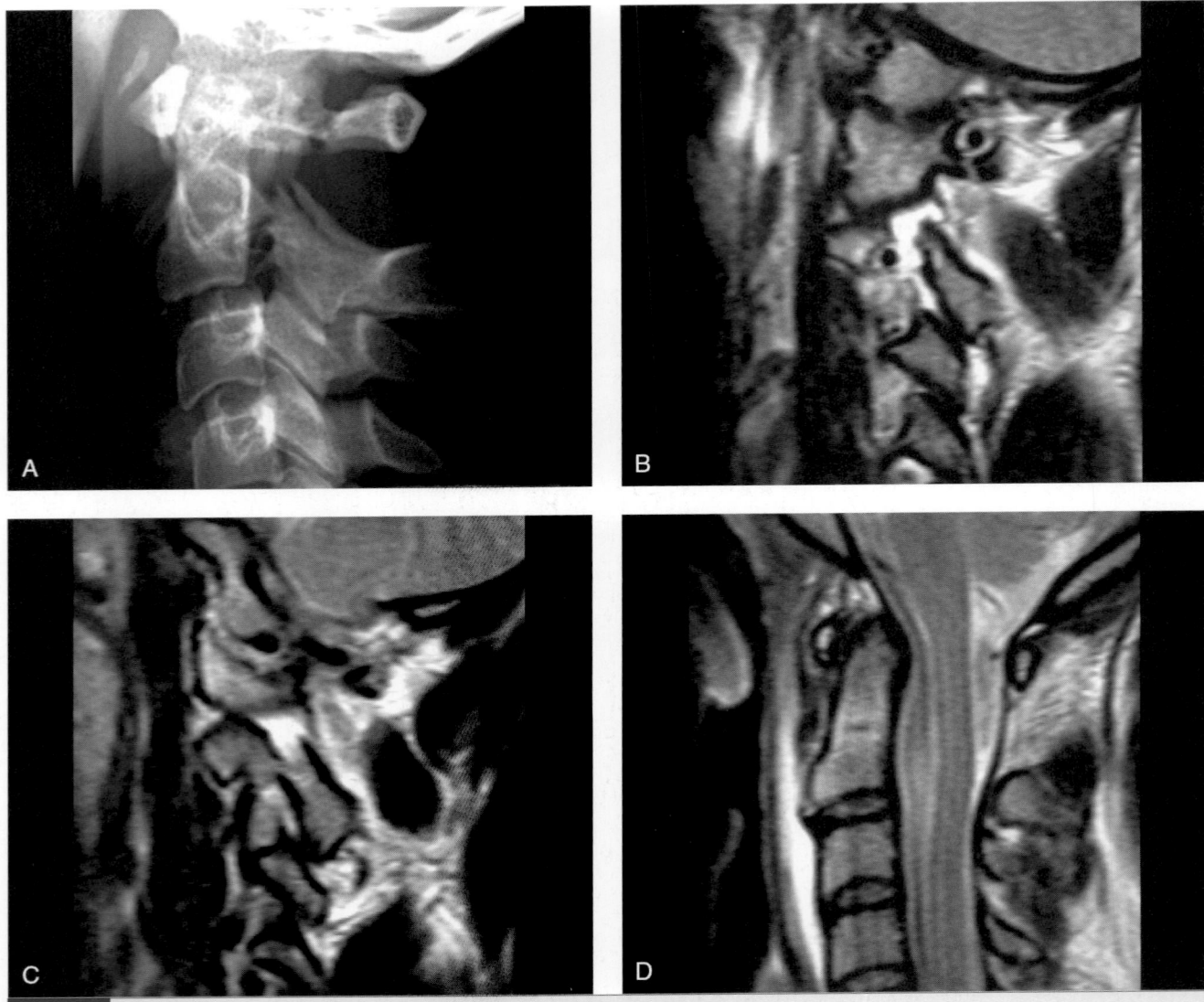

Figure 3 **A,** A 17-year-old girl sustained a type I C2 traumatic spondylolisthesis with an associated C1 posterior arch fracture in a motor vehicle collision. Left (**B**) and right (**C**) parasagittal T2-weighted images show the fractures of the pars interarticularis. **D,** Midsagittal fat-suppressed MRI demonstrates anterior soft-tissue edema and injury to the ALL. The C2-3 disk and PLL are preserved. The patient was treated with halo immobilization.

C2 Hangman's Fractures (C2 Traumatic Spondylolisthesis)

Bilateral C2 pars interarticularis fractures are commonly referred to as hangman's fractures based on the resemblance of this fracture pattern to fractures created by judicial hanging.[13] Type I fractures have less than 3 mm of C2-3 subluxation and heal reliably after 6 to 12 weeks in an orthosis (**Figure 3**).

Type II fractures have more than 3 mm of C2-3 subluxation with minimal angulation. This pattern is considered potentially unstable. Traditionally, treatment consisted of prolonged reduction traction for days to weeks, followed by 12 weeks of halo immobilization. However, because these fractures healed predictably despite moderate residual fracture displacement, short-term traction (for 1 to 3 days) or immediate halo im-

mobilization has been advocated. Successful treatment with hard collar immobilization alone has also been reported.

In contradistinction to type II fractures, type IIa fractures have C2-3 kyphotic angulation and disk space distraction without significant subluxation. This pattern is unique in that it tends to displace in traction, and therefore is reduced with gentle extension and compression. Type IIa fractures are also considered potentially unstable and are treated by immediate halo vest application.

With halo vest immobilization of type II and IIa fractures, outcome is generally good with restoration of stability after predictable healing of the pars fractures and/or C2-3 ankylosis. However, recent data from a small series suggest that persistent neck pain after bony

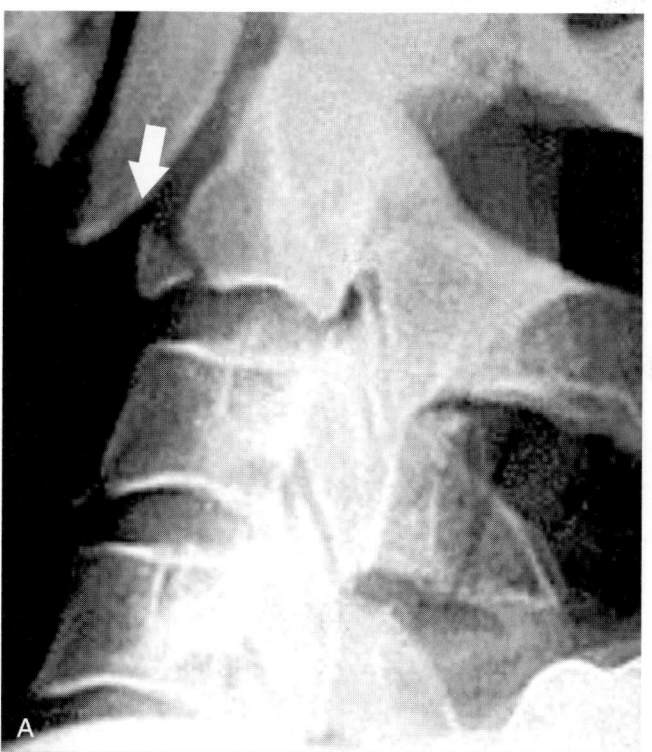 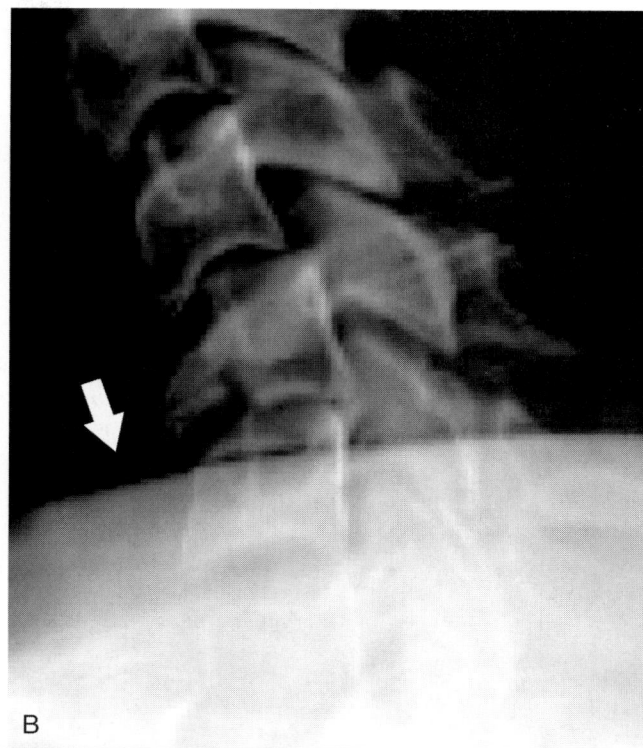

Figure 4	A, Stable avulsion fractures involving a small portion of the anterior-inferior vertebral body are called "extension teardrop" fractures (*arrow*). These should not be confused with flexion-compression (teardrop) fractures (**B**), which can be very unstable (*arrow*).

union may be related to residual kyphosis, residual translation, and fracture extension into the C2 inferior facet.[14]

In patients who cannot tolerate a halo, there is considerable debate as to which type II and IIa fractures are stable enough to be treated in an orthosis versus requiring surgical treatment. No generally accepted criteria to determine fracture instability currently exist. Surgery involves direct osteosynthesis of the C2 fracture with a lag screw through the pars interarticularis with or without posterior C2-3 fusion or anterior C2-3 fusion.[15]

The rare type III fractures are associated with C2-3 facet dislocation and are severely unstable. The C2-3 disk, ALL, PLL, and facet joints are all disrupted. The dislocation is irreducible via closed means and surgical treatment with posterior open reduction and C2-3 fusion is necessary.

C2 Avulsion (Extension Teardrop) Fracture

Avulsion fractures involving a small portion of the anterior-inferior vertebral body are often referred to as "extension teardrop" fractures (**Figure 4**). These benign fractures are caused by an extension mechanism and most commonly occur at C2 or C3. This fracture should not be confused with the subaxial flexion-compression teardrop fracture, which is very unstable and associated with devastating SCIs. Extension avul-

sion fractures are stable and can be treated with a hard collar.

Odontoid Fractures

Odontoid fractures occur from high-energy trauma in younger patients and from low-energy falls in the elderly.[16] In the elderly population, this injury is associated with an in-hospital mortality rate of 35%.

Type I odontoid fractures are avulsion fractures of the alar ligament and occur at the tip of the odontoid process. C1-2 stability is preserved because the injury occurs above the transverse ligament. Avulsion odontoid fractures are rare and, if present, concomitant occipitocervical dissociations must be ruled out. When they occur in isolation, type I odontoid fractures are treated with a hard collar.

Type II odontoid fractures are the most common type of odontoid fracture and occur at the junction of the odontoid base and the C2 body. The fracture occurs inferior to the C1 ring and does not extend caudally into the C2 superior articular facet. Closed treatment with halo vest immobilization leads to successful union in 66% of patients.[17] However, because of the high complication rates associated with halo treatment in the elderly, an orthosis or open surgical treatment should be considered in this population. Orthosis treatment alone should be undertaken with the expectation of a nonunion and is reserved for elderly patients with

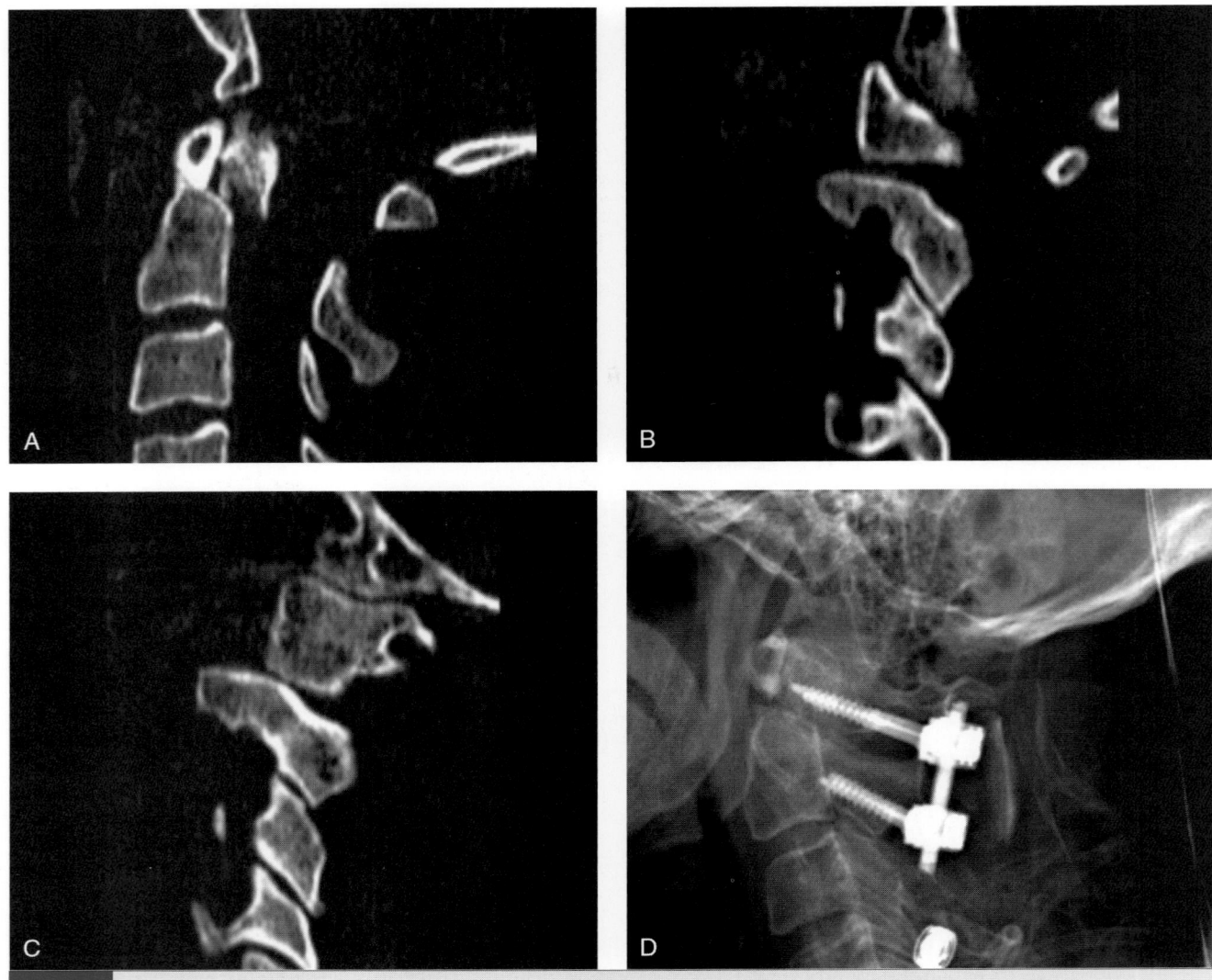

Figure 5   **A,** CT scan of a 61-year-old man who sustained a type II posteriorly displaced odontoid fracture after a fall out of a tree stand. Parasagittal CT views demonstrate the C1-2 subluxation (**B** and **C**). The patient was neurologically intact, and the fracture was irreducible via closed means. He underwent posterior C1-2 fusion and instrumentation using the Harms technique (C1 lateral mass screws and C2 isthmus screws) and structural iliac crest autograft (**D**).

low functional demand. The long-term implications of a stable or mobile nonunion are largely unknown, but likely have no effect on elderly patients.[18]

Higher rates of odontoid nonunion have also been observed in fractures with initial displacement greater than 5 mm, angulation greater than 10°, posterior displacement, and in patients older than 50 years; as a result, surgical treatment should be strongly considered. The surgical options include anterior screw fixation and posterior C1-2 fusion. Anterior screw fixation of acute odontoid fractures results in healing rates of approximately 90% and preserves C1-2 motion. However, anterior screw fixation requires near-anatomic fracture reduction, absence of significant comminution, and good bone quality; it is also contraindicated in the presence of a transverse ligament rupture and an anterior-inferior to posterior-superior fracture pattern.

Posterior C1-2 fusion provides immediate C1-2 stability but eliminates approximately 50% of cervical rotation. Posterior C1-2 fusion can be accomplished using classic wiring techniques, transarticular Magerl screws, or the Harms technique. Wiring techniques have high rates of success but require an intact C1 posterior arch and use of postoperative halo immobilization. Use of transarticular Magerl screws provides rigid fixation and is associated with high rates of success, but requires near-anatomic reduction, endangers the vertebral artery, and is technically challenging. The Harms technique provides rigid fixation, has a high rate of success, allows for open C1-2 reduction, and can be performed with minimal risk to the vertebral artery (Figure 5).

Based on these treatment considerations, subclassification of type II fractures into subtypes A, B, and C has been suggested[19] (Figure 6). Type IIA is nondisplaced and can be treated with external immobilization. Type IIB has an anterior-superior to posterior-inferior pattern and is amenable to anterior screw fixation. Type IIC has an anterior-inferior to posterior-superior pattern or is comminuted, and is best treated with posterior C1-2 fusion.

Type III odontoid fractures occur within the cancellous C2 body and extend into the C2 superior articular facet. These fractures are relatively stable and have a high rate of union after reduction and external immobilization in a halo vest. Orthosis treatment is associated with malunion and nonunion, and is recommended only for patients with minimally displaced fractures or elderly patients.

Subaxial Cervical Injuries and Treatment

Cervical Compression Fractures

Cervical compression fractures occur via compressive failure of the anterior vertebral body with preservation of the posterior body, PLL, and the posterior column. The vertebral body is wedged, but there is minimal kyphosis and no canal compromise. Patients are usually neurologically intact and, in the absence of significant deformity, can be treated in an orthosis for 6 to 12 weeks.

Cervical Burst Fractures and Compression-Flexion (Teardrop) Fractures

Cervical burst fractures occur via a primarily axial load with subsequent compressive failure of the vertebral body and bony retropulsion into the spinal canal (Figure 7). The fracture pattern is similar to burst fractures in the thoracolumbar spine. They are usually unstable and associated with SCI.

In contrast, compression-flexion (teardrop) fractures occur via an axial load with a concomitant flexion force. Compression-flexion fractures occur in varying degrees of severity.[20] The compression-flexion force creates a large triangular bony fragment off the anterior-inferior aspect of the vertebral body with tensile failure of the posterior osteoligamentous complex, kyphosis, and retrolisthesis of the remaining vertebral body into the spinal canal (Figure 8). When severe, these injuries are highly unstable and associated with a high incidence of SCI.

Treatment decision making for cervical burst and compression-flexion fractures is similar, and is primarily

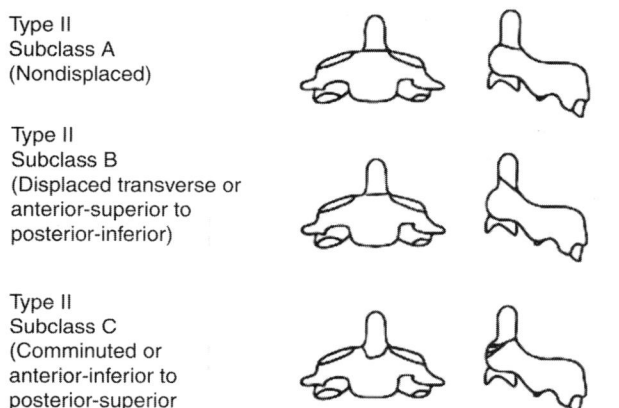

Type II
Subclass A
(Nondisplaced)

Type II
Subclass B
(Displaced transverse or anterior-superior to posterior-inferior)

Type II
Subclass C
(Comminuted or anterior-inferior to posterior-superior

Figure 6 Subclassification of type II odontoid fractures. *(Reproduced with permission from Maak TG, Grauer JN: The contemporary treatment of odontoid injuries. Spine 2006;31(11 suppl): S53-S60.)*

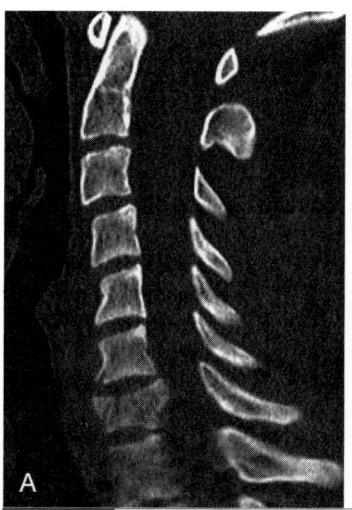 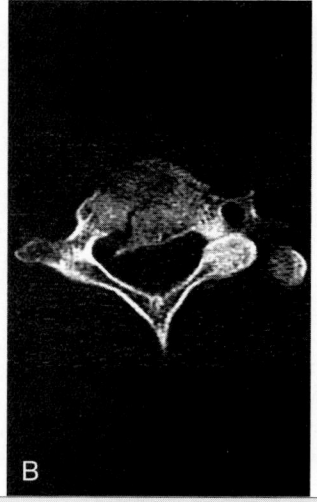 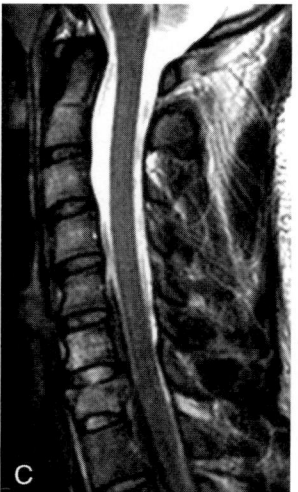 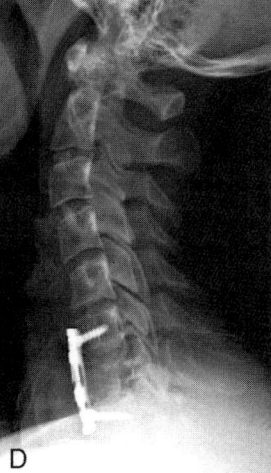

Figure 7 A 20-year-old man sustained a C7 burst fracture in a high-speed motor vehicle collision. He was neurologically intact. Midsagittal (**A**) and axial (**B**) CT scans demonstrate compressive failure of the vertebral body with bony retropulsion into the canal. MRI demonstrated no spinal cord compression (**C**). The patient was treated with C7 corpectomy and anterior fusion (**D**).

5: Spine

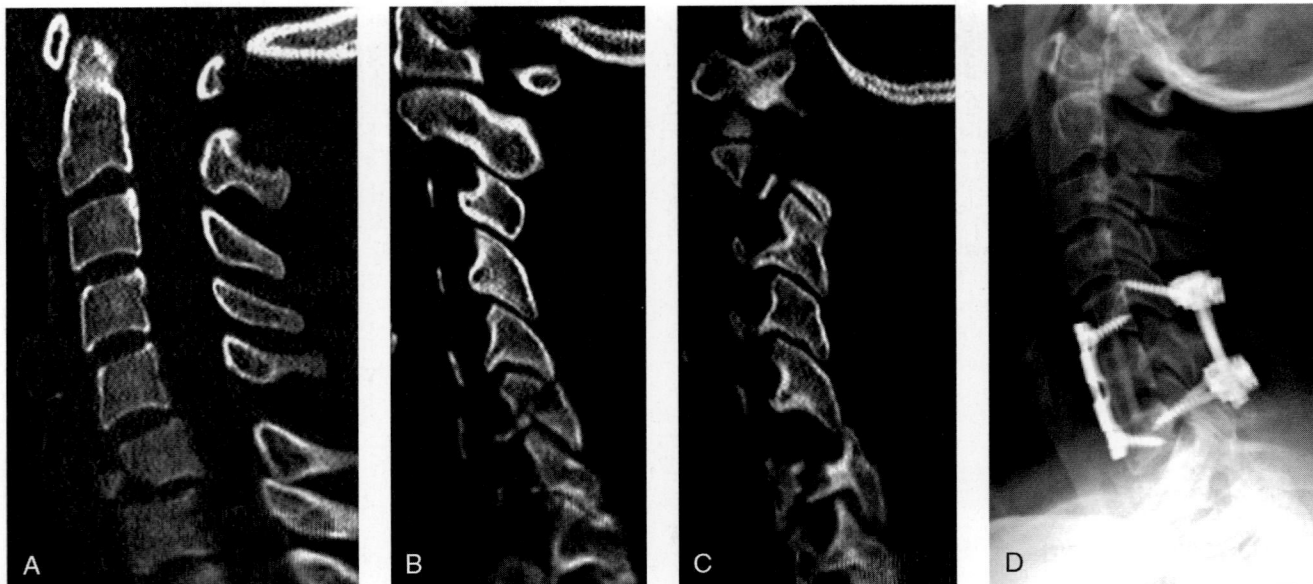

Figure 8 A 32-year-old man involved in a rollover motor vehicle collision sustained a C6 compression-flexion teardrop fracture (**A**) accompanied by a left C6 facet fracture (**B**) and right C5-6 dislocation with a C6 pedicle fracture (**C**). He had an incomplete SCI. He underwent anterior C6 corpectomy followed by posterior reduction and instrumentation using C5 lateral mass screws and C7 pedicle screws (**D**).

based on neurologic status and the estimation of mechanical stability. In the past, many of these fractures were managed nonsurgically with days to weeks of prolonged traction in an SCI bed, followed by delayed halo immobilization. Traction was required because halo vests are not capable of maintaining axial distraction. However, because of the morbidity associated with prolonged bed rest and the advent of modern instrumentation techniques, these methods have become largely obsolete. In fractures associated with neurologic injury, instability is inferred and surgical treatment is generally recommended. In the neurologically intact patient, treatment decisions are based solely on the estimation of mechanical stability. Unfortunately, there are currently no universally accepted criteria to determine mechanical stability. The degree of kyphosis, amount of vertebral body height loss, severity of posterior osteoligamentous injury, and amount of anticipated patient loading all contribute to the estimation of mechanical instability. Fractures deemed stable are treated with an orthosis or halo vest, with or without an attempt at reduction with short-term traction. Current surgical treatment of unstable burst and unstable compression-flexion fractures generally involves anterior corpectomy, structural grafting, and rigid plate fixation with possible posterior stabilization. Supplemental posterior stabilization should be strongly considered in patients with osteopenia and in fractures associated with frank disruption of the posterior osteoligamentous complex.

Facet Dislocations

Facet dislocations are the result of a high-energy flexion-distraction force. They represent a broad spectrum of bony and soft-tissue injury, ranging from subluxation to dislocation, with involvement of one or both facet joints, and with or without fractures. Unilateral dislocations are associated with 25% vertebral subluxation and unilateral radiculopathy. Bilateral dislocations are associated with 50% vertebral subluxation and SCI.

Treatment of facet dislocations has remained controversial. The initial step in management is consideration for closed reduction using cranial tong traction. Closed reduction is effective and safe, but should only be attempted in alert and cooperative patients. Imaging studies should be carefully reviewed to rule out a noncontiguous injury cephalad to the level of dislocation. An initial 10 to 15 lb of weight is applied and sequentially increased in 5- to 10-lb increments. A neurologic examination is performed and radiographs are obtained after each incremental weight increase to ensure that the patient's neurologic status is stable and that the level of injury is not overdistracted. Although safe closed reduction has been reported with weights up to 150 lb, reduction is usually achieved after 40 to 70 lb. The decision to apply more weight depends on surgeon comfort and experience.

The main area of controversy in the treatment of facet dislocations pertains to whether MRI is required before closed reduction. The primary advantage of rapid closed reduction without MRI is that it allows immediate indirect decompression of the spinal cord to maximize neurologic recovery. This advantage is amplified in patients who are seen within 4 hours after injury and at institutions where MRI requires more time. The major disadvantage of rapid closed reduction without MRI is the potential for an unrecognized disk herniation to cause neurologic deterioration. A significant disk herniation has the potential to be forced posteriorly into the spinal canal during reduction, causing further compression of the spinal cord. Because of this concern, MRI before closed reduction is considered. If a significant disk herniation is found, closed reduction can be avoided and an anterior diskectomy can be performed before reduction. However, prereduction MRI usually can demonstrate variable degrees of disk injury, bulge, hematoma, and/or herniation. The clinical significance of these prereduction MRI findings is unknown. No generally accepted criteria exist for a "significant disk herniation" that has the potential to cause neurologic deterioration.[21] There is also no correlation between the presence of prereduction or postreduction disk herniations and the occurrence of neurologic deterioration. A recent study of MRI-guided closed reductions demonstrated that traction reduction leads to progressive return of herniated disk material into the intervertebral space, with subsequent improvement in canal dimensions.[22]

The prereduction MRI scan, therefore, provides imperfect and equivocal information that has the potential to cause patient morbidity. MRI evidence of a herniated disk may unnecessarily compel the surgeon to perform a three-stage procedure: anterior diskectomy, followed by posterior reduction and fusion, and return anteriorly for fusion. With a successful closed reduction, the surgeon usually only needs to perform one procedure, either anteriorly or posteriorly.

With these concerns and the available clinical evidence in mind, immediate closed reduction in awake and alert patients with complete motor and sensory loss is recommended. For patients who are neurologically intact or have an incomplete SCI, treatment depends on surgeon preferences and individual injury characteristics. For incomplete SCIs in alert patients seen within 4 hours of injury, strong consideration should be given to perform rapid closed reduction without MRI. For patients who are neurologically intact or have radiculopathy alone, strong consideration should be given to prereduction MRI (Figure 9).

In general, closed reductions in the awake patient are preferred over open reductions under anesthesia. The ability to perform frequent neurologic examinations in the awake patient is superior to any currently available neurophysiologic monitoring methods. Neurologic deterioration has also been reported more commonly after open reductions under general anesthesia in comparison with closed reductions in awake patients.[23] In addition, once the fracture has been reduced and immobilized, the definitive surgical treatment can be performed in a semielective controlled setting rather than on an urgent basis. MRI can be done after successful closed reduction to direct definitive surgical treatment. The presence of a postreduction compressive disk herniation necessitates an anterior decompression and fusion, with or without supplemental posterior stabilization.

If open reduction is required, preoperative MRI is necessary. If there is no disk herniation, posterior re-

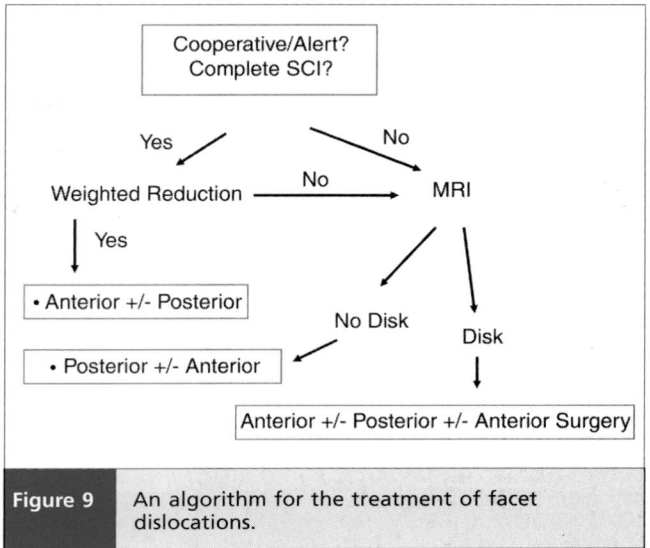

Figure 9 An algorithm for the treatment of facet dislocations.

duction and stabilization can be used; posterior reduction requires less force and is more reliably successful than anterior reduction. MRI scans can be obtained after posterior open reductions to determine if a supplemental anterior decompression is required (Figure 10). If, however, the preoperative MRI scan demonstrates disk material protruding posterior to the subadjacent vertebral body, an anterior approach is first required to evacuate the disk, followed by a gentle attempt at anterior reduction using Caspar pins and/or traction. If anterior reduction is successful, the injury is stabilized anteriorly and supplemental posterior instrumentation can be added as needed. If anterior reduction is unsuccessful, the patient is positioned prone for posterior reduction and posterior stabilization, followed by return to the supine position for anterior stabilization. All surgical reductions are performed using neurophysiologic monitoring.

Facet Fractures
Facet fractures are common and easily missed on plain radiography. The superior facet is involved in 80% of affected patients. Inferior facet fractures tend to begin at the base of the lamina and are associated with laminar fractures. Most facet fractures are unilateral, small, nondisplaced, and without subluxation. Fractures without significant subluxation or kyphosis can usually be successfully treated with an orthosis for 6 to 12 weeks. Unilateral facet fractures with more than 40% of the height of the lateral mass involved or with associated injuries to the discoligamentous complex seen on MRI scans may be unstable and predict failure of nonsurgical treatment.[24] Bilateral fractures are also associated with shear injuries across the disk and may be unstable.

Unlike most facet fractures, the floating lateral mass fracture is highly unstable and warrants special consideration. The lamina and ipsilateral pedicle of the same segment are fractured, leading to a free-floating lateral

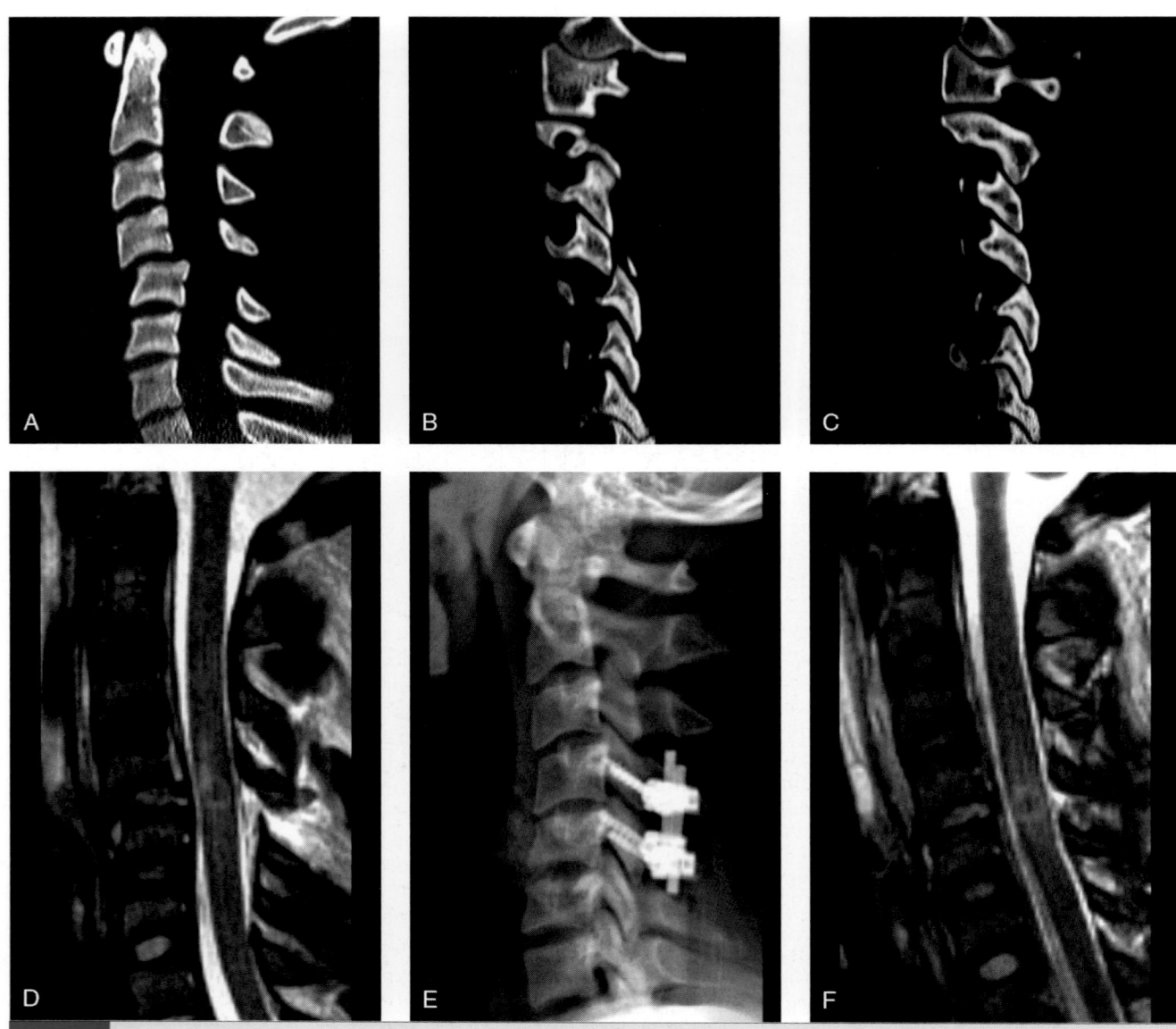

Figure 10 **A** through **C**, CT scans of a 19-year-old man with a left C4-5 facet fracture-dislocation and right C4-5 facet subluxation from a fall from 15 feet. He had an incomplete SCI. After an emergent laparotomy, he was taken directly from the operating room to the MRI suite. MRI revealed a small disk bulge and spinal cord contusion (**D**). He returned immediately to the operating room and underwent posterior open reduction and stabilization (**E**). **F**, MRI performed immediately after surgery revealed reduction of the disk herniation and indirect spinal cord decompression.

mass (Figure 11). This fracture is also commonly referred to as a lateral mass dissociation or fracture-separation. Traumatic radiculopathy is common. In 80% of patients, the floating lateral mass is associated with subluxation at the caudal interspace (for example, a C6 floating lateral mass with a C6-7 subluxation). This fracture pattern was originally described as a two-level injury with need for a two-level stabilization.[25] However, when the soft-tissue injury demonstrated on MRI scan is clearly at one level with preservation of the adjacent level, a single-level stabilization is adequate[26] (Figure 11).

Distraction-Extension Injuries (Diffuse Idiopathic Skeletal Hyperostosis/Ankylosing Spondylitis)

Distraction-extension injuries are associated with ankylosing conditions of the spine such as ankylosing spondylitis, diffuse idiopathic skeletal hyperostosis (or Forestier's disease), and multilevel ankylosed spondylosis in elderly patients. The stabilizing ligaments of the spine are ossified and fracture leads to complete structural compromise despite minimal displacement. The fused cervical spine behaves more like a long bone when fractured and severe instability results because of

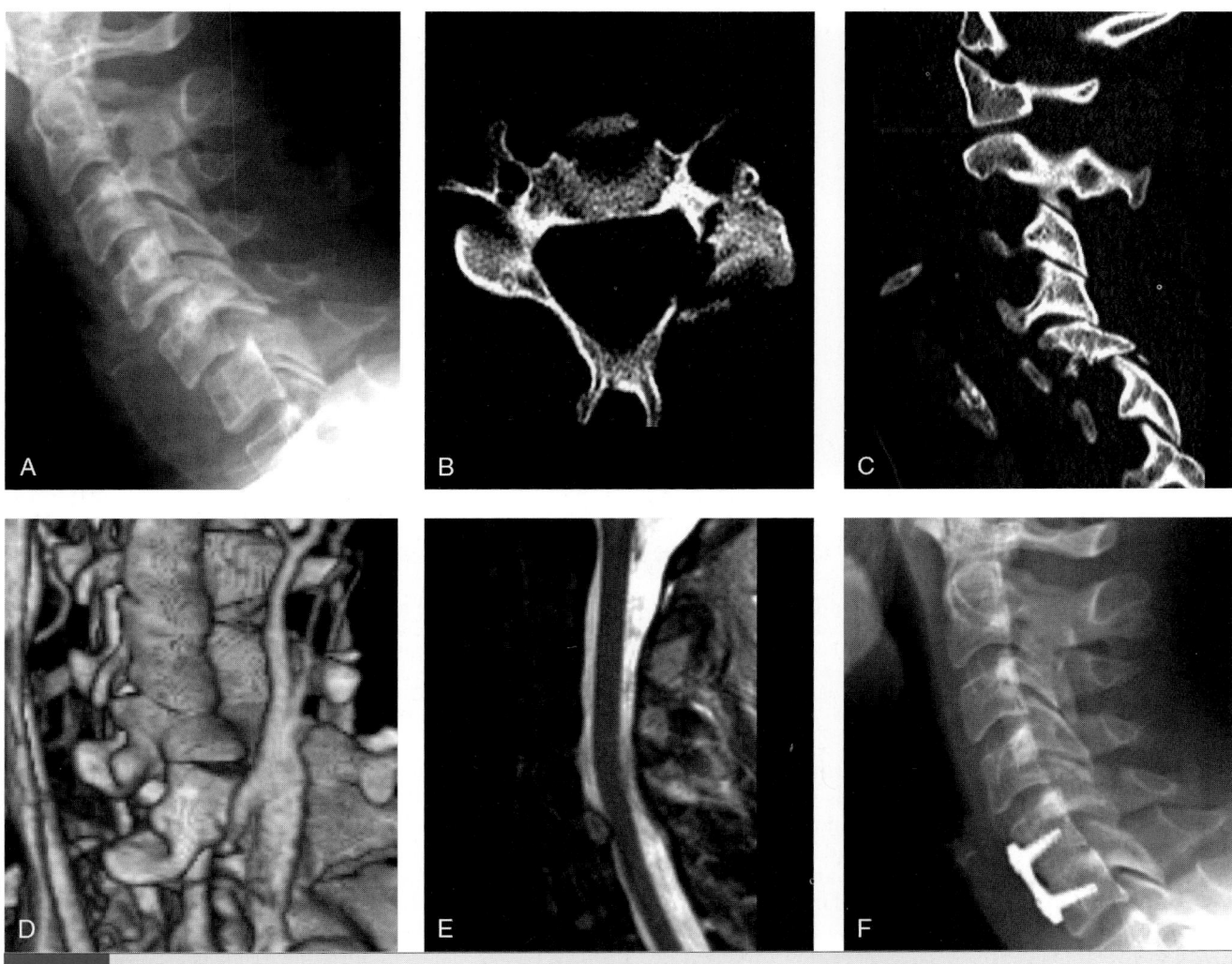

Figure 11 Imaging studies of a 25-year-old man with a left C5 floating lateral mass fracture, C5-6 anterolisthesis (**A**), and left C6 radiculopathy. Axial (**B**), parasagittal (**C**), and three-dimensional reconstruction (**D**) CT views reveal the C5 ipsilateral pedicle and lamina fracture with a malrotated lateral mass. MRI revealed no injury to the C4-5 disk (**E**). **F,** The patient underwent anterior C5-6 diskectomy and fusion.

the long lever arms adjacent to the injury. These injuries occur most commonly at the cervicothoracic junction. They are frequently missed because they occur via low-energy falls and radiographs are often inadequate or benign-appearing because of osteopenia. When the diagnosis is missed, attempts at mobilizing the patient without proper immobilization can lead to devastating neurologic deterioration. In addition, patients with inflammatory ankylosing conditions are prone to bony bleeding, and neurologic deterioration can result from a compressive epidural hematoma.

Imaging and immobilization of patients with ankylosing conditions of the spine should be aggressive after even minor trauma with minor neck pain. Plain radiographs alone are inadequate; CT and/or MRI are required. Imaging of the entire spine should be done because noncontiguous injuries are also common. Once the condition is recognized, the patient should be ag-

gressively immobilized. Cervical traction should be avoided. Surgical treatment is recommended for most patients in whom it can be tolerated.[27] Extreme care should be used during positioning to prevent iatrogenic fractures and to account for any preexisting kyphosis. A posterior approach is usually preferred for reduction and stabilization (**Figure 12**). Instrumentation is extended to multiple levels above and below the injury to counteract long lever arms and compensate for poor bone quality. Supplemental anterior instrumentation is also often required.

Summary

Because the cervical spine is susceptible to a broad spectrum of bony, soft-tissue, and neurologic injury patterns, a high index of suspicion should be main-

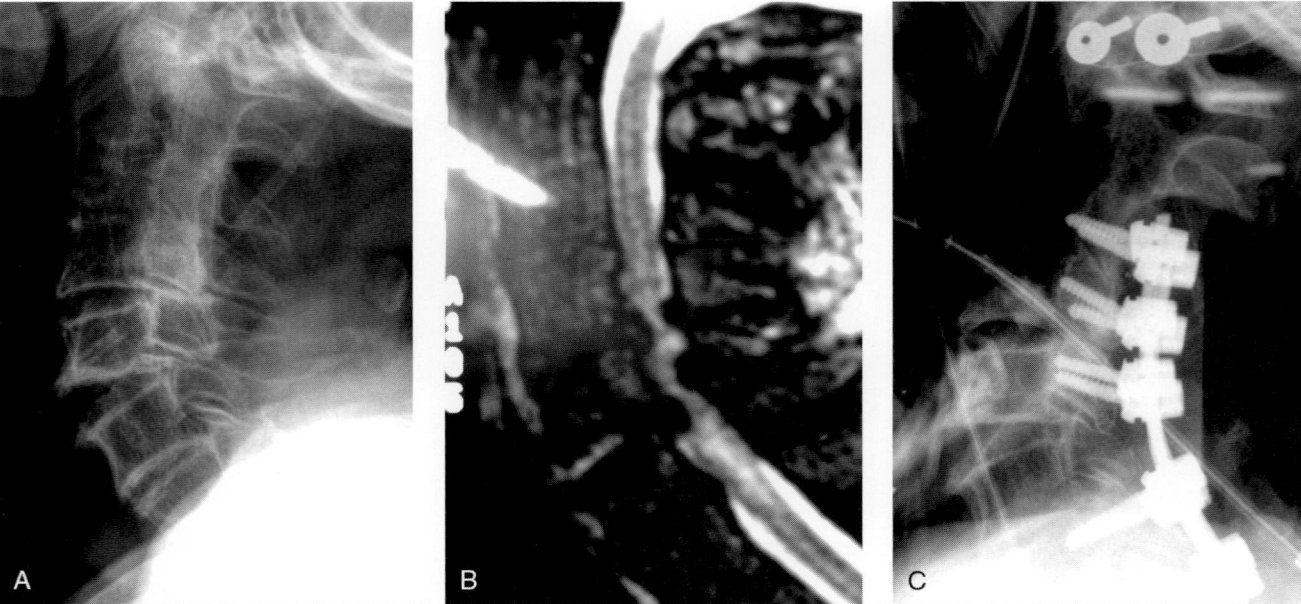

Figure 12   A 75-year-old man with no prior known history of ankylosing spondylitis had a complete SCI from a fall from a standing position. **A,** Plain radiograph revealed a distraction-extension injury at C5-6. **B,** Fat-suppressed sagittal MRI revealed anterior soft-tissue swelling, high signal through the C5-6 disk, and spinal cord compression at C4-5 and C5-6. The patient underwent posterior stabilization from C3 to T1, using lateral mass screws at C3-5 and pedicle screws at C7 and T1. **C,** After stabilization, a laminectomy from C3 to C6 was performed.

tained in patients with high-energy trauma, particularly if a thorough physical examination is prohibited by altered mental status. Advanced imaging studies can help estimate mechanical stability and guide treatment. Contemporary instrumentation systems and techniques allow for rigid stabilization and avoidance of prolonged bed rest.

Annotated References

1. Fisher CG, Noonan VK, Smith DE, Wing PC, Dvorak MF, Kwon BK: Motor recovery, functional status, and health-related quality of life in patients with complete spinal cord injuries. *Spine* 2005;30:2200-2207.

   A retrospective review of 70 patients with truly complete SCIs demonstrated that motor recovery does not occur below the zone of injury.

2. Oleson CV, Burns AS, Ditunno JF, Geisler FH, Coleman WP: Prognostic value of pinprick preservation in motor complete, sensory incomplete spinal cord injury. *Arch Phys Med Rehabil* 2005;86:988-992.

   A multicenter retrospective review of 131 patients with motor complete/sensory incomplete SCI demonstrated an improved prognosis for ambulation in patients with preserved baseline lower extremity or sacral pin-prick sensation.

3. Stiell IG, Wells GA, Vandemheen KL, et al: The Canadian C-spine rule for radiography in alert and stable trauma patients. *JAMA* 2001;286:1841-1848.

4. Stiell IG, Clement CM, McKnigh RD, et al: The Canadian C-spine rule versus the NEXUS low-risk criteria in patients with trauma. *N Engl J Med* 2003;349:2510-2518.

5. Majercik S, Tashjian RZ, Biffl WL, Harrington DT, Cioffi WG: Halo vest immobilization in the elderly: A death sentence? *J Trauma* 2005;59:350-356.

   A trauma registry-based retrospective review of more than 400 patients showed a 40% mortality rate in patients older than 65 years who were treated with halo vest immobilization for a cervical spine fracture.

6. Anderson PA, Montesano PX: Morphology and treatment of occipital condyle fractures. *Spine* 1988;13:731-736.

7. Hanson JA, Deliganis AV, Baxter AB, et al: Radiologic and clinical spectrum of occipital condyle fractures: Retrospective review of 107 consecutive fractures in 95 patients. *AJR Am J Roentgenol* 2002;178:1261-1268.

8. Bellabarba C, Mirza SK, West GA, et al: Diagnosis and treatment of craniocervical dislocation in a series of 17 consecutive survivors during an 8-year period. *J Neurosurg Spine* 2006;4:429-440.

   A retrospective review of 17 patients with craniocervical dissociation revealed that an average 2-day delay in diagnosis was associated with profound neurologic deterioration in nearly one third of patients. At average 2-year follow-up, 76% of the patients had useful motor function in the extremities.

9. Traynelis VC, Marano GD, Dunker RO, Kaufman HH: Traumatic atlanto-occipital dislocation: Case report. *J Neurosurg* 1986;65:863-870.

10. Vaccaro AR, Lim MR, Lee JY: Indications for surgery and stabilization techniques of the occipito-cervical junction. *Injury* 2005;36(suppl 2):B44-B53.

    The authors provide a review of the historical evolution of occipitocervical stabilization with a discussion of contemporary techniques and instrumentation systems.

11. Levine AM, Edwards CC: Fractures of the atlas. *J Bone Joint Surg Am* 1991;73:680-691.

12. Kontautas E, Ambrozaitis KV, Kalesinskas RJ, Spakauskas B: Management of acute traumatic atlas fractures. *J Spinal Disord Tech* 2005;18:402-405.

    This article presents a prospective review of 29 patients with atlas fractures. Isolated nondisplaced C1 fractures or nondisplaced C1 fractures combined with nondisplaced C2 fractures were treated with a rigid cervical collar alone. Isolated displaced C1 fractures or nondisplaced C1 fractures with accompanying displaced C2 fractures were immobilized with a halo vest. Solid fusion was achieved in 96% of the patients.

13. Levine AM, Edwards CC: The management of traumatic spondylolisthesis of the axis. *J Bone Joint Surg Am* 1985;67:217-226.

14. Watanabe M, Nomura T, Toh E, Sato M, Mochida J: Residual neck pain after traumatic spondylolisthesis of the axis. *J Spinal Disord Tech* 2005;18:148-151.

    Radiographic analysis and telephone interviews were conducted in a small series of nine patients treated nonsurgically for C2 traumatic spondylolisthesis. The authors suggested that persistent neck pain after bony union may be related to residual kyphosis, residual translation, and fracture extension into the C2 inferior facet.

15. Bristol R, Henn JS, Dickman CA: Pars screw fixation of a hangman's fracture: Technical case report. *Neurosurgery* 2005;56:E204.

    This article provides a technical description of direct C2 osteosynthesis via lag screw across the pars interarticularis.

16. Anderson LD, D'Alonzo RT: Fractures of the odontoid process of the axis. *J Bone Joint Surg Am* 1974;56:1663-1674.

17. Clark CR, White AA III : Fractures of the dens: A multicenter study. *J Bone Joint Surg Am* 1985;67:1340-1348.

18. Hart R, Saterbak A, Rapp T, Clark C: Nonoperative management of dens fracture nonunion in elderly patients without myelopathy. *Spine* 2000;25:1339-1343.

19. Grauer JN, Shafi B, Hilibrand AS, et al: Proposal of a modified, treatment-oriented classification of odontoid fractures. *Spine J* 2005;5:123-129.

    Moderate interobserver agreement was found for a contemporary treatment-oriented subclassification system for type II odontoid fractures.

20. Allen BL Jr, Ferguson RL, Lehmann TR, O'Brien RP: A mechanistic classification of closed, indirect fractures and dislocations of the lower cervical spine. *Spine* 1982;7:1-27.

21. Vaccaro AR, Falatyn SP, Flanders AE, Balderston RA, Northrup BE, Cotler JM: Magnetic resonance evaluation of the intervertebral disc, spinal ligaments, and spinal cord before and after closed traction reduction of cervical spine dislocations. *Spine* 1999;24:1210-1217.

22. Darsaut TE, Ashforth R, Bhargava R, et al: A pilot study of magnetic resonance imaging-guided closed reduction of cervical spine fractures. *Spine* 2006;31:2085-2090.

    The authors report a prospective study of 17 patients with facet dislocations who underwent closed reduction using serial MRI guidance. Pretraction MRI showed disk disruption in 88% of patients and posterior herniation in 24%. Traction led to the return of herniated disk material toward the disk space in all patients. The process of reduction was gradual, with progressive improvement in canal dimensions occurring before achieving anatomic realignment.

23. Initial closed reduction of cervical spine fracture-dislocation injuries. *Neurosurgery* 2002;50(3 suppl):S44-S50.

24. Spector LR, Kim DH, Affonso J, Albert TJ, Hilibrand AS, Vaccaro AR: Use of computed tomography to predict failure of nonoperative treatment of unilateral facet fractures of the cervical spine. *Spine* 2006;31:2827-2835.

    This retrospective review of 24 patients with unilateral facet fractures showed that fractures involving greater than 40% of the absolute height of the intact lateral mass or an absolute height greater than 1 cm are at increased risk for failure of nonsurgical treatment.

25. Levine AM, Mazel C, Roy-Camille R: Management of fracture separations of the articular mass using posterior cervical plating. *Spine* 1992;17:S447-S454.

26. Kotani Y, Abumi K, Ito M, Minami A: Cervical spine injuries associated with lateral mass and facet joint fractures: New classification and surgical treatment with pedicle screw fixation. *Eur Spine J* 2005;14:69-77.

    In this retrospective review, 31 patients with lateral mass fractures were classified into four types: separation, comminution, split, and traumatic spondylolysis. In the separation type (floating lateral mass), a single-level posterior fusion using pedicle screw fixation was successfully performed in half the patients. More comminuted patterns required two-level fusion. The split and traumatic spondylolysis patterns all required two-level fusion.

27. Einsiedel T, Schmelz A, Arand M, et al: Injuries of the cervical spine in patients with ankylosing spondylitis:

5: Spine

Experience at two trauma centers. *J Neurosurg Spine* 2006;5:33-45.

This retrospective review reported on 37 patients with ankylosing spondylitis treated surgically for cervical fractures over a 15-year period. Patients with a delayed diagnosis had greater neurologic deficits and had less postoperative improvement. There was a 50% failure rate of anterior-alone stabilization.

Chapter 47

Thoracolumbar Trauma

Ravi K. Ponnappan, MD   Joon Y. Lee, MD

Introduction

Although the worldwide incidence of spine fractures (estimated to be between 9 and 22 cases per 1,000 people annually) has remained stable, the mechanisms of injury and the patient demographics have shown subtle changes. Fractures involving the thoracolumbar spine occur in approximately 6% of patients experiencing blunt trauma, with most occurring at the thoracolumbar junction (T12-L1). Bimodal distribution of thoracolumbar fractures is associated with patient age and the amount of energy required to produce the injury. High-energy mechanisms typically affect a younger patient population and include motor vehicle collisions, falls from heights, sports participation, and, more recently, thrill-seeking activities. Approximately 15% of thoracolumbar fractures are associated with concomitant spine injuries at other noncontiguous levels, reflecting the severity of trauma required to produce them. Low-energy injuries, such as a fall from the standing position, occur in older patients with osteoporosis. As the median age of the general population continues to increase, osteoporotic vertebral compression fractures (VCFs) have become an expanding clinical problem.[1] Although approximately 25% of patients with VCFs present clinically with significant pain, most can be adequately managed with nonsurgical measures.[2] Treatment of high-energy injuries and VCFs differs based on the mechanism of injury, fracture pattern, concomitant soft-tissue injury, and bone quality.

Anatomic Considerations

Anatomic characteristics unique to the thoracic and lumbar spine may influence the pattern of injury resulting from trauma. The thoracic spine is relatively rigid and has 20° to 50° (an average of 35°) of kyphosis. Coronally oriented facet joints allow torsional and lateral bending movements with minimal flexion or extension motion. In addition, each thoracic vertebra is further stabilized by its costovertebral articulations, which are anchored anteriorly to the sternum. The diameter of the osseous midthoracic spinal canal is relatively narrow with minimal tolerance to accommodate canal disruption or intrusion.

Normal lumbar lordosis is in the range of 30° to 50° (an average of 40°) and occurs primarily between L4 and S1. Flexion and extension constitute the primary motion of the lumbar spine and occur through the sagittally oriented facet joints. The thoracolumbar junction is localized to the T11-L2 spinal levels and represents the transition zone between a rigid thoracic spine and a mobile lumbar spine. In addition, the weight-bearing axis shifts from kyphosis to lordosis at the T12-L1 intervertebral disk.

The adult spinal cord typically extends from the foramen magnum to the L1 vertebral body level and is at risk for injury at any of these levels. One anterior spinal artery and two posterior spinal arteries perfuse the thoracic spinal cord. Both the anterior and posterior spinal arteries receive their supply in a segmental fashion from the radicular arteries, which originate from the posterior intercostal arteries. It is postulated that in 10% to 16% of patients, there is a dominant anterior radicular artery (artery of Adamkiewicz) originating from one of the left T8-L2 intercostal arteries. This may provide a major portion of the vascular supply to the anterior thoracolumbar spinal cord.

Injury Assessment

Field

Treatment of thoracolumbar fractures, as with all spinal injuries, begins with recognition and assessment. The systematic universal approach to all trauma patients as dictated by the Basic Life Support and Advanced Trauma Life Support guidelines should be instituted. Primary responders in the field should secure the airway, ensure respiration with supplemental oxygen, and support circulation. Bradycardia associated with hypotension in the trauma setting is indicative of neurogenic shock and is often associated with concomitant spinal cord injury (SCI). Patients experiencing neurogenic shock may exhibit circulatory collapse secondary to loss of sympathetic tone resulting from the SCI. Precautionary immobilization using in-line manual traction, a hard cervical collar, and a rigid backboard are mandatory before transportation. Field assessments of injury mechanism, energy, and gross neurologic status are critical to initiating the appropriate algorithm of care. Transportation to the nearest facility with the resources to treat acute trauma and spine injury should be facilitated as soon as possible. Optimal outcomes are achieved with a multidisciplinary team approach.

5: Spine

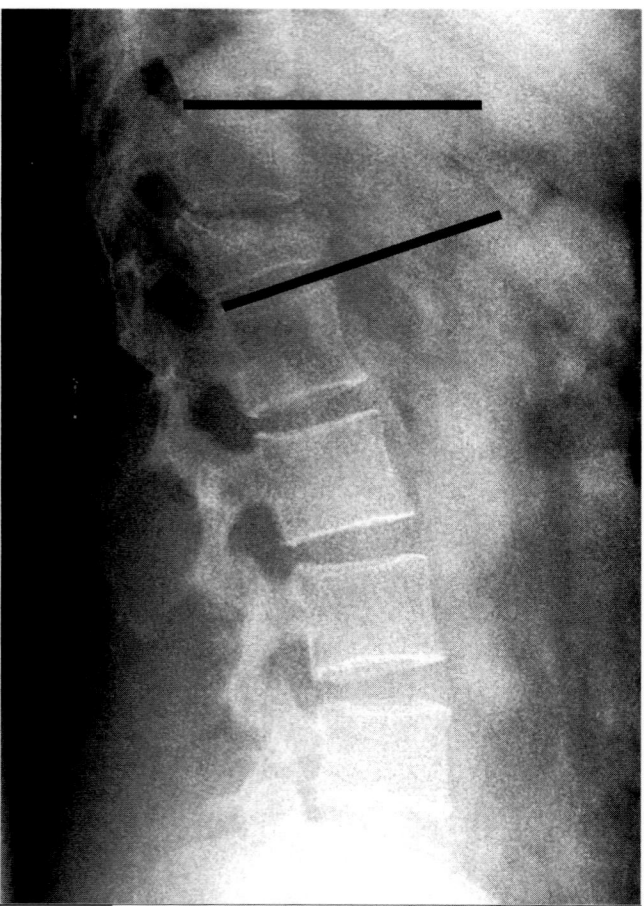

Figure 1	The sagittal alignment of the thoracolumbar junction can be assessed using the Cobb method. Tangential lines to the end plates of the adjacent noninjured levels are drawn and the angle between them is measured (black lines). Alternatively, the anterior and posterior vertebral body height can be measured at the injured level and compared with that of the adjacent noninjured level.

Physical Examination

Initial evaluation of patients with thoracolumbar fractures should include a detailed assessment of neurologic function. A thorough neurologic examination should include motor, sensory, reflex, and rectal examinations and is usually quantified using either the Frankel Impairment Scale or the American Spinal Injury Association (ASIA) form. These tools help to monitor patient progress, standardize care, and evaluate outcomes. The initial ASIA scale score has been shown to be a reliable predictor of long-term outcome in patients with cervical or thoracic SCI. In the patient with incomplete SCI, sacral nerve root sparing (detected by a normal sacral sensation or rectal examination) has been shown to be a positive prognostic factor for potential SCI recovery.

Documentation of the spine examination should include the status of the overlying skin and soft tissues. Spinal levels corresponding to the areas of tenderness and palpable step-offs should be noted. It has been reported that persistent localized tenderness after trauma to the thoracolumbar spine without obvious radiographic findings is indicative of underlying occult spinal fracture in 30% of patients. In the multiply injured patient, an altered level of consciousness or head trauma should prompt more detailed spine examination. Concomitant patterns of injury such as multiple rib fracture, pulmonary contusion, abdominal bruising, visceral injury, and bilateral calcaneus fractures may indicate occult thoracic or lumbar spine trauma. Associated spinal injuries are missed on initial examination in 50% of patients, and delays in diagnosis can lead to potential and preventable neurologic deterioration.

Imaging Evaluation
Standard radiographs of the thoracic or lumbar spine should include orthogonal AP and lateral views. Traditionally, advanced imaging modalities such as MRI or CT were reserved to detail injury morphology *after* screening plain films. Recent trauma literature, however, has questioned the economic and diagnostic value of screening radiographs, citing the delays in care and diagnostic inaccuracy from poor quality films and multiple film attempts.[3] Current imaging technology allows for rapid screening helical CT scans of the head, thorax, abdomen, and pelvis (usually obtained as part of the routine trauma evaluation), which can then be reformatted to evaluate the entire spine. Studies have shown increased sensitivity, specificity, and predictive value of CT in detecting spinal injury compared with traditional radiography.[3,4] In addition, CT scans are particularly useful in evaluating areas difficult to visualize with standard radiographs (for example, cervicothoracic junction and fractures in obese patients). Axial imaging with coronal and sagittal reconstructions allows for quantification of canal encroachment as well as assessment of sagittal and coronal alignment.

Plain Radiographic Evaluation
Sagittal alignment can be quickly screened on the lateral view. When making an assessment of the sagittal alignment with initial trauma radiographs, the physician should be aware that screening films are usually taken with the patient in the supine position. Often, the alignment will worsen when weight-bearing radiographs are taken. At the thoracolumbar junction, the sagittal alignment is normally neutral. Any kyphotic alignment at the thoracolumbar junction can be quantified using the Cobb method (Figure 1), which involves measuring the angle between the superior end plate of the nearest uninjured cranial vertebra and the inferior end plate of the nearest uninjured caudal vertebra. Vertebral body height loss can also be used to quantify the amount of injury. Anterior and posterior vertebral body height is measured at the injured and uninjured level, and the loss of height is expressed in percentage. Anterior loss of height greater than 50% may be suggestive of a more significant posterior ligamentous complex (PLC) injury.

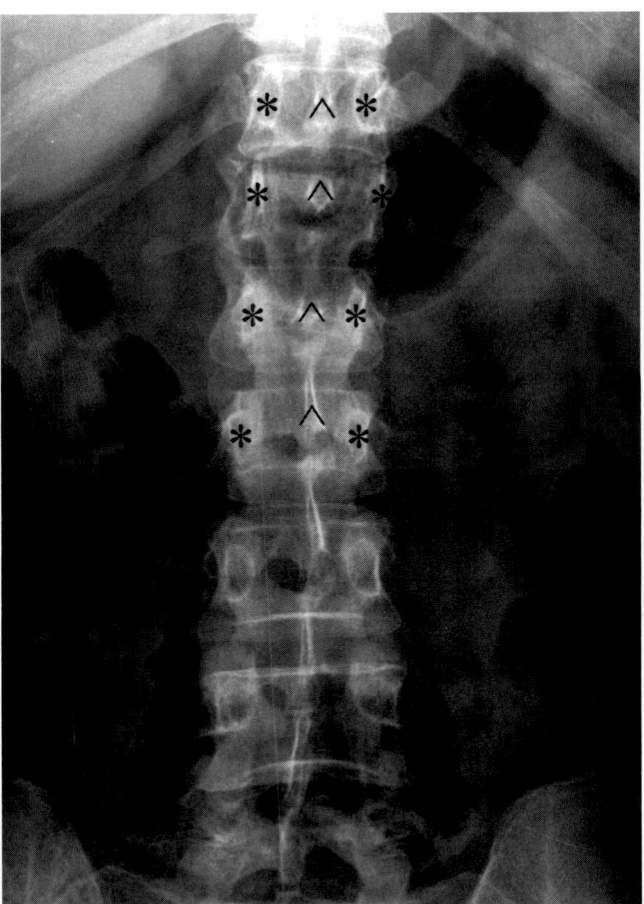

Figure 2 The AP plain radiograph should be scrutinized for the interpedicular distance (*) and the alignment of the spinous processes (^). If the interpedicular distance is abnormally widened, an axial compression mechanism should be suspected, and a burst-type injury may be present. If the interspinous process is abnormally widened, a flexion component to the injury may also be present.

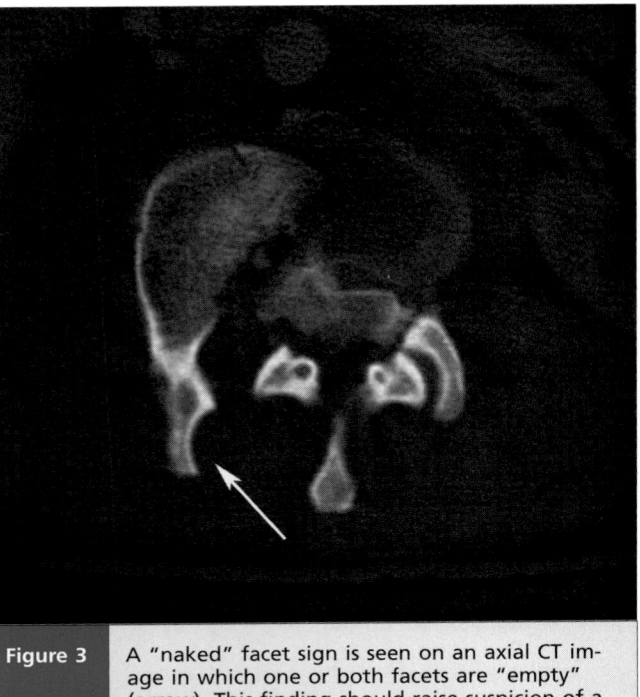

Figure 3 A "naked" facet sign is seen on an axial CT image in which one or both facets are "empty" (*arrow*). This finding should raise suspicion of a facet dislocation.

The AP view is useful to assess coronal alignment (Figure 2). Each spinous process should align with the corresponding cephalad and caudad levels. If the distance between spinous processes is increased, a flexion-type injury should be suspected. If a spinous process is misaligned to one side, a rotational type of injury should be suspected. Interpedicular distance at each level should also be scrutinized because acute increase in interpedicular distance may indicate a burst fracture. The presence of focal scoliosis may also indicate a more unstable injury.

CT Evaluation

As noted, rapid helical CT may ultimately replace initial screening plain radiography in the trauma setting. Once an injury is detected, a more detailed thin-cut (2-mm) image can be obtained at the level of the injury.

CT is particularly useful for evaluation of the spinal canal, posterior facets, and the integrity of the vertebral body. Canal encroachment can be quantified with either midsagittal views or axial views. The midsagittal technique (comparing the diameter of the canal at the injured level with that of the uninjured subjacent level) can be misleading if there are bony fragments not visualized on the midsagittal cut, or if the patient has a scoliotic deformity. The actual amount of canal compromise can be underestimated or overestimated. Alternatively, the use of axial images to evaluate canal compromise may underestimate injury severity in patients with translational or rotational-type injuries. Posterior facet fractures and dislocations can be easily detected on axial views. Asymmetry of right and left facets should be noted because any widening of the facets may indicate a flexion, rotation, or distraction type of injury. A frank dislocation of the facet may be indicated by an "empty" or "naked" facet sign (Figure 3).

MRI Evaluation

MRI is invaluable in assessing the integrity of nonosseous spine structures (intervertebral disks, ligamentous structures, and the spinal cord) and occult fractures. Current indications for obtaining an MRI scan following thoracolumbar trauma include suspected intervertebral disk or ligamentous injury, neurologic impairment, and/or occult fractures. The sensitivity for detecting PLC injury by physical examination alone (spinous process step-off, tenderness to palpation, and degloving injury) has been shown to be low. T2-weighted MRI is useful in detecting disruptions in the

5: Spine

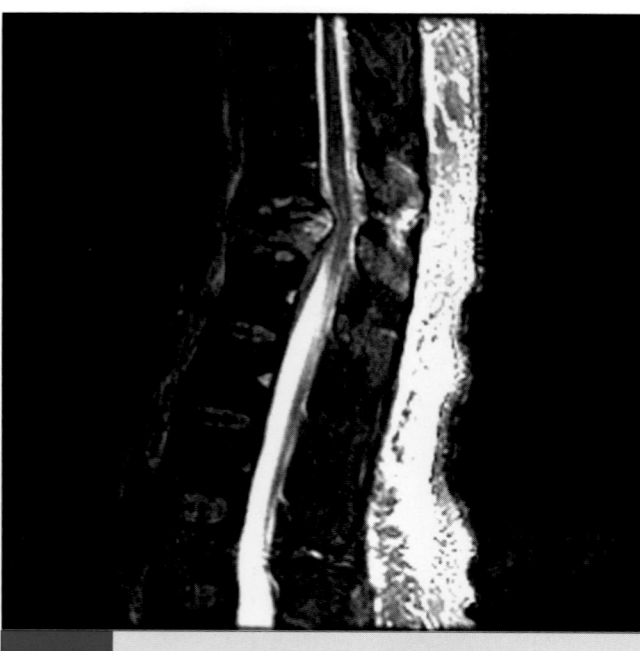

Figure 4 Increased signal on T2-weighted MRI scan at the posterior ligamentous complex (in this instance in the interspinous ligament) represents injury to the posterior stabilizing elements. This may signify a more unstable fracture pattern.

PLC (supraspinous and interspinous ligaments, ligamentum flavum, and facet capsules), which may indicate a more unstable injury pattern. In particular, fat-suppressed T2-weighted MRI can further increase the sensitivity of injury detection by suppressing normal adipose tissue enhancements. A PLC injury will show an increased signal on T2-weighted MRI scans, indicating edema or frank disruption (**Figure 4**). Injury to one or all components of the PLC should alert the treating physician to a potentially more serious mechanism of injury. Similarly, a disruption of the intervertebral disk will be indicated by a bright signal through the anterior longitudinal ligament, the disk, and/or the posterior longitudinal ligament (PLL) on T2-weighted MRI scans. This finding is often associated with a more unstable fracture pattern (rotational or distraction mechanism).

Injury to the spinal cord may be indicated by bright signal within the substance of the spinal cord on T2-weighted MRI scans. This finding indicates spinal cord hemorrhage and edema, and is a poor indicator for neurologic recovery. MRI evaluation of the spinal cord is particularly useful in evaluating neurologic status in obtunded patients or those unable to cooperate with a neurologic examination.

Occult fractures, especially the noncontiguous injuries, can be readily visualized with MRI. Sagittal T2-weighted reconstruction MRI scans will indicate bony edema by displaying bright signals within the vertebral body or the end plates. These can indicate subtle compression fractures that are often missed on plain radiographs or CT. This is particularly important for pa-

tients in whom surgical fixation is used to treat a more severe adjacent level injury, as the inclusion of occult injury in the fixation construct should be considered.

Defining Spinal Stability and Recognizing the Pattern of Injury

The concept of spinal stability is difficult to define. Spinal instability has been described as the loss of the ability of the spine under physiologic loads to maintain its pattern of displacement so that there is no initial or additional neurologic deficit, no major deformity, and no incapacitating pain. Any injury to the thoracolumbar junction, because of its unique transitional anatomy, can alter the equilibrium between the kyphotic thoracic spine and the lordotic lumbar spine. Often, the decision whether to treat these injuries nonsurgically or surgically depends on determining initial instability and predicting future mechanical failure. The first step in this decision-making process should begin with analyzing the mechanisms of injury that lead to distinct patterns of injuries.

Flexion
Flexion injuries typically involve anterior compression and posterior tensile loads. In the three-column model, the anterior column fails in compression and the middle and posterior columns remain intact. The resultant wedging of the anterior column may impart significant tensile forces on the posterior column. When there is greater than 50% loss of anterior vertebral body height, an injury to the PLC may also be present.

Axial Compression
Axial compression injuries typically involve the anterior and middle columns. The typical burst fracture pattern results from axial load causing end-plate fracture and then subsequent failure of the vertebral bodies. Sagittal posture at the time of load may also determine whether compression or burst fracture occurs, with increased propensity for burst fracture morphology with extension posture.

Lateral Compression (Focal Scoliosis)
Asymmetric collapse similar to the anterior wedge compression fracture can occur on either side of the vertebral body. This results from compressive force on half of the body and tension on the opposite side. The resultant laterally wedged compression fracture can be chronically unstable, causing painful deformity and focal scoliosis.

Flexion Rotation
Flexion rotation injuries can involve all three columns and are considered unstable. Typically, the anterior column fails with flexion and the middle and posterior columns fail with shear. These injuries are most notable on AP spine radiographs, which may show subtle lateral listhesis at the injured level.

5: Spine

Flexion-Distraction (Chance)

In flexion-distraction injuries (typically seen with seat-belt injuries), the axis of rotation typically lies anterior to the vertebral body, resulting in tensile failure of the anterior, middle, and posterior columns. Distinction is made whether the failure occurs entirely through the bony or ligamentous elements. The axis of rotation can also occur through the middle column, causing failure of the anterior column in compression and tensile disruption of the posterior elements.

Extension

Extension injuries typically result in failure of the anterior column in tension and compression failure of the posterior column. Significant displacement can be seen with distractive forces through all three columns, resulting in highly unstable shear injuries. This is particularly evident in conditions that cause ankylosis of the adjacent spine segments (diffuse idiopathic skeletal hyperostosis or ankylosing spondylitis).

Fracture Classifications

Historically, there have been abundant attempts to create fracture classifications to link either mechanistic, anatomic, or biomechanical features of the injury to prognostic factors. Early classification systems (Watson-Jones, Nicoll, and Holdsworth) were useful in categorizing spine injuries based on morphology, but they were unreliable in determining instability, prognosis, and optimal treatment. As newer classification systems (Ferguson and Allen, Magerl) attempt to become more inclusive, they have increased in complexity, resulting in difficult practical application and poor reliability.[5,6] The most recent attempt to guide treatment algorithms resulted in the Thoracolumbar Injury Classification and Severity Score (TLICSS).[7]

Holdsworth Classification

The early column concept of spine biomechanics was first described by Holdsworth in the 1960s. The original two-column model separated the spine into the solid anterior column (consisting of the vertebral bodies, intervertebral disks, and the associated longitudinal ligaments) and the hollow posterior neural arches (consisting of the pedicles, laminae, facet joints, spinous processes, and associated ligaments). This classification did not provide much guidance to prognostic factors or treatment algorithms.

Denis Classification

The most popular and cited system was described in 1983 based on injury patterns in 412 patients. This system was a modification of the two-column concept in which the anterior column was divided into two columns (anterior and middle) to allow better prediction of spinal stability. Denis first stratified thoracolumbar fractures into major and minor injuries. Minor injuries included fractures of the transverse or spinous processes, lamina, or the pars interarticularis. Major injuries included compression fractures, burst fractures, flexion-distraction injuries, and fracture-dislocations. Within this classification, Denis further subclassified burst fracture into five types based on involvement of the specific end plate and rotational and/or eccentric load. Flexion-distraction injuries were divided based on levels of involvement and the involvement of bone versus ligamentous structures. Fracture-dislocations were subclassified into six types based on number of levels involved and whether the injured elements were bony or ligamentous.

McAfee Classification

This classification evolved from the Denis system, in an attempt to more accurately predict mechanism of failure of the middle column. This system was based on analysis of CT scans and plain radiographs of 100 consecutive thoracolumbar injuries, which revealed that the middle column could fail by axial compression, axial distraction, or translation. The McAfee classification distinguishes injuries resulting primarily from distractive force from those resulting from compressive force, recognizing that some injuries will displace with exaggerated compression or distraction. This understanding can aid in surgical reduction and fixation of some fracture patterns. However, this classification is criticized by some to be inadequate in describing all types of fracture patterns, and it has yet to be validated for its prognostic value.

Magerl (AO) Classification

Based on the analysis of more than 1,400 thoracolumbar fractures, the Magerl (AO) classification divides injuries into either compression (type A), distraction (type B), or rotation (type C) injuries. Injuries are further classified based on the disruption pattern (morphology) of the various spine "elements," primarily distinguishing bony disruption and ligamentous injuries. The Magerl (AO) classification is the most comprehensive of the systems; however, the interobserver and intraobserver reliability has been a problem. One recent study revealed that both the Magerl (AO) and Denis classifications had only moderate reliability and repeatability. The intraobserver agreement (repeatability) was 82% and 79% for the Magerl (AO) and Denis types, respectively, and 67% and 56% for the Magerl (AO) and Denis subtypes, respectively.[6]

Thoracolumbar Injury Classification and Severity Score

TLICSS is the most recent evolution in the attempt to integrate morphologic and mechanistic aspects of thoracolumbar injury with prognosis and treatment.[7] Although the ultimate treatment should depend on either initial or predicted instability, the method for determining this "instability" remains controversial.

An example of this continued controversy is the confusion regarding the treatment of a simple burst fracture. In the Holdsworth two-column model, the pri-

Table 1

Use of the TLICSS to Determine Fracture Stability and Guide Nonsurgical Versus Surgical Treatment

Fracture Morphology/Mechanism	Qualifier	Points
Compression		1
	Lateral angulation > 15°	1
	Burst	1
Translational/rotational		3
Distraction		4
Neurologic Involvement		
Intact		0
Nerve root		2
Cord, conus medullaris	Incomplete	3
	Complete	2
Cauda equina		3
Posterior Ligamentous Complex Status		
Intact		0
Injury suspected/indeterminate		2
Injured		3
Management		
Nonsurgical		0 to 3
Nonsurgical or surgical		4
Surgical		≥ 5

(Reproduced with permission from Lee JY, Vaccaro AR, Lim MR, et al: Thoracolumbar classification system and injury severity score: A new paradigm for the treatment of thoracolumbar spine trauma. J Orthop Sci 2005;10:671-675.)

mary determinant of instability in burst fractures is disruption of the posterior column. A cadaveric biomechanical study analyzing sequential disruption of the anterior, middle, and posterior columns confirmed that there is greater flexion instability when the PLC is disrupted.[8] This finding supports the clinical correlation of a two-column stability model and stresses the functional importance of the posterior tension band when the anterior column is disrupted. However, some studies have shown that isolated posterior injury without middle column injury remains stable. Thus, the proponents of the three-column model propose that injuries involving two or more columns should be considered unstable.

Although conceptually appealing, the three-column description of thoracolumbar fractures has not been substantiated clinically. With the exception of penetrating trauma, isolated PLC injury is rarely seen clinically. In addition, the concept of a stable burst fracture is contradictory to this model. Numerous clinical outcome reports of successful nonsurgical treatment of stable burst fractures have been published. A prospective randomized study showed that burst fractures in neurologically intact patients can be treated surgically or nonsurgically with minimal difference in clinical outcome (anatomic or functional).[9] Conversely, the two-column model is inadequate to account for instability in the coronal plane, such as focal scoliosis from a lateral compression fracture in which the PLC is intact. In general, older classification systems attempted to base treatment decisions on theoretical instability of specific fracture patterns, which is not always clinically applicable.

Because of these inadequacies, the Spine Trauma Study Group, combining the clinically relevant concepts of previous systems and incorporating neurologic impairment, has recently introduced a new classification system of thoracolumbar fractures. The TLICSS uses three primary criteria to determine stability— fracture morphology, neurologic injury, and status of the PLC[10,11] (Table 1). This scoring system serves as an algorithm to assign points for each of these criteria, and determines a severity score for the patient that then can be used to decide treatment[7] (Figure 5).

Fracture morphology is determined primarily by plain radiographs and CT scans. It is divided into three classes of compression, translation/rotation, or distraction, and is meant to reflect the mechanism of injury. Burst injury is a subcategory of compression morphology. TLICSS assumes that the presence of a neurologic injury indicates a higher mechanism of injury. Hence, the presence of a neurologic deficit, particularly the incomplete type, will result in a higher score, leading to a surgical treatment. T2-weighted MRI scans (particularly fat-suppressed images) are used to determine the integrity of the PLC. A disrupted PLC is given a higher score, leading to surgical intervention.[12]

Surgery is recommended for a score ≥ 5, and nonsurgical management is warranted for a score ≤ 3. It should be noted that this algorithm is not yet fully validated by a prospective randomized study, and is derived primarily through a conglomerate of current understanding of the injury pattern and historical treatments of thoracolumbar fractures. The reliability scores for the TLICSS system have been promising. In one study, surgeons agreed with the TLICSS recommendation 96.4% of the time. Intrarater kappa coefficients were 0.57 ± 0.04 for injury mechanism, 0.93 ± 0.02 for neurologic status, 0.48 ± 0.04 for PLC status, 0.46 ± 0.03 for TLICSS total, and 0.62 ± 0.04 for treatment recommendation. These results compared favorably with other contemporary classification systems.[13]

Treatment Options and Guidelines

Treatment options for thoracolumbar fractures can be broadly divided into nonsurgical and surgical interventions. Whether to choose one option over another is, again, dependent on characteristics of the fracture and determination/prediction of initial and future instability. As suggested previously, no standard algorithm exists on how instability is determined on initial presentation. The new scoring method using the TLICSS system may help, but its usefulness remains to be validated in a large prospective trial.

Nonsurgical

Nonsurgical treatment can be used for stable thoracolumbar injuries that include Denis' minor injury types, compression fractures, stable burst fractures, or those with a TLICSS ≤ 3. Treatment modalities include analgesics, bed rest, bracing, and/or extension casting. Patients with stable injuries can be mobilized after several days of bed rest and analgesia with either a thoracolumbosacral orthosis (TLSO) or Risser-like body cast applied with the spine in hyperextension. Although extension casting provides greater immobilization than a removable orthotic device, patients tolerate a TLSO better than casting. Immobilization is recommended for a minimum of 10 to 12 weeks to allow for bony union. Frequent clinical and radiographic evaluation is recommended to assess for fracture healing and maintenance of spinal alignment.

Progressive improvement in pain, return to function, and radiographic evidence of union imply fracture healing. In a prospective randomized trial comparing nonsurgical versus surgical management of stable burst fractures in 53 patients, nonsurgical management showed equivalent functional results to surgical treatment with fewer reported complications, significantly lower pain and disability scores, and lower cost.[9] Failure of nonsurgical management is defined as patient intolerance to casting or brace treatment, progressive loss of spinal alignment, persistent pain, and progressive neurologic impairment.

Surgical

Surgical treatment is strongly indicated for patients in whom initial nonsurgical treatments have failed. Other strong indications for surgery include incomplete neurologic impairment with kyphosis or canal compromise, fracture-dislocations, and multiple noncontiguous spinal injuries. Relative indications for surgical treatment include fracture of the anterior and middle column in conjunction with PLC injury (as seen on MRI scans), other nonspinal injuries (such as visceral or extremity injuries) necessitating frequent surgical care or patient manipulation, or comorbidities (such as morbid obesity) that preclude brace/cast treatment.

Surgical care can be subdivided into anterior only, posterior only, or combined procedures. The type of surgical treatment can be influenced by the fracture pattern, neurologic status, and surgeon's preference. Currently, there are a limited number of studies that compare anterior, posterior, or combined surgical approaches.

Anterior Surgery

Incomplete neurologic injury with spinal canal compromise is a strong indication for anterior surgery. Patients with thoracolumbar fractures often present with injury to the conus medullaris or cauda equina, with impingement from retropulsed bone or kyphotic alignment. If

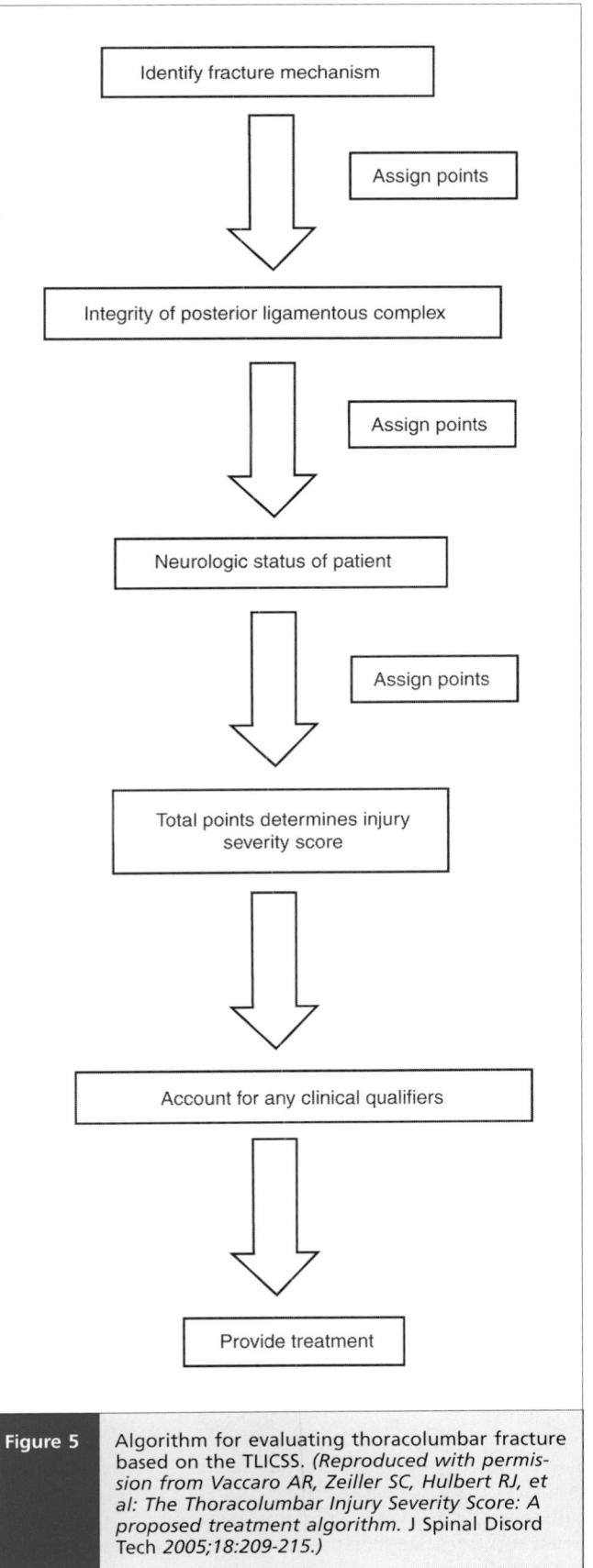

Figure 5 Algorithm for evaluating thoracolumbar fracture based on the TLICSS. (Reproduced with permission from Vaccaro AR, Zeiller SC, Hulbert RJ, et al: The Thoracolumbar Injury Severity Score: A proposed treatment algorithm. J Spinal Disord Tech 2005;18:209-215.)

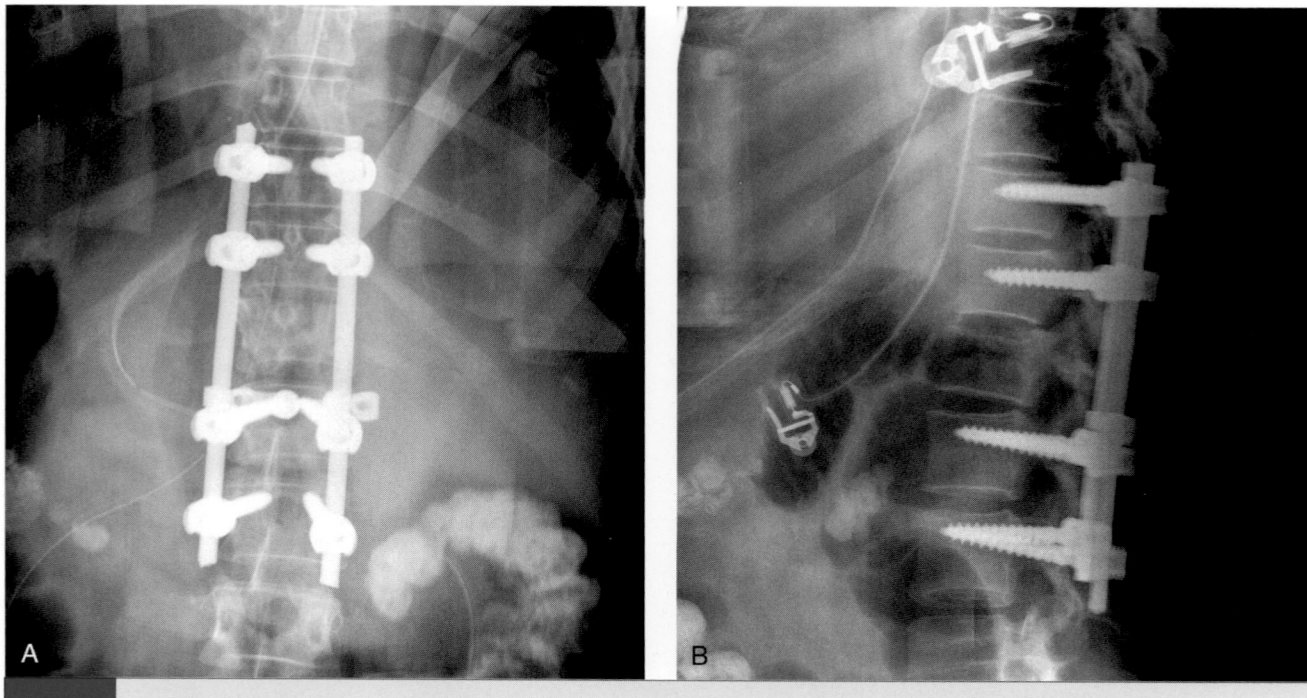

Figure 6 AP **(A)** and lateral **(B)** radiographs of a patient who underwent posterior fixation for a burst fracture.

an associated incomplete neurologic injury is present, then anterior decompression of the spinal canal should be strongly considered. Often full or partial corpectomy of the retropulsed body is required to decompress the canal, and the decompressed space can be filled with either a cadaveric bone (allograft femur, humerus, or fibula) or a cage construct.

Whether anterior decompression and stabilization alone (without posterior fixation) is sufficient is still a subject of controversy. The most common fracture pattern that is amenable to anterior-only surgery is a burst fracture with partial neurologic injury, without evidence of PLC injury. In a study of 150 consecutive patients with thoracolumbar burst fractures treated with a single-stage anterior decompression, grafting, and instrumentation, researchers found a 93% fusion rate, with improvement of at least one Frankel grade in 142 of 150 patients.[14] One recent study retrospectively evaluated 40 patients who underwent anterior decompression and two-segment instrumentation reconstruction. No patients had neurologic deterioration, and 30 patients (91%) with incomplete neurologic deficits improved by at least one modified Frankel grade. Mean preoperative segmental kyphosis of 22.7° was improved to 7.4°. Most importantly, the loss of kyphosis at the latest follow-up averaged only 2.1°.[15]

Posterior Surgery
The posterior approach can be used for stabilization and indirect or direct decompression of thoracolumbar fractures. Posterior instrumentation with either a segmental hook/rod construct or a pedicle screw/rod construct is the most common method to stabilize various thoraco-

lumbar fracture types (**Figure 6**). The hook/rod construct is becoming less popular as more surgeons are becoming comfortable with placement of thoracic and lumbar pedicle screws. Pedicle screws also allow for short-segment fixation to stabilize compression and burst-type injuries. A theoretic advantage of short-segment instrumentation and arthrodesis (one level above and below the injury) is that more segments of the mobile lumbar spine are left out of the fusion construct. However, recent reviews have shown that short-segment constructs can lead to instrumentation failure and progressive kyphosis. One prospective randomized study of 20 patients showed progressive kyphosis or screw breakage in 50% of patients treated with short-segment instrumentation.[16] Another study comparing short- and long-segment posterior fixation concluded that short constructs had a higher failure rate (55%) as defined by progressive kyphosis and anterior vertebral body height loss, although significant clinical difference could not be determined.[17] A recent review of biomechanical studies of short-segment fixation indicates that loss of anterior column integrity may place significant stress on the short fixation, which may lead to instrumentation failure.[18] Therefore, current literature seems to support the notion that short-segment posterior fixation is best when combined with anterior column reconstruction or with fracture patterns without much anterior column loss (flexion-distraction or Chance-type injuries). Otherwise, long-segment fixation (two or more levels above and below the injury) should be used.

Indirect decompression of the spinal canal can be achieved through a posterior approach if the PLL is intact. Indirect decompression is achieved by longitudinal distraction and postural reduction of the sagittal alignment, leading to ligamentotaxis and reduction of the fracture fragment. One recent retrospective study using CT scans of 157 consecutive thoracolumbar fractures showed 23% improvement in the mean canal cross-sectional area following posterior indirect decompression. At 5-year follow-up, remodeling of the residual bone fragment occurred, with the mean canal cross-sectional area measuring 87% of normal.[19] The consensus of the literature seems to support that the fracture patterns most amendable to indirect decompression are compression fractures and burst fractures with intact PLL as seen on MRI scans.

Some have advocated direct decompression of the anterior bone fragment using the posterior approach. The technique involves removal of the facet/lamina/pedicle complex to gain access to the posterior vertebral body. The proponents of this method state that the patient morbidity of a separate anterior approach may be obviated using this technique. The critics of this method indicate that removal of posterior bony elements in the setting of significant anterior column compromise will further destabilize the spine and predispose to mechanical failure. One recent retrospective study using a modification of this method showed neurologic improvement in 23 of 28 patients in the group, but with a high rate (17.8%) of pseudarthrosis.[20] Regardless of approach, adequately stabilized burst fractures have shown the ability to heal, remodel, and resorb retropulsed bone fragments even when decompression is not performed, thereby questioning the need for decompression in neurologically intact patients. However, in the presence of incomplete spinal cord injury, adequacy of canal clearance has been shown to correlate with improved neurologic recovery and should be considered when associated with significant canal encroachment. When burst fractures are associated with a concomitant lamina fracture at the same level, there have been reports of a high incidence of trapped neural elements and dural tears. In these instances, initial posterior exploration is indicated to decompress, reduce, and repair the neural structures prior to anterior decompression.

Combined Anterior and Posterior Surgery

Definitive indications for a combined anterior and posterior approach are still a matter of debate. The disadvantage of combined surgery is that the patient is exposed to the morbidity of both anterior and posterior approaches. The theoretic advantage of this method is that it combines the direct anterior decompression of the spinal canal with structural reconstruction of both anterior and posterior spinal elements (**Figure 7**). Mechanism of injury that includes axial compression (compression fracture, burst fracture) with posterior distraction, rotation, or translation will often result in canal compromise and dislocation of the spine. Therefore, a strong indication for the combined surgery will include thoracolumbar injuries with incomplete

neurologic injury, canal compromise (bone retropulsion), and severe injury to the posterior bony elements or PLC. There is some experimental biomechanical evidence[21] and clinical evidence[22] that combined approaches for severe injuries give superior structural rigidity as well as radiographic outcome, but no randomized prospective study exists to validate the theoretic advantages.

Osteoporotic VCFs

Recent epidemiologic reviews have shown an increasing incidence of vertebral insufficiency fractures secondary to osteoporosis proportional to the aging population. It is estimated that in the United States, VCFs occur in 20% of people 70 years of age or older, leading to a potential 700,000 new fractures each year and $17 billion in direct costs annually.[23]

Fortunately, most VCFs will respond to nonsurgical brace treatment. When nonsurgical management is unsuccessful, either open surgical intervention or percutaneous cement augmentation may be required. Open treatment of VCFs may be indicated if either the associated kyphosis or bone retropulsion into the spinal canal causes neurologic deficit. Optimal fixation of instrumentation in osteoporotic bone may include increasing points of fixation (additional levels), sublaminar wiring, larger pedicle screws for better fill, and cement screw augmentation.[24]

Often, patients with VCFs have comorbid medical conditions that preclude prolonged anesthesia. Newer minimally invasive alternatives to posterior spinal fusion such as kyphoplasty and vertebroplasty have offered improved symptom relief with minimal surgical morbidity. Vertebroplasty uses percutaneous transpedicular injection of low-viscosity polymethylmethacrylate (PMMA) cement into fractured vertebral bodies under fluoroscopic guidance to decrease pain and prevent further body collapse. Kyphoplasty is a variation of vertebroplasty, which uses a balloon tamp to create a void within the vertebral body before injecting the viscous PMMA cement. Both procedures have reported excellent success rates for pain relief (60% to 100%), with kyphoplasty showing the added benefit of an average of 30% anterior height restoration and 50% midbody height restoration at approximately 2 years postprocedure (average 21 months follow-up) and an average 14° reduction of focal kyphosis.[25] Although outcome analysis for each shows a slightly better safety profile for kyphoplasty with decreased risk of cement extravasation, there is no proven long-term clinical benefit of kyphoplasty over vertebroplasty to date to reflect the increased cost of kyphoplasty.[23] The risk of subsequent vertebral insufficiency fractures without treatment, after vertebroplasty, and after kyphoplasty ranges from 19% to 52%. Although there are theoretic benefits of restoration of spinal alignment, the clinical benefit of vertebral height restoration remains unclear. Neither vertebroplasy nor kyphoplasty is indicated for fractures that extend into the posterior vertebral body (burst fractures) or fractures that in-

5: Spine

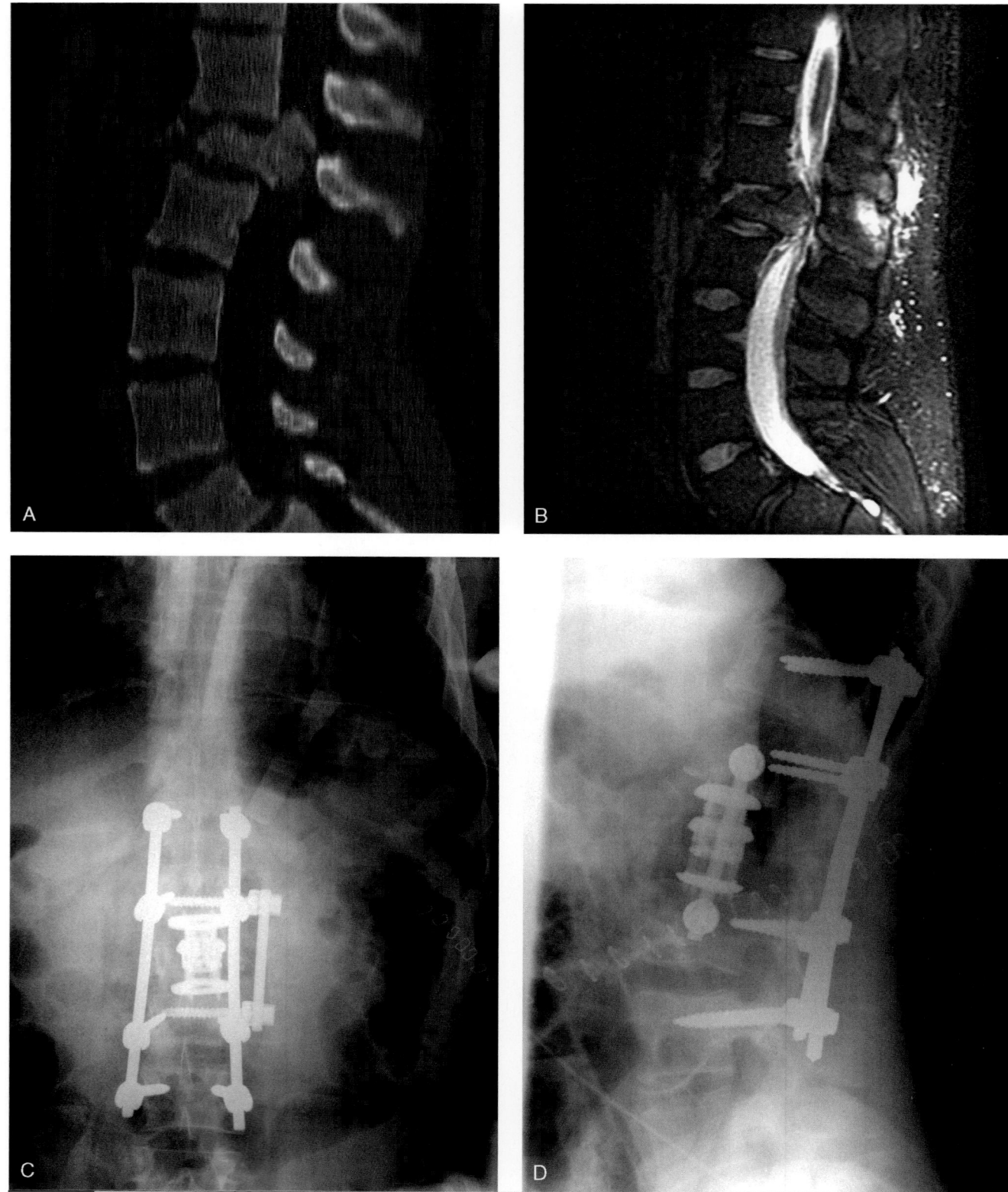

Figure 7 **A,** Sagittal CT reconstruction of a patient who had a burst fracture with injury to the PLC shows severe spinal canal compromise. **B,** T2-weighted MRI scan shows edema of the PLC indicating posterior element instability. AP **(C)** and lateral **(D)** postoperative radiographs showing decompression of the spinal canal with a corpectomy. The reconstruction of the anterior column was performed with an expandable cage, and the reconstruction of the posterior spine was performed with a pedicle screw/rod construct.

5: Spine

volve the pedicle because of the concern of cement extravasation into the spinal canal.

Emerging Concepts

The treatment of thoracolumbar fractures has evolved as the improved description and classification of the injuries has provided a rationale for surgical decision making. Early recognition of thoracolumbar injury with detailed physical and radiographic (or CT) evaluation allows for accurate preoperative injury assessment. MRI evaluation to recognize PLC injury is becoming more common and integral in the management of these injuries.

A new scoring system (TLICSS) has been introduced to improve on the classification and decision making when treating these fractures. Injury morphology, neurologic status, and PLC integrity are critical to the assessment of fracture stability and the TLICSS score. Treatment decisions based on accurate assessment instability may help maximize successful surgical outcomes and patient satisfaction. Both surgical and nonsurgical treatments of thoracolumbar fractures have been shown to yield satisfactory results in appropriately selected patients. Surgical approach, reconstruction, and construct are based on mechanism and morphology of injury. Success of treatment is gauged on the maintenance of spinal alignment without additional neurologic deficit or debilitating pain.

Annotated References

1. Fisher CG, Noonan VK, Dvorak MF: Changing face of spine trauma care in North America. *Spine* 2006;31 (11 suppl):S2-S8.

   In this multidisciplinary, evidence-based review and summary of literature, the authors discuss the clinical, epidemiologic, and research issues influencing spine trauma care. They also summarize epidemiologic trends in spine trauma care over the past decade.

2. Rao RD, Singrakhia MD: Painful osteoporotic vertebral fracture: Pathogenesis, evaluation, and roles of vertebroplasty and kyphoplasty in its management. *J Bone Joint Surg Am* 2003;85:2010-2022.

3. Berry GE, Adams S, Harris MB, et al: Are plain radiographs of the spine necessary during evaluation after blunt trauma? Accuracy of screening torso computed tomography in thoracic/lumbar spine fracture diagnosis. *J Trauma* 2005;59:1410-1413.

   The authors undertook a retrospective review of 103 blunt trauma patients' clinical and imaging records to evaluate sensitivity, specificity, and utility of chest/abdomen/pelvis CT scans obtained in the trauma setting to diagnose thoracolumbar fractures. CT proved to be more sensitive and as equally specific as traditional radiography. The authors assert that although there may

be a slight increase in cost, omission of plain radiography and utilization of CT to evaluate spine trauma may expedite care without sacrificing accuracy. Level of evidence: III.

4. Inaba K, Munera F, McKenney M, et al: Visceral torso computed tomography for clearance of the thoracolumbar spine in trauma: A review of the literature. *J Trauma* 2006;60:915-920.

   This recent literature review looks at studies analyzing the use of CT of the abdomen and torso to evaluate for spine injuries. The authors conclude that all of the referenced studies found CT to be more accurate, faster, and cost-effective in evaluating spine trauma. Level of evidence: III.

5. Mirza SK, Mirza AJ, Chapman JR, Anderson PA: Classifications of thoracic and lumbar fractures: Rationale and supporting data. *J Am Acad Orthop Surg* 2002;10: 364-377.

6. Wood KB, Khanna G, Vaccaro AR, Arnold PM, Harris MB, Mehbod AA: Assessment of two thoracolumbar fracture classification systems as used by multiple surgeons. *J Bone Joint Surg Am* 2005;87:1423-1429.

   The authors report a case-controlled study comparing the reproducibility and repeatability of the Denis and AO classification systems for assessing thoracolumbar trauma using 31 case examples evaluated by 19 trained spine surgeons. Surgeons were asked to re-evaluate cases 3 months later. Interobserver and intraobserver agreement using kappa values were determined at best to be moderate for both systems. Level of evidence: III.

7. Lee JY, Vaccaro AR, Lim MR, et al: Thoracolumbar injury classification and severity score: A new paradigm for the treatment of thoracolumbar spine trauma. *J Orthop Sci* 2005;10:671-675.

   This article describes a new classification system (TLICSS) incorporating fracture morphology, neurologic injury, and PLC status to assign an injury severity score for thoracolumbar fractures. The TLICSS score can be used to determine the need for surgical intervention. The authors outline the rationale and application of the scoring system.

8. James KS, Wenger KH, Schlegel JD, Dunn HK: Biomechanical evaluation of the stability of thoracolumbar burst fractures. *Spine* 1994;19:1731-1740.

9. Wood K, Buttermann G, Mehbod A, et al: Operative compared with nonoperative treatment of a thoracolumbar burst fracture without neurological deficit: A prospective, randomized study. *J Bone Joint Surg Am* 2003;85:773-781.

10. Vaccaro AR, Lehman RA Jr, Hurlbert RJ, et al: A new classification of thoracolumbar injuries: The importance of injury morphology, the integrity of the posterior ligamentous complex, and neurologic status. *Spine* 2005; 30:2325-2333.

    This is another article on the new classification system (TLICSS) incorporating fracture morphology, neurologic

5: Spine

injury, and PLC status to assign an injury severity score for thoracolumbar fractures. The authors describe the background, rationale, and application of the scoring system.

11. Vaccaro AR, Lim MR, Hurlbert RJ, et al: Surgical decision making for unstable thoracolumbar spine injuries: Results of a consensus panel review by the Spine Trauma Study Group. *J Spinal Disord Tech* 2006;19:1-10.

    This article presents results and discussion of a consensus panel review of surgical criteria and treatment algorithms used by 22 experienced spine trauma surgeons based on their responses to 6 clinical case scenarios. Three critical elements of thoracolumbar trauma were identified: neurologic status, fracture morphology, and integrity of the PLL. A systematic framework for surgical decision making is proposed.

12. Vaccaro AR, Lee JY, Schweitzer KM Jr, et al: Assessment of injury to the posterior ligamentous complex in thoracolumbar spine trauma. *Spine J* 2006;6:524-528.

    This article presents analysis of the survey results from the members of the Spine Trauma Study Group asked to rank the most important diagnostic criteria to determine PLC injury. A list of 12 diagnostic criteria was provided and ranked. Vertebral body translation on plain radiographs was most commonly identified as the most important indicator of posterior ligament injury. The accuracy of MRI in evaluating ligamentous injury is discussed and a recent literature review of diagnostic criteria is provided.

13. Vaccaro AR, Baron EM, Sanfilippo J, et al: Reliability of a novel classification system for thoracolumbar injuries: The Thoracolumbar Injury Severity Score. *Spine* 2006;31(11 suppl):S62-S69.

    This prospective study assessing the inter- and intra-observer reliability of the TLICSS scoring system. Five surgeons evaluated 71 clinical cases and repeated their evaluations 1 month later. Kappa coefficients were calculated and showed moderate interrater agreement for injury mechanism, PLC status, and TLICSS. Excellent agreement was noted for neurologic status and overall treatment plan agreement. The authors concluded that TLICSS compares favorably with other recent classification systems. Level of evidence: II.

14. Kaneda K, Taneichi H, Abumi K, Hashimoto T, Satoh S, Fujiya M: Anterior decompression and stabilization with the Kaneda device for thoracolumbar burst fractures associated with neurological deficits. *J Bone Joint Surg Am* 1997;79:69-83.

15. Sasso RC, Best NM, Reilly TM, McGuire RA Jr: Anterior-only stabilization of three-column thoracolumbar injuries. *J Spinal Disord Tech* 2005;18(suppl): S7-S14.

    This article presents a retrospective review of 40 patients with unstable thoracolumbar fractures that were treated with single-stage anterior decompression and fusion, with modern instrumentation techniques. The authors report a 95% fusion rate with only one construct failure. Most patients with neurologic deficits (91%) improved at least one Frankel grade and maintained kyphotic correction. The authors concluded that single-

stage anterior stand-alone techniques may be a feasible treatment option for thoracolumbar burst fractures. Level of evidence: III.

16. Alanay A, Acaroglu E, Yazici M, Aksoy C, Surat A: The effect of transpedicular intracorporeal grafting in the treatment of thoracolumbar burst fractures on canal remodeling. *Eur Spine J* 2001;10:512-516.

17. Tezeren G, Kuru I: Posterior fixation of thoracolumbar burst fracture: Short-segment pedicle fixation versus long-segment instrumentation. *J Spinal Disord Tech* 2005;18:485-488.

    This prospective study of 18 patients with thoracolumbar burst fractures compared short-segment fixation (one level above and below fracture level) and long-segment fixation (claw construct two levels above and pedicle screws two levels below). The authors found an increased failure rate with short-segment constructs (55%) and prolonged surgical time with long-construct usage. Interestingly, there was no significant difference in outcome scores between the two groups. Level of evidence: III.

18. McLain RF: The biomechanics of long versus short fixation for thoracolumbar spine fractures. *Spine* 2006;31 (11 suppl):S70-S79.

    In this literature review, the author discusses the mechanics of long- versus short-segment pedicle instrumentation in the treatment of thoracolumbar fractures.

19. Wessberg P, Wang Y, Irstam L, Nordwall A: The effect of surgery and remodelling on spinal canal measurements after thoracolumbar burst fractures. *Eur Spine J* 2001;10:55-63.

20. Kaya RA, Aydin Y: Modified transpedicular approach for the surgical treatment of severe thoracolumbar or lumbar burst fractures. *Spine J* 2004;4:208-217.

    The authors conducted a retrospective review of 28 cases of thoracolumbar fractures associated with neural canal compromise that were treated with a modified transpedicular approach for spinal canal decompression and found improved neurologic status after the procedure. Level of evidence: III.

21. Wilke HJ, Kemmerich V, Claes LE, Arand M: Combined anteroposterior spinal fixation provides superior stabilisation to a single anterior or posterior procedure. *J Bone Joint Surg Br* 2001;83:609-617.

22. Been HD, Bouma GJ: Comparison of two types of surgery for thoraco-lumbar burst fractures: Combined anterior and posterior stabilisation vs. posterior instrumentation only. *Acta Neurochir (Wien)* 1999;141:349-357.

23. Manson NA, Phillips FM: Minimally invasive techniques for the treatment of osteoporotic vertebral fractures. *J Bone Joint Surg Am* 2006;88:1862-1872.

    The authors of this review article discuss the epidemiology, treatment, and outcomes of osteoporotic compression fractures. They review the indications, comparison, and adverse outcomes of kyphoplasty and vertebro-

5: Spine

plasty, and include a detailed description of surgical technique for kyphoplasty.

24. Hu SS: Internal fixation in the osteoporotic spine. *Spine* 1997;22(24 suppl):43S-48S.

25. Majd ME, Farley S, Holt RT: Preliminary outcomes and efficacy of the first 360 consecutive kyphoplasties for the treatment of painful osteoporotic vertebral compression fractures. *Spine J* 2005;5:244-255.

This article discusses the safety and efficacy of kyphoplasty in patients with osteoporotic vertebral compression fractures based on the results of a retrospective, single-arm cohort study.

5: Spine

Chapter 48

Infections of the Spine

Jonathan N. Grauer, MD   Peter Whang, MD

Introduction

Infections of the spine comprise a spectrum of pathologic conditions with significant potential local and systemic sequelae. There are several different types of spinal infections that demonstrate various modes of transmission. Postoperative infections, for example, generally arise from direct inoculation of a wound at the time of surgical intervention, whereas diskitis and epidural infections most commonly result from hematogenous seeding. Different types of spinal infections are associated with specific pathogens. Because there are no clinical or radiographic findings pathognomonic for spinal infection, a high level of suspicion must always be maintained to identify infection and initiate appropriate management.

Postoperative Infections

Incidence and Microbiology

Postoperative infections occur almost exclusively from inoculation of a surgical site with skin flora at the time of surgical intervention and are less likely caused by hematogenous seeding from another source. The incidence of postoperative infections is relatively low; however, this complication dramatically alters the treatment course of the affected patient.

Multiple procedural and patient-related variables may influence the incidence of postoperative infections.[1] More extensive surgeries and those that involve longer surgical times are associated with an increased risk of infection. The risk of infection following lumbar diskectomy, for example, is less than 1%, whereas posterior instrumented fusions have consistently demonstrated infection rates of approximately 6% in several large published series. Specific surgical risk factors for infection include a posterior approach, longer hardware constructs, the use of instrumentation or an operating microscope, longer duration of surgery, and increased blood loss. Each of these variables increases the potential for wound contamination.

Certain patients are at greater risk for developing postoperative infections. Most of these patients are immunocompromised. Poor nutritional status may be one of the strongest risk factors, as malnourished patients are 16 times more likely to develop an infection after spinal procedures. Obese patients with a body mass index greater than 35 are becoming increasingly commonplace, and are five times more likely to develop an infection than patients of normal weight. Other risk factors are advanced patient age, diabetes mellitus, smoking, alcohol abuse, use of steroids, malignancy, and neurologic deficit. Similarly, previous spinal surgery or local radiation to the surgical field can also compromise local wound healing. Other less important patient factors include a history of trauma and presentation with a neurologic deficit.

Clinical Presentation

Increased pain and tenderness around the surgical site are the most common clinical symptoms of a postoperative spinal infection. In some instances, patients may present with systemic reports of fever, chills, or malaise. Incisional erythema, dehiscence, or persistent or recurrent wound drainage are also common findings. However, a tight fascial closure may allow deep-seeded infections to fester without any obvious superficial manifestations.

Unfortunately, there is often a delay of 1 week or longer after surgery before a wound infection is apparent. Accordingly, any clinical suggestion of infection warrants close monitoring or even presumptive treatment.

Diagnostic Studies

Laboratory studies may be helpful in establishing the diagnosis of postoperative spinal infection. White blood cell (WBC) counts may be elevated, but are less sensitive than the Westergren erythrocyte sedimentation rate (ESR) and C-reactive protein (CRP) level. The ESR normally peaks within 5 days of surgery but may be increased for more than 40 days after surgery. In contrast, the CRP level normally peaks after approximately 2 days, but this value may be elevated for more than 14 days after surgery. Elevated values beyond these periods should raise the suspicion for infection. Once baseline laboratory studies are obtained for a patient with a possible wound infection, a gradual return to normal levels would be expected for an unaffected individual; however, continued elevation of these laboratory values would be expected in the presence of infection.

Plain radiographs of the surgical site should be considered in any patient returning with symptoms suggestive of postoperative infection to rule out underlying structural abnormalities that might account for the symptoms. In the absence of any findings, cross-sectional

5: Spine

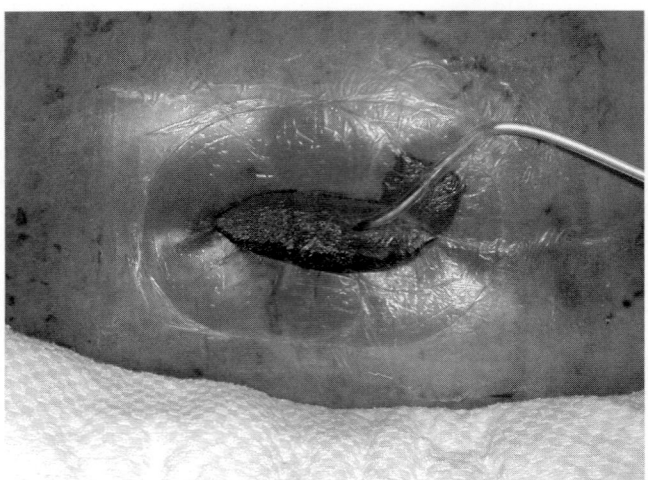

Figure 1 Lumbar spine of a patient in the lateral position showing VAC over a wound that had been irrigated and débrided for postoperative infection.

imaging such as CT or MRI may be indicated if the diagnosis of infection cannot be made clinically. Nonetheless, even with these advanced imaging modalities, the diagnosis of a wound infection may be difficult to differentiate from normal postoperative changes. For example, increased bone resorption may be seen with rhBMP-2 in early postoperative images.[2] Even contrast enhancement may also be nonspecific in nature.

Superficial wound cultures are generally not indicated after surgery because this patient population is at significant risk for skin flora contamination. Blood cultures should be drawn if a systemic infection is suspected. In equivocal clinical scenarios, a needle biopsy may be a reasonable option to access deep fluid loculations that cannot be differentiated from postoperative hematomas. Nonetheless, intraoperative cultures demonstrate the greatest sensitivity and specificity for confirming the presence of an active wound infection and identifying the pathogen involved.

Prophylactic Antibiotics

Perioperative prophylactic antibiotics have demonstrated efficacy in reducing the incidence of postoperative wound infections by up to 60%. Based on these data, it is widely recommended that a single parenteral dose of antibiotics be given 30 to 60 minutes before incision to allow for systemic distribution and tissue penetration.[3]

First generation cephalosporins (for example, cefazolin) are frequently used because they provide good coverage of gram-positive organisms including *Staphylococcys aureus* and *Staphylococcus epidermidis*, two of the most common skin contaminants. In patients with sensitivities to cephalosporins or those known to be colonized with methicillin-resistant *S aureus* (MRSA), an alternative antibiotic such as vancomycin should be considered.

For prolonged surgical procedures, additional doses of antibiotics should be administered at intervals one to two times the half-life of the medication during the operation; redosing may also be warranted in patients with significant blood loss or gross contamination. Although many spine surgeons continue prophylactic antibiotics in the postoperative period, this practice is not supported by any level I or II evidence and may actually be detrimental by selecting for resistant organisms with greater virulence. Irrigation of a surgical wound is also advocated to dilute pathogens and remove potential nonviable debris. Diluted betadine has been suggested with irrigation.[4]

Management

A suspected superficial postoperative spinal infection may be considered for medical management in the absence of a frank abscess or fluid collection evident on imaging studies. However, any suspected wound infection treated with antibiotics alone must be followed with extreme vigilance to rule out any disease progression or involvement of the deeper tissues. In addition to the superficial appearance of the incision, the patient's response to medical treatment may also be monitored with laboratory studies.

The mainstay of treatment of postoperative spinal infections is surgical irrigation and débridement. If there is sufficient clinical suspicion for a wound infection, this surgical intervention could be performed on a presumptive basis and not delayed for confirmatory imaging studies. After obtaining superficial and deep wound cultures, a thorough irrigation and débridement is routinely performed.

Strategies for managing instrumentation and bone graft are a matter of some controversy. Certainly the presence of instrumentation or bone graft may act as a nidus of infection. Nonetheless, many surgeons will leave spinal instrumentation in place because the stability afforded by internal fixation is not only presumed to be important for the underlying spinal pathology, but may also facilitate the eradication of infection. Instrumentation that has clearly loosened is generally removed. Loose bone graft in the surgical site is usually removed, whereas any material that is adherent to the surrounding bony structures is often left in place.

Once irrigation and débridement has been completed (a decision based on appearance of the wound), many surgeons will close the wound, primarily over drains. Alternatively, a grossly infected wound may be left open for serial irrigation and débridement until there is no evidence of contamination and cultures are negative, at which point delayed wound closure may be performed. More recently, various suction/irrigation and vacuum-assisted closure systems have been described in the literature and may be useful for the treatment of these infections (**Figure 1**).[5,6] Broad-spectrum antibiotics are typically initiated postoperatively. Coverage is then tailored according to the results of the intraoperative wound cultures. Antibiotics are routinely continued for at least 6 weeks, and any subsequent changes in medical management are based on the clinical response and laboratory profile of each patient.[7]

Hematogenous Diskitis and Osteomyelitis

Incidence and Microbiology

Pyogenic infections of the spine that are not introduced at the time of a surgical procedure most frequently develop secondary to hematogenous seeding from distant sites, although direct extension from adjacent structures may also occur.[8] Hematogenous spinal infections represent approximately 2% to 7% of all cases of pyogenic osteomyelitis. The age distribution of spinal infections is classically bimodal, with a small peak between 10 and 20 years of age and another larger peak in the elderly. In all age groups, males are more commonly affected than females, accounting for 60% to 80% of these types of infections.

Over the past several years, the incidence of pyogenic spinal infections appears to be increasing, which may be related to an escalation in the number of invasive medical procedures being performed as well as to any number of patient-related factors, including advanced age, an immunocompromised state, and the presence of other significant medical comorbidities. Pyogenic infections are also becoming more common in young adults, most likely because of increased rates of human immunodeficiency virus infection and intravenous drug use. Each of these risk factors has the potential to decrease the host response to transient bacteremia, originating in other organ systems as is seen with urinary tract infections or pneumonias and rendering an individual even more prone to developing subsequent infections in the spine.

In hematogenously spread spinal infections, the pathologic organisms usually emanate from the vascular end plates into the relatively avascular disk space, ultimately spreading to the adjacent vertebral bodies. Infections were initially thought to spread to the spine in a retrograde fashion via the rich network of valveless venous channels of the epidural space known as Batson's venous plexus. This theory has been largely abandoned because the abdominal pressures required to produce significant retrograde flow through this system would need to be extremely high and are essentially nonphysiologic. Alternatively, it has been shown that the cartilaginous end plates of the vertebral bodies contain multiple small, low-flow vascular anastomoses that provide an ideal environment for the inoculation and growth of microorganisms. As the infection progresses, necrosis of the end plates allows these infectious agents to penetrate the avascular disk space, where they are shielded from host defenses.

Diskitis most commonly occurs in the lumbar spine (50% to 60% of spinal infections), followed by the thoracic (30% to 40%) and cervical spines (10%). Up to 17% of these patients with infections will present with neurologic deficits resulting from compression of the neural elements secondary to the progressive collapse of the vertebral column or from the direct extension of the infection itself.

S aureus has been shown to be the most common pathogen responsible for pyogenic spinal infections and is isolated in up to 65% of these patients. Gram-negative enteric bacteria may also be responsible for another 20% of vertebral osteomyelitis and diskitis cases. As the prevalence of drug-resistant organisms continues to increase, MRSA species are being identified as the causative agents in a greater proportion of these types of spinal infections.

Clinical Presentation

Diskitis or vertebral osteomyelitis may be difficult to differentiate from degenerative spondylotic disease or sprain/strain types of spinal injuries. With axial spine pain nearly ubiquitous in modern society, detecting the warning signs indicative of nondegenerative causes of spinal pain is key to initiating the proper care for these potentially more serious conditions. Patients should be routinely questioned regarding any history of night pain, fever, chills, and unexpected weight loss, which may raise the possibility of an infection or malignancy. Inquiring about any recent illnesses, spinal procedures, and travel may also be helpful for establishing this diagnosis.

However, in many patients these various clinical findings may not be evident even after obtaining a complete history and performing a physical examination; for example, only approximately one third of patients with diskitis will report a history of fever. Because the clinical presentation of diskitis and vertebral osteomyelitis may be nonspecific, most of these patients will exhibit some signs and symptoms of their spinal infection for more than 3 months before the correct diagnosis is made.

Diagnostic Studies

As with postoperative spinal infections, laboratory studies such as the WBC, ESR, and CRP level may also be suggestive of diskitis or vertebral osteomyelitis. As many of these infections are indolent in nature, the WBC may be normal; however, the ESR and CRP level are elevated in 90% of patients with diskitis. In most patients the CRP level should be expected to rise more acutely with the onset of the infection and normalize more quickly than the ESR as it resolves. Thus, these values are not only important for establishing the initial diagnosis but may also be helpful for measuring the response to treatment.

As always, the initial imaging study for a patient with axial spine pain should be plain radiography. Plain radiographs may be helpful in assessing structural pathology of the spine and may also reveal evidence of end-plate erosions or sclerosis, destruction of disk spaces, or collapse of the vertebral bodies. All of these may be suggestive of a more aggressive process.

Because findings suggestive of infection may not be apparent on plain radiographs for weeks or even months, CT is another effective tool for evaluating a patient with a suspected spinal infection. CT provides more information about bony cross-sectional anatomy and may demonstrate pathologic changes earlier in the disease than plain radiography. With the addition of contrast, CT also facilitates the visualization of psoas or epidural fluid collections. Plain radiographs or CT

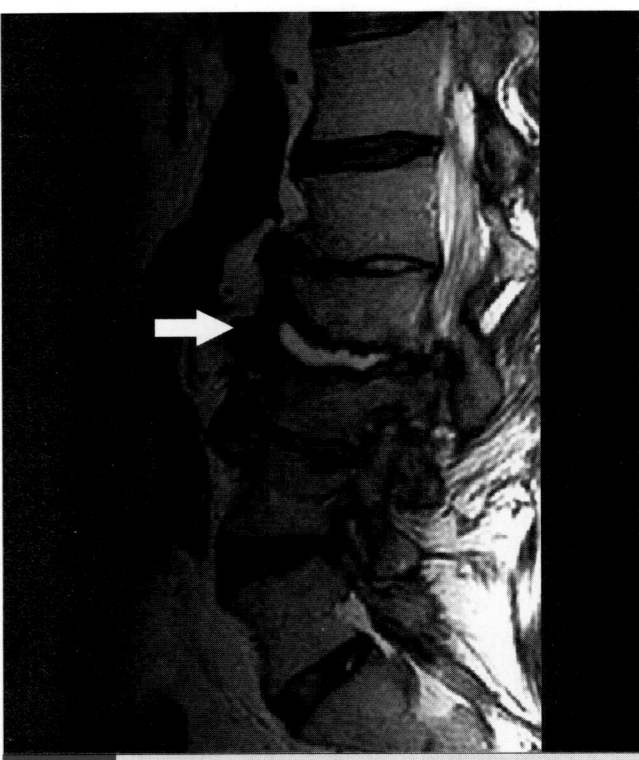

Figure 2 MRI scan of a 60-year-old patient with diabetes and isolated back pain. MRI findings were consistent with multilevel degenerative changes as well as fluid in the disk and collapse at L2-L3 (*arrow*). Needle biopsy revealed *S aureus*; the patient was treated with bracing and a 3-month course of antibiotics.

scans may also reveal air within the disk space, a phenomenon referred to as a "vacuum disk"; this finding is believed to represent degenerative disease rather than infection, which is more likely to demonstrate fluid within the evacuated disk space.

MRI is the primary imaging modality for confirming the diagnosis of infectious diskitis (**Figure 2**). As part of the normal degenerative cascade, the intervertebral disk initially exhibits low signal on sagittal T2-weighted images before the appearance of other degenerative findings such as Modic end-plate changes. In the setting of an infection, the fluid-filled disk is brighter on T2-weighted images, as is any edema that subsequently develops in the adjacent vertebral bodies. Moreover, paraspinal and epidural enhancement may also be observed with the administration of gadolinium. Unlike most malignancies in which the tumor primarily involves the vertebral body, with infection the nidus is typically located within the disk space, a characteristic that may be used to differentiate an infectious process from other potential diagnoses.

If MRI is not possible or the images prove to be inconclusive, various nuclear medicine studies including technetium-99 bone scanning and indium-111 tagged WBC scanning may be useful in the setting of suspected diskitis. Although these nuclear medicine techniques are extremely sensitive, they are not specific for a diagnosis of infection. Other pathologic processes such as degenerative spondylosis may yield similar findings.

Blood cultures should be routinely assessed in patients with suspected hematogenous osteomyelitis and diskitis. These cultures are positive in approximately 33% of patients with pyogenic spinal infections and correctly identify the causative pathogen in approximately 85%. The likelihood of isolating a specific organism is greater if the cultures are drawn before the administration of antibiotics and the patient is actively febrile. CT-guided biopsy of the lesion may be used to confirm the diagnosis and provide tissue for culture and sensitivity testing, the results of which are important for guiding subsequent antibiotic therapy.

Management

Most patients with vertebral osteomyelitis or diskitis are managed nonsurgically with antibiotics, immobilization, and other supportive care. Broad-spectrum parenteral antibiotics should be administered empirically until a specific pathogen is isolated from blood or tissue cultures, at which point antibiotics may be modified according to the susceptibilities of the organism. Treatment with intravenous antibiotics is usually continued for a minimum of 4 to 6 weeks. Response to antibiotics should be monitored with serial clinical evaluations and laboratory studies. Imaging may be significantly delayed in demonstrating response to treatment. After completion of a course of parenteral antibiotics, oral antibiotics for variable lengths of time may be considered.

Spinal immobilization is believed to help with the treatment of spinal infections. Not only may this procedure provide symptomatic relief, but the stability may also be helpful in the management of the infection itself and limit the development of deformity.

Surgical intervention may be considered in the management of vertebral osteomyelitis or diskitis if there is a neurologic deficit, need for diagnosis (considered when percutaneous biopsy is not successful), or failure of medical management. Elderly individuals or those with compromised immune function are most likely to fail to respond to conservative therapy and may therefore require surgical intervention.

Because vertebral osteomyelitis and diskitis typically affect the anterior column, these lesions are generally addressed with an anterior débridement from anterior or posterior approaches. Regardless of the surgical approach, the primary objectives of surgical treatment are débridement of the infectious region, decompression of the neural elements, and stabilization of any resultant spinal deformity or instability that may be present. An anterior débridement resulting in a significant defect in the anterior column may be supported with a strut graft or interbody implant. Patients with significant instability or severe deformities may also require supplementary posterior instrumentation concurrently or in a staged fashion to achieve a solid ar-

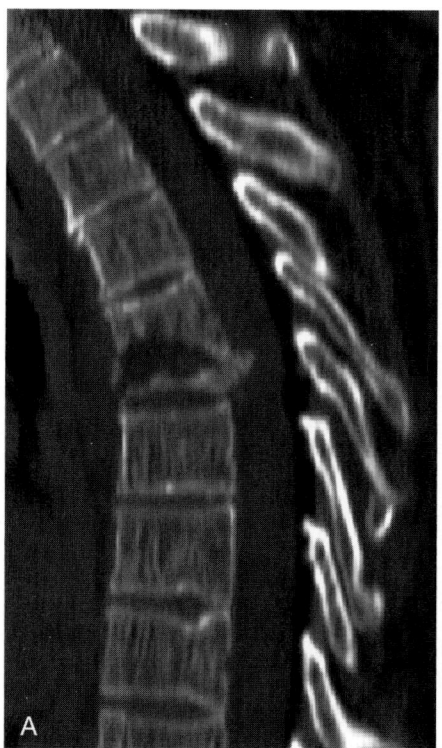
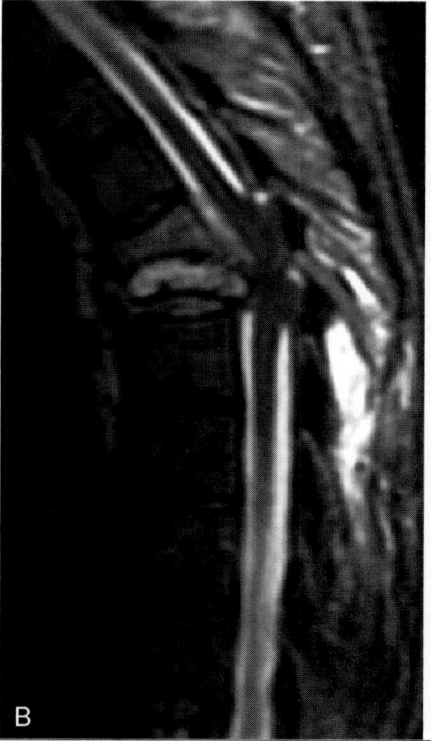
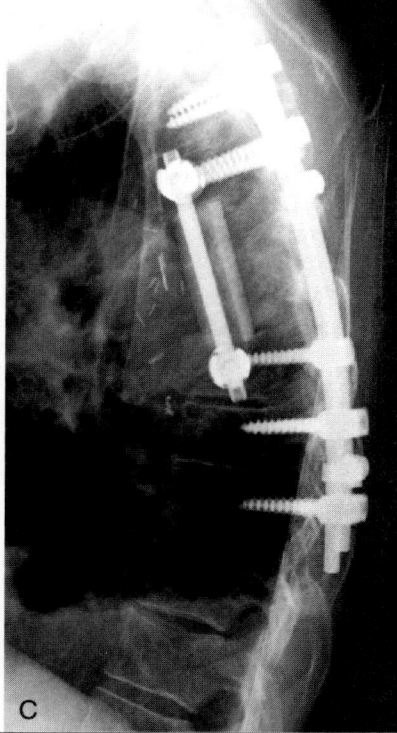

Figure 3 CT **(A)** and MRI **(B)** scans of a 55-year-old immunocompromised alcoholic patient with thoracic pain, loss of lower extremity function, and a recent history of pneumonia revealed destruction and collapse at T5-T6. Anterior corpectomies with allograft reconstruction and instrumentation were followed by a posterior instrumented fusion in a staged fashion **(C)**. Cultures isolated the same organism that had been identified with the prior pneumonia. The patient returned to baseline function and completed the antibiotic course.

throdesis of the diseased segments (Figure 3). Although autograft has been the gold standard graft material, especially in the setting of infection, there is increasing evidence that allograft and/or metallic implants may be acceptable to achieve stability as necessary.[9,10]

Granulomatous Infections

Incidence and Microbiology

Granulomatous infections of the spine, also known as atypical or nonpyogenic infections, are caused by certain atypical bacteria, fungi, or spirochetes. Although collectively these types of infections include a variety of disparate organisms, they are often classified together because of their similar clinical and histologic features. Compared with pyogenic infections, atypical infections are rare in the United States and other developed countries. As the number of immunocompromised hosts has increased, however, so has the incidence of nonpyogenic infections.

Historically, the most common cause of granulomatous spinal infections has been *Mycobacterium tuberculosis*. Approximately 15% of tuberculosis infections disseminate to extrapulmonary sites, with at least 5% affecting the spine. The spinal column is the most common site of extrapulmonary bone involvement. This colonization generally occurs by hematogenous spread, although it may also result from direct extension from visceral lesions.

Granulomatous infections may also be generated by fungal species such as *Aspergillus, Blastomyces, Coccidioides, Histoplasma,* and *Cryptococcus,* all of which are endemic to different regions of the United States. Atypical bacterial species and spirochetes (for example, *Actinomyces israelii* and *Treponema pallidum*) are responsible for an even smaller proportion of granulomatous infections. Although these other pathogens are exceedingly rare compared to *M tuberculosis*, they should be considered in the differential diagnosis when evaluating patients with granulomatous spinal infections.

Atypical infections may also be classified according to the anatomic area of the spine that is involved. The most common scenario is peridiskal disease, in which the focus of infection originates in the metaphysis of a vertebral body and subsequently extends underneath the anterior longitudinal ligament to adjacent spinal segments. Unlike the more typical pyogenic infections, the nidus of infection is established in the middle of the vertebral body, where it remains isolated and the disks are relatively spared. Because of their anatomic pattern, these lesions are often mistaken for tumors and may often lead to deformity secondary to collapse of the diseased vertebral body.

Clinical Presentation
Patients with granulomatous spinal infections will typically present with thoracic discomfort, which is the most common site of involvement. These individuals also usually report a history of fever, weight loss, malaise, night sweats, or other systemic complaints. In particular, these constitutional signs and symptoms may be difficult to interpret in immunocompromised patients who are predisposed for developing these infections. The diagnosis of nonpyogenic infections may be further complicated by the tendency of pain to be a relatively late finding that may only become apparent once significant vertebral collapse and deformity have already occurred. In the absence of any pathognomonic clinical features, a high index of suspicion should always be maintained for a patient with risk factors for atypical spinal infections.

Diagnostic Studies
Laboratory studies may be suggestive of infection in the setting of granulomatous infections, but are generally nonspecific. Although the WBC count, ESR, and CRP level may suggest a reactive process, these values may be normal in as many as 25% of affected patients. In general, these indicators of systemic inflammation are usually less elevated in patients with atypical infections when compared with indicators in patients with pyogenic diskitis or osteomyelitis. Individuals with active tuberculosis or previous exposure to *Mycobacterium* will normally exhibit a positive tuberculin purified protein derivative (PPD) skin test, but this test result may be falsely negative in an anergic patient (and can be assessed with control skin tests).

Sputum specimens collected from subjects with pulmonary disease may also reveal acid-fast bacilli (AFB). However, cultures may be negative by the time remote involvement is declared. An absolute diagnosis of tuberculosis requires a tissue biopsy of the spinal lesion itself, which should be sent for AFB stains and cultures. The detection of other atypical bacteria and fungal species also necessitates special stains and tissue preparations.

Other than a chest radiograph, which should be obtained for any patient suspected of having tuberculosis, the radiographic evaluation of atypical spinal infections is similar to that of pyogenic disease. Given the insidious nature of granulomatous infections, any changes on plain radiographs may be slow to develop. Even when present, radiographic signs may be subtle and include findings such as peridiskal disease and scalloping of the anterior aspects of the vertebral bodies. However, because the onset of back pain and other clinical symptoms may be delayed in patients with these types of infections, the initial screening radiographs of the spine may reveal significant bony destruction and collapse of the affected segments associated with a focal kyphotic deformity.

MRI remains the imaging modality of choice for evaluating granulomatous infections and provides the most information regarding the extent of both bony and soft-tissue involvement. The pathologic signal changes are similar for both atypical and pyogenic infections, although there is generally relative sparing of the intervertebral disks with granulomatous lesions. The addition of gadolinium is useful for distinguishing between an abscess that will only demonstrate peripheral enhancement and an accumulation of granulation tissue, characterized by a more global increase in signal intensity throughout the entire soft-tissue lesion.

Management
Pharmacotherapy directed at the causative pathogen is the most effective treatment of granulomatous infections, but the effective medical management of these infections has become more difficult with the emergence of more atypical organisms and worsening drug-resistant patterns.

The standard empirical treatment of tuberculosis calls for the long-term administration of isoniazid, rifampin, pyrazinamide, and either streptomycin or ethambutol. It is possible that some of these medications may be able to be discontinued based on the results of culture and sensitivity testing. Patients with active disease usually undergo a minimum of 6 to 12 months of therapy, although the final duration of treatment will ultimately be dictated by their subsequent response to medical management. Most fungal species are adequately covered with either one or a combination of antifungal agents, such as amphotericin B and ketoconazole.

Because of the chronic nature of nonpyogenic infections, urgent surgical intervention is rarely required except for situations marked by progressive neurologic decline. In these instances, surgical decompression has been shown to bring about greater neurologic recovery than chemotherapy alone. Otherwise, surgery is considered for abscesses, deformity, or failure of medical management.

The surgical treatment of granulomatous infections varies according to the specific anatomic site of involvement and extent of vertebral collapse. The current recommendations for anterior lesions include débridement followed by reconstruction. Anterior column support is critical for restoring alignment and limiting the development of a late kyphotic deformity. The stability of the vertebral column may be restored using a strut graft with or without supplementary internal fixation. These are often complex surgical interventions, with significant potential morbidity. Fortunately, persistent colonization of metal implants is far less common with granulomatous infections than it is with pyogenic infections.

Epidural Infections

Incidence and Microbiology
An epidural abscess is an infection outside the dura but within the bony spinal canal in the area of the epidural adipose tissue. This occurs most commonly as an extension of adjacent vertebral osteomyelitis or diskitis; however, hematogenous seeding of bacteria and direct

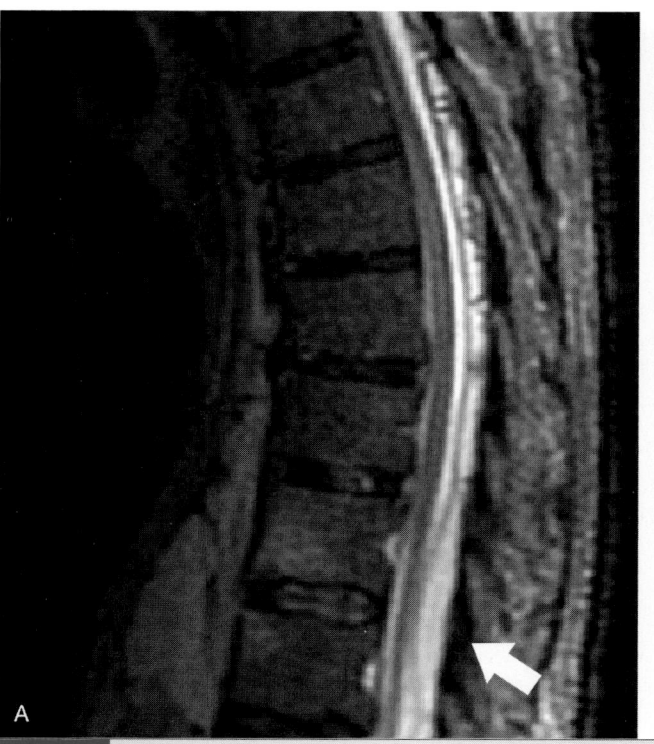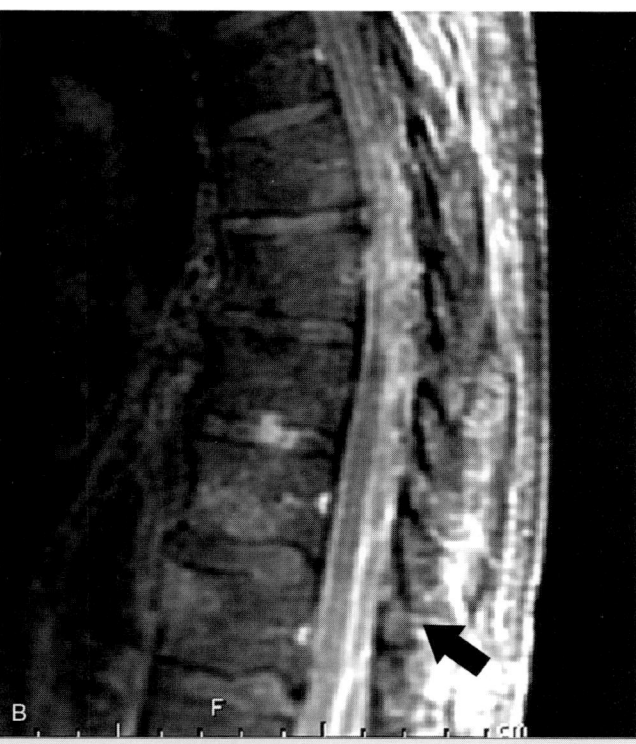

Figure 4 | T2-weighted MRI scan of an 87-year-old man with diffuse back pain and gradual decline in ambulation revealed a thoracolumbar posterior epidural abscess (**A**, *arrow)*, which was rim-enhanced with gadolinium (**B**, *arrow)*. The patient was treated with laminectomy. Broad-spectrum antibiotics were initiated and tailored once bacteria was isolated.

inoculation during spinal procedures are also potential etiologies of epidural infection. Epidural abscesses currently account for approximately 7% of all spinal infections, and their incidence has continued to rise over the past decade, due in part to the increased population of immunocompromised patients and the growing number of invasive spinal procedures. Epidural abscesses usually occur in adults 60 years of age or older and affect both genders equally.

Most spinal epidural abscesses occur in the thoracic (51%) and lumbar (35%) spine and tend to be in the posterior epidural space. To a much lesser extent, epidural abscesses occur in the cervical spine and tend to be in the anterior epidural space. Although these infections may be focal, epidural abscesses frequently extend over three to four motion segments. *S aureus* is identified as the causative agent in more than 60% of these cases, whereas gram-negative rods are responsible for another 20%.

Clinical Presentation

As with other types of spinal infections, the clinical presentation of an individual with an epidural abscess is highly variable, which is why these lesions may be initially misdiagnosed in as many as 50% of patients. Intractable neck or back pain is the most common complaint associated with these infections, and patients with acute epidural abscesses generally report more constitutional symptoms consistent with a systemic illness than do those with vertebral osteomyelitis or disk-

itis. Of note, chronic infections may be present in compromised hosts or with organisms of lesser virulence and associated with lesser symptoms.

Over time, neurologic deficits may develop secondary to direct compression of the neural elements by the focus of infection. In the absence of appropriate treatment, patients with epidural infections may even progress to complete paralysis. Neurologic deficit may be present more than expected based on the degree of neural element compression, which is believed to be related to the vascular effect of infections in this region.

Diagnostic Studies

As with other spinal infections, patients with epidural abscesses may exhibit leukocytosis and generally have elevated ESR and CRP levels. Blood cultures are positive in 60% of affected patients. A definitive diagnosis is best established by obtaining tissue or fluid specimens directly from the abscess; cultures of this material have been shown to have a sensitivity of at least 90%.

Plain radiographs of the spine often appear unremarkable, unless there is a concurrent vertebral osteomyelitis or diskitis that is sufficiently advanced to produce radiographic abnormalities. As with radiography, CT has limited utility for the detection of epidural abscesses. Because of its ability to visualize the soft tissues and fluid collections, MRI with gadolinium is considered to be the imaging modality of choice for identifying epidural abscesses (**Figure 4**).

Management

Once the diagnosis of an epidural abscess has been confirmed, a proper treatment plan must be instituted immediately to prevent further deterioration in the patient's condition. The primary goal of treatment is preservation or improvement of neurologic function, eradication of the infection, relief of axial pain, and maintenance of spinal stability.

Surgical intervention is the mainstay of treatment of patients with epidural abscesses. Recent studies have suggested that patients who are neurologically intact may be considered for nonsurgical treatment with antibiotics alone, but any evidence of progressive neurologic decline or lack of response warrants emergent surgical intervention.[11] However, with the exception of these rare considerations (for example, patients not deemed to be suitable surgical candidates), it is recommended that most patients with epidural abscesses undergo surgical decompression of the affected levels followed by antibiotic therapy.

The specific surgical approach is again dependent on the anatomic location of the epidural abscess. Because most of these lesions are based posteriorly, a laminectomy is often required to adequately decompress the infection. When an abscess arises secondary to vertebral osteomyelitis, an anterior or circumferential decompression may be required. Fusion with or without instrumentation is also indicated if spinal stability is compromised either by the infection itself or as a result of any subsequent decompression or débridement of the abscess.

As with other types of spinal infections, the wound may be closed primarily over drains, left open for serial débridements, or managed with specialized wound care systems (such as suction/irrigation or vacuum-assisted closure.

Annotated References

1. Fang A, Hu SS, Endres N, Bradford DS: Risk factors for infections after spinal surgery. *Spine* 2005;30:1460-1465.

   In a retrospective review, 48 spinal infections were evaluated. Age older than 60 years, smoking, diabetes, previous surgical infection, increased body mass index, and alcohol abuse were preoperative risk factors. Staged anterior/posterior fusions were the most common type of surgery. Level of evidence: III.

2. Hansen SM, Sasso RC: Resorptive response if rhBMP2 simulating infection in an anterior lumbar interbody fusion with a femoral ring. *J Spinal Disord Tech* 2006;19:130-134.

   Recombinant bone morphogenetic proteins are being used with increased frequency for on- and off-label uses. This case report highlights the potential resorptive effect around such implants and the importance of recognizing that this may mimic the appearance of infection. Level of evidence: IV.

3. Brown EM, Pople IK, de Louvois J, et al: Spine update: Prevention of postoperative infection in patients undergoing spinal infection. *Spine* 2004;29:938-945.

   The authors review the incidence, prophylaxis, and management of postoperative spine infections. Level of evidence: III.

4. Cheng MT, Chang MC, Wang ST, Ye WK, Liu CL, Chen TH: Efficacy of dilute betadine solution irrigation in the prevention of postoperative infection of spinal surgery. *Spine* 2005;30:1689-1693.

   Patients undergoing spinal surgery were randomized to undergo irrigation with dilute betadine (3.5%) or saline. Decreased infections were observed in the experimental group, and this practice was advocated, particularly in patients with increased infection risk. Level of evidence: I.

5. Brown MD, Brookfield KFW: A randomized study of closed wound suction drainage for extensive lumbar spine surgery. *Spine* 2004;29:1066-1068.

   Patients undergoing significant spinal surgery were randomized to receive a postoperative drain or no drain. There were no significant differences in rates of infection, epidural hematoma, or new neurologic deficits. The use of postoperative drains could not be supported by these data. Level of evidence: II.

6. Mehbod AA, Ogilvie JW, Pinto MR, et al: Postoperative deep wound infections in adults after spinal fusion: Management with vacuum-assisted wound closure. *J Spinal Disord Tech* 2005;18:14-17.

   Vacuum-assisted wound closure has been used more commonly in the management of spinal infections. A series of patients with postoperative spine infections were treated with vacuum-assisted wound closure dressings and delayed wound closure. All patients went on to clear their infections without removal of instrumentation. Level of evidence: IV.

7. Khan MH, Smith PN, Rao N, Donaldson WF: Serum C-reactive protein levels correlate with clinical response in patients treated with antibiotics for wound infections after spinal surgery. *Spine J* 2006;6:311-315.

   The authors of this study assessed patients undergoing treatment of postoperative spine infections and reported that C-reactive protein levels improved during the treatment course. However, the erythrocyte sedimentation rate did not show the same correlation, despite improvement in C-reactive protein levels and clinical picture. Level of evidence: IV.

8. An HS, Seldomridge JA: Spinal infections: Diagnostic tests and imaging studies. *Clin Orthop Relat Res* 2006;444:27-33.

   The diagnosis of spinal infections can be challenging. This article reviews the workup of patients presenting with a clinical picture suggestive of spinal infection. Level of evidence: V.

9. Dimar JR, Carreon LY, Glassman SD, Campbell MJ, Hartman MJ, Johnson JR: Treatment of pyogenic vertebral osteomyelitis with anterior debridement and fusion

followed by delayed posterior spinal fusion. *Spine* 2004; 29:326-332.

Patients with pyogenic vertebral osteomyelitis were treated with anerior débridement and fusion followed by delayed posterior spinal fusion. All patients had resolution of their infections and no evidence of recurrence. This is a common treatment course for patients who have not responded to medical management of this condition. Level of evidence: IV.

10. Korovessis P, Petsinis G, Koureas G, Iliopoulos P, Zacharatos S: Anterior surgery with instrumentation of titanium mesh cage and posterior instrumented fusion performed sequentially on the same day under one anesthesia for septic spondylitis of thoracolumbar spine: Is the use of titanium mesh cages safe? *Spine* 2006;31:

1014-1019.

Patients with pyogenic vertebral osteomyelitis were treated as described in the article title. Patient outcomes were acceptable, and this treatment was proposed as a surgical option. Level of evidence: IV.

11. Savage K, Holton PD, Zalavras CG: Spinal epidural abscess: Early clinical outcome in patients treated medically. *Clin Orthop Relat Res* 2005;439:56-60.

Epidural abscesses have traditionally been managed surgically. This retrospective study evaluated patients with no systemic sepsis and a normal or stable neurologic examination who were treated medically. This appeared to be a viable management option in selected patients with close clinical following. Level of evidence: IV.

5: Spine

Chapter 49

Adult Spinal Deformity

*Anthony Rinella, MD   *Clifford Tribus, MD   Patrick J. Cahill, MD

Adult Scoliosis

Adult spinal deformity encompasses a wide range of spinal pathologies and is defined by multiple parameters. Some authors prefer a broad chronologic definition, such as the onset of scoliosis of more than 10° after skeletal maturity. Others prefer a definition that includes a specific age, such as scoliosis recognized in a patient older than 25 years. Both definitions have limitations—the former because the timing of skeletal maturity can be difficult to ascertain and varies between genders, and the latter because of the considerable unlabeled time gap between adolescent idiopathic scoliosis and adult scoliosis. No specific age has yet been standardized for adult scoliosis. Adult idiopathic scoliosis is a complex condition with a wide age distribution that is complicated by an increased likelihood of segmental or global alignment decompensations, symptomatic lumbar spondylosis or spinal stenosis, or significant medical comorbidities.

Classification Systems

The most basic classification system separates adult spinal deformity into two subgroups: new-onset (de novo) scoliosis and preexisting idiopathic scoliosis that progresses into adulthood. The two groups can often be difficult to distinguish and the distinction has limited clinical value. Less common types of spinal deformities include posttraumatic, iatrogenic, paralytic, neuromuscular, or congenital deformities, or curves related to severe osteoporosis.

The Adult Deformity Committee of the Scoliosis Research Society developed the most complete radiographic classification of adult spinal deformity based on standing, full-length (14 in × 36 in) radiographs in the coronal and sagittal planes.[1] The goal was to establish a universal classification system to provide a radiographic framework for categorizing complex adult spinal deformities, to provide insight into treatment strategies, and to facilitate the comparison of various treatment methods. Important changes were made to the Lenke classification system of adolescent idiopathic scoliosis, including the addition of a seventh major category (primary sagittal deformity), a regional sagittal modifier (upper thoracic, main thoracic, thoracolumbar, and lumbar), a lumbar degenerative modifier (degenerative disk disease, listhesis, and fractional lumbosacral curve), and a global balance modifier (sagittal and coronal).[2]

Disease Burden

The incidence of scoliosis in the general adult population is estimated to be 2.9% based on a review of 5,000 intravenous pyelograms.[3] Although most curves are between 10° to 24°, a correlation has been noted between curves of more than 45° and the presence of back pain. The prevalence of back pain, however, seems to be somewhat age-dependent. In another recent study, the incidence of scoliosis was found to be much higher (68%) in a group of healthy volunteers with an average age of 70.5 years.[4]

Several studies have shown that scoliosis has a negative impact on the overall health of adult patients. In a series of studies with long-term follow-up, an increased frequency, intensity, and duration of back pain was found in adults with untreated adult scoliosis compared with an age-matched control group.[5] Sixty-one percent of adults with untreated scoliosis reported chronic back pain compared with 35% in the control group; however, most patients reported only little or moderate back pain. Outcomes studies further objectify these findings. A 2003 study showed the significant negative impact of adult scoliosis on Medical Outcomes Study 36-Item Short Form Health Survey (SF-36) scores and on Scoliosis Research Society-22 scores.[6] However, the data did not show any relationship between severity of the disability and radiographic markers. Another study also found a significant decrease in SF-36 scores in adults with scoliosis.[4] The SF-36 scores were also lower than those of adults with sciatica but without scoliosis. Although these outcomes data are important for understanding adult scoliosis, clear clinical recommendations have not yet been elucidated.

Several studies have shown the strongly negative ef-

*Anthony Rinella, MD or the department with which he is affiliated has received research of institutional support from Medtronic DePuy and Synthes. Clifford Tribus, MD or the department with which he is affiliated has received research or institutional support from Danek (Medtronic), miscellaneous nonincome support, commercially derived honoraria, or other nonresearch related funding from Danek (Medtronic), royalties from Stryker Spine, holds stock or stock options in St. Francis Medical, and is a consultant or employee for St. Francis Medical and Stryker Spine.

5: Spine

fects of fixed positive sagittal imbalance. In the largest of these studies, the authors found positive sagittal imbalance to be the greatest predictor of symptomatology, and also found that coronal imbalance of more than 4 cm was predictive of pain.[7] The presence of thoracolumbar or lumbar deformity was a greater predictor for lower outcome scores than thoracic deformity. The same group of authors demonstrated an inverse linear relationship between outcome measures and sagittal imbalance.

A 1983 study demonstrated the natural history of idiopathic scoliosis and identified risk factors for curve progression after skeletal maturity.[8] Curves with a magnitude of less than 30° did not progress. Thoracic curves greater than 50°, with apical vertebral rotation greater than 30°, or a Mehta angle greater than 30° tended to progress. Lumbar and thoracolumbar curves of more than 30° with apical vertebral rotation greater than 30° or with translatory shifts tended to progress. The relationship of the fifth lumbar vertebra to the iliac crest and the direction of the curve were also predictive of progression in lumbar curves. Thoracic curves progress at a rate of approximately 1° per year until they reach 75°, at which point progression slows to 0.3° per year. Lumbar curves progress at a rate of 0.3° to 0.4° per year. In combined curves, the thoracic component progresses at a rate of 0.3° per year and the lumbar component progresses at 0.3° to 0.6° per year. Based on these findings, surgical stabilization in curves of more than 50° is often indicated. Curves from 30° to 50° should be evaluated every 3 to 5 years (or sooner if symptomatic) to document the rate and type of progression.

Patient Evaluation
Patient History
A detailed patient history is the most crucial element in the evaluation of an adult patient with spinal deformity. Back pain is the most common and chief reported problem, but symptoms related to neurogenic claudication are also common. The patient history should focus on establishing a time line for the disorder and sorting the origins of axial back and radicular pain generators. Similarly, it is important to distinguish tenderness related to spinal curvature from sacroiliac or hip disease, and to distinguish peripheral from central nerve impingement syndromes. Symptoms often vary considerably with patient age; therefore, adult deformity should be approached as a continuum instead of a homogenous group. For example, patients younger than 40 years often have disease characteristics that are more similar to those of patients with adolescent idiopathic scoliosis than patients with more pronounced degenerative changes. The effect of the condition on the patient's vocational and daily activities is important. Because prior radiographs are often unavailable, clues about the progression of the deformity may be determined from information about changes in height, trunk position, and clothing size and fit. Increases in the frequency or severity of episodes of back pain may also be

an indication of a worsening deformity. Other important considerations include details of prior surgeries and the benefits of prior nonsurgical management (physical therapy, injections, and medications).

Physical Examination
A thorough physical examination is needed because multiple pain generators or areas of spinal deformity may be present. A basic examination includes evaluation of any rib prominence, lumbar or trapezial fullness, asymmetry of shoulder heights, pelvic obliquity, and the relationship of the rib cage to the pelvis. Musculoskeletal examination should include evaluation of gait, and amount/quality of lower extremity range of motion. Contractures and dysfunction in any of these joints or limb-length inequality may lead to compensatory alterations in spinal alignment. Conversely, a longstanding spinal deformity or sagittal imbalance may be compensated for by hip and/or knee flexion. It is helpful to assess the flexibility of individual curves and the degree of difficulty the patient has in attaining neutral alignment with their hips and knees in full extension. A complete neurologic and distal lower extremity vascular evaluation is essential. When examining the lumbosacral junction (a common area of concern), special attention should be directed to areas of midline, paraspinal, sacroiliac, gluteal, groin, and peritrochanteric tenderness to help distinguish spinal pain generators from sacroiliac, hip, or radicular pain generators.

Imaging
Upright, 36-in, long-cassette, PA and lateral radiographs are the front-line studies used to evaluate adult spinal deformity. PA radiographs as opposed to AP radiographs are recommended to limit radiation exposure to the neck and chest. The lateral radiograph should be taken with the knees fully extended to properly evaluate sagittal balance. Cobb angles can be measured on the PA radiograph to quantify the degree of deformity. The PA radiograph may also reveal signs of spondylosis, the extent of apical rotation, and areas of segmental olisthesis (rotational step-offs) or asymmetric facet collapse (Figure 1). Common areas of neural impingement include vertical foraminal compression or lateral recess stenosis in the concavity of the lumbar or fractional lumbosacral curves; or central, lateral recess, or foraminal stenosis in areas of olisthesis, asymmetric facet degeneration, or spondylolisthesis. Lateral radiographs should also be evaluated for evidence of disk space narrowing, spondylolisthesis, and spondylosis. Supine PA and bending radiographs are useful for predicting curve flexibility before surgery. The supine radiographs may help define pedicle anatomy and patient alignment during surgery. Traction or bolster views also may be helpful in assessing flexibility. MRI scans are usually obtained to assess disk degeneration and areas of neural compression. A CT myelogram also may be used in patients who were previously treated with instrumentation, or when MRI is contraindicated. A myelogram may show areas of neural compression in the upright

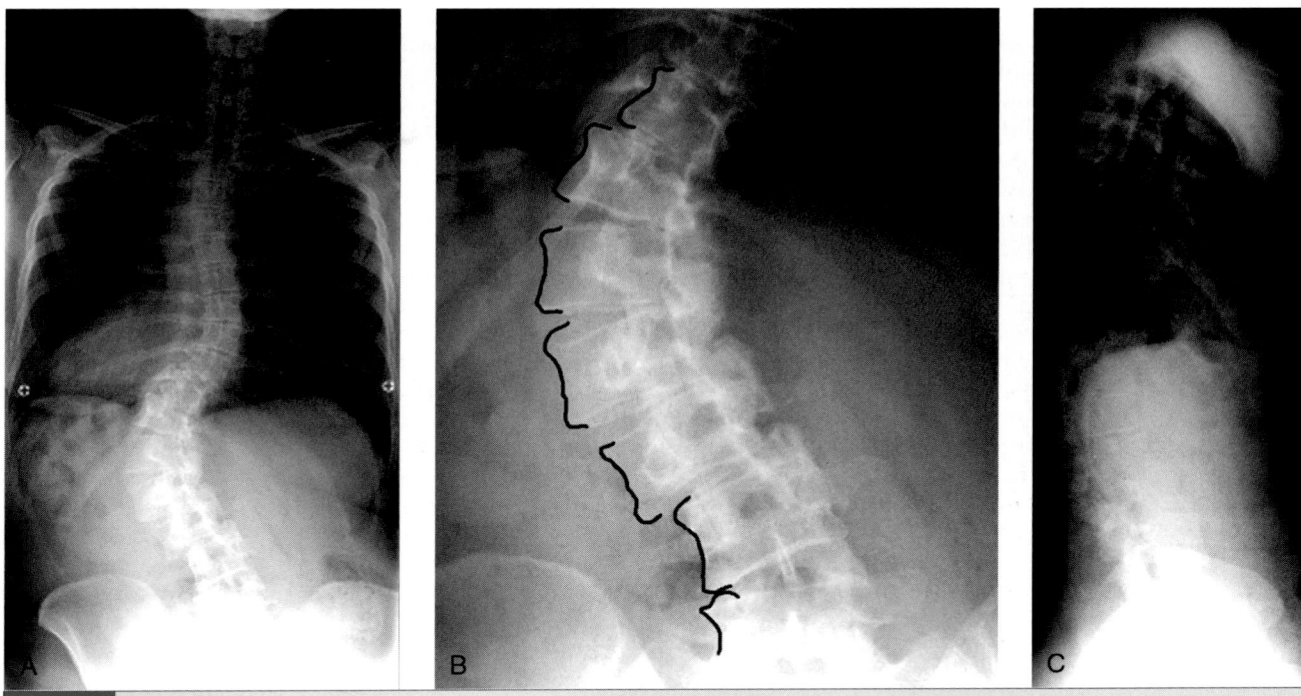

Figure 1 Radiographs of a 60-year-old woman with lumbar back pain. **A**, AP radiograph shows a primary lumbar curve with compensatory thoracic and lumbosacral curves. **B**, A magnified AP view shows significant apical rotation; olisthesis at T11-12, L2-3, and L3-4; and asymmetric degenerative changes on the left at L4-5. **C**, Lateral radiograph shows that the patient has neutral sagittal balance, but thoracolumbar kyphosis and compensatory lower thoracic lordosis.

position that may not be as clear on a standard supine CT scan.

Nonsurgical Treatment

The goal of nonsurgical treatment of adult spinal deformity is to limit the severity and frequency of pain, improve quality of life, and maximize overall function. To effectively achieve this goal, it is important to understand the source(s) of pain. Front-line treatments for axial back pain, muscular fatigue, and mild radicular symptoms include activity modification, physical therapy, and anti-inflammatory drug regimens. It is important to understand the type and quality of past physical therapy and long-term patient compliance. Anti-inflammatory drug regimens may be limited by a history of gastric ulcers, renal insufficiency, or patient intolerance. If sacroiliac, peritrochanteric, or radicular pain is the primary symptom or will significantly limit participation in a core strengthening program, various injections of steroids and local anesthetics may be considered. The goals of these injections are both diagnostic and therapeutic. A short-term improvement in the level of radicular pain after an epidural steroid injection may be interpreted as failed treatment by the patient, but can provide valuable information about the relative contribution to pain generation of a specific area of neural compression. Close communication with the physician who is performing the injections is necessary to maximize the goals of nonsurgical management of adult spinal deformity. The timing of administration

of these various modalities must be tailored to the relative contributions of various pain generators, patient motivation, and concerns. Bracing has limited value in this patient population because it may contribute to atrophy of the core musculature. Chronic pain syndromes may benefit from a multidisciplinary approach that includes pain specialists, physiatrists, and acupuncture specialists. The period of nonsurgical treatment should also be used to gain a deeper sense of the patient's motivation, secondary gains, and social structure.

Surgical Treatment

Typical indications for surgery are chronic pain and/or disability that nonsurgical treatment has failed to improve, progression of the spinal deformity in curves of more than 50°, progressive neurologic compromise, and the development of poor spinal balance causing functional difficulties. The necessity for a thorough course of nonsurgical management cannot be overstated, except in rare instances of rapid neurologic deterioration or myelopathy. Information gained from evaluating injection treatments, when appropriate, is helpful in setting patient expectations for relief from various pain generators.

Prior to surgical intervention, it is critical to determine if the patient is a surgical candidate. Algorithmic assessment of radiographic evidence is not appropriate because of the high physiologic stress of surgery and the relatively high risk of complications. An assessment of the patient's physiologic age is more important than chronologic age; however, healthy elderly patients may not have the physiologic reserves necessary for recuperation. Medical clearance of the patient is typically recommended; however, it is important for the clearing physician to understand the length of surgery, anticipated blood loss, and rehabilitation period. Preoperative nutritional status must be maximized, and perioperative nutrition must also be considered to minimize complications (especially in staged procedures).[9] An understanding of the patient's psychology and support network are also important. Some authors recommend a formal psychological evaluation as part of the multidisciplinary treatment regimen.

The goals of surgical treatment of adult scoliosis are to alleviate and prevent worsening of symptoms by restoring stability and balance to the spine and decompressing neural elements. These goals are best achieved with rigid fixation that may diminish or obviate the need for postoperative external immobilization, allow more rapid and aggressive rehabilitation, and improve the likelihood for a solid bony fusion. It is important to understand the biomechanics of various regions of the spine, accommodate transitions into compensatory curves, and limit the potential for transition syndromes. Transition syndrome is a term used to describe changes to the levels immediately adjacent to a fusion, either proximally or distally. At times, rapid degeneration or loss of correction may occur (Figure 2). The restoration of spinal balance, especially in the sagittal plane, cannot be overemphasized.

Thoracic Deformities

Thoracic deformities are less likely to require stabilization than lumbar curves because of the inherent stability of the rib cage. However, large curves (> 75°) with significant rotational abnormalities may contribute to restrictive lung disease. Single curves can be treated with anterior or posterior instrumentation, or a combined approach. Important considerations in the decision process are the patient's pulmonary function and flexibility of the curves.

Thoracolumbar and Lumbar Curves

In young patients with a single structural thoracolumbar or lumbar curve and flexible compensatory curves, anterior-only surgery may be considered. Possible advantages of anterior surgery in this setting are the inclusion of fewer segments, lower infection rates, and higher fusion rates. The disadvantage of anterior surgery is the decreased ability to decompress the neural elements and diminished pulmonary function if the diaphragm is incised. If neural decompression is required, or if instrumentation must be extended to L5 or S1, a posterior or combined approach is required. Combined approaches, either single-day or staged, may also be used to maintain or improve sagittal correction, release rigid anterior structures, or improve fusion rates. Anterior support can be performed from a separate anterior or flank approach, lateral approach (extreme lateral interbody fusion), or transforaminal/posterior interbody

fusion. Posterior approaches may provide greater flexibility to decompress neural elements, achieve adequate stability (especially in the low lumbar and lumbosacral regions), and correct sagittal deformities.

It is important to have realistic goals for curve correction and to prioritize the various objectives of surgery. The primary goals remain a well-balanced spine, not a straight spine, and adequate decompression of necessary neural elements. Excessive corrective forces may compromise screw purchase and increase the likelihood of instrumentation failure. For longer surgical procedures, estimating the amount of surgery a patient can safely tolerate and the amount of surgery the surgeon can safely perform is important. Alternate plans that can adapt to surgical aberrations and complications should always be considered. Regular discussions are needed with the anesthesiologist and the team monitoring neurologic function to maximize patient safety throughout the procedure.

Individualized treatment plans should be formulated for adults with two or more structural curves. The plan should consider the severity, flexibility, and overall effect on balance caused by the deformity. In general, when more than one structural curve is present, a posterior or combined approach is required.

Lumbosacral Fixation

One of the more difficult decisions concerns extending the fusion of a lumbar curve construct to the sacrum. Stopping a long construct at L5 requires less surgical time than extending the instrumentation to the sacrum and/or pelvis, but leaves a potential pain generating level and may lead to sagittal decompensation over time. The indications for extending the fusion to the sacrum include pelvic obliquity caused by an unbalanced lumbosacral curve; or disk degeneration, spinal stenosis, or spondylolisthesis at the L5-S1 level. In a recent study, a matched cohort analysis was used to compare the outcomes of patients who had a long fusion to the lowest instrumented vertebra of either L5 or S1.[10] Results showed higher complication rates (including pseudarthrosis, sacroiliitis, and sacral fracture) in patients treated with fusion to the sacrum. However, in the group with spinal fusion to L5, subsequent disk degeneration was common and may be associated with a forward shift in sagittal balance. In another study, long posterior fixation for adult scoliosis was stopped at L5.[11] The authors noted a 38% incidence of radiographic degeneration of L5-S1, with a 19% rate of resurgery in a relatively short follow-up period (average, 32 months). Patients with good preoperative sagittal balance, preserved lumbar lordosis, and good postoperative fractional curve correction are most likely to avoid degeneration at L5-S1. Long fusions that extend distally to L4 or higher do not have predictable rates of disk degeneration immediately below the fusion, but transition syndrome is slightly more common when comparing distal fusion levels of T11-L2 with those at L3-4.[12]

Several important technical considerations should be

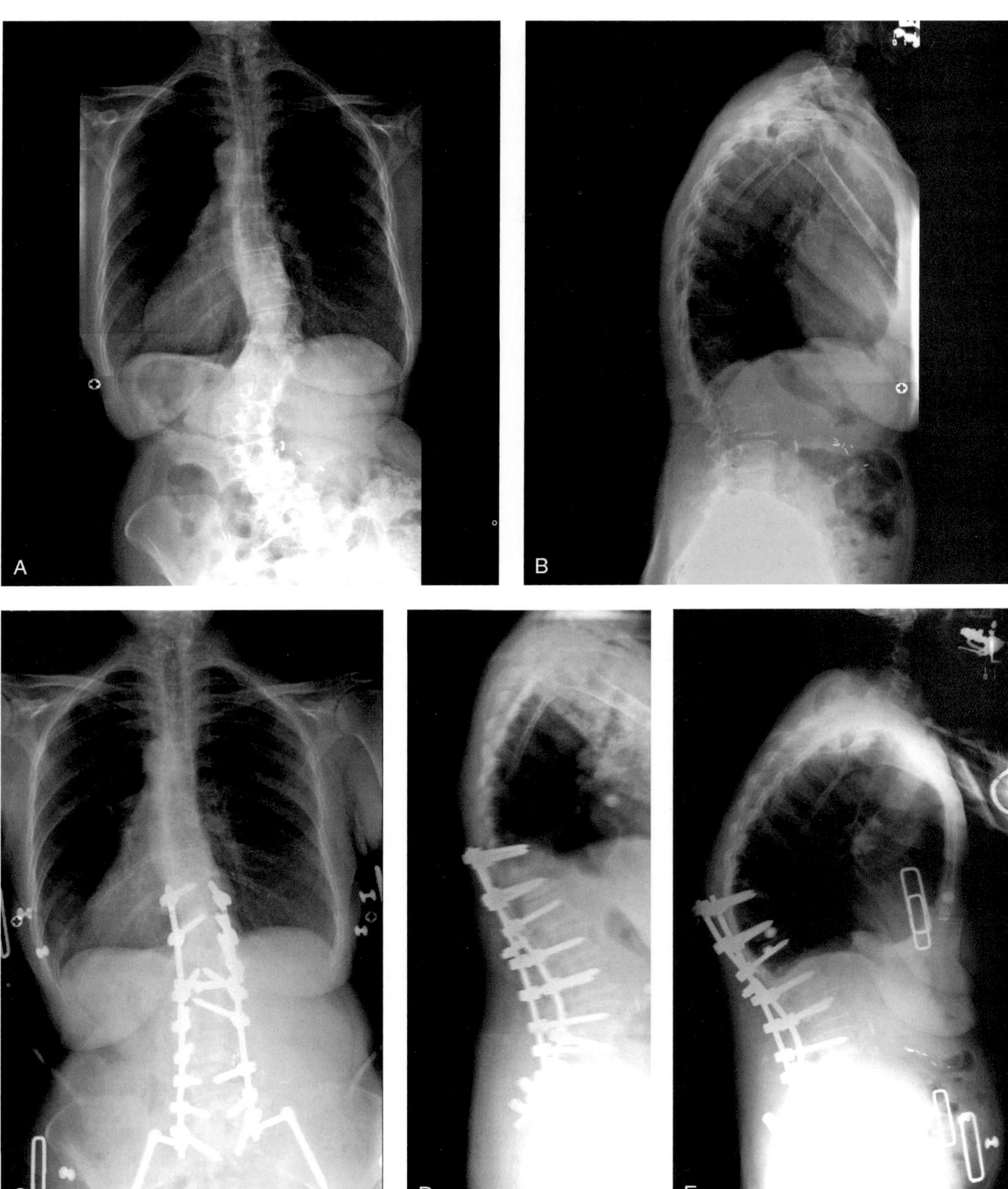

Figure 2 Radiographs of a 58-year-old woman with progressive lumbar back pain. **A,** Preoperative PA view. **B,** Preoperative lateral view showing positive sagittal balance. **C,** Postoperative PA view. **D,** Postoperative lateral view. **E,** Lateral view 6 weeks after surgery demonstrating severe transition syndrome. Although the preoperative radiographs are similar, the lateral views show that the curve patterns shown in Figures 1 and 2 are different. Figure 1 shows a lordotic thoracic spine and neutral sagittal balance, whereas Figure 2 shows a hyperkyphotic thoracic spine and positive sagittal balance.

5: Spine

made when performing lumbosacral fusion. Both anterior and posterior instrumented fusion should be considered to minimize the potential for pseudarthrosis. This goal can be achieved with separate anterior and posterior approaches or with transforaminal or posterior lumbar interbody fusion. A separate anterior lumbar approach offers a twofold advantage: easier exposure to adjacent disks, and lordotic cages can be inserted. Maintaining lordosis in the lower lumbar spine is important because two thirds of lumbar lordosis occurs through the lowest two segments. A posterior interbody technique avoids the time and complications of using an anterior approach. It should be noted that these techniques are technically more difficult to perform in this setting because there is more blood in the surgical field.

In long fusions to the sacrum, the S1 screws should be backed up with appropriate secondary instrumentation. In a 2002 study using a calf spine model, several types of supplementary fixation to S1 screws were tested.[13] All types of secondary instrumentation provided considerable additional stability; however, iliac screws were the most biomechanically sound because they provided the greatest reduction of S1 strain and catastrophic failure.

Intraoperative Monitoring and Management
Adult scoliosis surgery frequently is associated with significant blood loss and fluid resuscitation. The anesthesiologist and surgical team must communicate regularly to minimize the likelihood of hemodynamic instability. Whether to use autologous or homologous blood is a decision that should be made by the patient and surgeon. For neurologic spinal cord monitoring, somatosensory- and motor-evoked potentials and electromyography may be used. If evidence of neurologic compromise is encountered, a source must be actively sought and corrected. Active communication between the monitoring and anesthesia teams is necessary to ensure that monitoring changes are not caused by the type of anesthesia used, anemia, or hypothermia. When doubt exists, a wake-up test remains the gold standard to ensure unimpaired neurologic function. If complications occur during correction or thereafter, the instrumentation must be released and the neurologic condition subsequently reevaluated.

Proximal Fusion Levels
Controversy remains concerning whether to set the upper-instrumented vertebra for primary lumbar curves at the upper lumbar spine (L1-L2), the lower thoracic spine (T8-12), or upper thoracic spine (T2-T4). Stopping the construct at L1 avoids disruption of the thoracolumbar junction, but places considerable stress on this region. Extending the instrumentation to T10 avoids this situation, but moves the upper-instrumented vertebra closer to the thoracic apex of kyphosis. Decompensation at this level may lead to severe junctional kyphosis in osteoporotic patients (Figure 2). Extending the instrumentation to the upper thoracic spine avoids midthoracic decompensation, but moves the transition

zone more proximally and extends surgical time. Ongoing studies are attempting to determine the ideal types of instrumentation (hooks, pedicle screws, hybrid constructs) to minimize the risks of transition and pseudarthrosis.

Outcomes
Fusion for adult scoliosis is a reliable method of treating pain symptoms related to spinal curvature. One study showed that a reduction in pain symptoms of 70% or more can be expected, and another study found an improvement in pain symptoms in 74% of adult scoliosis patients treated with surgery.[14,15] The overall patient satisfaction rate was 87%. An accurate diagnosis of the source of pain leads to improved outcomes. Normal postoperative sacral inclination and a C7 plumb line lead to decreased radiographic evidence of adjacent-level degeneration.

Complications frequently occur following surgical treatment for adults with scoliosis. The results of one study showed complication rates as high as 40%.[16] However, most complications are minor and have no impact on final outcome. Neurologic injury is rare but potentially devastating. Risk factors for neurologic injury in adults undergoing surgery for scoliosis include extreme kyphosis, combined anterior and posterior surgery, and the presence of large, rigid curves.[17] Pulmonary embolism can occur and is most frequent in elderly patients who undergo anterior surgery. The placement of prophylactic inferior vena cava filters in high-risk patients to reduce the likelihood of pulmonary embolism is recommended by some authors.[18] Infection rates of 1% to 8% have been reported.

The most common long-term complication related to poor outcomes is pseudarthrosis. In a study of 96 adult scoliosis patients, the authors found a strong negative correlation between pseudarthrosis and outcomes as measured by Scoliosis Research Society-24 scores.[19] The authors reported a positive correlation for pseudarthrosis with the number of surgical levels (> 12) and patient age (older than 55 years). The authors also noted that pseudarthrosis usually occurred between the T9 and L1 levels, at sites of cross-links or dominoes, and occurred over multiple levels. In a larger study, the authors noted a 24% rate of pseudarthrosis in long fusion down to the sacrum.[20] Thoracolumbar kyphosis, osteoarthritis of the hip, use of the thoracoabdominal approach (versus a paramedian approach), positive sagittal balance of 5 cm or more, patient age of 55 years or older, and incomplete sacropelvic fixation significantly increased the likelihood of pseudarthrosis.

Sagittal Plane Deformity

Sagittal plane deformity is a condition of spinal imbalance in which the patient is unable to maintain an upright posture in the sagittal plane. The condition can lead to functional and social deficits and thus can have a profound effect on quality of life. Before treating sagittal imbalance, the surgeon must identify and quantify the patient's condition, ultimately determining whether the potential gain in quality of life is sufficient to warrant the risks of surgery.

Etiology

Loss of lumbar lordosis most commonly results from degenerative disk disease associated with aging; this condition usually does not lead to sagittal imbalance. The most common cause of fixed sagittal imbalance is iatrogenic flat back secondary to distraction instrumentation used in treating scoliosis in the lower lumbar spine. Other iatrogenic causes of sagittal imbalance include anterior instrumented fusion performed in compression (with or without interbody support), multilevel lumbar laminectomy, posterior interbody fusion performed with cylindrical cages (with or without posterior transpedicular stabilization), instrumented posterior lumbar fusion performed in or settled into a position of kyphosis (using, for example, the Andrews frame), multilevel lumbar pseudarthroses, junctional kyphosis, and spondylolisthesis adjacent to a previous fusion. The noniatrogenic causes of sagittal imbalance include thoracolumbar trauma leading to posttraumatic deformity, multilevel compression fracture, and congenital kyphoscoliosis.

The treatment of flat back has evolved from surgical techniques developed to correct ankylosing spondylitis. Ankylosing spondylitis is an enthesopathy characterized by inflammation leading to calcification and ossification of the points of attachment to bone of ligaments, tendons, and joint capsules. In the spine, the disease occurs in the outer layers of the anulus fibrosus of the disk and ultimately leads to the classic bamboo or autofused spine, frequently in kyphotic imbalance.

Classification

No validated classification system exists for sagittal imbalance. Table 1 presents an etiologic classification system that includes modifying factors affecting treatment decisions.

Sagittal balance should not be confused with sagittal deformity. Sagittal balance refers to the global position of the spine relative to the sacrum. Sagittal deformity refers to a segment of the spine that is outside the normal range, such as 20° to 45° for the thoracic spine. In normal alignment, the head is aligned directly over the sacrum (Figure 3). Sagittal imbalance occurs when a sagittal deformity in one area of the spine cannot be compensated for by the rest of the spine. Clinically positive sagittal imbalance is the inability of the patient to stand upright because the head position is in front of the pelvis. On a long-cassette lateral radiograph, this condition is seen if the C7 plumb line lies anterior to the sacral promontory.

A sagittal deformity that is well compensated for within the spinal column, such as Scheuermann's kyphosis, is termed congruent. Sagittal balance is normal when the hips and knees are extended. An incongruent

Table 1

Causes of Fixed Sagittal Imbalance

Iatrogenic Causes

Distraction instrumentation used in scoliosis treatment, extending to the lower lumbar spine

Anterior instrumented fusion performed in compression or without adequate interbody support

Multilevel lumbar laminectomy

Posterior interbody fusion performed in cylindrical cages, with or without posterior transpedicular stabilization

Instrumented posterior lumbar fusions performed in a position of kyphosis (for example, with an Andrews frame)

Settling after long instrumented fusions, leading to hypolordosis or lumbar kyphosis

Multilevel lumbar pseudarthroses

Junctional kyphosis or spondylolisthesis adjacent to a previous fusion

Noniatrogenic Causes

Ankylosing spondylitis

Congenital kyphoscoliosis

Thoracolumbar trauma

Multilevel compression fractures

Nonspinal Causes

Hip flexion contracture

Knee flexion contracture

Modifying Factors

Spinal congruency

Compensation

Dynamic or fixed (segmental or global) characteristics

Solid anterior column

sagittal deformity occurs when the sagittal deformity is not compensated for within the spinal column (Figure 4). The hips and knees must be flexed to bring the sagittal plumb line back to the sacral promontory. Spinal balance that can be maintained by flexion of the hips and knees is termed incongruent and compensated. Finally, incongruent, uncompensated spinal balance results when the combination of knee and hip flexion is not sufficient to bring the sagittal plumb line into alignment.[21]

Just as the alignment of the segments of the spine changes with age, the body's ability to compensate for sagittal deformity changes with age. A well-compensated spinal deformity can become decompensated over time. A flexible or dynamic sagittal deformity can lead to a functional sagittal imbalance that causes fatigue or pain. A dynamic or segmental deformity can be overcome by positioning and patient effort, but a fixed or global deformity cannot be overcome.

5: Spine

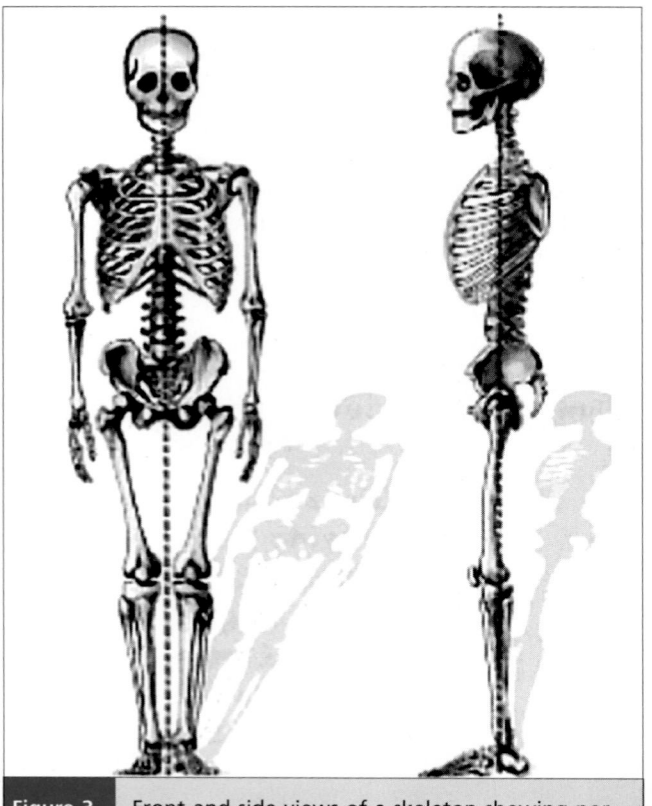

Figure 3 Front and side views of a skeleton showing normal coronal and sagittal balance with a central line of gravity. *(Reproduced with permission from Knight R, Jackson R, Killian J, Stanley E, Lowe T, Winter R: Scoliosis Research Society white paper on sagittal plane alignment. Milwaukee, WI, Scoliosis Research Society, 2003. Available at: www.srs.org/professionals/resources/sagittal_plane_white_paper.pdf. Accessed October 22, 2007.)*

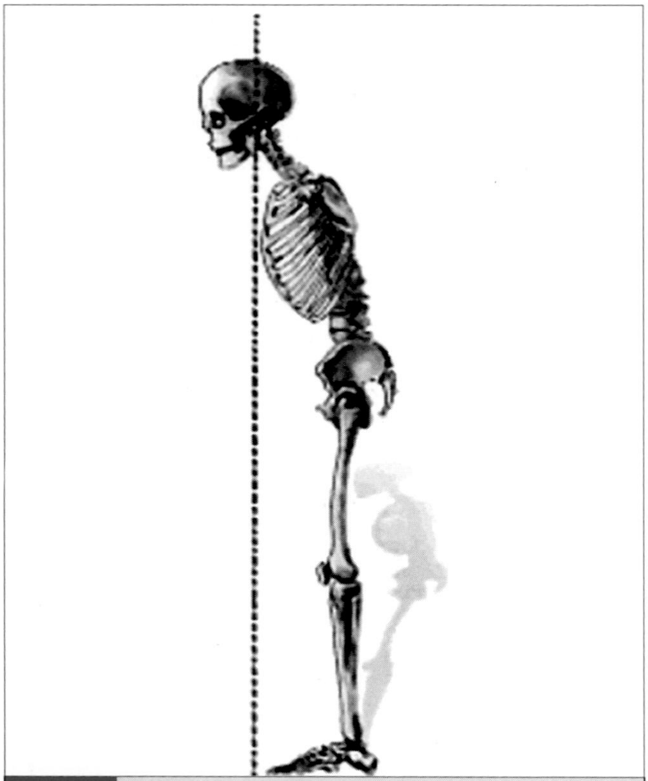

Figure 4 Side view of a skeleton showing an incongruent sagittal deformity. The plumb line is shifted anteriorly. Compensation could be obtained with knee flexion and hip extension. *(Reproduced with permission from Knight R, Jackson R, Killian J, Stanley E, Lowe T, Winter R: Scoliosis Research Society white paper on sagittal plane alignment. Milwaukee, WI, Scoliosis Research Society, 2003.. Available at: www.srs.org/professionals/resources/sagittal_plane_white_paper.pdf. Accessed October 22, 2007.)*

Disease Burden

Fixed sagittal imbalance has the most negative impact on quality of life of all adult spinal deformities. In an evaluation of 48 patients with lumbar kyphosis, 28 were treated with reconstructive surgery; the remaining 20 did not undergo realignment surgery, although 16 of them underwent minor procedures. Of this conservatively treated group, only 27% had long-term positive outcomes, and these patients originally had only mild sagittal imbalance (plumb line > 4 cm positive).[22]

A study of 172 patients who had not undergone previous surgery and 126 patients who had previous surgery found that the extent of positive sagittal balance was most predictive of symptoms. In both groups, the patients with positive sagittal balance reported greater pain and lower self-image, as well as lower social and overall functioning, compared with those who had neutral or negative sagittal balance (as measured using the Scoliosis Research Society-22 and Oswestry Disability Index instruments).[23] A subsequent study of 352 patients with positive sagittal balance ranging from 1 mm to 271 mm found a correlation between sagittal imbalance and deterioration in health (as measured using the Medical Outcomes Study 12-Item Short Form Health Survey physical health composite score; the Scoliosis Research Society-29 pain, activity, and total domains; and the Oswestry Disability Index). A decline in health measure scores was correlated with increasingly positive sagittal balance and a more distal deformity.[24]

Assessment

Clinical History

A thorough medical history must be obtained. Pain is frequently an important component of a patient's complaints, and it should be pursued by the physician. However, declining function may be more important as an objective measure. The physician should attempt to understand the adaptations the patient has made. Knowledge of pastimes or sports the patient has given up, as well as the patient's tolerance of walking and standing, can provide insight into the condition. Fatigue during standing and walking can result when the patient compensates for the deformity by flexing the knees and extending the hips and thoracic spine while adducting the scapula. The patient should be considered a candidate for surgery only in the presence of a compelling story of decline and frustration as well as pain. The use of outcomes instruments such as the Oswestry Disability Index and SF-36 can be a useful adjunct to discussion.

The patient's spinal history, particularly a history of ankylosing spondylitis or spinal surgery, should be explored. The physician must understand the indications for any earlier spinal surgeries. A patient who has undergone multiple spine fusions may have entirely iatrogenic pathology. For example, surgery to correct pseudarthrosis and flat back may have been considered successful, but the patient is still reporting pain. The history of any lower extremity neurologic complaints must also be understood to establish the likelihood of future relief of pain.

The correction of a major spinal deformity is a substantial undertaking, and the expectations and trade-offs must be discussed with the patient. Patients frequently develop remarkable compensations for their deformity, and dramatic changes in posture without restoration of motion can introduce complications. After realignment surgery, the patient may have difficulty achieving independence in bathroom use and other aspects of personal hygiene.

The patient's general health, nutritional status, smoking history, and comorbidities can affect the surgical outcome. They must be defined and addressed preoperatively.

Physical Examination
The physical examination of a patient with a sagittal deformity should attempt to define the extent of the deformity and rule out other possible contributors to sagittal imbalance. A thorough evaluation of the patient's lower extremities is necessary. Hip flexion contractures, in particular protrusion of the acetabulum seen in people with ankylosing spondylitis, must be ruled out. Knee and ankle deformities and contractures must be defined. Lower extremity deformities should be addressed first in any attempt to reestablish sagittal balance. Correcting these deformities may obviate the need for spinal surgery or simplify the recovery from surgery.

Patients should be asked to stand as upright as possible and then demonstrate their typical posture. The physician should pay close attention to the position of the hips and knees, as well as that of the thoracic spine and shoulders. The following questions should be answered: Is the sagittal deformity fixed or flexible? What are the compensatory mechanisms? Is the spinal balance congruent or incongruent? Is it compensated or uncompensated? Is there a coexisting coronal deformity?

The chin-brow angle, best measured on a clinical photograph, is defined by the intersection of the line of the floor with a line drawn from the patient's brow to the chin. The two lines should be perpendicular. This measurement is of particular importance in patients with ankylosing spondylitis who frequently have a stiff cervical spine and a limited ability to maintain a horizontal gaze. Sagittal imbalance leads to a positive chin-brow angle because the brow is pitched forward over the chin. This angle should be addressed in preoperative planning to avoid an overcorrection. After surgery, patients who have a chin-brow angle of less than −10° have great difficulty in achieving a horizontal gaze, as well as great dissatisfaction with the surgical result.[25]

Sitting balance should be assessed. If the sitting balance is normal, a hip flexion contracture may be the primary cause of the deformity. A sitting imbalance often represents a more severe deformity. If the patient has sagittal imbalance in the sitting position, marked by slouching to achieve a neutral visual angle, the physician should look closely at the cervical and thoracic spine to assess its relative contribution to overall sagittal balance.

When the deformity is present only in the lumbar spine, the patient is able to lie supine with the shoulders and head flat. If the head, shoulders, or both remain above the examining table, the cervical and thoracic spine is likely to be contributing to the sagittal imbalance.

Finally, the skin and soft-tissue coverage of the posterior spine must be assessed. Soft-tissue coverage is often compromised in patients who have undergone multiple spine surgeries or have ankylosing spondylitis.

Imaging
Weight-bearing AP and lateral radiographs taken on a 36-inch cassette can best define the deformity and determine how much correction is necessary. The knees should be extended to allow the radiographs to show the true deformity. Cobb measurements of the lumbar spine and plumb line should be recorded. If the patient has leg symptoms, an imaging study is needed. MRI is adequate if no instrumentation is present; a CT myelogram is necessary if the patient has instrumentation. Instrumentation placement and the health of junctional disks, as well as the presence of a solid anterior column fusion, junctional stenosis, or pseudarthrosis, should be documented.

Nonsurgical Management
Nonsurgical care is important in the management of sagittal imbalance. The underlying goal is to restore function while minimizing pain and the impact of care. The treatment options include education, medication, injections, behavioral modification, physical therapy, bracing, and self-guided exercise programs. Through nonsurgical management and continuing follow-up, the physician can observe the impact of the patient's condition over time. Tolerance of sagittal imbalance varies widely among patients, and the physician must curb the desire to fix a deformity until it is clear that the deformity represents an important deficit in the patient's quality of life.

Physical therapy to strengthen the posterior musculature can be beneficial to the patient with dynamic in-

5: Spine

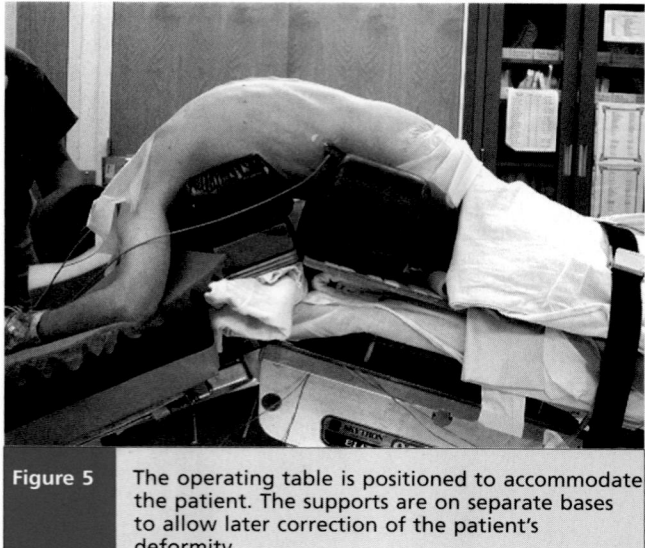

Figure 5 | The operating table is positioned to accommodate the patient. The supports are on separate bases to allow later correction of the patient's deformity.

stability. Bracing is not likely to be of significant benefit, particularly in a patient with a fixed deformity. Injection therapy directed toward areas of neural compromise can alleviate leg pain and help restore function, although the benefit is often short lived. Injection therapy can provide the physician with information about the source of the patient's pain, as well as the potential of the neural elements to recover. Providing the patient with education about treatment options and a general exercise plan can be useful in establishing a maintenance program. Over time, the patient and physician can both gain insight into the potential need for surgical care.

Surgical Management

Surgery to correct sagittal imbalance should be considered in the presence of refractory pain, deformity progression, severe functional deficit, or neurologic loss. Communicating with the patient about surgical expectations and outcomes is of critical importance. The patient may be more interested in subjective improvement of pain than in the objective deficit.

The results of surgical care are negatively affected by coexistent medical comorbidities, residual sagittal imbalance, and pseudarthrosis.[26] Therefore, patient selection is important; surgical care may not be appropriate for a patient with comorbidities. Aggressiveness in correcting the sagittal imbalance is also important because the incidence of pseudarthrosis is lessened with restoration of sagittal balance. The use of adjunctive interbody fusion must be considered, particularly when adding on to existing levels of fusion from previous surgery. Considering adjunctive levels in the fusion is particularly important in two scenarios: the fixation points through the previous fusion mass are inadequate above or below the planned osteotomy, or the junctional disks above or below the earlier fusion appear to be degenerating.[27]

Choosing a Procedure
The patient best suited to undergo a pedicle subtraction osteotomy has a sagittal deformity and a solid anterior column, either from previous fusion or ankylosing spondylitis. In addition, patient positioning during surgery is an important factor (Figure 5). A pedicle subtraction osteotomy can be performed in a patient with open disk spaces, although the proximal and distal aspects of the wedged vertebral body will be left unattached to the hardware and therefore difficult to control. Multilevel Smith-Peterson osteotomies should also be considered, with or without an anterior fusion. A subtle coronal imbalance can be treated with a pedicle subtraction osteotomy, although imbalance in the coronal plane can also be made worse by a pedicle subtraction osteotomy. If a concomitant coronal imbalance greater than 6 cm exists, then a vertebral resection should be considered (Figure 6).

Planning an Osteotomy
Standing lateral radiographs can be traced to create a template for the osteotomy. The ability to correct the sagittal balance to posterior translation of C7 over the sacral promontory is a function of the level chosen and the amount of posterior element resected. A pedicle subtraction osteotomy is not intended to lengthen the anterior column. A Smith-Peterson osteotomy can be performed behind an open disk space, and, during correction of the deformity, the anterior column can be lengthened by opening the disk space. If the disk space was completely disrupted, the correction can be quite dramatic. However, theoretic concerns have been expressed about lengthening the great vessels and possibly causing rupture or attenuated blood flow. Planning for a pedicle subtraction osteotomy should include maintenance of anterior column height and shortening of the posterior column. Two reports have found that pedicle subtraction osteotomy results in an average 30° correction per level and Smith-Peterson osteotomy results in an average 10° correction per level.[28,29] The effect on posterior translation and the resulting improvement in sagittal balance are increased when the osteotomy is relatively distal. This benefit must be balanced against compromised distal fixation. A typical one-level pedicle subtraction osteotomy is performed at L3 or L4 if more effective correction is required and excellent bone quality is anticipated.[30-33]

Pedicle Subtraction Osteotomy
The pedicle subtraction osteotomy is a posterior-only three-column resection and shortening of the spinal column that is performed to effect a correction in the sagittal plane. Important aspects of this technically demanding procedure are listed in Table 2.

Smith-Peterson Osteotomy
The Smith-Peterson osteotomy can be combined with an anterior release and fusion or performed separately as a posterior procedure. Resection of the facet joint, lateral fusion mass, or both is combined with a lami-

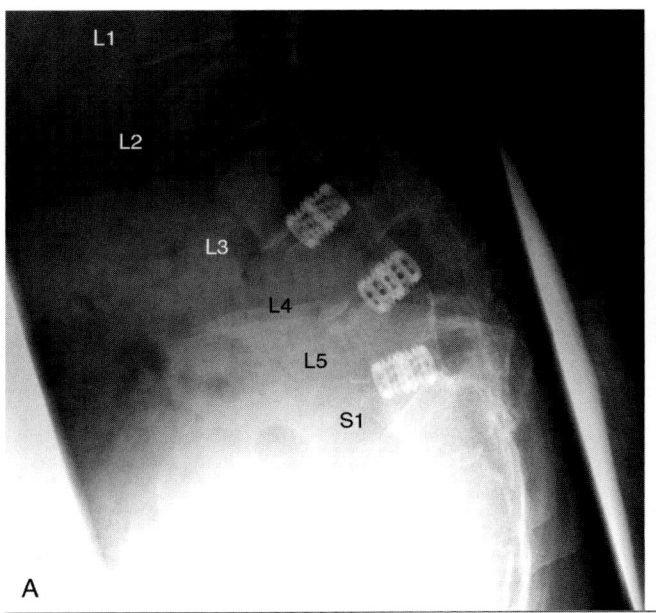
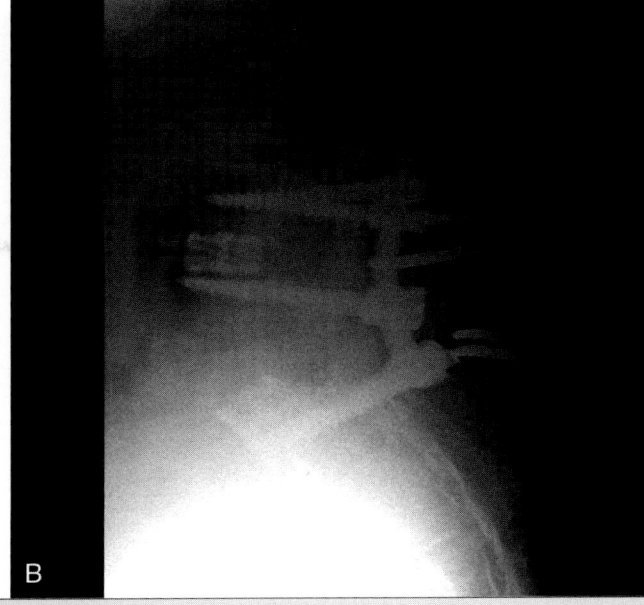

Figure 6 **A,** Lateral radiograph taken before a standard pedicle subtraction osteotomy combined with an interbody fusion. **B,** Lateral radiograph showing that the L4-5 threaded cylindrical cage has been removed, and a small vertically oriented cage has been placed in the anterior disk space to act as a fulcrum.

nectomy to prevent neural impingement during correction. The pedicle is not resected, and the correction is obtained anteriorly through the disk space. In a patient who has a combined sagittal and coronal deformity with the shoulder angulation tilted into the concavity, an anterior release followed by a posterior fusion with multilevel Smith-Peterson osteotomies can be useful. The combined anterior and posterior approach using multiple Smith-Peterson osteotomies can provide sagittal correction similar to that obtained with a pedicle subtraction osteotomy. The advantage of a Smith-Peterson osteotomy is less blood loss, but the disadvantage is the additional anterior exposure required.[31]

Vertebral Resection

Vertebral resection uses a combined anterior and posterior approach in which the vertebral column is resected at the apex of the deformity, allowing the corrective maneuvers of spinal shortening and translation to rebalance the spine (Figure 7). The rare patient for whom this procedure is recommended has severe fixed kyphoscoliosis with sagittal or coronal imbalance and shoulders parallel to the pelvis or tipping to the convex side of the deformity.[28,29]

Complications and Postoperative Management

The critical care needs of the postsurgical patient should be anticipated. Continuing fluid resuscitation and evaluation with frequent monitoring may be accompanied by overnight intubation. Early complications include atelectasis, pressure sores, thrombosis, and ileus. Wound infections are usually subacute or late

Table 2

Planning a Pedicle Subtraction Osteotomy

Fiberoptic intubation should be considered for anesthesia administration if ankylosing spondylitis is present.

The patient should be placed on the operating table in a well-padded, unstressed position, and the planned osteotomy site should be placed directly over the hinge on the operating table.

Neurologic monitoring is of varying usefulness, depending on the level of the osteotomy.

The procedure requires a posterior exposure. Three levels of fixation above and below the osteotomy should be planned, if possible. Fixation points proximal and distal to the planned osteotomy should be obtained before the spine is destabilized.

The osteotomy resection begins with a wide laminectomy extending proximal and distal to the planned wedge resection; this important step allows neural buckling and prevents neural compression upon closure of the osteotomy. Next, the lateral mass and pedicles are removed. A wedge is resected from the posterior vertebral body using a burr or curets. The posterior cortex is pushed into the created void. The anterior cortex is greensticked at time of closure. A temporary rod can be placed to prevent premature closure of the osteotomy.

To close the osteotomy, the table should be reflexed slowly while the surgeon directly inspects the osteotomy site and neural elements, watching for translation of the osteotomy.

When the hardware has been tightened, the table should be returned to a flat position to decrease pressure on the patient's legs and chest.

5: Spine

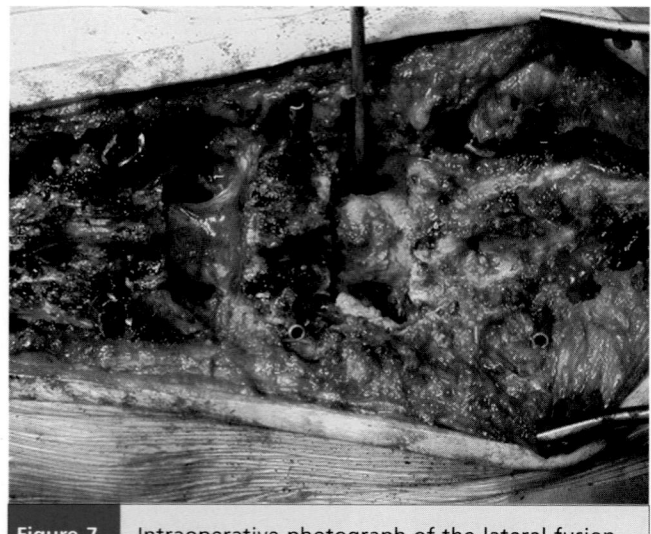

Figure 7 Intraoperative photograph of the lateral fusion mass, pedicles, and wedge of vertebral body resected at both L2 and L4. The neural elements are widely exposed.

complications, whereas the rare nonunion presents late. Neurologic complications should be evaluated aggressively. The occasional single-nerve radiculopathy may be transient, but a high index of suspicion must be maintained because the neural elements may be trapped in the osteotomy site closure. This complication can be avoided by vigilant preparation of the laminectomy and resection of the entire pedicle.

A postsurgical brace may be needed. The patient should wear a thoracolumbosacral orthosis, with or without a combined thigh cuff, for 6 to 8 weeks during all out-of-bed activities. The patient should be instructed to avoid flexing the hip more than 45°, and a bed pan should be used if bone quality is in question. As an alternative to bracing, a tilt table can be used to help the patient stay upright without flexing the hips. Once in an upright position, the patient is free to walk without the brace. This option can allow the patient more independence, but it requires a prolonged stay at a skilled nursing facility.

Annotated References

1. Lowe T, Berven SH, Schwab FJ, Bridwell KH: The SRS classification for adult spinal deformity: Building on the King/Moe and Lenke classification systems. *Spine* 2006; 31(suppl 19):S119-S125.

   Nineteen surgeons evaluated 25 adults with spinal deformity to validate the Scoliosis Research Society Classification of Adult Spinal Deformity. Substantial interobserver reliability for curve types, regional sagittal modifiers, and degenerative lumbar modifiers were noted. When choosing fusion levels, there was substantial agreement for the lower instrumented vertebra, but only moderate agreement for the upper instrumented vertebra.

2. Lenke LG, Betz RR, Harms J, et al: Adolescent idiopathic scoliosis: A new classification to determine extent of spinal arthrodesis. *J Bone Joint Surg Am* 2001;83-A: 1169-1181.

3. Kostuik JP, Bentivoglio J: The incidence of low-back pain in adult scoliosis. *Spine* 1981;6:268-273.

4. Schwab F, Dubey A, Gamez L, et al: Adult scoliosis: Prevalence, SF-36, and nutritional parameters in an elderly volunteer population. *Spine* 2005;30:1082-1085.

   The authors present a prospective analysis of adult scoliosis in 75 volunteers older than 60 years. The overall rate of curves of more than 10° was 68%. There were no significant correlations between radiographic measurements and visual analog scale scores or nutritional status.

5. Weinstein SL, Dolan LA, Spratt KF, Peterson KK, Spoonamore MJ, Ponseti IV: Health and function of patients with untreated idiopathic scoliosis: A 50-year natural history study. *JAMA* 2003;289:559-567.

6. Berven S, Deviren V, Demir-Deviren S, et al: Studies in the modified Scoliosis Research Society Outcomes Instrument in adults: Validation, reliability, and discriminatory capacity. *Spine* 2003;28:2164-2169.

7. Glassman SD, Bridwell K, Dimar JR, Horton W, Berven S, Schwab F: The impact of positive sagittal balance in adult spinal deformity. *Spine* 2005;30:2024-2029.

   A retrospective review of 752 patients with adult spinal deformity who were enrolled in a prospective database is presented. The authors found that progressive positive sagittal imbalance correlated with a linear increase in the severity of symptoms.

8. Weinstein SL, Ponseti IV: Curve progression in idiopathic scoliosis. *J Bone Joint Surg Am* 1983;65:447-455.

9. Lapp MA, Bridwell KH, Lenke LG, Baldus C, Blanke K, Iffrig TM: Prospective randomization of parenteral hyperalimentation for long fusions with spinal deformity: Its effect on complications and recovery from postoperative malnutrition. *Spine* 2001;26:809-817.

10. Edwards CC II, Bridwell KH, Patel A, Rinella AS, Berra A, Lenke LG: Long adult deformity fusions to L5 and the sacrum: A matched cohort analysis. *Spine* 2004;29: 1996-2005.

    Ninety-five patients with adult spinal deformity whose spines were fused to either L5 or the sacrum were classified and precisely matched into two cohorts. Correction of sagittal imbalance was superior for the patients who had fusion to the sacrum; however, these patients required more surgical procedures and had a greater frequency of major complications and medical morbidities compared with the group with spinal fusion to L5. In contrast, the L5 group had a high rate (67%) of L5-S1 disk degeneration that may be associated with a forward shift in sagittal balance.

11. Brown KM, Ludwig SC, Gelb DE: Radiographic predictors of outcome after long fusion to L5 in adult scoliosis. *J Spinal Disord Tech* 2004;17:358-366.

The authors evaluated 16 patients with adult scoliosis who had spinal fusion to L5. Sixty-two percent had no evidence of subjacent disk degeneration, whereas 38% did. Patients with good preoperative sagittal balance, preserved lumbar lordosis, good postoperative fractional curve correction, and L5-S1 disk height preservation had the best outcomes without sacral fusion.

12. Rinella A, Bridwell K, Kim Y, et al: Late complications of adult idiopathic scoliosis primary fusions to L4 and above: The effect of age and distal fusion level. *Spine* 2004;29:318-325.

In this study, 67 patients with adult spinal deformity were classified into two groups based on their distal fusion level (T11-L2 versus L3-4). Both groups had similar pseudarthrosis rates, but higher rates of transition syndrome occurred when the distal fusion was at L3-4 compared with T11-L2.

13. Lebwohl NH, Cunningham BW, Dmitriev A, et al: Biomechanical comparison of lumbosacral fixation techniques in a calf spine model. *Spine* 2002;27:2312-2320.

14. Simmons ED, Kowalski JM, Simmons EH: The results of surgical treatment for adult scoliosis. *Spine* 1993;18:718-724.

15. Ali RM, Boachie-Adjei O, Rawlins BA: Functional and radiographic outcomes after surgery for adult scoliosis using third-generation instrumentation techniques. *Spine* 2003;28:1163-1169.

16. Grubb SA, Lipscomb HJ, Suh PB: Results of surgical treatment of painful adult scoliosis. *Spine* 1994;19:1619-1627.

17. Bridwell KH, Lenke LG, Baldus C, Blanke K: Major intraoperative neurologic deficits in pediatric and adult spinal deformity patients: Incidence and etiology at one institution. *Spine* 1998;23:324-331.

18. Rosner MK, Kuklo TR, Tawk R, Moquin R, Ondra SL: Prophylactic placement of an inferior vena cava filter in high-risk patients undergoing spinal reconstruction. *Neurosurg Focus* 2004;17:E6.

The authors present the results of a pilot study of 22 patients who were considered high-risk for major spine reconstruction and underwent prophylactic inferior vena cava filter placement. No patients had pulmonary embolisms; however, two patients had deep venous thrombosis. A follow-up study evaluated 74 patients who met one or more of the following criteria: a history of thromboembolism, diagnosed thrombophilia, diagnosed malignancy, patient was bedridden more than 2 weeks before surgery, patient had staged procedures or procedures at multiple levels, patient had surgery that combined anterior/posterior approaches, there was an expected need for significant iliocaval manipulation during exposure, and single-stage anesthetic time of more than 8 hours was required. The authors reported 1 pulmonary embolism and 27 instances of deep venous thrombosis (frequently at the inferior vena cava filter placement site).

19. Kim YJ, Bridwell KH, Lenke LG, Cho KJ, Edwards CC II, Rinella AS: Pseudarthrosis in adult spinal deformity following multisegmental instrumentation and arthrodesis. *J Bone Joint Surg Am* 2006;88:721-728.

Of 232 patients with adult spinal deformity treated at a single institution, 40 developed pseudarthrosis. Factors that increased the incidence of kyphosis were preoperative thoracolumbar kyphosis of more than 20°, age greater than 55 years, distal fusion to S1 (versus L5), and arthrodesis of more than 12 vertebrae. Clinical outcome was negatively impacted by the presence of pseudarthrosis.

20. Kim YJ, Bridwell KH, Lenke LG, Rhim S, Cheh G: Pseudarthrosis in long adult spinal deformity instrumentation and fusion to the sacrum: Prevalence and risk factor analysis of 144 cases. *Spine* 2006;31:2329-2336.

A retrospective review of 144 adult patients with spinal deformity showed a 24% rate of pseudarthrosis in long fusions extended to the sacrum. Risk factors that increased the incidence of pseudarthrosis included thoracolumbar kyphosis, osteoarthritis of the hip, the use of a thoracoabdominal approach (versus paramedian approach), positive sagittal balance of 5 cm or more, patient age of 55 years or older, and incomplete sacropelvic fixation.

21. Knight R, Jackson R, Killian J, Stanley E, Lowe T, Winter R: Scoliosis Research Society white paper on sagittal plane alignment. Milwaukee, WI, Scoliosis Research Society, 2003. Available at: www.srs.org/professionals/resources/sagittal_plane_white_paper.pdf. Accessed March 2, 2007.

22. Farcy JP, Schwab FJ: Management of flatback and related kyphotic decompensation syndromes. *Spine* 1997;22:2452-2457.

23. Glassman SD, Berven S, Bridwell K, Horton W, Dimar JR: Correlation of radiographic parameters and clinical symptoms in adult scoliosis. *Spine* 2005;30:682-688.

In 298 patients, positive sagittal balance was the most reliable predictor of clinical symptoms. Significant coronal imbalance of greater than 4 cm was associated with deterioration in pain and function scores for patients who did not undergo surgery but not in patients who previously had surgery.

24. Glassman SD, Bridwell K, Dimar J, Horton W, Berven S, Schwab F: The impact of positive sagittal balance in adult spinal deformity: Clinical case series. *Spine* 2005;30:2024-2029.

Although even mildly positive sagittal balance is detrimental, the severity of symptoms increases in a linear fashion with progressive sagittal imbalance. Kyphosis is better tolerated in the upper thoracic region than in the lumbar spine.

25. Suk KS, Kim KT, Lee SH, Kim JM: Significance of chin-

brow vertical angle in correction of kyphotic deformity of ankylosing spondylitis patients. *Spine* 2003;28:2001-2005.

26. Bridwell KH, Lewis S, Lenke L, Baldus C, Blanke K: Pedicle subtraction osteotomy for the treatment of fixed sagittal imbalance. *J Bone Joint Surg Am* 2003;85:454-463.

27. Kwon BK, Elgafy H, Keynan O, et al: Progressive junctional kyphosis at the caudal end of lumbar instrumented fusion: Etiology, predictors, and treatment. *Spine* 2006;31:1943-1951.

Potential fixation failure at the caudal end of lumbar-instrumented fusion should be considered in patients with progressive sagittal decompensation. The high potential for failure of L5 pedicle screws after the index surgery warrants serious consideration of extending such fusions into the sacrum and ilium.

28. Bridwell KH: Decision making regarding Smith-Petersen vs. pedicle subtraction osteotomy vs. vertebral column resection for spinal deformity. *Spine* 2006;31(suppl 19): S171-S178.

Smith-Petersen osteotomy, pedicle subtraction, and vertebral column resection have specific applications and potential complications. As the extent of the resection increases, the ability to correct deformity and the risk of complications also increase.

29. Bradford DS, Tribus CB: Current concepts and management of patients with fixed decompensated spinal deformity. *Clin Orthop Relat Res* 1994; 306:64-72.

30. Cho KJ, Bridwell KH, Lenke LG, Berra A, Baldus C: Comparison of Smith-Petersen versus pedicle subtraction osteotomy for the correction of fixed sagittal imbalance. *Spine* 2005;30(18):2030-2038.

In a comparison of 14 patients who had undergone three or more Smith-Peterson osteotomies and 41 patients who had undergone one pedicle subtraction osteotomy, the correction in kyphosis was found to be nearly identical. The likelihood of decompensating the patient to the concavity was significantly greater with three or more Smith-Peterson osteotomies than with a single pedicle subtraction osteotomy ($P < 0.02$). The blood loss was substantially greater in the pedicle subtraction osteotomy group ($P < 0.001$).

31. Potter BK, Lenke LG, Kuklo TR: Prevention and management of iatrogenic flatback deformity. *J Bone Joint Surg Am* 2004;86-A:1793-1808.

The treatment of flatback syndrome involves corrective pedicle subtraction or Smith-Peterson osteotomies with segmental instrumentation. Polysegmental osteotomies and vertebral column resection can be used for patients with sloping global sagittal imbalance and related severe coronal imbalance, respectively.

32. Murrey DB, Brigham CD, Kiebzak GM, Finger F, Chewning SJ: Transpedicular decompression and pedicle subtraction osteotomy (eggshell procedure): A retrospective review of 59 patients. *Spine* 2002;27:2338-2345.

33. Kim KT, Suk KS, Cho YJ, Hong GP, Park BJ: Clinical outcome results of pedicle subtraction osteotomy in ankylosing spondylitis with kyphotic deformity. *Spine* 2002;27:612-618.

Chapter 50

Spondylolysis and Spondylolisthesis

R. Shay Bess, MD   Alpesh A. Patel, MD

Introduction

Spondylolysis is a disruption or insufficiency of the bony connection between the superior and inferior articular facets of the posterior spinal arch (the pars interarticularis). Spondylolisthesis is an anterior vertebral translation, or slippage, in relation to the caudal vertebra. This chapter focuses on developmental spondylolisthesis. Acquired, and especially degenerative, spondylolisthesis is discussed in the lumbar spinal stenosis section of chapter 45, Degenerative Disease of the Lumbar Spine.

Spondylolysis

The traditional definition of spondylolysis as a bony defect of the pars interarticularis has been expanded to include a spectrum of other pathologies, such as stress reaction, stress fracture, pars fracture, and pars nonunion. A stress reaction occurs as intraosseous edema with associated sclerosis of the pars interarticularis, lamina, or pedicle, without cortical or trabecular disruption. A stress fracture is a disruption of pars trabecular or cortical bone without diastasis between the fracture fragments. A pars fracture is a disruption of the pars interarticularis with associated displacement. The most common spondylolytic defect is chronic nonunion of the pars interarticularis, with associated bony sclerosis and fibrous tissue.

Symptoms

Patients typically report midline low back pain. Radicular symptoms, including pain and numbness, may be present, caused by either nerve root compression and fibrous tissue hypertrophy within the pars defect or foraminal stenosis resulting from an associated spondylolisthesis. The symptoms are often exacerbated by extension-based activities.

The differential diagnosis is based primarily on symptoms and patient age. In patients age 18 years or younger, primary spinal neoplasms and infection must be ruled out. Older patients may have degenerative disk disease, facet arthrosis, infection, or a malignancy. Intra-abdominal, intrapelvic, and psychological sources of pain also must be considered.

Diagnostic Imaging

Radiographic assessment should begin with AP and lateral plain images. Defects in the pars interarticularis can usually be seen on AP radiographs, and, if the spondylolysis is bilateral, it can be seen on lateral radiographs. Plain radiographs can also reveal a coexisting condition such as degenerative disk disease or spondylolisthesis and help rule out the presence of fracture, tumor, or infection. Oblique radiographs show defects or sclerosis of the pars interarticularis that are not visible on AP or lateral images. Standing 36-inch cassette radiographs can reveal global sagittal balance, thoracic kyphosis, lumbar lordosis, pelvic incidence, sacral slope, and pelvic tilt.

CT is useful in detecting subtle pars defects that are difficult to see on routine radiographs (Figure 1). Because axial images may not reveal spondylolytic defects that lie in the plane of the axial cuts, sagittal and coronal reconstructions should always be obtained. CT can also reveal facet arthrosis and alignment, which may alter the treatment plan. A technetium bone scan can be useful in establishing the diagnosis, treatment, and prognosis. Single photon emission CT has been reported to aid in the diagnosis of spondylolysis by showing abnormal uptake in the pars interarticularis despite normal plain radiographs.

MRI can be used to define the relevant neuroanatomy as well as to identify any coexistent pathology. It has been used to describe edema patterns in the pars interarticularis, ipsilateral pedicle, and lamina. These stress patterns are believed to precede the development of pars defects. Relief of symptoms has been associated with resolution of MRI edema patterns. Additionally, MRI edema patterns may hold prognostic value in the treatment of spondylolysis. A postsurgical review of 37 patients with 68 pars defects found that the presence of high signal changes in the ipsilateral pedicle was correlated with pars union, and the absence of signal changes was correlated with pars nonunion.[1]

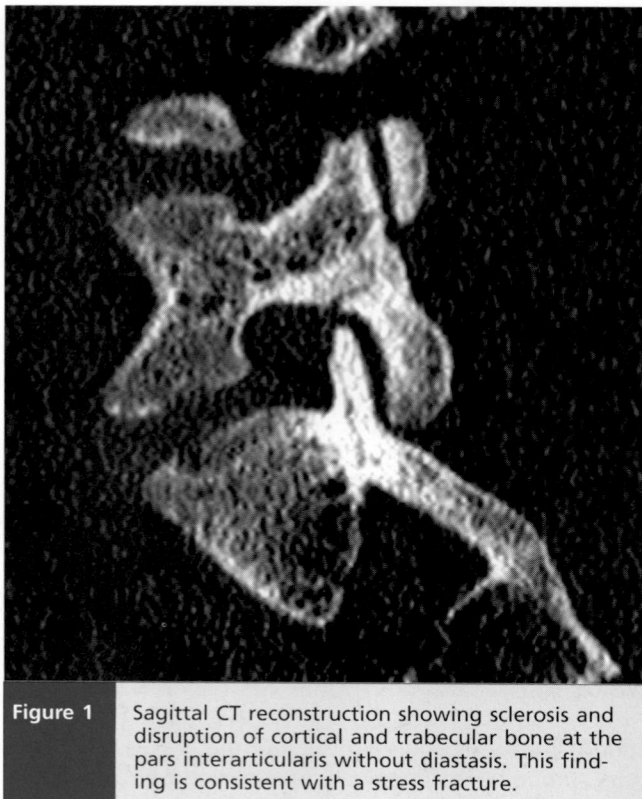

Figure 1 Sagittal CT reconstruction showing sclerosis and disruption of cortical and trabecular bone at the pars interarticularis without diastasis. This finding is consistent with a stress fracture.

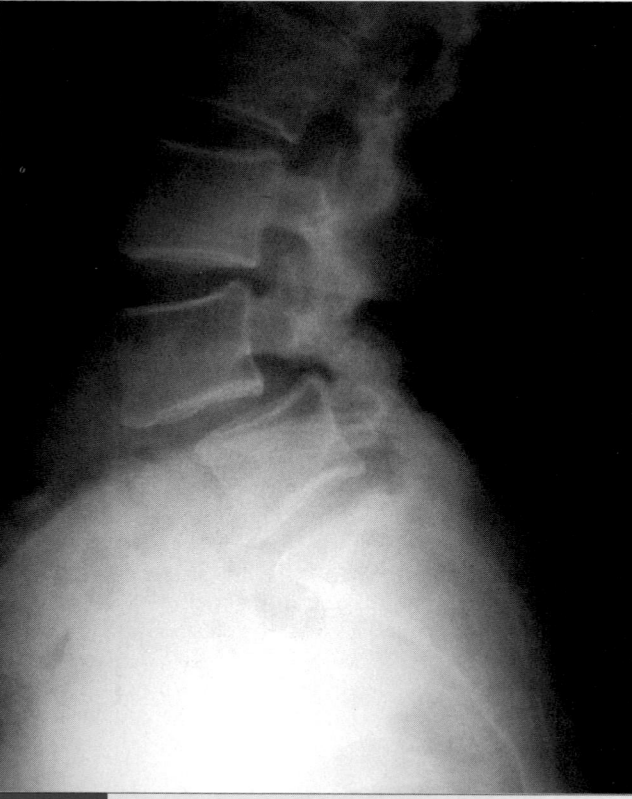

Figure 2 Lateral radiograph of the lumbar spine showing a 45% slippage, classified as Meyerding grade II, Wiltse iatrogenic, or Marchetti and Bartolozzi acquired spondylolisthesis.

Spondylolisthesis

Classification

Several systems for classifying spondylolisthesis have been described[2-4] (**Figure 2, Table 1**). The Meyerding system describes slippage as a percentage of the caudal vertebral end plate; slippage of more than 100% is defined as spondyloptosis (grade V spondylolisthesis). Grades I and II are referred to as low grade; grades III through V are referred to as high grade. The Meyerding system is widely used but has prognostic limitations.

The Wiltse classification system describes five types of spondylolisthesis (dysplastic or congenital, isthmic, degenerative, traumatic, pathologic) based on their etiology. Isthmic spondylolisthesis has three subtypes: lytic defect (spondylolysis), pars elongation resulting from repeated fracture and healing, and acute pars fracture. Traumatic spondylolisthesis results from trauma to the posterior elements outside of the pars interarticularis. The Wiltse system also has prognostic limitations.

The Marchetti and Bartolozzi classification system organizes spondylolisthesis by anatomic etiology and prognosis. The two primary categories distinguish between developmental slips, which are at high risk of progression, and acquired slips, which are relatively stable. Developmental spondylolisthesis is further divided into high-dysplastic or low-dysplastic categories, based on the concept that dysplastic changes in the spinal anatomy can lead to instability and slip progres-

sion. Examples of dysplastic abnormalities include incompetence of the posterior arch (the pedicle, lamina, and pars interarticularis), an abnormal structure or orientation of the facets, a trapezoidal L5 body, and a rounded S1 superior end plate (**Figure 3**). Spondylolisthesis that occurs in the setting of normal spinal morphology is classified as acquired. In the Marchetti and Bartolozzi system, the acquired (postsurgical or iatrogenic) classification and three of the Wiltse categories (degenerative, traumatic, and pathologic) are considered subcategories of acquired spondylolisthesis, because they are similar in prognosis (specifically, slip progression) and treatment.

Symptoms

The symptoms often vary with the type of spondylolisthesis. In addition to back pain, patients with acquired spondylolisthesis (especially degenerative spondylolisthesis) may have symptoms consistent with neurogenic claudication. Patients with developmental spondylolisthesis typically have back pain beginning in adolescence. Neurologic symptoms also may be present. The L5 nerve roots are usually affected in an L5-S1 slip. Occasionally, compression of the cauda equina occurs when the posterior bony arch is intact. Hamstring contractures and postural and gait disturbances (a

5: Spine

Table 1

Spondylolisthesis Classification Systems

System	Type	Descriptors
Meyerding	Radiographic	Grade I (0 to 25%)
		Grade II (26% to 50%)
		Grade III (51% to 75%)
		Grade IV (76% to 100%)
		Spondyloptosis (> 100%)
Wiltse	Etiologic	Congenital
		Isthmic
		Degenerative
		Traumatic
		Pathologic
Marchetti and Bartolozzi	Etiologic and radiographic	Developmental
		High dysplastic
		Low dysplastic
		Acquired
		Traumatic
		Degenerative
		Pathologic
		Postsurgical

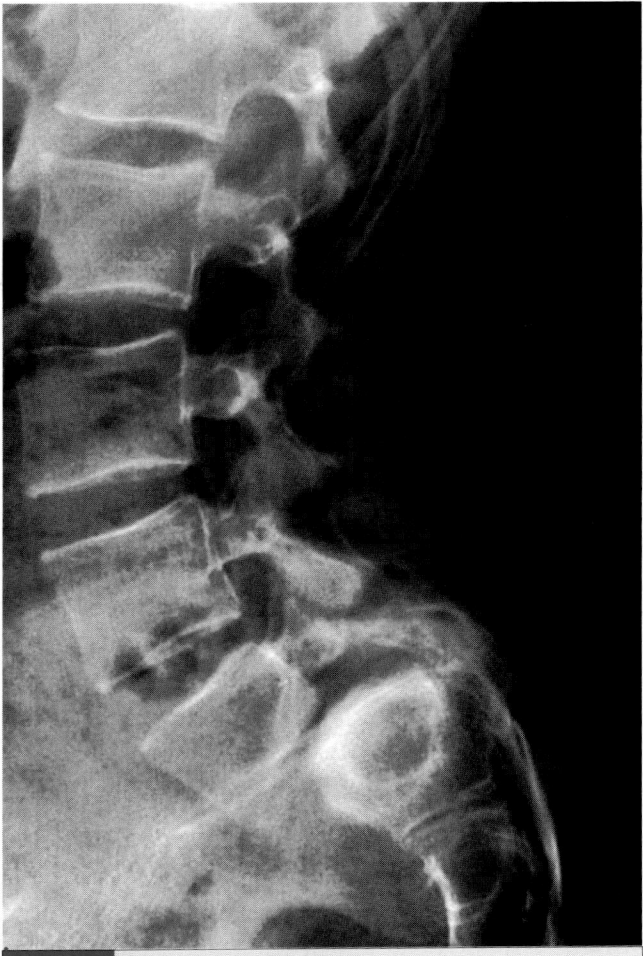

Figure 3 Lateral radiograph of high-grade (grade IV) dysplastic spondylolisthesis, showing a trapezoidal L5 body and dome-shaped S1 end plate.

crouched gait) may occur, especially in a patient who has high-grade dysplastic spondylolisthesis.

Diagnostic Imaging

Radiographic assessment begins with standing AP and lateral plain film images. Supine radiographs fail to reveal spondylolisthesis in as many as 20% of patients. Lateral radiographs show the degree of dysplasia, as well as slippage, which is graded using the Meyerding classification. Plain films also allow measurement of the associated slip angle, or focal kyphosis. A Ferguson view, which is an AP radiograph angled at approximately 30° cephalad, can provide a true AP view of the L5-S1 level in high-grade spondylolisthesis. Plain radiographs also can help define coexistent disk degeneration. Flexion and extension images may reveal subtle or unstable slips that are accentuated by flexion and reduced in extension. Dynamic radiographs offer information about the stability of the slip. Although a strict definition of slip stability does not exist, the presence or absence of large changes in vertebral positioning can influence treatment. Standing 36-inch cassette radiographs allow measurement of global sagittal balance, thoracic kyphosis, lumbar lordosis, pelvic incidence, sacral slope, and pelvic tilt. Many of these measurements, especially pelvic incidence, may be closely related to the potential for slip progression.

CT scans show bony anatomy more clearly than plain radiographs. The combination of thin-cut axial images (1 to 2 mm) with sagittal reconstructions can further define the dysplastic features of the anterior and posterior columns. However, because CT images are taken in the supine position, the degree of spondylolisthesis is often underestimated.

MRI is used to define the relevant neuroanatomy and reveal any coexisting pathology. Stenosis of the central canal, lateral recess, and foramen can be caused by facet overgrowth, ligamentum hypertrophy and buckling, or vertebral translation (**Figure 4**). MRI can also show degenerative changes in adjacent segments that appear normal on CT images and plain radiographs. Upright dynamic MRI may show stenosis that is underestimated on routine supine MRI. Postmyelography CT can be useful when MRI use is limited (in patients with severe deformity, prior surgery, or prior in-

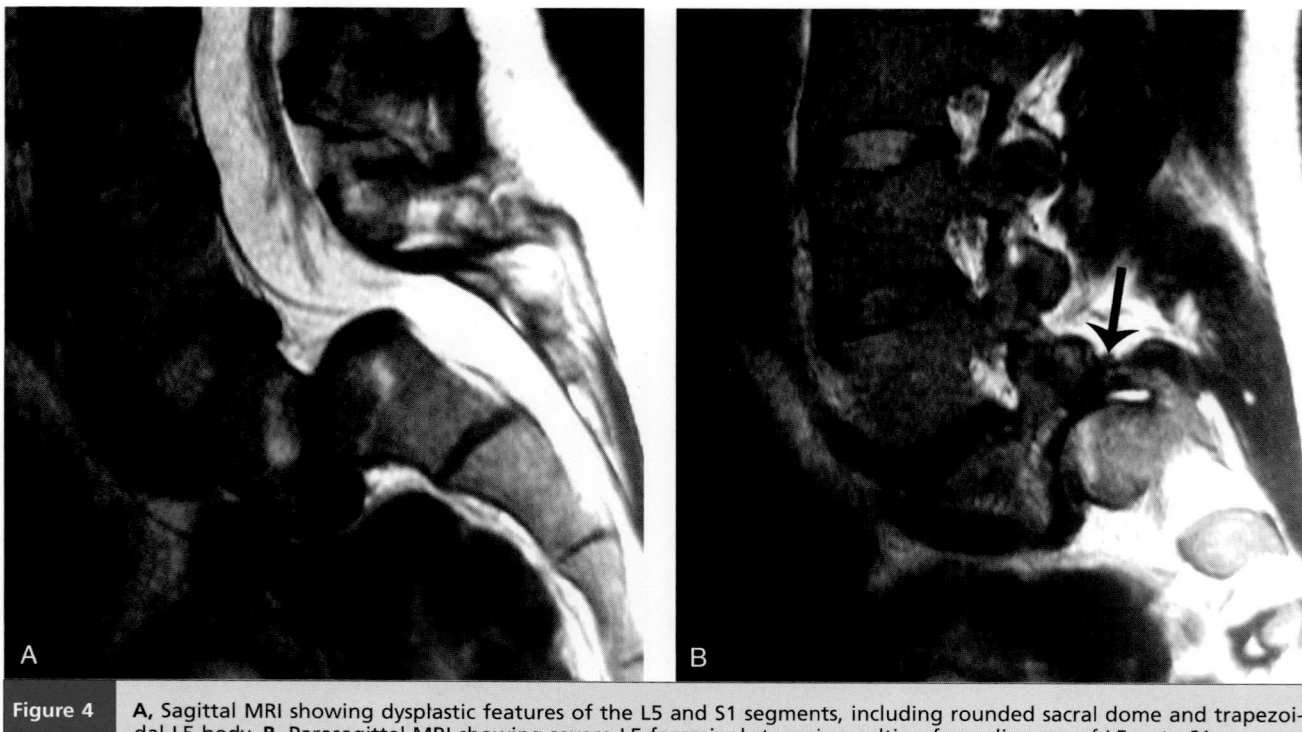

Figure 4 **A,** Sagittal MRI showing dysplastic features of the L5 and S1 segments, including rounded sacral dome and trapezoidal L5 body. **B,** Parasagittal MRI showing severe L5 foraminal stenosis resulting from slippage of L5 onto S1 (*arrow*).

strumentation) or when MRI use is prohibited (in patients with a cardiac defibrillator or pacemaker).

Spinopelvic Alignment

There is increasing interest in the relationship between the alignment of the pelvis and spine and the development and progression of spondylolysis and spondylolisthesis. The techniques for measuring lumbar lordosis, sacral slope, pelvic tilt, and pelvic incidence have been well described[5] (Figure 5), and adult and pediatric normal values have been published[6] (Table 2). These parameters are believed to be linked and to affect both global sagittal balance and focal spinopelvic alignment. Pelvic incidence is an anatomic constant; the other parameters vary with position but are constrained by the pelvic incidence. The relationship among them is stated as pelvic incidence equals sacral slope plus pelvic tilt (PI = SS + PT). A larger pelvic incidence results in a more horizontally oriented sacrum, and, therefore, a greater compensatory lumbar lordosis is required to establish spinal balance.

A review of 82 patients found that those with spondylolysis or low-grade spondylolisthesis had significantly greater pelvic incidence and lumbar lordosis than unaffected individuals.[7] A review of 214 patients with developmental spondylolisthesis found that they had significantly higher values for pelvic incidence, sacral slope, pelvic tilt, and lumbar lordosis than control group patients.[8] A linear relationship was found between pelvic incidence, sacral slope, pelvic tilt, lumbar lordosis, and degree of slip.

The relationship between spinopelvic measurements and spondylolisthesis led to the development of a new classification scheme for pediatric spondylolisthesis based on degree of slip, degree of dysplasia, and sagittal spinopelvic balance.[9] Two spinopelvic types of low-grade slips were defined: nutcracker type (low pelvic incidence, low sacral slope) and shear type (high pelvic incidence, high sacral slope). A large pelvic incidence is usually seen in high-grade slips, which are divided into two types: balanced pelvis (high sacral slope, low pelvic tilt) and retroverted pelvis (low sacral slope, high pelvic tilt) (Figure 6). A surgical treatment strategy based on this classification scheme was proposed, but it has not yet been validated.

Treatment

Surgical Versus Nonsurgical Treatment

The reported incidence of spondylolysis or spondylolisthesis is 3% to 10%. Although the condition is commonly believed to primarily affect athletes and adolescents, according to a recent cross-sectional survey of 4,151 adults in Denmark, a higher prevalence of spondylolysis at both L4 and L5 was directly correlated with increasing age and obesity.[10] Despite the relatively high incidence of the condition, a radiographic finding of a pars defect or vertebral slippage is not well correlated with clinical symptoms.[11]

In a study of more than 500 patients who received pelvic and abdominal CT scans for reasons unrelated to the lumbar spine, it was determined that the incidence of spondylolysis was 6% and the incidence of spondylolisthesis was 3%.[12] A 45-year study to determine risk factors and rate of slip progression as well as development of symptoms among patients with a pars defect, with or without spondylolisthesis, found that those with a unilateral pars defect did not develop spondylolisthesis, had minimal degenerative changes on MRI, and, at most, reported mild or intermittent low back pain.[11,13] The average slip progression for patients with bilateral pars defects was 11%; of these patients, 18% did not develop spondylolisthesis. Slip progression occurred most often during the first decade of follow-up, and it was not related to slip angle or lumbar index. Disk degeneration found on MRI was directly correlated with the amount of vertebral slip (slippage > 15% was associated with 100% disk degeneration). Vertebral slip progression was not associated with increased low back pain. No significant difference was found between the Medical Outcomes Study 36-Item Short Form scores of the study group and those of the general population of the same age.

Few studies have compared surgical and nonsurgical treatments of symptomatic spondylolisthesis. Superior clinical outcomes were found at 2-year follow-up for adult patients randomly assigned to surgical treatment (instrumented or noninstrumented posterolateral fusion) compared with patients treated with an exercise program.[14,15] Long-term follow-up, averaging 9 years, of the same patient population found limited but persistent improvement among the surgically treated patients. Another study confirmed the efficacy of surgical treatment, finding significant postoperative functional improvement among adult patients who underwent arthrodesis for spondylolisthesis with pars defect.[16]

Despite the reported benefits of surgical treatment of spondylolisthesis, controversy exists about the preferability of instrumented or noninstrumented spinal fusion, the risks and benefits of spondylolisthesis reduction using spinal instrumentation, the role of interbody fusion, the usefulness of decompression combined with fusion rather than fusion alone, and the benefits of pars

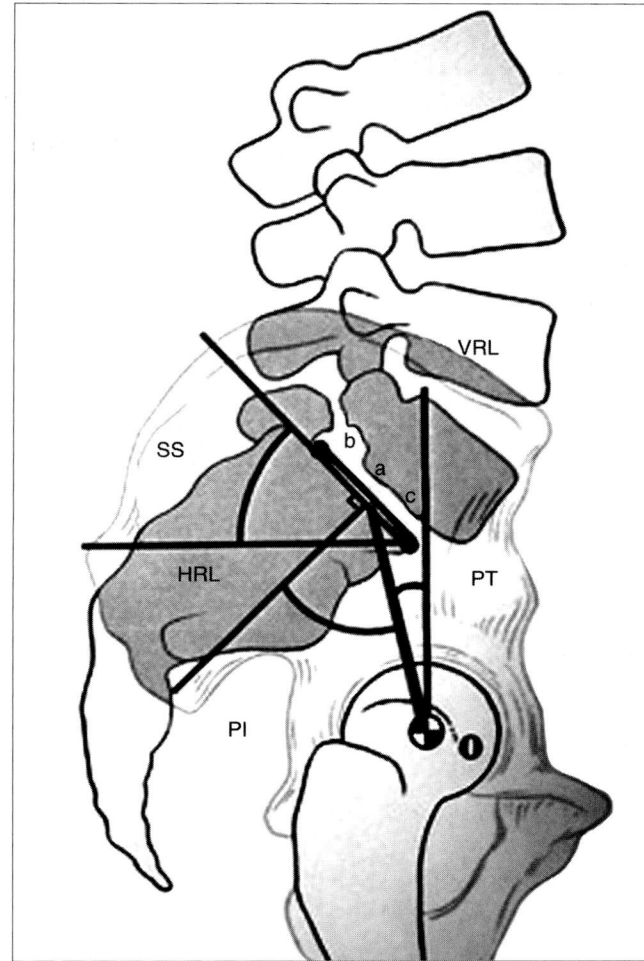

Figure 5 Pelvic incidence (a), sacral slope (b), and pelvic tilt (c). SS = sacral slope; HRL = horizontal reference line; PI = pelvic incidence; PT = pelvic tilt; VRL = vertical reference line. (*Reproduced with permission from O'Brien MF, Kuklo TR, Blanke KM, et al: Radiographic Measurement Manual: Spinal Deformity Study Group. Memphis, TN, Medtronic Sofamor Danek, 2004.*)

Table 2			
Normal Values for Pelvic Incidence, Sacral Slope, and Pelvic Tilt			
Population	**Radiographic Parameters (in degrees)**		
	Pelvic Incidence	Sacral Slope	Pelvic Tilt
Children and adolescents (ages 3 to 18 years)			
Male	49.2 ± 11.2	41.7 ± 8.4	49.2 ± 11.2
Female	49.7 ± 10.7	41.2 ± 8.0	8.5 ± 8.3
Adults (ages 19 to 50 years)			
Male	53.2 ± 10.3	41.9 ± 8.7	11.9 ± 6.6
Female	48.2 ± 7.0	38.2 ± 7.8	10.3 ± 4.8

5: Spine

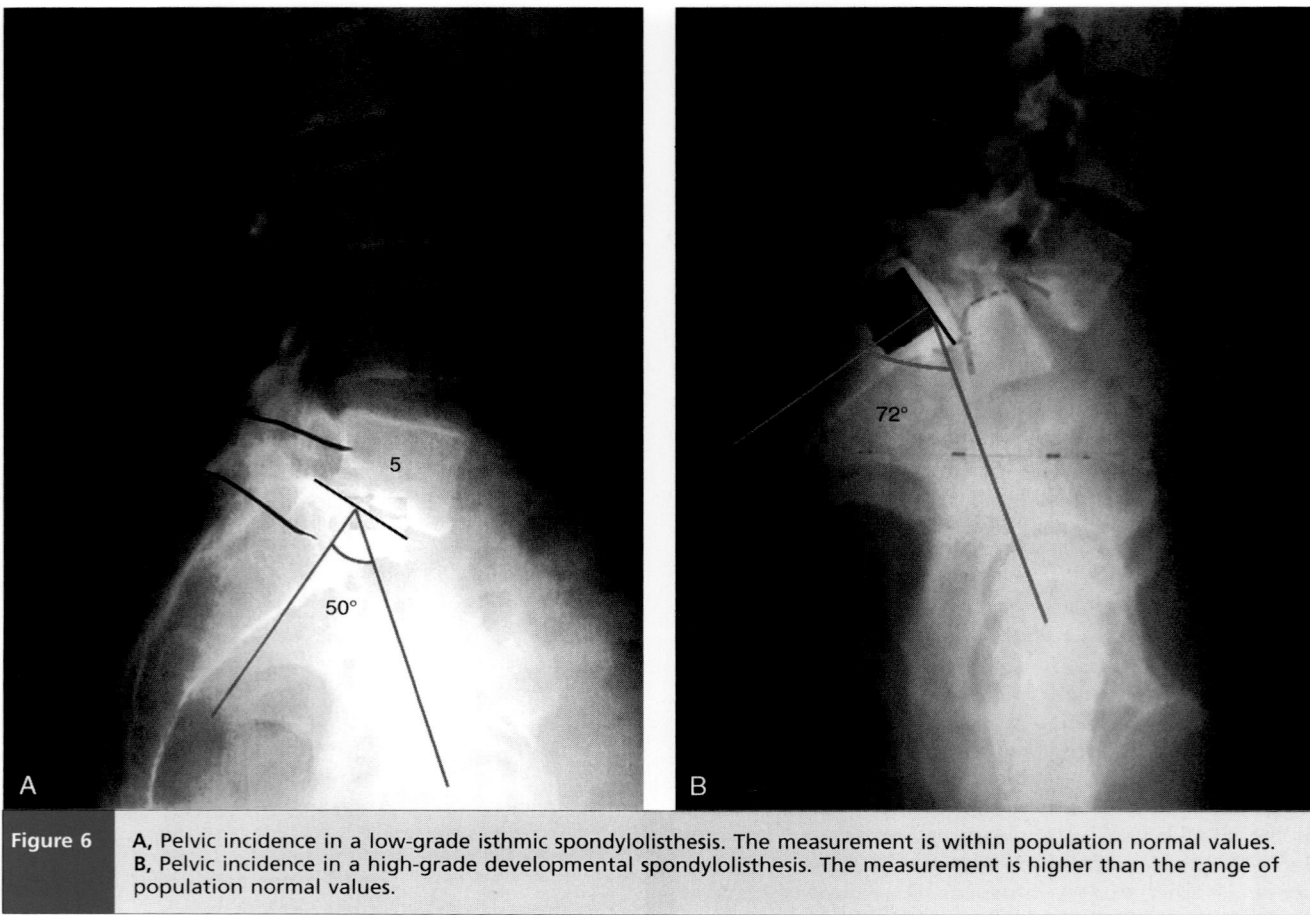

Figure 6   **A,** Pelvic incidence in a low-grade isthmic spondylolisthesis. The measurement is within population normal values. **B,** Pelvic incidence in a high-grade developmental spondylolisthesis. The measurement is higher than the range of population normal values.

repair for low-grade spondylolisthesis or vertebral resection for high-grade spondylolisthesis.

Instrumented or Noninstrumented Fusion

Spinal instrumentation is widely accepted for the treatment of developmental spondylolisthesis with spondylolysis. However, few reports have demonstrated instrumented spinal fusion is beneficial compared with noninstrumented fusion when treating spondylolisthesis with an associated pars defect. One study found no difference in clinical outcomes or fusion rate at 2-year and 9-year follow-up of 77 adults randomly assigned to instrumented or noninstrumented fusion for spondylolisthesis with an associated pars defect.[14,15] A subgroup analysis of adult patients randomly assigned to instrumented or noninstrumented fusion for treatment of spondylolysis with a pars defect found better clinical outcomes in patients treated without instrumentation and no difference in fusion rates between the instrumented and noninstrumented fusion groups at 5-year follow-up.[17]

Some proponents of spinal instrumentation claim that it achieves slip reduction and restores sagittal balance so that fusion occurs in a more anatomic alignment. Despite the neurologic risks, several authors have recently reported good results using spondylolisthesis reduction maneuvers. Temporary fixation into L4 to reduce focal lumbosacral kyphosis, followed by L5-S1 monosegmental fusion and interbody fusion, achieved good results in 27 patients with high-grade, high-dysplastic developmental L5-S1 spondylolisthesis. The authors reported 86% slip correction, reduction of slip angle, and restoration of L5-S1 lordosis. Six patients had L5 nerve root complications, five of which resolved at 2-year follow-up.[18] Good results were also reported using posterior instrumentation for L4-through-S1 fusion and partial (50%) slip reduction in 44 patients with high-grade L5-S1 spondylolisthesis.[19] Twenty-two of 44 patients received supplementary anterior spinal fusion. Neural decompression was not performed before reduction. Twenty-one complications developed. Five patients had postoperative neurologic deficits; all were unilateral L5 deficits that developed 2 to 10 days postoperatively, following a normal wake-up test during surgery. Three of these patients had complete resolution of the deficit from 1 month to 1 year after surgery. Two patients demonstrated a residual deficit (one motor and one sensory) at last follow-up. Neurologic complications developed in 19% of the patients who had combined AP fusion, compared with 5% of patients who had posterior fusion alone. Pseudarthroses developed in five patients, of whom four received AP fusion.

Despite the good results reported following spondylolisthesis reduction, slip reduction has not demonstrated long-term clinical benefit compared with in situ fusion. Comparison of 11 adolescents treated with posterior spinal instrumentation and reduction followed by anterior fusion with 11 adolescents treated with in situ AP fusion demonstrated at average 14-year follow-up that the in situ fusion group had significantly better scores than the reduction group on the Oswestry Disability Index and, Scoliosis Research Society Outcomes Instrument. The reduction group had almost 50% slip reduction compared with 2% slip reduction in the in situ fusion group.[20] Neurologic complications and pseudarthrosis each occurred in 18% of the reduction group; no patients in the in situ fusion group had neurologic complications or pseudarthrosis. MRI taken at the last follow-up showed less disk degeneration in the in situ fusion group.

Interbody Fusion

Several authors have advocated the use of anterior column support in treating high-grade spondylolisthesis. At a mean 17-year follow-up, adolescents with high-grade dysplastic spondylolisthesis treated with noninstrumented in situ AP fusion had better clinical and radiographic outcomes than those treated with noninstrumented in situ posterior fusion.[21] According to another report, adolescents treated with posterior instrumented fusion combined with either anterior lumbar interbody fusion (ALIF) or posterior lumbar interbody fusion (PLIF) had better clinical outcomes, and higher fusion rates, than those treated with only posterior instrumented or noninstrumented fusion.[22] The incidence of neurologic complications in the interbody and the posterior-only instrumented groups was 15% (reduction maneuvers were used for both groups), compared with no neurologic complications in the posterior in situ fusion group. Good results were also reported for 23 of 27 patients with high-grade dysplastic spondylolisthesis who were treated with slip reduction and posterior and interbody fusion (19 received PLIF and 8, ALIF).[18] In 18 adolescent patients treated with posterior L5-S1 instrumentation, slip reduction, and PLIF for high-grade dysplastic spondylolisthesis, the fusion rate was 100% and no neurologic complications were reported;[23] the authors stressed the importance of anterior column support using titanium mesh PLIF cages filled with autograft to create a favorable biomechanical environment for reduction maintenance and fusion.

Fibula dowel (autograft or allograft) can also be used in high-grade spondylolisthesis for interbody fusion. The dowel can be placed in either a posterior-to-anterior or anterior-to-posterior direction to secure L5 to S1. Initial reports of the use of autograft fibula dowel and noninstrumented posterior spinal fusion in two patients demonstrated good results.[24] In a subsequent study of 11 patients who underwent decompression and fibular dowel interbody fusion, a 100% fusion rate and postoperative improvement in neurologic symptoms were reported.[25] Using a similar transsacral interbody fusion

technique, a titanium mesh cage filled with autograft was used in 15 patients.[26] The interbody graft was supplemented with L4-through-S1 posterior spinal fusion and instrumentation and L4-L5 PLIF in 13 patients, and only L5-S1 instrumentation in 2 patients. The authors reported a 100% fusion rate and neurologic complications in one patient. The technique included partial slip reduction using distraction between L2 and the sacrum. In another study, 17 patients were treated with posterior spinal decompression and fusion (15 of the patients received spinal instrumentation) followed by fibula dowel grafting (autograft or allograft) using a posterior-to-anterior approach (2 patients) or an anterior-to-posterior approach via a separate anterior incision (15 patients).[27] Sixteen of the 17 patients had solid fusion at an average 4-year follow-up. No significant difference was found in the incorporation rate of autograft and allograft fibula (6 and 11 patients, respectively). The dowel graft fractured in one patient who had received noninstrumented posterior spinal fusion.

Although the benefits of interbody fusion are well documented for high-grade spondylolisthesis, the need for anterior column support for low-grade spondylolisthesis is debatable. A comparison of adult patients with grade I or II spondylolisthesis and an associated pars defect treated with AP fusion using ALIF for anterior column support or treated with posterior fusion alone found that the AP fusion group had better early clinical outcomes.[28] However, the outcome differences between the two groups diminished after 6 months, and were similar at 2-year follow-up. Patients in the AP fusion group had more complications. A meta-analysis of surgical treatment for low-grade spondylolisthesis in adults revealed that patients receiving interbody fusion (with ALIF, PLIF, or transforaminal LIF) had improved clinical and radiographic outcomes.[29] However, the authors noted a lack of high-quality studies; most studies were single institution case series describing the use of one technique, and the average follow-up time was less than 2 years. Conversely, several studies have found similar or worse outcomes and higher complication rates when using interbody fusion compared with posterior fusion alone for patients with low-grade spondylolisthesis with lysis.[30] The high failure rate of stand-alone interbody fusion devices is especially notable. A growing number of reports have cited high complication rates and cage migration after spondylolisthesis treatment with stand-alone ALIF or PLIF.[31] The use of supplemental posterior instrumentation is strongly recommended in conjunction with interbody fusion for spondylolisthesis.

Interbody fusion is most likely not advisable for all patients with low-grade spondylolisthesis with lysis, although anterior column support may provide increased stability for patients at risk for failure of a stand-alone posterior fusion. Risk factors include smoking and a large disk space. An increased incidence of instrumentation failure and pseudarthrosis was reported in patients who had a preoperative disk more than 20% higher than the superior adjacent vertebra or a loss of lordosis (focal kyphosis) at the affected segment.[32] The authors of this study stipulated that pedicle screw instrumentation may be unable to control motion at an interspace with maintained disk height and focal kyphosis, and the patient may benefit from the added stability of interbody fusion.

Fusion Versus Decompression and Fusion

Partial or complete laminectomy is commonly performed for treatment of low-grade or high-grade spondylolisthesis with lysis to decompress nerve roots compressed by the hypertropic bone and fibrous tissue formed at the pars defect. Some authors have argued that the radiculopathy caused by spondylolisthesis is a dynamic stenosis that can be relieved when the abnormal motion segment is stabilized and the hypertropic material formed at the pars defect may resorb with a solid fusion. Additionally, the retained lamina may provide more posterior substrate for solid fusion. Lower fusion rates and worse clinical outcomes were reported in patients randomly assigned to treatment with decompression and fusion compared with patients treated with fusion alone.[33] However, a meta-analysis showed that decompressive laminectomy did not significantly impair clinical outcomes or fusion rates for low-grade spondylolisthesis with lysis.[29]

Pars Defect Repair

Several techniques have been described for repair of the pars interarticularis defect in low-grade spondylolisthesis with lysis, including defect bone grafting and compression instrumentation across the defect. The theoretic benefits of using pars interarticularis defect repair rather than segmental fusion include reduction of stress and degeneration of adjacent segments. A three-dimensional, nonlinear, finite element model showed that creation of a pars defect increases disk stresses at the cranial and caudal adjacent levels; spondylolysis repair restored normal stress to both disk levels.[34] In a calf spine model, increased motion was demonstrated at the cranial segment adjacent to a spondylolysis defect.[35] Pars repair decreased abnormal adjacent-segment motion, however, and pedicle screw segmental fixation increased cranial adjacent segment motion by decreasing motion at the fused segment. Consequently, pars repair may restore physiologic segmental motion adjacent to a spondylolytic defect and may reduce adjacent-level mechanical stresses compared with pedicle screw-rod segmental fixation.

Vertebral Resection

Grade V spondylolisthesis (spondyloptosis) is uncommon. The treatment is challenging, because by definition the affected vertebra is situated below the level of the caudal adjacent vertebra. One treatment option is L5 vertebrectomy and reduction of L4 onto S1. Long-term results with this procedure were recently discussed.[36] All patients were satisfied with the procedure, reported relief of back and leg pain, and had improved posture. Twenty-three of 30 patients had temporary postoperative deficits in one or both of the L5 nerve roots. Neurologic recovery was achieved in 6 weeks to 3 years. Two of the 23 patients had persistent L5 motor weakness, and one had chronic postoperative dysesthetic pain requiring pain management. No patients had postoperative bowel, bladder, or sexual dysfunction, although one patient reported retrograde ejaculation likely associated with the anterior portion of the procedure. Intraoperative somatosensory-evoked potentials were not predictive of postoperative neurologic deficits. It was concluded that, although prevention of injury is the best management, treatment of fixed spondyloptosis with vertebral resection is effective.

Summary

Spondylolysis and spondylolisthesis are relatively common; however, the presence of these conditions does not imply that the patient has symptoms. The clinical and radiographic course of the most common forms of spondylolysis and spondylolisthesis appears to be benign. However, high-dysplastic conditions are at risk for progression and are best treated early before they develop into high-grade spondylolisthesis. The Marchetti and Bartolozzi classification system allows identification of slips that are at risk of progression. Research on spinopelvic balance has provided some understanding of the biomechanical factors that can lead to spondylolisthesis and may help identify patients at risk for slip progression. Future research may lead to treatment guidelines. Several surgical treatment options are available for low-grade and high-grade spondylolisthesis, although few high-quality studies have directly compared these options.

Annotated References

1. Sairyo K, Katoh S, Takata Y, et al: MRI signal changes of the pedicle as an indicator for early diagnosis of spondylolysis in children and adolescents: A clinical and biomechanical study. *Spine* 2006;31:206-211.

   Thirty-seven patients with 68 pars defects on CT were included in this clinical review of pediatric patients with lumbar spondylolysis. High signal changes (HSC) of the pedicles on axial T2-weighted MRI were compared with CT-based stages of the defect. The correlation between high stresses in the pedicle and the corresponding HSC suggests that signal changes in MRI could be used as an early indicator of spondylolysis. Furthermore, HSC may indicate whether a bony union will result from conservative treatment.

2. Meyerding HW: Spondylolisthesis. *Surg Gynecol Obstet* 1932;54:371-377.

3. Marchetti PG, Bartolozzi P: Spondylolisthesis: Classification of spondylolisthesis as a guide for treatment, in Bridwell KH, DeWald RL (eds): *The Textbook of Spinal*

Surgery, ed 2. Philadelphia, PA, Lippincott-Raven, 1997, pp 1211-1254.

4. Wiltse LL, Newman PH, Macnab I: Classification of spondylolysis and spondylolisthesis. *Clin Othop Relat Res* 1976;117:23-29.

5. Legaye J, Duval-Beaupere G, Hecquet J, Marty C: Pelvic incidence: A fundamental pelvic parameter for three-dimensional regulation of spinal sagittal curves. *Eur Spine J* 1998;7:99-103.

6. Mac-Thiong JM, Labelle H, Berthonnaud E, Betz RR, Roussouly P: Sagittal spinopelvic balance in normal children and adolescents. *Eur Spine J* 2007; 16:227-234.

    Sagittal spinopelvic balance in the pediatric population was characterized and correlations between spinopelvic parameters evaluated.

7. Roussouly P, Gollogly S, Berthonnaud E, Labelle H, Weidenbaum M: Sagittal alignment of the spine and pelvis in L5-S1 isthmic lysis and spondylolisthesis. *Spine* 2006;31:2484-2490.

    In 82 patients with spondylolysis and low-grade spondylolisthesis, pelvic incidence and lumbar lordosis was increased but there was less segmental extension between L5 and S1 compared with normal subjects.

8. Labelle H, Roussouly P, Berthonnaud E, et al: Spondylolisthesis, pelvic incidence, and spinopelvic balance: A correlation study. *Spine* 2004;29:2049-2054.

    Results from this study indicate that the anatomy of the pelvis directly influences the development of spondylolisthesis.

9. Mac-Thiong JM, Labelle H: A proposal for a surgical classification of pediatric lumbosacral spondylolisthesis based on current literature. *Eur Spine J* 2006;15:1425-1435.

    This classification, the first specifically designed to guide surgical treatment of L5-S1 spondylolisthesis in children and adolescents, is based on degree of slippage, degree of dysplasia, and sagittal spinopelvic balance.

10. Sonne-Holm S, Jacobsen S, Rovsing HC, Monrad H, Gebuhr P. Lumbar spondylolysis: A life long dynamic condition? A cross sectional survey of 4,151 adults. *Eur Spine J 2007;16:821-828.*

    A cross-sectional survey of lumbar radiographs and general epidemiological data from the Copenhagen Osteoarthritis Study cohort of 4,151 subjects found that men were significantly more at risk for L5 spondylolysis (*P* = 0.002). No sex-specific differences appeared regarding lumbar spondylolysis incidence at the L4 level. This study conflicts with commonly held views that the prevalence of lumbar spondylolysis increases throughout life and is not restricted to adolescence. The cross-sectional nature of the study prevents an exact estimate of age at onset. Age, obesity, lordotic angle, and pelvic inclination were found to be risk factors for lumbar spondylolysis.

11. Fredrickson BE, Baker D, McHolick WJ, Yuan HA, Lubicky JP: The natural history of spondylolysis and spondylolisthesis. *J Bone Joint Surg Am* 1984;66:699-707.

12. Belfi LM, Ortiz AO, Katz DS: Computed tomography evaluation of spondylolysis and spondylolisthesis in asymptomatic patients. *Spine* 2006;31:E907-E910.

    Abdominal and pelvic CT scans of 510 patients with clinical conditions other than back pain were analyzed in a retrospective study. Twenty-nine patients (5.7%) had spondylolysis at L5; of the 23 with bilateral spondylolysis, 16 also had spondylolisthesis (13 had grade I, and 3 had grade II).

13. Beutler WJ, Fredrickson BE, Murtland A, Sweeney CA, Grant WD, Baker D: The natural history of spondylolysis and spondylolisthesis: 45-year follow-up evaluation. *Spine* 2003;28:1027-1035.

14. Moller H, Hedlund R: Instrumented and noninstrumented posterolateral fusion in adult spondylolisthesis: A prospective randomized study. Part 2. *Spine* 2000;25:1716-1721.

15. Moller H, Hedlund R: Surgery versus conservative management in adult isthmic spondylolisthesis: A prospective randomized study. Part 1. *Spine* 2000;25:1711-1715.

16. L'Heureux EA Jr, Perra JH, Pinto MR, Smith MD, Denis F, Lonstein JE: Functional outcome analysis including preoperative and postoperative SF-36 for surgically treated adult isthmic spondylolisthesis. *Spine* 2003;28:1269-1274.

17. Bjarke Christensen F, Stender Hansen E, Laursen M, Thomsen K, Bunger CE: Long-term functional outcome of pedicle screw instrumentation as a support for posterolateral spinal fusion: Randomized clinical study with a 5-year follow-up. *Spine* 2002;27:1269-1277.

18. Ruf M, Koch H, Melcher RP, Harms J: Anatomic reduction and monosegmental fusion in high-grade developmental spondylolisthesis. *Spine* 2006;31:269-274.

    In a retrospective review of 27 consecutive patients with severe developmental spondylolisthesis at L5-S1 who were treated with surgical slip reduction via temporary instrumentation of L4 and monosegmental fusion of L5-S1, 23 patients were pain free at latest follow-up and 4 had moderate pain. All radiographic parameters had improved: mean slippage improved from 74% before surgery to 11% after surgery and 10% at latest follow-up. Slip angle improved from 36.6° before surgery to 8.1° after surgery and 7.6° at latest follow-up. One superficial infection occurred, and six patients had L5 root symptoms (five resolved, and one patient had a persistent sensory deficit). Four patients had decompensation at L4-L5; two revisions were required.

19. Sailhan F, Gollogly S, Roussouly P: The radiographic results and neurologic complications of instrumented reduction and fusion of high-grade spondylolisthesis without decompression of the neural elements: A retrospective review of 44 patients. *Spine* 2006;31:161-169.

5: Spine

According to the results of this retrospective review of all patients with high-grade spondylolisthesis treated by one surgeon between 1991 and 2003, there was an average L5-S1 reduction from 64% to 38%. At 2-year minimum follow-up, five patients (11.4%) had pseudarthrosis or loss of reduction. The overall neurologic complication rate was 9.1%, with a 2.3% chance of a persistent motor deficit. At last follow-up and after revision procedures, 40 (90.9%) of 44 patients had good or fair clinical results.

20. Poussa M, Remes V, Lamberg T, et al: Treatment of severe spondylolisthesis in adolescence with reduction or fusion in situ: Long-term clinical, radiologic, and functional outcome. *Spine* 2006;31:583-590.

    This retrospective study evaluated 22 adolescents with severe (more than 60%) slippage who were treated with either slip reduction and fusion or in situ fusion. Oswestry Disability Index scores were significantly improved. Scoliosis Research Society Outcomes Instrument scores in the in situ fusion group were improved compared with that of the reduction and fusion group. MRI-evident disk degeneration above the fusion was more common in the reduction group. There was no difference in spinal mobility or trunk strength measurements between the groups.

21. Helenius I, Lamberg T, Osterman K, et al: Posterolateral, anterior, or circumferential fusion in situ for high-grade spondylolisthesis in young patients: A long-term evaluation using the Scoliosis Research Society questionnaire. *Spine* 2006;31:190-196.

    Clinical and radiographic outcomes were compared retrospectively in children and adolescents after posterolateral, anterior, or circumferential in situ fusion without instrumentation for high-grade spondylolisthesis. The mean follow-up was 17.2 years. The average Scoliosis Research Society Outcomes Instrument total score was 89.7 in the posterolateral, 93.2 in the anterior, and 100.0 in the circumferential fusion group ($P = 0.021$). Patients in the circumferential fusion group had better values for pain ($P = 0.023$) and function from back condition domains ($P = 0.079$) than patients in the posterolateral or anterior groups. The average Oswestry Disability Index score was 9.7 in the posterolateral, 8.9 in the anterior, and 3.0 in the circumferential fusion group ($P = 0.035$).

22. Molinari RW, Bridwell KH, Lenke LG, Ungacta FF, Riew KD: Complications in the surgical treatment of pediatric high-grade, isthmic dysplastic spondylolisthesis: A comparison of three surgical approaches. *Spine* 1999;24:1701-1711.

23. Shufflebarger HL, Geck MJ: High-grade isthmic dysplastic spondylolisthesis: Nonsegmental surgical treatment. *Spine* 2005;30:S42-S48.

    In a prospective evaluation of 18 adolescents with high-grade isthmic dysplastic spondylolisthesis treated with distraction reduction, PLIF and posterior compression improved slip from 77% to 13%. Slip angle improved from 35° to 3.8° initially and was 4.3° at final follow-up. Sacral inclination improved from 28° to 39°. No neurologic or infectious complications or overt instrumentation failures appeared. Arthrodesis was achieved in all cases. Two patients had structural complications, neither of which required revision.

24. Bohlman HH, Cook SS: One-stage decompression and posterolateral and interbody fusion for lumbosacral spondyloptosis through a posterior approach: Report of two cases. *J Bone Joint Surg Am* 1982;64:415-418.

25. Smith MD, Bohlman HH: Spondylolisthesis treated by a single-stage operation combining decompression with in situ posterolateral and anterior fusion: An analysis of eleven patients who had long-term follow-up. *J Bone Joint Surg Am* 1990;72:415-421.

26. Bartolozzi P, Sandri A, Cassini M, Ricci M: One-stage posterior decompression-stabilization and trans-sacral interbody fusion after partial reduction for severe L5-S1 spondylolisthesis. *Spine* 2003;28:1135-1141.

27. Hanson DS, Bridwell KH, Rhee JM, Lenke LG: Dowel fibular strut grafts for high-grade dysplastic isthmic spondylolisthesis. *Spine* 2002;27:1982-1988.

28. Swan J, Hurwitz E, Malek F, et al: Surgical treatment for unstable low-grade isthmic spondylolisthesis in adults: A prospective controlled study of posterior instrumented fusion compared with combined anterior-posterior fusion. *Spine J* 2006;6:606-614.

    A prospective controlled trial comparing single-level posterolateral instrumented fusion with combined anterior and posterolateral instrumented fusion in sequential matched cohorts of patients with radiographically unstable isthmic spondylolisthesis found improved outcomes in the anteroposterior cohort in all measures at 6 months and 12 months. Three nonunions occurred in the posterior-alone cohort, and one appeared in the combined group. Rates of serious complication and revision were similar in the two groups. Between-group differences were attenuated after 6 months.

29. Kwon BK, Hilibrand AS, Malloy K, et al: A critical analysis of the literature regarding surgical approach and outcome for adult low-grade isthmic spondylolisthesis. *J Spinal Disord Tech* 2005;18(suppl):S30-S40.

    This systematic review of the literature on radiographic and clinical outcomes of adult patients undergoing surgery for low-grade isthmic spondylolisthesis found that only 4 of 34 reports were prospective randomized controlled studies; the remainder were retrospective case series. Patients with combined anterior and posterior procedures were most likely to achieve a solid fusion and successful clinical outcome. Spinal fixation also increased the chance of fusion and successful clinical outcome.

30. Madan S, Boeree NR: Outcome of posterior lumbar interbody fusion versus posterolateral fusion for spondylolytic spondylolisthesis. *Spine* 2002;27:1536-1542.

31. Button G, Gupta M, Barrett C, Cammack P, Benson D: Three- to six-year follow up of stand-alone BAK cages implanted by a single surgeon. *Spine J* 2005;5:155-160.

    A retrospective review of 3- to 6-year clinical outcomes,

including fusion rate, revision rate, complications and functional status of patients who underwent stand-alone ALIF with a Bagby and Kuslich (BAK) cage performed by a single surgeon found a 22% revision rate. Ten patients (22%) had 14 total complications not requiring revision surgery; 70% of patients had a fair or poor outcome as assessed by the Prolo rating system, and 58% had, at a minimum, severe disability as measured on the Oswestry Disability Index. Fifty percent of patients were satisfied with their surgery. The authors concluded that clinical outcomes after stand-alone BAK cage surgery were significantly worse than previously reported and that the use of stand-alone BAK cages should be reconsidered.

32. Suda K, Ito M, Abumi K, Haba H, Taneichi H, Kaneda K: Radiological risk factors of pseudoarthrosis and/or instrument breakage after PLF with the pedicle screw system in isthmic spondylolisthesis. *J Spinal Disord Tech* 2006;19:541-546.

A retrospective analysis of 101 patients with isthmic spondylolisthesis who underwent pedicle screw instrumented posterior spinal fusion revealed that posterior instrumented spinal fusion provided satisfactory results with a high fusion rate. However, preoperative disk height and slip angle were the most crucial factors leading to pseudarthrosis or instrument failure.

33. Carragee EJ: Single-level posterolateral arthrodesis, with or without posterior decompression, for the treatment of isthmic spondylolisthesis in adults: A prospective, randomized study. *J Bone Joint Surg Am* 1997;79:1175-1180.

34. Sairyo K, Goel VK, Faizan A, Vadapalli S, Biyani S, Ebraheim N: Buck's direct repair of lumbar spondylolysis restores disc stresses at the involved and adjacent levels. *Clin Biomech (Bristol, Avon)* 2006;21:1020-1026.

A three-dimensional nonlinear finite element model of the intact ligamentous L3-through-S1 segment with bilateral lumbar spondylolysis was simulated by creating bilateral pars defects with a 1.0 mm gap at L5. Buck's direct repair model was simulated with 4.0 mm cannulated titanium screws placed bilaterally across the defect. Von Mises stresses in the anulus fibrosus and nucleus pulposus at L4-L5 (cranial adjacent) and L5-S1 (caudal adjacent) disk levels were analyzed in flexion, extension, lateral bending, and axial rotation. After spondylolysis, anulus fibrosus and nucleus pulposus stresses at L4-L5 increased to 111% and 120%, respectively. After treatment with Buck's technique, they recovered to 102% and 105%, respectively. At L5-S1, anulus fibrosus stress increased to 168% and nucleus pulposus stress, to 155%. After treatment with Buck's technique, the stresses recovered to 125% and 120%, respectively.

35. Mihara H, Onari K, Cheng BC, David SM, Zdeblick TA: The biomechanical effects of spondylolysis and its treatment. *Spine* 2003;28:235-238.

36. Gaines RW: L5 vertebrectomy for the surgical treatment of spondyloptosis: Thirty cases in 25 years. *Spine* 2005;30:S66-S70.

This is a retrospective review by a single surgeon of long-term results, complications, and predictability of L5 vertebrectomy and reduction of L4 onto S1 for the surgical treatment of fixed spondyloptosis.

Chapter 51

Thoracic Disk Herniations

Peter G. Whang, MD   Jonathan N. Grauer, MD

Epidemiology

Abnormalities of intervertebral disk are encountered much less frequently in the thoracic spine than in the cervical and lumbar regions. Although MRI studies have suggested that incidental thoracic disk herniations (TDHs) may be present in up to 37% of adults, most of these are of little clinical significance and do not require treatment.[1] Less than 1% of symptomatic disk herniations occur in the thoracic spine. The overall incidence of symptomatic TDH has been estimated to be approximately 1 in 1 million patient-years.

TDHs are most common in the fourth to sixth decades of life, with no gender predilection. These herniations are most typically observed between T8 and L1, with only a small fraction detected above the T4-5 level. Although multiple thoracic segments may exhibit radiographic evidence of degenerative changes, it is uncommon for more than one of these levels to be symptomatic. Most thoracic disk pathology is located either centrally or paracentrally, but can also be posterolateral or more foraminal in nature.

Etiology

Even though almost one half of all patients with symptomatic TDH report a history of trauma or recall an inciting event before the onset of their symptoms, it is widely believed that these pathologic changes arise more as a result of the natural degenerative processes that affect cervical and lumbar disks in a similar fashion.[2]

The mobility of the thoracic spine is limited by multiple factors, including the stabilizing effects of the rib cage and costovertebral articulations as well as the vertical orientation of the facet joints in the coronal plane. By resisting motion in all directions, these anatomic constraints limit the forces applied to thoracic disks and minimize their risk of subsequent degeneration. This protective mechanism not only accounts for the decreased incidence of TDH in comparison with other regions of the spine but may also explain why the more flexible lower thoracic segments generally demonstrate greater disease involvement than the stiffer segments of the upper thoracic spine, which are subjected to less stresses and loads.

Despite the relative paucity of symptomatic TDH, there are several anatomic features that predispose patients with thoracic disk abnormalities to neurologic dysfunction. Although the diameter of the spinal cord is smallest in the thoracic spine, the cord-to-canal ratio is actually larger in this region because of the undersized dimensions of the canal itself, leaving little space for the neural elements. The physiologic kyphosis of the thoracic spine may also exacerbate compression of the spinal cord or nerve roots by draping these structures over prominences originating from the posterior aspects of the vertebral bodies or disk spaces. In addition, the more tenuous vascular supply to the thoracic spinal cord creates a watershed area particularly susceptible to ischemic injury, which may compound any neurologic deficits brought about by compressive pathology.

Clinical Presentation

Patients with TDH may initially report varied symptoms that are frequently subtle or vague; therefore, this condition may not be recognized until later in the disease course. Establishing a definitive diagnosis is made even more difficult by the high prevalence of incidental TDH and the extensive differential diagnosis that exists for this often nonspecific clinical presentation. For this reason, it is critical that the treating physician maintain an index of suspicion for TDH while ruling out all other potential causes of these symptoms[3] (Table 1).

The most common symptom is axial pain based in the thoracolumbar spine, but many individuals will experience radicular discomfort that radiates to the anterior chest wall in a dermatomal distribution. Sensory changes may also be present in these patients. In some instances, myelopathic findings may already be evident at the time of diagnosis, characterized by changes in bowel or bladder function, gait abnormalities, spasticity, or other long-tract signs.

The pattern of symptoms that each patient exhibits is largely dependent on the position of the pathology within the spinal canal and the neural structures that are being compressed. Lateral protrusions that only encroach on the nerve roots are more likely to produce radicular pain, whereas midline and paramedian herniations are more likely to result in myelopathy. Although TDH may give rise to considerable morbidity in a small percentage of these individuals, there are currently no reliable methods for predicting which thoracic lesions will ultimately become symptomatic.

5: Spine

Table 1

Differential Diagnosis for Thoracic Pain, Radicular Symptoms, and/or Myelopathy

Nonspinal Etiologies
  Visceral
    Intrathoracic
    Intra-abdominal
  Musculoskeletal
    Muscle strains
    Inflammatory arthritides
    Rheumatologic conditions
  Neurologic
    Herpes zoster
    Intercostal neuralgia
  Metabolic
  Psychosocial
Spinal Etiologies
  Thoracic disk herniation
  Degenerative
    Spondylosis
    Spinal stenosis
    Degenerative disk disease
  Infectious
  Neoplastic
  Traumatic
  Vascular
  Deformity

(Adapted from Vanichkachorn JS, Vaccaro AR: Thoracic disk disease: Diagnosis and treatment. J Am Acad Orthop Surg 2000;8:159-169.)

Diagnostic Imaging

When a patient's history and physical examination are suggestive of TDH, appropriate imaging modalities are used to corroborate this diagnosis. Screening radiographs are important for evaluating the sagittal and coronal alignment of the thoracic spine and are useful for excluding other more obvious disorders such as fractures or malignancies. In addition to displaying osteophytes, disk-space narrowing, and other degenerative changes, radiographs may also reveal calcification of TDHs; however, in most instances these calcified lesions are not readily apparent on plain films.

MRI remains the gold standard technique for evaluating TDH[3] (Figure 1, A). In addition to identifying and defining compressive pathology, these studies can be helpful in ruling out other thoracic pathologies.

CT may be considered to determine whether TDHs are calcified, particularly if surgery is being considered (Figure 1, B and C). Calcification suggests that a disk may be more difficult to mobilize because of associated dural adhesions or possible intrathecal extension of disk fragments. CT myelography may also be performed as an alternative to MRI. In addition to providing the information evident on standard CT scans, a CT myelogram is useful for evaluating compression of the neural elements.

Because incidental disk abnormalities are routinely noted on these advanced neuroimaging studies, corre-

lating radiographic pathology with the clinical presentation remains a formidable challenge. Diskography is a controversial diagnostic procedure that can be considered to identify a discogenic pain generator in certain patients who present with predominantly axial discomfort and no neurologic symptoms. However, the sensitivity and specificity of thoracic diskography have not been established, and there is no definitive evidence to suggest that this technique improves clinical outcomes following surgery. As a result, it is difficult to justify the regular use of diskography for patients with thoracic symptoms.

Nonsurgical Management

The natural history of TDH is similar to that of herniations in the cervical and lumbar spines in that most of these lesions are benign and follow a self-limiting course.[4] Longitudinal studies have shown that asymptomatic TDHs do not typically demonstrate significant changes in size over time and seldom result in clinical symptoms.

Patients who seek treatment for their symptoms will usually respond favorably to a combination of conservative measures, including a medical regimen comprising anti-inflammatory medications or oral steroids, activity modification, physical therapy, bracing, or epidural/foraminal injections. Given that the implementation of these nonsurgical therapies ordinarily brings about significant clinical improvement without any long-term sequelae, it has been estimated that fewer than 2% of TDHs necessitate subsequent surgical intervention.

Even individuals with early or stable myelopathy with no appreciable functional impairment may be initially managed conservatively, although they must be closely observed for persistent neurologic symptoms or any evidence of neurologic decline.

Surgical Management

Each year only 1% of all the spinal procedures that are performed to address intervertebral disk pathology are related to the treatment of TDH. The primary indication for surgery in these patients is myelopathy or neurologic deterioration, but surgical management may also be considered for disabling radicular symptoms or axial back pain that has proved to be refractory to conservative therapies.

Successful surgical outcomes are clearly contingent on meticulous preoperative planning, which is essential for determining the morphology and anatomic location of a TDH. In particular, the specific level of pathology must be definitively established to ensure that a normal disk space is not inadvertently violated. Although the ribs and prominent osteophytes may serve as distinguishing landmarks on plain radiographs, the most precise method for identifying the correct spinal segment involves counting from C2 or the sacrum on the sagit-

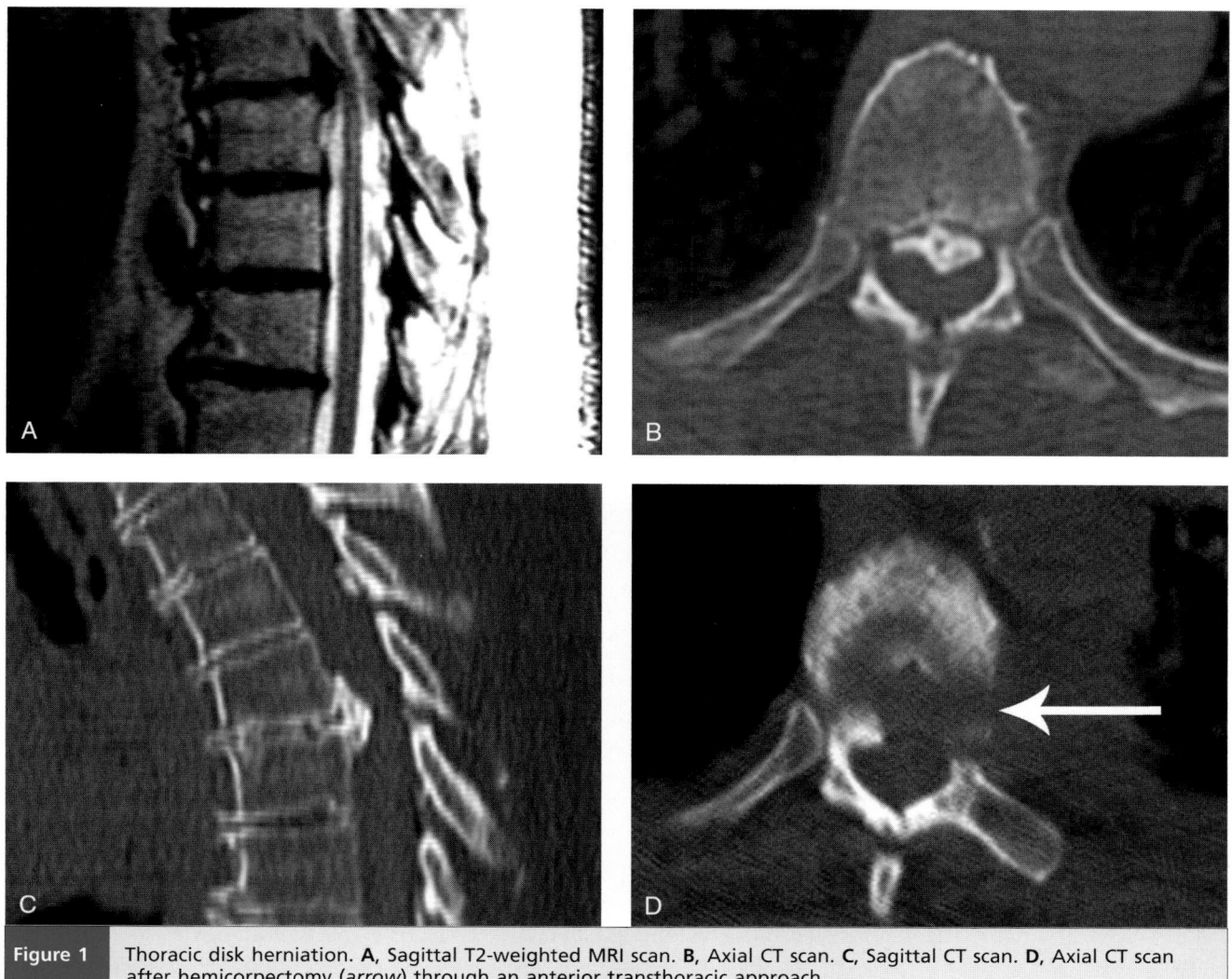

Figure 1 Thoracic disk herniation. **A,** Sagittal T2-weighted MRI scan. **B,** Axial CT scan. **C,** Sagittal CT scan. **D,** Axial CT scan after hemicorpectomy (*arrow*) through an anterior transthoracic approach.

tal images of MRI or CT myelography. To that end, one must make sure that preoperative cross-sectional studies allow visualization from one end of the spine to the desired pathology. These findings should also be matched to plain radiographs, which may be more readily compared with intraoperative films. The level of interest must then be confirmed intraoperatively, using radiographs or fluoroscopy to localize a radiographic marker. With anterior surgical approaches the rib heads may be directly counted as a confirmatory measure.

The surgical strategy originally described for the treatment of TDHs consisted of thoracic laminectomy followed by excision of the compressive lesion, similar to techniques used in the lumbar spine. However, this direct posterior approach has largely fallen out of favor because the retraction of the spinal cord required to gain access to the disk material was associated with an unacceptably high rate of postoperative neurologic problems.

Anterior thoracotomy has been used as an alternative approach to laminectomy, allowing for a direct line

of sight for visualization of ventral disk pathology without requiring manipulation of the neural elements[5,6] (**Figure 1,** *D*). In performing this procedure, after the patient is placed in the lateral position, a thoracotomy is made and the rib head is resected so that the disk can be accessed. The posterior vertebral bone above and below the disk can be resected and the disk gently drawn away from the neural elements into the cavity that is created.

Certainly, the thoracotomy approach is associated with morbidity.[7] Besides generally necessitating postoperative chest tube drainage, opening the thoracic cavity may compromise respiratory function to the extent that patients with pulmonary disorders or a previous thoracotomy may not be appropriate candidates for this technique. And, although rare, vascular or visceral injuries may be encountered. Furthermore, disk spaces cephalad to the T4 vertebra or caudal to the thoracolumbar junction may not be accessible by this method secondary to the anatomic constraints of the heart and diaphragm.

5: Spine

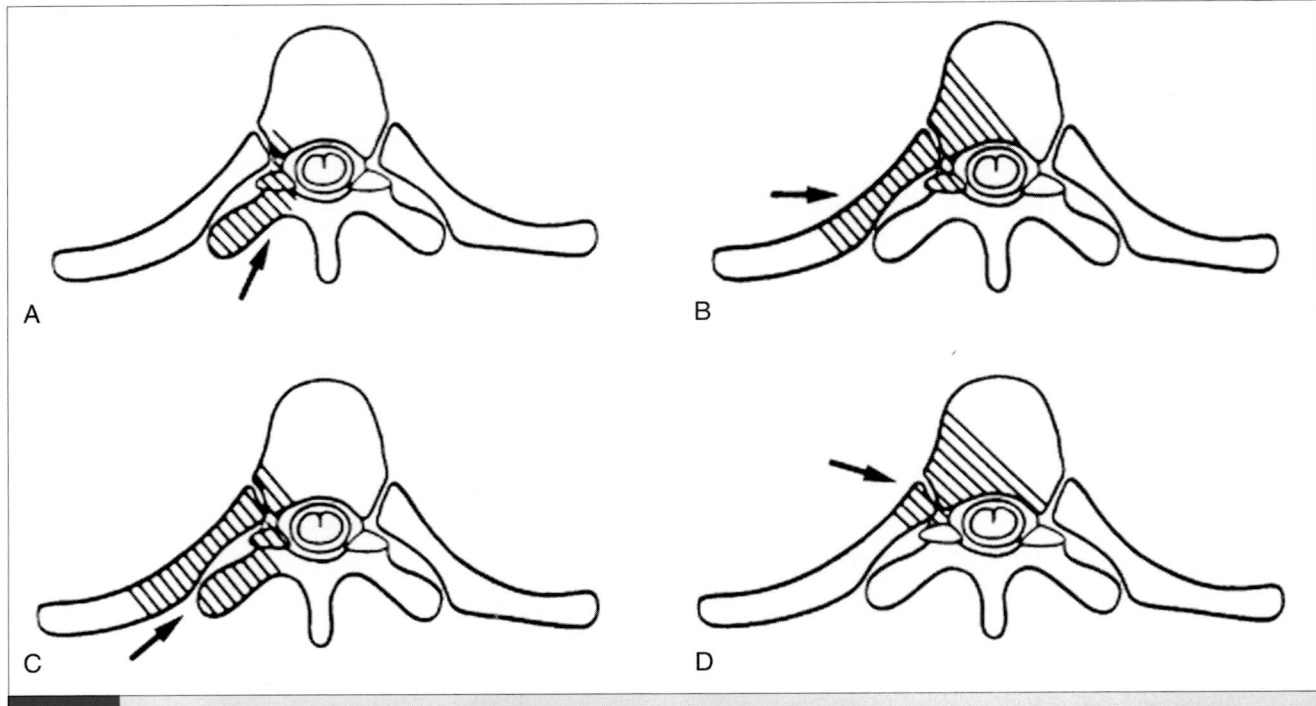

Figure 2 Different surgical approaches for addressing thoracic disk pathology: transpedicular **(A)**, lateral extracavitary **(B)**, costotransversectomy **(C)**, and transthoracic **(D)**. *(Reproduced with permission from Cybulski G: Thoracic disc herniation: Surgical technique. Contemp Neurosurg 1992;14:1-6.)*

Video-assisted thoracoscopic surgery is a minimally invasive strategy that may be considered an alternative surgical approach to thoracic disk pathology. Although technically demanding, requiring specialized instruments, and associated with a learning curve, multiple studies have reported that video-assisted thoracoscopic surgery may yield clinical outcomes that are comparable to those observed following an open thoracotomy with lower rates of pulmonary complications and intercostal neuralgia.[8,9]

Because many surgeons prefer to avoid the anterior approaches if possible, other more laterally based posterior approaches have been developed to allow access to thoracic disk pathology while minimizing manipulation of the neural elements (**Figure 2**). These approaches are generally best for more laterally based TDHs that are not calcified.

The transpedicular approach is somewhat similar to the posterior laminectomy approach; however, bone is taken down along the path of the pedicle to allow for greater visualization of the underlying disk. Nevertheless, limited additional visualization is afforded with this technique, which is generally reserved for soft, lateral protrusions. There is less soft-tissue disruption than with other approaches, but excessive resection of the facets and other posterior elements may lead to segmental instability in these patients.

The costotransversectomy approach moves the dissection more laterally and entails removal of the transverse process and its articulation with the medial rib, along with the adjacent pedicle, facet joint, and the su-

perolateral portion of the caudal vertebral body. The lateral extracavitary approach is based even more laterally than a costotransversectomy and calls for the removal of the same structures with the exception of the transverse process and potentially the medial facet to gain entry to the disk space. Both of these extrapleural strategies facilitate the decompression of the neural elements by providing an enhanced view of the thecal sac and the posterior aspect of the spinal column that is superior to the exposure generated by the transpedicular method. Even with their more lateral trajectories, these approaches may also not be suitable for more central or calcified disk herniations. Additionally, the greater bone resection may increase the destabilizing effect of these procedures.

The exact role of arthrodesis after removal of a TDH continues to be a matter of some debate. After anterior thoracotomy, many surgeons will place rib or other graft in the cavity of resected bone. This may be done with or without instrumentation. Posteriorly based procedures may require fusion if sufficient bone is removed, raising concerns for possible instability. Posterior fusions are generally performed with posterior instrumentation.

Emerging Concepts

Although these decompressive procedures represent a well-accepted treatment for symptomatic disk herniations in the thoracic spine, a variety of minimally invasive surgical approaches have recently been developed.[10,11] By avoiding much of the morbidity associated with conventional surgical strategies, these novel techniques may have the potential to facilitate patient recovery and improve clinical outcomes.

Annotated References

1. Wood KB, Garvey TA, Gundry C, Heitoff KB: Magnetic resonance imaging of the thoracic spine: Evaluation of asymptomatic individuals. *J Bone Joint Surg Am* 1995; 77:1631-1638.

2. Linscott MS, Heyborne R: Thoracic intervertebral disk herniation: A commonly missed diagnosis. *J Emerg Med* 2007;32:235-238.

    In the largest single study of TDHs, the medical records of 78 patients with symptomatic lesions were reviewed. Injury was associated with disk herniation in approximately one half of the patients, a rate much higher than reported previously. Back pain was the most common presenting symptom (73% of patients), and weakness was the most common physical finding (42% of patients). Eighty-five percent of patients demonstrated either a history of or physical findings consistent with neuropathy; 26% of patients had multiple TDHs. Level of evidence: IV.

3. Vanichkachorn JS, Vaccaro AR: Thoracic disk disease: Diagnosis and treatment. *J Am Acad Orthop Surg* 2000;8:159-169.

4. Brown CW, Deffer PA Jr, Akmakjian J, Donaldson DH, Brugman JL: The natural history of thoracic disc herniation. *Spine* 1992;17:S97-S102.

5. Bohlman HH, Zdeblick TA: Anterior excision of herniated thoracic discs. *J Bone Joint Surg Am* 1988;70: 1038-1047.

6. Ohnishi K, Miyamoto K, Kanamori Y, et al: Anterior decompression and fusion for multiple thoracic disc herniation. *J Bone Joint Surg Br* 2005;87:356-360.

    In this case series, 12 patients with multilevel TDHs were treated with anterior decompression and fusion through a transthoracic approach. Postoperatively, two patients improved by two Frankel grades (C to E), one patient improved by one grade (C to D), and nine pa-

tients who had been classified as grade D had no change. The Japanese Orthopaedic Association scores improved significantly after surgery, with a mean recovery rate of 44.8% +/− 24.5%. These findings indicate that this technique may bring about satisfactory results in patients with this relatively rare condition. Level of evidence: IV.

7. Currier BL, Eismont FJ, Green BA: Transthoracic disc excision and fusion for herniated thoracic discs. *Spine* 1994;19:323-328.

8. Regan JJ, Ben-Yishay A, Mack MJ: Video-assisted thoracoscopic excision of herniated thoracic disc: Description of technique and preliminary experience in the first 29 cases. *J Spinal Disord* 1998;11:183-191.

9. Anand N, Regan JJ: Video-assisted thoracoscopic surgery for thoracic disc disease: Classification and outcome study of 100 consecutive cases with a 2-year minimum follow-up period. *Spine* 2002;27:871-879.

10. Issacs RE, Podichetty VK, Sandhu FA, et al: Thoracic microendoscopic discectomy: A human cadaver study. *Spine* 2005;30:1226-1231.

    The authors describe a novel method of percutaneous posterolateral thoracic microendoscopic diskectomy, which was validated in a human cadaver model. From these preliminary results, it is possible that the effective treatment of TDHs through a minimally invasive posterolateral approach may avoid the morbidity associated with entry into the thoracic cavity and expedite patient recovery.

11. Lidar A, Lifshutz J, Bhattacharjee S, et al: Minimally invasive, extracavitary approach for thoracic disc herniation: Technical report and preliminary results. *Spine J* 2006;6:157-163.

    The purpose of this investigation was to assess the feasibility, safety, and early outcomes associated with a minimally invasive extracavitary approach for TDHs. After this technique was attempted in cadavers, 10 patients with thoracic myelopathy secondary to herniated disks were treated using this strategy. All of the disk herniations were successfully removed and no complications were documented. Patients had significant improvement in multiple subjective and objective clinical outcomes measures, suggesting that a minimally invasive extracavitary approach may be a valuable surgical option for managing symptomatic TDHs.

Chapter 52

Spine Tumors

*Rex Marco, MD

Introduction

The evaluation and treatment of patients with primary and metastatic spinal column tumors is diverse and complex. The type of tumor (Tables 1 and 2), the level of spinal column involvement, the location within the vertebrae, the presence of spinal cord compression with or without neurologic deficits, the physiologic stability of the spine, the responsiveness of the tumor to adjuvant treatment, and the patient's medical condition must be considered before proceeding with definitive treatment. A multidisciplinary team composed of a radiologist, pathologist, oncologist, and spine surgeon with expertise in the treatment of primary and metastatic spinal column tumors is required to provide optimal care for the patient.

Primary bone tumors of the spinal column usually present as a solitary lesion. A thorough history and physical examination, as well as appropriate radiologic studies, are performed before diagnostic tissue is obtained. Benign primary bone tumors are more common in children, whereas malignant primary bone tumors are more common in adults. Pain is the most common presenting symptom. Neurologic deficits are less commonly identified. Plain radiographs evaluate the level of the lesion, local anatomy, and overall spinal alignment. A staging bone scan helps confirm the solitary nature of the tumor. CT defines bony architecture and can demonstrate characteristic findings of hemangioma, osteoid osteoma, and osteochondroma. A staging CT scan of the chest, abdomen, and pelvis is obtained to evaluate for areas of distant metastases. MRI evaluates soft-tissue extension, compression of the neural elements within the vertebra, and location of metastases. Fluid-fluid levels are often seen on MRI if the tumor has a component of an aneurysmal bone cyst.

The histologic diagnosis and the physiologic stability of the spine direct appropriate treatment of patients with primary and metastatic spinal column tumors.[1] A biopsy is obtained before performing the definitive procedure, even if a patient has a progressive neurologic deficit with spinal cord compression. Fortunately, most patients do not present with a progressive neurologic

deficit even in the presence of severe spinal cord compression with a baseline neurologic deficit (Figure 1). A stable, nonprogressive neurologic examination with or without a baseline neurologic deficit provides the practitioner with time to obtain a biopsy before proceeding with definitive treatment. In the presence of spinal cord compression, corticosteroids usually maintain the patient's neurologic function and provide improved pain control. However, the oncolytic effect of corticosteroids on myelogenous tumors such as myeloma and lymphoma can decrease the likelihood of obtaining diagnostic tissue. To expedite the diagnostic process and treatment, an urgent biopsy followed by administration of corticosteroids is thus warranted for patients with spinal cord compression associated with a solitary lesion. The corticosteroids can stabilize or improve neurologic function while the final histologic diagnosis is determined. A core needle biopsy minimizes contamination more than an open biopsy. Minimizing contamination preserves most surgical options, including en bloc excision. If the core needle biopsy is not diagnostic, then a carefully planned open biopsy is indicated.

Occasionally, a patient will present with spinal cord compression and a progressive neurologic deficit. A biopsy is still warranted before proceeding with definitive treatment. An emergent posterior decompression with a frozen section analysis simultaneously decompresses the spine and provides diagnostic tissue. Additionally, a posterior approach does not expose vascular and visceral structures to contamination with tumor cells, which in turn probably decreases the likelihood of local recurrence and preserves treatment options such as en bloc excision. If the pathologist identifies metastatic carcinoma, then performance of an intralesional excision and definitive stabilization should be considered (Figure 2). However, if a primary bone tumor is suspected, then a spine surgeon with expertise in the treatment of spinal column tumors should be consulted before definitive treatment is started. If the spinal column is rendered unstable by the decompression, then provisional posterior spinal instrumentation can be placed to stabilize the spine until the diagnosis is confirmed. If a primary bone tumor is identified, then appropriate adjuvant therapy can be administered before proceeding with definitive surgical intervention.

Surgical staging of bone tumors is prognostic and can facilitate subsequent treatment. Enneking developed a staging system for both benign and malignant primary

---

*Rex Marco, MD is a consultant or employee for DePuy Spine and Synthes.

5: Spine

Table 1

Benign Primary Bone Tumors

Tumor	Tissue Type	Incidence of Spine Involvement Relative to All Benign Bone Tumors	Age	Sex	Clinical Presentation
ABC	Unknown	< 1%	2nd decade	F > M	Pain; neurologic symptoms usually mild
GCT	Unknown	3.50%	3rd decade	F > M	Pain; radicular pain or weakness common
LCH	Unknown	2%	1st or 2nd decade	M = F	Pain; torticollis common with cervical involvement
Osteoid osteoma	Bone	10%	2nd decade	M > F	Night pain relieved by NSAIDs Painful scoliosis
Osteoblastoma	Bone	2%	2nd decade	M > F	Night pain and painful scoliosis common
Osteochondroma	Bone and cartilage	1%	2nd decade	M > F	Usually asymptomatic, but pain common when neural compression is present

ABC = aneurysmal bone cyst; GCT = giant cell tumor; LCH = Langerhans cell histiocytosis; OGS = osteogenic sarcoma; RBCs = red blood cells; NSAIDS = nonsteroidal anti-inflammatory drugs

bone tumors. Arabic numbers designate the stages of benign tumors (Table 3), whereas malignant tumors are designated by Roman numerals. Histologic grade (low [I] or high [II] grade), compartmentalization within the bone (intracompartmental [A] or extracompartmental [B]) and presence (III) or absence of metastases are factors used to stage malignant primary bone tumors (Table 4). The most commonly used staging system in the spine is based on the location and local extension of the tumor in the vertebra. The vertebra is divided into 12 sectors similar to the face of a clock (Figure 3).

Benign Primary Bone Tumors

Aneurysmal Bone Cyst

Intralesional excision, en bloc excision, direct injection of calcitonin combined with corticosteroids, selective arterial embolization, and radiation therapy have been successfully used, alone or in combination, to treat aneurysmal bone cysts.[2] If the spine is physiologically stable, then less invasive techniques such as selective arterial embolization or direct injection with calcitonin

Table 1

Benign Primary Bone Tumors (cont)

Radiologic Findings	Level	Location	Histology	Treatment of Choice	Local Recurrence
Lytic, expansile lesion on CT scan Fluid-fluid levels on MRI	10% cervical 40% thoracic 20% lumbar 30% sacral	Posterior +/– anterior columns	Cavernous spaces containing RBCs; often arising in association with other primary bone tumors (GCT, chondroblastoma, osteoblastoma, telangiectatic OGS)	Selective arterial embolization; en bloc excision if located in spinous process or lamina; intralesional excision	5% to 10%
Often lytic with soft-tissue extension	10% cervical 15% thoracic 10% lumbar 65% sacral	Vertebral body	Multinucleated osteoclast-like giant cells with mononuclear cells	Intralesional, extracapsular excision	83% when treated before referral to tertiary center 18% when treated initially at tertiary center
Vertebral plana	20% to 45% cervical 14% to 32% thoracic 10% to 23% lumbar	Vertebral body	LCH, eosinophils	Nonsurgical	Uncommon
Scoliosis with convex away from side of lesion, CT scan with nidus surrounded by sclerotic rim	10% cervical 30% thoracic 40% lumbar 20% sacral	Posterior elements	Osteoid forming nidus surrounded by sclerotic rim of bone	NSAIDs or marginal excision if symptoms persist	10%
> 1.5 cm lesion CT scan demonstrates cortical rim or hypervascular area	30% cervical 20% thoracic 30% lumbar 20% sacral	Posterior elements	Similar appearance as osteoid osteoma	En bloc excision, when feasible. Consider preoperative selective arterial embolization if hypervascular area noted on CT scan	5% to 10% if cortical outline present on CT scan; 20% if hypervascular area present on CT scan
Cartilaginous cap seen on CT and MRI	40% cervical 30% thoracic 20% lumbar 10% sacral	Posterior elements	Osseous base with cartilaginous cap	Marginal en bloc excision of cartilaginous component	

combined with corticosteroids should be considered. Methylprednisolone may be angiostatic and inhibit fibroblast formation, whereas calcitonin inhibits osteoclastic activity, which may promote bone formation. Lesions located entirely within the lamina or spinous process can be treated with an en bloc excision if nonsurgical measures fail or are not indicated. Patients with physiologic instability (progressive neurologic deficits, progressive or unacceptable deformity, or intractable pain) may benefit from surgery. Patients with a physiologically unstable spine with a tumor involving the lamina or spinous process are treated with en bloc

excision with spinal stabilization and fusion, whereas those with vertebral body or pedicle involvement can be treated with preoperative embolization followed by an intralesional extracapsular excision, stabilization and fusion. Malignant transformation of aneurysmal bone cysts has been described in patients previously treated with irradiation. Radiation therapy is thus not usually recommended for these patients.

Giant Cell Tumor
Intralesional extracapsular or en bloc marginal excision is recommended for giant cell tumor involving the mo-

Table 2

Malignant Primary Bone Tumors

Tumor	Tissue Type	Incidence of Spine Involvement Relative to All Malignant Primary Bone Tumors	Age	Sex	Clinical Presentation
Chondrosarcoma	Cartilage	2%	4th to 6th decade	M = F	Pain; commonly originating from a benign tumor
Chordoma	Notochordal remnant	4%	6th decade	M > F	Pain; obstipation can occur with large sacral tumors
Ewing's sarcoma	Unknown	1%	2nd decade	M > F	Pain; neurologic deficit common
Lymphoma	Hematopoietic	2%	6th or 7th decade	M > F	Pain
Myeloma	Hematopoietic	5%	6th to 8th decade	M > F	Often asymptomatic unless presenting with pathologic fracture or spinal cord compression
Osteogenic sarcoma	Bone	1%	2nd decade	M > F	Pain; two thirds of patients present with neurologic deficits

bile spine and sacrum. Surgical excision at a tertiary care center is associated with a decreased incidence of local recurrence compared with surgical excision performed before referral (83% versus 18%).[3] Optimal treatment is determined by the spinal level and location within the vertebra.

En bloc marginal excision is recommended for lesions involving vertebra from T2 to T12. Nerve roots at these levels can be sacrificed without significant functional impairment. Transection of the nerve roots and mobilization of the tumor from the aorta facilitates en bloc excision at these levels. An en bloc excision with planned contamination within the pedicle may be required for lesions involving the vertebral body, pedicle, and lamina because complete en bloc excision without some contamination is nearly impossible when the tumor involves the pedicle and lamina.

Giant cell tumors involving the cervical spine, T1, or lumbar spine are usually treated with an intralesional, extracapsular excision. En bloc excision at these levels is more complex than at the thoracic level because of the proximity of the tumor to functional nerve roots and less mobile vascular structures such as the vertebral and iliac arteries and veins. Additionally, acceptable local control rates are obtained with an extracapsular excision. Tumor contamination must be minimized and removal of the entire capsule should be performed to decrease the likelihood of local tumor recurrence. En bloc excision is considered for recurrent giant cell tumor at these levels or for lesions that are deemed amenable to en bloc excision. Preoperative embolization probably decreases intraoperative blood loss and may decrease the incidence of local recurrence. Bisphosphonates and interferon may prove to be useful adjuncts to help decrease the likelihood of local recurrence or treat unresectable tumors.

Table 2

Malignant Primary Bone Tumors (cont)

Radiologic Findings	Level	Primary Location	Histology	Treatment of Choice	Local Recurrence
Mixed lytic and blastic lesion with soft-tissue mass	20% cervical 30% thoracic 20% lumbar 20% sacral	Vertebral body; posterior elements when associated with osteochondroma	Varies based on grade of tumor	En bloc excision	20% after en bloc excision; 100% after intralesional excision
Mixed lytic and blastic; soft-tissue mass common Satellite lesions in gluteus maximus seen with sacral tumors	10% cervical 5% thoracic 10% lumbar 75% sacral	Vertebral body	Physaliferous cells	En bloc excision	33% after en bloc excision; 75% to 100% after intralesional excision
Lytic lesion with large soft-tissue mass	5% cervical 5% thoracic 25% lumbar 65% sacral	Vertebral body	Small round blue cells with 11:22 translocation	Neoadjuvant or adjuvant chemotherapy with definitive local control with en bloc excision or radiation therapy	25% following chemotherapy plus radiation therapy; presumably lower incidence with en bloc excision
Large soft-tissue mass commonly seen on MRI	70% mobile spine 30% sacral	Vertebral body	Small round blue cells plus lymphoma markers	High-dose corticosteroids plus chemotherapy	Uncommon
Marrow replacement common on MRI	10% cervical 55% thoracic 20% lumbar 15% sacral	Vertbral body	Small round cells resembling plasma cells	High-dose corticosteroids plus chemotherapy	Uncommon
Blastic; ivory body sometimes seen	20% cervical 25% thoracic 25% lumbar 30% sacral	Vertebral body	Spindle cells surrounded by osteoid matrix	Neoadjuvant or adjuvant chemotherapy with definitive local control with en bloc excision	20% after en bloc excision; 60% after intralesional excision

Giant cell tumor involving the sacrum is usually treated with serial, selective arterial embolization or intralesional, extracapsular excision.[4] En bloc excision should be reserved for some recurrent tumors and tumors caudal to S2. En bloc excision of the proximal sacrum is not usually recommended because of the morbidity associated with lumbosacral dissociation and sacral nerve root transection. Radiation therapy is associated with the development of postradiation sarcoma and is not recommended for most patients with giant cell tumor.

Hemangioma

Vertebral hemangiomas are relatively common lesions consisting of vascular channels (capillary, cavernous, arteriovenous, or venous) lined with endothelial cells. Based on postmortem studies, hemangiomas are present in about 11% of spines. These lesions are usu-ally asymptomatic and identified as an incidental finding on MRI. Hemangiomas have an intermediate signal on both T1- and T2-weighted images. Symptomatic lesions without spinal cord compression can be treated with percutaneous cement augmentation using a vertebroplasty or kyphoplasty technique. Patients with spinal cord compression may require posterior decompressive surgery with spinal stabilization and vertebral body cement augmentation with or without spinal instrumentation, or anterior decompressive surgery with spinal reconstruction.

Langerhans Cell Histiocytosis

Patients with Langerhans cell histiocytosis sometimes have vertebral plana. The differential diagnosis of lesions causing vertebral plana includes osteomyelitis, Ewing's sarcoma, lymphoma, aneurysmal bone cysts, acute leukemia, metastatic rhabdomyosarcoma or neu-

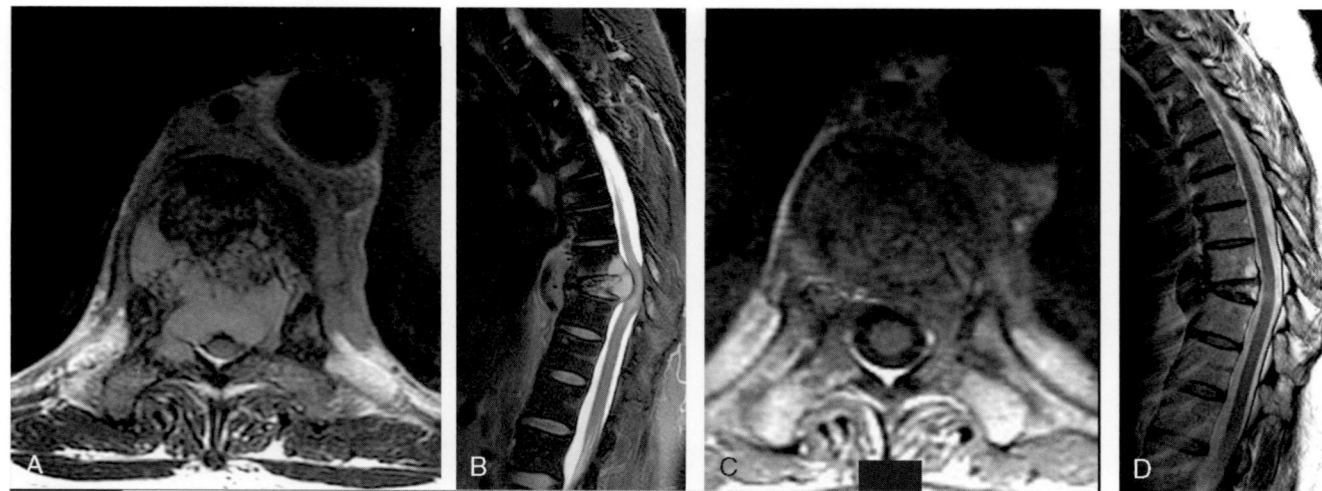

Figure 1 Imaging studies from a 65-year-old woman with paraparesis (Frankel C) and spinal cord compression from a solitary lesion at T10. **A**, Axial, and **B**, sagittal T2-weighted MRI scans. The patient presented with weakness, but her neurologic deficit was not progressive. An urgent needle biopsy was performed and corticosteroids were subsequently administered. Multiple myeloma was diagnosed. MRI scans showed minimal kyphosis and disk-on-disk findings suggestive of spinal stability. Chemotherapy, corticosteroids, and radiation therapy were administered. The patient regained full motor strength and maintained satisfactory coronal and sagittal alignment. T1-weighted axial **(C)** and T2-weighted sagittal **(D)** MRI scans at 9-month follow-up demonstrate resolution of the spinal cord compression with nonsurgical management.

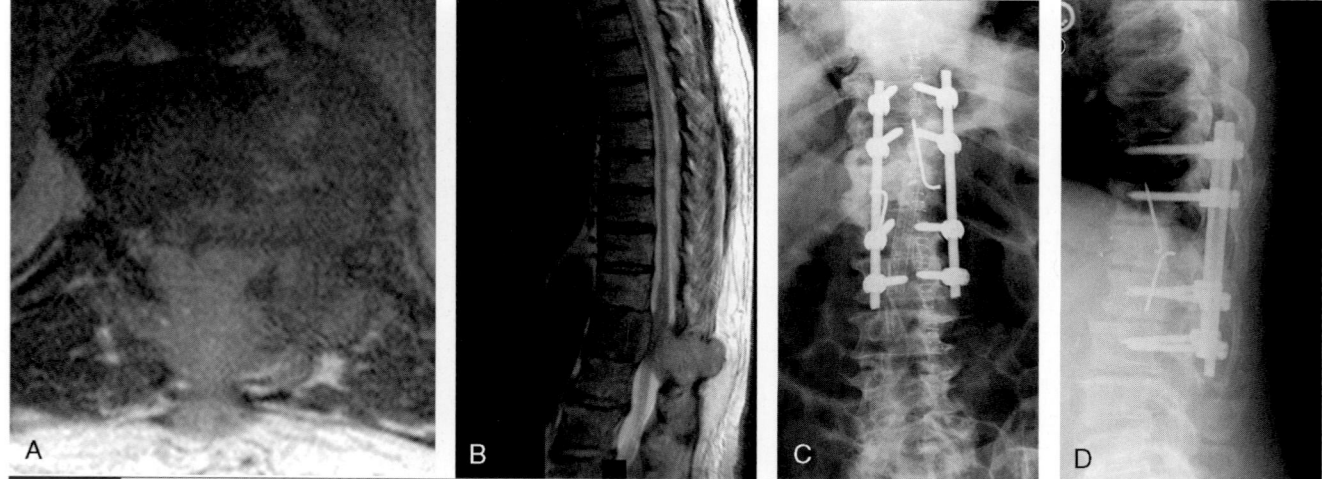

Figure 2 Imaging studies of a 62-year-old man with a solitary lesion at T12 and a remote history of thyroid carcinoma. He had normal neurologic function but reported severe, disabling pain. Axial **(A)** and sagittal **(B)** T2-weighted images show severe, near-circumferential compression of the conus medullaris. The patient was started on intermediate-dose corticosteroids. Ideally, a biopsy should be performed before intervention. However, the interventional neuroradiologist would not perform the biopsy because of the high degree of compression and high risk of potential bleeding. An open biopsy through a limited incision was performed, and frozen section analysis was consistent with thyroid carcinoma. A transpedicular excision with corpectomy and anterior column reconstruction with posterior stabilization was performed through a posterior-only approach as seen on the AP **(C)** and lateral **(D)** plain radiographs.

roblastoma, metastatic carcinoma, and plasmacytoma. Obtaining diagnostic tissue with a CT-guided needle biopsy is thus warranted. Cytologic examination can be performed while the needle remains within the lesion. If the cytologic examination is consistent with Langerhans cell histiocytosis, then an intralesional corticoster-oid injection can be performed[5] (**Figure 4**). This treatment is both diagnostic and therapeutic. The procedure is ideally performed at a tertiary care center with expertise in the fields of interventional radiology, musculoskeletal oncology and pathology. Other treatment options for Langerhans cell histiocytosis involv-

Table 3

Enneking System for Staging of Benign Bone Tumors

Stage	Definition	Behavior
1	Latent	Remains static or heals spontaneously
2	Active	Progressive growth, but limited by natural barriers
3	Locally aggressive	Progressive growth, not limited by natural barriers

Table 4

Enneking System for Staging of Malignant Primary Bone Tumors

Stage	Grade	Site	Metastases
IA	G1 (low)	T1 (intracompart-mental)	M0 (none)
IB	G1	T2 (extracom-partmental)	M0
IIA	G2 (high)	T1	M0
IIB	G2	T2	M0
IIIA	G1 or G2	T1	M1 (regional or distant)
IIIB	G1 or G2	T2	M1

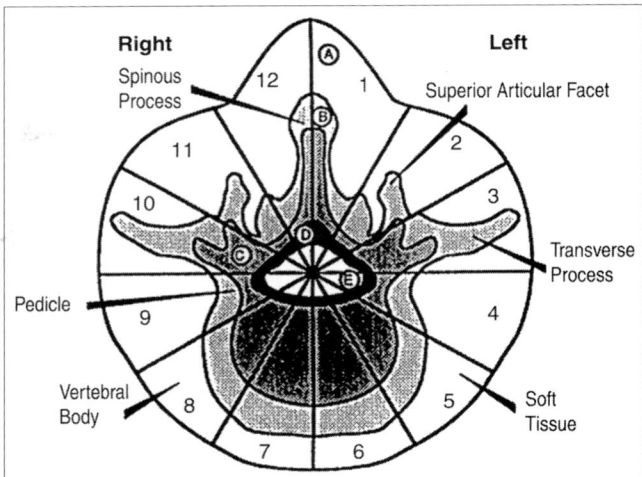

Figure 3 Proposed surgical staging system for spine tumors. **A** = extraosseous soft tissues, **B** = intraosseous (superficial), **C** = intraosseous (deep), **D** = extraosseous (extradural), and **E** = extraosseous (intradural). Numbers 1 through 12 represent location of tumor. (*Reproduced with permission from Boriani S, Weinstein JN, Biagini R: Primary bone tumors of the spine. Spine 1997;22:1036-1044.*)

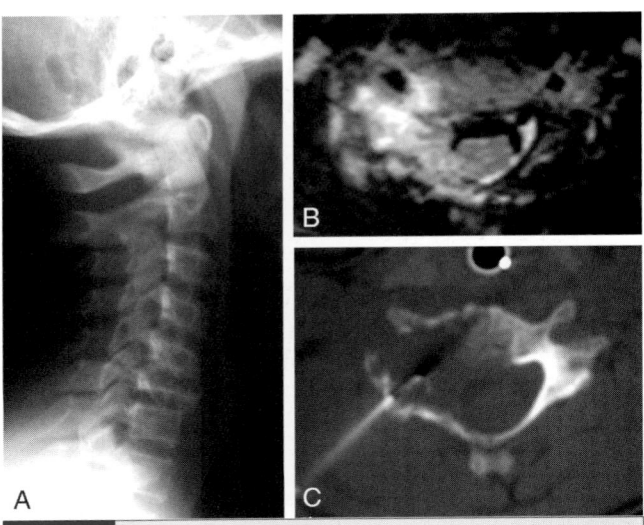

Figure 4 Imaging studies of a 9-year-old boy with a C6 lesion and decreased neck range of motion. Plain radiographs demonstrate vertebral plana **(A)**, whereas MRI **(B)** shows a lesion that surrounds the vertebral artery and compresses the lateral thecal sac. A percutaneous CT-guided needle biopsy **(C)** was performed. Immediate cytologic examination was performed while the needle remained within the lesion. Langerhans cell histiocytosis was diagnosed and intralesional corticosteroids were administered. Symptoms resolved and no local recurrence occurred.

ing the spinal column include observation, oral corticosteroids, chemotherapy, and low-dose radiation therapy.[6]

Neurofibroma

Neurofibromas are unencapsulated tumors consisting of a mixture of Schwann cells, perineural cells, and fibroblasts. Intraspinal neurofibromas usually arise from a posterior nerve root and are usually entirely intradural. However, intradural and extradural dumbbell-shaped lesions can occur. The extradural component can extend through the vertebral foramen and result in enlargement of the foramen. Symptomatic neurofibromas are treated with a marginal excision.

Spinal deformities are common in patients with neurofibromatosis 1. These patients usually present with periosteal neurofibromas rather than intraspinal lesions. Progressive scoliosis, penciling of one or more ribs, and scalloping of the vertebra are commonly seen. Progressive scoliosis should be treated with spinal fusion and instrumentation. Patients with scoliosis and neurofibromatosis have an increased incidence of pseudarthrosis following posterior fusion alone compared with treatment with a combined anterior and posterior spinal fusion. Posterior segmental fixation with pedicle screws may decrease the incidence of pseudarthrosis in comparison with hook-and-rod constructs, which in turn may obviate the need for anterior spinal fusion.

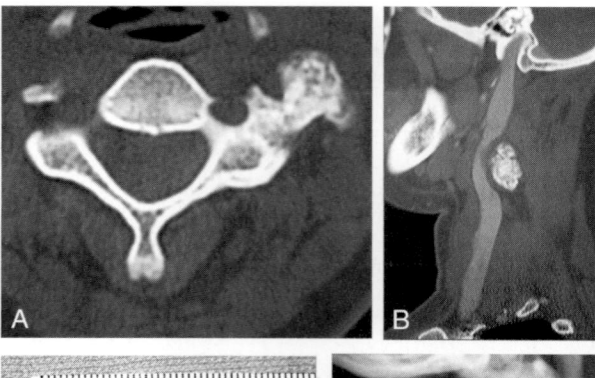

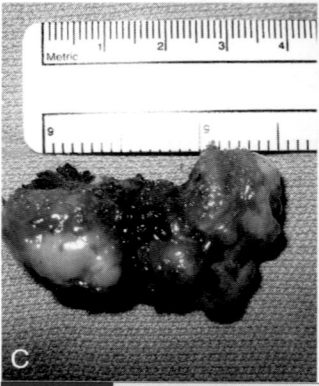
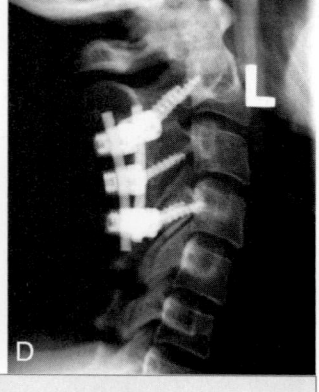

Figure 5 Imaging studies of a 38-year-old woman with a recurrent C3 osteochondroma, which was previously removed with an intralesional excision. **A** and **B**, Axial and sagittal reconstruction CT scans, respectively, demonstrate the proximity of the lesion to the vertebral foramen and internal jugular vein. En bloc excision with stabilization was performed. **C**, Excised tissue. **D**, Stabilization of the spine.

Osteoid Osteoma

Patients with osteoid osteoma are often treated long term with nonsteroidal anti-inflammatory drugs.[7] Excision of the tumor is recommended for patients with persistent pain. Marginal excision with complete removal of the nidus is recommended for these patients. En bloc excision is preferred for lesions located entirely within the lamina. Spinal fusion and stabilization are recommended if more than 50% of the cervical or lumbar facet joint is removed. Preoperative CT-guided needle placement can be used to localize lesions within the sacrum, pedicle, or vertebral body. Radiofrequency ablation is not commonly used for osteoid osteoma of the spine because the lesions are in close proximity to neural or vascular structures, which can be injured with this technique. However, lesions located entirely within the pedicle or vertebral body may be treated with radiofrequency ablation.

Osteoblastoma

Osteoblastoma resembles osteoid osteoma on histologic examination, but is usually larger (> 1.5 cm), more aggressive, and more likely to recur after excision.[8] A CT scan helps direct the ideal form of treatment by evalu-

ating the surrounding rim of tissue. Lesions with a reactive cortical outline can be treated with an intralesional excision. However, lesions surrounded by a hypervascular area may be more aggressive. These lesions have higher local recurrence rates following an intralesional excision. Preoperative selective arterial embolization may decrease blood loss and enhance local tumor control. En bloc excision of these tumors, when feasible, is warranted to decrease the likelihood of local recurrence, which in turn reduces the morbidity associated with re-excision of recurrent tumors.

Osteochondroma

Osteochondroma of the spinal column is usually asymptomatic unless it protrudes into the spinal canal. En bloc excision is recommended to decrease contamination of local tissue with the cartilaginous component of the tumor (**Figure 5**). Minimizing tumor contamination probably decreases the likelihood of local tumor recurrence.[9]

Malignant Primary Bone Tumors

Chondrosarcoma

Chondrosarcomas often arise in the posterior elements in association with a preexisting osteochondroma or as a primary lesion arising in the vertebral body. En bloc excision is recommended because intralesional excision is associated with a higher incidence of local recurrence and death compared with en bloc excision.[10] Chondrosarcoma is resistant to most protocols of radiation therapy and chemotherapy. Proton-beam radiation therapy may slow local progression of chondrosarcomas that are not amenable to en bloc excision.

Chordoma

Chordoma is a slow-growing, malignant primary bone tumor that usually arises from the clivus, odontoid, or sacrum. En bloc excision is recommended because there is a high incidence of local recurrence after intralesional excision.[11] However, en bloc excision of tumors involving the upper cervical spine and proximal sacrum is associated with functional impairment that may not be acceptable to the patient. Additionally, en bloc excision of tumors involving the tip of the odontoid is almost impossible because the vertebral arteries, spinal cord, hard palate, and ligamentous structures impede complete en bloc removal unless the tumor is unilaterally located in the caudal aspect of the odontoid. Extensive preoperative counseling regarding the expected functional impairment after total sacrectomy or odontoid resection helps prepare patients for the inevitable consequences of sacral nerve root transection, iliosacral dissociation, and mandibular-splitting transoral approaches. Bowel, bladder, and sexual dysfunction are common after a partial or total sacrectomy. Near-normal bowel, bladder, and sexual function are expected if bilateral S2 nerve roots or unilateral S2, S3, and S4 nerves are spared. Iliosacral ligament function is

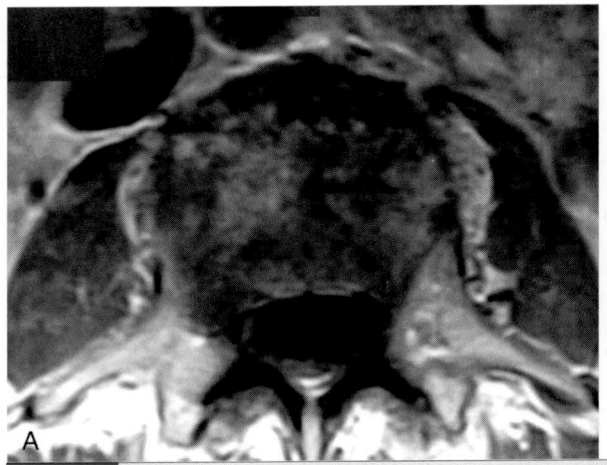
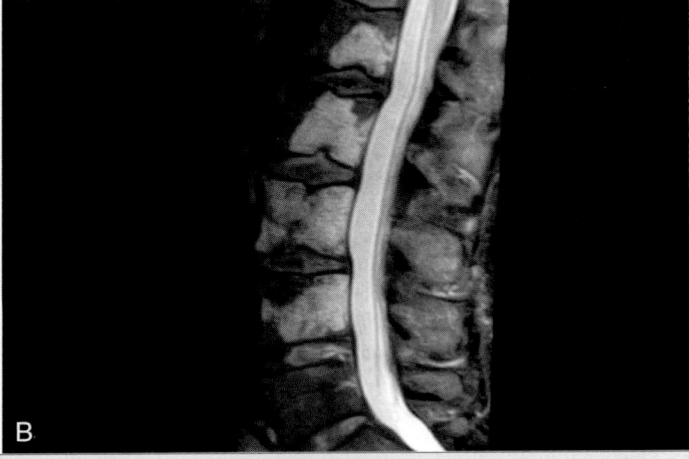

Figure 6 A 57-year-old woman with multilevel lumbar ecchordosis (notochordal rests). T1-weighted axial **(A)** and T2-weighted sagittal **(B)** MRI scans show multilevel involvement. No soft-tissue mass or cortical disruption is noted. Histology demonstrated notochordal tissue without features consistent with chordoma.

usually maintained if 1.5 cm of the cephalad portion of the sacrum is spared. Pain and poor ambulatory function are common after total sacrectomy. Sparing the iliolumbar ligament with or without subsequent lumbopelvic reconstruction may improve functional outcomes. Gluteal advancement flaps are sometimes used to cover the resultant soft-tissue defect and reconstruction. However, there are often satellite lesions in the gluteal muscles, which require excision of medially located gluteal muscle. The resultant soft-tissue defect is often extensive. In these situations, a pedicled myocutaneous rectus abdominis flap usually provides satisfactory coverage, as well as improved visualization of the anterior neurovascular and visceral structures during the flap harvest and anterior mobilization stage of the sacrectomy.

Occasionally, large notochordal remnants are identified within the vertebral column.[12] This tumor is differentiated from chordoma both radiologically and histologically. Bone destruction and soft-tissue extension are absent on CT and MRI scans (**Figure 6**). Histologically, there is uniform cell proliferation without lobularity or variability, lack of pleomorphism, necrosis or mucinous pools, and absent mitotic activity. This tumor is termed ecchordosis physaliphora, notochordal rest, or giant notochordal rest. Ecchordosis is usually an incidental finding on radiographs. A biopsy confirms the presence of notochordal tissue without morphologic features of chordoma. Close observation with periodic imaging is recommended. Patients with disabling symptoms or enlarging, destructive tumors should be treated with an en bloc excision when feasible.

Ewing's Sarcoma

Neoadjuvant chemotherapy followed by definitive local tumor control with radiation therapy or en bloc excision is recommended for patients with Ewing's sarcoma of the spine or sacrum. En bloc excision probably decreases the incidence of local recurrence compared with radiation therapy alone or intralesional excision combined with radiation therapy. Progressive kyphosis and radiation-associated myelopathy are common complications associated with the use of radiation therapy for definitive local control.[13] En bloc excision obviates the need for radiation therapy, which in turn may decrease the incidence of radiation-associated myelopathy and radiation-associated sarcoma. A multidisciplinary conference with the patient involving the oncologist, radiation oncologist, and spine tumor surgeon is required to optimize treatment. Neoadjuvant chemotherapy usually results in significant reduction of the soft-tissue component of the tumor. En bloc excision is sometimes feasible for lesions located in the vertebrae from T2 to L5 and distal sacrum. Spinal fusion with instrumentation probably decreases the incidence of progressive kyphosis. Radiation therapy is usually used to provide definitive local tumor control for patients with cervical, T1, and proximal sacral lesions. Stereotactic radiotherapy may decrease the incidence of radiation-associated myelopathy.

Myeloma and Lymphoma

Nonsurgical treatment with high-dose corticosteroids, bisphosphonates, and chemotherapy are recommended for most patients with spinal cord compression associated with myeloma or lymphoma.[14,15] Epidural compression is dramatically decreased by the administration of corticosteroids. Improved pain control and neurologic function are expected with the combination treatment of corticosteroids and chemotherapy, even in the presence of profound neurologic deficits (**Figure 1**). Bracing is recommended to prevent further collapse of the vertebral body. Radiation therapy is considered, but not always required. Most patients heal without any progression of deformity. Some patients continue to have mechanical back pain with mobilization. These patients can be treated with percutaneous cement augmentation of the vertebral body with a vertebroplasty or a kyphoplasty. Bisphosphonates decrease the likelihood of developing additional pathologic compression fractures.

Solitary plasmacytoma of bone is an uncommon entity. The diagnosis is made when there are no other skeletal lesions, the bone marrow biopsy is negative, and there is no persistent protein abnormality in the serum or urine. The treatment of choice is radiation therapy. Local recurrence is uncommon. Surgery is reserved for patients with a physiologically unstable spine.

Osteogenic Sarcoma

Neoadjuvant chemotherapy followed by en bloc excision is recommended for patients with osteogenic sarcoma of the spine. However, the location and extent of the tumor may render performance of a wide or marginal en bloc excision impractical. Neoadjuvant or adjuvant multiagent chemotherapy combined with intralesional excision is a reasonable treatment option for these patients. Although the role of radiation therapy is unclear, proton beam or stereotactic radiation is considered following an aggressive intralesional excision. Radiation therapy is not usually recommended following an en bloc excision unless tumor contamination is encountered during the resection.

Pagetic Sarcoma

The spinal column is affected in 50% of patients with Paget's disease. Spinal stenosis and compression fractures are common; sarcomatous degeneration is uncommon. Males are affected more often than females. Pagetic sarcoma most commonly arises within the sacrum.[16] Back pain, radiculopathy, and weakness are common signs and symptoms. Osteogenic sarcoma is the most commonly associated malignant tumor followed by chondrosarcoma and malignant fibrous histiocytoma. Median patient survival is less than 6 months. Radiation therapy or surgery may provide palliative pain control.

Surgical Treatment and Challenges

Giant cell tumor, osteoblastoma, symptomatic osteochondroma, chondrosarcoma, chordoma, osteogenic sarcoma, and accessible Ewing's sarcoma are usually treated with surgical resection. The optimal resection is dependent on the type, location, and extent of the tumor. En bloc excision without tumor contamination is possible for tumors located completely within the vertebral body, at the distal portion of the sacrum, or within the spinous process. However, en bloc excision is not practical for tumors located within the tip of the odontoid, tumors involving both vertebral artery foramen, tumors involving both pedicles, or tumors extending from the vertebral body through the pedicle and into the lamina. Tumors located in these areas are probably best treated with an intralesional, extracapsular excision or an en

bloc excision, with intentional contamination through the anatomic structures impeding a "true" en bloc excision. Chondrosarcoma, chordoma, and osteogenic sarcoma that are unilaterally located in the lower cervical and cervicothoracic vertebra with minimal extension into the pedicle can be treated with an en bloc excision. Preservation of the functionally important cervical and T1 nerve roots, as well as the vertebral arteries, impedes the ability to complete an en bloc resection.

In contrast, tumors located in the thoracic and thoracolumbar region are more amenable to en bloc excision because transection of these nerve roots can be performed without significant functional loss. Multilevel laminectomy combined with pedicle removal and bilateral nerve root transection facilitates en bloc excision. Sectioning of appropriate ribs and a threadwire saw facilitates removal of the tumor from a posterior-only approach, if desired. Wide excision with en bloc removal of the tumor surrounded by a cuff of normal tissue (pleura, psoas, posterior longitudinal ligament, or dura) probably decreases the incidence of local recurrence compared with marginal en bloc excision or intralesional, extracapsular excision. Ligation and transection of the spinal cord or cauda equina is considered for patients with massive malignant or aggressive benign tumors presenting with extensive epidural tumor, and concomitant long-standing paralysis.[17] This type of resection further enhances surgical margins.

The lumbar nerve roots are usually spared during en bloc excisions at these levels. These tumors are thus more difficult to remove using a posterior-only approach compared with a combined posterior and subsequent anterior approach. Tumors located below the S2 level can be removed using a posterior-only approach, whereas proximal sacral tumors are usually removed with a combined anterior and posterior approach.

Radiation Therapy

Radiation therapy is not recommended for most patients with a primary bone tumor. Satisfactory local control of benign primary bone tumors is usually obtained using nonsurgical measures or an appropriate excision without adjuvant radiation therapy. There is a small risk of developing a radiation-associated malignancy following administration of radiation.

Chondrosarcoma, chordoma, and osteosarcoma are relatively radioresistant tumors; therefore, conventional external beam radiation therapy is not recommended for patients with these tumors. However, proton beam or stereotactic radiation therapy is considered for patients with residual microscopic tumor following an appropriate surgical excision with inadvertent or intentional contamination or for patients with inoperable tumors.[18,19] External beam radiation therapy or intensity-modulated radiotherapy (IMRT) may decrease the incidence of local recurrence for patients with Ewing's sarcoma who have residual microscopic disease following an oncologic excision or for patients who are not surgical candidates. IMRT and stereotactic radiosurgery precisely deliver high doses of radiation to the tumor or tumor bed with less radiation exposure to the spinal cord and surrounding tissue.[20] Patients with myeloma or lymphoma are usually initially treated with corticosteroids and chemotherapy, followed by radiation therapy if deemed necessary.

Metastatic Disease

Controversy exists regarding the optimal treatment of patients with spinal cord compression associated with metastatic disease. Overall medical condition, ambulatory status, tumor type, spinal level, extent of disseminated disease, physiologic spinal stability, and response to adjuvant therapy must be considered before initiating definitive therapy.[21] Most patients with metastatic disease are ideally treated with corticosteroids, radiation therapy, and a brace. Patients in poor medical condition are usually treated expectantly and rarely benefit from decompressive surgery. Patients with extremely radiosensitive tumors (lymphoma, leukemia, multiple myeloma, and germ-cell tumors) are usually treated with corticosteroids and chemotherapy with or without radiation therapy rather than surgery. Percutaneous cement augmentation with vertebroplasty or kyphoplasty is considered for patients with these tumors who continue to have persistent mechanical back pain despite nonsurgical treatment. Patients with multilevel spinal cord compression are ideally treated nonsurgically. Patients with extensive visceral metastases or metastatic lung, gastric, or unknown carcinoma usually have a limited life expectancy and may be best treated with corticosteroids and radiation therapy rather than surgery. Patients with metastatic prostate and breast carcinoma respond well to adjuvant chemotherapy, hormonal therapy, and radiation therapy. Recently developed antiangiogenic agents combined with stereotactic radiotherapy may decrease the incidence of decompressive surgery for the treatment of patients with spinal cord compression associated with metastatic renal cell carcinoma and other relatively radioresistant tumors. Ambulatory patients with spinal cord compression usually remain ambulatory after treatment with corticosteroids, radiation therapy, chemotherapy, and a brace.

There are subsets of patients with spinal cord compression who benefit from decompressive surgery and stabilization. Healthy patients with limited disease (solitary lesion with minimal visceral involvement) who have locally recurrent disease, persistent mechanical instability, intractable pain, or progressive or severe kyphotic deformity probably benefit from decompressive surgery, spinal stabilization and postoperative radiotherapy.[22,23] En bloc spondylectomy is considered for selected patients with solitary lesions.

Complications

Complications related to the treatment of spinal column tumors commonly occur. Accurate preoperative assessment and diagnosis increase the likelihood of providing optimal treatment. A careful history and physical examination can identify coexisting premorbid conditions, which may require further evaluation before surgical intervention. Obtaining diagnostic tissue using minimally invasive techniques decreases local tumor contamination. A multidisciplinary team approach of surgical, medical, and radiation oncologists, combined with experienced radiologists and pathologists, helps optimize patient care. The goals of surgical intervention for patients with spinal tumors are pain control, maintenance or improvement of neurologic function, eradication of the tumor, and maintenance of spinal stability and normal coronal and sagittal alignment. Attention to details and appropriate goal-oriented intervention should help decrease the incidence of complications related to spinal surgery.[24]

Annotated References

1. Clayer M, Duncan W: Importance of biopsy of new bone lesions in patients with previous carcinoma. *Clin Orthop Relat Res* 2006;451:208-211.

   Fifty patients with new metastases to bone after a previous diagnosis of localized visceral carcinoma were identified. A biopsy on the new lesion was performed. A new tumor was identified in nine patients (15%), necrotic tissue in two patients, and normal tissue in one patient. The authors recommend performing a biopsy for patients with a history of carcinoma who present with a new bone lesion. Level of evidence: IV.

2. Boriani S, De Iure F, Campanacci L, et al: Aneurysmal bone cyst of the mobile spine: Report on 41 cases. *Spine* 2001;26:27-35.

3. Hart RA, Boriani S, Biagini R, Currier B, Weinstein JN: A system for surgical staging and management of spine tumors: A clinical outcome study of giant cell tumors of the spine. *Spine* 1997;22:1773-1782.

4. Lackman RD, Khoury LD, Esmail A, Donthineni-Rao R: The treatment of sacral giant-cell tumours by serial arterial embolization. *J Bone Joint Surg Br* 2002;84: 873-877.

5. Yasko AW, Fanning CV, Ayala AG, Carrasco CH, Murray JA: Percutaneous techniques for the diagnosis and treatment of localized Langerhans-cell histiocytosis (eosinophilic granuloma of bone). *J Bone Joint Surg Am* 1998;80:219-228.

6. Garg S, Mehta S, Dormans JP: Langerhans cell histiocytosis of the spine in children: Long-term follow-up. *J Bone Joint Surg Am* 2004;86:1740-1750.

Twenty-six children with biopsy-proven Langerhans cell histiocytosis involving the spine were treated. Most (24 of 26) patients (92%) healed without surgical intervention. Level of evidence: IV.

7. Kneisl JS, Simon MA: Medical management compared with operative treatment for osteoid-osteoma. *J Bone Joint Surg Am* 1992;74:179-185.

8. Boriani S, Capanna R, Donati D, Levine A, Picci P, Savini R: Osteoblastoma of the spine. *Clin Orthop Relat Res* 1992;278:37-45.

9. Samartzis D, Marco RAW: Osteochondroma of the sacrum: A case report and review of the literature. *Spine* 2006;31:E425-E429.

10. Boriani S, De Iure F, Bandiera S, et al: Chondrosarcoma of the mobile spine: Report on 22 cases. *Spine* 2000;25:804-812.

11. Boriani S, Bandiera S, Biagini R, et al: Chordoma of the mobile spine: Fifty years of experience. *Spine* 2006;31:493-503.

Forty-eight patients with chordoma involving the mobile spine were evaluated. Fourteen of these patients who received radiation alone, intralesional excision, or a combination had a local recurrence and died. Intralesional, extracapsular excision combined with radiation therapy resulted in local recurrence in 12 of 16 patients (75%), whereas only 6 of 18 patients (33%) who underwent en bloc excision had a local recurrence. Level of evidence: III.

12. Kyriakos M, Totty WG, Lenke LG: Giant vertebral notochordal rest: A lesion distinct from chordoma. discussion of an evolving concept. *Am J Surg Pathol* 2003;27:396-406.

13. Marco RAW, Gentry JB, Rhines LD, et al: Ewing's sarcoma of the mobile spine. *Spine* 2005;30:769-773.

Twelve patients with Ewing's sarcoma of the mobile spine were treated with multiagent chemotherapy combined with radiation therapy for definitive local control. Local recurrence (23%) and progressive deformity (40%) occurred frequently. Current spinal resection and reconstruction techniques may decrease the incidence of local recurrence and progressive deformity. Level of evidence: IV.

14. Rao G, Ha CS, Chakrabarti I, Feiz-Erfan I, Mendel E, Rhines LD: Multiple myeloma of the cervical spine: Treatment strategies for pain and spinal instability. *J Neurosurg Spine* 2006;5:140-145.

The authors report the results of radiotherapy and surgical treatment of patients with myeloma involving the cervical spine. The authors suggest that external-beam radiation can effectively treat most patients with clinical or radiographically documented instability. Level of evidence: III.

15. Hayes FA, Thompson EI, Hvizdala E, O'Connor D, Green AA: Chemotherapy as an alternative to laminec-

tomy and radiation in the management of epidural tumor. *J Pediatr* 1984;104:221-224.

16. Sharma H, Mehdi SA, MacDuff E, Reece AT, Jane MJ, Reid R: Paget sarcoma of the spine: Scottish Bone Tumor Registry experience. *Spine* 2006;31:1344-1350.

These authors evaluated the clinical, radiologic, and histologic features of Paget's sarcoma of the spine. Level of evidence: IV.

17. Keynan O, Fisher CG, Boyd MC, O'Connell JX, Dvorak MF: Ligation and partial excision of the cauda equina as part of a wide resection of vertebral osteosarcoma: A case report and description of surgical technique. *Spine* 2005;30:E97-E102.

The authors describe the indications and surgical techniques for wide excision of a vertebral osteosarcoma, including ligation and resection of a portion of the cauda equina and conus medullaris. Level of evidence: IV.

18. Hug EB, Fitzek MM, Liebsch NJ, Munzenrider JE: Locally challenging osteo- and chondrogenic tumors of the axial skeleton: Results of combined proton and photon radiation therapy using three-dimensional treatment planning. *Int J Radiat Oncol Biol Phys* 1995;31:467-476.

19. Suit HD, Goitein M, Munzenrider J, et al: Definitive radiation therapy for chordoma and chondrosarcoma of base of skull and cervical spine. *J Neurosurg* 1982;56:377-385.

20. Bilsky MH, Yamada Y, Yenice KM, et al: Intensity-modulated stereotactic radiotherapy of paraspinal tumors: A preliminary report. *Neurosurgery* 2004;54:823-830.

This study evaluated 16 patients with metastatic and primary tumors. High tumoral doses of radiation were administered to both metastatic and primary tumors (20 Gy and 70 Gy, respectively), while minimizing the dose of radiation to the spinal cord (6 Gy and 16 Gy, respectively). IMRT effectively treated pain and improved function. Level of evidence: IV.

21. Tokuhashi Y, Matsuzaki H, Oda H, Oshima M, Ryu J: A revised scoring system for preoperative evaluation of metastatic spine tumor prognosis. *Spine* 2005;30:2186-2191.

The accuracy of a revised scoring system used to predict prognosis and suitability of subsequent treatment. The system evaluated the following items: (1) general condition, (2) number of extraspinal bone metastases, (3) number of metastases in the vertebral body, (4) presence or absence of metastases to major internal organs, (5) site of the primary lesion, and (6) severity of neurologic deficit. The scoring system was useful for determining appropriate treatment and survival. Level of evidence: IV.

22. Wang JC, Boland P, Mitra N, et al: Single-stage posterolateral transpedicular approach for resection of epidural metastatic spine tumors involving the vertebral body with circumferential reconstruction: Results in 140 pa-

tients. Invited submission from the Joint Section Meeting on Disorders of the Spine and Peripheral Nerves. *J Neurosurg Spine* 2004;1:287-298.

A single-stage posterolateral transpedicular decompression and circumferential stabilization was performed in 140 patients with metastatic spine tumors. Ninety-six percent of patients experienced improved pain control and improvement or stabilization of neurologic status. Adequate circumferential decompression with anterior and posterior stabilization was performed through a single-stage posterior approach without the morbidity associated with an anterior approach. Level of evidence: IV.

23. Patchell RA, Tibbs PA, Regine WF, et al: Direct decompressive surgical resection in the treatment of spinal cord compression caused by metastatic cancer: A randomised trial. *Lancet* 2005;366:643-648.

A prospective, randomized trial comparing decompressive surgery to radiotherapy for spinal cord compression caused by metastatic cancer located in a single area. Patients with radiosensitive tumors (lymphoma, leukemia, multiple myeloma, and germ-cell tumors) were excluded. More patients in the surgery group (42 of 50,

84%) than in the radiotherapy group (29 of 51, 57%) were able to walk after treatment. Additionally, 10 of 16 patients (62%) in the surgery group versus 3 of 16 (19%) in the radiotherapy group regained the ability to walk. These data suggest that healthy patients with a solitary area of spinal cord compression who present with inability to ambulate probably benefit more from decompressive surgery than radiation therapy. However, definitive conclusions regarding optimal treatment of ambulatory patients with or without a stable spine cannot be made from these data. Level of evidence: IV.

24. Marco R, An HS: Complications of surgical and medical care: Anticipation and management, in McLain RF, Lewandrowski KU, Markman M, Bukowski RM, Macklis R, Benzel EC (eds): *Current Clinical Oncology: Cancer in the Spine. Comprehensive Care*. Totowa, NJ, Humana Press, 2005, pp 323-336.

These authors discuss the anticipation, prevention, and management of medical and surgical complications associated with the care of patients with tumors of the spinal column.

5: Spine

Chapter 53

New Technologies in Spine Surgery

Thomas N. Scioscia, MD   *Arya Nick Shamie, MD   Jeffrey C. Wang, MD

Introduction

Many of the new products being developed for spinal pathologies represent a spectrum of motion-preserving technologies. Although fusion is an acceptable procedure in many instances, ways to improve results are constantly sought. Motion-sparing devices may theoretically decrease the risk of adjacent segment disease, and obviate the nonunions and donor-site morbidity that are currently associated with fusion procedures. Many of the products discussed in this chapter represent motion-sparing alternatives. Because preliminary published results of these devices are industry-financed, the data must be critically analyzed. Further prospective randomized studies are important in eliminating bias and will be required to truly demonstrate efficacy. Some of these implants may prove to be beneficial and may change the manner in which spinal pathologies are treated, whereas many will be proven inferior to current techniques. Perhaps the greatest concern about these novel implants is the inevitable failure of at least a certain percentage of these devices, while the treatment strategies and outcomes are as yet to be determined. The new technologies covered in this chapter are cervical disk replacement, lumbar total disk arthroplasty/replacement (TDA/TDR), lumbar dynamic stabilization, facet replacement, and interspinous distraction spacers. In general, novel devices used to treat simple conditions usually fare better than devices developed to treat difficult-to-treat diseases.

Cervical Disk Arthroplasty

Cervical disk arthroplasty is a novel motion-preserving procedure that provides an alternative to fusion. Arthroplasty was designed to maintain cervical motion, prevent or reduce adjacent segment degeneration, and eliminate nonunion and donor-site morbidity. The incidence and prevalence of adjacent segment degeneration in the cervical spine recently has been studied. Data collected show a 9% to 17% prevalence and an annual incidence of approximately 3% of adjacent-level disease developing following anterior cervical diskectomy and fusion.

This rate is equivalent to the reported incidence of adjacent-level disease in patients who had nonfusion foraminotomies and also those patients who had no surgery. Although increased adjacent-segment disease as a sequela of fusion makes theoretic sense, the increase still has not been shown to be greater than the natural history of progressive degeneration.

Unlike lumbar TDR, which has been used to treat axial back pain, cervical disk replacement was developed to treat primarily neural compressive disorders such as radiculopathy and possibly myelopathy. The criteria used for disk replacement in the US Food and Drug Administration (FDA) investigational device exemption (IDE) clinical trials to date have included radiculopathy caused by disk herniations or osseous foraminal stenosis, and myelopathy caused by soft-disk herniation. Cervical TDA is not currently recommended in the treatment of axial neck pain. Cervical TDA is contraindicated for the treatment of cervical deformity or for patients with cervical instability. Other relative contraindications include rheumatoid arthritis, osteoporosis, renal failure, corticosteroid use, and history of infection.

Replacement Options and Results

The number of cervical disk implants is growing rapidly. The first implant was approved by the FDA in 2007. Those mentioned in this chapter are the most studied to date. Most designs comprise two metal end plates that are fixed to the vertebral body by a press fit, with or without supplemental screw fixation or keel stabilization. Between these end plates, there is an articulation combining metal-on-metal or metal-on-polyethylene surfaces. A few products use a one-piece design. There are multiple uncontrolled clinical studies in the literature evaluating the use of cervical disk arthroplasties.[1] Most conclude that cervical disk replacements are performing well at the 2-year follow-up point. There have been two controlled prospective studies reporting equivalent results between anterior cervical disk fusion and cervical disk arthroplasty with follow-up at 2 years.[2] Another study notes a significantly higher incidence of adjacent segment degeneration in the fusion group determined by radiographic osteophyte progression in the rostral disk space. Disk replacements were found to preserve preoperative motion but not to restore normal motion. Segmental kyphosis was noted to progress in some studies but this finding did not correlate with clinical results.[3]

*Arya Nick Shamie, MD is a consultant or employee of St. Francis Medical Technologies.

5: Spine

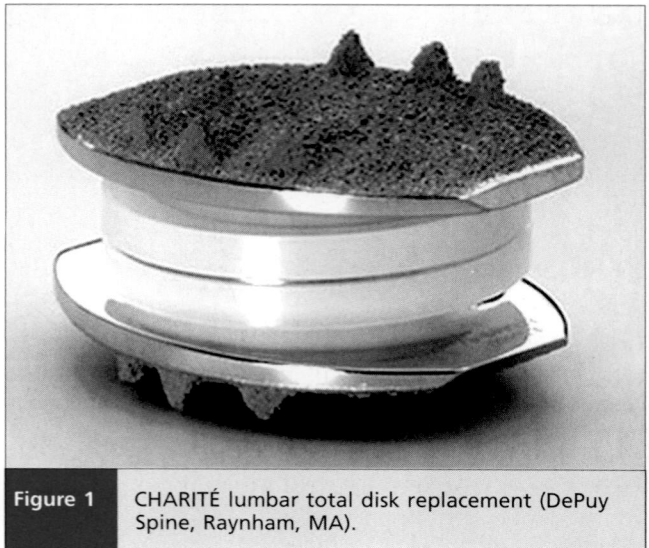

Figure 1 CHARITÉ lumbar total disk replacement (DePuy Spine, Raynham, MA).

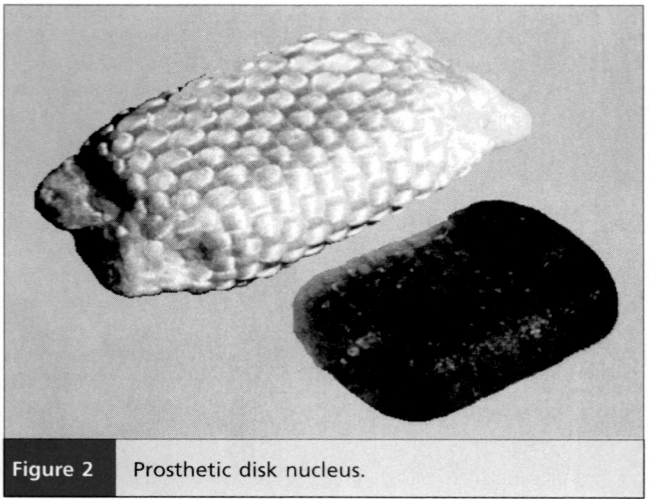

Figure 2 Prosthetic disk nucleus.

The disadvantage of disk arthroplasty is the potential for failure. Wear debris is phagocytized by multinucleated cells and macrophages that produce cytokines. There is some concern that the activation of these cytokines may incite an inflammatory response, leading to pain or irritation of the nerves and surrounding tissues. These chemicals also may cause osteoclasts to resorb bone and may lead to osteolysis and loosening of the implants. Catastrophic failure is also an issue and can be caused by instability, failure of ingrowth, or mechanical failure of the prosthesis.

The decision to use cervical TDR must be critically contemplated and examined for the proper indications and the absence of any contraindications. If performed, the proper technique and follow-up are essential to prevent potentially devastating complications. Anterior cervical fusion is an extremely successful procedure and has minimal risk for failure once fusion has occurred. Only time will tell if cervical disk replacement offers a better alternative to fusion surgery for the cervical spine. The answer will also depend on whether disk replacement will decrease the incidence of adjacent segmental disease and need for subsequent surgeries, while providing long-term survivorship at the site of index surgery.

Lumbar Disk Arthroplasty

Lumbar disk replacement was first attempted in the 1950s using the Fenstrom steel-ball endoprosthesis. In recent years, more than 100 implant designs have been developed but only a few have made it to clinical use. Two primary design principles are generally represented in current designs. Some prostheses aim to replace the motion characteristics of the entire disk in the functional spinal unit (generally fabricated from metal and polyethylene) (**Figure 1**), whereas other designs intend to replicate the normal viscoelastic properties of only the nucleus and are usually made from synthetic polymers (nucleus replacement, **Figure 2**). In the United States, disk replacement is currently outpacing nucleus replacement. The disk replacement design has many IDE clinical trials, whereas studies involving nucleus replacement are in their infancy. In Europe, some nucleus replacement studies have shown promise, but dislodgement is a problem that has slowed progress. Proponents of TDR view it as a technology to treat back pain while attempting to decrease adjacent segment disease. Early results have shown equivalent outcomes with fusion and preservation of motion, especially at the L4-5 level.

The early excitement generated by lumbar disk arthroplasty has been tempered by a host of factors. First, surgeons are realizing that identifying the specific causative origin of back pain is difficult, and that there is an inherent limited success in general for treating patients with mechanical lumbar back pain. Because of this, some patients achieve only modest improvements after surgery and up to 75% of patients continue to use narcotics for pain control. Despite the continued use of narcotics for pain control, the results can be quite good in the properly selected patient. Careful attention should be directed to the patient's psychosocial situation during the selection process because this can influence treatment outcomes. Second, the reports of mechanical failures are becoming more frequent. Third, there have been problems with reimbursement to hospitals and physicians for these costly devices and procedures, which can typically involve the use of an additional approach surgeon.

The indications for TDR are similar in some aspects to the indications for lumbar fusion. Patients should have back pain with MRI degenerative changes and a concordant diskogram, and have been treated with nonsurgical therapy for 6 months to 1 year. Contraindications to TDR include facet disease, previous laminectomy, pars fracture, deformity, and instability. Most of these patients are better served with interbody and posterior lateral fusion techniques.

Replacement Options and Outcomes

There are a variety of implant designs with different materials used in each. The first approved implant consists of two concave metal end plates and an unconstrained biconvex polyethylene core. The back of the end plates are polished and rely on small spikes to assist with fixation, although modifications to a porous ingrowth surface are being considered. This prosthesis is unconstrained in rotation and semiconstrained in most other motions. The second device to be approved is semiconstrained and consists of two metal end plates, one of which has an attached concave polyethylene inlay and the other has a metal convex articulating surface (**Figure 3**). Fixation is assisted by a small keel. There are other designs, one of which consists of a metal-on-metal prosthesis with large center keels. The center of rotation of these devices varies and also contributes to the motion and stability of the designs. There have been multiple studies assessing the performance of these devices, including FDA IDE multicenter studies.

The short- to intermediate-term pain relief using the lumbar disk replacements is similar to fusion surgery.[4,5] Long-term retrospective studies seem to demonstrate maintenance of pain relief. Many patients continue to need narcotics after surgery, indicating that pain relief is often incomplete. The hospital stay is slightly shorter in TDR patients compared with that of fusion patients. The rate of return to work is similar between the TDR and fusion surgeries. The range of motion after TDR is similar to preoperative motion in the degenerative segment, and normal motion of the spine is not fully restored.

Adjacent segment disease also has been evaluated. Currently there is little evidence that TDR decreases adjacent segment disease compared with fusion, and the complication rates of TDR and fusion appear to be the same. Early case studies and reports of the initial use of lumbar disk arthroplasty actually showed an increased incidence of adjacent segment disease, although the prospective randomized studies are showing no differences.[4,5] These early studies demonstrating inferior results with regard to adjacent segment disease may reflect the critical importance of patient selection, regardless of the technology used.

There are a host of possible disadvantages to lumbar TDR. Facet disease or progressive foraminal stenosis may cause symptomatic pain in the future. The absence of improvement of back pain is the most common complication after TDR. Failure of the prosthesis may be of greater concern in the younger population because they will generate more force on the components for a longer period of time. Failure can be caused by osteolysis, implant fracture or wear, vertebral body fracture, failure of ingrowth, or instability with dislocation. Unlike failure in the cervical spine, lumbar failure presents a difficult revision exposure because of the extensive scarring in the anterior abdominal area. Revision surgery in this location is difficult, with a higher risk of injury to the surrounding

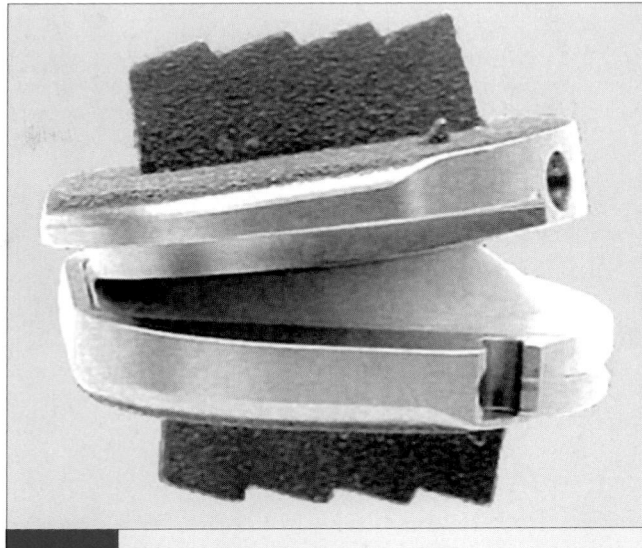

Figure 3   ProDisc lumbar total disk replacement (Synthes, Paoli, PA).

anatomic structures. A vascular injury in this location may place a patient's limbs or life in jeopardy. Revision strategies include a revision anterior approach and implant removal with fusion or posterior instrumented fusion. The revision approach must be carefully planned with the possible placement of ureteral stents, pulse oximetry monitoring of the lower extremities, and the use of a highly experienced approach surgeon who is familiar with the anatomy.

Lumbar TDR has several advantages and pitfalls, and currently its future is still unknown. In the short and intermediate term, the implants tend to preserve preoperative motion (but do not restore regular motion) and have performed equivalent to fusion. The disadvantage is unpredictable failure, which requires technically difficult revision surgery that can be life-threatening. Device-related complications may present a larger problem than adjacent segment disease seen after fusion surgery (which has not yet been proven to be eliminated with TDR). It must also be remembered that any surgery for axial lumbar pain may not benefit the patient because of the inability to identify the true pain generator.

Dynamic Stabilization

Dynamic stabilization systems were first developed as fusion devices. The first FDA-approved device was approved as a fusion stabilization device. As the interest in nonfusion technology developed, investigators began using these systems for dynamic stabilization without fusion. The rationale behind these products stems initially from the results of noninstrumented fusion in stenosis patients. Despite developing radiographic nonunions, the patients still did as well as those with complete union of the fusion mass. It is postulated that the

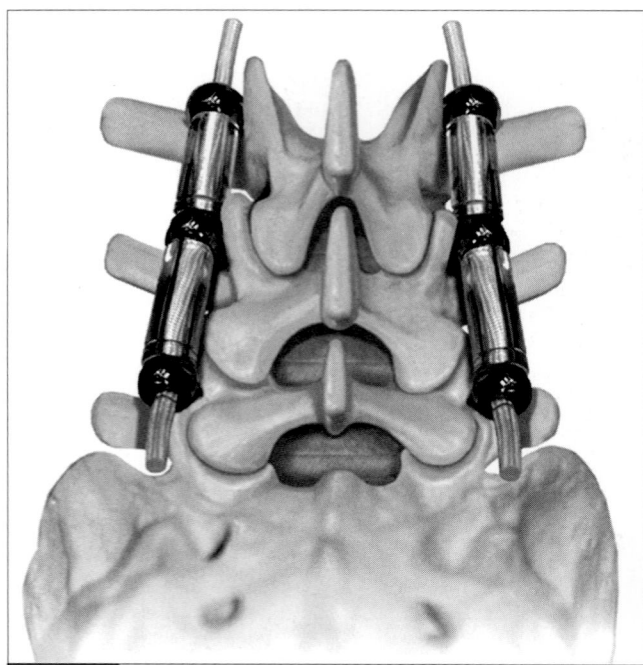

Figure 4   Dynesys Dynamic Stabilization System (Zimmer, Warsaw, IN).

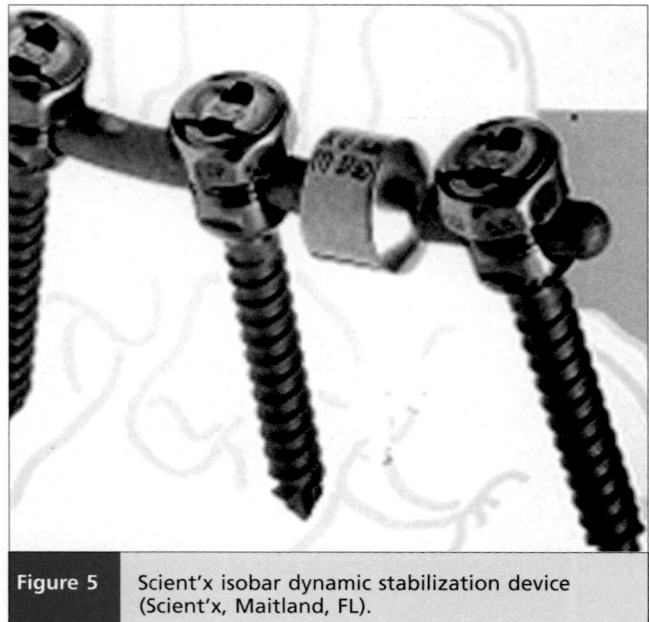

Figure 5   Scient'x isobar dynamic stabilization device (Scient'x, Maitland, FL).

pseudarthrosis "stiffened" the symptomatic level enough to prevent further instability. The theory is that dynamic stabilization could potentially stiffen the symptomatic level while preserving some motion, which in theory decreases the risk of adjacent segment disease. Dynamic stabilization is currently being used in four types of lumbar spine diseases. It is most commonly used to stabilize spondylolisthesis after laminectomy as an alternative to fusion. Another use is to protect a degenerated disk above a fusion to prevent the progression of adjacent segment disease. It has also been used after diskectomy to protect the disk against further degeneration. In addition, it is being used for mechanical back pain resulting from degenerative disk disease.

The first approved device is the most studied of these systems (Figure 4). It consists of pedicle screws that are attached by a rope and a plastic cylinder. The rope is threaded through the cylinder and tensioned to 300 N. The rope and cylinder decrease the amount of flexion and extension at the instrumented motion segment. Results of the use of this system for a variety of spine disorders were retrospectively analyzed in two European studies. One study demonstrated good results, recommending dynamic stabilization as an option to fusion in spondylolisthesis. Another study stated that use of this device was associated with poor results and it should not be used. Both of these studies showed a 17% hardware failure or loosening rate, which is quite alarming.[6,7] Currently this system is being used in the United States for the four spinal disorders noted above; however, there are no data at this time that conclusively demonstrate its efficacy. There have been no published

IDE prospective studies using dynamic stabilization as a nonfusion device. Other constructs have also been developed for dynamic stabilization of the lumbar spine. Most of these constructs involve pedicle screws with soft or jointed rods that allow some motion (Figure 5). Hybrid soft and stiff rods with pedicle screws can allow fusion at one level and dynamic stabilization at a degenerated level above or below the rigid fusion in hopes of preventing adjacent segment disease.

Facet Replacement

The newest arthroplasty technology being pioneered is facet replacement. The functional spinal unit is made up of three joints, including two facets and one disk. An inherent criticism of disk replacement is that it substitutes for only one articulation. Facet replacement replaces both facet joints, and in conjunction with TDR, all three pain generators would potentially be eliminated. Two types of designs have been the basis of the prototypes developed. The first is a relatively unconstrained anatomic design in which two unlinked components articulate with each other and rely on its anatomic design for its motion and stability (Figure 6). The second design is a linked system that attempts to reproduce the stability and motion properties but is anatomically different from normal facets.

Indications for facet replacement are still evolving but are similar to those of dynamic stabilization. The approved IDE studies are focusing on use in spinal stenosis patients. The rationale behind its use is that facets can be removed for wide decompression while maintaining stability and obviating the need for a fusion. Patients with grade I spondylolisthesis are also included in these studies to assess whether these implants can afford enough spinal stability after decom-

5: Spine

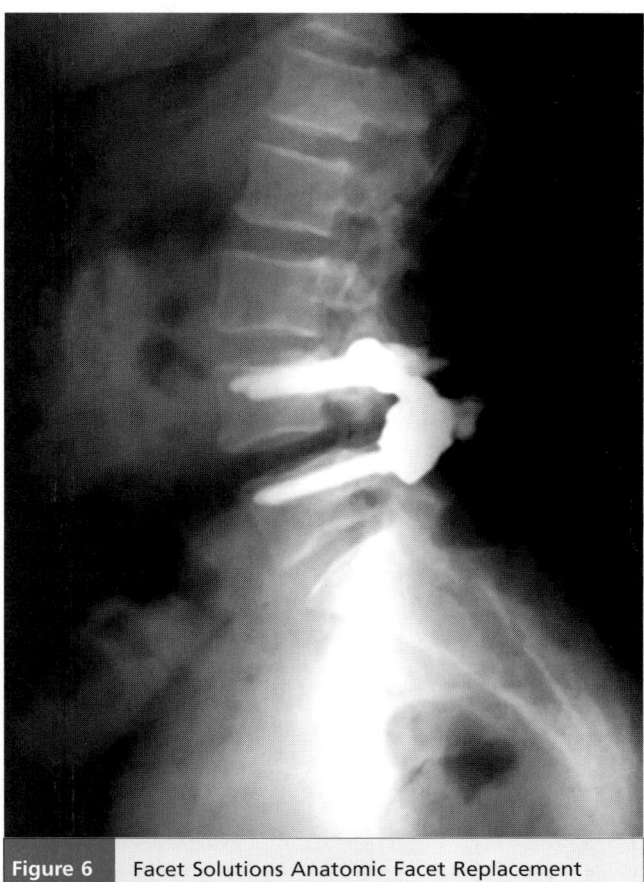

| Figure 6 | Facet Solutions Anatomic Facet Replacement System (AFRS) (Facet Solutions, Logan, UT). |

sions can be drawn on the efficacy and safety of facet replacement.

Interspinous Spacer Technology

Patients with intermittent neurogenic claudication (INC) are commonly treated in a spine practice, with an estimated 2 million doctor visits annually. Most patients describe symptomatic relief in a seated or flexed position. Many state that leaning over a shopping cart at the grocery store relieves their symptoms. Standing upright for these patients is typically the most symptomatic position. The positional symptomatic relief created in relative lumbar flexion is caused by the posterior column distraction that increases canal and foramen diameter. As the lamina and the facet joints move away from each other, the redundant ligamentum flavum stretches and moves away and posteriorly from the neural elements. Furthermore, the distraction of the facet joints and the pedicles may relieve some of the foraminal and lateral recess stenosis. If left untreated and followed for 5 years, INC symptoms worsen in 60% of patients and improve in 20% of patients. Additional adverse events ensue with the immobility of INC, including osteoporosis, depression, and cardiovascular impairment.

The standard treatment options remain nonsurgical management, including nonsteroidal anti-inflammatory drugs, activity modification, weight loss, and epidural steroid injections. Most patients gain long-term benefits from nonsurgical management. Those patients whose condition does not improve may be candidates for surgical intervention, which traditionally has been lumbar laminectomy with possible fusion if the patient has preoperative or iatrogenic instability. Lumbar laminectomy in these patients is generally successful in several long-term studies, but laminectomy has potential complications. Anesthesia complications, wound hematoma, iatrogenic dural leak, and neural injury are possible.

An interspinous spacer implant is placed between the adjacent spinous processes and distracts the lamina, recreating the flexed and symptom-free position of patients with INC. The implantation of the spacer can be performed without general anesthesia and with conscious sedation and local anesthesia. Because laminectomy is avoided, potential injury to the dura or the nerves is eliminated. The spacer is placed through the interspinous ligament of the affected level using a 5- to 8-cm incision and minimal paraspinal muscle injury. Not unlike most spinal surgery procedures, proper indications predict the success rate of patients receiving the interspinous implant.

Early results of interspinous technology have been encouraging. A large 2-year follow-up study shows results similar to laminectomy. A 4-year follow-up of 18 implantations has shown 78% satisfactory results.[8] Patients who benefit most from this technology are the ones whose symptoms are relieved when in a seated position. In fact, if the patients do not experience relief of their symptoms in a seated position or if they have

pression. The control arm of these studies will be instrumented fusion patients with or without instability. Other possible indications for facet replacement may be for axial back pain for primary facet disease, although this subset of patients may be quite small because discogenic pain is usually the prominent pain generator in the lumbar spine. The last potential indication for this technology may be in combination with disk replacement to replace all the degenerated and painful articulations of the functional spinal unit. The cost of the complete procedure may be the limiting factor for this application because two implants would be used.

There are inherent problems with facet replacement that are similar to dynamic stabilization as the two technologies are almost identical in their indications and very similar in their theoretic benefits. The goal of both technologies is to achieve stabilization without fusion from a posterior approach, while allowing decompression of the neural elements. After a certain number of loading cycles in the human body, implant loosening or failure can become problematic. Current fixation methods use pedicle fixation with screws into the pedicles in the rostral and caudal vertebrae. Subluxation also may occur in unconstrained models. Loosening may become more prevalent in the presence of osteoporosis. Further research is needed before conclu-

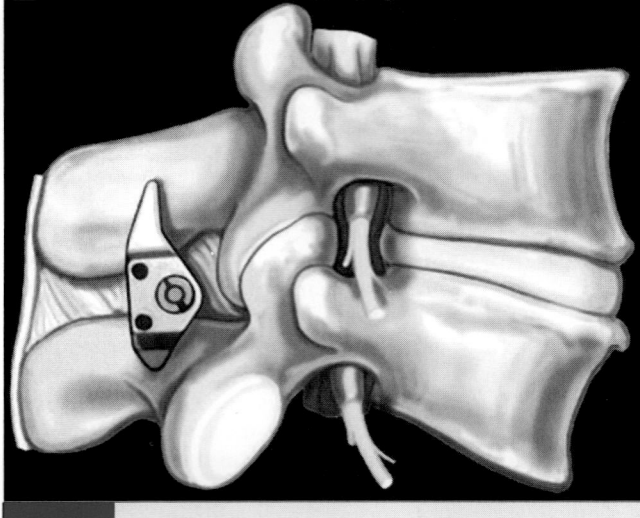

Figure 7 X STOP interspinous spacer technology (Medtronic, Minneapolis, MN).

fixed neurologic deficits, then implantation is contraindicated. Patients with fixed stenosis that is not relieved with positional change should undergo laminectomy with foraminotomies to decompress their neural elements. Biomechanical studies have shown that the spacer has numerous benefits at the implanted level without having any significant effect on the adjacent levels above and below the implant. These benefits include increase in the canal area by 18% and foraminal area by 25%,[9] decrease in the posterior anulus fibrosus pressures in extension by 63%, and decrease in mean facet loads by 39% and contact area by 47%.[10] The implant has been shown to cause an average 1.8° of kyphosis when two adjacent levels have been implanted. However, the overall change in lumbar lordosis was insignificant as measured by an in vivo dynamic MRI study.[10] The first interspinous device approved by the FDA for the treatment of INC was approved in November 2005 (**Figure 7**). Many other interspinous devices are under clinical investigation for treatment of stenosis and back pain associated with degenerative disk disease. These devices are believed to improve back pain by providing some stability while attaching to the posterior elements but still preserving some mobility.

Summary

Motion-preservation or nonfusion technologies are rapidly being developed in the spine field. Disk replacement may be conceptually better in the cervical spine. The role of lumbar disk replacement is still evolving. Dynamic stabilization and facet replacement should be prospectively studied before any conclusions can be made about their efficacy and safety. The early results of interspinous spacer technology are promising; this may become a viable alternative to laminectomy and fusion surgery for patients with INC.

Annotated References

1. Bertagnoli R, Duggal N, Gwynedd EP, et al: Cervical total disc replacement, part two: Clinical results. *Orthop Clin North Am* 2005;36:355-362.

   This article focuses on the outcomes of three prostheses (the Bryan Cervical Disk [Spinal Dynamics, Mercer Island, WA], the Bristol Disk [Medtronic Sofamor Danek, Memphis, TN], and the ProDisc-C). Development, design, and biomechanical characteristics of each prosthesis are given and surgical indications and clinical results are summarized and analyzed.

2. Hacker RJ: Cervical disc arthroplasty: A controlled randomized prospective study with intermediate follow-up results. *J Neurosurg Spine* 2005;3:424-428.

   Forty-six patients with single-level discogenic cervical radiculopathy and/or myelopathy were randomized to undergo arthroplasty or fusion as part of an FDA medical device study. Patients were followed for 1 year and had equivalent results. Level of evidence: II.

3. Robertson JT, Metcalf NH: Long-term outcome after implantation of the Prestige I disc in an end-stage indication: 4-year results from a pilot study. *Neurosurg Focus* 2004;17:E10.

   The authors conducted clinical and radiographic examinations at 3 and 4 years postoperatively to evaluate the long-term performance of the Prestige I device (Medtronic). The Prestige I disk maintained motion at the treated segment at 3 and 4 years postoperatively. Level of evidence: IIB.

4. Blumenthal S, McAfee PC, Guyer RD, et al: A prospective, randomized, multicenter Food and Drug Administration investigational device exemptions study of lumbar total disc replacement with the CHARITÉ artificial disc versus lumbar fusion: Part I. Evaluation of clinical outcomes. *Spine* 2005;30:1565-1575.

   This prospective, randomized, multicenter study demonstrated lumbar total disk replacement with the CHARITÉ artificial disk are equivalent to clinical outcomes with anterior lumbar interbody fusion. Level of evidence: II.

5. Delamarter RB, Bae HW, Pradhan BB: Clinical results of ProDisc-II lumbar total disc replacement: Report from the United States clinical trial. *Orthop Clin North Am* 2005;36:301-313.

   This study states the clinical results of the IDE clinical trial of the ProDisc-II prosthetic disk at one site and deems it equivalent to 360° of fusion. Level of evidence: II.

6. Schnake KJ, Schaeren S, Jeanneret B: Dynamic stabilization in addition to decompression for lumbar spinal stenosis with degenerative spondylolisthesis. *Spine* 2006;31:442-449.

   In this retrospective study, the authors advocate the use of Dynesys for dynamic stabilization after laminectomy in grade I spondylolisthesis despite a loosening rate of 17% at 2 years. Level of evidence: IV.

5: Spine

7. Grob D, Benini A, Junge A, Mannion AF: Clinical experience with the Dynesys semirigid fixation system for the lumbar spine: Surgical and patient-oriented outcome in 50 cases after an average of 2 years. *Spine* 2005;30: 324-331.

    The authors evaluate retrospectively the use of Dynesys system for a variety of lumbar disorders and report disappointing clinical results. Level of evidence: IV.

8. Kondrashov DG, Hannibal M, Hsu KY, Zucherman JF: Interspinous process decompression with the X-STOP device for lumbar spinal stenosis: A 4-year follow-up study. *J Spinal Disord Tech* 2006;19:323-327.

    This article reports a 78% satisfactory result in 18 patients followed for average of 4.2 years after X STOP implantation. Level of evidence: II.

9. Richards JC, Majumdar S, Lindsey DP, Beaupre GS, Yerby SA: The treatment mechanism of an interspinous process implant for lumbar neurogenic intermittent claudication. *Spine* 2005;30:744-749.

    Lumbar specimens (L2-5) were evaluated using MRI before and after X STOP implantation at L3-4 level. Spinal canal and neural foramina dimension changes are described.

10. Siddiqui M, Karadinas E, Nicol M, et al: Effects of X-STOP device on sagittal lumbar spine kinematics in spinal stenosis. *J Spinal Disord Tech* 2006;19:328-333.

    The objective of this study is to understand the sagittal kinematics in vivo of the lumbar spine at the instrumented and adjacent levels. The X STOP device does not affect the sagittal kinematics of the lumbar spine in vivo, including disk pressures.

Section 6

Pediatrics

SECTION EDITOR:

JOHN M. FLYNN, MD

Chapter 54

Shoulder, Upper Arm, and Elbow Trauma: Pediatrics

James F. Mooney III, MD

Introduction

Fractures of the shoulder, upper arm, or elbow resulting from trauma are common in children and adolescents. Diagnosis and subsequent management can be difficult because of the growth plates and multiple centers of ossification in these areas. The presence of an associated neurovascular injury affects the relative urgency and choice of treatment, and the varying ability and rate of remodeling of the injured structure must also be considered. For example, because remodeling of a proximal humerus fracture continues until the child's teenage years, relatively large degrees of regional displacement and angulation are acceptable, depending on the age of the patient at the time of injury. In contrast, fractures near the elbow have limited potential for remodeling; therefore, less residual deformity can be tolerated.

A general evaluation of the patient is the first step in treating an upper extremity injury. Tenderness, deformity, and range of motion must be assessed, and a careful, well-documented neurovascular examination must be performed. Radiographic evaluation should include, at a minimum, AP and lateral views of the injured area as well as the joints proximal and distal to the injured bone. Oblique images can be useful in assessing a possible fracture near the elbow. In rare instances, MRI may be necessary to clarify the nature of certain fractures of the proximal or distal humerus.

Sternoclavicular Injuries

Injuries to the sternoclavicular joint account for fewer than 5% of pediatric clavicle fractures. The mechanism of injury is usually axial compression of the shoulder. The patient will have pain, swelling, and tenderness over the medial portion of the clavicle. Because of the relative strength of the joint capsule compared with the physis, and the fact that the medial clavicular physis usually remains open into adulthood (until the early 20s), most sternoclavicular joint injuries are physeal fractures rather than true joint dislocations.

The direction of displacement of the lateral fragment can be either anterior or posterior. A patient with an anteriorly displaced fracture has localized pain and an obvious anterior prominence. A patient with a posterior fracture may have signs and symptoms associated with compression of the trachea, esophagus, or underlying great vessels. Specialized plain radiographs, including the Hobb or serendipity view, can be helpful in establishing the diagnosis. However, CT is more useful for viewing both sternoclavicular joints (**Figure 1**).

Management of nondisplaced and most anteriorly displaced fractures is symptomatic. Although closed reduction of an anterior-directed injury can be attempted, redisplacement often occurs. Significant remodeling can be expected in most instances. The fracture is unlikely to cause long-term difficulty, although a cosmetically unattractive prominence is possible. Acceptable functional results have been reported after surgical management of symptomatic, unstable anterior injuries using autologous woven tendon grafts.[1] Reduction of a posterior sternoclavicular joint injury should be attempted, particularly in the presence of symptoms of compression of mediastinal structures. A thoracic surgeon should be available for attempted reduction of a posteriorly displaced fracture. Fixation of an unstable posterior fracture or dislocation can be accomplished through a variety of suture or wiring techniques. Smooth implants should not be used because of the risk of migration.

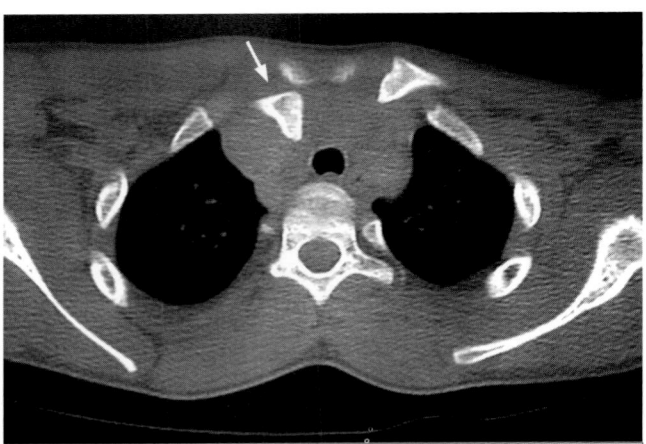

Figure 1 CT scan of a patient with a posterior sternoclavicular dislocation (arrow).

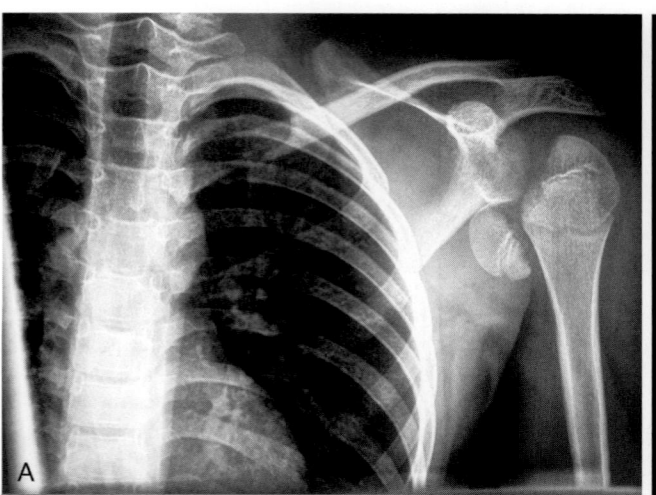
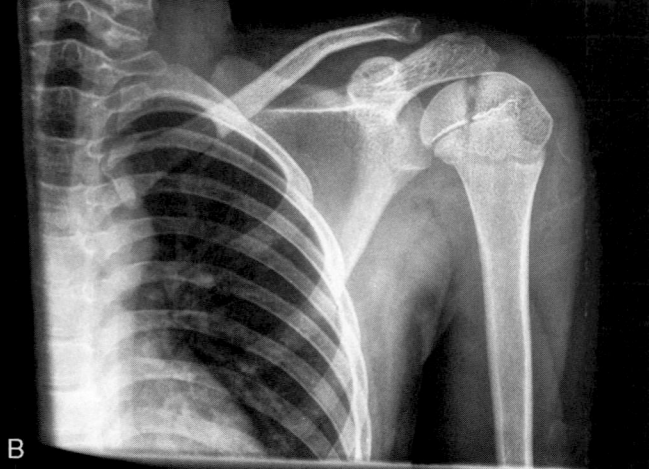

Figure 2   **A,** AP radiograph of a 5-year-old patient before reduction of a Salter-Harris type IV fracture of the proximal humerus. **B,** AP radiograph of the same patient after closed reduction of the fracture.

Clavicle Fractures

Clavicle fractures occur as a result of birth trauma in approximately 5 of every 1,000 live births. Although these fractures usually are associated with vaginal delivery, they also have been reported after cesarean section. The risk factors include shoulder dystocia, large birth weight, prolonged gestation, and forceps delivery. Approximately 9% of patients with a neonatal clavicle fracture have an associated brachial plexus injury. Neonatal clavicle fractures require little or no treatment beyond supportive care, and they heal readily without sequelae.

In older children, 85% of clavicle fractures occur in the midshaft of the clavicle, and most are either nondisplaced or minimally displaced. A history of a fall onto a shoulder or outstretched hand, with resulting tenderness and swelling over the midshaft, is usually sufficient to establish a diagnosis. Confirmatory radiographs are sometimes helpful. Radiographic confirmation of a nondisplaced fracture may not be possible until new callus formation becomes visible in 10 to 14 days.

Clavicle fractures are managed with a sling or figure-of-8 splint for comfort. The patient's activities should be limited until the pain is resolved and use of the extremity returns. Internal fixation is rarely necessary for pediatric clavicle fractures. However, some unstable, widely displaced fractures may benefit from surgical treatment, particularly if the overlying skin is at risk. Surgical treatment also may be indicated for open fractures and those with associated vascular injury. Although plate fixation is the standard method of surgical repair, intramedullary fixation with titanium elastic nails also has been reported.[2]

Proximal Humerus Fractures

Proximal humerus fractures represent approximately 0.45% of all pediatric fractures and 3% of all epiphyseal injuries. In children, proximal humerus fractures often involve the growth plate. Salter-Harris type I fractures are most common in patients younger than age 5 years, and Salter-Harris type II fractures are most common in those older than age 11 years. Metaphyseal fractures without epiphyseal involvement predominate in patients who are 5 to 11 years of age. Salter-Harris type III and IV fractures occur only rarely (**Figure 2**).

A proximal humerus fracture can be difficult to diagnose in a neonate, who may have diminished motion in the extremity and apparent paralysis. A proximal humerus fracture must be differentiated from brachial plexus injury, clavicle fracture, shoulder joint sepsis, and osteomyelitis of the humerus. Plain radiographs may not provide adequate information, because the proximal humeral epiphysis does not begin to ossify until approximately 6 months of age. MRI, ultrasound, or arthrogram may be necessary to determine the diagnosis. A proximal humerus fracture in an older child or adolescent typically is the result of a fall onto an outstretched arm or shoulder. If significant fracture displacement has occurred, the patient has pain on palpation and apparent deformity. Plain radiographs are almost always sufficient to establish the diagnosis.

Because of the proximity of the humeral growth plate and the significant remodeling potential of the proximal humerus, most proximal humerus fractures can be managed by closed reduction. The acceptable angulation and displacement vary with the patient's age. For a child younger than 5 years of age, as much as 70° of angulation and 100% displacement can be ac-

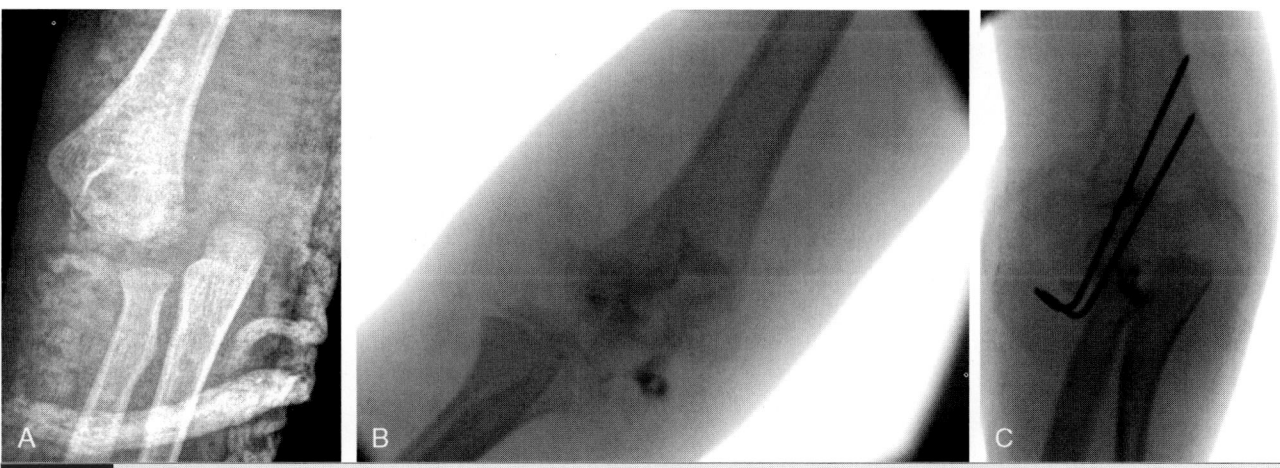

Figure 3   **A,** AP radiograph of an 18-month-old patient with a transphyseal distal humerus fracture. **B,** Intraoperative arthrogram showing the displaced transphyseal fracture. **C,** Arthrogram after closed reduction and percutaneous pinning showing anatomic reduction and stable fixation.

by appropriate fixation of displaced fractures. Some authors have recommended fixation of nonunions having more than 1 cm of displacement. Open reduction without soft-tissue stripping and fixation in a nonanatomic position is recommended. The risk of osteonecrosis can be minimized by limiting posterior dissection of the fracture fragment during the initial fixation or repair of a nonunion.

Medial Epicondyle Fractures

Fractures of the medial epicondyle account for fewer than 10% of all pediatric elbow fractures. Most result from a valgus stress to the elbow that generates an avulsion of the flexor-pronator origin and medial collateral ligament. Sometimes these fractures are associated with dislocation of the elbow. Patients have swelling over the medial aspect of the elbow and elbow pain. Instability to valgus stress may be evident. Radiographs usually are sufficient to confirm the diagnosis, although the fragment may not be visible in a younger patient with an unossified apophysis or a patient with a retained intra-articular fragment after spontaneous or manipulative reduction of an associated elbow dislocation.

Management of medial epicondyle fractures is controversial. Surgical treatment is indicated for fractures in which the fragment is trapped within the joint after elbow dislocation, fractures with associated ulnar neuropathy, fractures in throwing athletes when clinical evidence of valgus instability appears, and fractures displaced more than 1 cm. Excision of the fragment and soft-tissue reconstruction should be avoided during the acute injury phase.[18] At the surgeon's discretion, screws or smooth pins can be used for fracture fixation. Radiographic nonunion may occur, particularly after nonsurgical management.

Medial Condyle Fractures

Medial condyle fractures are rare, accounting for fewer than 2% of all pediatric elbow fractures. Radiographic diagnosis may be difficult if the patient's medial condylar ossification center is not yet present. Plain radiographs may show a metaphyseal fragment, although MRI or arthrography may be necessary to fully assess any intra-articular displacement. Fractures with little or no joint line displacement can be managed with closed reduction and cast immobilization. Fractures with displacement should be treated with open reduction and internal fixation. Complications can include delayed union or nonunion, osteonecrosis of the trochlea, and loss of elbow range of motion.

Transphyseal Distal Humerus Fractures

Transphyseal distal humerus fractures are uncommon injuries that are rarely seen in patients older than 2 years of age and may be associated with child abuse. They can be difficult to diagnose; apparent malalignment between the distal humerus and the proximal radius and ulna may be the only finding on standard radiographs. MRI, ultrasonography, or arthrography can help in determining the final diagnosis and the treatment. Displaced fractures should be treated with closed reduction and percutaneous pinning. An intraoperative arthrogram during fixation provides visualization of the distal fragment for reduction and pinning (**Figure 3**).

Elbow Dislocations

Dislocations account for approximately 3% of all pediatric elbow injuries. Most occur in adolescents; the highest incidence is between 13 and 15 years of age.

6: Pediatrics

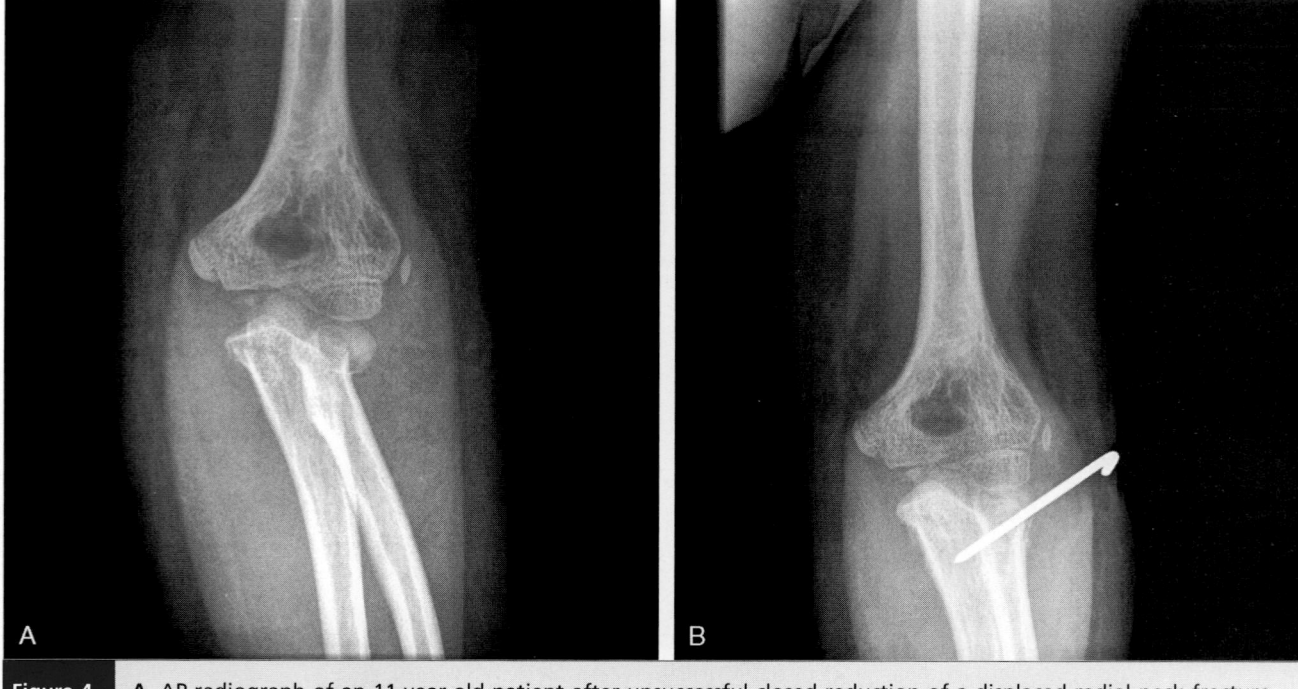

Figure 4   **A,** AP radiograph of an 11-year-old patient after unsuccessful closed reduction of a displaced radial neck fracture. **B,** AP radiograph 3 weeks after percutaneous joystick reduction and pinning.

Posterior dislocations are the most common, and anterior dislocations are rare. The mechanism of posterior dislocation is usually a fall onto an outstretched hand. Diagnosis is confirmed by standard radiographs. Care must be taken to distinguish an elbow dislocation from a distal humeral physeal separation, particularly if the patient is very young.

Closed reduction and splint or cast immobilization is usually sufficient. Postreduction radiographs must be scrutinized for evidence of residual joint space irregularity, which can indicate the presence of an entrapped bone fragment. The most frequently entrapped fragments are from the medial epicondyle or coronoid process. The presence of entrapped fragments, failure to obtain or maintain an adequate closed reduction, and significant joint instability are indications for surgical management. Immobilization should be limited to 2 to 3 weeks to minimize the risk of stiffness. Complications of elbow dislocation include heterotopic ossification, loss of terminal flexion or extension, and chronic instability.

Elbow Contractures

Most children rapidly regain full range of motion after an elbow trauma. A recent study found that physical therapy was unnecessary for children after surgical fixation of supracondylar humerus fractures.[19] However, a small percentage of patients do not obtain a functional arc of motion. For these patients, noninvasive methods such as physical therapy and splinting are the initial methods of treatment. Open capsular releases have been reported as successful after all noninvasive methods have failed. Gradual distraction using external fixation, both with and without soft-tissue release, was recently reported as having mixed success.[20-22]

Olecranon Fractures

Approximately 5% of all pediatric elbow fractures involve the olecranon, and as many as half of the patients also have other elbow fractures. The combination of injuries may be more important in the outcome than the severity of the olecranon fracture itself. Patients with osteogenesis imperfecta tarda are at particular risk of displaced olecranon sleeve fractures. Most olecranon fractures involve the metaphyseal region and are intra-articular. Closed treatment may be suitable for olecranon fractures with less than 2 mm of intra-articular displacement. Those with greater displacement require open reduction and fixation. Several types of fixation have been recommended. A recent report described excellent clinical and radiographic results after open reduction and fixation using percutaneously placed smooth pins and absorbable suture in a tension-band fashion. The authors found that this method maintained reduction and avoided the need for a second procedure to remove retained hardware.[23]

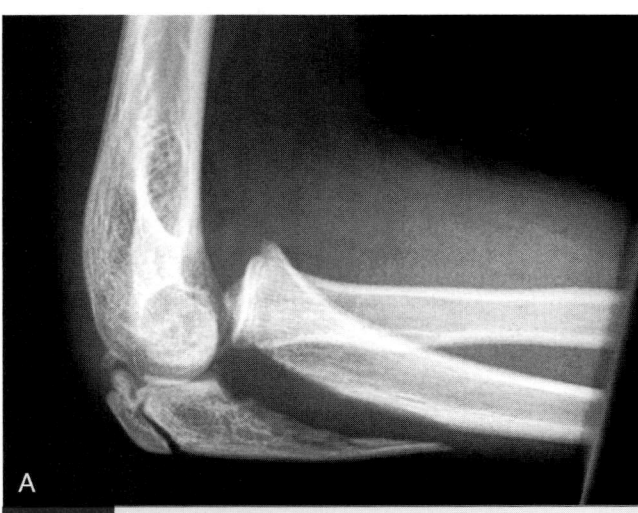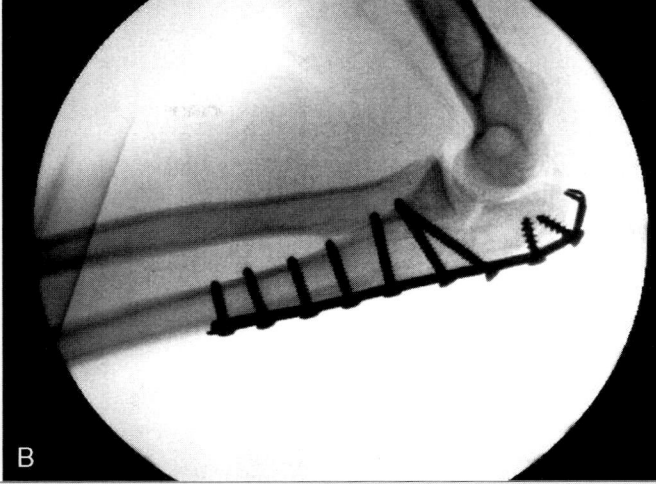

Figure 5 **A,** Lateral radiograph of a patient with a Bado type III Monteggia fracture. **B,** Lateral radiograph after open reduction and internal fixation of the proximal ulna fracture, showing spontaneous reduction of the radial head dislocation.

Proximal Radius Fractures

Fractures of the proximal radius are relatively rare in children. Fractures through the radial neck are most common, and the fracture sometimes involves the radial head. Although anatomic alignment should be the goal of treatment, radial neck fractures with less than 3 mm of displacement or less than 30° of angulation can be managed with short-term immobilization and early motion. Fractures with greater residual displacement, angulation or significant residual translation of the fragment after attempted closed reduction are best treated with surgical reduction and internal fixation. Percutaneous manipulation of the fragment with smooth pins or small instruments (joystick reduction) can be attempted (**Figure 4**). Indirect reduction and stabilization with retrograde intramedullary nails also has been used with success. In a recent multicenter study of 66 patients, 78% had good or excellent results after open or closed reduction and subsequent intramedullary fixation.[24] If all other methods fail to achieve an acceptable position, displaced radial neck fractures should be treated with open reduction and fixation, usually with smooth pins. Radial head fractures, if displaced, should be reduced anatomically because of their intra-articular nature. `

Monteggia Fractures

A true Monteggia fracture combines a proximal ulna fracture, either complete or with plastic deformation, and a radial head dislocation. The Bado classification (I through IV) and the known equivalent injuries are applicable to pediatric fractures. The most common Monteggia fractures in children are classified as Bado types I and III. Because overlooking a Monteggia injury can have significant consequences, including pain, deformity, and limited range of motion, complete radiographic evaluation of the elbow and forearm of every patient with an apparently isolated ulna fracture or radial head dislocation must be performed.

Closed reduction is usually successful in children, although maintaining the reduction can be difficult. Fixation of the ulna may be necessary using closed or open intramedullary pinning or open plating of the ulna. Generally, the radial head remains in place after stable fixation of the ulna (**Figure 5**).

Management of a chronic radial head dislocation associated with a previous acute Monteggia injury is controversial. Significant complications, including loss of motion, redislocation of the radial head, and compartment syndrome, have been reported. However, more favorable results were noted in a recent study of 15 patients after delayed reconstruction. The authors reported improvement of carrying angle and functional arc of motion with no evidence of neural injury after annular ligament reconstruction of chronic Monteggia injuries, although four patients experienced recurrent but asymptomatic radial head subluxation. These authors stressed the need for annular ligament reconstruction using the Bell Tawse procedure, with ulnar osteotomy if needed, to attain anatomic reduction of the radial head.[25]

Annotated References

1. Bae DS, Kocher MS, Waters PM, Micheli LM, Griffey M, Dichtel L: Chronic recurrent anterior sternoclavicular joint instability. *J Pediatr Orthop* 2006;26:71-74.

6: Pediatrics

The authors reviewed the functional results of surgical management for patients with recurrent anterior sternoclavicular joint instability. Level of evidence: III.

2. Kubiak R, Slongo T: Operative treatment of clavicle fractures in children: Review of 21 years. *J Pediatr Orthop* 2002;22:736-739. Level of evidence: III.

3. Beaty JH: Fractures of the proximal humerus and shaft in children. *Inst Course Lect* 1992; 41:369-372. Level of evidence: IV.

4. Beringer DC, Weiner DS, Noble JS, Bell RH: Severely displaced proximal humerus epiphyseal fractures: A follow-up study. *J Pediatr Orthop* 1998;18:31-37. Level of evidence: III.

5. Lucas JC, Mehlman CT, Laor T: The location of the biceps tendon in completely displaced proximal humerus fractures in children. *J Pediatr Orthop* 2004;24: 249-253.

   The common belief that biceps tendon entrapment can lead to failure of closed reduction of a displaced proximal humerus fracture is challenged in this report of four pediatric patients evaluated with MRI, with additional study of an adult cadaver model. Level of evidence: III.

6. Shaw BA, Murphy KM, Shaw A, Oppeheim WL, Myracle MR: Humerus shaft fractures in young children: Accident or abuse? *J Pediatr Orthop* 1997;17:293-297. Level of evidence: III.

7. Sarwark JF, King EC, Luhmann SJ: Proximal humerus, scapula and clavicle, in Beaty J, Kasser J (eds): *Rockwood and Wilkins Fractures in Children, ed 6*. Philadelphia, PA, Lippincott Williams and Wilkins, 2006, pp 713-771.

   This book is an updated version of the classic pediatric fracture text. This chapter discusses essentially all issues relevant to the management of fractures of the humerus, scapula, and clavicle, including complications of injury and treatment. Level of evidence: IV.

8. Leitch KK, Kay RM, Femino JD, Tolo VT, Storer SK, Skaggs DL: Treatment of multidirectionally unstable supracondylar humerus fractures in children: A modified Gartland type IV fracture. *J Bone Joint Surg Am* 2006; 88:980-985.

   The authors report on nine patients with supracondylar humerus fractures believed to be unstable in both flexion and extension and propose a modified method of closed reduction and percutaneous pinning. Level of evidence: III.

9. Gupta N, Kay RM, Leitch K, Femino JD, Tolo VT, Skaggs DL: Effect of surgical delay on perioperative complications and need for open reduction in supracondylar humerus fractures in children. *J Pediatr Orthop* 2004;24:245-248.

   This retrospective review found that a delay of more than 12 hours in treating pediatric supracondylar fractures did not lead to more perioperative complications or open reductions compared with more urgent treatment. Level of evidence: III.

10. Sibinski M, Sharma H, Bennet GC: Early versus delayed treatment of extension type-3 supracondylar fractures of the humerus in children. *J Bone Joint Surg Br* 2006; 88:380-381.

    A comparison of patients managed less than 12 hours after injury and those treated more than 12 hours after injury found no statistical difference in perioperative complications. Level of evidence: III.

11. Walmsley PJ, Kelly MB, Robb JE, Annan IH, Porter DE: Delay increases the need for open reduction of type-III supracondylar fractures of the humerus. *J Bone Joint Surg Br* 2006;88:528-530.

    The rate of open reduction after attempted closed reduction was significantly increased in patients for whom treatment was delayed more than 8 hours after injury compared with those who were treated in less than 8 hours. Level of evidence: III.

12. Ay S, Akinci M, Kamilglu S, Ercetin O: Open reduction of displaced pediatric supracondylar humeral fractures through the anterior cubital approach. *J Pediatr Orthop* 2005;25:149-153.

    The authors describe their experience with open reduction of pediatric supracondylar fractures using a transverse antecubital incision through an anterior approach. Level of evidence: III.

13. Ponce BA, Hedequist DJ, Zurakowski D, Atkinson CC, Waters PM: Complications and timing of follow-up after closed reduction and percutaneous pinning of supracondylar humerus fractures. *J Pediatr Orthop* 2004;24: 610-614.

    The authors found no association between late follow-up and complications after closed reduction and percutaneous pinning and concluded that initial postoperative evaluation can be delayed until pin removal. Level of evidence: III.

14. Rasool MN: Ulnar nerve injury after K-wire fixation of supracondylar humerus fractures in children. *J Pediatr Orthop* 1998;18:686-690. Level of evidence: III.

15. Pankaj A, Dua A, Malhotra R, Bhan S: Dome osteotomy for posttraumatic cubitus varus. *J Pediatr Orthop* 2006;26:61-66.

    The described osteotomy technique for cubitus varus reconstruction appeared to minimize generation of lateral condylar prominence in 12 patients. Level of evidence: III.

16. Abraham E, Gordon A, Abdul-Hadi O: Management of supracondylar fractures of the humerus with condylar involvement in children. *J Pediatr Orthop* 2005;25:709-716.

    Closed reduction and percutaneous pin fixation using a specific crossed-pin technique is recommended in this review of 22 patients with a complex supracondylar humerus fracture. Level of evidence: III.

17. Remia LF, Richards K, Waters PM: The Bryan-Morrey triceps-sparing approach to open reduction of T-condylar humeral fractures in adolescents. *J Pediatr Orthop* 2004;24:615-619.

    A retrospective review of nine patients who underwent surgical management of T-condylar fractures found that the triceps-sparing approach can be safely used in adolescent patients. Level of evidence: III.

18. Farsetti P, Potenza V, Caterini R, Ippolito E: Long-term results of the treatment of fractures of the medial humeral epicondyle in children. *J Bone Joint Surg Am* 2001;83:1299-1305. Level of evidence: III.

19. Keppler P, Salem K, Schwarting B, Kinzl L: The effectiveness of physiotherapy after operative treatment of supracondylar humeral fractures in children. *J Pediatr Orthop* 2005;25:314-316.

    Physiotherapy did not improve patients' range of motion 1 year after open reduction and fixation of a displaced supracondylar humerus fracture. Level of evidence: I.

20. Gausepohl T, Mader K, Pennig D: Mechanical distraction for the treatment of posttraumatic stiffness of the elbow in children and adolescents. *J Bone Joint Surg Am* 2006;88:1011-1021.

    Treatment using closed distraction and range of motion with a hinged monolateral external fixator was successful in patients with posttraumatic stiffness compared with other methods. Level of evidence: III.

21. Ayoub K, Gibbons P, Bradish CF: Compass elbow hinge: Short-term results in five adolescents. *J Pediatr Orthop B* 2004;13:395-398.

    Five patients with elbow contractures were managed using open release, distraction, and immediate range of motion with the compass hinge device with acceptable short-term results. Level of evidence: III.

22. Wang AA, Hutchinson D: Use of the elbow compass universal hinge in pediatric patients. *J Pediatr Orthop* 2006;26:58-60.

    The results and complications of pediatric use of the compass hinge device are reported for a wide range of indications, including elbow contractures. Level of evidence: III.

23. Gortzak Y, Mercado E, Atar D, Weisel Y: Pediatric olecranon fractures: Open reduction and internal fixation with removable Kirschner wires and absorbable sutures. *J Pediatr Orthop* 2006;26:39-42.

    Olecranon fractures were fixed using percutaneous pins and absorbable suture to minimize the need for hardware removal. Good results and no complications were noted. Level of evidence: III.

24. Schmittenbecher PP, Haevernick B, Herold A, Knorr P, Schmid E: Treatment decision, method of osteosynthesis, and outcome of radial neck fractures in children: A multicenter study. *J Pediatr Orthop* 2005;25:45-50.

    A prospective case collection study found that the use of elastic-stable intramedullary nailing for stabilization of displaced radial neck fractures yielded good or excellent results for most patients. Level of evidence: III.

25. Gyr BM, Stevens PM, Smith JT: Chronic Monteggia fractures in children: Outcome after treatment with the Bell-Tawse procedure. *J Pediatr Orthop B* 2004;13: 402-406.

    All 15 patients managed with the Bell Tawse procedure for chronic Monteggia injury regained functional flexion and extension. Ulnar osteotomy was needed for most patients requiring reconstruction. Level of evidence: III.

6: Pediatrics

Chapter 55

Forearm, Wrist, and Hand Trauma: Pediatrics

Charles T. Mehlman, DO, MPH

Epidemiology

Overview

Pediatric fractures of the forearm (including the wrist region) and hand represent two of the top ten reasons for pediatric orthopaedic hospitalization and collectively account for about half of all fractures in children.[1] Approximately 75% of forearm shaft fractures, distal radius/ulna fractures, and finger/hand fractures occur in children 8 years of age and older. Among hand injury patients, distal phalanx fractures predominate in children 8 years of age and younger, proximal phalanx injuries (of the small finger) are most common in those 9 to 12 years of age, and teenagers most frequently present with fractures of the neck of the fifth metacarpal.[2]

Increasing Fracture Rates

An American population-based study spanning a 30-year period documented a 32% increase in distal radius/ulna fracture rates for boys and a 56% increase for girls.[3] Precise explanations for such increased fracture rates are lacking, but several possible factors exist. Sports participation may have a major impact. Approximately 25% of all childhood soccer injuries are fractures; forearm fractures have been shown to be strongly associated with certain childhood activities such as trampoline and monkey bar use.[4] In comparison with falls from a standing height, falls from playground equipment were associated with a nearly four times greater risk of requiring fracture reduction.[5] Childhood obesity or increased body mass index is another precipitating factor for increased fracture rates. Even falls from standing height have been shown to be dangerous for obese children, with almost twice the risk of forearm fracture.[6] Other researchers also have found an increased risk of forearm fracture in obese children.[7,8]

Multiple studies have confirmed that children who avoid milk (and other dairy products) have an increased risk of fracture.[9] However, a recent meta-analysis of randomized controlled trials showed that the use of calcium supplementation in otherwise normal children had no effect on bone mineral density.[10,11] Another meta-analysis focusing on the relationship between bone density and childhood fractures concluded that evidence of an association is limited and is predominantly based on case-control (retrospective) studies.[12] Increased body weight and decreased cross-sectional dimensions of the forearm bones also has been demonstrated in girls with forearm fractures. It also has been shown that during puberty girls demonstrate a differential and transient decrease in bone mineral density in the distal radius compared with the tibial shaft.[13]

Forearm

Pain Issues Related to Forearm Fractures

Parents and medical practitioners have been shown to be unable to accurately judge children's pain severity. One study found that more than one third of pediatric fracture patients did not receive documented pain medication in the emergency department.[14] Displaced forearm fractures are the single most common reason for sedation in pediatric patients in the emergency department. Sedation can be performed by several different methods. Propofol/fentanyl procedural sedation is associated with faster recovery time but higher rates of respiratory depression in comparison with ketamine/midazolam sedation.[15] A small randomized trial of children older than 8 years of age found no significant difference between axillary block and a ketamine/midazolam sedation protocol.[16] In a randomized trial of more than 100 children undergoing forearm fracture reduction, nitrous oxide plus hematoma block was shown to provide equivalent pain relief and fewer adverse effects than ketamine/midazolam sedation.[17] Two separate studies have found no evidence of racial disparity relative to pediatric forearm fracture care.[18,19] Waterproof cast liners have also been shown to be effective in the setting of stable fracture patterns.[20]

Forearm Fracture Classification

Pediatric forearm fractures may be divided into three anatomic regions: forearm shaft (between Lister's tubercle and the bicipital tuberosity, ulnar shaft fractures are defined according to their corresponding radial level); distal metaphyseal (from the physis to Lister's tubercle); and distal physeal (growth plate and epiphysis).

6: Pediatrics

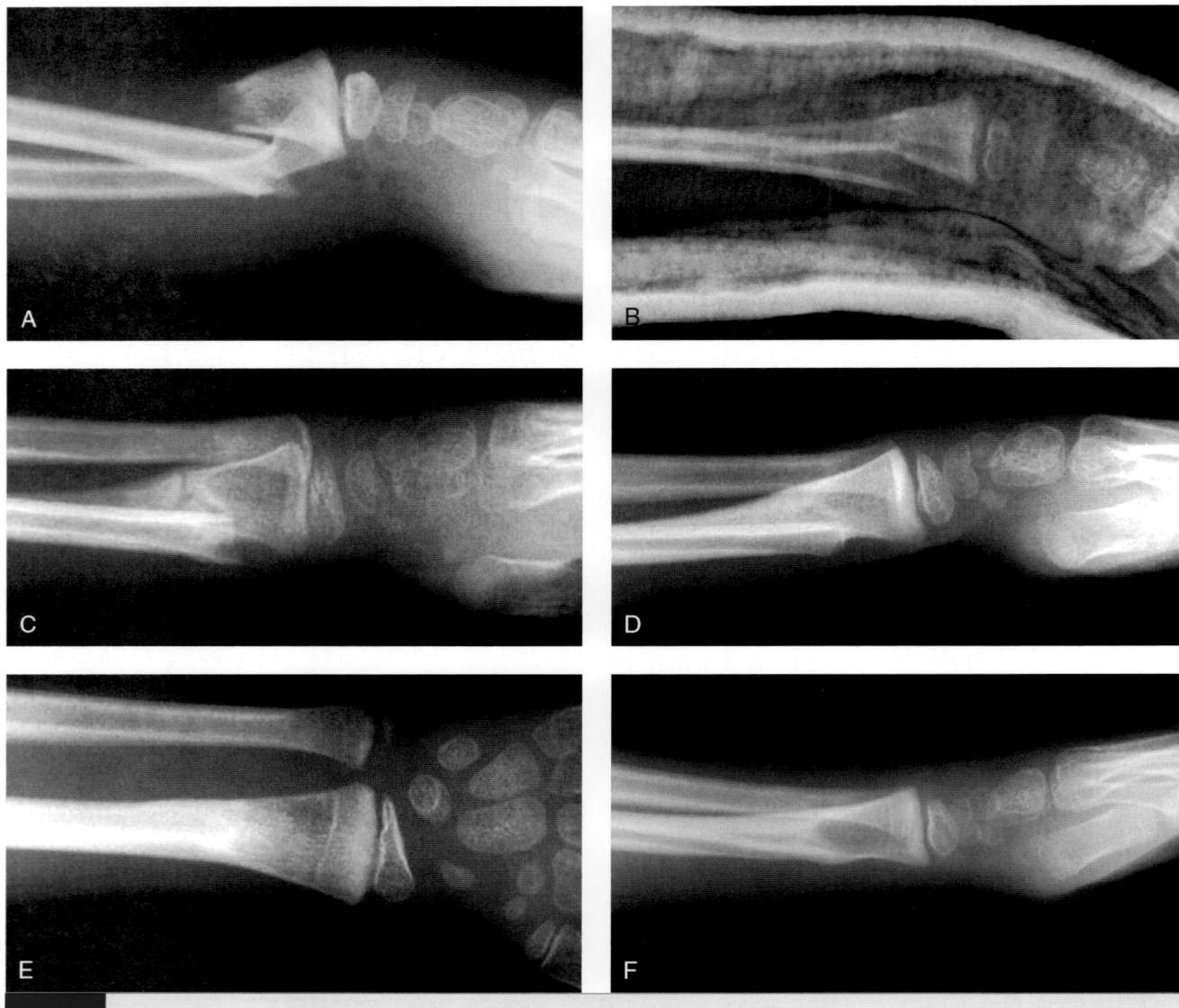

Figure 1 An example of healing and remodeling of a completely displaced metaphyseal fracture of the distal radius in conjunction with a greenstick fracture of the distal ulna in a 6-year-old boy is shown. **A,** Prereduction lateral radiograph. **B,** Ulnar alignment is improved following closed reduction but approximately 100% radial displacement persists. **C,** Follow-up lateral radiograph at 6 weeks. **D,** Follow-up lateral radiograph at 2.5 months. Follow-up AP radiograph **(E)** and follow-up lateral radiograph **(F)** both at 5 months, demonstrating essentially normal anatomy.

Distinct differences exist among these three different categories relative to decision making regarding treatment and likely complications. Complete forearm shaft fractures are associated with a higher rate of complications, especially in children older than 8 to 10 years,[21] and account for most of the poor results in reported studies of cast-treated patients. Complete metaphyseal fractures are associated with considerably less likelihood of complications in comparison with shaft fractures, because metaphyseal fractures demonstrate substantial remodeling potential (**Figure 1**). Displaced physeal fractures of the radius and ulna also demonstrate great remodeling potential but carry the added risk of growth disturbance (**Figure 2**).

Shaft Fractures of the Radius and Ulna

A practical classification of forearm shaft fractures can be applied by remembering two bones (radius and ulna), three levels (proximal, middle, and distal thirds), and four fracture patterns (plastic deformation, greenstick, complete, and comminuted). This fundamental information is necessary for deciding on treatment of forearm shaft fractures. In children younger than 8 to 10 years, most of these fractures are successfully treated using closed (cast) methods. Immobilization of such forearm fractures with the elbow in extension has been associated with lower rates of redisplacement.[22] In children older than 8 to 10 years, plastic deformation (al-

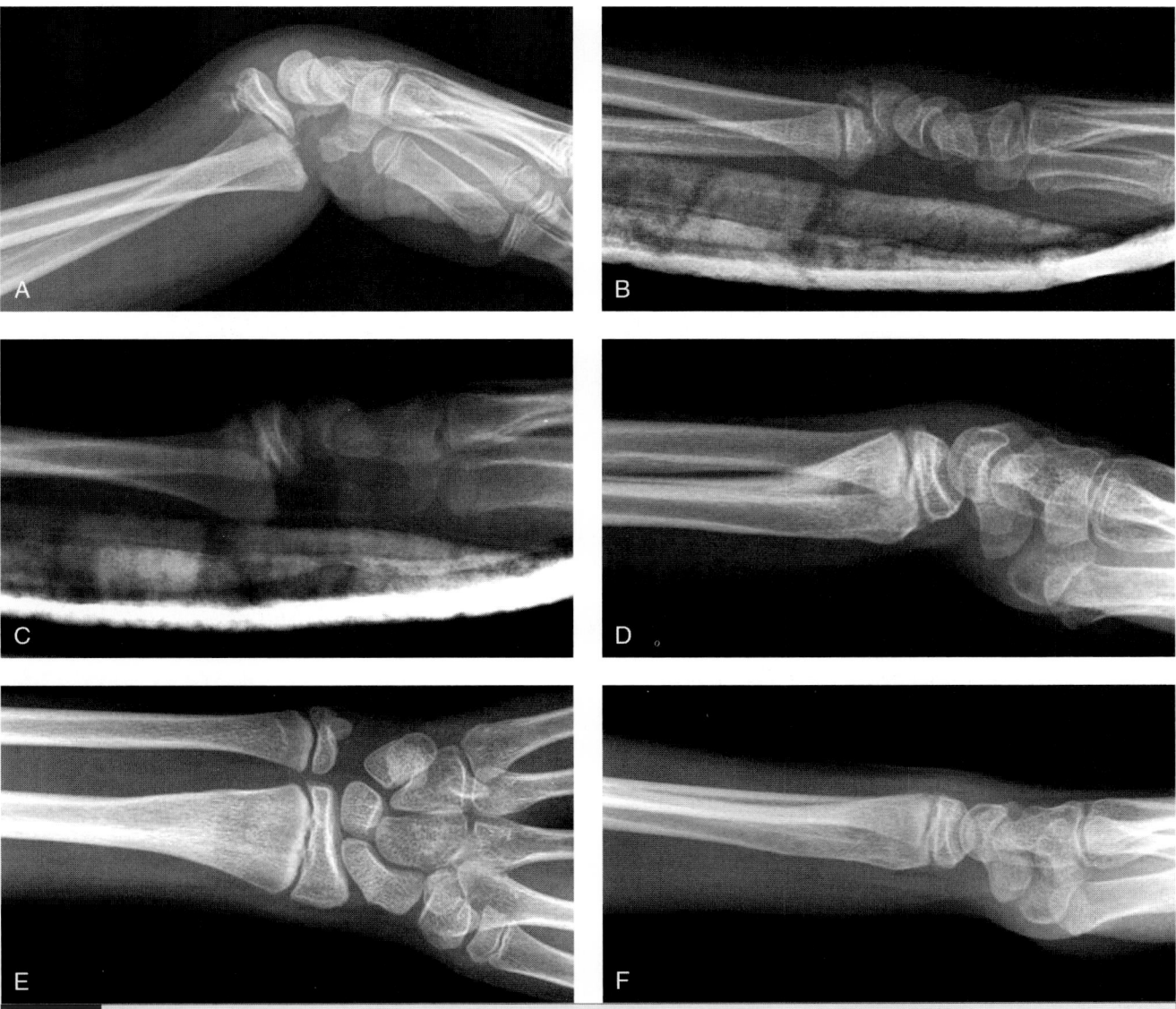

Figure 2	An example of healing and remodeling of a displaced Salter-Harris II fracture of the distal radius in a 10-year-old girl. **A,** Lateral radiograph obtained on the day of injury. **B,** Postreduction lateral radiograph. **C,** Follow-up lateral radiograph at 1 week. Loss of reduction is seen. **D,** Follow-up lateral radiograph at 4 months. Follow-up AP **(E)** and lateral **(F)** radiographs at 10 months show remodeling and no growth arrest.

though occasionally problematic) and greenstick fractures are best managed with closed treatment methods whereas complete and comminuted fractures are more likely to require fixation. Most authors agree that treatment is increasingly difficult as forearm shaft fractures progress from distal to proximal, and guidelines for children younger than 8 to 10 years regarding acceptable angulation steadily decrease accordingly (acceptable angulation: distal third, 20°; middle third, 15°; proximal third, 10°). For children older than 10 years, the acceptable angulation should be less than 10°. The potential for rotational malreduction must also be kept in mind, and clinical correlation is always important.[23] When closed reduction is not successful, flexible intramedullary nailing (usually of both bones) has be-

come a commonly used treatment[24-28] (**Figure 3**). Ulnar shaft fracture site distraction followed by delayed union and nonunion has been reported following flexible intramedullary nail fixation.[29] Because of compromise of the intramedullary canal as well as multiplanar deformity, surgical treatment of forearm shaft refractures or malunion still commonly involves plate fixation.[23,30]

Metaphyseal Fractures of the Distal Radius and Ulna

There are three main types of distal radial and ulnar metaphyseal fractures: torus or buckle (cortical wrinkling but no true cortical breach), greenstick (violation of one to three cortices), and complete fractures (viola-

6: Pediatrics

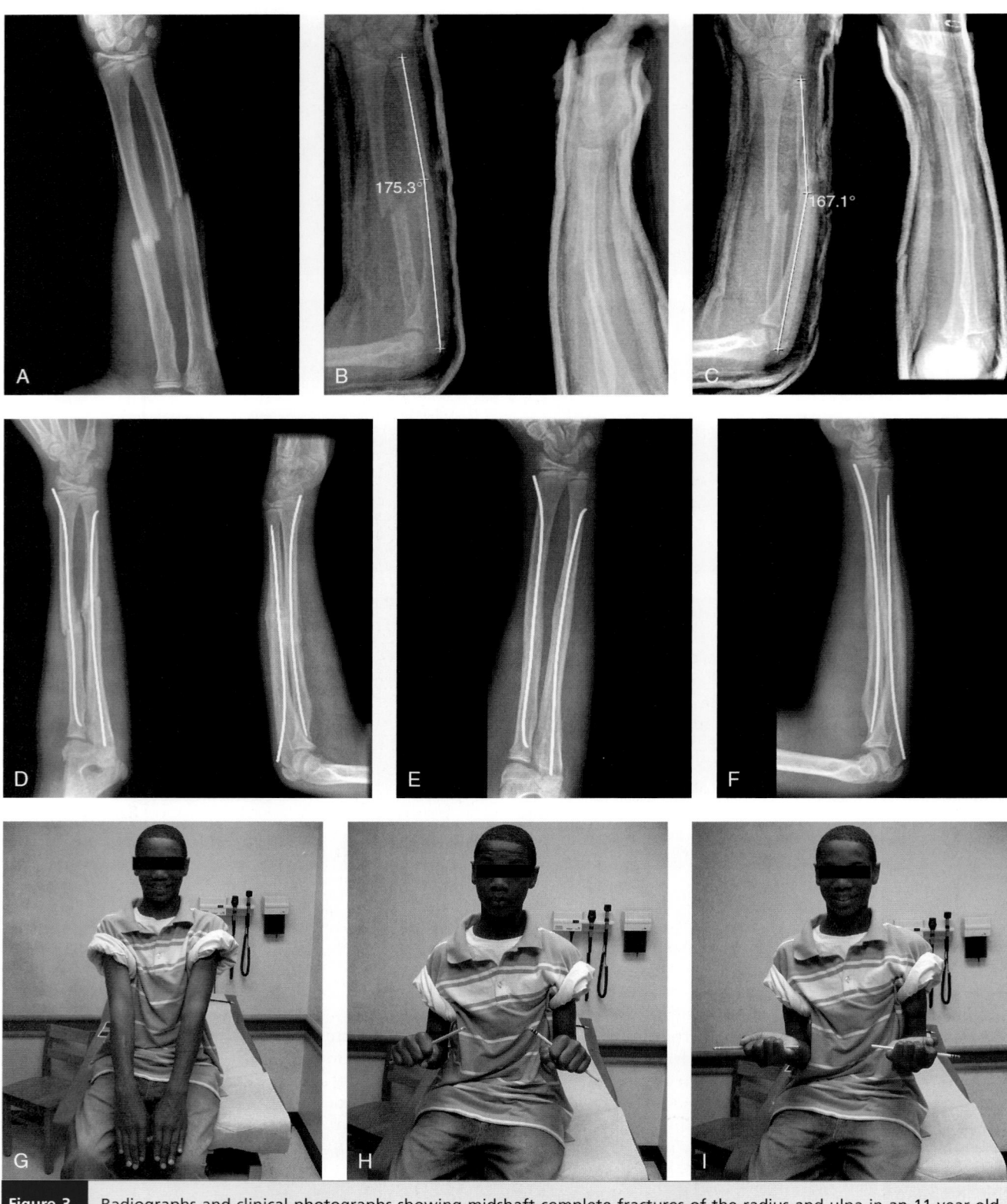

Figure 3 Radiographs and clinical photographs showing midshaft complete fractures of the radius and ulna in an 11-year-old boy. **A,** AP radiograph obtained on the day of injury. **B,** Postreduction radiographs showing 50% translation of the radius and 5° of angulation of the ulna. **C,** 1-week follow-up radiographs show 100% translation of the radius and 13° of angulation of the ulna. **D,** Postoperative AP and lateral radiographs after open reduction and internal fixation with flexible intramedullary nails. **E,** Six-month follow-up AP radiograph. **F,** Six-month follow-up lateral radiograph. **G,** Satisfactory axial alignment at 6-month follow-up. **H,** Symmetrical pronation at 6-month follow-up. **I,** Symmetrical supination at 6-month follow-up.

Table 1

Carpal Ossification Sequence

Carpal	Age of Appearance in Boys	Age of Appearance in Girls	Pneumonic Device
Capitate*	3 months	2 months	Cathy's
Hamate	4 months	3 months	Highwire
Triquetrum	2 years	1.5 years	Tricks
Lunate	4 years	2.5 years	Lacked
Scaphoid	5.5 years	4 years	Several
Trapezium+	6 years	4 years	Trapeze
Trapezoid	6 years	4 years	Talent
Pisiform	11 years	9.5 years	Points

*Capitate often present, at birth in both sexes
+Trapezium often appears ahead of scaphoid, especially in girls

tion of all four cortices). A series of published reports have demonstrated the success of minimalistic approaches to buckle fracture care, but precise radiographic diagnosis remains elusive and an incorrect diagnosis (for example, mistaking a greenstick fracture for a buckle fracture) can have consequences such as late displacement and malunion.[31-33] Growth arrest following buckle fractures, as well as other metaphyseal injuries, has been reported.

Fractures of the distal one third of the forearm continue to receive attention in the literature and these fractures have an excellent prognosis similar to that of metaphyseal fractures. Two separate randomized trials of distal third forearm fractures showed well-molded below-elbow cast immobilization to be equivalent or superior to above-elbow casting following fracture reduction.[34,35] After satisfactory closed reduction, the quality of the cast (as measured by indices such as the cast index and the gap index) has been shown to be important in maintaining reduction.[36,37] Management of completely displaced fractures of the distal radius was studied by randomly assigning supplementary percutaneous Kirschner wire fixation to some patients who underwent reduction and above-elbow casting under anesthesia. The additional Kirschner wire was shown to significantly decrease the need for fracture remanipulation ($P < 0.01$).[38] Previous work in this area has also suggested that the fracture pattern represented by a completely displaced distal radius fracture in conjunction with an intact ulna is also best treated with closed reduction and percutaneous pinning. Closed reduction and percutaneous pin fixation is also indicated for displaced distal radius fractures that occur in conjunction with supracondylar humeral fractures (floating elbow).

Physeal (Growth Plate) Fractures of the Distal Radius and Ulna

The Salter-Harris classification remains the standard for describing growth plate fractures of the distal radius and ulna; types I and II are the most common.

Table 2

Scapholunate Interval in Children at Selected Chronologic Ages

Age (years)	Boys' Measurement (range in mm)	Girls' Measurement (range in mm)
6	8.9 (5.8 to 11.9)	6.7 (4.2 to 9.2)
10	5.9 (2.9 to 8.9)	4.4 (2.0 to 6.9)
14	3.0 (0.6 to 6.0)	2.1 (0.5 to 4.7)

Closed reduction and cast treatment is usually successful for these fractures. Even when a previously satisfactory reduction is lost, nonsurgical treatment usually prevails because of the substantial remodeling capacity of the distal radial physis (**Figure 2**). Radiographic normalization is a common occurrence in children younger than 10 years, and asymptomatic mild radiographic abnormality is common in older children. Physeal fractures of the distal ulna are associated with higher rates of growth arrest (50%) than similar fractures of the distal radius (3% to 7%). Displaced intra-articular fractures such as Salter-Harris types III and IV are rare, but require anatomic reduction and stable fixation.

Galeazzi Fracture/Galeazzi Forearm Injury in Children

A lateral radiograph of the wrist should demonstrate the normal colinear relationship of the distal radius and ulna (maintained by the distal radioulnar joint (DRUJ)). Varying loss of this relationship (along with an appropriate clinical scenario) should prompt consideration of the diagnosis of Galeazzi fracture (radial shaft fracture along with DRUJ disruption) or Galeazzi-equivalent injury (for example, radial shaft fracture along with distal ulnar Salter-Harris fracture type I or II). Most of these injuries will respond to

6: Pediatrics

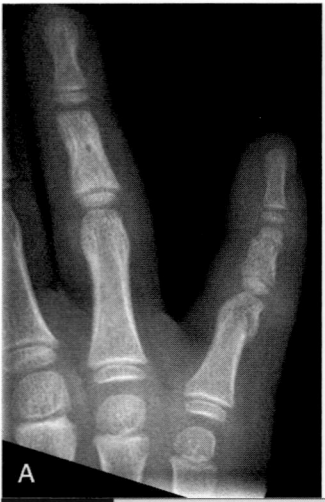
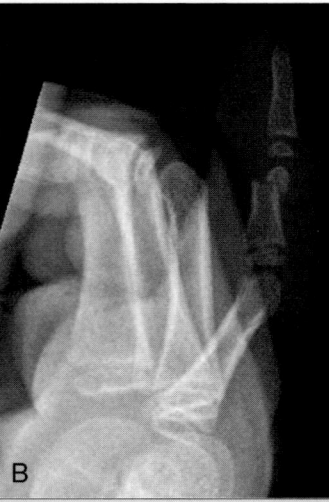
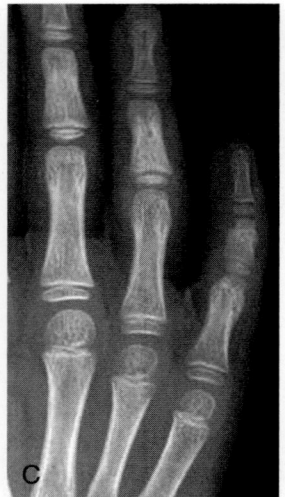
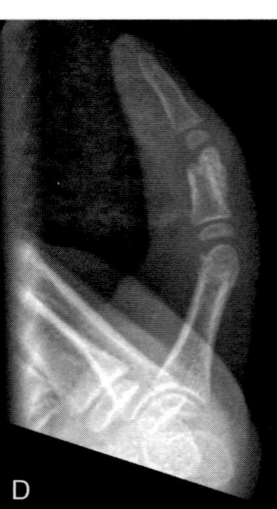

Figure 4	Radiographs of a 7-year-old boy with phalangeal neck fractures of both the proximal and middle phalanges of the same finger (small finger). AP radiograph (**A**) and lateral radiograph (**B**) obtained on the day of injury. AP radiograph (**C**) and lateral radiograph (**D**) obtained at 4-week follow-up.

closed reduction and immobilization in an above-elbow cast (with the forearm in supination for improved stability of the DRUJ). A rare Galeazzi fracture may require both internal fixation of the radius and pinning of the DRUJ to maintain satisfactory alignment. Distal radioulnar joint subluxation has also been reported following intramedullary nail fixation of pediatric forearm fracture. Ulnar styloid fractures are common in children and asymptomatic nonunion may occur in some instances. However, persistent posttraumatic ulnar-sided wrist pain should prompt appropriate evaluation and possible treatment of triangular fibrocartilage complex (TFCC) injury.

Wrist

Carpal ossification, a process that spans about a decade, has a remarkably consistent pattern that progresses from the capitate (often present at birth) toward the hamate, continuing in a rotational fashion and ending with the appearance of the pisiform (**Table 1**). Although uncommon, pediatric scapholunate (SL) ligament injuries do require special knowledge of age-adjusted norms for carpal measurements.[39-41] For instance, a 6-year-old boy may have a SL interval of almost 9 mm (**Table 2**). The most frequently occurring carpal fracture in children is the scaphoid, with only scattered reports of similar injury to the other carpal bones.[42,43] A high index of clinical suspicion and plain radiographs remain the cornerstones of diagnosis. Most acute scaphoid fractures in children are incomplete or nondisplaced and may be successfully treated with above-elbow thumb spica cast immobilization for 6 to 8 weeks.

Pain with palpation in the anatomic snuffbox and normal plain radiographs should prompt cast immobilization and repeat radiographs in several weeks to rule out a radiographically occult scaphoid fracture. Displaced fractures in children older than 10 years should prompt consideration of open reduction and internal fixation. Because of the scaphoid's inherently precarious blood supply as well as frequent delayed presentations, nonunions are common.[44-48] The absence of satisfactory bony healing after 3 months of immobilization has been suggested as a definition for scaphoid nonunion in children. Key components of scaphoid nonunion treatment include autogenous bone grafting and internal fixation. No clear role for MRI is apparent from the existing literature regarding either acute scaphoid fracture or scaphoid nonunion in children.[49]

Hand

Approximately one third of fractures of the metacarpals and phalanges represent true physeal fractures in children. Despite this high rate of physeal involvement, posttraumatic growth disturbance is rare, occurring in only about 1.5% of patients. Metacarpal fractures tend to occur in adolescents and teenagers via axial loading or bending mechanisms such as punching objects or people and from the hand being stepped on. To identify problematic rotational displacement, the alignment (cascade) of the digits of the injured and uninjured hand must be assessed in both extension and relative flexion. Angulation of up to 45° (apex dorsal) is routinely accepted in distal fourth and fifth metacarpal fractures (less for the other metacarpals). Angulation in this same range and up to about 50% displacement may also be accepted in Salter-Harris fracture types I and II of the proximal aspect of the thumb metacarpal. Multiple metacarpal shaft fractures as well as open and pathologic fractures remain indications for surgical stabilization in children.

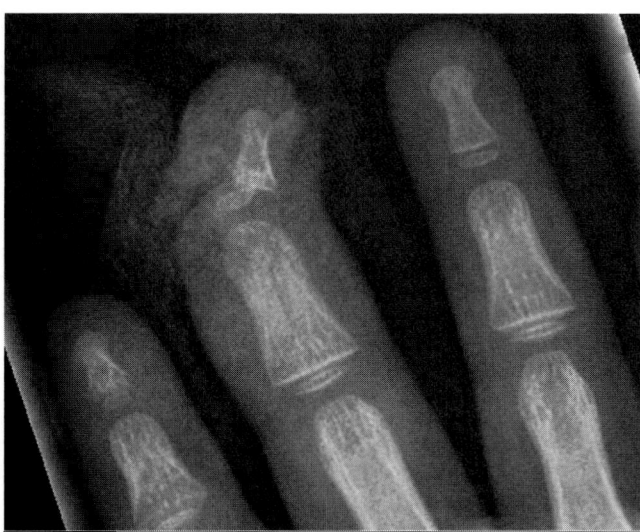

Figure 5 Seymour fracture of the distal phalanx long finger in a 3-year-old girl.

Fractures of the proximal and middle phalanges tend to occur either proximally (metaphyseal buckle fracture or Salter-Harris type I or II) or distally (phalangeal neck). Significantly displaced (apex radial) Salter-Harris type II fractures of the small finger proximal phalanx (juvenile extra octave fracture) usually warrant closed reduction facilitated by a stout pen placed into the webspace as a fulcrum. Growth plate injuries of the other proximal phalanges may be treated in a similar manner. Phalangeal neck fractures present special challenges to the treating orthopaedic surgeon because their radiographic appearance may be startling to both the doctor and the parents, although clinical deformity may be almost completely absent (**Figure 4**). For children age 5 years and younger, there may be little need for surgical intervention; remodeling of fractures with 100% displacement (bayonet apposition) has been documented.[50-52] Fractures with unacceptable clinical deformity, those in older patients, or rare injuries with intra-articular extension warrant reduction and stabilization, preferably using indirect reduction techniques and percutaneous fixation.[53]

Distal phalangeal growth plate fractures often present with subungual hematomas or frank nail bed disruption. This represents a subtle open fracture (Seymour fracture) that requires local wound care and possible antibiotic treatment.[54] Significantly displaced versions of the same injury may mimic a mallet finger and deserve similar wound care, antibiotic treatment, and sometimes reduction and fixation[55] (**Figure 5**). Crush injuries to the distal phalanx (tuft fractures) also occur and are usually closed injuries that do not affect the growth plate. Approximately 3 weeks of protective immobilization is usually adequate. Clinical signs of fracture healing (absence of pain to palpation at the fracture site, absence of motion at the site, and absence of increased temperature at the site) are much more important guides than the radiographs, which may not appear normal for many months.

Pediatric flexor tendon injuries have several remarkable distinctions from those of adults. Delayed presentation is more common in children, at times requiring staged flexor tendon reconstruction.[56] Three to 4 weeks of postoperative immobilization following acute repair is recommended in children as opposed to the early motion protocols used in adults with equivalent clinical outcomes. Temporary paralytic agents (botulinum toxin type A) have also been shown to facilitate the rehabilitation phase of flexor tendon care in very young children.[57]

Annotated References

1. Galano GJ, Vitale MA, Kessler MW, Hyman JG, Vitale MG: The most frequent traumatic orthopaedic injuries from a national pediatric inpatient population. *J Pediatr Orthop* 2005;25:39-44.

   A national pediatric inpatient database was reviewed. Most pediatric orthopaedic trauma was treated at non-children's hospitals.

2. Rajesh A, Basu AK, Vaidhyanath R, Findlay D: Hand fractures: A study of their site and type in childhood. *Clin Radiol* 2001;56:667-669.

3. Khosla S, Melton LJ III, Dekutoski MB, Achenbach SJ, Oberg AL, Riggs BL: Incidence of childhood distal forearm fractures over 30 years: A population-based study. *JAMA* 2003;290:1479-1485.

4. Adams AL, Schiff MA. Childhood soccer injuries treated in U.S. emergency departments. *Acad Emerg Med* 2006;13:571-574.

   The number of children treated in emergency departments for soccer-related injuries was evaluated and the types of injuries were described. Wrist and finger injuries were the most common.

5. Fiissel D, Pattison G, Howard A: Severity of playground fractures: Play equipment versus standing height falls. *Inj Prev* 2005;11:337-339.

   The authors conducted a retrospective study aimed at evaluating the relative severity of playground injuries secondary to falls from playground equipment (719) versus falls from standing height (351). Fractures resulting from falls from playground equipment were nearly four times more likely to require reduction.

6. Davidson P, Goulding A, Chalmers D: Biomechanical analysis of arm fracture in obese boys. *J Paediatr Child Health* 2003;39:657-664.

7. Goulding A, Jones IE, Taylor RW, Williams SM, Manning PJ: Bone mineral density and body composition in boys with distal forearm fractures: A dual-energy x-ray absorptiometry study. *J Pediatr* 2001;139:509-515.

8. Jones IE, Williams SM, Goulding A: Associations of birth weight and length, childhood size, and smoking

6: Pediatrics

with bone fractures during growth: Evidence from a birth cohort study. *Am J Epidemiol* 2004;159:343-350.

A cohort of more than 600 children were tracked from birth to 18 years of age. Tall and heavy children were at increased fracture risk as well as adolescents who smoked.

9. Goulding A, Rockell JE, Black RE, Grant AM, Jones IE, Williams SM: Children who avoid drinking cow's milk are at increased risk for prepubertal bone fractures. *J Am Diet Assoc* 2004;104:250-253.

Fifty children who did not drink milk were studied and were found to be more prone to fractures and low bone mineral density values.

10. Winzenberg T, Shaw K, Fryer J, Jones G: Effects of calcium supplementation on bone density in healthy children: Meta-analysis of randomized controlled trials. *BMJ* 2006;333:775.

11. Winzenberg TM, Shaw K, Fryer J, Jones G: Calcium supplementation for improving bone mineral density in children. *Cochrane Database Syst Rev* 2006;2: CD005119.

In the above two studies, 19 randomized controlled trials involving 2,859 healthy children were analyzed. All children were treated with calcium supplementation for at least 3 months and bone density was measured after at least 6 months follow-up. There was no effect on bone mineral density of the femoral neck or lumbar spine. There was a small effect on total body bone mineral content and upper limb bone mineral density that was considered unlikely to result in a clinically significant decrease in fracture risk. The results did not support the use of calcium supplementation in healthy children.

12. Clark EM, Tobias JH, Ness AR: Association between bone density and fractures in children: A systematic review and meta-analysis. *Pediatrics* 2006;117:e291-e297.

In a case-control study, the authors identified and analyzed healthy children younger than 16 years. Evidence for an association between low bone density and fracture was considered to be limited because of the nature of the study; however, the pooled data analysis revealed a 32% lower bone density ($P < 0.001$) in patients who sustained fractures compared with those without fractures.

13. Wang Q, Alen M, Nicholson P, et al: Growth patterns at distal radius and tibial shaft in pubertal girls: A 2-year longitudinal study. *J Bone Miner Res* 2005;20: 954-961.

The geometry and bone mineral density of 258 pubertal girls was assessed over a 2-year period via quantitative CT. A transient decrease in bone mineral density in the distal radius was noted as a result of asynchronous growth.

14. Cimpello LB, Khine H, Avner JR: Practice patterns of pediatric versus general emergency physicians for pain management of fractures in pediatric patients. *Pediatr Emerg Care* 2004;20:228-232.

The analgesic administration practices of pediatric and general emergency medicine physicians were found to be similar for treating fractures in children; however, general emergency medical physicians prescribed discharge pain medications and prescription analgesics more often.

15. Godambe SA, Elliot V, Matheny D, Pershad J: Comparison of propofol/fentanyl versus ketamine/midazolam for brief orthopedic procedural sedation in a pediatric emergency department. *Pediatrics* 2003;112:116-123.

16. Kriwanek KL, Wan J, Beaty JH, Pershad J: Axillary block for analgesia during manipulation of forearm fractures in the pediatric emergency department: A prospective randomized comparative trial. *J Pediatr Orthop* 2006;26:737-740.

Forty-one children older than 8 years of age were randomized to either axillary block (transarterial technique) or deep sedation via a ketamine/midazolam protocol. There was no significant difference between the groups (6.4 versus 7.5) using the Children's Hospital of Eastern Ontario Pain Scale (CHEOPS). The authors stated that their study had 80% power to detect a two-point change in CHEOPS between the groups. Axillary block was unsuccessful in 10% of children (2 of 20).

17. Luhmann JD, Schootman M, Luhmann SJ, Kennedy RM: A randomized comparison of nitrous oxide plus hematoma block versus ketamine plus midazolam for emergency department forearm fracture reduction in children. *Pediatrics* 2006;118:e1078-e1086.

One hundred two children (mean age, 9 years) undergoing forearm fracture reduction were randomized to two groups. All patients also received oral oxycodone at least 45 minutes before reduction. The procedures were videotaped and assessed via the Procedure Behavioral Checklist. The nitrous oxide/hematoma block group demonstrated fewer adverse sedation effects and significantly shorter recovery time.

18. Slover J, Gibson J, Tosteson T, Smith B, Koval K: Racial and economic disparity and the treatment of pediatric fractures. *J Pediatr Orthop* 2005;25:717-721.

The correlation between racial and economic factors and the treatment of long bone fractures in children was examined.

19. VanderBeek BL, Mehlman CT, Foad SL, Wall EJ, Crawford AH: The use of conscious sedation for pain control during forearm fracture reduction in children: Does race matter? *J Pediatr Orthop* 2006;26:53-57.

Retrospective study of 503 children (83% Caucasian, 17% African-American) with displaced forearm fractures requiring reduction indicated that race was not a predictor ($P = 0.1678$) of conscious sedation use (versus nonconscious sedation methods). Multivariate analysis showed that fracture translation ($P < 0.0001$), fracture angulation ($P < 0.0027$), and younger age ($P < 0.0059$) were predictors of conscious sedation use.

20. Shannon EG, DeFazio R, Kasser J, Karlin L, Gerbino P: Waterproof casts for immobilization of children's fractures and sprains. *J Pediatr Orthop* 2005;25:56-59.

The effectiveness of waterproof cast materials for short-arm, long-arm, and short-leg casts was studied, and these casts were found to allow acceptable immobilization with no additional risk of complications.

21. Zionts LE, Zalavras CG, Gerhardt MB: Closed reduction of displaced diaphyseal both-bone forearm fractures in older children and adolescents. *J Pediatr Orthop* 2005;25:507-512.

    Twenty-five children (8 to 15 years of age, mean 13 years) whose forearm shaft fractures were treated via closed methods were studied. Most fractures (22 of 25) were in the middle or proximal third of the forearm. The patients were followed for an average of more than 4 years. All fractures united and an average of 9° (0°-18°) residual angulation was noted for the radius and an average of 8° (0°-20°) for the ulna. Forearm supination loss averaged 4° (0°-20°) and pronation loss averaged almost 7° (0°-40°). Twelve percent (3 of 25) of the patients lost a total of 35° to 40° of forearm rotation and were classified as having achieved fair results.

22. Bochang C, Jie Y, Zhigang W, Weigl D, Bar-On E, Katz K: Immobilization of forearm fractures in children. *J Bone Joint Surg Br* 2005;87:994-996.

    A prospective cohort study of 111 children from two different medical centers demonstrated that 9 of 51 patients with flexed elbow casts experienced redisplacement (> 15°) in the first 2 weeks after fracture reduction whereas none of the 60 children immobilized with the elbow in extension lost position.

23. Hutchinson DT, Wang AA, Ryssman D, Brown NA: Both-bone forearm osteotomy for supination contracture: A cadaver model. *J Hand Surg Am* 2006;31:968-972.

    Ten fresh-frozen cadaveric forearms were used to ascertain the optimal method for treating a supination contracture (pronation deficit). Approximately 100° of correction was possible when first performing rotational osteotomy of the proximal ulna followed by similar osteotomy of the distal radius. Approximately 60° of correction was achievable with the distal radius osteotomy alone.

24. Yung PSH, Lam CYL, Ng BKW, Lam TP, Cheng JC: Percutaneous transphyseal intramedullary Kirschner wire pinning: A safe and effective procedure for treatment of displaced diaphyseal forearm fractures in children. *J Pediatr Orthop* 2004;24:7-12.

    The authors treated 84 patients (2 to 14 years of age, mean 7.5 years) via transphyseal Kirschner wire fixation (either 1.6 mm or 1.1 mm in diameter) followed by an average of 5 weeks in an above-elbow cast; 71% of patients underwent indirect reduction and internal fixation and 29% required open reduction and internal fixation. Pins were left proud and removed (on average) at the same time as the above-elbow cast. At an average follow-up of 70 months (and a minimum of 2 years) all patients had good functional results and none had nonunion, deep infection, or premature physeal closure.

25. Fernandez FF, Egenolf M, Carsten C, Holz F, Schneider S, Wentzensen A: Unstable diaphyseal fractures of both bones of the forearm in children: Plate fixation versus intramedullary nailing. *Injury* 2005;36:1210-1216.

    In a retrospective study, the results of plate fixation were compared with those of intramedullary fixation in the treatment of diaphyseal fractures. Intramedullary fixation and plate fixation resulted in similar radiologic and functional outcomes. Intramedullary fixation was deemed superior because of its minimally invasive nature.

26. Kapoor V, Theruvil B, Edwards SE, Taylor GR, Clarke NM, Uglow MG: Flexible intramedullary nailing of displaced diaphyseal forearm fractures in children. *Injury* 2005;36:1221-1225.

    In 47 children, flexibile intramedullary nailing of displaced diaphyseal forearm fractures led to early bone union and acceptable bony alignment.

27. Kanellopoulos AD, Yiannakopoulos CK, Soucacos PN: Flexible intramedullary nailing of pediatric unstable forearm fractures. *Am J Orthop* 2005;34:420-424.

    In this retrospective study, 23 patients treated with closed reduction and percutaneous stabilization experienced fracture healing without complications.

28. Smith VA, Goodman HJ, Strongwater A, Smith B: Treatment of pediatric both-bone forearm fractures: A comparison of operative techniques. *J Pediatr Orthop* 2005;25:309-313.

    Fifty-three forearm fractures were studied retrospectively (17 closed treatment, 15 plate fixation, 21 intramedullary nailing). There were a small number of open fractures in all of the treatment groups. Major complications were most common following plate fixation. Both surgical techniques demonstrated significantly more complications when compared to closed treatment methods. The authors state that the subset of both-bone forearm fractures (those in which cast efforts fail) carry a higher risk of complications.

29. Ogonda L, Wong-Chung J, Wray R, Canavan B: Delayed union and non-union of the ulna following intramedullary nailing in children. *J Pediatr Orthop B* 2004;13:330-333.

    Two 7-year-old boys and one 12-year-old girl (one boy had osteogenesis imperfecta and all of the children had closed forearm fractures) were studied. The authors used 2.0 to 2.5 mm flexible titanium nails and a smooth Steinmann pin to fix central third ulnar shaft fractures via olecranon starting points. The narrowest portion of the ulnar medullary canal is distal (not midshaft) and a narrow diameter intramedullary device (perhaps one without a curved tip) is considered best for ulnar fixation.

30. Price CT, Knapp DR: Osteotomy for malunited forearm shaft fractures in children. *J Pediatr Orthop* 2006;26:193-196.

    Treatment (and outcome) of nine children with a malunited forearm shaft fracture is described. The key aspect of the corrective osteotomy is to fluoroscopically determine the plane of maximum deformity in each bone and then perform a closing wedge osteotomy at the apex of the deformity.

6: Pediatrics

31. Plint AC, Perry JJ, Correll R, Gaboury I, Lawton L: A randomized controlled trial of removable splinting versus casting for wrist buckle fractures in children. *Pediatrics* 2006;117:691-697.

    Univariate analysis of 87 children (6 to 15 years of age) randomly assigned to either a below-elbow cast group or a removable splint group revealed no significant group differences in the primary outcome variable (14-day scores on Activities Scales for Kids) regarding pain ($P = 0.41$), but significantly better function in the splint group ($P < 0.001$). Radiographic outcomes were not tracked in this study. Fifteen patients with greenstick fractures were misdiagnosed by emergency department personnel as having buckle fractures, allowing the misclassification rate to be estimated at 17%. Eighty-six percent of patients were contacted via phone at 6-month follow-up; no refractures were reported.

32. van Bosse HJ, Patel RJ, Thacker M, Sala DA: Minimalistic approach to treating wrist torus fractures. *J Pediatr Orthop* 2005;25:495-500.

    In the 33 patients treated in this retrospective review, all fractures were healed with no notable clinical changes in angulation, and there were no complications.

33. Symons S, Rowsell M, Bhowal B, Dias JJ: Hospital versus home management of children with buckle fractures of the distal radius: A prospective randomised trial. *J Bone Joint Surg Br* 2001;83:556-560.

34. Bohm ER, Bubbar V, Yong Hing K, Dzus A: Above and below-the-elbow plaster casts for distal forearm fractures in children: A randomized controlled trial. *J Bone Joint Surg Am* 2006;88:1-8.

    One hundred two children (4 to 12 years of age) with displaced distal third forearm fractures were randomly allocated to above- and below-elbow plaster cast groups and analyzed via univariate and multivariate statistical techniques. Two patients were excluded because of inadequate radiographs. Open fractures and Salter-Harris fracture types III and IV were excluded. The authors did not control for forearm position (neutral, pronation, supination) in the above-elbow group. Rates of radiographic reduction loss were low and not significantly different between the two groups ($P = 0.27$). Similarly, the rates of fracture remanipulation did not significantly ($P = 0.38$) differ between above- and below-elbow groups (3 of 55, and 1 of 45 patients, respectively).

35. Webb GR, Galpin RD, Armstrong DG: Comparison of short and long arm plaster casts for displaced fractures in the distal third of the forearm in children. *J Bone Joint Surg Am* 2006;88:9-17.

    This study analyzed 113 children (4 to 16 years of age) with displaced distal third forearm fractures who had been randomized to either above- or below-elbow plaster cast immobilization. Study criteria were such that all displaced distal radius fractures (physeal, greenstick, complete) were included. The authors did not account for the rate of ulna fracture in the two groups or forearm position (neutral, pronation, supination) in the above-elbow group. Univariate statistical analysis demonstrated a significantly ($P = 0.045$) higher rate of loss of reduction (angulate 10° or translate 20%) in the above-elbow group (9 of 60) versus the below-elbow group (2 of 53).

36. Bhatia M, Housden PH: Re-displacement of paediatric forearm fractures: Role of plaster moulding and padding. *Injury* 2006;37:259-268.

    A retrospective cohort study of 142 children undergoing reduction of displaced forearm or wrist fractures is presented. Plaster molding and padding were assessed via the cast index, the padding index, and the sum of the two indices (Canterbury index). All indices were significantly ($P < 0.005$) greater in the portion of the cohort that suffered redisplacement. The authors suggest cast index of more than 0.8, padding index of more than 0.3, and Canterbury index of more than 1.1 as important risk factors for fracture re-displacement.

37. Malviya A, Tsintzas D, Mahawar K, Bache CE, Glithero PR: Gap index: A good predictor of failure of plaster cast in distal third radius fractures. *J Pediatr Orthop B* 2007;16:48-52.

    A case-control study (retrospective by definition) that contrasted 25 patients (all known to have required remanipulation) with 75 patients who had not required any repeat fracture manipulation. All were treated with above-elbow casts. The status of the cast index (lateral divided by anteroposterior cast diameter at the level of the radial fracture) and the gap index (similar measure that controls for the space between the cast and the skin) was analyzed for the two groups. A cast index of more than 0.8 was associated with a 6.8 times higher risk of loss of reduction whereas a gap index of more than 0.15 led to a 35 times higher risk. Interobserver and intraobserver reliability was shown to be acceptable for these measures (0.61 – 0.81 via Pearson correlation coefficient). Further validation in a prospective setting is needed.

38. McLauchlan GJ, Cowan B, Annan IH, Robb JE: Management of completely displaced metaphyseal fractures of the distal radius in children: A prospective randomized controlled trial. *J Bone Joint Surg Br* 2002;84:413-417.

39. Earp BE, Waters PM, Wyzykowski RJ: Arthroscopic treatment of partial scapholunate ligament tears in children with chronic wrist pain. *J Bone Joint Surg Am* 2006;88:2448-2455.

    Thirty-two children with an average age of 13.1 years (range, 6.7 to 17.3 years) injured their wrists, had pain for an average of 14.1 months; arthroscopy later showed partial SL ligament tears. Associated injuries (including short radiolunate ligament, lunotriquetral ligament, TFCC, and chondral injuries) were common; only one patient had an isolated SL partial tear. Preoperative MRI (28 of 32 patients) demonstrated 70% sensitivity and 0% specificity regarding SL and TFCC injuries. All patients had arthroscopic débridement of their SL tears and 14 of 32 had additional procedures (such as TFCC repair or ulnar shortening). Within the context of a minimum 2-year follow-up, 25% of patients (8 of 32) later required additional surgery because of persistent pain.

6: Pediatrics

40. Alt V, Gasnier J, Sicre G: Injuries of the scapholunate ligament in children. *J Pediatr Orthop B* 2004;13: 326-329.

Wrist arthroscopy in three children (9, 11, and 12 years old) with persistent dorsal wrist pain confirmed SL ligament injury and was immediately followed by open surgical repair of all lesions. At an average of 2.4 years follow-up, all patients were pain free and had full function.

41. Kaawach W, Eckland K, DiCanzio J, Zurakowski D, Waters PM: Normal ranges of scapholunate distance in children 6 to 14 years old. *J Pediatr Orthop* 2001;21: 464-467.

42. Kuniyoshi K, Toh S, Nishikawawa S, Kudo S, Ogawa T, Pegoli L: Long-term follow-up of a malunited isolated fracture of the capitate in a 6-year-old boy. *J Pediatr Orthop B* 2005;14:46-50.

Long-term follow-up studies of a 6-year-old boy with an isolated fracture of the capitate treated with immobilization indicate that there were no radiographic changes and that the capitate had regained an almost normal shape.

43. Mancini F, DeMaio F, Ippolito E: Pisiform bone fracture-dislocation and distal radius physeal fracture in two children. *J Pediatr Orthop B* 2005;14:303-306.

This artocle presents two case reports that are remarkable for their nonsurgical long-term follow-up of very unusual pediatric wrist trauma. Significant deformity (palmar prominence) and 5 mm of displacement in a 6-year-old boy with a capitate fracture remodeled completely by the time the child was 10.5 years old. At 11-year follow-up, the same child continued to have normal radiographs and normal function. Two boys (ages 12 and 13 years) were noted to have pisiform fracture-dislocations in addition to their minimally displaced Salter-Harris I or II fractures. Closed reduction and cast immobilization was used for all injuries and at 30- and 31-year follow-up, respectively, there was no clinical or radiographic evidence of abnormalities in either patient.

44. Duteille F, Dautel G: Nonunion fractures of the scaphoid and carpal bones in children: Surgical management. *J Pediatr Orthop B* 2004;13:34-38.

Surgical treatment of carpal bone fractures was studied. After minimum 1-year follow-up, 11 of 12 patients with fractures regained strength and mobility and experienced a near-total absence of pain.

45. Fabre O, DeBoeck H, Haentjens P: Fractures and nonunions of the carpal scaphoid in children. *Acta Orthop Belg* 2001;67:121-125.

46. Garcia-Mata S: Carpal scaphoid fracture nonunion in children. *J Pediatr Orthop* 2002;22:448-451.

47. Henderson B, Letts M: Operative management of pediatric scaphoid fracture nonunion. *J Pediatr Orthop* 2003;23:402-406.

48. Toh S, Miura H, Arai K, Yasumura M, Wada M, Tsubo K: Scaphoid fractures in children: Problems and treatment. *J Pediatr Orthop* 2003;23:216-221.

This article details the treatment of 83 scaphoid nonunions in children. Ninety-five percent of patients (79 of 83) were treated successfully with a variety of surgical techniques (some involving internal fixation) whereas 5% (4 of 83 patients) were successfully treated via cast immobilization alone. Several authors emphasize that late presentation is common in these pediatric scaphoid injuries.

49. Cook PA, Yu JS, Wiand W, Cook AJ II, Coleman CR, Cook AJ: Suspected scaphoid fracture in skeletally immature patients: Application of MRI. *J Comput Assist Tomogr* 1997;21:511-515.

50. Al-Qattan MM, Rasool MN, El Shayeb A: Remodeling in a malunited phalangeal neck fracture. *Injury* 2004; 35:1207-1210.

Remodeling of a phalangeal neck fracture is discussed in this study.

51. Cornwall R, Waters PM: Remodeling of phalangeal neck fracture malunions in children: Case report. *J Hand Surg Am* 2004;29:458-461.

The 5-year-old boy in this study with a malunion of a proximal phalanx neck fracture experienced near-complete remodeling.

52. Hennrikus WL, Cohen MR: Complete remodeling of displaced fractures of the neck of the phalanx. *J Bone Joint Surg Br* 2003;85:273-274.

53. Waters PM, Taylor BA, Kuo AY: Percutaneous reduction of incipient malunion of phalangeal neck fractures in children. *J Hand Surg Am* 2004;29:707-711.

Retrospective study of eight children (1 to 16 years old; mean age, 6 years) treated via an intrafocal (through the fracture site) Kirschner wire-pinning technique where the wire is used as a lever to reduce the fracture. All patients had a preoperative block to flexion secondary to fracture malalignment that obliterated the subcondylar fossa. Postoperatively all eight patients had complete fracture healing as well as normal motion and function. The authors offer the procedure as a minimally invasive method aimed at preventing flexion loss caused by malunion of the phalangeal subcondylar fossa.

54. Al-Qattan MM: Extra-articular transverse fractures of the base of the distal phalanx (Seymour's fracture) in children and adults. *J Hand Surg Br* 2001;26:201-206.

Eighteen children and adolescents with this periphyseal open fracture of distal phalanges of the hand were evaluated. The middle finger was most commonly involved. Clinically they presented with mallet deformity and nail bed lacerations. Cornerstones of treatment were local wound care and antibiotics along with reduction and splinting (internal fixation is rarely required). The author reiterated Seymour's own recommendation to maintain the patient's nail (reinserting it under the proximal nail fold) because it adds stability.

6: Pediatrics

55. Ganayem M, Edelson G: Base of distal phalanx fracture in children: A mallet finger mimic. *J Pediatr Orthop* 2005;25:487-489.

    The authors evaluated six children (4 to 10 years of age) with Seymour fractures (physeal or periphyseal open fracture) of the distal phalanx. The middle finger was most commonly involved. Local wound care (under regional anesthesia), intravenous antibiotics, nail preservation, and Kirschner wire fixation were recommended by these authors.

56. Darlis NA, Beris AE, Korompilias AV, Vekris MD, Mitsionis GI, Soucacos PN: Two-stage flexor tendon reconstruction in zone 2 of the hand in children. *J Pediatr Orthop* 2005;25:382-386.

    Severe zone 2 flexor tendon injuries in nine children were treated via a modified Hunter reconstruction using silicone rods in the first stage and an intrasynovial flexor digitorum sublimis grafting technique in the second stage. Ages ranged from 2 to 15 years with an average of 6.9 years. At an average of over 40 months follow-up, eight of nine patients had good or excellent results according to Buck-Gramcko and revised Strickland scales.

57. Tuzuner S, Balci N, Ozkaynak S: Results of zone II flexor tendon repairs in children younger than 6 years: Botulinum toxin type A administration eased cooperation during the rehabilitation and improved outcome. *J Pediatr Orthop* 2004;24:629-633.

    Seven children between 1 and 5 years of age had zone 2 flexor tendon rehabilitation augmented by intraoperative botulinum toxin type A injection aimed at the specific muscles associated with the tendon repairs. Rehabilitation was initiated on the second postoperative day with a Duran's passive motion program. Sufficient muscle relaxation was noted 48 to 72 hours after injection and continued for approximately 6 weeks. With a mean follow-up of 18 months, two patients had good and five had excellent results using the Strickland criteria.

Chapter 56

Upper Extremity Disorders: Pediatrics

Donald S. Bae, MD

Introduction

Congenital anomalies of the upper extremity can arise from genetic or developmental factors. The incidence is approximately 2 infants per 1,000 live births. The American Society for Surgery of the Hand and the International Federation of Societies for Surgery of the Hand have adopted universal categories of congenital anomalies of the upper extremity,[1] as shown in **Table 1.**

The upper limb bud appears during the fourth week of gestation and develops from the fifth to the eighth week of gestation. Several signaling centers are critical: the apical ectodermal ridge guides proximal to distal development and mediates interdigital necrosis, the zone of polarizing activity guides radioulnar development, and the Wnt signaling center guides dorsoventral development. In utero joint motion is required for development of the joints.

Brachial Plexus Birth Palsy

Despite advances in prenatal and obstetric care, the incidence of brachial plexus birth palsy remains 1 to 4 infants per 1,000 live births. Most affected infants recover spontaneously, but neurologic deficits persist in some infants and require surgical intervention. Controversy continues as to the timing of microsurgical reconstruction of the brachial plexus. Most authorities agree that microsurgery is indicated at 3 months for patients with total plexopathy associated with Horner's syndrome and between 3 months and 9 months for patients with upper trunk lesions and an absence of antigravity biceps function. Depending on the pattern of injury, surgical treatment typically involves brachial plexus exploration with neurolysis, nerve repair, neuroma excision and nerve grafting, or nerve transfers.[2,3]

A patient with upper trunk lesions (called Erb's palsy) and incomplete neurologic recovery may have limitations involving active shoulder abduction and external rotation, often accompanied by internal rotation contractures of the shoulder. Anterior release of the pectoralis major, subscapularis, or anterior capsule, combined with tendon transfers of the latissimus dorsi and teres major to the rotator cuff, can provide significant improvement in global shoulder function.[4] Persis-

tent muscular imbalance across the developing shoulder leads to progressive glenohumeral dysplasia, which is characterized by increased glenoid retroversion, humeral head flattening, and posterior humeral head subluxation[5,6] (**Figure 1**). Because glenohumeral deformity can begin in young patients, serial radiographic evaluation with ultrasound, arthrography, MRI, or CT is warranted. Extra-articular soft-tissue rebalancing with anterior releases and tendon transfers can halt, but not reverse, progressive glenohumeral dysplasia. However, glenohumeral remodeling is possible through tendon transfer with arthroscopic capsular release or open capsulorrhaphy.[7,8]

Although they are effective in younger patients, latissimus dorsi and teres major tendon transfers are not a viable option for older patients with severe glenohumeral joint deformity. For these patients, external rotation osteotomy of the humerus can provide improvement in global shoulder function.[9]

Efforts are underway to assess the natural history and functional outcomes of surgical treatment of patients with brachial plexus birth palsy. Several stan-

Table 1

American Society for Surgery of the Hand and International Federation of Societies for Surgery of the Hand Classification of Congenital Anomalies of the Upper Extremity

Category	Example
Failure of formation	Congenital below-elbow amputation Radial dysplasia
Failure of differentiation	Syndactyly
Duplication	Preaxial polydactyly Postaxial polydactyly
Overgrowth	Macrodactyly
Undergrowth	Poland's syndrome
Congenital constriction band	Constriction band syndrome
Generalized skeletal abnormalities	Arthrogryposis

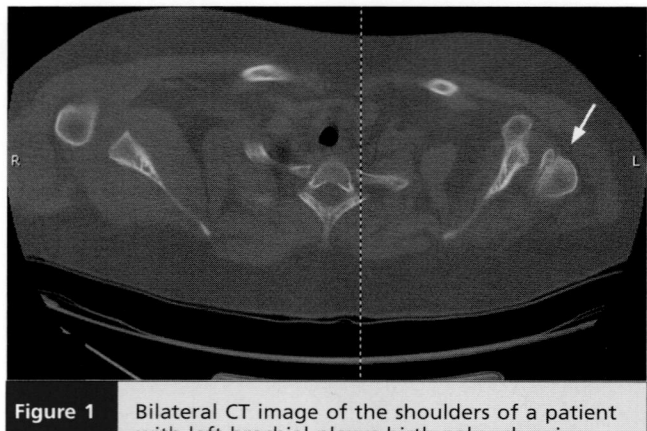

Figure 1   Bilateral CT image of the shoulders of a patient with left brachial plexus birth palsy, showing severe glenohumeral deformity (humeral head flattening, posterior glenoid dysplasia, and posterior instability of the glenohumeral joint). (Copyright Children's Orthopaedic Surgery Foundation, 2006.)

dardized outcomes instruments, including the Pediatric Evaluation of Disability Inventory and the Pediatric Outcomes Data Collection Instrument, are effective in measuring the effect of brachial plexus birth palsy and surgical treatment interventions.[10,11]

Sprengel's Deformity

Sprengel's deformity results from failure of scapular descent during embryologic development. The condition is clinically characterized by a hypoplastic, high-riding scapula with varying degrees of diminished scapulothoracic motion. The right and left scapulae are affected with equal frequency, and the condition is bilateral in 10% to 30% of patients. As many as 50% of patients have an abnormal fibrous, cartilaginous, or bony connection, called the omovertebral bar, between the superior scapular angle and the cervical spine. Sprengel's deformity is often seen in association with Klippel-Feil syndrome, scoliosis, torticollis, facial asymmetry, or pulmonary or renal disorders.

The Cavendish classification is used to describe the degree of deformity and guide treatment.[12] No treatment is recommended for a patient with a grade 1 deformity, in which the glenohumeral joints are level and no deformity is visible when the patient is dressed. In a grade 2 deformity, the glenohumeral joints are level but a prominence in the neck is visible when the patient is dressed. An aesthetically unpleasing scapular prominence can be resected with the omovertebral bar, if it is present. Grade 3 deformity represents moderate deformity, with a shoulder elevation of 2 cm to 5 cm compared with the contralateral side. Grade 4 denotes severe deformity in which the scapula lies at the level of the occiput.

For a grade 3 or grade 4 deformity associated with functional impairment, surgical treatment consists of excision of the superior margin of the scapula and the anomalous omovertebral connection, with derotation and caudal repositioning of the scapula. Several procedures have been proposed. The Woodward procedure involves detachment and relocation of the parascapular musculature. The Green procedure repositions the scapula by extraperiosteal detachment of the scapular musculature, caudal repositioning of the scapular with the use of wires or cables, and subsequent parascapular muscular reattachment. Vertical osteotomy of the scapula also has been proposed.[13,14] For older children, concomitant clavicular osteotomy or morcellation is advised during surgical correction to prevent iatrogenic neurovascular injury.

Glenoid Hypoplasia

The normal concave glenoid develops from consolidation of the secondary centers of ossification of the superior glenoid, inferior glenoid, and coracoid. Glenoid hypoplasia results from failure of the inferior glenoid to ossify. This rare condition can occur in isolation or in association with another condition such as a skeletal dysplasia, mucopolysaccharidosis, or Holt-Oram, Apert's, or Cornelia de Lange's syndromes. Glenoid hypoplasia is typically bilateral and symmetric. It can result in limited shoulder abduction and forward flexion, mild axillary webbing, and multidirectional instability. Radiography, MRI, or CT can confirm the diagnosis. Most patients have minimal functional limitations. Symptomatic patients can be treated with physical therapy; range-of-motion and strengthening exercises focus on the deltoid, rotator cuff, and parascapular muscles.

Congenital Pseudarthrosis of the Clavicle

Congenital pseudarthrosis of the clavicle results from failure of medial and lateral primary centers of ossification to unite during development.[15] The theory that vascular pulsations of the adjacent subclavian artery cause the failure of coalescence may explain the clinical observation that congenital pseudarthrosis of the clavicle occurs on the right side in more than 90% of patients (the right subclavian artery is more cephalad as it courses over the first rib). The vascular pulsation theory is also supported by the left-side involvement seen in patients with dextrocardia.

The diagnosis is usually made shortly after birth. Affected infants have a painless, subcutaneous prominence over the middle third of the clavicle. Radiography confirms the diagnosis. The absence of pain and lack of periosteal reaction or bony healing distinguish congenital pseudarthrosis of the clavicle from birth-related fracture. The absence of associated musculoskeletal abnormalities distinguishes congenital pseudarthrosis of the clavicle from neurofibromatosis, cleidocranial dysphasia, or another skeletal dysplasia.

Although spontaneous bony union does not occur, most children have normal shoulder motion with little to no pain or functional limitation. In rare instances,

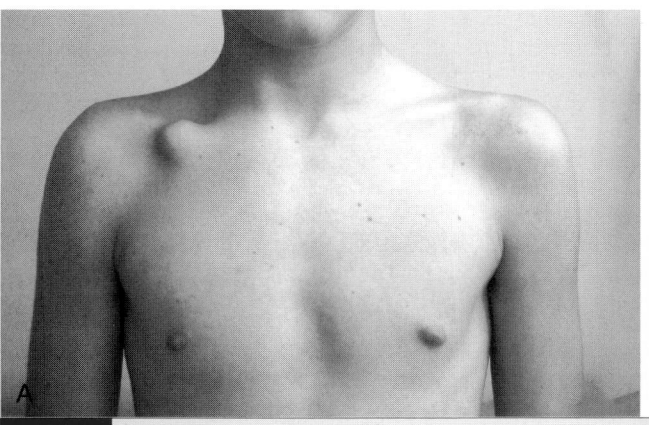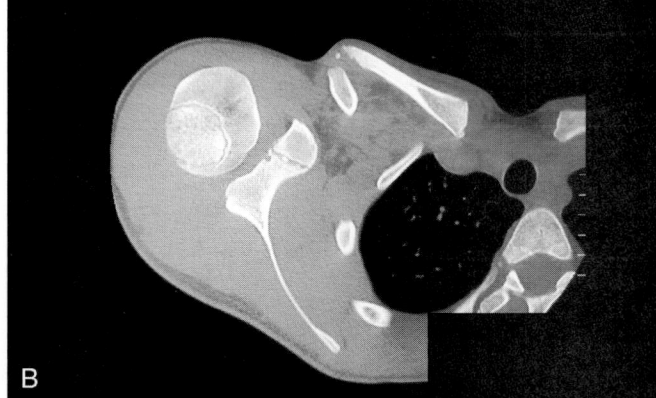

Figure 2 Congenital pseudarthrosis of the clavicle in a 14-year-old patient. **A,** Clinical photograph. **B,** Axial CT scan. (Copyright Children's Orthopaedic Surgery Foundation, 2006.)

discomfort at the site of the pseudarthrosis, shoulder asymmetry, decreased motion, and thoracic outlet syndrome develop as the patient grows older (**Figure 2**). For these reasons, the indications for surgery are not clear-cut. The choice of surgical treatment is predicated on the age of the child. For an infant or young child, resection of the fibrous tissue and sclerotic bone with periosteal preservation and suture reapproximation of the clavicular segments may suffice. For an older child, bone grafting and rigid internal fixation are required to achieve union after pseudarthrosis resection.

Congenital Radial Head Dislocation

Congenital radial head dislocation is often unrecognized until late childhood or adolescence, because most patients do not have symptoms or functional limitations. Patients may have a bony prominence on the lateral aspect of the elbow, with mild limitations in elbow flexion-extension or forearm rotation. The condition is often bilateral and may be associated with arthrogryposis or with Cornelia de Lange's, Klippel-Feil, Klinefelter's, nail-patella, or Silver's syndromes. Radiography can confirm the diagnosis. Typically, patients have flattening or hypoplasia of the capitellum, a convex or dome-shaped radial head, and mild bowing of the proximal ulna; these characteristics distinguish congenital radial head dislocation from an acquired posttraumatic condition. For a symptomatic patient at or near skeletal maturity, radial head excision is recommended. Bony regrowth of the proximal radius, wrist pain, and proximal migration of the radius have all been reported following radial head excision, although the long-term consequences have yet to be determined.[16,17]

Radioulnar Synostosis

Failure of differentiation between the radius and ulna can lead to congenital radioulnar synostosis. In most

instances, radioulnar synostosis is bilateral and affects males and females with equal frequency. Usually it occurs in isolation, although in one third of patients it appears to be associated with Apert's, Carpenter's, or Klinefelter's syndromes, arthrogryposis, or radial head dislocation. The radial head may be dislocated or absent, and the forearm is typically fixed in pronation. Elbow flexion-extension and wrist motion are generally not affected. For patients with severe fixed pronation and functional limitations, an osteotomy through the bony synostosis or distal radius can be performed to rotate the forearm into a more functional position (typically 10° to 20° of pronation).[18,19] Synostosis excision with free vascularized fascio-fat graft interposition has also been reported to separate the radius and ulna, restore motion, and prevent reformation of the synostosis.[20]

Radial Longitudinal Deficiency

Radial longitudinal deficiency is also called radial clubhand or radial dysplasia. The term refers to failure of formation of the radial side of the forearm, wrist, and hand. The condition is estimated to occur in 1 infant per 25,000 live births. It is associated with several congenital conditions, including thrombocytopenia-absent radius, Fanconi's anemia, Holt-Oram syndrome, and the vertebral-anal-cardiac-tracheal-esophageal-renal-radial-limb (VACTERRL) association.[21] Timely diagnosis of associated conditions is critical, because their presence may affect the timing of orthopaedic and medical interventions. Fanconi's anemia, which is an autosomal recessive disorder characterized by bone marrow failure and progressive pancytopenia, may be diagnosed with the mitomycin-C chromosomal challenge test; for these patients, bone marrow transplantation can be a life-saving and curative procedure.

The clinical features of radial longitudinal deficiency typically include elbow flexion contracture, shortened or bowed forearms, radial deviation of the wrist, and

6: Pediatrics

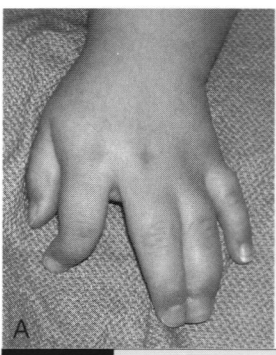
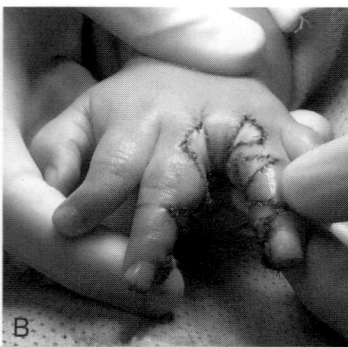

Figure 3   **A,** Simple complete syndactyly of the third web space. **B,** Intraoperative photograph after syndactyly release with full-thickness skin grafting. (Copyright Children's Orthopaedic Surgery Foundation, 2006.)

aplasia or hypoplasia of the thumb. Parallel deficiencies appear in radial soft-tissue structures (radial artery, median or radial nerves, flexor carpi radialis). The Bayne classification is used to characterize the deformity and guide treatment.[22] Bayne type I is characterized by the delayed appearance of distal epiphysis and a shortened radius. In type II, growth of the proximal and distal radius is deficient and the radius is very small.

Stretching exercises and serial casting or splinting are initiated shortly after birth. In patients with severe, stiff radial deviation of the wrist, progressive distraction using external fixation can be performed.[23] Patients with Bayne type III have a partial absence of the radius, typically of the distal portion. In type IV, the radius is completely absent. For patients with type III or type IV, centralization or radialization of the carpus is performed between 6 months and 12 months of age and is followed by index finger pollicization, if the patient has thumb aplasia. Radial lengthening procedures have also been proposed to rebalance the wrist.[24] Surgery is not recommended for severe elbow flexion contractures or for older patients who have adjusted to their deficiency. Long-term assessments of the outcomes of the centralization procedure have revealed a likelihood of recurrent deformity and limited hand function.[25]

Madelung's Deformity

Madelung's deformity is a characteristic abnormality of distal radial growth caused by disturbance of the volar and ulnar distal radial physis. It affects females more often than males and is often seen in association with a thick volar ligament (called Vicker's ligament) that tethers the lunate to the distal radius. This condition results in increased radial inclination, volar subluxation of the carpus, and apparent dorsal subluxation of the distal ulna.[26] Significant pain, weakness, or deformity often does not appear until early adolescence. A condition similar to Madelung's deformity can occur in conjunction with osteochondromatosis, or with a skeletal dys-

plasia such as Leri-Weill syndrome, or as a sequela of distal radial physeal arrest or infection.

Surgical treatment can be considered for patients with functionally limiting pain, weakness, or deformity. Physiolysis with release of Vicker's ligament has been proposed for treating younger patients who have skeletal growth remaining. In older, skeletally mature patients, combinations of completion epiphyseodesis, lateral closing wedge osteotomy, dome radial osteotomy, and ulnar shortening osteotomy may be performed.[27]

Central Deficiency

Central deficiency, also called cleft hand, is rare; the estimated incidence is 1 infant per 90,000 to 150,000 live births. Although most instances of central deficiency are unilateral and sporadic, it is sometimes inherited in an autosomal dominant pattern. Associated anomalies include cleft palate, cleft foot, syndactyly, polydactyly, deafness, heart defects, and anal atresia. Surgical treatment, when indicated, typically involves closure of the central deficiency and reconstitution of a functional first web space.[28]

Syndactyly

Syndactyly results from failure of interdigital necrosis of the developing hand paddle. It is among the most common congenital hand disorders, occurring in 1 infant per 2,000 to 2,500 live births. In approximately 40% of patients, the condition is inherited in an autosomal dominant pattern with variable penetrance. Associated conditions include Poland's syndrome (absent sternocostal head of the pectoralis major, upper limb hypoplasia, and symbrachydactyly), Apert's syndrome (acrocephalosyndactyly), and Carpenter's syndrome (acrocephalopolysyndactyly).

Syndactyly is classified by the extent of interdigital webbing (incomplete or complete) and the character of the conjoined tissue (simple, complex, or complicated). The third web space is most commonly affected, followed in order of frequency by the fourth, second, and first web spaces.

Because of the importance of independent digital motion, surgical release is recommended. When the syndactyly affects digits of different sizes (the first and fourth web spaces), the surgery is usually performed early to avoid deformity and growth disturbance. Only one side of the digit is operated on during a single procedure to avoid vascular embarrassment. Dorsal skin is used as a local advancement flap to reconstitute the interdigital commissure and avoid scar contracture or web creep in the reconstructed web space. The depth of the reconstructed web space may be limited by the location of the digital artery bifurcation. Because of the geometry of a complete syndactyly, full-thickness skin grafting is typically required to cover bare areas after separation (**Figure 3**). Graftless techniques of syndactyly release have also been proposed, using extended dorsal metacarpal island flaps as V-Y advancement flaps to reconstitute the web commissure and facilitate direct skin closure over the separated digits.[29]

Polydactyly

Preaxial polydactyly, also known as thumb polydactyly or thumb duplication, has been reported to occur in 1 infant per 1,000 to 10,000 live births. It affects males more often than females and Asian and white children more often than black children. Occurrence is usually sporadic, and associated congenital anomalies are rare. The Wassel classification is used to categorize preaxial polydactyly by level of duplication. Wassel type IV (duplicated proximal phalanges) (**Figure 4**) and type II (duplicated distal phalanges) are the most common.[30] Radial and ulnar thumbs both contain structures that must be preserved and reconstructed to provide a single, stable, mobile, and functional thumb. For this reason, simple excision of one of the thumbs is absolutely contraindicated. The radial thumb is usually more hypoplastic. Surgery consists of ablation of the radial thumb with reconstruction of the radial collateral ligament or advancement of the thenar insertions to the retained ulnar thumb or both. Chondroplasties or corrective osteotomies of the metacarpals or phalanges may be needed to reconstitute the longitudinal axis of the thumb. A late deformity develops in approximately 15% to 20% of patients. The causes include failure to recognize a pollex abductus, inadequate correction of the longitudinal thumb alignment, inadequate reconstruction of the collateral ligament, and failure to centralize the extensor or flexor tendons.[31]

Postaxial polydactyly refers to duplication of the ulnarmost digit. Inheritance is autosomal dominant, and the condition affects black children more often than white children. In black children, postaxial polydactyly is usually an isolated condition; as many as 30% of affected white children have associated organ system disorders. The duplicated digit can be fully developed (type A) or rudimentary and pedunculated (type B).[32] Type B can be treated with suture ligation in the newborn nursery, although infection, bleeding, and incomplete removal are commonly reported complications. Type A postaxial polydactyly may require collateral ligament and hypothenar muscle reconstruction similar to the procedures for preaxial polydactyly.

Camptodactyly

Camptodactyly refers to flexion contracture and deformity of a finger, typically the proximal interphalangeal joint of the small finger. Although the true incidence is unknown, it is estimated that up to 1% of the population may be affected. Camptodactyly is usually sporadic, but some patients have an autosomal dominance inheritance with variable penetrance. Abnormalities in

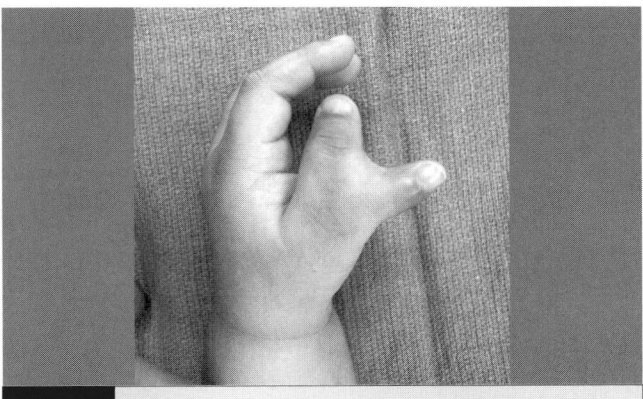

Figure 4 Wassel type IV preaxial polydactyly. (Copyright Children's Orthopaedic Surgery Foundation, 2006.)

lumbrical or flexor digitorum superficialis anatomy are most commonly cited as potential etiologies, but skin contracture, absent extensor tendon function, volar plate anomalies, and articular incongruity have also been considered.[33]

The classification is partly based on the age at presentation. Type I occurs in infancy, and type II occurs during adolescence. Type III occurs in the setting of an underlying syndrome. Splinting and stretching exercises are recommended for initial treatment. Camptodactyly rarely results in profound functional impairment, and surgical treatment should be considered only for severe contractures (> 45°) with functional loss. Multiple procedures have been proposed, but incomplete correction and recurrent deformity are common.

Clinodactyly

Clinodactyly is an angular deformity of a digit in the radioulnar plane. It is typically bilateral, and the small finger is most commonly affected. Inheritance is believed to be autosomal dominant; the many associated syndromes include trisomy 21, Rubenstein-Taybi syndrome, and Cornelia de Lange's syndrome. Clinodactyly is classified as simple (bony deformity alone) or complex (soft-tissue involvement) and as uncomplicated (< 45° angulation) or complicated (> 45° angulation, with rotation). Splinting and stretching exercises can be implemented, although they are not always successful. Clinodactyly is usually an aesthetic rather than a functional problem. Surgery is indicated only for severe deformity with functional compromise.

If the proximal physis of the phalanx is not perpendicular to the long axis of the bone, the result is a triangular- or trapezoidal-shaped bone with clinodactyly, called the delta phalanx. More precisely referred to as a longitudinal epiphyseal bracket (**Figure 5**), progressive angular deformity develops with skeletal growth; the shortened side of the phalanx contains the epiphyseal bracket.[34] Depending on the amount of growth remaining, the surgical options to correct sig-

6: Pediatrics

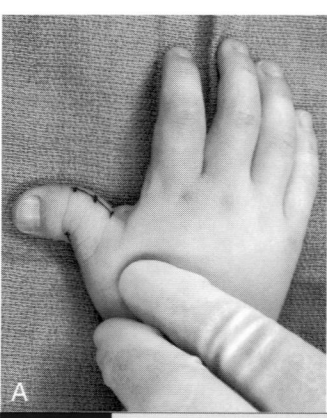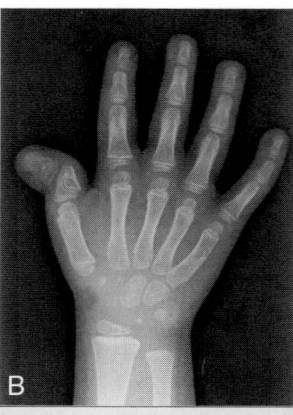

Figure 5 Clinodactyly of the thumb caused by a longitudinal epiphyseal bracket of the proximal phalanx. **A,** Clinical photograph. **B,** Radiograph. (Copyright Children's Orthopaedic Surgery Foundation, 2006.)

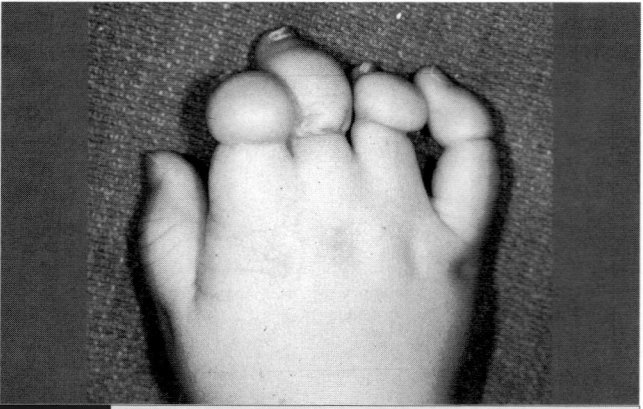

Figure 6 Constriction ring syndrome of the digits. (Copyright Children's Orthopaedic Surgery Foundation, 2006.)

nificant deformity and functional limitation include corrective osteotomy and physiolysis, in which the longitudinal portion of the epiphyseal bracket is excised and replaced with fat.

Constriction Ring Syndrome

Constriction ring syndrome, which is also called constriction band syndrome or amniotic disruption sequence, occurs in approximately 1 infant per 15,000 live births. Although the exact etiology is unknown, the prevailing theory is that amniotic disruption releases strands of membrane that circumferentially wrap the developing upper limb, resulting in a spectrum of congenital differences that range from mild skin dimpling to amputation of an affected digit (**Figure 6**). On clinical examination, bands are found perpendicular to the longitudinal axis of the limb or digit. More than 90% are distal to the wrist. Central digits are most commonly affected. In the absence of amputation, secondary syndactyly or bony fusions can occur. Clubfoot, cleft palate, and craniofacial defects are commonly associated with constriction ring syndrome.

The treatment is determined by the nature of the constriction. A patient with a constriction that is mild or associated with distal lymphedema can be simply observed, or excision of the constriction ring with local soft-tissue rearrangement can be considered. Syndactyly releases are performed if necessary. For patients with congenital amputation, hand function can be improved by reconstructive procedures including bone lengthening, web deepening, or free vascularized toe transfer. These procedures are possible because normal neurovascular and musculoskeletal anatomy exists proximal to the constriction. In rare instances, a constriction ring causes vascular insufficiency; release may need to be performed in the first few days of life to avoid digital necrosis.

Thumb Hypoplasia

Thumb hypoplasia lies within the spectrum of radial longitudinal deficiency, but it is classified as an undergrowth[35] (**Table 1**). The condition is often bilateral. Its reported incidence is 1 infant per 30,000 to 100,000 live births, and it affects males and females equally. Like radial longitudinal deficiency, it can occur in association with Holt-Oram syndrome, Fanconi's anemia, thrombocytopenia-absent radius, and VACTERRL association. It is classified using Buck-Gramcko's and Manske's modification of the Blauth classification, which guides the choice of treatment. Blauth type I thumbs are slightly smaller than normal thumbs but function well. Blauth type II thumbs are characterized by the absence of thenar muscles. Blauth type III thumbs lack both intrinsic and extrinsic motor function, and the thumb metacarpal is underdeveloped. They are subdivided into type IIIA, in which the carpometacarpal joint is stable, and type IIIB, in which the carpometacarpal joint is unstable or absent. Floating thumbs are classified as type IV. Type V refers to an absent thumb.

Type II and type IIIA thumbs are characterized by a tight first web space, interphalangeal joint stiffness, metacarpophalangeal joint instability, and thenar weakness. They are best treated with web space deepening, metacarpophalangeal joint stabilization, and opponensplasty. For type IIIB, type IV, and type V, thumb ablation and index finger pollicization is recommended.[36]

Congenital Trigger Digits

Trigger thumb is a relatively common condition having an estimated incidence of 3 infants per 1,000 live births.[37] Numerous studies have found that trigger thumb is an acquired, rather than congenital, condition. Its occurrence is sporadic, and as many as 30% of patients have bilateral involvement. On clinical examination, patients have a palpable nodule of the flexor pollicis longus tendon with either triggering or a fixed flexion contracture of the interphalangeal joint. The condition resolves itself before 1 year of age in 30% to 50% of patients, but the likelihood of spontaneous resolution diminishes as a child grows older. Surgical release of the A1 pulley is almost always successful and is recommended for patients who are older than 1 year.

Trigger fingers are much less common than trigger thumbs. They result from anomalous anatomy, such as abnormal lumbrical insertion or proximal decussation of the flexor digitorum superficialis tendon. Associated conditions include mucopolysaccharidosis, diabetes, and juvenile rheumatoid arthritis. Release of the A1 pulley alone may not suffice; the recurrence rate is as high as 50%.[38] Surgical treatment requires more extensile exposure and specific attention to the underlying pathoanatomy, with lumbrical, A1 pulley, and A3 pulley releases as well as excision of the slip of the flexor digitorum superficialis tendon.

Cerebral Palsy

Cerebral palsy is an irreversible, nonprogressive central nervous system disorder characterized by abnormal motor control and sensory and cognitive impairment. The upper extremity deformity in spastic cerebral palsy typically involves shoulder adduction and internal rotation, elbow flexion, forearm pronation, wrist flexion and ulnar deviation, digital flexion and swan-neck deformity, and thumb-in-palm deformity. Initial treatment is directed at maximizing upper limb and hand function by alleviating spasticity, preventing myostatic contractures, and preventing joint deformity. Splinting, stretching, and pharmacologic measures such as selective botulinum toxin A injections to spastic muscles are used to achieve these goals. Recently, interest has been renewed in treating young patients with constraint therapy, in which the unaffected limb is immobilized or restricted to encourage use of the affected upper extremity and hand.[39]

Surgical treatment can be considered to improve a patient's function or nursing care. The best surgical candidates are usually those with voluntary hand use, adequate sensibility, appropriate cognitive ability, and absence of dyskinetic or athetotic features. The three basic surgical procedures are tailored to the individual: soft-tissue release to loosen spastic muscles, tendon transfer to augment weak antagonistic muscles, and correction of otherwise irreversible bone or joint deformity. Validated, reliable functional outcome instruments are being developed to assess the results of these interventions.[40]

Arthrogryposis

Several congenital conditions characterized by symmetric, nonprogressive joint contractures and muscular weakness are referred to as arthrogryposis. Upper extremity involvement is characterized by shoulder inter-

nal rotation, elbow extension, and wrist flexion contractures, with stiff digits and thumb-in-palm deformity. Patients with arthrogryposis have normal intelligence, and they often have significant lower extremity involvement. Maximizing upper limb function can improve a patient's mobility and ability to complete activities of daily living. Surgical treatment is aimed at restoring joint motion, improving upper limb position, and when feasible, allowing active motion. The treatments proposed to meet these goals include internal rotation osteotomy of the humerus, triceps lengthening and posterior elbow capsulotomy, tendon transfer to restore elbow flexion, carpal wedge osteotomy, and release of the first web space.[41,42]

Congenital Upper Limb Deficiency

Transverse deficiency (congenital amputation) of the upper extremity is rare. It is typically sporadic, unilateral, and not associated with other conditions. Below-elbow amputation affecting the left upper extremity occurs most frequently. The usual recommendation is to fit the child with a passive terminal prosthesis at the age of 6 months and to fit a series of active terminal devices as the patient grows. Recent investigations have challenged accepted beliefs about patients' compliance with prosthesis use as well as the usefulness of prostheses for unilateral deficiencies.[43]

Pediatric Hand Infections

The most common infection of a toddler's hand is herpetic whitlow, which is caused by the herpes simplex virus. Digital sucking is the likely mode of transmission. Herpetic whitlow is characterized by the presence of vesicular eruptions over an erythematous base. It is a self-limiting disease for which surgical treatment is unnecessary. Antibiotic therapy is indicated only in the presence of bacterial superinfection.

Bacterial hand infections are common among children. *Staphylococcus aureus* and group A streptococcus are the most common causative organisms, but anaerobic or mixed infections may be seen in up to 30% of affected patients.[44] Early recognition and prompt treatment are essential. Treatment should include adequate wound management, antibiotic therapy, and appropriate immunization.

Annotated References

1. Swanson AB: A classification for congenital limb malformations. *J Hand Surg Am* 1976;1:8-22.

2. Birch R, Ahad N, Kono H, Smith S: Repair of obstetric brachial plexus palsy: Results in 100 children. *J Bone Joint Surg Br* 2005;87:1089-1095.
   Brachial plexus birth palsy microsurgery for repair or

reconstruction of C5, C6, C7, or C8-T1 lesions yielded good results in 33% to 57% of 100 patients (mean age, 7 months; average follow-up, 85 months). No difference was observed in C5 lesions treated with nerve grafting or nerve transfers. Level of evidence: IV.

3. Noaman HH, Shiha AE, Bahm J: Oberlin's ulnar nerve transfer to the biceps motor nerve in obstetric brachial plexus palsy: Indications and good and bad results. *Microsurgery* 2004;24:182-187.

    Five of seven patients with brachial plexus birth palsy and inadequate biceps recovery (average age, 16 months) obtained antigravity elbow flexion after Oberlin's procedure. This procedure is recommended for C5-C6 nerve root avulsion or for neuroma-in-continuity of the upper trunk with preserved preoperative shoulder function. Level of evidence: IV.

4. Pagnotta A, Haerle M, Gilbert A: Long-term results on abduction and external rotation of the shoulder after latissimus dorsi transfer for sequelae of obstetric palsy. *Clin Orthop Relat Res* 2004;426:199-205.

    Patients with mild preoperative shoulder dysfunction and C5-C6 lesions had better gains after tendon transfer for shoulder abduction and external rotation than those with C5-C6-C7 or complete palsies (203 children, evaluation to age 15 years). Functional improvement was not related to age at surgery. Progressive deterioration of abduction occurred after age 6 years. Level of evidence: IV.

5. Pearl ML, Edgerton BW: Glenoid deformity secondary to brachial plexus birth palsy. *J Bone Joint Surg Am* 1998;80:659-667.

6. Waters PM, Smith GR, Jaramillo D: Glenohumeral deformity secondary to brachial plexus birth palsy. *J Bone Joint Surg Am* 1998;80:668-677.

7. Waters PM, Bae DS: Effect of tendon transfers and extra-articular soft-tissue balancing on glenohumeral development in brachial plexus birth palsy. *J Bone Joint Surg Am* 2005;87:320-325.

    Anterior musculotendinous lengthenings and latissimus dorsi and teres major tendon transfers to the rotator cuff significantly improved global shoulder function in 25 patients (average 43-month follow-up). The procedures halted the progression of, but did not reverse, glenohumeral dysplasia. Level of evidence: IV.

8. Pearl ML, Edgerton BW, Kazimiroff PA, Burchette RJ, Wong K: Arthroscopic release and latissimus dorsi transfer for shoulder internal rotation contractures and glenohumeral deformity secondary to brachial plexus birth palsy. *J Bone Joint Surg Am* 2006;88:564-574.

    Arthroscopic anterior capsular release, with or without latissimus dorsi transfer, improved passive external rotation and glenohumeral deformity in 33 children (minimum 2 years clinical and radiographic follow-up). Level of evidence: IV.

9. Waters PM, Bae DS: The effect of derotational humeral osteotomy on global shoulder function in brachial plexus birth palsy. *J Bone Joint Surg Am* 2006;88:1035-1042.

    For 43 patients with severe glenohumeral joint deformity in the setting of internal rotation contracture and external rotation weakness, external rotation osteotomy of the humerus significantly improved global shoulder function (average follow-up, 3.7 years). Level of evidence: IV.

10. Ho ES, Curtis CG, Clarke HM: Pediatric Evaluation of Disability Inventory: Its application to children with obstetric brachial plexus palsy. *J Hand Surg [Am]* 2006; 31:197-202.

    The Pediatric Evaluation of Disability Inventory differentiated self-care activities performed by 45 children with differing severities of brachial plexus birth palsy. No differences were seen between patients with no hand impairment and their age-matched peers. Level of evidence: II.

11. Huffman GR, Bagley AM, James MA, Lerman JA, Rab G: Assessment of children with brachial plexus birth palsy using the Pediatric Outcomes Data Collection Instrument. *J Pediatr Orthop* 2005;25:400-404.

    Scores on the Pediatric Outcomes Data Collection Instrument were significantly lower among patients who were candidates for shoulder surgery compared with age-matched controls. The instrument may be useful in measuring baseline and postsurgical function of children with brachial plexus birth palsy. Level of evidence: I.

12. Cavendish ME: Congenital elevation of the scapula. *J Bone Joint Surg Br* 1972;54:395-408.

13. Aydinli U, Ozturk C, Akesen B, Ozer O: Surgical treatment of Sprengel's deformity: A modified Green's procedure. *Acta Orthop Belg* 2005;71:264-268.

    Twelve patients with Sprengel's deformity were treated with detachment of the parascapular muscles, omovertebral band excision, and suture fixation of the scapula into a pocket of the latissimus dorsi. All patients had improved shoulder motion and appearance. Level of evidence: IV.

14. McMurtry I, Bennet GC, Bradish C: Osteotomy for congenital elevation of the scapula (Sprengel's deformity). *J Bone Joint Surg Br* 2005;87:986-989.

    Appearance and shoulder abduction were improved with the use of vertical scapular osteotomy in 12 patients with Sprengel's deformity (average 10 years follow-up). Level of evidence: IV.

15. Gomez-Brouchet A, Sales de Gauzy J, Accadbled F, Abid A, Delisle MB, Cahuzac JP: Congenital pseudarthrosis of the clavicle: A histopathological study in five patients. *J Pediatr Orthop B* 2004;13:399-401.

    Examination of specimens from five patients revealed enchondral ossification on either side of the pseudarthrosis and thus supported the theory that congenital pseudarthrosis of the clavicle is caused by failure of the primary centers of ossification to unite. Level of evidence: IV.

6: Pediatrics

16. Campbell CC, Waters PM, Emans JE: Excision of the radial head for congenital dislocation. *J Bone Joint Surg Am* 1992;74:726-733.

17. Kelly DW: Congenital dislocation of the radial head: Spectrum and natural history. *J Pediatr Orthop* 1981; 1:295-298.

18. Ramachandran M, Lau K, Jones DH: Rotational osteotomies for congenital radioulnar synostosis. *J Bone Joint Surg Br* 2005;87:1406-1410.

    Derotational osteotomy for fixed pronation deformities improved the forearm position from a mean 68° pronation to the desired 10° supination in five patients. Bony union was achieved with no loss of correction. Level of evidence: IV.

19. Fujimoto M, Kato H, Minami A: Rotational osteotomy at the diaphysis of the radius in the treatment of congenital radioulnar synostosis. *J Pediatr Orthop* 2005; 25:676-679.

    Radioulnar synostosis was treated via rotational osteotomy through the distal radius, with bony healing and functional improvement for all four patients. Level of evidence: IV.

20. Kanaya F, Ibaraki K: Mobilization of a congenital proximal radioulnar synostosis with use of a free vascularized fascio-fat graft. *J Bone Joint Surg* 1998;80A:1186-1192.

21. Goldfarb CA, Wall L, Manske PR: Radial longitudinal deficiency: The incidence of associated medical and musculoskeletal conditions. *J Hand Surg Am* 2006;31: 1176-1182.

    A high incidence of associated medical or musculoskeletal abnormalities appeared in 164 patients with radial longitudinal deficiency; the percentage of associated conditions increased with the severity of radial longitudinal deficiency. The authors stress the importance of comprehensive screening and evaluation. Level of evidence: IV.

22. Bayne LG, Klug MS: Long-term review of the surgical treatment of radial deficiencies. *J Hand Surg Am* 1987; 12:169-179.

23. Sabharwal S, Finuoli AL, Ghobadi F: Pre-centralization soft tissue distraction for Bayne type IV congenital radial deficiency in children. *J Pediatr Orthop* 2005;25: 377-381.

    Four limbs were treated with gradual soft-tissue distraction using an Ilizarov external fixator before centralization. At average 26-month follow-up, the mean correction was 72° in hand-forearm angle and 19 mm in wrist-forearm position. No neurovascular or infection complications occurred. Level of evidence: IV.

24. Matsuno T, Ishida O, Sunagawa T, Suzuki O, Ikuta Y, Ochi M: Radius lengthening for the treatment of Bayne and Klug type II and type III radial longitudinal deficiency. *J Hand Surg Am* 2006;31:822-829.

    An external fixator device was used to achieve an aver-age of 28 mm of radial length in four patients with radial longitudinal deficiency. Multiple lengthening procedures were required, and deformity recurred with continued skeletal growth. Level of evidence: IV.

25. Goldfarb CA, Klepps SJ, Dailey LA, Manske PR: Functional outcome after centralization for radial dysplasia. *J Hand Surg Am* 2002;27:118-124.

26. McCarroll HR, James MA, Newmeyer WL, Molitor F, Manske PR: Madelung's deformity: Quantitative assessment of x-ray deformity. *J Hand Surg Am* 2005;30: 1211-1220.

    The severity of Madelung's deformity was reliably and reproducibly assessed by measuring ulnar tilt, lunate subsidence, and palmar carpal displacement in this study of 48 wrists. Level of evidence: III.

27. Harley BJ, Brown C, Cummings K, Carter PR, Ezaki M: Volar ligament release and distal radius dome osteotomy for correction of Madelung's deformity. *J Hand Surg Am* 2006;31:1499-1506.

    Vicker's ligament release and radial osteotomy led to pain reduction, improved radial inclination and lunate subsidence, and greater forearm supination and wrist extension in this retrospective study of 26 wrists of 18 patients with Madelung's deformity. Level of evidence: IV.

28. Manske PR, Halikis MN: Surgical classification of central deficiency according to the thumb web. *J Hand Surg Am* 1995;20:687-697.

29. Teoh LC, Lee JY: Dorsal pentagonal island flap: A technique of web reconstruction for syndactyly that facilitates direct closure. *Hand Surg* 2004;9:245-252.

    Use of the dorsal metacarpal island flap in syndactyly release obviated the need for skin grafting. No major complications occurred in 22 web spaces (33-month follow-up), although significant dorsal scarring was noted. Level of evidence: IV.

30. Wassel HD: The results of surgery for polydactyly of the thumb: A review. *Clin Orthop Relat Res* 1969;64:175-193.

31. Larsen M, Nicolai JP: Long-term follow-up of surgical treatment of thumb duplication. *J Hand Surg Br* 2005; 30:276-281.

    At an average 22 years after thumb-duplication reconstruction, 18 of 19 patients had satisfactory function, and 12 thumbs had an adequate appearance. Level of evidence: IV.

32. Watson BT, Hennrikus WL: Postaxial type-B polydactyly. *J Bone Joint Surg Am* 1997;79:65-68.

33. Smith RJ, Kaplan EB: Camptodactyly and similar atraumatic flexion deformities of the proximal interphalangeal joints of the fingers: A study of thirty-one cases. *J Bone Joint Surg Am* 1968;50:1187-1203.

6. Pediatrics

34. Light TR, Ogden JA: The longitudinal epiphyseal bracket: Implications for surgical correction. *J Pediatr Orthop* 1981;1:299-305.

35. James MA, Green HD, McCarroll HR, Manske PR: The association of radial deficiency with thumb hypoplasia. *J Bone Joint Surg Am* 2004;86:2196-2205.

   All 139 patients with radial or carpal deficiency (227 affected upper limbs) had thumb hypoplasia; the severity of thumb deficiency was directly proportional to the severity of radial deficiency. These findings supported the notion that thumb hypoplasia lies within the spectrum of radial longitudinal deficiency. Level of evidence: IV.

36. Staines KG, Majzoub R, Thornby J, Netscher DT: Functional outcome for children with thumb aplasia undergoing pollicization. *Plast Reconstr Surg* 2005;116:1314-1323.

   All 10 children assessed after index pollicization for thumb aplasia used their pollicized digit in a normal pattern, despite significant differences in grip strength, pinch strength, and functional dexterity. This study supported literature showing improved, but not normal, function after pollicization. Level of evidence: IV.

37. Kikuchi N, Ogino T: Incidence and development of trigger thumb in children. *J Hand Surg Am* 2006;31:541-543.

   None of the 1,116 infants examined at birth had any evidence of congenital trigger thumb, but the incidence of trigger thumb within the first year of life was 3.3 per 1,000 live births. Level of evidence: III.

38. Cardon LJ, Ezaki M, Carter PR: Trigger finger in children. *J Hand Surg Am* 1999;24:1156-1161.

39. Naylor CE, Bower E: Modified constraint-induced movement therapy for young children with hemiplegic cerebral palsy: A pilot study. *Dev Med Child Neurol* 2005;47:365-369.

   Supervised constraint therapy resulted in improved upper extremity function for nine children with spastic hemiplegia, as measured in this pilot study by the Quality of Upper Extremity Skills Test. Level of evidence: IV.

40. Davids JR, Peace LC, Wagner LV, Gidewall MA, Blackhurst DW, Roberson WM: Validation of the Shriners Hospital for Children Upper Extremity Evaluation (SHUEE) for children with hemiplegic cerebral palsy. *J Bone Joint Surg Am* 2006;88:326-333.

   The validity and reliability of this video-based assessment of upper extremity function were confirmed in a study of 11 patients with spastic hemiplegia. Level of evidence: III.

41. Lahoti O, Bell MJ: Transfer of pectoralis major in arthrogryposis to restore elbow flexion: Deteriorating results in the long term. *J Bone Joint Surg Br* 2005;87:858-860.

   Long-term evaluation of 10 pectoralis major to biceps transfers in 7 patients with arthrogryposis found progressive elbow flexion deformity with decreased arc of elbow motion. The authors advise that unilateral pectoralis-to-biceps transfers be considered to prevent functional loss. Level of evidence: IV.

42. Ezaki M, Carter PR: Carpal wedge osteotomy for the arthrogrypotic wrist. *Tech Hand Up Extrem Surg* 2004;8:224-228.

   The technique of carpal wedge osteotomy for flexion and ulnar deviation contractures of the wrist in arthrogryposis is described. Level of evidence: V.

43. James MA, Bagley AM, Brasington K, Lutz C, McConnell S, Molitor F: Impact of prostheses on function and quality of life for children with unilateral congenital below-the-elbow deficiency. *J Bone Joint Surg Am* 2006;88:2356-2365.

   A multicenter study of 489 children with unilateral below-elbow congenital amputations found that prosthetic use was not associated with higher function or quality of life, as measured by four outcomes instruments. Level of evidence: II.

44. Harness N, Blazar PE: Causative microorganisms in surgically treated pediatric hand infections. *J Hand Surg Am* 2005;30:1294-1297.

   In this review of 32 upper extremity infections requiring surgical treatment, *Staphylococcus aureus* was isolated in 37% of patients and Group A *Streptococcus pyogenes,* in 20%. Mixed aerobic-anaerobic species were isolated in 7 of 32 cultures. Level of evidence: IV.

Chapter 57

Spine Trauma and Disorders: Pediatrics

Peter O. Newton, MD   Vidyadhar V. Upasani, MD

Pediatric Spine Trauma

Injuries to the spine represent only 1% to 2% of all pediatric fractures.[1] A fracture that requires surgery in an adult may not in a child because of the child's elastic soft tissue, potential for remodeling, and normal bone mineralization. Most childhood spinal injuries are caused by a fall, motor vehicle crash, athletic activity, gunshot wound, birth trauma, or nonaccidental trauma.[2] The incidence of injury from each of these causes is unknown and may be underestimated in the literature. Boys have a bony injury more often than girls, although boys and girls have a similar incidence of nonosseous injury.

Because there is a 50% incidence of associated injuries in children with spine trauma[3] and 20% of children with spine trauma have a neurologic injury,[4] a thorough physical examination is essential. Examination of a young child may be difficult, and a high index of suspicion may be required to arrive at the correct diagnosis. Tenderness to palpation, swelling, limited range of motion, and a palpable posterior gap between the spinous processes are frequently the only objective findings. A series of motor and sensory examinations must be performed and clearly documented.

Anatomy and Radiographic Evaluation

Developing vertebrae form three primary ossification centers within a cartilaginous template: one for the vertebral body and one for either side of the neural arch (**Figure 1**). The fusion of the posterior arches by the age of 3 years precedes the fusion of the vertebral body and the lateral masses at the neurocentral synchondrosis, which takes place at approximately 7 years of age. Five secondary centers of ossification usually appear after puberty. In evaluating a child's spine radiographically, it is important to be aware of these physes to avoid mistaking them for fractures or overlooking fractures that occur through open physes.

Plain AP and lateral radiographs are useful in the initial evaluation of vertebral alignment and soft-tissue swelling. However, these radiographs may not show the full extent of the suspected injury. A complete cervical spine series must be taken for evaluation of the cervicothoracic junction. In addition, an odontoid open-mouth

view for evaluation of the atlantoaxial articulation and oblique radiographs for specific evaluation of the facet joints and the pedicles can sometimes be helpful. For children, CT scans are often used instead of these radiographic views.

A CT scan with sagittal and coronal reconstruction can be used to define bony structures, identify fractures poorly shown on radiographs, and evaluate the extent of canal impingement. MRI can best show soft-tissue structures; one study found MRI helpful in ruling out cervical spine injuries in obtunded patients.[5] A technetium bone scan may be helpful in diagnosing stress fractures in the spine or, when used with laboratory studies, in differentiating infectious or tumor etiology from trauma.

Spine Fracture Management

Early immobilization is an important factor in managing any suspected spinal injury, especially if the patient is unresponsive or unconscious. Appropriate immobilization of a child's cervical spine is difficult, because

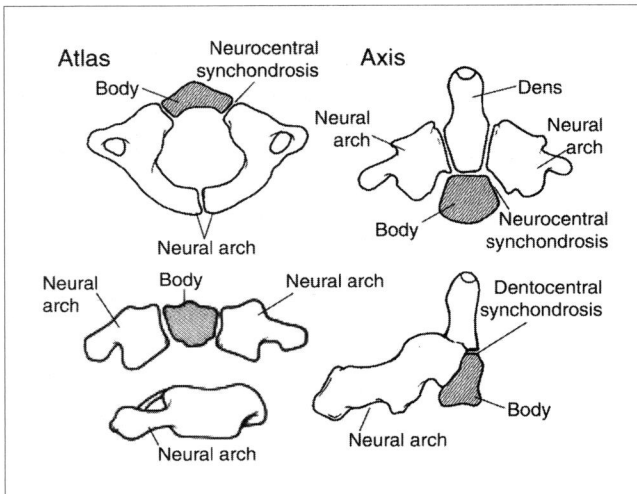

Figure 1   Ossification centers of the atlas and axis. *(Reproduced from Copley LA, Dormans JP: Cervical spine disorders in infants and children. J Am Acad Orthop Surg 1998;6:205.)*

6: Pediatrics

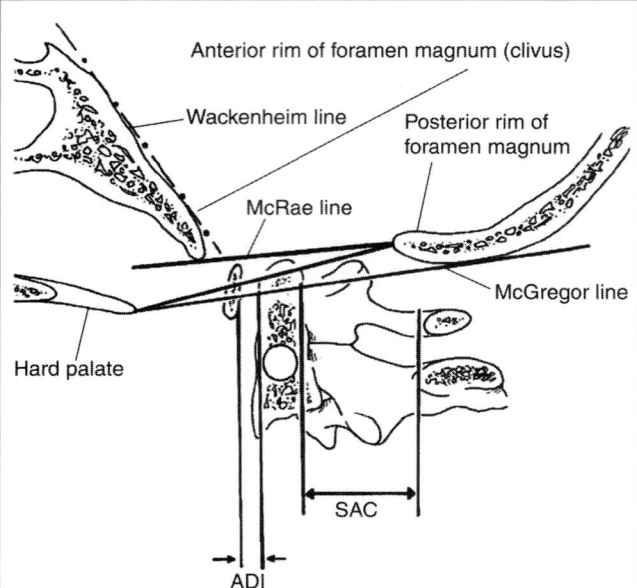

Figure 2 The lines commonly used to determine basilar impression and the measurements for determining atlantoaxial instability. ADI = atlanto-dens interval, SAC = space available for the cord. The Wackenheim line is drawn along the clivus into the cervical spinal canal and should pass just posterior to the tip of the odontoid. The McRae line defines the opening of the foramen magnum. The McGregor line is drawn from the upper surface of the posterior edge of the hard palate to the most caudal point of the occipital curve of the skull. *(Reproduced from Copley LA, Dormans JP: Cervical spine disorders in infants and children. J Am Acad Orthop Surg 1998;6:206.)*

commercial cervical collars do not fit properly. A spine board with an occipital recess or a split mattress that can accommodate the relatively large size of a child's head in relation to the trunk should be used to prevent excessive flexion of the cervical spine during transport. The paraspinal supporting soft tissues are immature in children and may allow an initial deformity to progress. However, the child's growth potential allows remodeling and reconstitution of the fracture over time.

Nonsurgical treatment will suffice in most instances, although an orthotic device may be required to maintain spinal alignment during walking. For more severe injuries, surgical treatment should permit the maximum neurologic recovery, restore spinal stability, and preserve as much spinal mobility as possible. The surgical options include reduction, fusion, decompression, and instrumentation of the fracture. The choice depends on the type of fracture, the presence of a neurologic deficit, and the surgeon's experience.

Cervical Spine Fractures
Odontoid Fractures
Fracture of the odontoid process in children is usually caused by a fall, motor vehicle crash, or minor trauma

and almost always occurs through the synchondrosis at the base of the dens. Neurologic deficits are rare in isolated odontoid fractures. The patient may have upper cervical or occipital pain, decreased range of motion, or muscle spasms. Radiographs may show an anterior angulation of the odontoid process; the fracture line through the physis can be difficult to see on a radiograph. If spontaneous reduction of the fracture has occurred, CT or MRI can be used to identify the injury.

Closed reduction by neck extension and immobilization using a cast, a brace, or halo traction for 6 to 8 weeks is usually sufficient to allow the fracture to heal. CT of the skull can show the thickness of the calvaria so that halo pins can be properly positioned and associated complications can be minimized. Insertion of as many as 12 pins at a lower torque is recommended for children younger than 4 years.[6]

Atlantoaxial Instability and Rotatory Subluxation
An atlanto-dens interval greater than 5 mm on a lateral radiograph suggests the presence of traumatic atlantoaxial subluxation secondary to rupture of the transverse ligament of the atlas[7] (**Figure 2**). An acute traumatic rupture can be treated with an immobilization trial of 8 to 12 weeks, although some ruptures require an arthrodesis to restore stability. Rotatory subluxation can result from trauma but more commonly occurs after an upper respiratory infection or an otolaryngologic procedure such as a tonsillectomy or pharyngoplasty. Rotatory fixation is classified into four types by the degree and direction of facet subluxation. Radiographs can show the superimposition of C1 onto C2 in a rotated position. Dynamic CT can show evidence of the loss of normal atlantoaxial rotation to confirm the diagnosis.[8]

Patients usually have only a painful torticollis, and neurologic involvement is rare. Treatment depends on the duration of symptoms. If diagnosed early, the condition is treated by immobilization in a soft collar, anti-inflammatory medications, and range-of-motion exercises. If symptoms are present longer than 1 week, cervical traction and muscle relaxants should be used until the spasms are resolved and the subluxation is reduced. This treatment is usually followed by 4 to 6 weeks of immobilization. For recurrent or persistent rotatory subluxation, surgical stabilization, either in situ or after attempted reduction, has been shown to be successful, with radiographic documentation of fusion and no incidence of neurologic complications.[9]

Occipitoatlantal Dislocation
Occipitoatlantal dislocation is often a fatal injury. It occurs more frequently in children than in adults because of their disproportionately large head size and higher level of physiologic motion. Several measurements on a lateral radiograph are useful in diagnosing this injury. The most notable is the Powers ratio[10] (**Figure 3**). The Powers ratio is sensitive to anterior occipitoatlantal dislocation and may be inaccurate if an atlas fracture or a foramen magnum congenital anomaly is present.

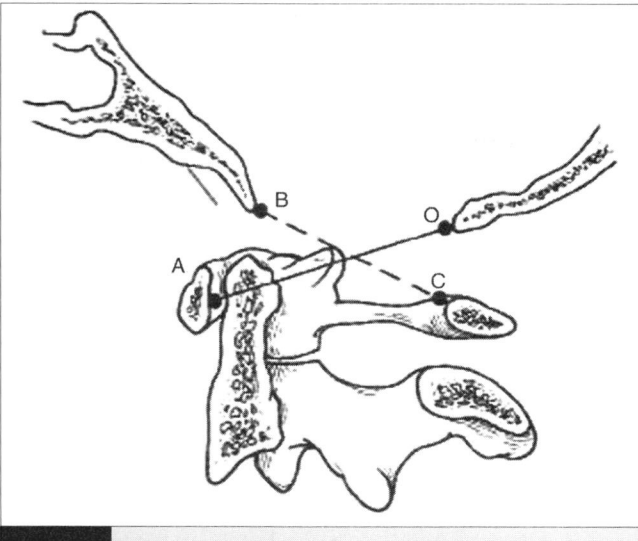

Figure 3 The Powers ratio is determined by drawing a line from the basion (B) to the posterior arch of the atlas (C) and a second line from the opisthion (O) to the anterior arch of the atlas (A). A BC:OA ratio of more than 1 indicates anterior atlantooccipital translation, and a ratio of less than 0.55 indicates posterior translation. *(Reproduced from Copley LA, Dormans JP: Cervical spine disorders in infants and children. J Am Acad Orthop Surg 1998;6:206.)*

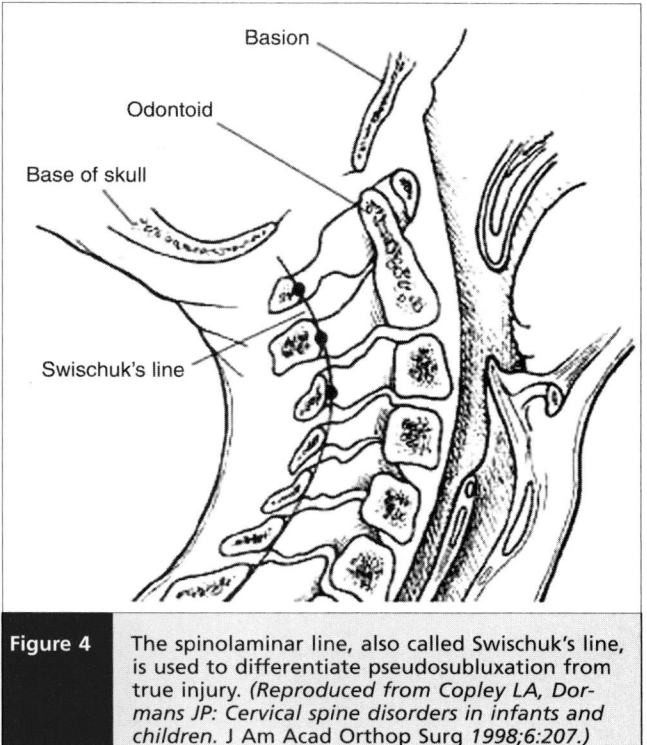

Figure 4 The spinolaminar line, also called Swischuk's line, is used to differentiate pseudosubluxation from true injury. *(Reproduced from Copley LA, Dormans JP: Cervical spine disorders in infants and children. J Am Acad Orthop Surg 1998;6:207.)*

Management of an occipitoatlantal dislocation is controversial. The recommendations include immobilization in a halo or Minerva cast (avoiding distraction of the occipitocervical junction) and a posterior fusion of the occiput to C1 or C2.[11]

Atlas Fractures
Burst fractures of the ring of C1 are infrequent in children or adults. An axial compressive force transmitted onto the lateral masses of the atlas through the occipital condyles is believed to cause one or more fractures of the ring as well as a rupture or avulsion injury to the transverse ligament. CT can permit diagnosis by revealing lateral displacement of the lateral masses. Nonsurgical treatment in a brace, cast, or cervical orthosis is recommended for as long as 3 months. At the end of treatment, flexion-extension radiographs can confirm stability of the atlantoaxial articulation.

Hangman's Fracture
Pathologic subluxation of C2 secondary to bilateral pedicle fracture is called hangman's fracture. It is believed to occur secondary to a forced distraction and hyperextension of the neck; nonaccidental trauma must be considered in younger children who have this injury. The fracture is usually difficult to see on radiographs, and it may be confused with neurocentral synchondroses that have yet to close. On a lateral radiograph, the spinolaminar (Swischuk's) line can help distinguish between pseudosubluxation and a true injury (**Figure 4**); anterior displacement of the posterior arch of C2

more than 2 mm from the spinolaminar line is believed to be indicative of an injury. The injury is treated with immobilization for 8 to 12 weeks.

Subaxial Injuries
Subaxial injuries to C3 through C7 are more common in children 9 years of age or older than in younger children. The injury patterns are similar to those found in adults.[12] A compression fracture from a flexion injury is most common. It can be treated surgically or with traction and immobilization. Separation of the vertebral end plate from the vertebral body because of an extension injury can also occur among children. In infants, these Salter-Harris type I injuries through the physis are believed to be extremely unstable, and may require surgical fixation.

Thoracolumbar Spine Injuries
The three-column spine theory allows for classification of adult or pediatric spine fractures based on their location.[13] Involvement of the three spinal columns depends on the forces of the injury. Minor injuries can cause isolated fractures of the posterior column. Major injuries can be classified as compression fractures, burst fractures, fracture-dislocations, or flexion-distraction injuries. Compression fractures are described as a failure of the anterior column with an intact middle column; they are frequently the result of a flexion mechanism of injury. Compression of 20% or less is common, and it may affect a span of several vertebral levels. Fractures that do not involve the apophyseal ring or posterior column and cause less than 50% collapse of

6: Pediatrics

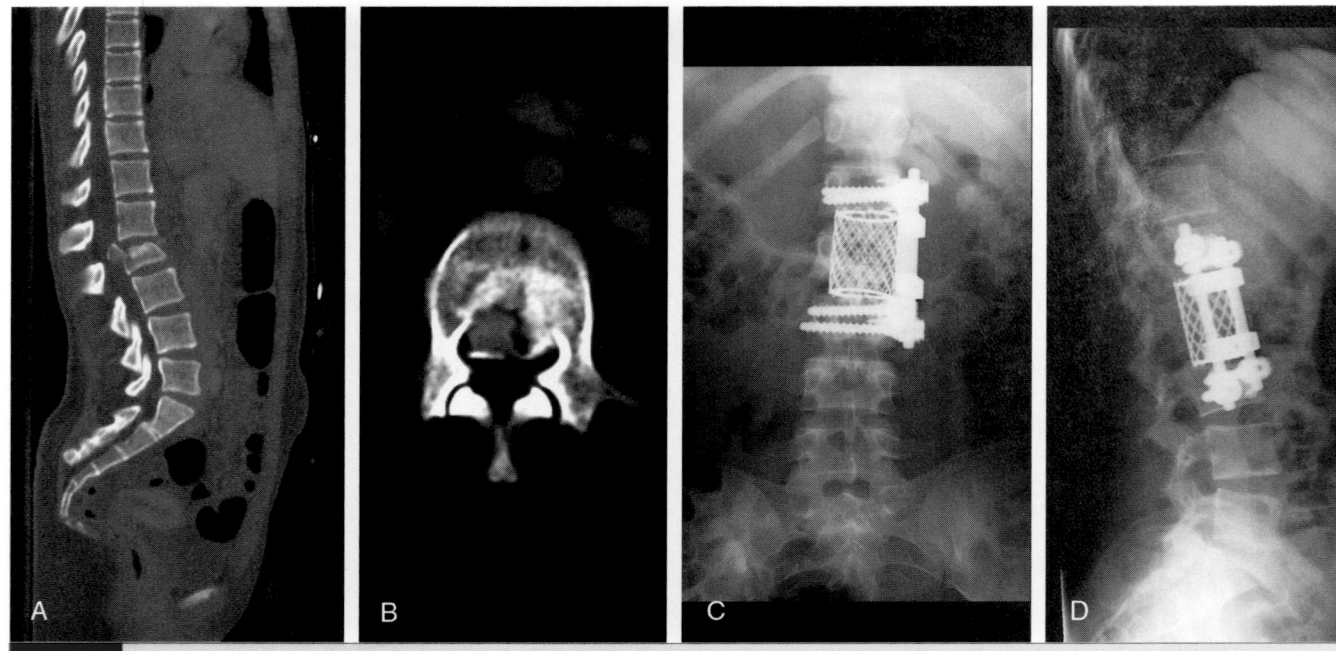

Figure 5 CT studies and radiographs of a 13-year-old girl with low back pain and left leg paresthesias. Sagittal (**A**) and transverse (**B**) CT images show a burst fracture at L2 with canal compromise. PA (**C**) and lateral (**D**) postoperative images after anterior L2 corpectomy, canal decompression, and L1 through L3 anterior spinal instrumentation and fusion.

anterior vertebral body height are usually stable mechanically and neurologically. They can be treated conservatively with Jewett brace immobilization and pain management, and they tend to heal without complication in 4 to 6 weeks. Posterior instrumentation may be necessary if a kyphotic deformity is present secondary to multiple compression fractures or if more than 50% loss of anterior height has occurred.

Burst fractures are described as failure of both the anterior and middle columns. They most commonly occur secondary to a compressive axial force (**Figure 5**). These fractures may be unstable and compromise the integrity of the spinal canal or neural foramina. CT can be used to evaluate middle column retropulsion and the extent of comminution. MRI is useful in determining whether posterior ligamentous or apophyseal avulsion injuries are present and ruling out nerve rootlet entrapment or a dural tear. Surgical treatment is recommended for a fracture associated with neurologic injury or kyphosis of more than 20°. Anterior grafting may be required if more than 60% of anterior body height is lost after reduction. Pedicle screw constructs usually extend one or two levels above and below the fracture. Anterior instrumentation may be necessary in patients with severe anterior angulation to restore vertebral height or achieve anterior decompression of the spinal canal. Stable burst fractures can be managed by use of an extension molded cast or a thoracolumbosacral orthosis for 8 to 12 weeks.

A flexion-distraction injury, also referred to as a seat belt or Chance fracture, is a compression injury to the anterior column, with distraction of the middle and posterior columns.[14] These fractures are classified based on the type of injury to the anterior column, the state of the vertebral body, and the injury to the posterior elements.[15] Children younger than 10 years are especially at risk for seat belt injuries. They have a high center of gravity because of their relatively large head size, and their underdeveloped anterior iliac crests are insufficient to anchor the lap belt. Intra-abdominal injury frequently occurs in conjunction with seat belt injuries. Fractures resulting from a flexion-distraction injury of bony elements can be treated in an extension cast or rigid orthosis if adequate reduction can be obtained. If the fracture involves the disk or posterior ligaments, surgical treatment with wiring or pedicle screw fixation one level above and below the injury is recommended.

Fracture-dislocation injury, the most severe type of thoracolumbar fracture, is a failure of all three columns. A shear injury is associated with rotation or distraction in these relatively uncommon fractures. They typically occur at the thoracolumbar junction and are accompanied by neurologic injuries. They almost always require surgical stabilization, with or without decompression.

Limbus or apophyseal fracture caused by heavy lifting or twisting is commonly seen in older children and adolescents. Patients describe feeling a popping sensation and report radicular symptoms. Plain radiographs are not usually sufficient to diagnose this injury. MRI or CT should be used to determine the exact location of the fracture. Nonsurgical management is rarely successful. A wide laminectomy with surgical excision of the limbus fragment is recommended if neurologic symptoms are present.

6: Pediatrics

Spinal Cord Injury Without Radiographic Abnormality

Spinal cord injury without radiographic abnormality occurs particularly in children younger than 8 years.[16] Plain radiography or CT does not reveal evidence of fracture or dislocation. MRI sometimes shows evidence of cord edema, epidural hematoma, or soft-tissue injury. The mechanism of injury is undetermined, although the elasticity of the immature spine may be a factor.[17] Other possibilities include vascular compromise with cord infarction, endplate separation, and transient subluxation.[18]

A thorough physical examination and radiographs are essential to evaluate spinal stability, and early immobilization is important for all patients. The neurologic injuries can be complete or incomplete. A complete lesion is characterized by immediate and total loss of motor and sensory function and segmental reflexes caudal to the injury during the period of spinal shock. The contused nerve roots may recover during a period of several months, although complete injuries rarely recover. Incomplete lesions are defined by patterns of partial neurologic loss. In general, the more distal the lesion, the better the prognosis for neurologic recovery.

Immobilization for at least 8 to 12 weeks is recommended. Surgical stabilization is required if an orthosis is unable to maintain a stable reduction or if instability appears after adequate immobilization. Long-term follow-up is important, because spinal and other orthopaedic deformities can occur after these injuries.

The National Acute Spinal Cord Injury Study recommends that methylprednisolone sodium succinate be administered for 23 hours, if started within 3 hours of the injury, or 48 hours, if started 3 to 8 hours after the injury (a 30 mg/kg bolus administered over 15 minutes followed by a maintenance infusion of 5.4 mg/kg per hour).[19] However, the value of high-dose steroids is controversial. A recent study concluded that the evidence is insufficient to support the use of methylprednisolone as a standard treatment for acute spinal cord injury.[20]

Pediatric Spine Disorders

Os Odontoideum

Os odontoideum is a rare anomaly in which a wide transverse gap exists in the tip of the odontoid process. It is probably caused by an injury to the vascular supply from an unrecognized odontoid fracture or damage to the epiphyseal plate during the first few years of life. Patients usually have localized neck pain, and they may also have transitory episodes of paresis, myelopathy, and brainstem ischemia. Radiography and CT can be used to identify an oval or round ossicle with sclerotic margins near the foramen magnum with a hypoplastic dens. Os odontoideum can lead to atlantoaxial instability and may require posterior cervical fusion for stabilization.[21] The indications for surgery include neurologic involvement, progressive instability, persistent

neck pain, an atlanto-dens interval of 10 mm or more, or space available for the cord restricted to 13 mm or less.

Klippel-Feil Syndrome

Klippel-Feil syndrome is characterized by a low posterior hairline, a short neck with limited range of motion, and congenital fusions of cervical vertebrae. Scoliosis, limb deficiency, deafness, cardiopulmonary dysfunction, and genitourinary abnormalities can also be present and are believed to result from the same unknown embryologic insult. A general pediatric evaluation and a renal ultrasound should be performed to discover associated congenital anomalies. Patients often require activity modification, because congenital cervical fusions increase the risk of spinal cord injury following forced flexion or a blow to the head. Later in life, arthrodesis is occasionally needed to manage neurologic symptoms caused by cervical instability at the unaffected motion segments.

Congenital Kyphosis and Scoliosis

Congenital kyphosis and scoliosis are deformities in spinal alignment caused by developmental vertebral anomalies. Their etiology is not known, although experiments in mice found that hypobaric hypoxia and carbon monoxide exposure were related to the development of vertebral malformations.[22] A defect in formation or segmentation of one or more vertebrae is believed to cause an imbalance in spinal growth and the development of a curve. Patients with congenital spinal anomalies may have associated malformations of the heart and genitourinary tract, as well as anomalies of the spinal cord. Early recognition of the deformity allows curve deterioration to be predicted and treatment to be initiated. In general, attempts to control a curve before it worsens are preferable to salvage procedures for a severe deformity.

Failures of segmentation can be unilateral or bilateral. A unilateral failure is much more common in congenital scoliosis than in congenital kyphosis. It results in the formation of a bar of bone through the disk spaces and facet joints. Rib fusions or other rib abnormalities can occur adjacent to this bar and affect the appearance of the deformity. In congenital scoliosis, curve deterioration depends on the growth potential of the curve convexity opposite the bar; the curve usually progresses approximately 5° a year. A unilateral unsegmented bar with a contralateral hemivertebra typically results in the most severe, rapidly progressing deformity. In congenital kyphosis, failure of segmentation of the anterior portion of one or more vertebral bodies leads to a slowly progressing deformity that imposes little neurologic risk. Bilateral failure of segmentation produces a shortened block segment with narrow or fused disk spaces like those in the cervical spines of children with Klippel-Feil syndrome. If longitudinal growth is symmetric, bilateral failure of segmentation causes little deformity.

Vertebral formation defects range in severity from

6: Pediatrics

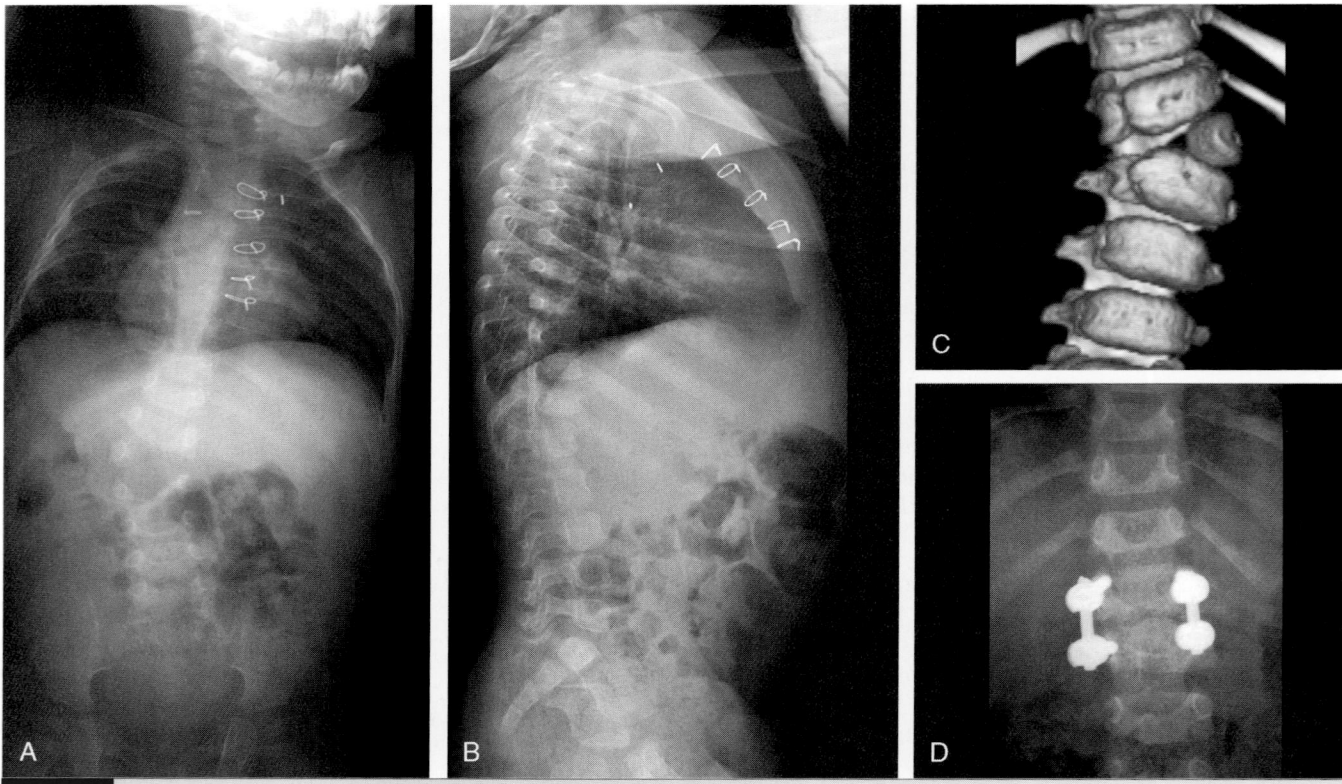

Figure 6 Imaging studies of a 21-month-old boy with a left L1 hemivertebra and congenital kyphoscoliosis. PA **(A)**, lateral **(B)**, and three-dimensional **(C)** CT images. **D,** Postoperative PA image after posterior L1 hemivertebra excision and T12 through L2 posterior spinal instrumentation and fusion.

mild wedge vertebra to hemivertebra. Wedge vertebrae usually do not cause significant congenital scoliosis, but they can require surgical treatment if more than one is present on the same side of the spine. A hemivertebra is one of the most common causes of congenital scoliosis (**Figure 6**). It consists of half a vertebral body, a single pedicle, and a hemilamina and can be fully segmented, semisegmented, or nonsegmented. Each of these types is associated with a different growth potential and severity of scoliosis. In congenital kyphosis, a partial or complete deficiency in the vertebral body may be associated with progressive paraplegia or sudden impingement of the spinal cord with posterior growth.

The prognosis for patients with congenital kyphosis or scoliosis depends on the site and type of the vertebral anomaly, the growth imbalance it causes, and the age of the patient at diagnosis. Spinal AP and lateral radiographs can be used to identify the vertebral anomaly and follow curve deterioration over time. MRI to reveal intraspinal or soft-tissue anomalies is required for surgical planning, and three-dimensional CT with sagittal and coronal reconstructions can be helpful in understanding the deformity.

The purpose of treatment is to prevent curve deterioration by balancing spinal growth. Bracing has been ineffective in controlling congenital curves, but it can be used postoperatively to control spinal alignment or compensatory curve development. Surgical treatment attempts to limit spinal growth on the convexity of the curve, maintain spinal canal integrity, or expand the volume of the thorax to allow adequate pulmonary development. Convex hemiepiphysiodeses, anterior and posterior or posterior-only curve correction with arthrodeses, spinal osteotomies, rib distractions, and hemivertebrectomies have all been described as ways to improve spinal alignment. Postoperative follow-up, including full-length radiographs, is important until the patient reaches skeletal maturity to ensure the correction has been maintained.

Spinal Dysraphisms

Spinal dysraphisms are disorders of the dorsal midline that result from abnormal early neural development. These malformations are often associated with congenital deformities of the spine and should be identified in the initial patient evaluation. Diastematomyelia occurs when a double neural tube is formed by a cleft along the spinal cord. Each half-cord contains only a single set of dorsal and ventral nerve roots, and midline bony, cartilaginous, or fibrous bands may be present between the two hemicords. A myelomeningocele results from a primary failure of neural tube closure, probably secondary to environmental, teratogenic, or genetic factors. The open neural tube with adjacent cutaneous ectoderm overlays a cerebrospinal fluid–filled sac. In contrast, a meningocele is a membrane-covered sac that contains no neural tissue and overlays a normal spinal cord; it is usually associated with normal neurologic function. A lipomyelomeningocele is a subcutaneous fatty mass attached to a tethered spinal cord, either through a dural defect or inside the thecal sac. It is believed to be caused by premature separation of cutaneous ectoderm before complete closure of the neural tube. Spina bifida occulta is caused by failure of posterior vertebral fusion. The underlying spinal cord is usually normal, but in rare instances becomes tethered in the bony malformations.

Spinal cord tethering associated with spinal dysraphism is a well-recognized cause of neurologic deterioration. In experimental animal models, progressive spinal cord ischemia because of cord tethering resulted in worsening neurologic symptoms.[23] In humans, growth of the vertebral column or even transient traction from flexion-extension movements of the spine can injure the spinal cord. Untethering procedures have been found to improve or stabilize neurologic function in patients with spinal deformities and should be considered before or in addition to orthopaedic management.[24]

Idiopathic Scoliosis

Idiopathic scoliosis is a common three-dimensional pediatric spine deformity. It is categorized based on age of onset: infantile (0 to 3 years of age), juvenile (4 to 10 years of age), and adolescent (11 years of age to maturity). The age of onset and the etiology of the curve seem to affect curve progression, cardiopulmonary impairment, and cosmetic appearance. Unlike congenital scoliosis, which is known to be caused by a failure of vertebral formation or segmentation, idiopathic scoliosis does not have a known etiology. Many theories have been proposed; central nervous system diseases, as well as disorders of the bones, muscles, and disks, have been associated with nonidiopathic scoliosis. Although several familial studies have demonstrated a polygenic inheritance pattern, the particular genes responsible for the deformity are unknown. Asymmetric spinal growth in the sagittal plane during the adolescent growth spurt is believed to cause spinal buckling and lead to curve formation.[25] Active research continues to discover a unifying theory for the development of idiopathic scoliosis.

A careful history and physical examination are essential to exclude the numerous other conditions associated with a spinal deformity and arrive at a diagnosis of idiopathic scoliosis. A detailed familial and surgical history, the presence of pain, the patient's recent growth, and a thorough review of systems should be documented. On examination, the patient's trunk shape and balance, pubertal development, limb lengths, and skeletal abnormalities should be noted. The Adams forward-bend test can be used to quantify the angle of trunk rotation in the upper thoracic, midthoracic, and lumbar regions of the spine. A complete neurologic examination is important to rule out intraspinal involvement.

Standing PA and lateral radiographs of the entire spine can be used to assess for scoliosis and follow curve progression. If surgical treatment is being considered, lateral-bending radiographs (supine or over a bolster), can be used to assess curve flexibility. MRI is indicated for idiopathic scoliosis patients with an infantile or juvenile curve, patients with an atypical left thoracic curve or neurologic abnormalities, or patients with substantial back pain of no obvious etiology.[26] Curve magnitude is determined by the Cobb method. To estimate the remaining growth potential of the spine, skeletal maturity can be determined radiographically by noting the state of the triradiate cartilage and the Risser stage of the iliac crest apophysis or assessing the ossification centers of the elbow or hand.

Infantile idiopathic scoliosis is relatively uncommon, and the ratio of males to females is 3:2. A neural axis abnormality, hip dysplasia, and congenital heart disease are often associated with the condition. Spontaneous correction frequently occurs. Curve progression can be predicted by the rib-vertebral angle difference or the phase of the rib head.[27] Rib overlap of the apical vertebral body or a rib-vertebral angle difference greater than 20° indicates that the curve is likely to progress. Curves that are greater than 30° or have progressed can be treated with an orthotic device or a Risser cast (**Figure 7**). Surgical treatment with anterior or posterior instrumentation and fusion, convex epiphysiodesis, or growing rods can be considered for curves greater than 50°, with definitive fusion delayed as long as possible to allow adequate growth and pulmonary development.

Juvenile idiopathic scoliosis curves are usually right sided. The condition tends to affect boys earlier than girls, although girls are more frequently affected than boys. These curves steadily progress, usually at the rate of 1° to 3° a year before the age of 10 years and dramatically faster after the age of 10 years. Bracing is used to treat curves greater than 25° to 30° that have progressed, although most patients with curves greater than 30° eventually require surgical treatment.[28] Anterior fusion is commonly required in addition to posterior treatment to prevent crankshaft rotation of the spine.

The development and progression of adolescent idiopathic scoliosis is associated with the peripubertal growth spurt, and severe curves occur more commonly in girls than boys. The growth potential of the patient should be assessed to determine the risk of curve progression. The time of peak growth velocity has been closely associated with the closure of triradiate cartilage, menarche, and the Risser stages occurring sequentially during the adolescent growth spurt. The Greulich and Pyle hand atlas and the modified Sauvegrain method (using four anatomic landmarks of the elbow) provide reproducible assessments of skeletal age during the pubertal growth spurt.[29] Curves less severe than 20° should be monitored with clinical examination and radiographs every 4 to 12 months until skeletal maturity. A curve that progresses during puberty and is greater than 30° for thoracolumbar curves and 40° for thoracic curves at maturity can be monitored approximately every 5 years, because in adulthood the risk of progression is low.

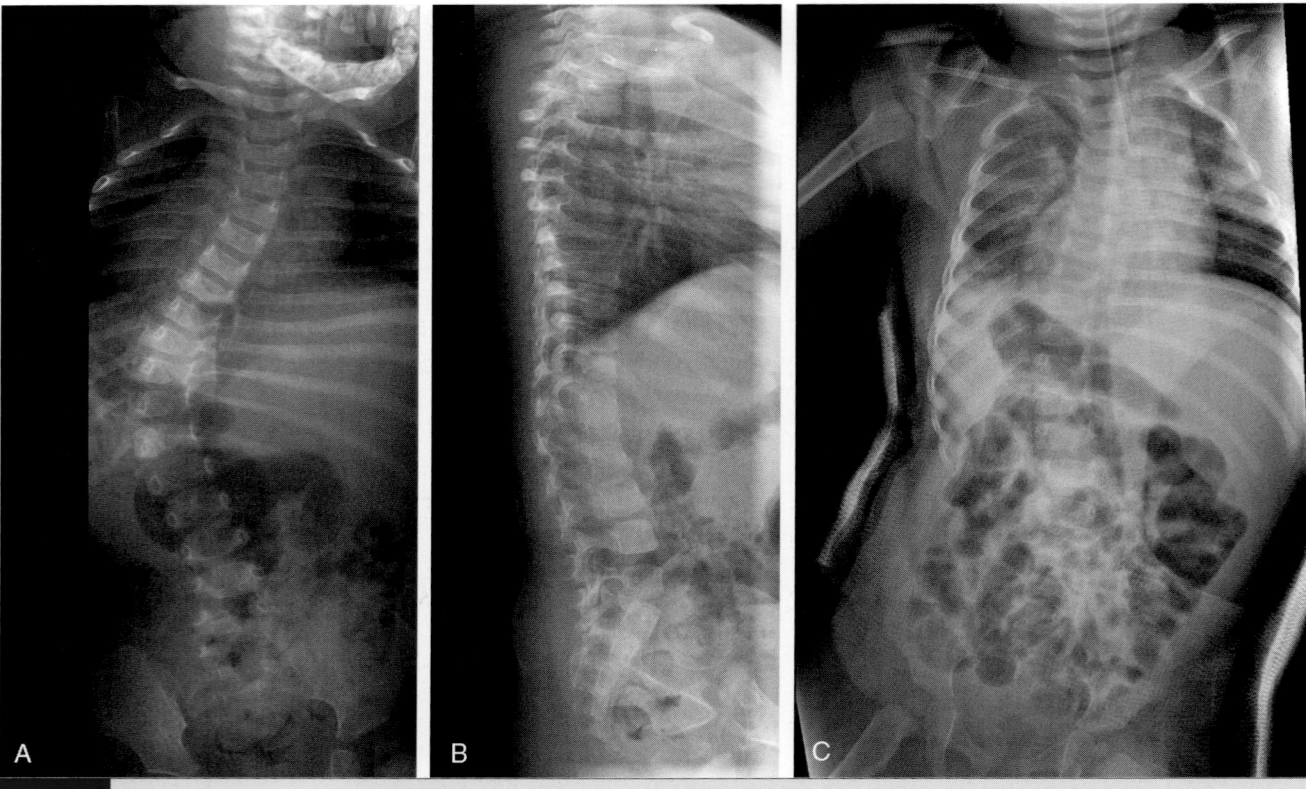

Figure 7   Radiographs of a 10-month-old girl with progressive infantile idiopathic scoliosis who was treated with a Risser cast. Supine PA **(A)** and lateral **(B)** radiographs show a 57° thoracolumbar curve. C, In-cast PA radiograph reveals curve improvement to 22°.

Orthotic treatment with a brace or a molded body cast is indicated for a patient with substantial growth potential (Risser ≤ 2) and a curve greater than 30° or for a patient with a curve greater than 20° to 25° with more than 5° of documented progression. The Scoliosis Research Society Prevalence and Natural History Committee finding of a direct relationship between prevention of curve progression and the number of in-brace hours (16 to 23 hours)[30] suggests that the more time the patient spends in the brace, the less likely the curve is to progress. However, braces are only capable of maintaining the existing curve. They may be relatively unsuccessful in applying corrective forces to the spine of a male patient with a muscular build or an obese patient with a large body mass. Optimal curve control also requires that the brace be well fitted, with pad adjustments by an experienced orthotist, with the goal of achieving at least a 30% and ideally a 50% reduction of the curve in the brace.

The goals of surgical correction are to improve spinal alignment and balance and prevent curve progression. Curve magnitude and pattern, the risk of curve progression (based on skeletal maturity), clinical deformity, and trunk balance and rotation must be considered in deciding whether surgery is indicated. In general, curves greater than 40° to 50° in skeletally immature patients should be considered for surgical treatment. New surgical instrumentation systems have

been developed since the Harrington rod and the Cotrel and Dubousset multihook system became available. Deformity correction and arthrodesis continue to be the primary process measures of surgical success.

Surgical planning should be based on the pattern of the curve, as described by the King-Moe or Lenke classification system.[31,32] Most curves are treated with posterior instrumentation, and every effort is made to spare the lumbar spine. The use of pedicle screw fixation (**Figure 8**) has improved the degree of correction while requiring less soft-tissue dissection at the distal level of fusion and possibly allowing greater control of the transverse plane and crankshaft growth. The correction obtained by posterior segmental pedicle screw constructs has been found to rival the correction obtained by combined anterior and posterior approaches.[33] The minimally invasive thoracoscopic anterior instrumentation approach recently was found to be successful for patients who met the weight, Cobb angle, and sagittal profile criteria.[34] The studied patients required postoperative bracing for 3 months, but they recovered from pain and regained pulmonary function more rapidly than patients who had an open thoracotomy approach. Dual-rod anterior constructs developed for the treatment of thoracolumbar scoliosis have been shown to provide a rigid and relatively short fusion with consistent results.[35]

The Scoliosis Research Society supported develop-

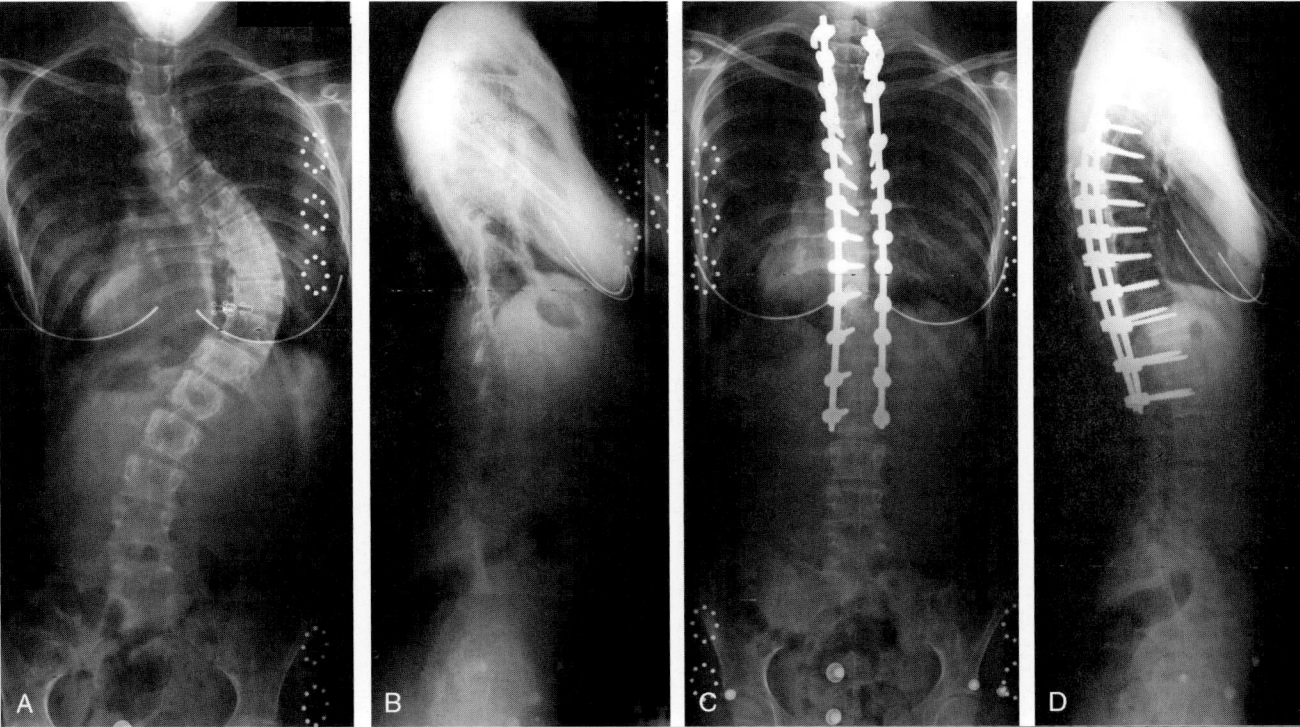

Figure 8 Imaging studies of a 14-year-old girl with progressive adolescent idiopathic scoliosis. PA (A) and lateral (B) radiographs demonstrate a 77° right thoracic curve. Postoperative PA (C) and lateral (D) radiographs after T2 through L2 segmental pedicle screw instrumentation and fusion.

ment of a disease-specific outcomes instrument to measure patient-determined success factors. Compared with preoperative scores on this instrument, adolescent patients' scores 24 months after surgery showed significant improvement in pain, function, general self-image, and level of activity.[36] Patients and their parents did not strongly agree on the cosmetic outcome of the surgery. Their perceptions were not well supported by radiographic and physical measurements of preoperative and postoperative deformity.[37]

Scheuermann Kyphosis

Scheuermann disease is a rigid juvenile kyphosis associated with a growth disturbance of the vertebral end plates. In the typical form, at least 5° of vertebral wedging is found in three or more consecutive vertebrae in the thoracic spine. The less common atypical form is found in the thoracolumbar or lumbar spine. The kyphosis usually begins during the prepubertal growth spurt (between 10 and 12 years of age) as the ring apophysis ossifies. The etiology of typical Scheuermann kyphosis is unknown, although genetic, vascular, metabolic, hormonal, and mechanical involvement has been proposed. The atypical form is believed to be caused by trauma to the immature spine, which leads to growth irregularities in the vertebral end plates. The kyphotic deformity progresses rapidly during the adolescent growth spurt; curve progression during adulthood is not well documented. In general, adult patients with

Scheuermann disease have mild functional limitations but no clinically significant restrictions. Some patients have an associated scoliosis, lumbar spondylolysis, endocrine abnormality, or inflammatory disorder.

Patients usually first report a postural deformity or pain over the kyphotic deformity. The pain tends to subside with the cessation of growth. On examination, the kyphosis is rigid and cannot be fully corrected with hyperextension. The neurologic examination is usually normal, because the kyphosis occurs gradually and over several segments. Lateral radiographs of the spine are used to evaluate vertebral wedging and measure the Cobb angle of the deformity; they may also reveal irregular vertebral end plates, narrowed disk spaces, and Schmorl's nodes. MRI is warranted to explore neurologic examination findings or rule out a disk herniation, if the patient is being considered for posterior surgical correction.

The indications for treatment of Scheuermann disease include pain, curve progression, and appearance of deformity. Exercise and physical therapy can be used to improve spine flexibility and strengthen the extensor muscles of the spine. Although few data exist to support casting or bracing, it can be used to treat a flexible, immature spine with more than 50° of kyphosis. Surgery may be considered to treat thoracic curves greater than 75° or thoracolumbar curves greater than 40° or to relieve pain that has failed to respond to nonsurgical measures (**Figure 9**). Posterior osteotomies and

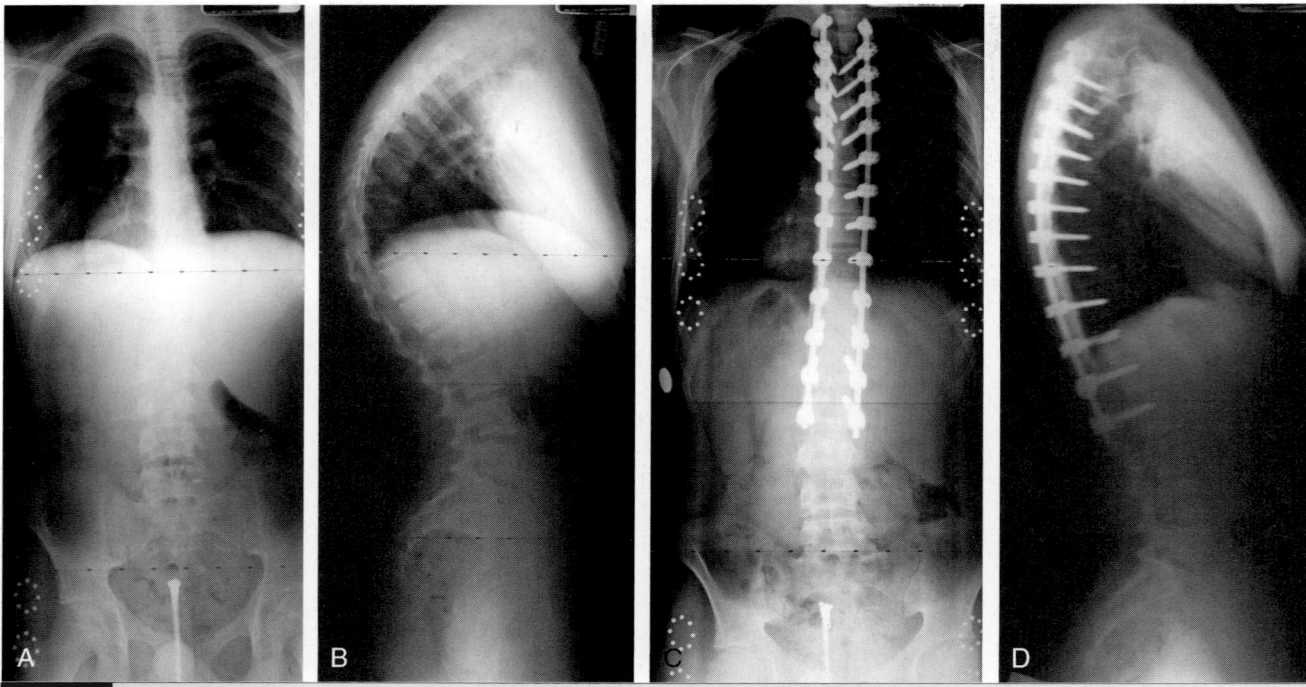

Figure 9   PA **(A)** and lateral **(B)** radiographs of a 16-year-old boy with 84° of Scheuermann kyphosis and multilevel anterior wedging. Postoperative PA **(C)** and lateral **(D)** radiographs after 10-level posterior spinal osteotomies and T2 through L2 posterior spinal instrumentation and fusion.

compression instrumentation have produced results similar to those of combined anterior release and posterior instrumentation.[38] Overcorrection of the deformity can lead to development of a junctional kyphosis, and, therefore, the postoperative kyphosis should rarely be less than 40°.

Spondylolysis and Spondylolisthesis

Spondylolysis is an isolated defect in the posterior elements of lumbar vertebrae that usually occurs at the L5 level. It can lead to spondylolisthesis, which is forward slippage of the vertebra onto the adjacent caudal vertebra. Only two of the five types of spondylolisthesis described in the literature have been reported in children: the dysplastic or congenital variety, in which the posterior bony arch is intact; and the more common isthmic variety, which is caused by a defect in the pars interarticularis.[39] Athletes, especially gymnasts whose activities accentuate lumbar lordosis, are at increased risk of spondylolisthesis. The intrinsic architecture of the pelvis and the stresses on the lumbosacral junction have been proposed as a mechanical etiology. A genetic factor may also be involved and may predispose certain patients to deterioration of bone healing capacity.[40]

Most patients with spondylolisthesis report localized low back pain that is exacerbated by activity and relieved by rest. However, spondylolisthesis can be asymptomatic, and it is sometimes discovered incidentally. The patient's symptoms and the physical examination findings usually determine the treatment. Radicular pain, which is uncommon in the pediatric patient,

may result from central or neuroforaminal stenosis at the level of the lytic defect. Worsening spondylolisthesis can lead to hamstring tightness or postural and gait changes.

A complete radiographic evaluation of the lumbosacral junction requires PA and spot lateral views. Right and left oblique views may also show the defect. CT can define bony anatomy and show defects in the transverse plane, and MRI is useful in identifying neural compression or a degenerated disk. The Meyerding and Boxall classification system can be used to grade the spondylolisthesis.[41] The slip angle, sagittal rotation, sacral inclination, and pelvic incidence can help determine the risk of slip progression.

Nonsurgical treatment can include observation, activity modification, exercise therapy, bracing, and pain management. Surgical options include reduction, decompression, instrumentation with repair of the defect, and single- or double-level fusion (**Figure 10**). Asymptomatic patients with low grade slip do not require treatment or activity modification. They should be followed radiographically every 6 months to 1 year until maturity. Symptomatic patients with low-grade slip should avoid contact sports and hyperextension of the back, and they should be treated with nonsurgical modalities.

High-grade slips (> 50%) require surgical stabilization. Significant debate exists regarding the optimal technique. For adolescents with a slip less than 50%, in situ fusion has been shown to be a safe and reliable procedure with high rates of arthrodesis.[42] Because slip

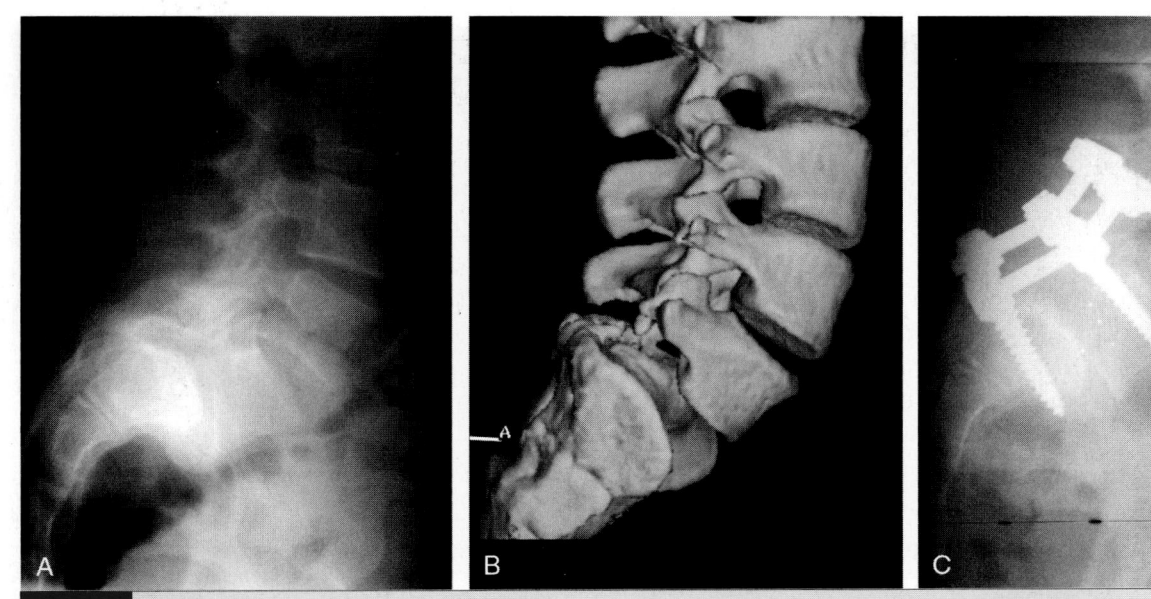

Figure 10 Imaging studies of a 15-year-old girl with low back and right posterior thigh pain. Lateral radiograph **(A)** and three-dimensional CT **(B)** revealed a grade III spondylolisthesis with a severe kyphotic deformity of L5-S1. **C,** Postoperative lateral radiograph after L5 bilateral laminectomy and decompression, L5-S1 interbody fusion, and L4 through S1 posterior spinal instrumentation and fusion.

progression and pseudarthrosis formation have been observed after in situ fusion, partial reduction of high-grade spondylolisthesis should be considered.[43] Kyphosis of L5 on S1 appears to be the most critical aspect of the deformity to correct. It is not necessary to reduce the slip completely, and doing so risks L5 nerve root stretch.[44] A partial reduction of high-grade spondylolisthesis generally includes L5 nerve root decompression and instrumentation as well as fusion from L4 to the sacrum. Anterior column support at L5-S1 can be accomplished using either an anterior or posterior approach.

Emerging Concepts and Future Directions

Pediatric spinal conditions differ from those in the adult population. Traumatic conditions require an understanding of the mechanisms of injury, as well as the healing and growth potential present. An area of active research is in the field of spinal cord regeneration. This field may be more promising in pediatric patients given their generally greater potential for healing. In addition, many questions remain in the field of pediatric spinal deformity, with regard to both etiology and long-term treatment outcomes. The genetic links to adolescent idiopathic scoliosis and Scheuermann kyphosis are clear; however, the responsible genes remain to be identified. Genetic markers for predicting curve progression are being sought that would allow more directed and early treatments to be developed. Unfortunately, many ultimate therapies in the spine involve a spinal fusion. This limits motion and concentrates stresses into adjacent nonfused segments that may result in premature degeneration. Advancements in motion-sparing solutions are required, particularly in pediatric populations who have many decades of life ahead.

Annotated References

1. Landin LA: Epidemiology of children's fractures. *J Pediatr Orthop B* 1997;6:79-83.

2. Finch GD, Barnes MJ: Major cervical spine injuries in children and adolescents. *J Pediatr Orthop* 1998;18:811-814.

3. McPhee IB: Spinal fracture and dislocations in children and adolescents. *Spine* 1981;6:533-537.

4. Carreon LY, Glassman SD, Campbell MJ: Pediatric spine fracture: A review of 137 hospital admissions. *J Spinal Disord Tech* 2004;17:477-482.

   Data from pediatric patients with spine injuries was reviewed. Age-related patterns of injury were noted.

5. Flynn JM, Closkey RF, Mahboubi S, et al: Role of magnetic resonance imaging in the assessment of pediatric cervical spine injuries. *J Pediatr Orthop* 2002;22:573-577.

6. Mubarak SJ, Camp JF, Vueltich W, et al: Halo application in the infant. *J Pediatr Orthop* 1989;9:612-614.

7. de Beer JD, Hoffman EB, Kieck CF: Traumatic atlanto-axial subluxation in children. *J Pediatr Orthop* 1990;10:397-400.

8. Hicazi A, Acaroqlu E, Alanay A, et al: Atlantoaxial rotatory fixation-subluxation revisited: A computed tomographic analysis of acute torticollis in pediatric patients. *Spine* 2002;27:27771-27775.

9. Subach BR, McLaughlin MR, Albright AL, et al: Current management of pediatric atlantoaxial rotatory subluxation. *Spine* 1998;23:2174-2179.

10. Powers B, Miller MD, Kramer RS, et al: Traumatic anterior atlanto-occipital dislocation. *Neurosurgery* 1979; 4:12-17.

11. Donahue DJ, Muhlbauer MS, Kaufman RA, Warner WC, Sanford RA: Childhood survival of atlanto-occipital dislocation: Underdiagnosis, recognition, treatment, and review of literature. *Pediatr Neurosurg* 1994; 21:105-111.

12. Dogan S, Safavi-Abbasi S, Theodore N: Pediatric subaxial cervical spine injuries: Origins, management, and outcome in 51 patients. *Neurosurg Focus* 2006; 20:E1.

    This study of 51 pediatric subaxial cervical spine injuries found that they are common in children 9 to 16 years of age and usually occur between C5 and C7. Most patients can be treated conservatively, although both anterior and posterior approaches are safe and effective.

13. Denis F: The three column spine and its significance in the classification of acute thoracolumbar spinal injuries. *Spine* 1983;8:817-831.

14. Davies KL: Buckled-up children: Understanding the mechanism, injuries, management, and prevention of seat belt related injuries. *J Trauma Nurs* 2004;11:16-24.

    This comprehensive overview of pediatric seat belt injuries includes exploration of the mechanisms responsible for typical patterns of injury, recognition of injuries during trauma assessment, diagnostic evaluation, and management of children with suspected or actual seat belt injuries.

15. Gertzbein SD, Court-Brown CM: Flexion-distraction injuries of the lumbar spine: Mechanisms of injury and classification. *Clin Orthop Relat Res* 1988;227:52-60.

16. Platzer P, Jaindl M, Thalhammer G, et al: Cervical spine injuries in pediatric patients. *J Trauma* 2007;62:389-396.

    This retrospective review was performed to determine the incidence and characteristics of pediatric cervical spine injuries after trauma. High rates of mortality and neurologic deficit in this patient population were reported.

17. Akbarnia BA: Pediatric spine fractures. *Orthop Clin North Am* 1999;30:521-536.

18. McCall T, Fassett D, Brockmeyer D: Cervical spine trauma in children: A review. *Neurosurg Focus* 2006;20:E5.

    This review of cervical spine injuries in children concludes that the unique biomechanics of the pediatric cervical spine lead to a different distribution of injuries and distinct radiographic features.

19. Bracken MB, Holford TR: Neurological and functional status 1 year after acute spinal cord injury: Estimates of functional recovery in National Acute Spinal Cord Injury Study II from results modeled in National Acute Spinal Cord Injury Study III. *J Neurosurg* 2002;96 (suppl 3):259-266.

20. Sayer FT, Kronvall E, Nilsson OG: Methylprednisolone treatment in acute spinal cord injury: The myth challenged through a structured analysis of published literature. *Spine J* 2006;6:335-343.

    This study evaluated the scientific basis for the use of methylprednisolone in acute spinal cord injury and found insufficient evidence to support its use as a standard treatment.

21. Sankar WN, Wills BP, Dormans JP, et al: Os odontoideum revisited: The case for a multifactorial etiology. *Spine* 2006;31:979-984.

    A retrospective analysis found two separate etiologies for os odontoideum: posttraumatic and congenital. The implication is that os odontoideum can develop without previous trauma in some children with a preexisting syndrome.

22. Farley FA, Loder RT, Nolan BT, et al: Mouse model for thoracic congenital scoliosis. *J Pediatr Orthop* 2001;21: 537-540.

23. Stiefel D, Shibata T, Meuli M, et al: Tethering of the spinal cord in mouse fetuses and neonates with spina bifida. *J Neurosurg* 2003;99(suppl 2):206-213.

24. Yamada S, Won DJ, Siddiqi J, et al: Tethered cord syndrome: Overview of diagnosis and treatment. *Neurol Res* 2004;26:719-721.

    The authors report on the basis of tethered cord syndrome as a stretch-induced spinal cord disorder, including pathophysiology, signs and symptoms, imaging diagnosis, indication for surgical treatment, and surgical procedures.

25. Guo X, Chau WW, Chan YL, et al: Relative anterior spinal overgrowth in adolescent idiopathic scoliosis: Results of disproportionate endochondral-membranous bone growth. *J Bone Joint Surg Br* 2003;85:1026-1031.

26. Benli IT, Uzumcugil O, Aydin E, et al: Magnetic resonance imaging abnormalities of neural axis in Lenke type 1 idiopathic scoliosis. *Spine* 2006;31:1828-1833.

    Preoperative MRI of 104 patients with Lenke type I scoliosis showed that age of onset and back pain can be used to predict neural axis abnormalities.

27. Mehta MH: The rib-vertebra angle in the early diagnosis between resolving and progressive infantile scoliosis. *J Bone Joint Surg Br* 1972;54:230-243.

28. Charles YP, Daures JP, de Rosa V, et al: Progression risk of idiopathic juvenile scoliosis during pubertal growth. *Spine* 2006;31:1933-1942.

A retrospective review of 205 patients with juvenile scoliosis found that curve pattern, Cobb angle at onset of puberty, and curve progression velocity were the strongest factors predicting curve progression.

29. Dimeglio A, Charles YP, Daures JP, et al: Accuracy of the Sauvegrain method in determining skeletal age during puberty. *J Bone Joint Surg Am* 2005;87:1689-1696.

The modified Sauvegrain method was shown to be simple, reliable, and reproducible. It complements the Greulich and Pyle hand atlas to assess skeletal age during the 2 years of the pubertal growth spurt.

30. Rowe DE, Bernstein SM, Riddick MF, et al: A meta-analysis of the efficacy of non-operative treatments for idiopathic scoliosis. *J Bone Joint Surg Am* 1997;79:664-674.

31. King HA, Moe JH, Bradford DS, et al: The selection of fusion levels in thoracic idiopathic scoliosis. *J Bone Joint Surg Am* 1983;65:1302-1313.

32. Lenke LG, Edwards CC II, Bridwell KH: The Lenke classification of adolescent idiopathic scoliosis: How it organizes curve patterns as a template to perform selective fusions of the spine. *Spine* 2003;28:S199-S207.

33. Potter BK, Kuklo TR, Lenke LG: Radiographic outcomes of anterior spinal fusion versus posterior spinal fusion with thoracic pedicle screws for treatment of Lenke Type I adolescent idiopathic scoliosis curves. *Spine* 2005;30:1859-1866.

A retrospective review of 40 patients with adolescent idiopathic scoliosis comparing curve correction and derotation following anterior spinal fusion versus posterior spinal fusion with thoracic pedicle screws found that posterior spinal fusion with thoracic pedicle screws provided superior results with, on average, only one additional spinal segment fused.

34. Newton PO, White KK, Faro F, et al: The success of thoracoscopic anterior fusion in a consecutive series of 112 pediatric spinal deformity cases. *Spine* 2005;30:392-398.

A review of 112 consecutive cases of thoracoscopic anterior release and fusion with open posterior instrumentation and fusion showed it to be a safe and effective procedure.

35. Hurford RK Jr, Lenke LG, Lee SS, et al: Prospective radiographic and clinical outcomes of dual-rod instrumented anterior spinal fusion in adolescent idiopathic scoliosis: Comparison with single-rod constructs. *Spine* 2006;31:2322-2328.

A retrospective review of 60 consecutive patients with adolescent idiopathic scoliosis comparing the results of anterior dual-rod instrumentation with a historical cohort of single-rod constructs found a similar amount of radiographic deformity correction with the absence of any pseudarthroses.

36. Merola AA, Haher TR, Brkaric M, et al: A multicenter study of the outcomes of the surgical treatment of adolescent idiopathic scoliosis using the Scoliosis Research Society (SRS) outcome instrument. *Spine* 2002;27:2046-2051.

37. Smith PL, Donaldson S, Hedden D, et al: Parents' and patients' perceptions of postoperative appearance in adolescent idiopathic scoliosis. *Spine* 2006;31:2367-2374.

This cross-sectional survey revealed that patients and parents did not strongly agree with one another on the cosmetic outcome of surgery to treat adolescent idiopathic scoliosis and that radiographic and physical measures of deformity were not highly correlated with patients' and parents' perceptions of appearance.

38. Papagelopoulos PJ, Klassen RA, Peterson HA, et al: Surgical treatment of Scheuermann's disease with segmental compression instrumentation. *Clin Orthop Relat Res* 2001;386:139-149.

39. Wiltse LL, Newman PH, Macnab I: Classification of spondylolysis and spondylolisthesis. *Clin Orthop Relat Res* 1976;117:23-29.

40. Komatsubara S, Sairyo K, Katho S, et al: High-grade slippage of the lumbar spine in a rat model of spondylolisthesis: Effects of cyclooxygenase-2 inhibitor on its deformity. *Spine* 2006;31:E528-E534.

Radiographic and histologic evaluation of spondylolisthesis in a rat model found that poor bone healing was one of the determinants of high-grade spondylolisthesis in children and adolescents.

41. Boxall D, Bradford DS, Winter RB, et al: Management of severe spondylolisthesis in children and adolescents. *J Bone Joint Surg Am* 1979;61:479-495.

42. Hensinger RN: Spondylolysis and spondylolisthesis in children and adolescents. *J Bone Joint Surg Am* 1989;71:1098-1106.

43. Lenke LG, Bridwell KH: Evaluation and surgical treatment of high-grade isthmic dysplastic spondylolisthesis. *Instr Course Lect* 2003;52:525-532.

44. Bradford DS, Gotfried Y: Staged salvage reconstruction of grade IV and V spondylolisthesis. *J Bone Joint Surg Am* 1987;69:191-202.

Chapter 58

Hip, Pelvis, and Femur Trauma: Pediatrics

Paul D. Sponseller, MD

Introduction

Injury to the pelvis or femur is common in children after major trauma. The treatment of children differs from that of adults with a similar injury because of the immature skeleton's small stature, growth potential, and mechanical properties.

Pelvic Fractures

Characteristics

Pediatric pelvic fractures most often occur when the child is involved in a motor vehicle accident, either as a passenger or a pedestrian. Iliac wing and single pelvic ring breaks account for more than 60% of pediatric pelvic fractures. Physical examination detects only 70% of pelvic fractures, so an AP pelvic radiograph is recommended for all pediatric blunt trauma patients.[1]

A significant force is required to cause a pelvic fracture, and, because a child's pelvis is more elastic than an adult's, it can more easily absorb the force. Most pediatric pelvic fractures are the result of lateral compression forces. Injury patterns in children are different from those in adults; instability and hemorrhage occur less often, and avulsion injuries, which are rare in adults, are common in children. In the immature pelvis, the bone apparently fails before the ligaments. At least partly as a result, unstable ring disruptions are rare in children. Vertically unstable or anteroposterior compression fractures are less common in children than adults. The mortality rate after a pelvic fracture is 5% for children and 17% for adults.[1]

Fracture patterns change significantly as the pelvis becomes more mature. One recent study found that patients with open triradiate cartilages had significantly fewer difficult fracture patterns (acetabular fractures or pubic or sacroiliac disruptions) than those with closed triradiate cartilages, and only patients with closed triradiate cartilages required surgery.[2] The triradiate cartilage closes at approximately age 12.5 years in girls and age 13.5 years in boys.

Treatment

Children with pelvic fractures have better outcomes when they are treated at a pediatric trauma center.[3] Those with minor injuries can be mobilized as tolerated, if their pelvic stability is not compromised. A spica cast can be used for an unstable unilateral pelvic fracture with minimal asymmetry. In an anteroposterior compression fracture of the open-book type, a diastasis of more than 2.5 cm should be reduced using external or internal fixation (**Figure 1**). Significant pelvic asymmetry should be reduced by surgical methods; anterior and posterior fixation is most likely to achieve reduction. In a child, the pins for an external fixator should be inserted through small incisions near the anterosuperior iliac spine. The cartilage apophysis complicates pin insertion; a small incision into the cartilage down to bone facilitates the insertion.

Complications

Limited remodeling may occur after a pediatric pelvic fracture, but it cannot be relied on to restore pelvic symmetry.[4] Complications after an imperfect reduction can include scoliosis, apparent limb-length inequality, low back pain, and abnormal gait. Triradiate cartilage injuries can cause acetabular undergrowth, but this complication is rare and only affects children injured when they were younger than 10 years.[3,4]

Acetabular Fractures

Characteristics and Imaging

Plain radiography, followed by thin-slice CT with multiplanar reconstruction, offers the most detailed view of acetabular fractures. The Watts classification of injuries to the pediatric acetabulum has been widely used for more than 30 years.[5] Watts type A is a dislocation with a small osteochondral fracture, type B is a linear nondisplaced fracture, type C is displacement of the weight-bearing dome, and type D is a central acetabular fracture or dislocation. Injury to the triradiate cartilage is a rare form of transverse acetabular fracture. After the triradiate cartilage closes, these injuries are classified, as they are for adults, as an anterior column, posterior column, or wall fracture.[6-8]

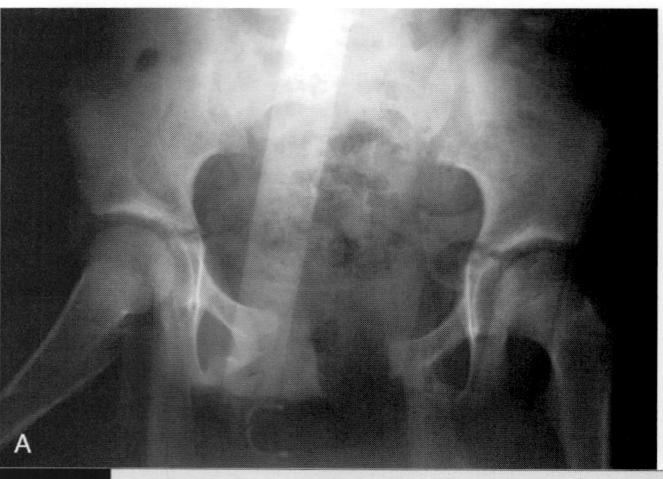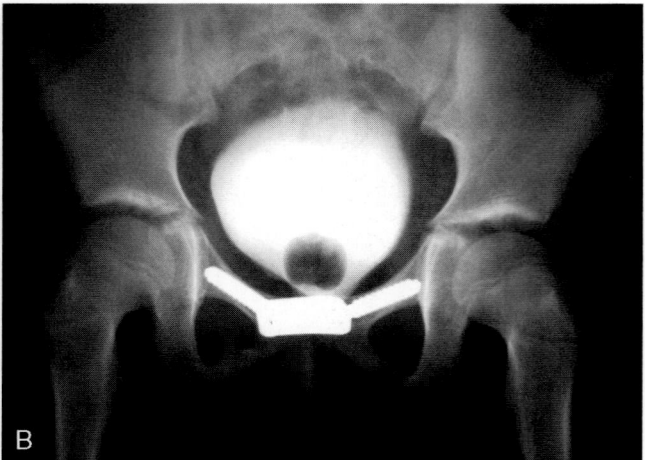

Figure 1   **A,** Radiograph showing AP compression fracture of the pelvis with 4.5 cm of widening in a 9-year-old girl. **B,** Postoperative radiograph showing plate fixation.

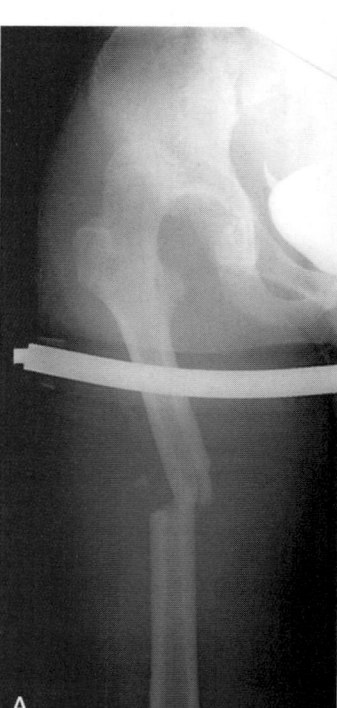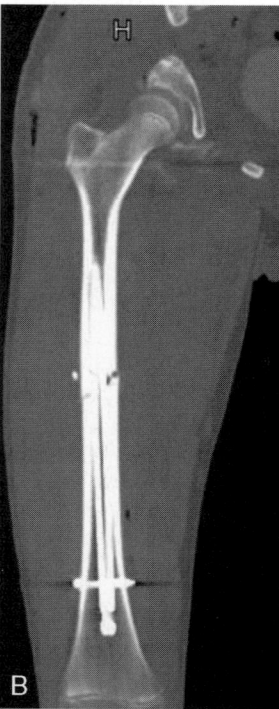

Figure 2   **A,** Fluoroscopic AP radiograph showing a fracture-dislocation of the femur in a 14-year-old boy. **B,** CT scan showing congruous reduction and no interposed fragments after reduction under general anesthesia and fluoroscopy, followed by internal fixation of the femur with a trochanteric nail.

Treatment

Closed reduction of a fracture-dislocation should be performed within 6 to 8 hours after injury, if possible. Plain radiography, CT, or both should be used to assess the congruity of the reduction, which may be compromised by interposed capsule, labrum, or osteochondral fractures. Intra-articular fractures that involve more

than 20% of the posterior wall and are displaced more than 2 mm are best treated with open reduction and internal fixation.

Complications

Osteonecrosis and stiffness or degeneration may occur after an acetabular fracture.[6] A posterior wall fracture may be missed and lead to late incongruity if the fracture allows subluxation of the femoral head.

Hip Dislocations

Characteristics and Treatment

Hip dislocations occur with less force in a young child than in a person who is skeletally mature, presumably because of the child's unossified acetabular cartilage and capsular laxity. A posterior dislocation is more common than an anterior dislocation. Before the teenage years, hip dislocations commonly result from play and sports activities. In teenagers, they more commonly result from a motor vehicle crash. A reduction should be performed within 6 hours of the trauma, to decrease the risk of osteonecrosis.[9] Epiphyseal separation during the reduction process has been reported numerous times in children older than 11 years; the cause is believed to be unrecognized physeal injury at the time of dislocation, leading to displacement during the reduction process.[10] For patients in this age range, the use of fluoroscopic visualization during reduction is recommended (Figure 2). If physeal widening is detected during the reduction maneuver, treatment is with internal fixation of the femoral head with a cannulated screw before reduction.

After reduction, a pelvic radiograph, arthrogram, or CT scan should be obtained to detect any intra-articular cartilaginous or osteocartilaginous fragments. These should be removed, if significant. A spica cast or brace is used for young children, and older children are

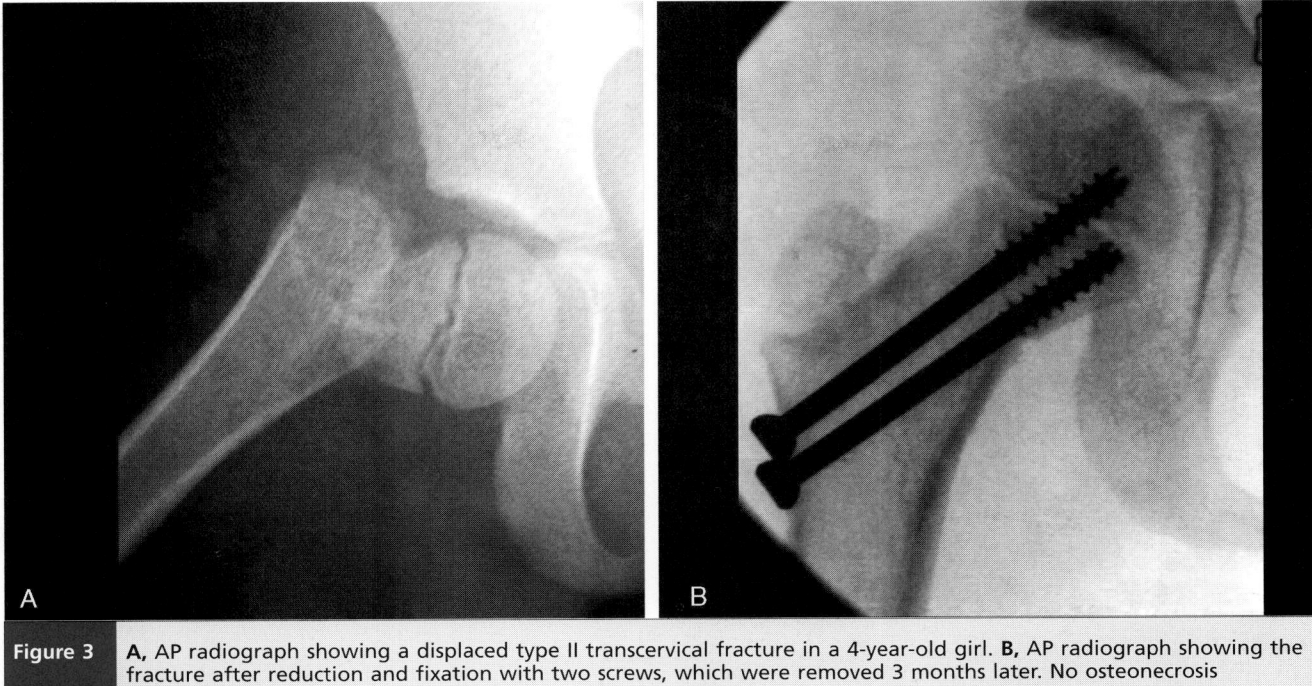

Figure 3 **A,** AP radiograph showing a displaced type II transcervical fracture in a 4-year-old girl. **B,** AP radiograph showing the fracture after reduction and fixation with two screws, which were removed 3 months later. No osteonecrosis occurred.

advised against full flexion or adduction. Monitoring for osteonecrosis should continue for 1 year. The risk of osteonecrosis is approximately 10%, and redislocation is rare.

Femoral Neck Fractures

Background and Classification

Hip fracture is rare in children, but it is noteworthy as a high-energy injury that is frequently accompanied by other injuries and has a risk of serious complications, such as osteonecrosis, nonunion, and malunion. The simple, widely known Delbet system classifies a hip fracture as type I (transphyseal separation), II (midcervical fracture), III (basicervical fracture), or IV (intertrochanteric fracture).[11]

A type I fracture, the rarest type, usually is seen in infants and in children age 2 to 6 years. It can occur as a result of a difficult childbirth or child abuse. In adolescents, a type I fracture often occurs during reduction of a hip dislocation. Hip dislocations and acetabular rim fractures are noted in approximately 50% of patients. Type II fractures occur in all age groups and are the most common type. The risk of osteonecrosis is approximately 50%.[11,12] In type III, the second most common, the risk of osteonecrosis is approximately 25%.[13] Coxa vara can occur, especially if anatomic reduction and stable fixation are not achieved. Type IV fractures are slightly more common than type I and have the best outcomes; the risk of osteonecrosis is small, and the remodeling potential is great.

Treatment

Anatomic reduction is essential for a type I, II, or III fracture.[11] In this area of pediatric trauma, stable fixation clearly improves results. The surgeon should not hesitate to place fixation across the physis in a child who is older than 12 years. In a younger child, casting for 6 weeks is usually recommended if fixation is stopped short of the physis.

A closed reduction of a type I fracture without dislocation, followed by internal fixation, can be performed under sedation or general anesthesia. Any intracapsular hematoma should be evacuated by aspiration or open means. Smooth Steinmann pins or cannulated screws can be used for fixation. Screws should be removed immediately after healing to promote continued physeal growth. Spica casting for 3 to 4 weeks can be used to protect Steinmann pins and promote healing. The presence of a hip dislocation increases the risk of osteonecrosis and decreases the likelihood of a successful closed reduction in a type I fracture. A single, careful attempt at closed reduction is acceptable, but if reduction is not achieved, open reduction from the direction of dislocation is necessary. Some surgeons believe that the blood supply is more likely to be preserved if open reduction is performed without closed manipulation.[11]

A type II fracture should be internally fixed even if nondisplaced, because of the risk of displacement and resulting coxa vara. Anatomic reduction often can be achieved by closed means and can be followed by percutaneous fixation (**Figure 3**). High-quality intraoperative imaging is needed. Hip aspiration may decrease the risk of osteonecrosis by lowering intracapsular pres-

6: Pediatrics

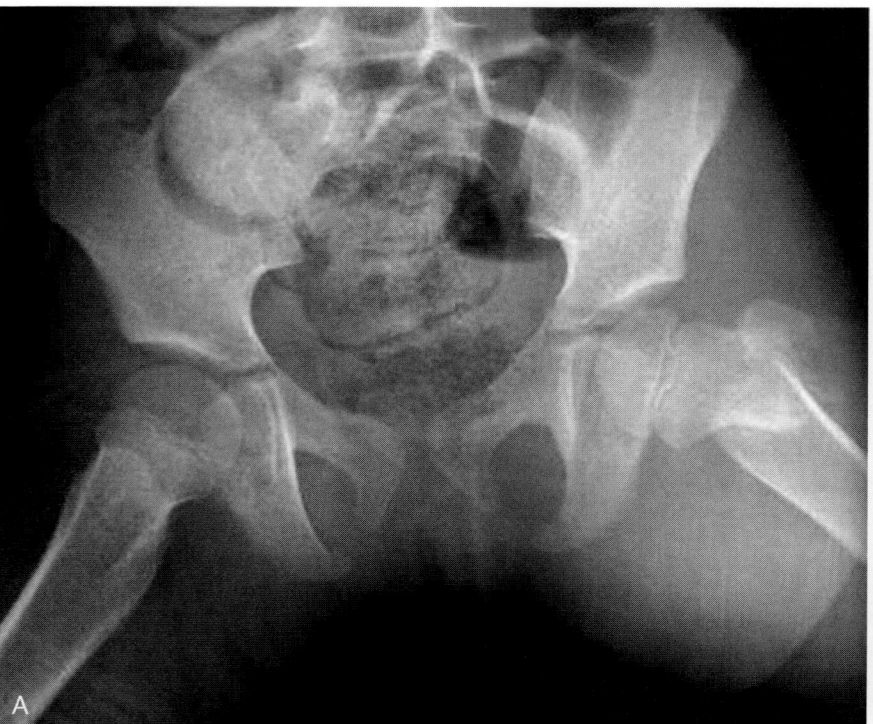
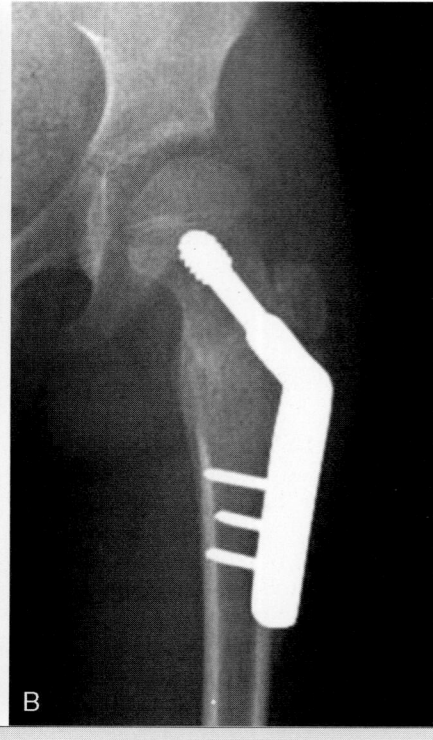

Figure 4　**A,** AP radiograph showing a displaced type IV cervicotrochanteric fracture in a 5-year-old girl. **B,** AP radiograph showing the fracture after open reduction and plate fixation.

sure. If anatomic reduction cannot be achieved by closed means, the surgeon should use open fracture reduction. A direct anterior Smith-Peterson approach to the fracture can be used, followed by percutaneous fixation; or a lateral Watson-Jones approach can be used for both the fracture and the fixation. The ideal fixation devices are cannulated screws. If the fracture is distal enough, fixation can stop short of the physis. However, adequate fixation is important, and crossing the physis is permissible if the surgeon believes it is necessary. Removal of the pin or the screw when the fracture heals should prevent compromise of the growth potential of the physis. The rigidity of the fixation also determines the need for postoperative immobilization. If fixation is not rigid or the screw is not placed across the physis, spica casting for 4 to 6 weeks is indicated.[14]

A type III fracture can be treated by open or closed reduction and stabilized with either a screw and side plate or two or three cannulated screws. Weight bearing should be restricted until the fracture has healed. For a type IV fracture, good results are achievable using traction followed by spica casting, immediate spica casting (if the displacement is minimal), or internal fixation (**Figure 4**). If a noninvasive treatment is chosen, the spica cast should be applied in the extended-abducted position, and less than 25° of coronal angulation should be accepted. For most patients, open reduction and internal fixation with a screw and side plate is used.

Complications

Osteonecrosis is progressively less likely to occur from type I to type IV fractures. However, the risk of osteonecrosis increases in all types of fracture with the degree of displacement and the patient's age.[13] The preferred treatment is protected weight bearing for at least 3 months, and for 6 to 9 months after a type I fracture. The early radiographic signs of osteonecrosis include the greater relative density of the epiphysis and a subchondral crescent seen on an AP or lateral view. Bone scanning with blood-pool images can be used 3 months after a high-risk femoral neck fracture to assess blood flow to the femoral head. If osteonecrosis is present and subchondral collapse occurs, the implant may need to be removed. No surgical treatment has been proved to alter the outcome if osteonecrosis occurs. However, in an older child (age 8 to 10 years), early core decompression, external distraction, or vascularized fibular grafting can be used before the femoral head collapses. The results of a collapse resemble those of Legg-Calvé-Perthes disease; the child may have several decades of satisfactory function. The surgeon should therefore try to maintain motion and alignment throughout the reossification phase rather than proceed immediately to arthrodesis or arthroplasty.

The likelihood of nonunion is related to the quality of the fixation. Nonunion should be treated quickly, with valgus osteotomy and improved fixation, with or without a dowel-type bone graft. Coxa vara or coxa valga can occur because of an imperfect reduction, loss of reduction, or later growth disturbance. Remodeling is possible after an imperfect reduction or loss of reduction, if the malposition is less than 25°. Premature physeal closure is of consequence only in a child younger than approximately 8 years; if limb-length inequality exceeds 2 cm, epiphysiodesis may be offered. A Trendelenburg gait may result from the relative trochanteric overgrowth. Trochanteric transfer is a late option, if the patient is bothered by the limp. Other complications include chondrolysis, late degeneration, and stress fracture resulting from a retained implant.

Subtrochanteric Femur Fractures

Characteristics
A subtrochanteric femur fracture in a child is defined as occurring below the lesser trochanter and within the proximal 10% of the femur.[15] These fractures tend to affect younger children and have some characteristics of hip fractures and shaft fractures. They have excellent rates of union and significant remodeling potential, as well as a tendency for femoral overgrowth similar to that of a diaphyseal fracture.

Treatment
Virtually all of the treatment options can produce satisfactory results.[15-17] In a young child, a spica cast should be used only if less than 3 cm of shortening or 30° of angulation is present, because shortening and angulation are difficult to control in a cast. A period of 2 to 3 weeks in traction followed by spica casting provides good control of length and angulation.[17] The hip should be in extension in a spica cast so that the alignment can be seen on radiographs. External fixation is feasible, because room is usually present for two or more pins, both proximally and distally. The fixator or a subsequent cast should be used until the fracture callus is well corticated. The use of retrograde elastic nails is successful if they are inserted high into the neck on the medial side and into the trochanteric apophysis on the lateral side.[15] Submuscular or open plate fixation produces good results, as does rigid pertrochanteric nailing in adolescents.

Femoral Shaft Fractures

Background
A femoral shaft fracture is the most common major pediatric condition that most orthopaedic surgeons encounter on a regular basis. The considerations differ by age group.[18,19]

Cortical thickness increases dramatically throughout childhood. As a result, a mechanism such as a fall is more likely to cause a fracture in an infant or young child than in an adult. As children grow older, falling, being struck by a vehicle, and being involved in a motor vehicle crash (as a passenger or driver) are successively the most common causes of a femoral shaft fracture.[20]

Nonaccidental injury, such as from child abuse, accounts for 25% to 50% of fractures in children younger than 1 year; the risk drops significantly after the child acquires walking and language skills.[18,21] The diagnosis of nonaccidental injury is rarely straightforward. Immediate diagnosis is possible only if the patient has multiple, simultaneous unexplained fractures or a physeal fracture with a metaphyseal corner extension. In all other patients, a careful history, complete physical examination, and, sometimes, evaluation of the family situation by a child protection team are necessary. A detailed history can be important in assessing the level of suspicion. For example, a careful analysis showed that the plausibility of stair falls as a cause of injury can be scored objectively.[22] A history of a true fall should include a description of the child's starting and ending position as well as the cause of the fall. The mechanism of injury should be consistent with the fracture pattern, and no unrelated soft-tissue injuries should be present. A buckle fracture is consistent with a child falling on his or her own leg, a spiral fracture is consistent with the child landing while in motion, and a transverse fracture is consistent with an older, heavier person falling onto the child. The caregiver should have sought medical attention promptly. By considering such factors, the orthopaedic surgeon should be able to develop an informed opinion about the likelihood of nonaccidental injury. It is important to avoid making unsubstantiated inferences about the mechanism of an injury or likelihood of abuse.

Characteristics
Femur fractures can be classified as transverse, oblique, spiral, greenstick, or comminuted. They can be further classified by location as proximal, midshaft, or distal. Pathologic fractures are uncommon, although they can occur because of nonossifying fibromas, fibrous dysplasia, or unicameral bone cysts. More rarely, they are caused by underlying generalized osseous fragility. All of these factors can affect the treatment selection.[18]

Treatment
Although the treatment options and their relative frequency of use continue to change, most of the options produce good results. The preferred treatments vary by patient age and fracture characteristics (**Table 1**). The following guidelines can be adjusted to fit the size and weight of the patient.

Spica Cast
Children 5 years of age or younger usually are best managed with early application of a spica cast. Some surgeons prefer to use a Pavlik harness for infants younger than 6 months.[23] If the fracture is expected to cause only modest shortening, the spica cast is appropriate for young children because these children weigh relatively little and are usually not in school full time. If the possibility of nonaccidental injury is being investigated, the child may need to be admitted for comprehensive evaluation before the cast is applied. Infants

Table 1

Age-Based Options for Treatment of Femoral Fractures

Ages 0 to 6 years

Early spica cast
If shortening is > 2.5 cm
    Flexible intramedullary nails
    External fixator
    Open plate
    Traction for 2 to 3 weeks, followed by spica cast

Ages 7 to 11 years

Flexible intramedullary nails
External fixator
Bridge plate
Open plate
Traction for 2 to 3 weeks, followed by spica cast

Ages 12 to 16 years

Transtrochanteric nail
External fixator
Plate (open or bridge)

can be immobilized in a Gore-Tex-lined spica cast for ease of cleaning. After a low-energy injury, a single-leg spica cast seems to provide adequate immobilization for a young child, with greater ease of management than a double-leg spica cast.[24] Because a spica cast does not control shortening well, other treatment methods should be considered for children with more than 3 cm overlap of the fracture at rest.[25]

A spica cast can be applied in the emergency department with the patient under sedation or in an operating room with the patient under general anesthesia (Figure 5). An infant with a low-energy fracture can be placed into a spica cast with the aid of simple analgesics. Cast application requires the assistance of at least one knowledgeable person. The long leg portion is typically applied, molded, and allowed to harden before the remainder of the cast is applied. A narrow medial-lateral mold helps to control angulation of the fracture. Alignment should be neutral to slight valgus, because the fracture may drift into varus with time. It is important to avoid excessive pressure from the cast onto the popliteal region of the injured leg.[25,26] The shortening should not exceed 1.5 cm at initial cast application or 2.5 cm at follow-up. The initial angulation should not exceed 10° in the coronal plane or 20° in the sagittal plane; increased angulation can usually be controlled within the first 3 weeks by wedging of the cast. A special vehicle restraint is necessary for safe automobile transport of the child. The time to healing ranges from 4 weeks in an infant to 8 weeks in an older child. Phys-

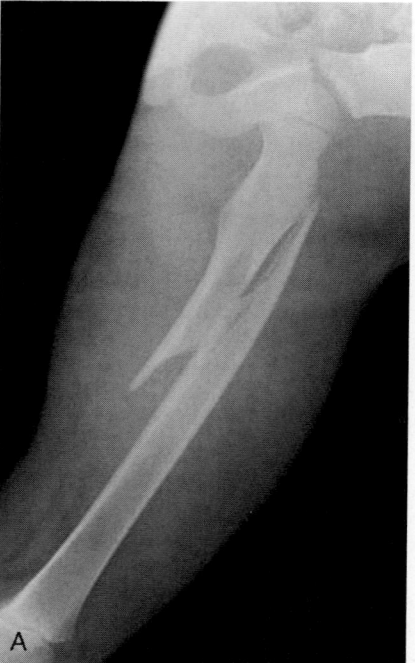
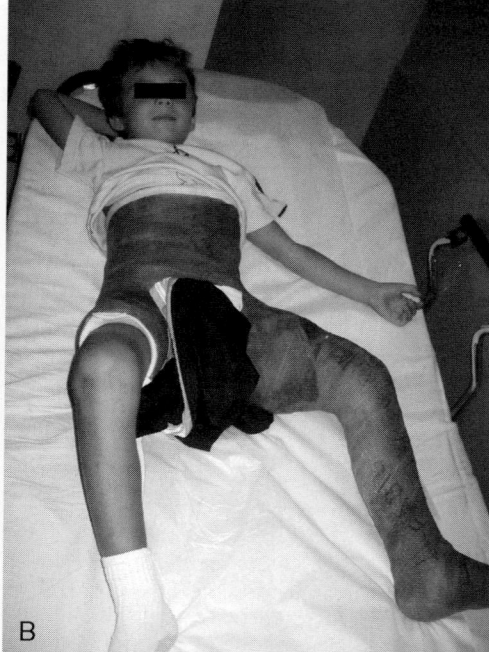
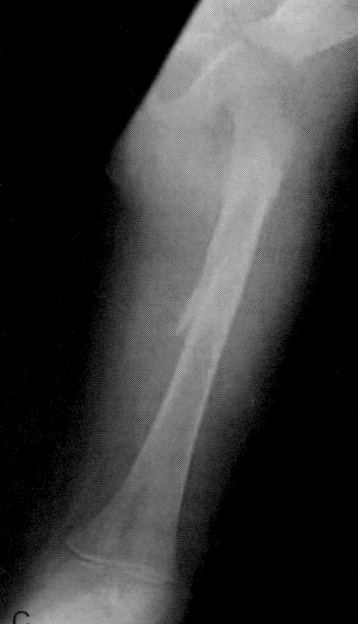

Figure 5 **A,** Lateral radiograph showing a spiral femur fracture in a 5-year-old boy. **B,** The patient after immediate outpatient treatment with a hip spica cast. **C,** AP Radiograph showing healing with 2 cm shortening; the patient had no limp after 2 months. Care was taken to keep knee flexion less than 90° in the spica cast and to contour the popliteal area smoothly.

ical therapy is not routinely necessary after cast removal.

For a child whose fracture has significant initial shortening or early shortening in the cast, skeletal traction can be applied after a traction pin is inserted into the distal femur. After early callus has formed at 2 to 3 weeks, a spica cast can be applied with little risk of shortening. If shortening in the cast exceeds 2.5 cm before consolidation, switching to another treatment method is recommended.

Spica cast treatment can produce pressure-related complications, such as popliteal skin breakdown, compartment syndrome, or palsy of the tibial or peroneal nerves.[25,26] The risk of complications can be minimized by keeping the popliteal region smoothly padded, avoiding flexion greater than 90°, and avoiding excessive traction through the cast. The patient's neurologic and vascular function, as well as comfort, should be checked before and after discharge.

Flexible Nails
Flexible (elastic) intramedullary nails are preferred for treating children between 6 and 11 years of age[18] (Figure 6). The bend in an elastic nail provides three-point contact inside the femur and allows rapid mobilization in carefully selected patients. The risk of complications is greater if the child weighs more than 100 lb or is older than 11 years, or if the child has osteoporosis, a very proximal or distal fracture, or a length-unstable fracture with a large butterfly fragment, long spiral, or additional cortical crack.[19,27,28]

The nails are inserted retrograde with the patient lying on a fluorolucent table. The diameter of the nail should be about 40% of the diameter of the femoral canal at the isthmus. The nails are introduced through small medial and lateral incisions, entering bone 1.5 to 2 cm proximal to the distal femoral physis. For proximal fractures, the nails should be advanced as far into the proximal femoral canal as possible. They should protrude to the level of the physis but not bend outward. An ideal transverse or short oblique fracture can be impacted and does not need external immobilization. For a borderline length-unstable fracture, a simple spica cast involving just the waist and the thigh can help prevent excessive shortening and angulation. The time required for union is approximately 10 weeks. Most surgeons recommend removal of the rod at healing.

Complications occur in as many as 17% of patients treated with flexible nails. They include wound infection, nail back-out, shortening, angulation, and nonunion. Complications are more common in older, heavier children and those with length-unstable fractures.[27,28] These patients may be better managed with a more rigid treatment option. The risk of wound complications can be minimized by ensuring that the incisions are large enough, protecting the skin during insertion, débriding damaged skin at the end of the procedure, and not allowing the rod ends to flare outward.

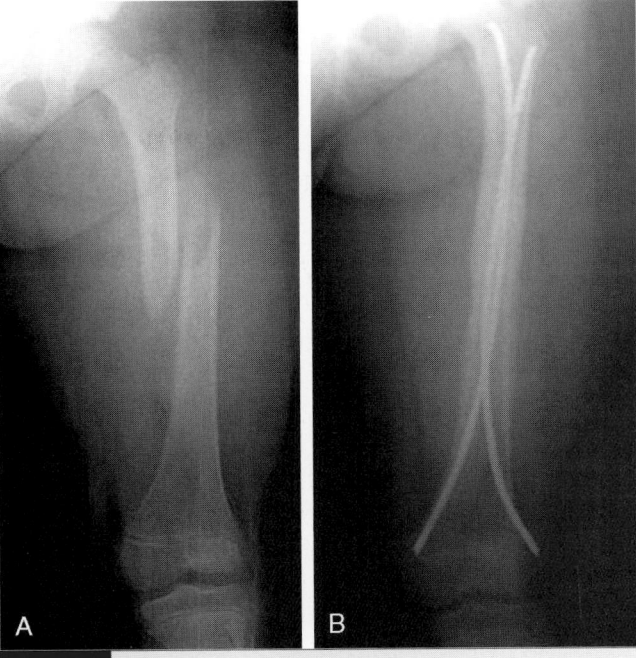

Figure 6 **A,** AP radiograph showing a femur fracture in a 7-year-old girl. **B,** AP radiograph showing fixation with titanium elastic nails, which were used because of the patient's age and length-stable fracture pattern.

External Fixation
Although external fixation is rarely a definitive treatment option for femur fractures in adults, it is a much better option for children, because of a child's ability to bridge osseous gaps even in the presence of stress shielding. External fixation is a versatile treatment method; satisfactory results have been reported in children of all ages and for most fracture locations and patterns.[29] Most femur fractures can be managed with two pins inserted into each fragment and a single monolateral bar. Older or larger patients may require additional fixation.

The mean healing time after external fixation is 11.5 weeks, which is more than other methods require. Pin tract infections are common, but they respond well to cleaning and oral antibiotics. The most important drawback to external fixation is the rate of refracture after removal, either through the small, weak callus or a pin hole. The risk is lower if the fracture has a large area of bone contact, as is found in a spiral or long oblique fracture. The risk can be minimized by delaying removal of the fixator until maturing of the callus can be observed as a smooth border on at least three of the four edges of combined AP and lateral radiographs.[30] If the fixator is removed before callus maturation is seen, refracture can be prevented by application for 1 month of a simple waist-to-thigh spica cast.

Compression Plate
Plate fixation has a high union rate, but a long incision is needed and significant blood loss often occurs. It is

6. Pediatrics

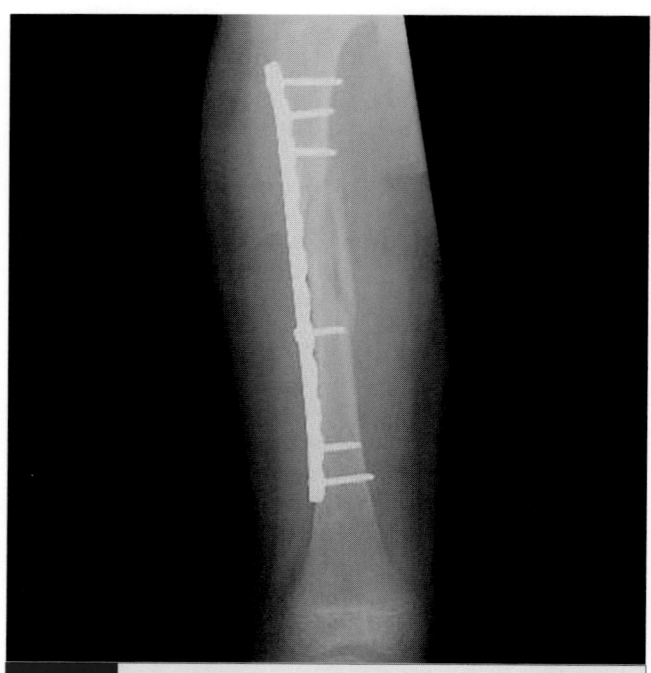

Figure 7 AP radiograph showing a proximal femur fracture with significant medial comminution in an 8-year-old boy. Because of the length-unstable pattern and the patient's age, the fracture was fixed with a submuscular bridge plate.

most useful if fluoroscopy is not available, as in a trauma emergency. At least six cortices of fixation above and below the fracture should be obtained. Refracture and plate failure have been reported in most large pediatric studies of patients treated with plate fixation.[31]

Submuscular Plate

Submuscular or bridge plating has biologic and mechanical advantages because it does not require fracture stripping or stress shielding. It is useful for treating length-unstable fractures and fractures in larger children (**Figure 7**).[32,33] The plate should have 12 to 15 holes. The use of locking plates is only necessary if osteoporosis is present. The plate is bent to the contour of the femur and introduced extraperiosteally from distal to proximal. After the reduction is held with Steinmann pins, three screws are dispersed widely on each side of the fracture. No weight bearing is allowed until callus can be seen on radiographs.

Rigid Intramedullary Rod Fixation

Rigid intramedullary rod fixation is the most stable option. Its only drawbacks are the reported risk of osteonecrosis and the potential effects on the growth of the proximal femur. Osteonecrosis has been reported in 1% of children younger than 15 years if a nail was inserted into the piriformis fossa. However, no risk has been reported if the nail was inserted through the trochanter, with a starting point lateral to the tip (**Figure**

2).[34,35] This method has no significant effect on the growth of the femur.[36] Several nails having small diameters are available for use in young patients; they are designed to be inserted through the trochanter. Experts differ on the age at which this method of fixation is preferred, but the range is 10 to 14 years.

Annotated References

1. Junkins EP, Nelson DS: A prospective evaluation of the clinical presentation of pediatric pelvic fractures. *J Trauma* 2001;51:64-68.

2. Silber JS, Flynn JM: Changing patterns of pediatric pelvic fractures with skeletal maturation: Implications for classification and management. *J Pediatr Orthop* 2002; 22:22-26. Level of evidence: IV.

3. Vitale MG, Kessler MG, Choe JC: Pelvic fractures in children: An exploration of practice patterns and patient outcomes. *J Pediatr Orthop* 2005;25:581-587.

    Using a national database, the authors showed that children with pelvic fractures had better outcomes if they were treated at a pediatric trauma center. Level of evidence: III.

4. Smith W, Shurnas P, Morgan S, et al: Clinical outcomes of unstable pelvic fractures in skeletally immature patients. *J Bone Joint Surg Am* 2005;87:2423-2431.

    After unstable pelvic fractures, children did not undergo significant remodeling of asymmetry present at the initial time of healing. Those with asymmetry greater than 1.1 cm had increased risk of pain, scoliosis, and dysfunction. Open reduction is indicated for children with fractures causing significant pelvic asymmetry. Level of evidence: III.

5. Trousdale RT, Ganz R: Posttraumatic acetabular dysplasia. *Clin Orthop Relat Res* 1994;305:124-132.

6. Heeg M: Acetabular fractures in children and adolescents. *Clin Orthop Relat Res* 2000;376:80-86.

7. Karunakar MA, Goulet JA, Mueller KL, Bedi A, Le TT: Operative treatment of unstable pediatric pelvis and acetabular fractures. *J Pediatr Orthop* 2005;25:34-38.

    Eighteen patients who were younger than 16 years and had acetabular or pelvic fractures were treated surgically at a single center. There were no growth arrests, infections, or wound complications. Level of evidence: III.

8. Liporace FA, Ong B: Development and injury of the triradiate cartilage with its effects on acetabular development: Review of the literature. *J Trauma* 2003;54: 1245-1249.

9. Mehlman CT, Hubbard DO, Crawford AJ, Roy DR, Wall EJ: Traumatic hip dislocation in children. *Clin Orthop Relat Res* 2000;376:68-79.

10. Herrera-Soto JA, Price CT, Preuss BL, Riley P, Kasser J,

Beaty J: Proximal femoral epiphysiolysis during reduction of hip dislocation in adolescents. *J Pediatr Orthop* 2006;26:371-374.

Five adolescents (mean age, 13 years; range, 12 to 15 years) had no reported evidence of injury to the upper femoral physis before reduction in the emergency department. All were discovered to have epiphyseal separation on postreduction radiographs, and all developed osteonecrosis within 15 months. The authors believe that the physeal injury occurred at the time of dislocation and that the reduction completed the separation. They recommend gentle reduction under fluoroscopy of all hip dislocations in this age group. Any physeal instability should be treated prophylactically before reduction. Level of evidence: III.

11. Beaty JH: Fractures of the hip in children. *Orthop Clin North Am* 2006;37:223-232.

This summary of state-of-the art treatment in a pediatric trauma center concludes that anatomic reduction and rigid fixation is almost always the best treatment choice.

12. Togrul E: Fractures of the femoral neck in children: Long-term follow-up in 62 hip fractures. *Injury* 2005; 36:123-130.

At a minimum 8-year follow-up of a large number of patients treated in Turkey, good results were obtained in 67%. The osteonecrosis rate was 14%, even in high-risk type II patients. Level of evidence: III.

13. Moon ES, Mehlman CT: Risk factors for avascular necrosis after femoral neck fractures in children: 25 Cincinnati cases and meta-analysis of 360 cases. *J Orthop Trauma* 2006;20:323-329.

Age and fracture type were the only variables predicting an increased risk of osteonecrosis. The osteonecrosis rate was 35% for Delbet type I hip fractures, 28% for type II, 18% for type III, and 5% for type IV. Level of evidence: III.

14. Flynn JM, Wong KL, Yeh GL, Meyer JS, Davidson RS: Displaced fractures of the hip in children: Management by early operation and immobilisation in a hip spica cast. *J Bone Joint Surg Br* 2002;84:108-112.

15. Pombo MW, Shilt JS: The definition and treatment of pediatric subtrochanteric femur fractures with titanium elastic nails. *J Pediatr Orthop* 2006;26:364-370.

The authors defined the subtrochanteric region of the femur in children as being within the proximal 10% of the femur length below the lesser trochanter. They found that titanium elastic nails provided good results if they were advanced far enough proximally. Level of evidence: III.

16. Jarvis J, Davidson D, Letts M: Management of subtrochanteric fractures in skeletally immature adolescents. *J Trauma* 2006;60:613-619.

Based on analysis of 13 subtrochanteric fractures in adolescents, the authors found that surgical treatment produced more satisfactory results than nonsurgical treatment. One case of osteonecrosis resulted from a nail

inserted medial to the tip of the trochanter in a location near the piriformis fossa. Level of evidence: III.

17. Jeng C, Sponseller PD, Yates A: Subtrochanteric femoral fractures in children. *Clin Orthop Relat Res* 1997;341: 170-174.

18. Flynn JM, Schwend RM: Management of pediatric femoral shaft fractures. *J Am Acad Orthop Surg* 2004;12: 347-359.

Current treatment options are reviewed, with a guide to decision making.

19. Moroz LA, Launay F, Kocher MS, et al: Titanium elastic nailing of fractures of the femur in children: Predictors of complications and poor outcome. *J Bone Joint Surg Br* 2006;88:1361-1366.

Evaluation of 234 femur fractures treated with flexible intramedullary nails at six pediatric trauma centers found poor results in 10%. Unacceptable angulation was the most common adverse outcome. Patient age more than 11 years and weight more than 49 kg were associated with a poorer outcome. Level of evidence: III.

20. Loder RT, O'Donnell PW, Feinberg JR: Epidemiology and mechanisms of femur fractures in children. *J Pediatr Orthop* 2006;26:561-566.

Examination of a nationwide database revealed slight differences in the incidence of fracture at different ages. Most of the fractures in young children resulted from falls, and motor vehicle crashes caused most fractures in older children. Level of evidence: IV.

21. Schwend RM, Werth C, Johnston A: Femur shaft fractures in toddlers and young children: Rarely from child abuse. *J Pediatr Orthop* 2000;20:475-481.

22. Pierce MC, Bertocci GE, Moreland M: Femur fractures resulting from stair falls among children: An injury plausibility model. *Pediatrics* 2005;115:1712-1722.

The authors developed a method for rating the plausibility of a stair-fall explanation of a femur fracture in an infant or toddler. The most useful information was derived from a detailed injury history that included the caregiver's ability to describe the child's position before and after the fall and the mechanics of the fall. Consistency with fracture type as well as time to seeking help were also included in the scoring. Level of evidence: III.

23. Podeszwa DA, Mooney JF III, Cramer K, Mendelow M: Comparison of Pavlik harness application and immediate spica casting for femur fractures in infants. *J Pediatr Orthop* 2004;24:460-462.

The authors used Pavlik harnesses to treat infants with a femur fracture, although the infants initially seemed uncomfortable in these devices. Level of evidence: III.

24. Epps HR, Molenaar E, O'Connor DP: Immediate single-leg spica cast for pediatric femoral diaphysis fractures. *J Pediatr Orthop* 2006;26:491-496.

The authors used a single-leg spica cast for 45 young children with a femur fracture. Mobility and ease of care were excellent. A tendency toward shortening appeared in patients who were older than 6 years or had a high-energy injury. Level of evidence: IV.

25. Weiss APC, Schenck R, Sponseller PD, et al: Peroneal palsy after early spica cast application for femoral fractures in children. *J Pediatr Orthop* 1992;12:25-28.

26. Mubarak SJ, Frick S, Sink E, et al: Volkmann contracture and compartment syndromes after femur fractures in children treated with 90/90 spica casts. *J Pediatr Orthop* 2006;26:567-572.

Nine children developed Volkmann contractures or pressure sores after treatment with a 90-90 spica cast. The authors recommend placing the leg in a less flexed position and avoiding use of a short leg cast for initial traction on the leg. Level of evidence: IV.

27. Ho CA, Skaggs DL, Tang C, Kay RM: Use of flexible intramedullary nails in pediatric femur fractures. *J Pediatr Orthop* 2006;26:497-504.

In this study of 93 patients with femur fractures treated using flexible intramedullary nails at a single trauma center, the overall complication rate was 17%. Complications requiring surgery were more common in children older than 10 years. The eventual results were good for most of these patients. Level of evidence: IV.

28. Sink EL, Gralla J, Repine M: Complications of pediatric femur fractures treated with titanium elastic nails: A comparison of fracture types. *J Pediatr Orthop* 2005;25:577-580.

A review of 39 consecutive children whose femur fractures were treated with flexible intramedullary nails found that length-unstable (comminuted or long spiral) fractures had a much higher complication rate than other types. Level of evidence: IV.

29. Blasier RD, Aronson J, Tursky EA: External fixation of pediatric femur fractures. *J Pediatr Orthop* 1997;17:342-346. Level of evidence: IV.

30. Skaggs DL, Leet AI, Money M: Secondary fractures associated with external fixation in pediatric femur fractures. *J Pediatr Orthop* 1999;19:582-586.

31. Caird MS, Mueller KA, Puryear A, Farley F: Compression plating of pediatric femoral shaft fractures. *J Pediatr Orthop* 2003;23:448-452. Level of evidence: IV.

32. Hedequist DJ, Sink E: Technical aspects of bridge plating for pediatric femur fractures. *J Orthop Trauma* 2005;19:276-279.

The use of bridge plating is recommended for patients with open physes having comminuted or length-unstable femur fractures. The authors believe that locked devices are not needed. At least three screws are needed above and below the fracture, spaced within each fragment as external fixator pins are spaced. The plates are eventually removed. Level of evidence: IV.

33. Sink EL, Hedequist D, Morgan SJ, Hresko T: Results and technique of unstable pediatric femoral fractures treated with submuscular bridge plating. *J Pediatr Orthop* 2006;26:177-181.

The authors provide valuable details on the technique of submuscular bridge plating. Level of evidence: IV.

34. Kanellopoulos AD, Yiannakopoulos CK, Soucacos PN: Closed, locked intramedullary nailing of pediatric femoral shaft fractures through the tip of the greater trochanter. *J Trauma* 2006;60:217-222.

Good results with no osteonecrosis were achieved in treating pediatric femoral shaft fractures with closed, locked intramedullary nailing. The nail was inserted through or lateral to the tip of the greater trochanter. Level of evidence: IV.

35. Tortolani PJ, Ain MC, Miller NH, Brumback R, Sponseller PD: Tibial nails for femoral shaft fractures in adolescents. *Orthopedics* 2001;24:553-557. Level of evidence: IV.

36. Gordon JE, Swenning TA, Burd TA, Schoenecker PL: Proximal femoral radiographic changes after lateral transtrochanteric intramedullary nail placement in children. *J Bone Joint Surg Am* 2003;85-A:1295-1301. Level of evidence: IV.

Chapter 59

Hip, Pelvis, and Femur Disorders: Pediatrics

Travis H. Matheney, MD   Young-Jo Kim, MD, PhD

Developmental Dysplasia of the Hip

Incidence and Risk Factors

The incidence of developmental dysplasia of the hip (DDH) is estimated to be 1 to 10 per 1,000 live births. The condition is relatively common in children of central European descent and uncommon in those of sub-Saharan African descent. Although DDH does not follow classic mendelian genetic inheritance patterns, a significant genetic component exists; the incidence of DDH in identical twins is 34%, compared with 3% in fraternal twins. In children with an affected sibling, the incidence rises to between 6% and 7%; it rises to 36% if both a parent and a sibling are affected.

In addition to genetic factors, the intrauterine mechanical environment is believed to affect the incidence of DDH. The condition is associated with a firstborn child, frank breech presentation, oligohydramnios, congenital muscular torticollis, metatarsus adductus, and congenital knee dislocation.[1]

Etiology

The etiology of DDH is unknown and appears to be multifactorial. The acetabulum and femoral head develop from the same primitive mesenchymal cells, and a cleft separating the two precartilage components develops in approximately the seventh week of gestation. The acetabulum grows in response to a concentrically reduced femoral head. Therefore, acetabular dysplasia can develop in response to a malpositioned femoral head or abnormal forces exerted by spastic muscles, as in neuromuscular hip dysplasia.

Diagnosis

Physical Examination

In the United States, neonatal physical examination with hip screening is the mainstay of diagnosis. The Ortolani test detects the presence of a dislocated but reducible hip in abduction. The Barlow test detects the presence of a subluxatable hip in adduction. When the infant reaches 3 to 6 months of age, the dislocated hip becomes contracted and these early signs may not be apparent. A positive Galeazzi sign (apparent femoral length discrepancy when the legs are held together with the hips and knees flexed), asymmetric thigh folds, and decreased hip abduction are also late indicators of a dislocated hip.

When the child reaches walking age, dislocation may be manifested as a flexion contracture of the affected side, a gluteus medius lurch, toe walking on the affected side, or increased lordosis with bilateral dislocation. If the dysplasia is mild and without dislocation, hip-groin pain consistent with labral pathology from overloading of the acetabular rim, as well as early arthritis, may develop in adolescence or young adulthood.

For infants who have a questionable diagnosis of DDH or are at high risk of DDH, the appropriateness of physical examination alone or in combination with close ultrasound surveillance is a topic of continued debate. Studies found that most hip abnormalities spontaneously resolve before the child reaches 6 months of age; the need for screening or treatment of infants who have stable hips on examination has been questioned.[2] One aspect of the controversy is the balance between accurate diagnosis and treatment; osteonecrosis was cited as a possible consequence of overtreatment. Because the natural history of DDH has not been fully elucidated, the initial physical examination by the primary care provider continues to be the mainstay of screening, and dynamic flexion/abduction bracing in a Pavlik harness continues to be the treatment of choice for most patients with DDH whose condition has been confirmed by ultrasound.

Ultrasound Imaging

Ultrasound is the best means of imaging the hip in children age 6 months or younger. Universal ultrasound screening is used in some European countries, but this practice has not been adopted in the United States. The standard coronal plane used in the United States is defined by the identification of a straight iliac line, the tip of the acetabular labrum, and the transition from the os ilium to the triradiate cartilage (**Figure 1**). The acetabular roof and labrum, as well as the femoral head, should be visible. The most commonly used measurements include the alpha (α) angle, which is formed by the straight iliac line and the bony acetabulum, and the percentage of the femoral head covered by the acetabulum. The normal α angle is greater than 60°, and it implies a more horizontal acetabular roof. The normal amount of femoral head coverage is 50% or more.

6: Pediatrics

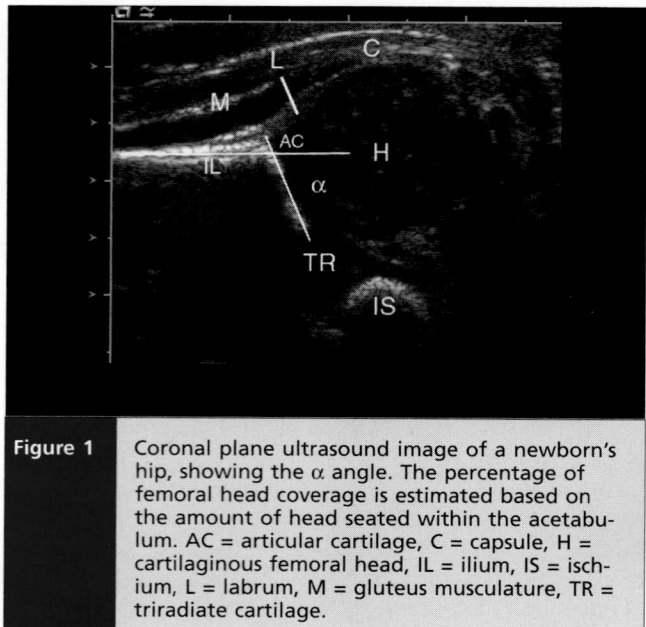

Figure 1 Coronal plane ultrasound image of a newborn's hip, showing the α angle. The percentage of femoral head coverage is estimated based on the amount of head seated within the acetabulum. AC = articular cartilage, C = capsule, H = cartilaginous femoral head, IL = ilium, IS = ischium, L = labrum, M = gluteus musculature, TR = triradiate cartilage.

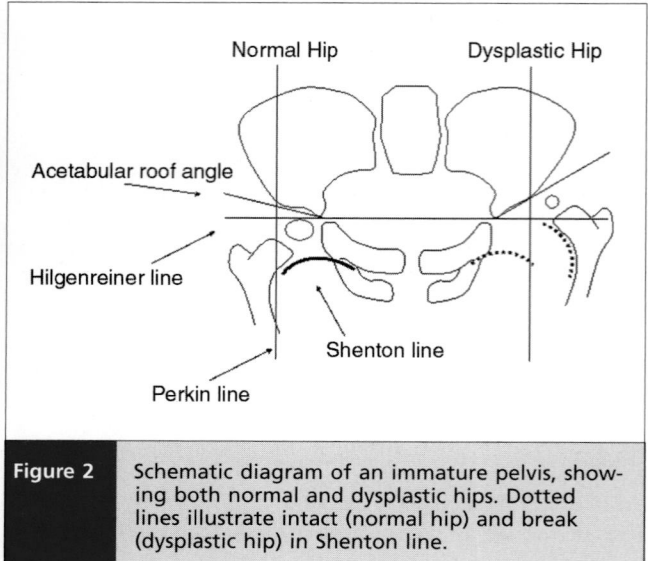

Figure 2 Schematic diagram of an immature pelvis, showing both normal and dysplastic hips. Dotted lines illustrate intact (normal hip) and break (dysplastic hip) in Shenton line.

Stress ultrasound views in the axial plane can determine the stability of the hip. Stability is assessed by dynamic imaging of the hip as axial compression and adduction forces are applied to the femoral head.[3,4]

The definition of a pathologic hip on ultrasound images is controversial. In general, an α angle of less than 50° is considered pathologic, and an angle between 50° and 60° is considered borderline pathologic in a child who is at least 3 months of age. An unstable hip in a child who is age 1 to 2 weeks or older is also considered pathologic.

Plain Radiography

Plain radiography is a better imaging modality than ultrasound after the femoral head begins to ossify at approximately 6 months of age. Several findings are typically noted on the standard AP radiograph of the pelvis. The dysplastic hip generally has a smaller femoral head epiphysis that is not located or is asymmetrically located within the acetabulum or is completely dislocated. Reference lines, including the Hilgenreiner, Perkin, and Shenton lines, are used because the adjacent bony landmarks are not completely ossified (**Figure 2**). The greater the subluxation or dislocation of the femoral head, the more the visible epiphysis will be lateral to the Perkin line or superior to the Hilgenreiner line. The obliquity of the acetabular roof is assessed as the angle subtended between the Hilgenreiner line and a line drawn through the visible acetabular roof. The normal value of the acetabular roof is less than 30°.

Arthrography, CT, and MRI

Arthrography and dynamic testing are used to check the stability of the infant hip and the quality of a reduction. Arthrography is commonly used after a closed reduction; it reveals structures blocking concentric reduc-

tion, such as a hypertrophic ligamentum teres, a capsular constriction, or a constricted iliopsoas tendon. CT and MRI are useful in assessing the adequacy of a closed or open reduction. Cross-sectional CT or MRI images can clearly show posterior subluxation that may not appear on plain radiographs. MRI has the additional advantages of avoiding further exposure of the child to ionizing radiation and, like arthrography, of showing soft structures that can block reduction.

Treatment

The primary goal of treatment for DDH is a concentrically reduced femoral head. Early diagnosis is essential, because a longer period of subluxation and dislocation typically results in a need for multiple greater interventions, including surgical reductions and possibly osteotomy.

Abduction Splinting

The Pavlik harness is the standard therapy for infants age 6 months or younger. The principle is to hold the hip in a flexed, abducted position that will allow gentle reduction and stabilization. The standard position for the brace is approximately 100° of flexion set by the anterior strap of the harness. The posterior strap should be adjusted to allow adduction of the leg only to a neutral position. This position minimizes the risks associated with overabduction and hyperflexion, which are associated with osteonecrosis and femoral nerve palsy.

The harness is initially worn 24 hours a day, until the hip is believed to be stable without support. It is worn part time until acetabular remodeling is adequate. A dislocated hip is monitored weekly using ultrasonography until the hip is located and stable. Pavlik harness treatment of a hip in a dislocated position for more than 3 weeks can lead to flattening of the posterior wall, which makes the subsequent closed reduction much more difficult.

If the Pavlik harness fails to provide adequate reduction within 3 to 4 weeks, or if the child is larger than the average 6-month-old, a rigid abduction orthosis or cast should be used, with ultrasound follow-up periodically or radiographs (if the patient is older than 6 months) every 2 to 4 weeks to assess the reduction. This transition in treatment has been shown in most patients to result in a concentrically reduced hip within 1 to 2 months and is recommended before treatment with closed reduction in the operating room.[5]

For unstable hips, early closed treatment using appropriate abduction bracing leads to excellent long-term outcomes. Results from a recent study of 223 unstable hips indicated that late dysplasia or dislocation did not occur after 6 weeks of abduction splinting.[6]

Closed and Open Reduction and Spica Cast Treatment

If bracing fails to provide adequate reduction, or if the infant is older than age 6 months and the hip is not easily reducible using the Ortolani maneuver, a closed or open reduction should be performed. In the past, these reductions were attempted after a period of traction and were not performed after the child reached 2 years of age unless an unforced reduction could be maintained. The currently preferred method of closed reduction uses general anesthesia and arthrography to confirm that reduction has occurred. If an adductor contracture or narrow stability zone is present, a percutaneous adductor tenotomy can be performed to allow greater abduction without the use of potentially harmful force. A cast is applied in the safe position, which is approximately 100° of flexion and an abduction angle within the stable zone. Abduction greater than 55° has been associated with the development of osteonecrosis. The presence of the ossific nucleus is believed to be protective of the femoral head from osteonecrosis after closed reduction. There is no current consensus on whether a closed reduction should be delayed until the ossific nucleus is formed to decrease the rate of osteonecrosis.

In children age 2 years or older or children age 18 months or older in whom closed reduction has failed, open reduction is an option to remove soft-tissue structures that prevent a concentric reduction. These structures include hypertrophied and inverted labrum, hypertrophied ligamentum teres, constricted transverse acetabular ligament, or constricted iliopsoas tendon and hip capsule. An anterior approach is most commonly used for the open reduction. It allows removal of all structures blocking reduction, as well as a capsulorrhaphy to help stabilize the hip. Medial and anteromedial approaches typically are more beneficial in children age 2 years or younger. These approaches do not allow capsulorrhaphy but help provide a good view of all impediments to reduction, except possibly the inverted labrum.

If the dislocation has been prolonged, a concomitant femoral shortening osteotomy may be necessary to improve the stability and decrease compressive forces on the femoral head. An acetabular osteotomy may be required, because the acetabulum invariably is more affected by dysplasia with prolonged dislocation. The Salter (innominate) osteotomy and the Pemberton and Dega acetabular osteotomies are commonly performed to help correct the anterolateral uncovering common in DDH.[7-11]

Achieving a concentrically reduced, stable hip is an absolute requirement. Either a femoral or pelvic osteotomy should be performed if necessary to produce a stable hip, but the age at which femoral and pelvic osteotomy is necessary is controversial. The patient's long-term prognosis is guarded if the hip requires additional treatment after bracing. These patients must be monitored until skeletal maturity because of the relatively high incidence of osteonecrosis and persistent acetabular dysplasia. Acetabular remodeling, if necessary, should occur within 18 months of the reduction. Persistent acetabular dysplasia should be treated with subsequent pelvic osteotomies.

Complications and Residual Deformities

Osteonecrosis

Osteonecrosis of the femoral head can occur after all forms of treatment of DDH and is associated with a poor long-term outcome. The precise cause of osteonecrosis after treatment of DDH is not known, but possible causes include excessive compression of an unossified femoral head, occlusion of the femoral head vasculature from positioning during bracing or casting, or disruption of the blood supply after surgery. The consequences of osteonecrosis range from a delay in ossification of the femoral head to growth arrest leading to varus or valgus deformity to complete femoral head necrosis. If osteonecrosis is detected, the hip should be monitored until skeletal maturity.

Persistent Acetabular Dysplasia

Residual hip dysplasia causes an overload on the acetabular labrum and articular edge and can result in early degeneration and tearing of the labrum and cartilage. The severity of dysplasia as seen on plain radiographs is associated with the development of osteoarthritis. On an AP pelvic radiograph, the lateral center-edge angle of Wiberg is a standard measure of dysplasia, and studies have shown that an angle less than 16° always leads to end-stage osteoarthritis by the sixth decade of life. In addition, the false profile view of Lequesne, which is a lateral projection of the acetabulum, may show mild residual dysplasia in the anterior acetabulum. MRI with arthrography is effective in diagnosing labral tears. Specialized imaging, such as delayed gadolinium-enhanced MRI of cartilage, can show early arthritis in dysplastic hips.[12] Residual dysplasia can be effectively treated with modern spherical or periacetabular osteotomies. The long-term results are good, if the preexisting arthritis in the joint was minimal.[13-15]

6: Pediatrics

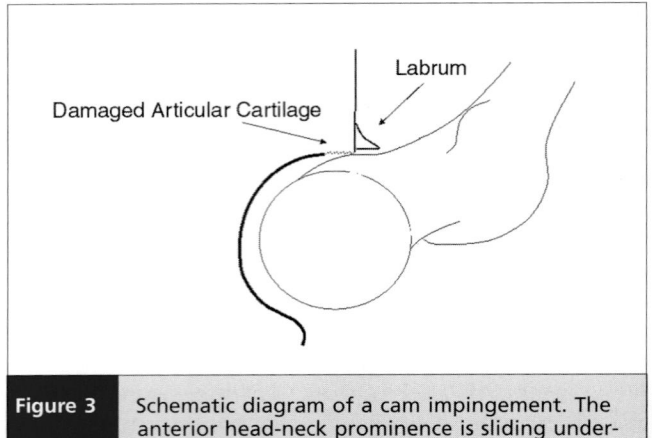

Figure 3 Schematic diagram of a cam impingement. The anterior head-neck prominence is sliding underneath the labrum and abrading against the acetabular articular rim.

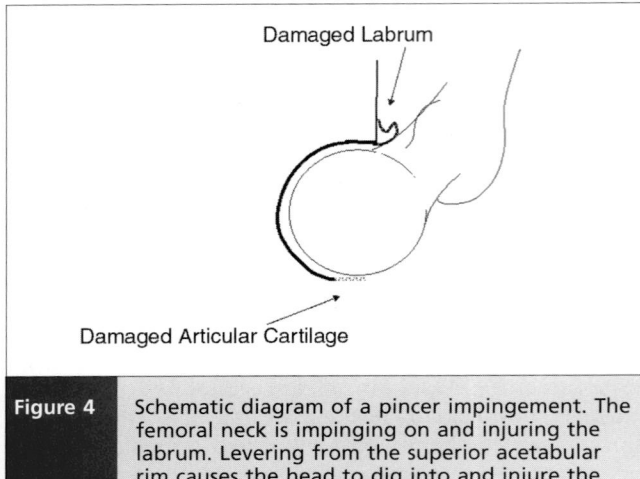

Figure 4 Schematic diagram of a pincer impingement. The femoral neck is impinging on and injuring the labrum. Levering from the superior acetabular rim causes the head to dig into and injure the posteroinferior acetabulum.

Femoroacetabular Impingement

Incidence and Etiology

The true incidence and etiology of femoroacetabular impingement is not known. A retroverted femoral head and a pistol grip deformity of the head-neck region have been highly associated with osteoarthritis in hips that were undergoing total joint arthroplasty.[16,17] These may be subtle developmental deformities related to slipped capital femoral epiphysis (SCFE). More recently, cam impingement associated with proximal femoral deformity and pincer impingement associated with acetabular deformity were described.[18-20] Cam impingement is associated with deformity of the anterolateral head and neck or a pistol grip appearance (**Figure 3**). The mechanism of injury is the prominent, increasingly aspherical head passing below the labrum and abrasion of the acetabular rim cartilage, leading to early degeneration of the cartilage or full-thickness flap tears. A labral tear can follow as part of the degenerative process. Pincer impingement usually results from overcoverage of the femoral head, which is caused by coxa profunda, protrusio acetabuli, or acetabular retroversion (**Figure 4**). The femoral neck impinges on, or pinches, the labrum, causing damage. In severe or chronic cases, the femoral neck can lever off the labrum and the anterosuperior acetabulum and cause a contrecoup injury to the posteroinferior acetabular cartilage. In the original description, cam impingement was more commonly seen in younger male athletes, and pincer impingement was more common in middle-aged female athletes.[21]

Diagnosis

The process of initial diagnosis begins with a history of symptoms similar to a labral tear. The initial diagnosis may be delayed because of the presence of smaller osseous prominences. The patient typically has groin pain that is worse with hip flexion, adduction, and internal rotation, or a positive impingement sign that brings the femoral neck into contact with the anterior acetabu-

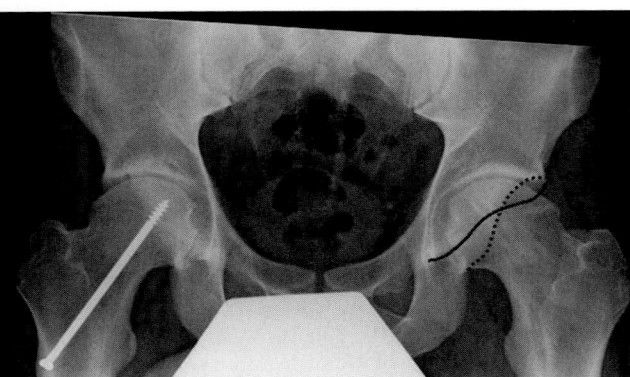

Figure 5 Anterior overcoverage and acetabular retroversion with cam-type impingement lesions. The solid line denoting the anterior acetabular wall "crosses over" the dotted line of the posterior wall, indicating anterior overcoverage and/or acetabular retroversion. The patient had percutaneous screw fixation of a mild SCFE at a younger age. Both femoral heads exhibit the head-neck prominences of cam impingement lesions.

lum. Plain radiography, CT, and MRI can aid in diagnosing and assessing the severity of both the deformity and the labral and articular cartilage damage. The plain radiographs should include an AP pelvic view and a true lateral view of the femur, with the hip internally rotated approximately 15°. In AP pelvic views, the coccyx should be in line with the pubic symphysis to minimize the effect of rotation. Loss of femoral head sphericity and anterior neck prominence can best be seen on the lateral views. Close inspection may reveal small herniation pits on the anterior neck, believed to indicate impingement. Anterior overcoverage or acetabular retroversion is indicated on AP pelvic views if the anterior acetabular wall shadow crosses over the posterior wall shadow (**Figure 5**). CT with three-dimensional reconstruction is useful in detecting subtle femoral head-neck junction prominences. MRI is useful in detecting labral tears, but it is not sensitive for detecting chondral lesions.

Treatment and Outcomes

Surgical treatment is performed through a surgical dislocation approach to allow full dynamic assessment of the impinging structures and complete treatment of the femoral as well as the acetabular abnormality.[21] For the common type of cam impingement, arthroscopic or limited open resection techniques are being developed to minimize the morbidity associated with the trochanteric osteotomy necessary for a surgical dislocation.

Only limited reports of surgical outcomes are available. In studies with short-term follow-up, clinical improvement was noted in hips with little or no arthritis on radiography.[22,23] Preservation of the labrum by reattachment after acetabular rim resection appeared to improve the outcome, compared with complete resection of the labrum.[24] It is not clear whether the benefits of a less invasive arthroscopic approach outweigh the disadvantage of a decreased ability for dynamic assessment of areas of impingement.[25]

Legg-Calvé-Perthes Disease

Epidemiology and Pathogenesis

Idiopathic osteonecrosis of the skeletally immature femoral head is called Legg-Calvé-Perthes (LCP) disease. The ratio of affected males to females is 4:1. The incidence is greater in children who have relatively short stature, delayed bone age, hyperactivity disorder, or exposure to secondhand smoke. The typical age of onset is 4 to 8 years, and the range is 2 to 12 years. Bilateral LCP disease occurs in 10% to 20% of patients and is rare among African-American children. Children of lower socioeconomic status are also at increased risk of LCP disease.[26-29] An association with abnormal clotting factors was described but not supported by recent studies.[30-32] The current belief is that LCP disease results from a vascular embarrassment early in development that blocks epiphyseal blood flow within the tenuous arterial plexus on the femoral neck. Femoral head collapse occurs during the fragmentation phase, and it may improve during the healing phase. The collapse was believed to occur secondary to applied stresses on the mechanically weak epiphysis, but increasingly the evidence indicates mechanical weakness is caused by an imbalance between osteoblastic and osteoclastic activity in the revascularization process.

Clinical Presentation

In the classic presentation, the child has a painless limp, which may be accompanied by a Trendelenburg gait. The child may also describe pain in the hip, thigh, or knee. Physical examination usually reveals a loss of abduction and internal rotation. The differential diagnosis in the early stages of the disease includes toxic synovitis, osteomyelitis, and septic arthritis. Plain radiography, including AP pelvic and frog-lateral views of the

hips, and routine laboratory tests, including white blood cell count, erythrocyte sedimentation rate, and C-reactive protein level, can help in differentiating early LCP disease from other causes of hip pain, such as septic arthritis, rheumatic disease, and osteomyelitis. The laboratory values are typically normal, although the erythrocyte sedimentation rate may be slightly elevated. Radionuclide bone scans with technetium-methylene diphosphonate can allow diagnosis earlier in the disease process. MRI is also useful in assessing early ischemia and can show changes in the femoral head months before they appear on plain radiographs.

The early stage of LCP disease is characterized by stiffness and contracture caused by joint synovitis. Activity restriction and nonsteroidal anti-inflammatory drugs can help relieve these symptoms. As the disease progresses and the femoral head heals, the synovitis resolves, but the loss of motion may become permanent if the femoral head is aspherical. Depending on the sphericity of the femoral head and its congruence with the acetabulum, premature osteoarthritis can develop in adulthood, leading to pain and disability.

Radiographic Stages

Radiographic abnormalities may not be obvious during the initial stage of LCP disease, although subtle signs may include a smaller, more radiodense ossific nucleus or an increased space between the medial femoral head and the acetabulum. After this early phase, the ossific nucleus is fragmented, and the subchondral plate fractures. Recent animal studies have shown that revascularization occurs during this stage. The third stage is reossification. Normal-appearing bone density returns, and the subchondral plate is re-formed. Often hip synovitis is resolved at this stage, but the femoral head deformity will persist. The final healing stage is characterized by the final appearance of the femoral head, with its residual deformity. This stage extends until skeletal maturity. If the shape of the femoral head is irregular, acetabular remodeling may continue throughout this stage.

Classification Systems

LCP disease can be classified using several systems based on radiographic findings. With the Salter and Thompson classification, the femoral head is classified as class A (less than 50% involvement) or class B (more than 50% involvement).[33] This system is simple, and the crescent sign used to assess the head involvement percentage is seen only in one third of cases. The crescent sign describes the appearance of a segment of subchondral bone with surrounding radiolucency in the femoral head. The Catterall classification divides epiphyseal involvement into four groups: less than 50% (in group 1, anterior head; or group 2, central and anterior head) or more than 50% (in group 3, most of the epiphysis; or group 4, the entire epiphysis).[34]

The lateral pillar system is most commonly used. The lateral pillar is the lateralmost 30% of the femoral head, as seen on an AP image of the hip. The original

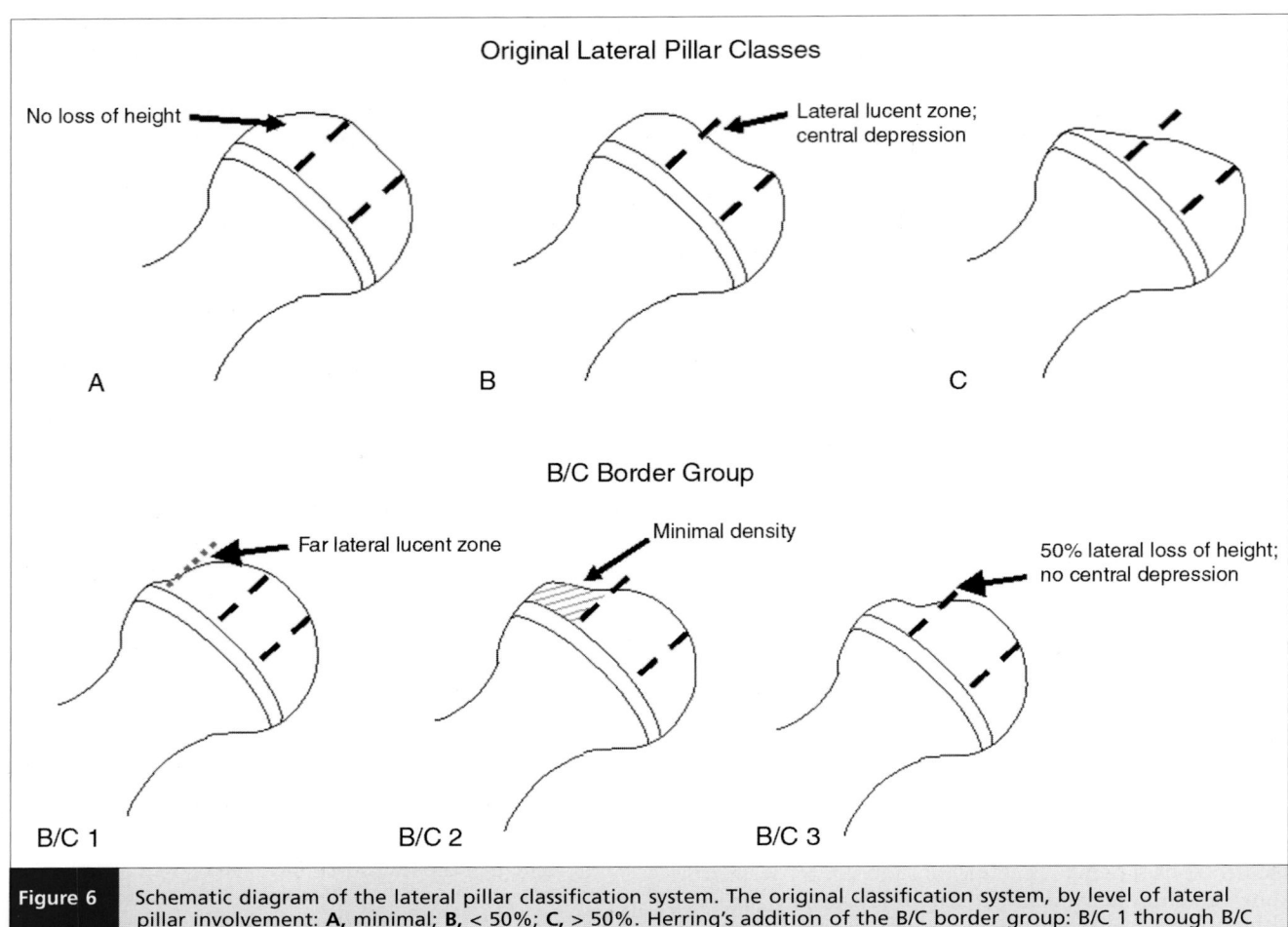

Original Lateral Pillar Classes

No loss of height

Lateral lucent zone; central depression

A

B

C

B/C Border Group

Far lateral lucent zone

Minimal density

50% lateral loss of height; no central depression

B/C 1

B/C 2

B/C 3

Figure 6	Schematic diagram of the lateral pillar classification system. The original classification system, by level of lateral pillar involvement: **A**, minimal; **B**, < 50%; **C**, > 50%. Herring's addition of the B/C border group: B/C 1 through B/C 3. B/C 1: lateral pillar has >50% height, but < 2 to 3 mm of width; B/C 2: lateral pillar > 50% height, but little ossification; B/C 3: 50% lateral height, but depressed relative to central column

lateral pillar system classified a hip into group A, B, or C; a later modification added the B/C border group (**Figure 6**). A hip in group A has no loss of height in the lateral pillar and no density changes; a group B hip has more than 50% of the original pillar height, a column width more than 3 mm, and substantial ossification. A group C hip has greater than 50% lateral column loss of height. In the B/C border group, the pillar has more than 50% of its original height and less than 2 to 3 mm of its width; more than 50% of its height but little ossification; or 50% or less of its original height but is depressed relative to the central pillar.[35]

Treatment and Containment

Much of the treatment of LCP disease is based on studies that showed the association between femoral head shape and congruence with the acetabulum and the development of osteoarthritis.[27] These studies showed that aspherical incongruent hips develop rapid premature arthritis and that they are relatively problem free into mid life.[36-41]

The treatment algorithm for early LCP disease is directed toward producing a spherical and congruent

joint, if possible. Nonsurgical management includes initial bed rest, range-of-motion exercises, and adductor stretching. It may include nonsteroidal anti-inflammatory medication. Abduction casting can be used for continued stretching, but full-time casting is not commonly used. It is accepted that physical therapy and bracing programs do not affect the natural history of the disease.[38] Therefore, they are no longer part of primary treatment but are used as adjuncts to observation or surgical treatment.

The indications for containment surgery were determined primarily on the basis of multiple long-term outcome studies. Most studies found an association between earlier onset of disease and better outcomes. Patients younger than 8 years at onset and with hips classified as lateral pillar group B did well regardless of treatment. Patients older than 8 years at onset and with hips classified as lateral pillar group B or B/C border group had better outcomes with surgical than with nonsurgical treatment. Patients with hips classified as lateral pillar group C had poor outcomes, regardless of age or treatment.[36,40,41]

The primary surgical treatment method for early

LCP disease is femoral or rotational pelvic osteotomy, or both, to keep the femoral head contained within the acetabulum. Containment strategies work only if performed during the fragmentation stage, when femoral head remodeling can still occur. Both femoral and pelvic osteotomies require the femoral head to move within the acetabulum, with no hinge abduction. Presurgical traction, bracing, and physical therapy may be necessary. If concentric motion cannot be restored, containment can be achieved using acetabular augmentation procedures, such as a shelf acetabuloplasty, with or without a valgus-extension femoral osteotomy.

Hips with poor sphericity or congruence may become symptomatic before the onset of end-stage osteoarthritis. The symptoms often result from impingement and poor range of motion caused by the misshapen femoral head. Often a femoral osteotomy can place the limb into a more functional position. The femoral head pathology may be accompanied by acetabular dysplasia. Joint congruence sometimes must be maintained by combining pelvic and femoral osteotomies. These salvage procedures can improve the symptoms, but it is not known whether they alter the long-term outcome.[42,43]

Slipped Capital Femoral Epiphysis

Etiology and Epidemiology

SCFE occurs if the proximal femoral epiphysis is displaced from the femoral neck through the hypertrophic zone of the adjacent physis. The etiology is unknown, although several theories have been proposed and several risk factors have been identified. The risk factors include African-American descent, renal failure, endocrine abnormalities (such as hypothyroidism or growth hormone deficiency), an associated vertical physis, and recent radiation or chemotherapy. The 60% average body mass index of SCFE patients is at or above the 95th percentile for age. Patients younger than 10 years with an SCFE should probably be assessed to rule out an endocrinopathy.[44-47]

The epiphyseal displacement is most commonly posterior and inferior onto the neck. However, the epiphysis actually remains seated in the acetabulum, and the femoral neck and shaft are displaced anteriorly and laterally. SCFE is the most common adolescent hip disorder, with prevalence estimated at 1 in 1,000 to 1 in 10,000. The ratio of affected males to females is 1.5:1. The mean age of occurrence is approximately the age of peak height velocity: 12 years in girls and 13.5 years in boys. SCFE is most commonly seen as a unilateral slip in which the slip on the left side is greater than the slip on the right. It is bilateral in approximately 20% of patients. The risk of subsequent slip in the contralateral hip is 30% to 60%.[44-47] A modification of the Oxford Bone Age scale was found to strongly predict SCFE in the contralateral hip. The scale assigns numeric values to maturation in five areas of the pelvis and proximal femur (femoral head, greater and lesser trochanters, triradiate cartilage, and iliac apophysis), as seen on AP and frog-lateral views. The sum of these values indicates the overall level of maturity and a correspondingly increased risk of contralateral SCFE.[48]

Clinical Findings

A patient with SCFE typically has a history of nonradiating, dull, aching, and chronic or intermittent pain in the hip, groin, thigh, or knee. The pain generally increases with physical activity. Often there is no antecedent trauma. In unstable SCFE, the patient will refuse to bear weight on the affected side. In more chronic, stable SCFE, the patient may have only a limp. A Trendelenburg gait and an external rotation to foot progression may be noted on physical examination. Limb length can be affected, with as much as 3 cm of shortening. Range-of-motion testing of the affected side typically reveals restricted internal rotation, abduction, and flexion, although these do not appear in the relatively rare valgus SCFE. Patients with more advanced slips have obligatory external rotation and abduction with hip flexion. Often the only symptom present is pain around the knee, which may cause a delay in diagnosis.

Imaging

Plain radiography should be performed first. The standard radiographs should include an AP pelvic view of both hips and a lateral view of each hip. If it is not possible to obtain the frog-lateral view of an unstable SCFE, a shoot-through lateral radiograph should be performed.

The Klein line, which is a line drawn along the superior border of the femoral neck that should intersect the epiphysis, can be assessed on an AP pelvic radiograph. Even mild slips can be diagnosed by looking at the variance between the affected side and the unaffected contralateral side. A widened and irregular physis or a decreased head-to-trochanter distance can also be seen. The Southwick epiphyseal-diaphyseal slip angle is the angle between a line drawn down the shaft of the femur and the perpendicular line to the transepiphyseal line (**Figure 7**). The angle on the side of the unaffected hip is subtracted from the angle on the affected side, and the difference is used to determine the slip magnitude. (If the SCFE is bilateral, 10° can be used as normal hip value.) A difference of 33° or less is a grade I slip, a 34° to 50° difference is a grade II slip, and a difference of more than 50° is a grade III slip. MRI is popular for assessment of the painful hip for a possible preslip appearance to the physis. The appearance of a preslip on MRI is determined by increased T2 signal and/or widening at the proximal femoral physis.

Classification

The classification schemes to define types of SCFE and predict outcome are based on severity and stability. Classification based on severity designates a slip as mild (displacement less than one third of the neck diameter or a less than 30% slip angle difference), mod-

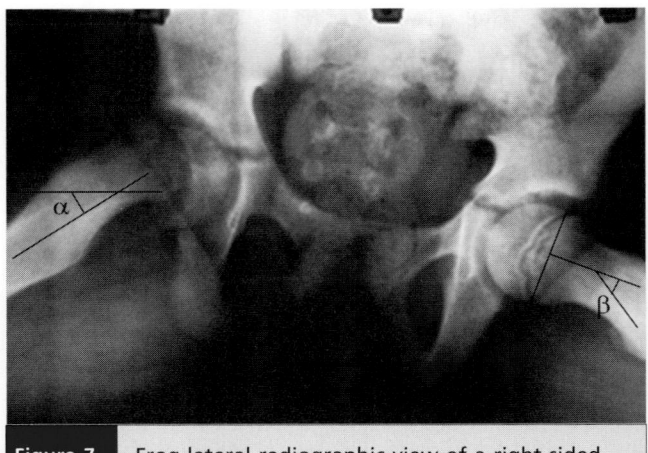

Figure 7 Frog-lateral radiographic view of a right-sided SCFE. The slip angle is computed as the difference between the epiphyseal-diaphyseal angles of the affected and nonaffected sides.

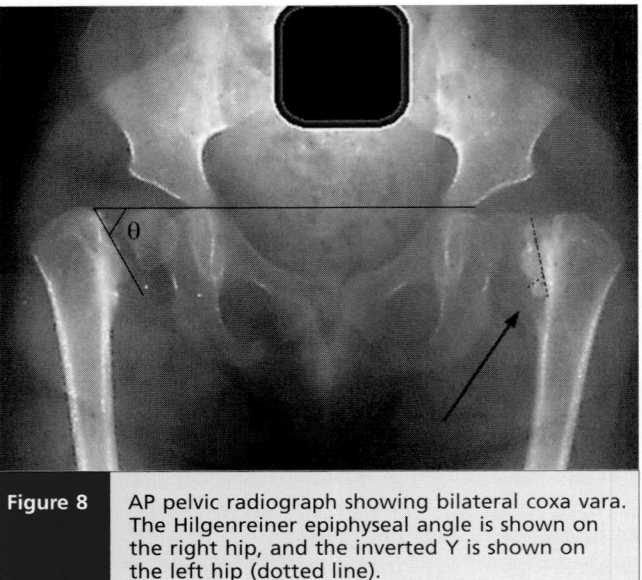

Figure 8 AP pelvic radiograph showing bilateral coxa vara. The Hilgenreiner epiphyseal angle is shown on the right hip, and the inverted Y is shown on the left hip (dotted line).

erate (displacement one third to one half of the neck diameter or a 30% to 50% slip angle difference), or severe (displacement greater than one half the neck diameter or a more than 50% slip angle difference). The most commonly used classification system is based on the presumed stability of the slip. A slip is classified as stable if the child is able to bear weight on the leg or unstable if the child is not able to bear weight.

Treatment

The primary goal of initial treatment is prevention of further slippage or deformity. Complications such as osteonecrosis and chondrolysis should be avoided during treatment. Spica casting was formerly used, but outcomes generally were poor, and the incidence of chondrolysis was 17%. The preferred treatment is in situ single screw fixation. Care must be taken to place the screw into the middle of the epiphysis. Fluoroscopic images should be obtained to verify that the screw has not penetrated the joint. A second screw can be added to provide additional support, particularly of an unstable hip, or prevent possible rotation of the proximal fragment. The use of a second screw has been shown to greatly increase the resistance to torsional forces.[49]

A stable SCFE should not be reduced. The incidence of osteonecrosis is inherently high in an unstable SCFE, although gentle closed reduction and percutaneous screw fixation can be attempted. Open reduction with subcapital osteotomy has been used, but its role in SCFE treatment is controversial. The original technique was associated with a risk of osteonecrosis as high as 40%, although studies with a lower rate of osteonecrosis have been reported.

In moderate to severe SCFE, limitations in range of motion may persist. For these patients, the corrective intertrochanteric osteotomy may be able to improve range of motion.[50] However, improvement in long-term development of osteoarthritis has yet to be demonstrated.

Prophylactic pinning of the unaffected hip is also controversial. Patients with risk factors should be considered as candidates. Several authors reported low complication rates at long-term follow-up, but others found that close, careful observation and avoidance of prophylactic surgery are more reliable.[51]

Coxa Vara

Incidence and Etiology

Coxa vara can be a congenital condition noted at birth, a progressive developmental autosomal dominant disorder, or a disorder acquired as a result of trauma, LCP disease, SCFE, or metabolic or neoplastic conditions.[52-54] The congenital form is believed to result from a limb bud abnormality or another intrauterine process. It is often associated with other limb deficiencies, such as proximal femoral focal deficiency or fibular hemimelia. Congenital coxa vara has an incidence of approximately 1 in 25,000. It affects males and females equally, with no predilection for the right or left side, and occurs bilaterally in 30% to 50% of patients. Most patients first have painless waddling or a Trendelenburg gait between 2 and 6 years of age; a decrease in hip abduction and a limb-length discrepancy, if the condition is unilateral, may also be present.[53]

Imaging

Plain radiographs of both hips, including AP pelvic and frog-lateral views, are usually sufficient. An inverted Y pattern may be seen at the proximal femoral physis, with a resulting fragment at the inferior neck that is sometimes referred to as the Fairbanks fragment.[52] Radiographic measurements should include femoral neck shaft angles and the Hilgenreiner epiphyseal angle (**Figure 8**). A neck shaft angle of less than 90° is considered an indication for corrective osteotomy. The Hilgen-reiner angle is subtended between the Hilgenreiner line on the AP pelvic radiograph and a line drawn through the proximal femoral physis. A child with a limp and a Hilgenreiner angle greater than 60°, or 45° to 60° with documented progression of varus deformity, should be treated.[53]

Treatment

The goal of treatment is to restore a more anatomic alignment and improve the hip range of motion and mechanics. A corrective intertrochanteric or subtrochanteric valgus osteotomy is the preferred treatment to restore the Hilgenreiner angle to approximately 25°, overcorrect the neck shaft angle to between 150° and 160°, and convert shear forces across the neck into compressive forces across the osteotomy site. A method of performing this osteotomy percutaneously has been described.[55] Additional treatment can include a concomitant adductor tenotomy and proximal femoral shortening to reduce pressure on the femoral head and to reduce the force of correction.

Several complications have been described, including premature physeal closure in as many as 90% of patients, greater trochanter overgrowth, recurrence of the deformity, possibly as a result of undercorrection, osteonecrosis, limb-length discrepancy, or degenerative osteoarthritis.[53]

In long-term studies, the predictors of improved clinical and radiographic outcomes include age younger than 9 years at the time of surgery and overcorrection of the neck-shaft angle to minimize the rate of recurrent deformity.[53]

Annotated References

1. Weinstein SL, Ponseti IV: Congenital dislocation of the hip. *J Bone Joint Surg Am* 1979;61:119-124.

2. Shipman SA, Helfand M, Moyer VA, Yawn BP: Screening for developmental dysplasia of the hip: A systematic literature review for the US preventative services task force. *Pediatrics* 2006;117:e557-e576.

   A large meta-analysis of screening and treatment for DDH is presented. The authors found poor support for universal ultrasound screening; ultrasound screening was recommended for high-risk infants and those with positive examination findings. Otherwise, all infants should have serial clinical examinations.

3. Graf R: Fundamentals of sonographic diagnosis of infant hip dysplasia. *J Pediatr Orthop* 1984;4:735-740.

4. Harcke HT, Kumar SJ: The role of ultrasound in the diagnosis and management of congenital dislocation and dysplasia of the hip. *J Bone Joint Surg Am* 1991;73:622-628.

5. Hedequist D, Kasser J, Emans J: Use of an abduction brace for developmental dysplasia of the hip after failure of Pavlik harness use. *J Pediatr Orthop* 2003;23:175-177.

6. Lauge-Pedersen H, Gustafsson J, Hagglund G: 6 weeks with the von Rosen splint is sufficient for treatment of neonatal hip instability. *Acta Orthop* 2006;77:257-261.

   Plastazote splint therapy for 223 clinically unstable hips at one institution during a 9-year period was evaluated at last radiographic follow-up (5 to 15 years). No residual dysplasia was found.

7. Pemberton PA: Pericapsular osteotomy of the ilium for treatment of congenital subluxation and dislocation of the hip. *J Bone Joint Surg Am* 1965;47:65-86.

8. Salter RB, Dubos JP: The first fifteen years' personal experience with innominate osteotomy in the treatment of congenital dislocation and subluxation of the hip. *Clin Orthop Relat Res* 1974;98:72-103.

9. Tönnis D, Behrens K, Tscharani F: A modified technique of the triple pelvic osteotomy: Early results. *J Pediatr Orthop* 1981;1:241-249.

10. Chiari K: Medial displacement osteotomy of the pelvis. *Clin Orthop Relat Res* 1974;98:55-71.

11. Staheli LT, Chew DE: Slotted acetabular augmentation in childhood and adolescence. *J Pediatr Orthop* 1992;12:569-580.

12. Cunningham T, Jessel R, Zurakowski D, Millis MB, Kim YJ: Delayed gadolinium-enhanced magnetic resonance imaging of cartilage to predict early failure of Bernese periacetabular osteotomy for hip dysplasia. *J Bone Joint Surg Am* 2006;88:1540-1548.

   The standard measures for assessing cartilage quality yield an incomplete evaluation. This article details an innovative new technique for assessing cartilage quality before and after periacetabular osteotomy. An unsuccessful procedure was associated with worse preoperative arthrosis, more subluxation, and poorer cartilage quality as assessed by the preoperative score.

13. Ganz R, Klaue K, Vinh TS, Mast JW: A new periacetabular osteotomy for the treatment of hip dysplasias: Technique and preliminary results. *Clin Orthop Relat Res* 1988;232:26-36.

14. Leunig M, Parvizi J, Ganz R: Nonarthroplasty surgical treatment of hip osteoarthritis. *Instr Course Lect* 2006;55:159-166.

   This article provides a thorough review of nonarthroplasty options for treatment of hip osteoarthritis as well as a review of DDH and femoroacetabular impingement.

15. Yasunaga Y, Ochi M, Terayama H, Tanaka R, Yamasaki T, Ishii Y: Rotational acetabular osteotomy for advanced osteoarthritis secondary to dysplasia of the hip. *J Bone Joint Surg Am* 2006;88:1915-1919.

   After rotational acetabular osteotomy, patients older

6: Pediatrics

than 40 years had improved functional and pain scores at an average 8.5-year follow-up, with a projected 10-year survivorship of 71%.

16. Murray RO: The aetiology of primary osteoarthritis of the hip. *Br J Radiol* 1965;38:810-824.

17. Stulberg SD, Harris WH: Acetabular dysplasia and development of osteoarthritis of hip, in Harris WH (ed): *The Hip: Proceedings of the Second Open Scientific Meeting of the Hip Society.* St. Louis, MO, Mosby, 1974, pp 82-93.

18. Ganz R, Parvizi J, Beck M, Leunig M, Notzli H, Siebenrock KA: Femoroacetabular impingement: A cause for osteoarthritis of the hip. *Clin Orthop Relat Res* 2003; 417:112-120.

19. Nötzli HP, Wyss TF, Stoecklin CH, Schmid MR, Treiber K, Hodler J: The contour of the femoral head-neck junction as a predictor for the risk of anterior impingement. *J Bone Joint Surg Br* 2002;84:556-560.

20. Beck M, Kalhor M, Leunig M, Ganz R: Hip morphology influences the pattern of damage to the acetabular cartilage: Femoroacetabular impingement as a cause of early osteoarthritis of the hip. *J Bone Joint Surg Br* 2005;87:1012-1018.

    Specific articular injury patterns associated with the two main types of femoroacetabular impingement (cam and pincer) are described.

21. Lavigne M, Parvizi J, Beck M, Siebenrock KA, Ganz R, Leunig M: Anterior femoroacetabular impingement: Part I. Techniques of joint preserving surgery. *Clin Orthop Relat Res* 2004;418:61-66.

    This is the first of two articles describing a technique for treating femoroacetabular impingement.

22. Beck M, Leunig M, Parvizi J, Boutier V, Wyss D, Ganz R: Anterior femoraoacetabular impingement: Part II. Midterm results of surgical treatment. *Clin Orthop Relat Res* 2004;418:67-73.

    Results are reported for the first 19 patients treated for femoroacetabular impingement by surgical dislocation. These patients (mean age, 36 years) had improved pain and function at an average 4.7 years after surgery.

23. Peters CL, Erickson J: Treatment of femoro-acetabular impingement with surgical dislocation and debridement in young adults. *J Bone Joint Surg Am* 2006;88:1735-1741.

    At follow-up less than 3 years after surgical dislocation performed on 30 hips for impingement, the hips with worse arthrosis at the time of surgery were found to be less likely to gain long-term benefit. Almost one half of the patients had undergone or were planning conversion to total hip arthroplasty.

24. Espinosa N, Rothenfluh DA, Beck M, Ganz R, Leunig M: Treatment of femoro-acetabular impingement: Preliminary results of labral refixation. *J Bone Joint Surg Am* 2006;88:925-935.

    At initial evaluation of patients undergoing femoral head-neck osteoplasty for impingement, the authors found that for patients with a labral tear, those who had a labral repair had better results than those who had a labral tear resection.

25. Philippon MJ, Schenker M: Arthroscopy for the treatment of femoroacetabular impingement in the athlete. *Clin Sports Med* 2006;25:299-308.

    The use of arthroscopy is described to treat both cam and pincer impingement by femoral head-neck contouring and acetabular rim trimming.

26. Herring JA, Lundeen MA, Wenger DR: Minimal Perthes' disease. *J Bone Joint Surg Br* 1980;62-B:25-30.

27. Stulberg SD, Cooperman DR, Wallensten R: The natural history of Legg-Calve-Perthes disease. *J Bone Joint Surg Am* 1981;63:1095-1108.

28. Guille JT, Lipton GE, Szoke G, Bowen JR, Harcke HT, Glutting JJ: Legg-Calve-Perthes disease in girls: A comparison of the results with those seen in boys. *J Bone Joint Surg Am* 1998;80:1256-1263.

29. Gordon JE, Schoenecker PL, Osland JD, Dobbs MB, Szymanski DA, Luhmann SJ: Smoking and socioeconomic status in the etiology and severity of Legg-Calve-Perthes' disease. *J Pediatr Orthop B* 2004;13:367-370.

    An investigation of the effect of secondhand smoke on the risk of developing LCP found an increased risk for a child who lived with a smoker or had increased exposure to secondhand smoke.

30. Eldridge J, Dilley A, Austin H, et al: The role of protein C, protein S, and resistance to activated protein C in Legg-Perthes disease. *Pediatrics* 2001;107:1329-1334.

31. Hresko MT, McDougall PA, Gorlin JB, Vamvakas EC, Kasser JR, Neufeld EJ: Prospective reevaluation of the association between thrombotic diathesis and Legg-Perthes disease. *J Bone Joint Surg Am* 2002;84-A:1613-1618.

32. Mehta JS, Conybeare ME, Hinves BL, Winter JB: Protein C levels in patients with Legg-Calve-Perthes disease: Is it a true deficiency? *J Pediatr Orthop* 2006;26:200-203.

    An investigation of the possible link between low levels of protein C, possibly causing a hypercoagulable state, and LCP disease found lower but normal levels of protein C in the LCP group. The authors hypothesize that a connection may exist, despite evidence to the contrary.

33. Salter RB, Thompson GH: Legg-Calve-Perthes disease: The prognostic significance of the subchondral fracture and a two-group classification of the femoral head involvement. *J Bone Joint Surg Am* 1984;66:479-489.

34. Catterall A: Natural history, classification, and x-ray signs in Legg-Calve-Perthes' disease. *Acta Orthop Belg* 1980;46:346-351.

35. Herring JA, Kim HT, Browne R: Legg-Calve-Perthes disease: Part I. Classification of radiographs with use of the modified lateral pillar and Stulberg classifications. *J Bone Joint Surg Am* 2004;86-A:2103-2120.

    An intraobserver and interobserver reliability assessment system is presented for modified versions of both the lateral pillar and Stulberg classifications of LCP. The authors found excellent reliability and generalizability in these two classifications systems.

36. Herring JA, Kim HT, Browne R: Legg-Calve-Perthes disease: Part II. Prospective multicenter study of the effect of treatment on outcome. *J Bone Joint Surg Am* 2004;86-A:2121-2134.

    In an evaluation of multiple factors to assess outcome in LCP disease, the authors found that age at onset and lateral pillar classification are strongly correlated with outcome.

37. Nathan Sambandam S, Gul A, Shankar R, Goni V: Reliability of radiological classifications used in Legg-Calve-Perthes disease. *J Pediatr Orthop B* 2006;15:267-270.

    Radiologists evaluated the intrarater and interrater observer reliability of the Salter-Thompson, lateral pillar, and Catterall classification systems and found the lateral pillar system to have the best intrarater and interrater reliability.

38. Meehan PL, Angel D, Nelson JM: The Scottish Rite abduction orthosis for the treatment of Legg-Perthes disease: A radiographic analysis. *J Bone Joint Surg Am* 1992;74:2-12.

39. Reinker KA: Early diagnosis and treatment of hinge abduction in Legg-Perthes disease. *J Pediatr Orthop* 1996; 16:3-9.

40. Weinstein SL: Legg-Calve-Perthes disease: Results of long-term follow-up. *Hip* 1985:28-37.

41. Kim WC, Hiroshima K, Imaeda T: Multicenter study for Legg-Calve-Perthes disease in Japan. *J Orthop Sci* 2006;11:333-341.

    A survey study of the Japanese population similar to the one conducted by Herring and associates examined factors that may affect outcome in LCP disease. The authors found that the lateral pillar classification system and age at diagnosis were predictive of outcome. They also found that surgically treated hips have better outcomes but stated that the optimal treatment method could not be determined by the study.

42. Grzegorzewski A, Synder M, Kozlowski P, Szymczak W, Bowen RJ: The role of the acetabulum in Perthes disease. *J Pediatr Orthop* 2006;26:316-321.

    The deformity of the acetabulum associated with LCP disease and the effect of its final shape on the appearance of the mature femoral head are described. A worse acetabular appearance at maturity was correlated with poorer femoral head appearance; only surgical treatment improved the appearance.

43. Domzalski ME, Glutting J, Bowen JR, Littleton AG: Lateral acetabular growth stimulation following a labral support procedure in Legg-Calve-Perthes disease. *J Bone Joint Surg Am* 2006;88:1458-1466.

    A review of 65 hips with unilateral disease found an advantage to surgically providing increased femoral head coverage and improving containment in hips with LCP, rather than performing a proximal femoral osteotomy alone. This shelf procedure had increased coverage and depth at 3-year follow-up. Level of evidence: Therapeutic level III.

44. Lehmann CL, Arons RR, Loder RT, Vitale MG: The epidemiology of slipped capital femoral epiphysis: An update. *J Pediatr Orthop* 2006;26:286-290.

    A review of pediatric discharge reports from 1997 and 2000 as well as US census databases to determine the epidemiology of SCFE in the United States found a higher incidence among Hispanics, African Americans, and males. There also may be an increased incidence in the Northeast and West regions.

45. Loder RT, Starnes T, Dikos G: Atypical and typical (idiopathic) slipped capital femoral epiphysis: Reconfirmation of the age-weight test and description of the height and age-height tests. *J Bone Joint Surg Am* 2006;88: 1574-1581.

    The authors reaffirm the accuracy of the age-weight and height tests to detect atypical SCFE, and they introduce the age-height test for the same purpose. All three tests provide good to excellent sensitivity and excellent negative predictive value when used to assess the need for further work for atypical SCFE. Level of evidence: Diagnostic level I.

46. Bhatia NN, Pirpiris M, Otsuka NY: Body mass index in patients with slipped capital femoral epiphysis. *J Pediatr Orthop* 2006;26:197-199.

    In an evaluation of body mass index and its relationship to bilateral involvement in SCFE, the 16 patients with bilateral SCFE had a significantly higher body mass index than patients with unilateral SCFE.

47. Loder RT, Starnes T, Dikos G, Aronsson DD: Demographic predictors of severity of stable slipped capital femoral epiphyses. *J Bone Joint Surg Am* 2006;88:97-105.

    A study of 328 stable slips found that early detection of SCFE can prevent increased severity and worse outcome. Older age and longer duration of symptoms were significant predictors of increased severity of slip.

48. Loder RT, Starnes T, Dikos G: The narrow window of the bone age in children with slipped capital femoral epiphysis: A reassessment one decade later. *J Pediatr Orthop* 2006;26:300-306.

    A reevaluation of the Oxford Bone Age scale found that lower bone age was correlated with increased risk of bilateral SCFE.

49. Segal LS, Jacobson JA, Saunders MM: Biomechanical analysis of in situ single versus double screw fixation in a nonreduced slipped capital femoral epiphysis model.

6: Pediatrics

J Pediatr Orthop 2006;26:479-485.

An evaluation of stiffness and resistance to torsional load in immature bovine femurs with one-screw or two-screw fixation found as much as 312% increased resistance to torsional load with two-screw fixation.

50. Diab M, Hresko MT, Millis MB: Intertrochanteric versus subcapital osteotomy in slipped capital femoral epiphysis. *Clin Orthop Relat Res* 2004;427:204-212.

A review of 15 intertrochanteric osteotomies and 11 subcapital osteotomies to correct proximal femoral deformity following severe SCFE found that intertrochanteric osteotomy was preferable for restoring proximal femoral anatomic relationships and had a lower reoperation rate.

51. Kocher MS, Bishop JA, Hresko MT, Millis MB, Kasser JR: Prophylactic pinning of the contralateral hip after unilateral slipped capital femoral epiphysis. *J Bone Joint Surg Am* 2004;86-A:2658-2665.

Decision analysis revealed that careful observation was the optimal choice after unilateral SCFE, unless the estimated probability of contralateral slip was higher than 27% or reliable follow-up was not feasible.

52. Fairbank HA: Coxa vara due to congenital defect of the neck of the femur. *J Anat* 1928;62:232-237.

53. Weinstein JN, Kuo KN, Millar EA: Congenital coxa vara: A retrospective review. *J Pediatr Orthop* 1984;4:70-77.

54. Aarabi M, Rauch F, Hamdy RC, Fassier F: High prevalence of coxa vara in patients with severe osteogenesis imperfecta. *J Pediatr Orthop* 2006;26:24-28.

Coxa vara in patients with severe osteogenesis imperfecta is not rare. The authors recommend routine assessment for progressive deformity of the proximal femur.

55. Sabharwal S, Mittal R, Cox G: Percutaneous triplanar femoral osteotomy correction for developmental coxa vara: A new technique. *J Pediatr Orthop* 2005;25:28-33.

The outcome of percutaneous triplanar proximal femoral osteotomy and acute correction of coxa vara at 2-year follow-up is described. A low-profile Ilizarov external fixator was used in six hips, achieving excellent correction with no nonunions.

Chapter 60

Knee, Leg, Ankle, and Foot Trauma: Pediatrics

R. Dale Blasier, MD, FRCS(C)

Distal Femur

Supracondylar Fractures

Fractures within approximately 3 inches of the distal femoral physis are called supracondylar fractures. In children 2 to 6 years of age, these fractures are often greenstick fractures. In children older than 6 years, the fracture is often complete and displaced.

In many ways, treatment of these fractures is similar to treatment of supracondylar fractures of the elbow. The fracture can be challenging to hold in a cast, and internal fixation may be required. For stable fractures, closed reduction and casting is appropriate. For unstable fractures, closed reduction and pinning should be considered. Often an extension component requires knee flexion to be reduced. Smooth pins are generally drilled from distal (femoral condyle) to proximal (distal metaphysis). Pins may protrude from the knee, although this position risks infection into the knee joint; or they may protrude proximally (**Figure 1**). Some fractures are too unstable or too proximal for fixation with pins and require open reduction and internal fixation with plate and screws, external fixation, or flexible intramedullary nailing from above (**Figure 2**).

The prognosis for healing is good. Residual angulation in flexion or extension will remodel, but varus and valgus are less well tolerated. Postoperative stiffness is rare.

Distal Femoral Physeal Fractures

A direct blow to the knee, which in an adult might be expected to cause injury to the medial collateral ligament or the anterior cruciate ligament, is more likely to displace the distal femoral epiphysis in a child. The Salter-Harris classification is generally useful in assessing these fractures, although the possibility of late growth disorders can be underestimated. A Salter-Harris type I or type II fracture can be termed distal femoral physeal separation. Truly nondisplaced and stable fractures can be managed with a cast and monitored for displacement. Displaced fractures should be reduced and fixed under general anesthesia (**Figure 3**). Fixation usually requires crossed smooth wires or transverse screws placed through the Thurston-Holland fragment.[1]

Separations of the distal femur may result in growth derangement because of shearing off of the remarkable undulations of the growth plate or scuffing of the growth plate by the metaphysis during displacement and replacement of the epiphysis.[2] Parents must be warned that physeal damage causes late growth derangement (stunted growth or angular deformity) in as many as 56% of patients.

Salter-Harris type III and type IV distal femoral epiphyseal fractures are of interest because they involve the growth plate and are intra-articular. CT may be indicated if plain radiography does not reveal the displacement or rotation of fracture fragments. Because of the mechanism of injury, it is likely that the cruciate ligaments are also injured. Preoperative MRI evaluation of the knee (before placement of metallic implants) may prove useful in delineating ligament or meniscal injuries. A stable, nondisplaced fracture can be managed by simple immobilization in a long-leg cast, provided the fracture is followed to check for displacement. All displaced intra-articular fractures must be anatomically reduced and fixed in a manner that will not disrupt growth. The prognosis is good for healing, although there is a risk of growth derangement.

Patellar Sleeve Fractures

Patellar sleeve fracture is an avulsion injury peculiar to children. It occurs during a strong contraction of the quadriceps against the fixed lower leg, when a sleeve of soft tissue consisting anteriorly of periosteum and posteriorly of articular cartilage is avulsed from the inferior pole of the patella. The patella is displaced superiorly, and active knee extension is lost.

The diagnosis can be made from plain radiographs, if a fragment of bone pulled away from the patella within the sleeve is seen distal to a high-riding patella. The injury is easily seen on MRI scans. It is repaired surgically with strong sutures through the patella.

Tibia

Proximal Tibial Epiphyseal Injuries

Proximal tibial epiphyseal injuries are uncommon. They typically result from a direct blow to the knee or,

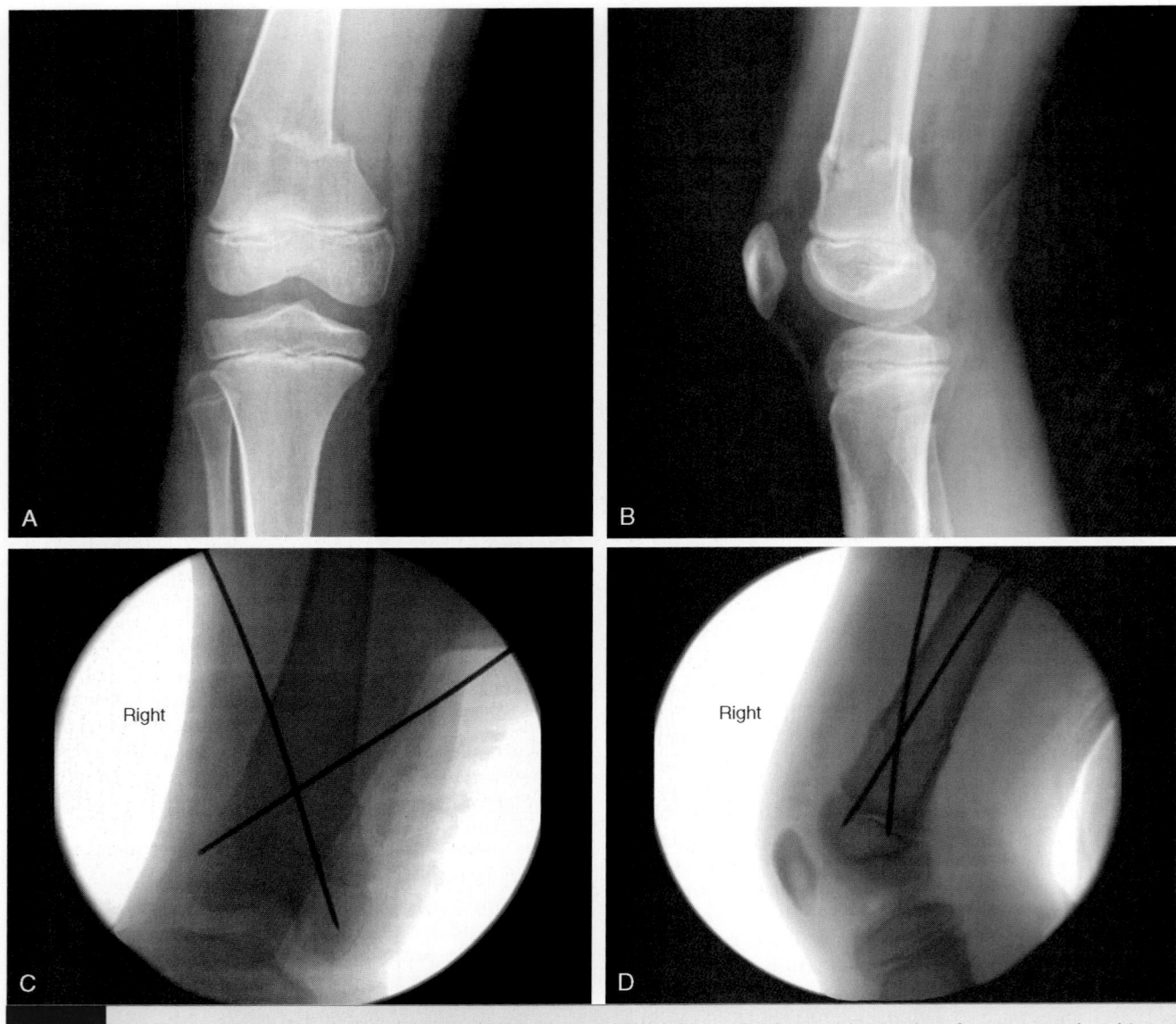

Figure 1 Supracondylar fracture of the femur. AP **(A)** and lateral **(B)** radiographs show an incomplete fracture angulated into varus. AP **(C)** and lateral **(D)** radiographs show results of reduction and pinning. The pins are brought out proximally through the skin to avoid articular contamination along pin tracts.

less frequently, an indirect injury to the knee, such as a hyperextension or twisting injury of the limb. The two main types are proximal tibial physeal separation and intra-articular fracture.

Because the epiphysis is spanned rather than attached to the collateral ligaments at the proximal tibia, avulsion fractures are unusual. The forces necessary to fracture the proximal tibial epiphysis must be unusual or severe. Plain radiography is usually sufficient to evaluate proximal tibial physeal separations. Intra-articular fractures that cannot be well visualized on plain radiographs should be evaluated with CT or MRI to assess displacement, step-off in the articular surface or physis, and possible joint depression. Arteriography should be considered if distal pulses are diminished after reduction of a proximal tibial physeal separation.

A true nondisplaced fracture, whether it is a physeal separation or intra-articular fracture, can be managed by simple immobilization in a long-leg cast. Displaced physeal separations must be reduced with the patient under general anesthesia. The reduction is rarely stable, and fixation with crossed smooth wires is usually necessary. The presence of interposed soft tissue must be suspected if closed reduction is not successful, and an open reduction should be performed. A displaced intra-articular fracture (Salter-Harris type III or type IV) should be managed by anatomic reduction and fixation (**Figure 4**). Rarely, an avulsion of the proximal fibular epiphysis is present. If it is widely displaced (more than 1 cm), it should be reduced and fixed. The possibility of late growth derangement should be explained to the parents at the time of injury.

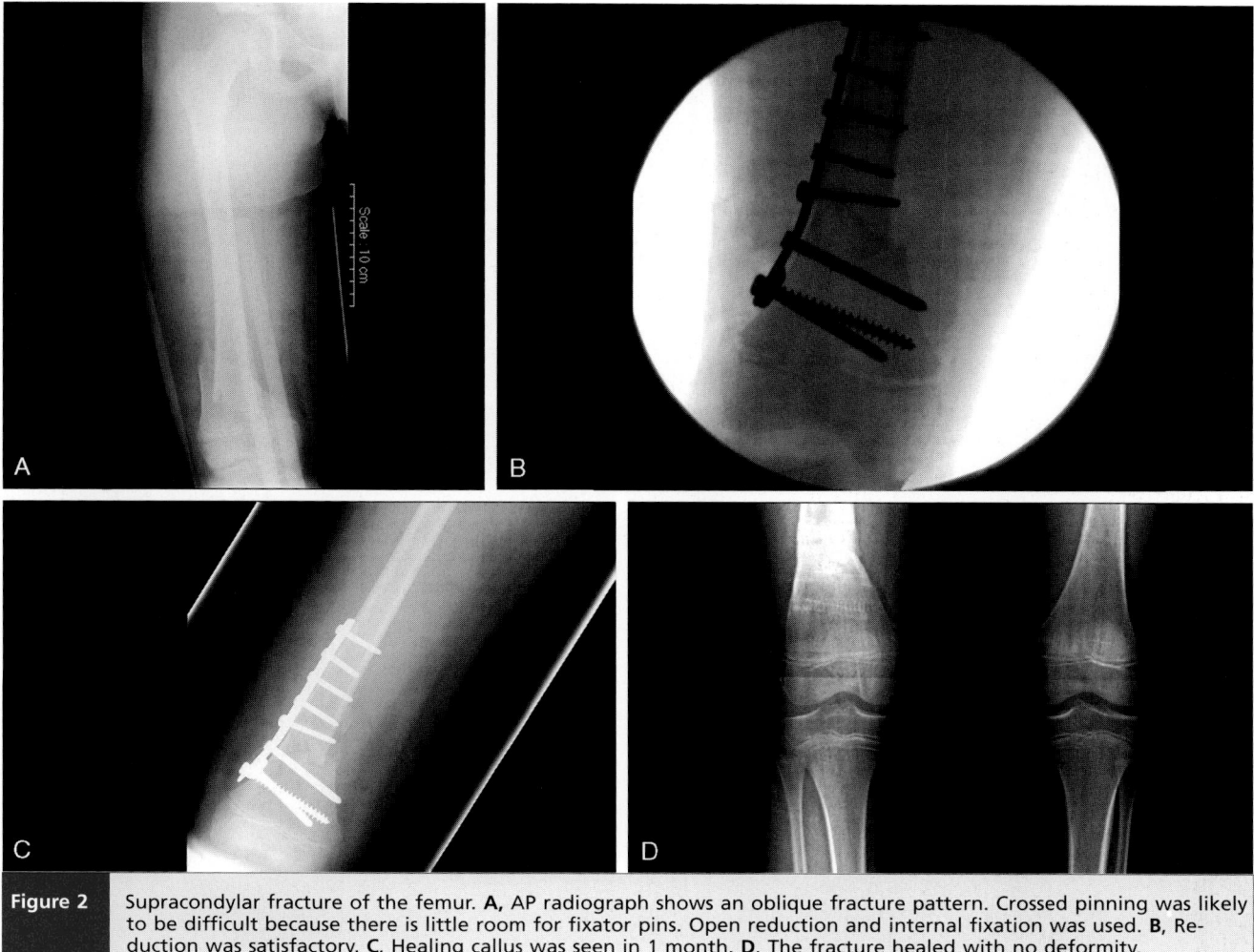

Figure 2   Supracondylar fracture of the femur. **A,** AP radiograph shows an oblique fracture pattern. Crossed pinning was likely to be difficult because there is little room for fixator pins. Open reduction and internal fixation was used. **B,** Reduction was satisfactory. **C,** Healing callus was seen in 1 month. **D,** The fracture healed with no deformity.

Fractures of the Tibial Tubercle

Fractures of the tibial tubercle are avulsion injuries that occur as the result of a strong concentric contraction during a jump or an eccentric contraction during landing. Portions of the tibial tubercle and the unfused anterior tibial epiphysis are pulled upward by the force of the quadriceps and, by necessity, the extensor retinaculum is also avulsed from the anterior tibia. Plain radiographs are generally sufficient for diagnosis of the injury. If intra-articular separation is a possibility, CT may be useful.

These fractures have been divided into three types based on fragment size and the extent of displacement.[3] In a type I injury, a small fragment is proximally displaced. In a type II injury, the secondary center of ossification has coalesced with the proximal tibial epiphysis, and the fracture is at this junction. The articular surface remains intact. In a type III injury, the fracture extends through the articular surface. Nondisplaced and type I fractures can be managed by immobilization with a comfortable degree of knee extension. Minimally displaced fractures may respond to closed reduction by direct pressure over the tubercle. If the tubercle

fragment tents the skin or if the tubercle fragment and patella have migrated proximally after attempted reduction, the fracture should be opened and fixed. A type II or type III tibial tubercle fracture requires open reduction and internal fixation. Fixation is best accomplished by placing one or two screws through the tibial tubercle into the proximal tibia or entirely within the epiphysis (**Figure 5**). Comminution and meniscal disruption may be present in type III fractures. If fluoroscopy suggests that the fracture is displaced, arthrotomy or arthroscopy can be used to visualize and explore the fracture. Anatomic reduction of the joint surface should be the goal. Cannulated screws are well suited for this repair. With type II and III fractures, the soft tissues avulsed from the proximal tibia should be reapproximated as completely as possible. Growth arrest is uncommon, because this fracture usually occurs at the end of bone growth.[4] Compartment syndrome may develop with this injury.

Proximal Tibial Metaphyseal Fractures

Fractures of the proximal tibial metaphysis are relatively common in young children (2 to 6 years of age)

6: Pediatrics

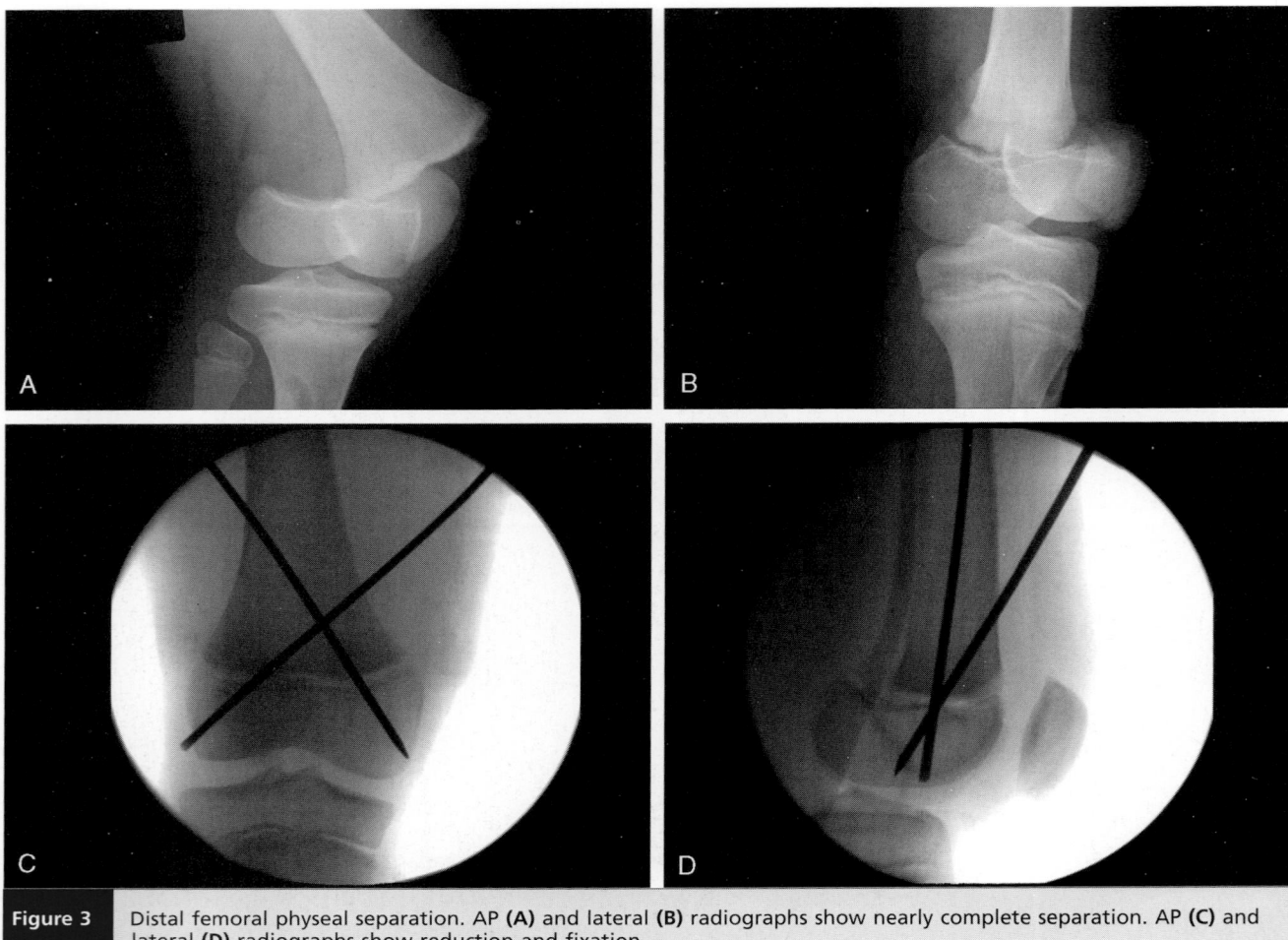

Figure 3 Distal femoral physeal separation. AP **(A)** and lateral **(B)** radiographs show nearly complete separation. AP **(C)** and lateral **(D)** radiographs show reduction and fixation.

as the result of a fall from a height or a direct blow to the lateral aspect of the knee. In young children, this low-energy injury typically is minimally displaced or nondisplaced. Commonly, it is a transverse impaction fracture or a valgus greenstick fracture that leaves the lateral cortex intact. The seemingly benign fracture has an unpredictable tendency to develop a valgus deformity months after the original injury. Therefore, these incomplete fractures are best treated by reducing or overreducing the valgus deformity. The reduction should be maintained in a long-leg cast with the knee in extension to control varus-valgus deformity. The fracture will heal in approximately 3 weeks. The patient should be followed to check for late valgus deformity. Parents should be warned at the time of injury about the possibility of valgus deformity.

In children older than 6 years, the fracture typically results from a high-energy injury that was caused by a direct blow (such as occurs during a motor vehicle crash). The fracture may be complete, displaced, or open. In a displaced fracture, the proximity of the trifurcation of the popliteal artery and the peroneal nerve must be considered. A high-energy fracture that is well aligned and has no associated soft-tissue injury can be managed in a cast. A fracture that cannot be well aligned with closed treatment or has associated soft-tissue or neurovascular injuries should be surgically stabilized with pins, plate, and screws or with an external fixator. If the fracture is complicated by late valgus deformity, the best course is observation until adolescence, because the valgus deformity often will improve with growth.[5] Valgus deformity is likely to recur after early osteotomy of the proximal tibia. Bracing has not been shown to have a beneficial effect. If surgical treatment is necessary, it should be delayed until near the end of bone growth. Correction can be obtained by osteotomy or a well-timed medial hemiepiphysiodesis.

Tibial Shaft Fractures

Tibial shaft fractures, which result from a direct blow to the leg or from a twisting injury, are common in ambulatory children. Sometimes these fractures are open. Often the fibula is also fractured. A nondisplaced fracture of a toddler's relatively plastic tibia is called a toddler's fracture.

Plain radiographs are generally sufficient to diagnose a fracture of the tibia or fibula, although a toddler's fracture may not be easily seen on plain radiographs

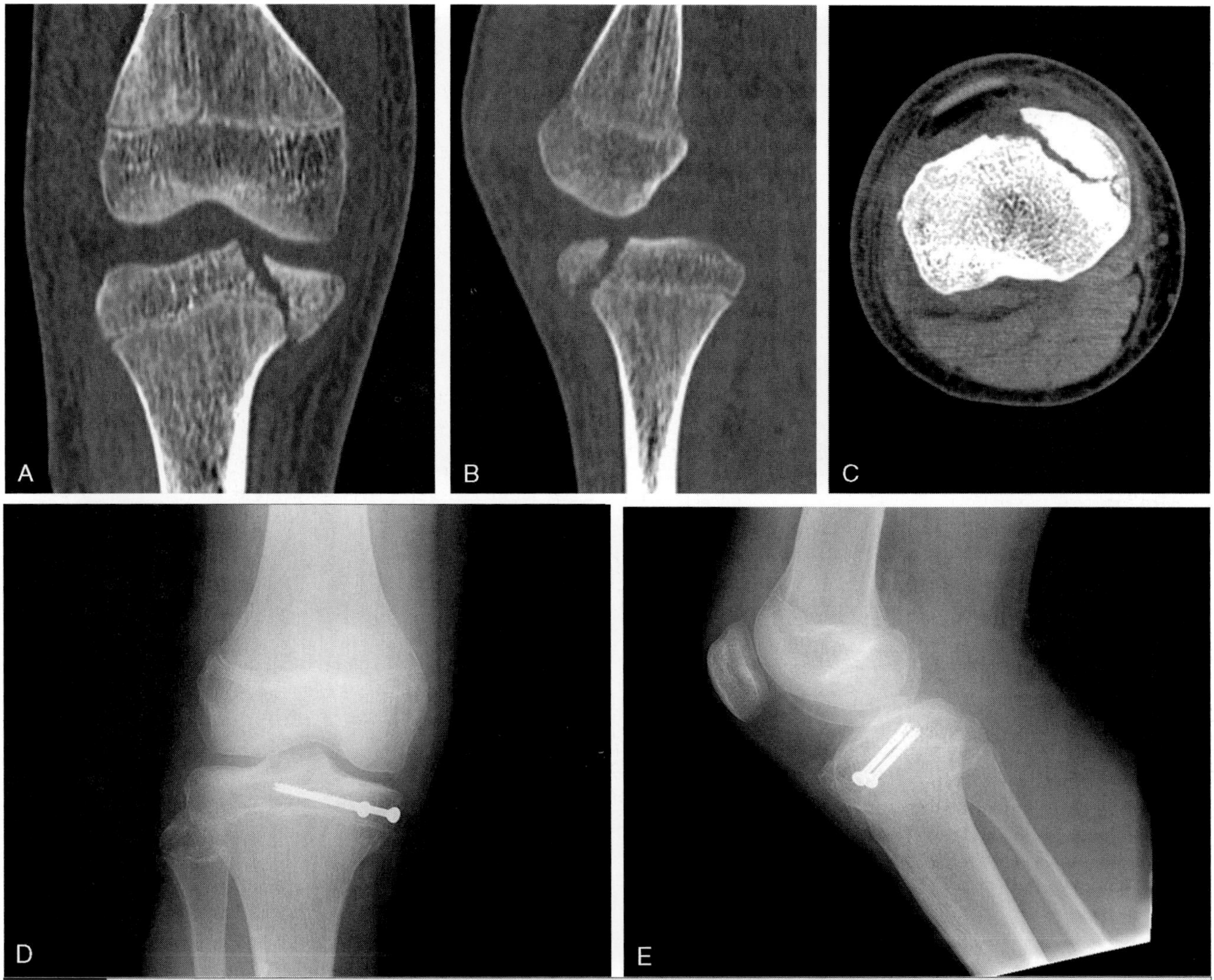

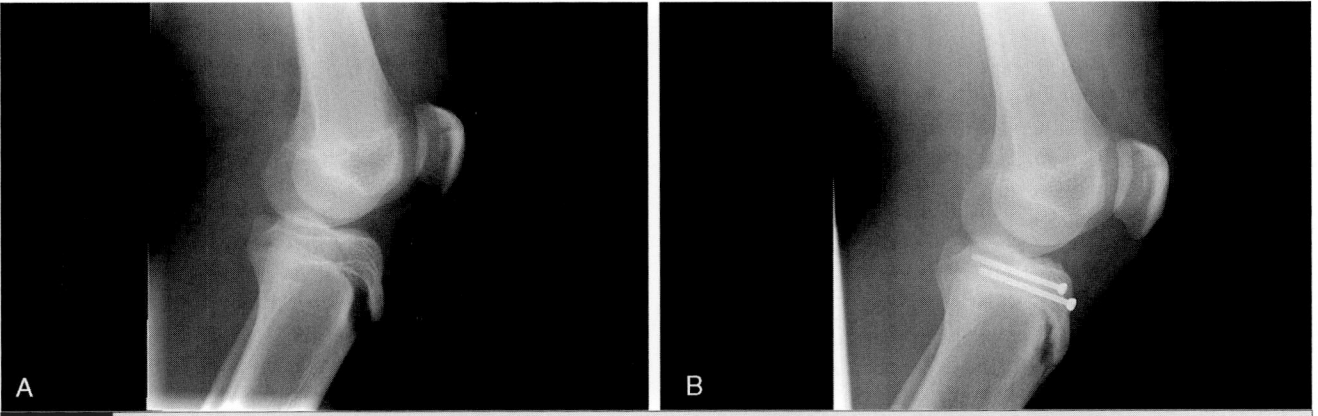

Figure 4   Fracture of the proximal tibia. Coronal **(A)**, sagittal **(B)**, and axial **(C)** CT cuts show a displaced intra-articular fracture. The fracture was lagged together with cannulated screws. AP **(D)** and lateral **(E)** radiographs show healing 2 months after screw fixation.

Figure 5   Lateral radiographs showing tibial tubercle avulsion fracture. **A,** Displacement is seen proximally. Interposed periosteum, which prevented closed reduction, was removed at surgery. **B,** Screws did not violate the physis. Healing was uneventful.

6: Pediatrics

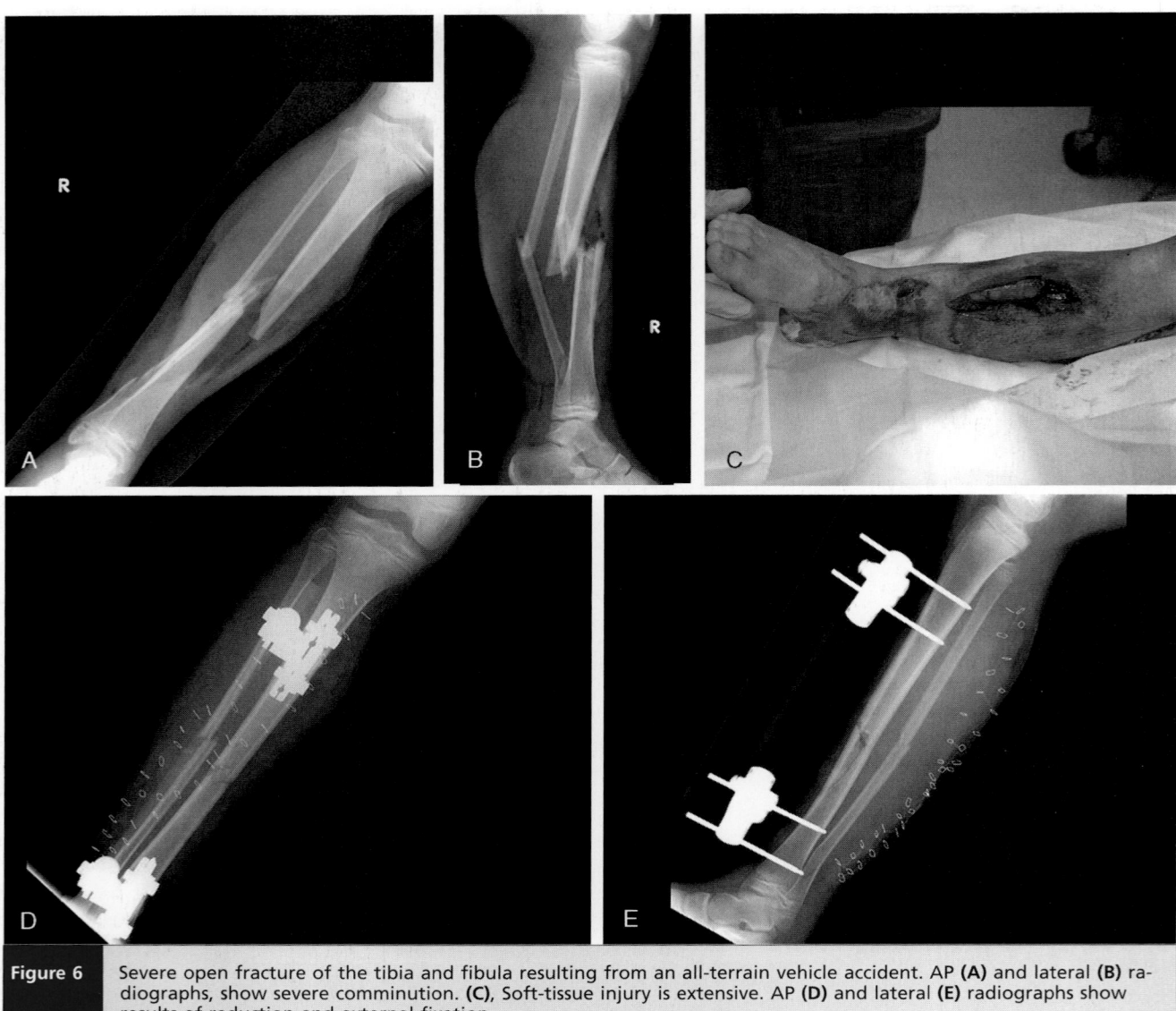

Figure 6 Severe open fracture of the tibia and fibula resulting from an all-terrain vehicle accident. AP **(A)** and lateral **(B)** radiographs, show severe comminution. **(C)**, Soft-tissue injury is extensive. AP **(D)** and lateral **(E)** radiographs show results of reduction and external fixation.

until callus begins to form. Closed treatment in an above-knee cast is appropriate for almost all tibial shaft fractures. Displaced fractures should be manipulated to within 10° of residual angulation as seen on AP and lateral images in children younger than 8 years. Angulation should be 5° or less in children older than 8 years.[6] If the fibula is intact (not fractured), reducing the tibial fracture out of varus may be difficult. Attention should be paid to rotation to avoid asymmetry after healing.

Surgical fixation is required for fractures in which adequate closed reduction cannot be obtained or maintained, fractures in a multiple trauma patient, or fractures complicated by wounds or burns that preclude casting. Several fixation choices are available. Standard plates and screws should be avoided because of the extensive soft-tissue stripping required for insertion, and the stress-riser effect. External fixation is suitable for

an open fracture or a fracture associated with skin disorders that would make internal fixation risky (**Figure 6**). Flexible intramedullary nails are useful in fixation of closed or low-grade open tibial shaft fractures[7,8] (**Figure 7**).

Healing is to be expected, unless the fracture was open or surgically exposed. Slight overgrowth sometimes occurs, and shortening may occur after a comminuted or long oblique fracture.[9] Nonunion, which is rare, usually responds to posterolateral bone grafting.

Compartment Syndrome

Compartment syndrome in the leg most commonly occurs after a closed tibial shaft fracture, although it can also occur after an open fracture. Reperfusion must be considered as a cause of compartment syndrome, even in the absence of fracture. The key to diagnosing compartment syndrome is to maintain a high degree of clin-

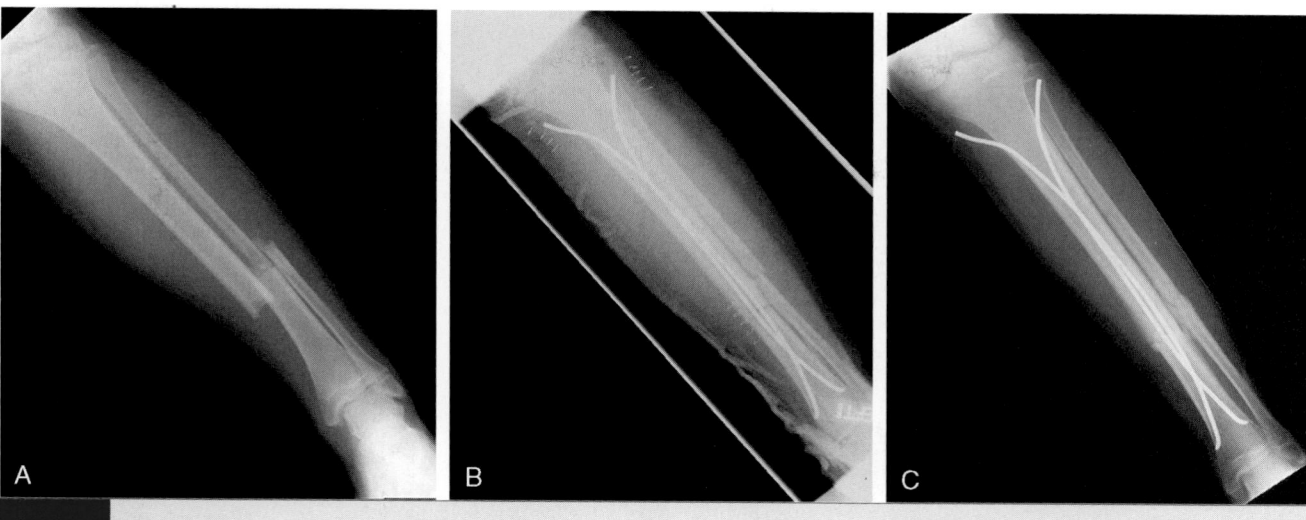

Figure 7 AP radiographs showing a fracture of the tibia and fibula resulting from a biking accident. **A,** The fracture involves the distal shaft. **B,** The fracture was reduced and fixed with nails. **C,** Callus is seen at approximately 6 weeks.

ical suspicion after an injury that has the typical physical findings. Pressure measurements can confirm the diagnosis. The treatment is emergent decompression by fasciotomy.[10-12]

Distal Tibial Metaphyseal Fractures

Distal tibial metaphyseal fractures usually to occur in children age 2 to 6 years who sustain a direct blow or a fall that results in injury to the distal tibia just above the ankle. Most commonly the result is a torus or greenstick fracture with mild recurvatum and a varus or valgus deformity. These fractures are rarely complete, and they tend to heal rapidly. For a fracture with little angulation, treatment consists of simple immobilization in a below-knee cast. For a fracture with significant angulation, closed reduction under general anesthesia is generally required to disimpact the fracture. Equinus immobilization may be necessary to prevent recurvatum at the fracture site.

Ankle

Distal Tibial Physeal Injuries

Distal tibial physeal injuries are relatively common and generally occur as a result of adduction or external rotation injuries. These Salter-Harris type I or type II injuries can be considered distal tibial physeal separations, and are more likely to cause growth derangement than other epiphyseal separations. Displaced fractures should be treated with closed reduction; an anesthetic is usually administered. The fracture is reduced by reversal of the mechanism of injury. For a stable fracture after closed reduction, immobilization in an above-knee cast is indicated (**Figure 8**). If the fracture is unstable after closed reduction, it can be stabilized with smooth Kirschner wires until healed. Residual gapping at the

physeal fracture line may be the result of interposed periosteum; open extraction of the periosteal flap can reduce the possibility of late growth derangement.[13]

Distal Tibial Epiphyseal Injuries

Distal tibial epiphyseal fractures are relatively uncommon. They tend to occur around the medial malleolus but can occur laterally (the lateral form is called juvenile Tillaux fracture). Injuries of the medial malleolus usually occur as a result of adduction force at the ankle. Often the fibula is also injured.

The significance of these Salter-Harris type III and type IV fractures is twofold: they are intra-articular, and they involve the physis. CT is indicated if any question exists as to the amount of displacement in the fracture. For nondisplaced fractures, simple immobilization may be sufficient for healing. Displaced fractures require open or closed reduction and internal fixation to realign the physis and the articular surface (**Figure 9**). Fixation with cannulated screws that cross the fracture parallel to the growth plate is preferred.[14] Although the prognosis is good, the possibility of late growth arrest exists.[15] With concomitant injuries of the fibula, observation or closed reduction is indicated.

Transitional Fractures of the Distal Tibia

Transitional fractures occur when the growth plate is beginning to close. Closure starts anteromedially, progresses posteriorly and laterally, and finishes anterolaterally. During this transitional period, fracture of portions of the distal tibial epiphysis may occur rather than complete separation of the distal tibial epiphysis. Transitional fractures of the distal tibia sometimes occur in adolescents nearing skeletal maturity. The unique sequence of closure of the distal tibial physis (central, medial, lateral, and anterolateral) causes the unusual fracture patterns of this injury.

6: Pediatrics

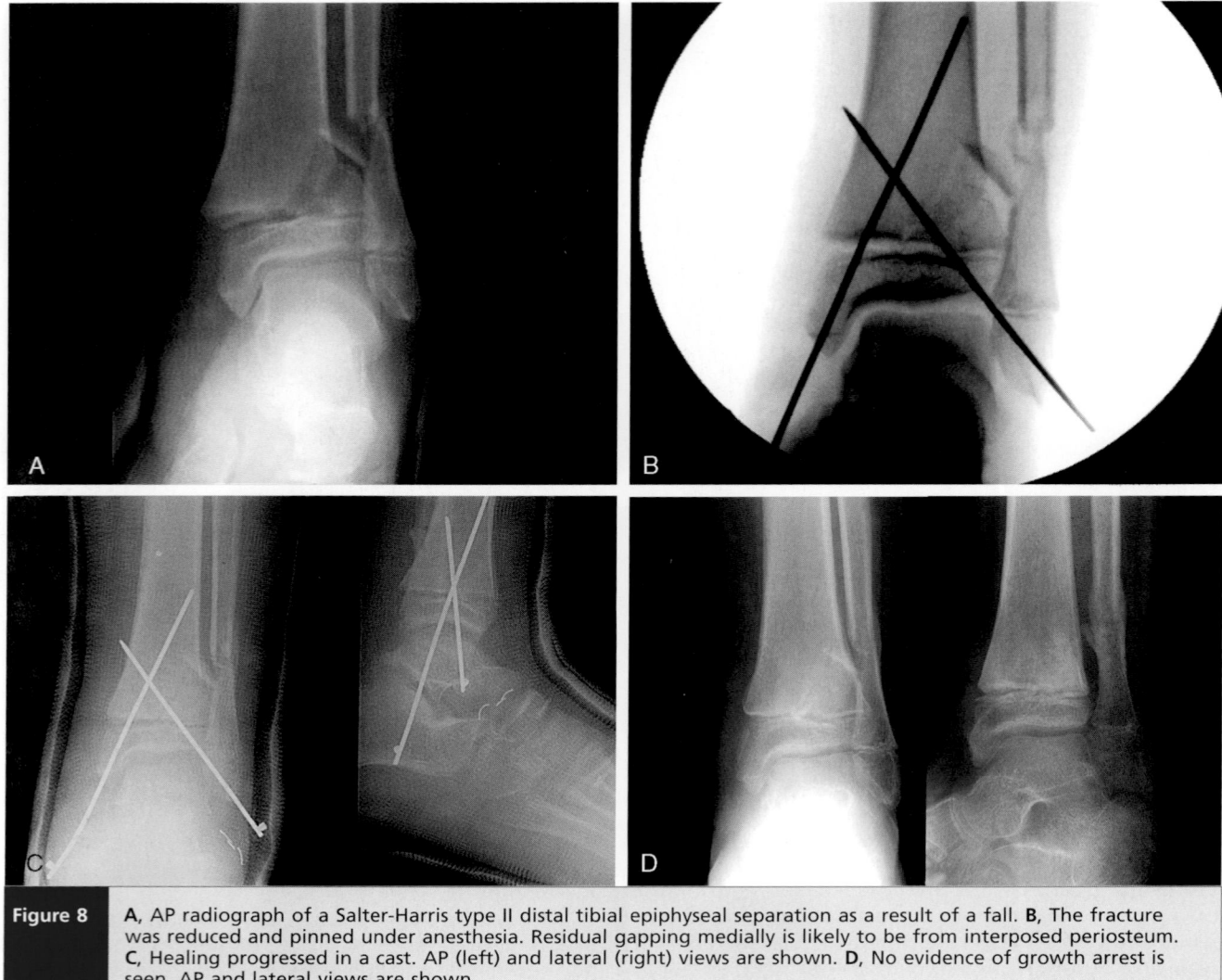

Figure 8   **A,** AP radiograph of a Salter-Harris type II distal tibial epiphyseal separation as a result of a fall. **B,** The fracture was reduced and pinned under anesthesia. Residual gapping medially is likely to be from interposed periosteum. **C,** Healing progressed in a cast. AP (left) and lateral (right) views are shown. **D,** No evidence of growth arrest is seen. AP and lateral views are shown.

The Tillaux fracture is an isolated fracture of the anterolateral portion of the distal tibial epiphysis. It occurs in early adolescence, when the medial half of the growth plate has closed but the lateral portion remains open. The fracture tends to occur as a result of a strong external rotation force. The anterior tibiofibular ligament, which is attached to the anterolateral portion of the tibial epiphysis, avulses the anterolateral quarter of the epiphysis. The result is a Salter-Harris type III fracture. If displacement is significant, gapping of the joint surface and late instability in external rotation may be present. Plain radiographs can suggest the diagnosis, but CT is needed to show the fracture's extent and displacement. If CT shows the fracture to be completely nondisplaced, treatment with closed immobilization alone may be possible. A fracture displaced more than 2 mm should be reduced open or closed and fixed with cannulated screws. Late growth derangement is unlikely because these fractures occur near the end of growth.

Triplane Fractures

The triplane fracture also tends to occur near the end of growth. Although variations are possible, the typical fracture line crosses the epiphysis in the sagittal plane, the physis in the transverse plane, and the distal tibial metaphysis in the coronal plane. There may be two to four fracture fragments with different degrees of displacement. CT is useful to determine the number of fragments and their displacement in order to plan surgery. The exact classification of these fractures is probably not as important as reconstitution of the joint surface and reattachment of the joint surface to the distal tibia. A closed reduction should be attempted. Fractures that cannot be reduced anatomically should be reduced open. Fixation is best achieved with cannulated screws (**Figure 10**).

Fractures of the Distal Fibula

Fractures of the distal fibula are relatively common and usually occur as isolated injuries resulting from inver-

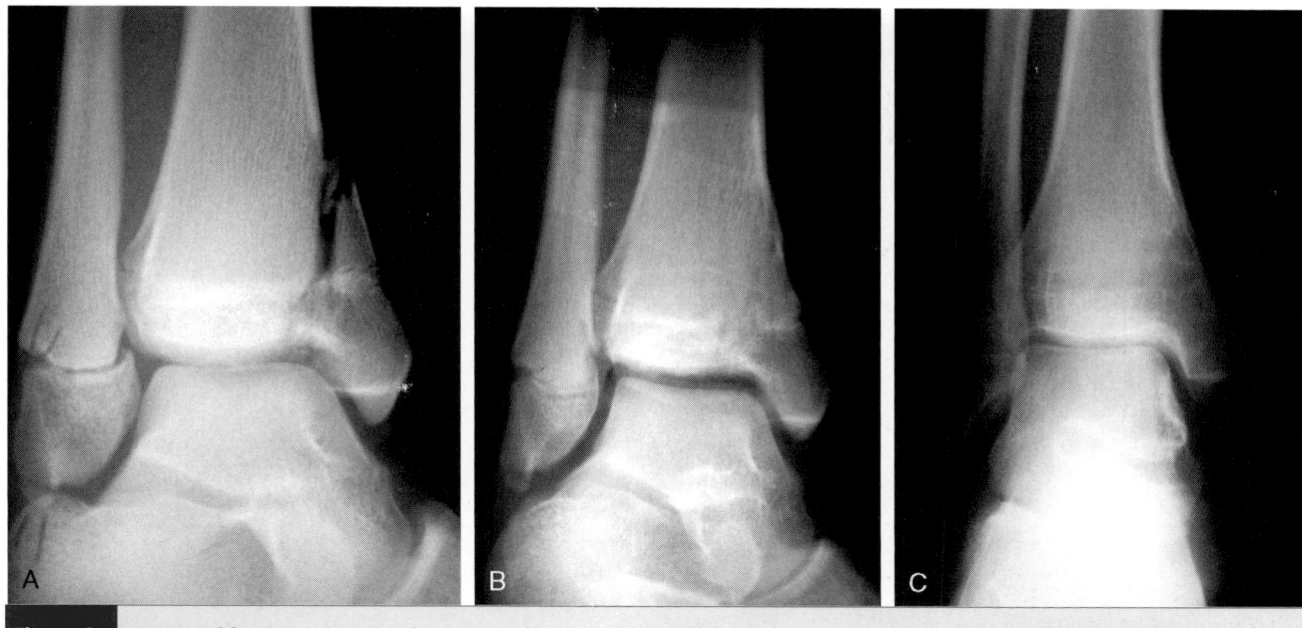

Figure 9 **A**, An adduction injury resulted in a Salter-Harris type IV fracture around the medial malleolus and a distal fibular physeal separation. **B**, The fracture around the medial malleolus was fixed with two resorbable screws that paralleled the physis. The distal fibula was reduced closed. **C**, Healing was uneventful. AP views are shown.

sion or external rotation at the ankle. They can also occur in association with fractures of the medial malleolus. The most common are classified as Salter-Harris type I or type II distal metaphyseal fractures. The ankle mortise is rarely disrupted. Treatment is generally by closed means, and manipulation is usually not needed. Open treatment and pinning with Kirschner wires is rarely necessary.

Foot

Fractures of the Talus

Fractures of the talus are rare in children. They can occur through the talar neck, as a compression fracture of the dome, or as a medial or lateral process fracture. These high-energy injuries usually result from a motor vehicle crash or a fall from a height. CT is indicated to resolve questions about the extent of the injury or displacement. The treatment of a nondisplaced fracture is simple immobilization. Process fractures generally can be managed by simple immobilization, unless the displacement is severe. Displaced fractures of the talar neck are anatomically reduced and fixed, usually with a medial approach; occasionally, an anterolateral approach is also needed. Medial malleolar osteotomy presents risks for growing children. The prognosis is generally good for these fractures, although possible complications include stiffness and late pain.

Fractures of the Calcaneus

Causes of a fracture of the calcaneus include stress, avulsion as a result of pull by the Achilles tendon on the tuberosity, a fall from a height causing a fracture of the tuberosity or body of the calcaneus, or direct injury as a result of a lawn mower accident or a gunshot wound, for example.

The calcaneus is almost entirely cancellous. The Achilles tendon is inserted at the posterior aspect of the large calcaneal apophysis, and the superior aspect of the calcaneus comprises a large portion of the subtalar joint. These injuries usually can be seen on plain radiographs, although CT is helpful if displacement or intra-articular involvement must be investigated.

Treatment depends on the nature of the injury. The priorities are to maintain the shape and weight-bearing surfaces of the calcaneus and to preserve the insertion of the Achilles tendon and the integrity of the subtalar joint. Avulsion fractures of the calcaneus involving the Achilles tendon generally should be reduced and fixed to maintain the competence of the gastrocnemius-soleus complex. Simple nondisplaced fractures to the metaphyseal bone can be managed by immobilization. Management of open fractures and those resulting from a penetrating injury must encompass wound management and hygiene. Displaced intra-articular fractures of the subtalar joint should be anatomically reduced and fixed, especially in an older child who is unlikely to undergo significant growth or remodeling[16] (**Figure 11**). If fixation is required, the approach should be through a lateral L-type incision similar to the incision used for adults.

The prognosis for healing is good. Intra-articular fractures can be complicated by late stiffness, and injury to the calcaneal apophysis, particularly as it occurs in lawn mower injuries, can result in late growth derangement.

6: Pediatrics

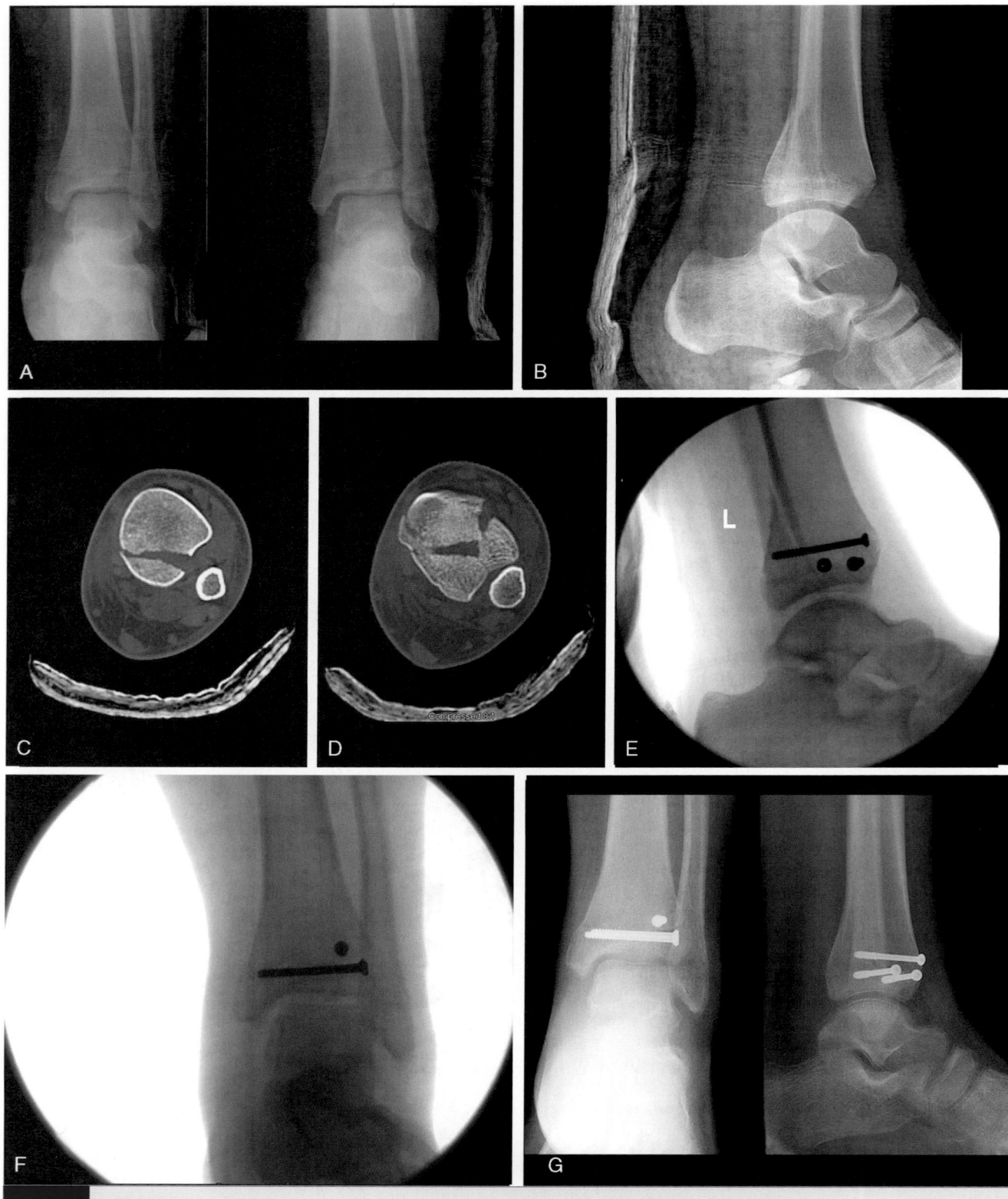

Figure 10   A twisting injury resulted in a triplane fracture of the distal tibia. **A,** AP radiographs show a fracture in the sagittal plane through the epiphysis. **B,** A lateral radiograph shows a fracture through the metaphysis in the coronal plane. **C,** An axial CT cut through the metaphysis shows displacement of the Thurston-Holland fragment. **D,** An axial CT cut through the epiphysis shows intra-articular separation. **E** and **F,** The fracture was reduced and fixed with cannulated screws only. **G,** The physis has closed and healing is complete at 6 weeks. AP (left) and lateral (right) views are shown.

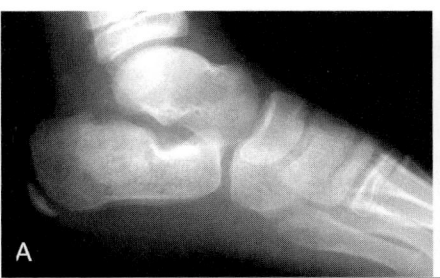 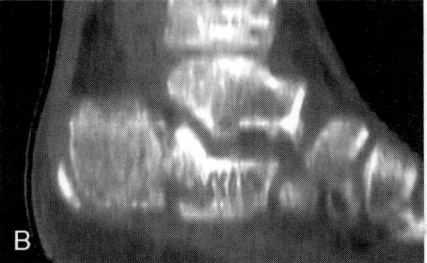 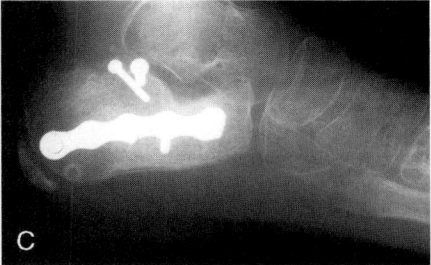

Figure 11 **A,** Lateral radiograph showing a fracture of the calcaneus caused by a fall from a height. **B,** A sagittal CT scan shows separation of the tuberosity and depression of the subtalar joint. **C,** After open reduction and internal fixation, recovery was complete. A lateral view is shown.

Fractures of the Midfoot

Injuries to the midfoot are rare.[17] They tend to occur as a result of sudden forceful twisting of the foot, a direct trauma such as a blow to the foot, or a penetrating injury. The most common injury is an avulsion fracture of the dorsal lip of the navicular by the attached capsule. Fractures of the cuboid, navicular, or cuneiform occur but are rarely displaced. In a toddler, a nondisplaced fracture may be identified as the cause of a limp; if plain radiographs are negative, a bone scan may identify a midfoot fracture.

For an avulsion or nondisplaced fracture, treatment consists of simple immobilization. Any fracture likely to permanently alter the shape or mobility of the foot should be treated with open or closed reduction and internal fixation. The treatment of a penetrating injury is generally dictated by the management of the wound. The prognosis is good if the foot architecture and joint alignment are maintained. Long-term complications can include joint stiffness and malalignment of the foot.

Tarsometatarsal Injuries

Tarsometatarsal injuries are rare in children, but they become more common as children approach adulthood. The midfoot breaks as a result of sudden, forceful flexion. The hallmark of injury is migration of the base of the second metatarsal away from the first cuneiform. This injury is the childhood equivalent of the adult Lisfranc fracture.

Tarsometatarsal instability is the feared consequence of a tarsometatarsal fracture. The tarsometatarsal joint is stabilized by ligaments, and the keystone contains the base of the second metatarsal within the mortise of the first and second cuneiforms. If the metatarsals are forcefully torn from this mortise, instability of the midfoot can result and a painful valgus flatfoot may develop. Truly nondisplaced injuries at the tarsometatarsal level can be immobilized but should be watched for late displacement. Disruption of the tarsometatarsal joint, characterized as lateral migration of the lesser metatarsals, should be anatomically reduced and fixed with smooth pins or screws. If the anatomy is fully restored, the prognosis is good; if not, late pain and stiffness are likely.

Fractures of the Forefoot

Fractures and dislocations of the forefoot and toes include fractures of the metatarsals and phalanges as well as dislocations of the toe joints. They are a common result of a direct blow or a stubbing, crushing, or penetrating injury. Minor fractures that do not result in an alteration of the shape or stability of the foot can be treated by simple immobilization in a cast or fracture shoe. If the shape of the foot has been altered, reduction with or without fixation is indicated to restore the bony alignment. Fractures that result in visible deformity of the digits should be reduced. Although isolated metatarsal fractures can simply be immobilized, multiple fractures of the metatarsals may require fixation to restore length and bony alignment. Dislocations are rare and usually involve the interphalangeal or metatarsophalangeal joints. Closed reduction should be attempted, but open reduction is indicated if the dislocation cannot be reduced closed. Fractures of the first ray occasionally require special attention, because the first ray is the mainstay of the arch of the foot. If the arch is deranged because of a fracture of the first metatarsal, it should be reduced and fixed. Salter-Harris type IV fractures can occur, involving the base of the first metatarsal or the base of the proximal phalanx. Displacement here may result in late growth derangement. To lessen this possibility, consideration should be given to anatomic reduction and fixation with small screws or smooth wires. The wound associated with an open injury should be managed by immediate wound débridement and repair. A fracture of the epiphysis of the distal phalanx may involve the nail bed; it must be recognized and treated as an open fracture. The prognosis is generally good for healing and a full return to function.

It is important to remember that compartment syndrome may complicate a foot injury, especially a high-energy or crushing injury. Tense swelling, unremitting pain, and pain out of proportion to the injury are key indicators of compartment syndrome. If necessary, compartment pressures should be measured and the compartments released.

Traumatic Amputations

Traumatic amputations most commonly occur as result of a high-energy injury, usually involving a motorized device such as a lawn mower, a piece of farm equipment, or an all-terrain vehicle. These injuries typically require multiple surgeries. The purpose of the first several surgeries is wound hygiene, and the next several are for wound closure.[18] The final surgeries are for reconstruction or revision.

Weight-bearing prominences or the soft tissues that protect them are often lost, and growth plates and growth centers are damaged. Tendons that normally balance the foot are often damaged asymmetrically; dynamic deformities are caused by the remaining functioning musculotendinous units.

Children and their families are often psychologically scarred by the injury and subsequent events. Many such injuries affect children at an age when they have difficulty tolerating dressing changes and other manipulations. Most children can return to full function with a partial foot. For some patients, the foot becomes stiff, insensate, unbalanced, painful, or chronically ulcerated. Amputation at a level higher than the injury with a prosthetic fitting can allow the patient a better return to function.

Complications include possible pain from altered weight-bearing surfaces and function. Late skin breakdown over bony prominences and painful stump overgrowth are also possible. Unbalanced muscle function can cause dynamic and late fixed deformity of the foot or ankle.

Tendon Injuries

Pediatric tendon injuries of the foot are surprisingly uncommon. They occur as a result of penetrating wounds of the foot or ankle with direct laceration of tendons. On clinical examination, abnormal posturing or motor function can suggest the presence of tendon laceration. Sometimes clinical examination is difficult, and exploration of the wound is necessary to determine what has been cut.

These injuries are described by the tendon involved, the location of the laceration, and the extent of the injury to the tendon. If a substantial portion of the tendon is intact, the laceration can be treated with simple immobilization. Complete laceration of a large tendon such as the tibialis posterior, tibialis anterior, Achilles tendon, or peroneal tendon should be repaired, primarily to prevent late weakness and foot deformity. Lesser but important tendons such as the extensor or flexor hallucis longus can be repaired acutely if the gain in function is determined to be worth the unavoidable tissue trauma. Late rerupture is possible after repair. Laceration to lesser toe flexors and extensors probably should not be treated. The prognosis for healing and a return to function is generally good.

Foot Puncture Wounds

Foot puncture wounds are common in children. The classic cause is stepping on a nail. A puncture wound is usually sore for a few days. However, contaminated material that reaches the depths of the foot can introduce an aggressive infection, typically by *Pseudomonas*

aeruginosa, which can damage the cartilage of joints and growth plates. If pain increases and swelling develops, possibly with drainage, open débridement is necessary to eradicate the infection. Cultures should be taken, and empiric antibiotic coverage for *Pseudomonas* should be started. The duration of antibiotic coverage depends on the clinical response. The wound should be kept open to promote drainage until clinical improvement occurs. Late joint stiffness or growth derangement is possible.

Annotated References

1. Butcher CC, Hoffman EB: Supracondylar fractures of the femur in children: Closed reduction and percutaneous pinning of displaced fractures. *J Pediatr Orthop* 2005;25:145-148.

   Eight children with displaced supracondylar fractures were treated with closed reduction and pinning. Seven patients had a satisfactory result. One patient had a valgus deformity, but none had growth plate arrest or limb length discrepancy. Level of evidence: IV.

2. Riseborough EJ, Barrett IR, Shapiro R: Growth disturbances following distal femoral fracture-separations. *J Bone Joint Surg Am* 1983;65:885-893. Level of evidence: IV.

3. Watson-Jones R: *Fractures and Joint Injuries,* ed 6. New York, NY, Churchill Livingstone, 1982. Level of evidence: V.

4. Mosier SM, Stanitski CL: Acute tibial tubercle avulsion fractures. *J Pediatr Orthop* 2004;24:181-184.

   Most tibial tubercle fractures in this review were sports injuries, particularly from basketball. The fractures were treated by open reduction and internal fixation or closed reduction and cast immobilization. The final outcome was good for all patients, regardless of fracture type or treatment. Level of evidence: V.

5. Zionts LE, MacEwen GD: Spontaneous improvement of post-traumatic tibial valga. *J Bone Joint Surg Am* 1986;68:680-687. Level of evidence: IV.

6. Mashru RP, Herman MJ, Pizzutillo PD: Tibial shaft fractures in children and adolescents. *J Am Acad Orthop Surg* 2005;13:345-352.

   Union of pediatric diaphyseal tibial fractures occurs in approximately 10 weeks; nonunion occurs in fewer than 2% of cases. Some clinicians consider sagittal deformity angulation >10° to be malunion and indicate that 10° of valgus and 5° of varus may not reliably remodel. Level of evidence: V.

7. Kubiak EN, Egol KA, Scher D, Wasserman B, Feldman D, Koval KJ: Operative treatment of tibial fractures in children: Are elastic stable intramedullary nails an improvement over external fixation? *J Bone Joint Surg Am* 2005;87:1761-1768.

   The functional outcomes of the intramedullary nailing

group were significantly better than those of the external fixation group. Level of evidence: Therapeutic level III.

8. O'Brien T, Weisman DS, Ronchetti P, Piller CP, Maloney M: Flexible titanium nailing for the treatment of the unstable pediatric tibial fracture. *J Pediatr Orthop* 2004;24:601-609.

   Sixteen tibia fractures in 14 patients were treated with flexible nails. Closed injuries healed in an average of 8 weeks, and the three open fractures healed in an average of 15 weeks. There was no malunion, growth arrest, remanipulation, or refracture. Level of evidence: IV.

9. Goodwin RC, Gaynor T, Mahar A, Oka R, Lalonde FD: Intramedullary flexible nail fixation of unstable pediatric tibial diaphyseal fractures. *J Pediatr Orthop* 2005;25:570-576.

   In 19 patients, fracture union occurred after flexible intramedullary nail fixation. Five patients had complications, but none required reoperation. Two angular deformities (≥ 10) occurred with the medial C-and-S construct, and none occurred with the double-C construct. Level of evidence: IV.

10. Whitesides TE, Haney TC, Morimoto K, Harada H: Tissue pressure measurements as a determinant for the need of fasciotomy. *Clin Orthop Relat Res* 1975;113:43-51. Level of evidence: IV.

11. Matsen FA III, Winquist RA, Krugmire RB: Diagnosis and management of compartment syndromes. *J Bone Joint Surg Am* 1980;62:286-291. Level of evidence: V.

12. Mubarak SJ: A practical approach to compartment syndromes: Part II. Diagnosis. *Instr Course Lect* 1983;32:92-102. Level of evidence: V.

13. Barmada A, Gaynor T, Mubarak SJ: Premature physeal closure following distal tibia physeal fractures: A new radiographic predictor. *J Pediatr Orthop* 2003;23:733-739.

    Salter-Harris types III and IV medial malleolar fractures accounted for 38% of premature physeal closures (seen in 27% of pediatric distal tibial fractures), types I and II for 36%, and triplane fractures for 21%. Anatomic reduction resulted in a lower premature closure rate. A residual physeal gap after reduction was associated with a 60% premature closure rate. Level of evidence: IV.

14. Charlton M, Costello R, Mooney JF, Podeszwa DA: Ankle joint biomechanics following transepiphyseal screw fixation of the distal tibia. *J Pediatr Orthop* 2005;25:635-640.

    Forces and contact pressures within the tibiotalar joint were measured in a cadaver study. Local peak contact pressures increased significantly after screws were placed in the epiphysis. Screw removal led to a net decrease in force and peak pressure values. Level of evidence: II.

15. Nenopoulos SP, Papavasiliou VA, Papavasiliou AV: Outcome of physeal and epiphyseal injuries of the distal tibia with intra-articular involvement. *J Pediatr Orthop* 2005;25:518-522.

    Varus deformity ranging from 10° to 15° occurred in 4 of the 83 reviewed intra-articular fractures of the distal tibia. One patient had limited ankle motion, and two had overgrowth of the medial malleolus. Level of evidence: IV.

16. Pickle A, Benaroch TE, Guy P, Harvey EJ: Clinical outcome of pediatric calcaneal fractures treated with open reduction and internal fixation. *J Pediatr Orthop* 2004;24:178-180.

    Outcomes of open reduction and internal fixation to treat pediatric intra-articular calcaneal fractures were reviewed. All patients were pain free in normal activities. All had full ankle motion, but five had decreased subtalar motion. None had complications, shoe wearing problems, or peroneal tendinitis. Level of evidence: IV.

17. Ribbans WJ, Natarajan R, Alavala S: Pediatric foot fractures. *Clin Orthop Relat Res* 2005;432:107-115.

    Displaced fractures of the talus and calcaneus and tarsometatarsal dislocations are rare in children, and the outcome is generally good. Repeated clinical examination and special imaging techniques such as bone scanning and MRI may be needed to establish a diagnosis. Level of evidence: V.

18. McClure SK, Shaughnessy WJ: Farm-related limb amputations in children. *J Pediatr Orthop* 2005;25:133-137.

    In this study, farm machinery accidents caused 12 limb amputations. Treatment consisted of débridement, antibiotics, attempted replantation, and wound closure. Infections developed in all patients who underwent attempted replantation. Replantation was successful in fewer than 20% of patients. Level of evidence: IV.

Chapter 61

Lower Limb and Foot Disorders: Pediatrics

Kenneth J. Noonan, MD

Normal Limb Alignment

Most lower limb rotational differences in young children are considered to be within normal limits. The normal spectrum is difficult to quantify, because the foot progression angle can vary with gait in children younger than 5 years. Most infants have external hip rotation because of residual muscle contractures from intrauterine positioning. Outtoeing is common in toddlers who are just beginning to walk, and intoeing also is seen.

Persistent intoeing can be the result of residual metatarsus adductus, persistent internal tibial torsion, or excessive femoral anteversion. On average, an infant's tibia is rotated internally to -5°; the average 10-year-old child has 10° of external rotation. Internal tibial torsion can be seen with physiologic genu varum (bow-leg deformity). Excessive femoral anteversion typically is seen in children 3 years of age or older. Although fetal anteversion can be as much as 50°, by maturity the anteversion has remodeled to approximately 20° and, therefore, the incidence of intoeing is reduced.

Most infants are born with varus knees, which straighten to a neutral position by age 18 months, progress to maximal valgus by age 2 to 3 years, and slowly remodel to a physiologic valgus of 6° to 7° during the next 5 years.

Genu varum is common because of the high incidence of physiologic varus. Its undesirable cosmetic appearance and the perception of diminished function are cause for parental concern. Physiologic varus has a worse cosmetic appearance when accompanied by internal tibial torsion. The pathologic causes of varus deformities include infantile Blount's disease, metabolic bone disease, and skeletal dysplasia.[1] Metabolic bone disease and skeletal dysplasia are rare and are usually found in children with height below the 10th percentile for their age or those with continued, progressive bowing of the legs. Radiographs are indicated for patients older than 2 years or those who have a progressive painful deformity. To successfully manage physiologic bowing, it is important to acknowledge the deformity, educate the family about its benign natural history, and inform the family that nonsurgical treatment methods to correct torsional or angular deformities are futile and that the patient should return for treatment if the deformity progresses.

Assessment of Limb Alignment in Normal and Pathologic Conditions

Understanding a pediatric lower limb deformity requires a patient medical history, physical examination findings, and, for some patients, a review of standard radiographs. It is important to determine whether the deformity is progressive, stable, or painful. In addition to neurologic and circulatory function, children are examined for scoliosis and foot deformity, conditions that may contribute to lower leg deformity. Discrepancies in leg length are noted; hip and knee joint motion are assessed for limiting joint contractures. An observational gait analysis is performed to document foot progression angle and antalgic gait and to rule out global pathologic conditions marked by limb scissoring, hyperlordotic gait, or a Trendelenburg gait. The patient's static rotational profile is determined in the prone position by documenting the amount of internal and external hip rotation, the thigh-foot axis, and the presence of any foot abnormalities.

If necessary, a standing alignment radiograph is obtained to document the direction and magnitude of the deformity. It is critical that the patella, not the foot, points forward. Standing lateral radiographs of the femur and tibia are taken to confirm a sagittal plane deformity.

The analysis of a deformity can be broken down into several simple steps. First, the radiographs are examined to document the presence of any obvious anatomic coronal or sagittal limb deformities, such as bowing of the bones. The coronal mechanical axis of the limb is drawn on the alignment film from the center of the hip to the center of the ankle (**Figure 1**). This line should pass within 1 cm of the tibial spines in both knees and if symmetric, is considered normal. Any deviation from this is the mechanical axis deviation.

Second, if an anatomic or mechanical deformity is present, the clinician must determine whether it is in the femur, the tibia, or both bones. The coronal mechanical axes of the normal-side and affected and contralateral sides of the femur and tibia are constructed and compared. If the disease is bilateral, the comparison is made with established norms. For example, the mechanical axis of the femur is drawn from the center of the hip to the center of the knee; this line normally

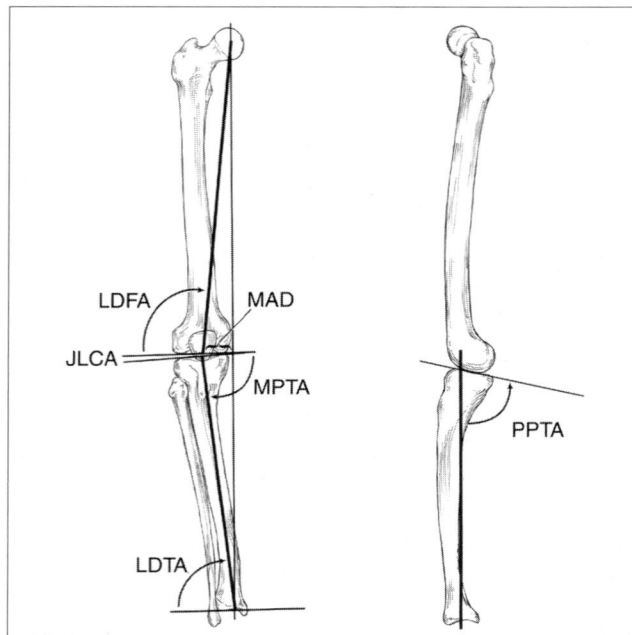

Figure 1 Schematic coronal plane illustrations of the determination of the mechanical axis, showing mechanical axis deviation (MAD). The lateral distal femoral angle (LDFA), the joint line congruency angle (JLCA), and the medial plateau tibial angle (MPTA) can be measured and compared with published norms or the contralateral side to document deformity in the distal femur, joint, or proximal tibia. Similarly, the lateral distal tibial angle (LDTA) and the posterior proximal tibial angle (PPTA) can also be assessed. (*Reproduced with permission from Gordon JE, Heidenreich FP, Carpenter CJ, Kelly-Hahn J, Schoenecker PL: Comprehensive treatment of late-onset tibia vara. J Bone Joint Surg Am 2005;87:1561-1570.*)

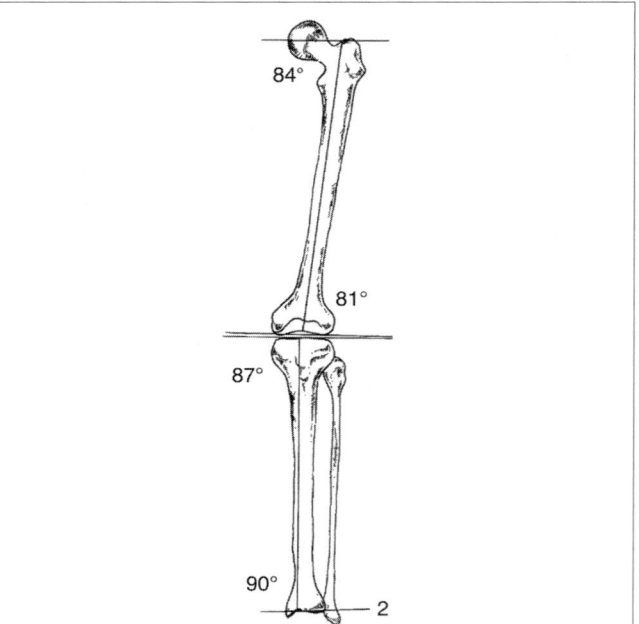

Figure 2 Average anatomic joint angle measurements in the coronal plane. (*Reproduced with permission from Price CT, Izuka BH: Osteotomy planning using the anatomic method: A simple method for lower extremity deformity analysis. Orthopedics 2005;28:20-25.*)

intersects the articular surface of the distal femur to produce a lateral distal-femoral angle of 87°. Similarly, the tibial mechanical axis is drawn as a line from the center of the knee to the center of the ankle; this line normally intersects the articular surface of the proximal tibia to produce a medial proximal tibia angle of 87°. The distal tibial articular surface normally is 90° with the mechanical axis of the tibia. Drawing and analyzing these values enables the clinician to determine whether a deformity exists in either of the two bones. Deformity in the knee is confirmed if the lines along the articular surfaces of the distal femur and proximal tibia are not parallel. Third, after the existence of a bone deformity has been confirmed, its exact location must be determined by drawing the normal mechanical axes of the proximal and distal ends of the bone. For example, in patients with Blount's disease the normal medial plateau tibial angle of 87° and the normal distal tibial axis are drawn. In the tibia, the distal axis is essentially parallel to the anatomic axis of the tibial shaft. The point at which these two lines intersect is considered the site of deformity or the center of rotation and angulation.

A similar approach is applied on lateral radiographs and can be used for assessment of sagittal plane deformity.

A similar methodology using the anatomic axes of the femur and the tibia has been described.[2] The normal proximal femoral angle is 84°; however, this is difficult to construct and thus a neck-shaft angle of 130° is used, the lateral distal femoral anatomic angle is 81°, the medial proximal tibial anatomic angle is 87°, and the distal tibial articular surface is at a 90° angle from the tibial shaft (**Figure 2**). In the lateral plane, the angle subtended by the femoral shaft and Blumensaat line is normally 83°, the tibial plateau is sloped posteriorly at 80° to the shaft of the tibia, and the tibial plafond is sloped anteriorly at 80°. If abnormal articular angles are measured, it can be concluded that a deformity exists within that bone. As mentioned above, constructing the normal anatomic axis of the proximal and distal ends of the bone in both the coronal and sagittal planes reveals the location of the center of rotation and angulation (**Figure 3**).

This methodology has important corollaries. If the standing alignment radiograph reveals an obvious anatomic deformity, although the mechanical axis line is intact, a compensatory deformity must exist. For example, correction of an anatomically obvious femoral varus malunion may produce a valgus limb because of a previously unrecognized distal femoral valgus orientation, which had compensated for the long-standing deformity. Or, if proximal and distal constructed axes

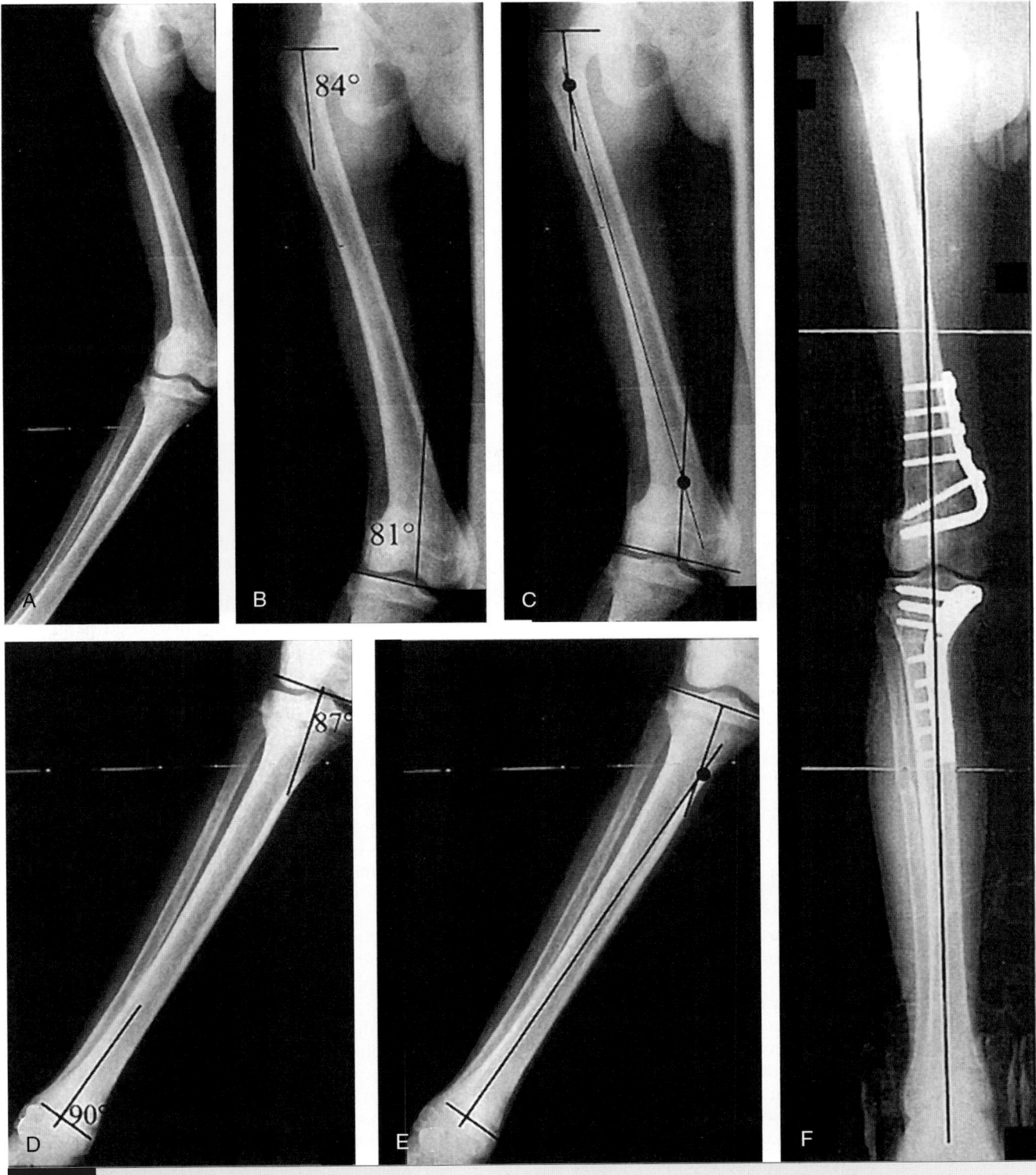

Figure 3 Deformity analysis of severe genu valgum using the anatomic method. **A,** Severe genu valgum. **B,** Proximal and distal femoral joint angles are constructed. **C,** Because the axes do not intersect, the intermediate axis of the femoral shaft is constructed and the intersection of the three axes shows two centers of rotation and angulation. **D,** The proximal and distal tibial axes are constructed. **E,** The intersection of these two axes reveals the center of rotation and angulation in the tibia. **F,** Correction is obtained at the knee by distal femoral and proximal tibial osteotomy. The proximal femoral varus was not corrected in this patient. (*Reproduced with permission from Price CT, Izuka BH: Osteotomy planning using the anatomic method: A simple method for lower extremity deformity analysis. Orthopedics 2005;28:20-25.*)

do not intersect, as outlined above, or do not intersect at an obvious deformity, another deformity must be present. Therefore, an intermediate axis must be drawn; the point at which the three lines intersect is the site of the multiple centers of rotation and angulation. This method can be more easily used with anatomic deformity analysis.[2]

Although the deformity is best corrected at the centers of rotation and angulation, doing so may not be feasible because of anatomic constraints. An osteotomy is performed at a location away from the focus and produces transitory deformity that must be compensated for during the correction.

Surgically Guided Growth

Angular deformity can increase the likelihood that degenerative arthritis eventually will develop. To treat angular deformity, either the abnormal bone is realigned via osteotomy or the forces within the growth plate are harnessed to correct the deformity via asymmetric growth.[3,4] Hemiepiphysiodesis is a well-accepted method of correcting long bone deformity in children who have significant remaining bone growth. Compared with osteotomy, which can have complication rates approaching 20%, guided growth is an elegant way to correct deformities with minimal morbidity. It can be achieved surgically by removing portions of the actively growing physis or using implants such as metal screws that cross the physis, or staples that bridge the physis. The application of a two-hole plate and screws on one side of the growth plate is a novel surgical technique that is gaining popularity to achieve unilateral tethering of the growth plate. Provided enough growth potential remains, these devices retard growth on the long side of the bone and gradually correct the deformity.

Metabolic Bone Deformity

The causes of angular deformities include congenital deficiency, developmental conditions, skeletal dysplasia, inflammation from arthritis or infection, trauma, and metabolic disease. Children with metabolic bone disease are usually of short stature, and the bones may be gradually bowed throughout their length; other radiographic evidence can include cupping and flaring of the metaphysis and widening of the growth plate. The serum and urine levels of electrolytes, calcium, phosphorus, and alkaline phosphatase are useful in investigating the possibility of metabolic bone disease, although more sophisticated evaluation is best performed with the help of a pediatric endocrinologist.

Progressive pathologic varus deformities of the limb usually result from congenital or early-onset disease. In an infant with nutritional or genetic (hypophosphatemic) rickets, normal physiologic varus deformity progresses to anterolateral bowing of the entire femur and varus bowing of the tibia. Conversely, a child in

whom metabolic disease develops (such as from an acquired renal deficiency or following a transplant) after attaining a normal valgus alignment can expect the valgus alignment to gradually worsen.

A progressive, painful deformity caused by metabolic abnormality should be corrected with surgery. Osteotomy and guided growth may be an option for a patient with excessive genu vara. Guided growth for a growing patient with a valgus deformity can be performed above and below the knee joint, with expected resolution of the deformity. Osteotomy is needed for a patient with a considerable deformity who has reached skeletal maturity and thus is not suitable for guided growth via hemiepiphysiodesis. For these patients, the deformity should be corrected gradually with external fixation to avoid peroneal nerve palsy, which can occur in patients with extreme valgus deformity who are undergoing acute correction.

Infantile Tibia Vara

It is difficult to differentiate between early infantile tibia vara, also called infantile Blount's disease, and extreme cases of physiologic genu varus, which improves with time. Blount's disease is diagnosed in children with apparent physiologic genu varus that fails to improve within 2 to 3 years. Infantile Blount's disease probably develops from an extreme case of physiologic genu vara that has progressed because of growth disturbance in the posteromedial tibial physis. Children with infantile Blount's disease are typically large for their age and walk at a relatively early age. The combination of large size and excessive varus because of early walking leads to compression of the physis on the medial side of the tibia, leading to growth retardation and progressive varus deformity. This disorder is most common in children of African decent.

Radiographs of a child with infantile tibia vara show sloping of the medial metaphysis and fragmentation of the epiphysis. Measurement of the metaphyseal-diaphyseal and metaphyseal-epiphyseal angles is helpful in predicting further progression and eventual diagnosis of infantile Blount's disease. Toddlers at high risk for infantile Blount's disease are likely to have a metaphyseal-diaphyseal angle greater than 16° or both a metaphyseal-diaphyseal angle greater than 10° and a metaphyseal-epiphyseal angle greater than 20°. Conversely, patients with physiologic genu vara are likely to have a metaphyseal-diaphyseal angle less than 9° or both a metaphyseal-diaphyseal angle less than 10° and a metaphyseal-epiphyseal angle less than 20°. Determination of these angles and an early diagnosis of Blount's disease may be beneficial so that orthotic management can be considered.

The natural history of infantile Blount's disease is not known with certainty. Ethnic or racial differences may exist. As many as 50% of patients improve with time, although some studies predict certain progression after Langenskiöld stage 3 changes occur.[5] The treatment of progressive infantile Blount's disease can include bracing, hemiepiphyseal stapling, or tibia and fibula osteotomy. Treatment of patients with early, mild Blount's disease with a long knee-ankle-foot orthosis without a knee joint is controversial, because orthotic treatment may not improve the natural history of the disease. A medially based strap is applied to the brace to provide a valgus moment. A pelvic band can be used to prevent internal rotation of the orthotic device. It must be worn during the day rather than at night to unload the compressive side of the cartilage. Surgically guided growth can be considered for a patient with infantile Blount's disease that has been confirmed based on its progression of metaphyseal sloping and epiphyseal fragmentation (Langenskiöld changes). Tibia and fibula osteotomy can be considered in a child who is younger than 4 years and has progressive varus and well-defined Langenskiöld changes without the presence of a bony bar. The child is immobilized until healing occurs, then carefully monitored to detect any recurrence of the deformity.

Children with severe uncorrected or relapsed infantile tibia vara (Langenskiöld V and VI changes are accompanied by bone growth arrest) have posteromedial joint depression and probably a physeal bar that predisposes them to a recurrence of the deformity. A combination of osteotomy, growth arrest, and limb lengthening may be needed to correct the deformity. Hemiplateau elevation can be considered. A preoperative CT scan can show the location of the deformity.[6]

Late-Onset Tibia Vara

Late-onset tibia vara occurs in both boys and girls and can be classified as juvenile (in a child 4 to 9 years of age) or adolescent (in a child age 10 years or older). The juvenile form may be a continuation of infantile tibia vara that has not improved. These patients have narrowing of the epiphysis, widening of the medial growth plate, and occasional widening of the lateral distal femoral physis. Late-onset tibia vara is a result of growth retardation of the proximal tibia medial physis and, occasionally, the distal femoral medial physis, although the femoral deformity is usually only 50% of the deformity present at the proximal tibia or 30% of the total deformity.[7]

Patients with adolescent tibia vara are usually large for their age or overweight and have unilateral involvement. In contrast to the infantile form, bilateral involvement, if present, is usually asymmetric. Patients with late-onset tibia vara have deformity progression and sometimes pain with weight bearing on the lateral side of the knee. Patients may also have a limb-length discrepancy in the affected leg because of growth retardation and the functional discrepancy of the varus positioning. The discrepancy may be 2 to 4 cm compared with the contralateral side and may appear in the femur, tibia, or both.

The natural history of late-onset tibia vara is not completely known, although progressive deformity can

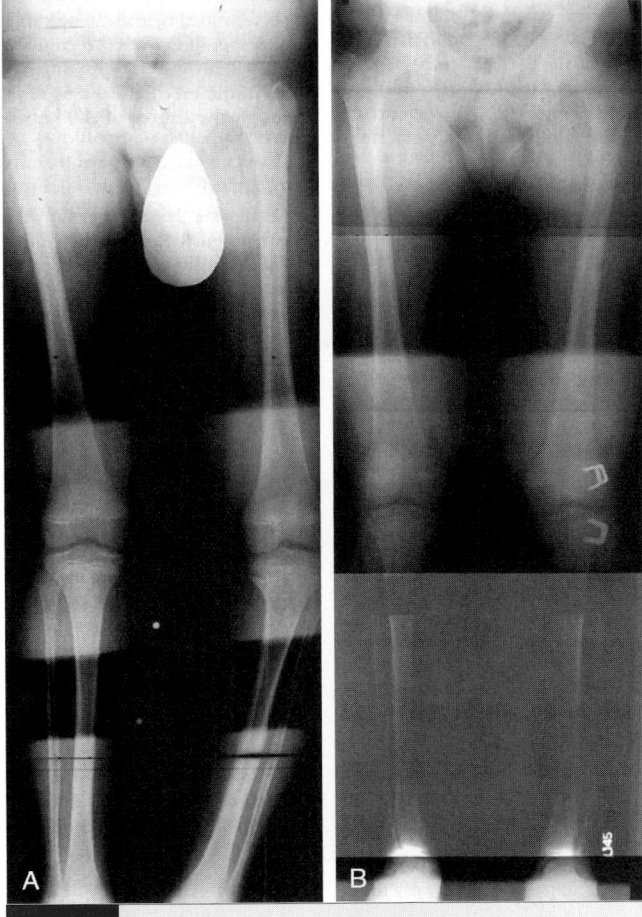

Figure 4 **A,** Standing radiograph showing adolescent tibia vara with distal femoral and proximal tibial deformity. **B,** Correction obtained via guided growth above and below the knee joint. (*Reproduced with permission from Park SS, Gordon JE, Luhmann SJ, Dobbs MB, Schoenecker PL: Outcome of hemiepiphyseal stapling for late-onset tibia vara. J Bone Joint Surg Am 2005;87:2259-2266.*)

be expected to lead to an increased rate of degenerative arthritis of the knee. Treatment of adolescent tibia vara involves surgically guided growth or osteotomy with deformity correction. Guided growth is chosen for patients who have either minimal deformity or several years of remaining bone growth, to permit correction of the deformity (**Figure 4**). Patients who have reached the end of bone growth or have a significant internal rotational deformity benefit from osteotomy. Guided growth cannot be expected to correct internal rotational deformities and is of limited use in patients with extreme deformity and little remaining growth. The decision to perform an osteotomy and correction above and below the knee depends on the magnitude of the femoral deformity. Children with a distal femoral varus deformity of 8° or greater should undergo osteotomy or guided growth at this level, in addition to tibia correction.[8] Failure to correct for excessive distal femoral deformity and overcorrection of the tibia leads to shear stresses at the knee.

Valgus Deformity

Excessive valgus deformity in a child older than 4 years may be associated with numerous conditions, including idiopathic genu valgus, skeletal dysplasia, metabolic bone disease, and renal abnormalities. The treatment of these deformities includes guided growth or osteotomy with deformity correction. Unilateral, progressive valgus deformity at the tibia, known as Cozen phenomenon, may follow a minimal fracture of the proximal tibia metaphysis.

Limb-Length Discrepancy

Limb-length discrepancy of as much as 1 cm has been reported in as many as 70% of adult patients.[9] Children with a discrepancy greater than 2 cm can compensate by walking on their toes or, as they grow older, vaulting over the short leg. The causes of limb-length discrepancy include changes in bone length, such as those following fracture malunion, changes in growth rate, or a combination of these factors. Limb-length discrepancy is associated with conditions such as congenital short femur, infection, paralysis, tumor, mechanical factors, vascular inflammation, and skeletal dysplasia. Traumatic injury to the growth plate can lead to a bar and limb-length discrepancy. Trauma in the metaphyseal region can lead to angular deformities, such as tibia valgus or overgrowth, and a longer limb.

It is important to predict the extent of limb-length discrepancy at skeletal maturity. A discrepancy with a congenital cause does not change proportionately, and therefore the discrepancy at maturity can be readily estimated. For other patients, the history and physical examination, as well as analysis of radiographic bone length data, are useful in making the prediction. Patients who have paralysis or require an orthotic device ultimately benefit from a 1 to 2 cm length discrepancy, which facilitates clearing of the weak foot during the swing phase of gait.

During physical examination, it is important to look for an ankle, knee, or hip flexion contracture or pelvic obliquity, which can make an anatomic discrepancy even more functionally apparent. Using a tape measure, anatomic limb lengths are measured from the medial malleolus to the anterosuperior iliac spine. Two radiographic methods are commonly used to assess limb-length discrepancy. A teloradiogram allows assessment of angular deformity, using a single exposure of both lower extremities; the patient is standing, and a radiopaque ruler may be positioned. A scanogram, commonly used to assess limb-length discrepancy, is helpful in accurately assessing total limb lengths and has the advantage of using a relatively short film. CT also can be used to assess lengths and is especially useful if the deformity is in the sagittal plane or is a joint contrac-

ture. It is important to assess a patient's current level of skeletal maturity; boys generally stop growing at age 16 years and girls generally stop growing at 14 years, although considerable variability exists. A PA radiograph of the left hand can be compared with data in the Greulich and Pyle atlas of normal standards to estimate the child's bone age.[10] This method is not useful for some patients, including those with upper extremity deficiencies. Wide variability exists in interobserver and intraobserver assessment of younger age groups, and it is difficult to extrapolate data to different ethnic groups. Despite these limitations, comparison with the Greulich and Pyle atlas is the predominant method by which clinicians assess skeletal age. Four methods are used to predict the discrepancy at maturity: the arithmetic method, the growth-remaining method, the multiplier method, and the straight line graph of Moseley.[9] The decision to treat limb-length discrepancy depends on the predicted discrepancy at skeletal maturity. A patient with a predicted discrepancy of less than 2 cm requires no treatment, although a 1 to 2 cm shoe lift can be used. A wedge placed on the bottom of the shoe may also be required. A predicted discrepancy between 2 and 6 cm can be treated with a shoe lift, epiphysiodesis, and skeletal shortening. Limb lengthening by distraction osteogenesis should be performed for a patient with a predicted discrepancy between 6 and 17 cm at skeletal maturity; this is performed by osteotomy of the short bone and gradual lengthening with internal or external devices. Treatment of a predicted discrepancy greater than 17 cm may require a prosthetic fitting.

One major objection to limb lengthening is the extent of external fixator time required for the bone to consolidate. Two recent advances include bone lengthening using external fixation over a standard intramedullary nail and bone lengthening from within using intramedullary nails.[11,12] The use of lengthening intramedullary nails appears to be a reasonable alternative to external fixation for limb lengthening, and it has the benefit of decreased pin tract complications and elimination of exposed hardware. These methods are useful for patients with minimal growth potential or closed growth plates.

Congenital Femoral Deficiency

The congenital abnormalities of the femur include congenital short femur, proximal femoral focal dysplasia, femoral hypoplasia, mini femur, and congenital coxa vara. The incidence of congenital anomalies of the femur is about 1 in 10,000 live births. Bilateral abnormalities occur in approximately 15% of patients.

Femoral hypoplasia is a common limb deficiency. Other skeletal abnormalities may be present with femoral hypoplasia, including proximal femoral retroversion and coxa vara. At the knee, lateral femoral condyle hypoplasia with patellar subluxation or congenital absence of cruciate ligaments may be present.[13] One half to two thirds of patients with congenital short femur have fibular hemimelia, and many of these patients also have a congenital absence of foot rays, ball-

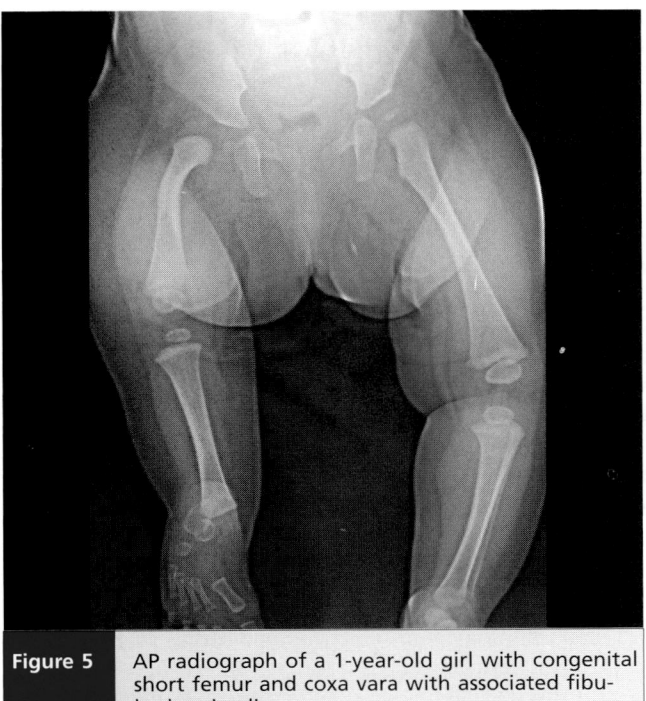

Figure 5 AP radiograph of a 1-year-old girl with congenital short femur and coxa vara with associated fibular hemimelia.

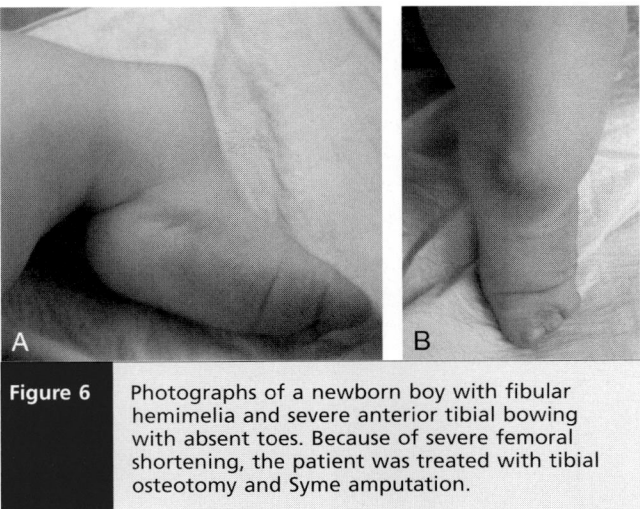

Figure 6 Photographs of a newborn boy with fibular hemimelia and severe anterior tibial bowing with absent toes. Because of severe femoral shortening, the patient was treated with tibial osteotomy and Syme amputation.

in-socket ankle, and tarsal coalition (**Figure 5**).

The treatment of femoral hypoplasia is based on a prediction of the limb-length discrepancy at skeletal maturity, as well as an assessment of the associated abnormalities. The options include limb reconstruction and lengthening or an early prosthetic fitting, possibly facilitated by surgery. Limb lengthening is generally recommended for children who have a projected discrepancy at skeletal maturity of less than 17 cm and who have a stable hip and knee with good foot and ankle function. Because of the congenital nature of the abnormality, families should be made aware that multiple lengthenings and complications can be expected during the child's early life. Patients with a predicted discrepancy greater than 17 cm may benefit from foot ablation and prosthetic fitting, with or without knee fusion. Rotationplasty, with or without hip fusion, is another option.

Fibular Hemimelia

Fibular hemimelia is a complete or partial absence of the fibula that can be proximal or distal. It is the most common congenital long bone deficiency, and it occurs in boys twice as often as girls. Affected individuals may have a normal-appearing but short foot and leg, or the limb may be severely deformed and nonfunctional. The tibia is shorter than normal and may be anteriorly bowed (**Figure 6**). A concurrent congenital deficiency of the femur or genu valgum may be present. Significant associated foot abnormalities include absence of the lateral rays of the feet, tarsal coalitions, ball-in-socket

ankle, and valgus positioning of the ankle. The different classification systems are based on the extent of fibular deficiency, the percentage of limb-length discrepancy compared with the contralateral side, and the presence of any concurrent foot abnormalities.

Fibular hemimelia is treated with amputation and prosthetic fitting or limb reconstruction and lengthening. Syme or Boyd amputation is considered for patients who have a nonfunctional foot with severe valgus positioning or fewer than three rays, as well as a projected limb-length discrepancy greater than 30% compared with the contralateral side. Amputation and prosthetic fitting are also strongly indicated for a patient with bilateral fibular hemimelia who has normal upper extremity function. Children treated with amputation and prosthetic fitting have good function, and long-term studies found athletic and psychological function similar to that of unaffected children.[9] Limb lengthening is considered for children who have a projected length discrepancy of less than 10%, compared with the contralateral side, as well as the potential for good foot function after ankle and foot reconstruction. Children with a discrepancy of between 10% and 30%, compared with the contralateral side, can be managed with either amputation and prosthetic fitting or limb reconstruction and lengthening. The decision is based on the preference of the treating physician and the family.

Tibial Hemimelia

Congenital deficiencies of the tibia are extremely rare; the incidence is 1 in 1 million. The deficiency is bilateral in 30% of patients, and between 60% and 70% of affected individuals have concurrent musculoskeletal disorders, including equinovarus foot, congenital short femur, and congenital dislocation of the hip or a cleft hand. Tibial deficiency is a unique congenital deficiency because of its genetic tendency for deformities in later generations.

6: Pediatrics

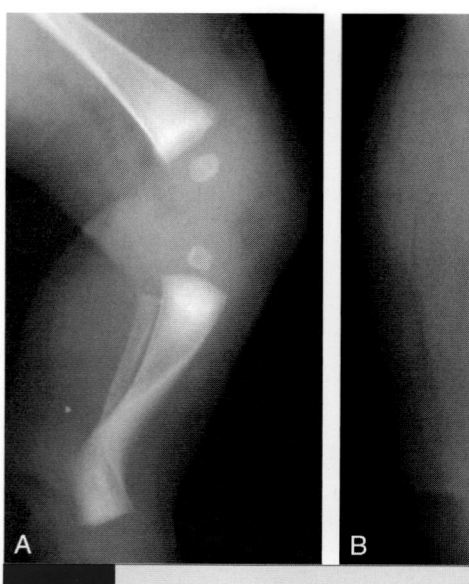
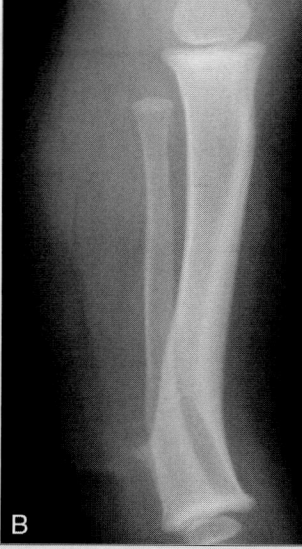

Figure 7 **A,** Oblique radiograph of a newborn child with posteromedial bowing of the tibia. **B,** AP radiograph shows that the deformity has improved at 14 months of age. Continued improvement can be expected with time.

The key feature of the classification system for tibial hemimelia is the presence of a proximal tibia and, hence, a functional quadriceps mechanism.[14] In a type I deficiency, no tibia is seen on radiographs, although a cartilage tibia anlage may appear on ultrasonography or MRI, with later ossification expected. In a type II deficiency, the child has an absent distal tibia but a normal proximal tibia and knee joint articulation. In a type III deficiency, the child has distal tibia and fibula diastasis.

Treatment of type I deficiency is usually with transarticular amputation. Fibular centralization should not be considered, unless an intact quadriceps mechanism is present. Treatment of a type II deficiency is with a Syme amputation of the dysfunctional foot and a proximal tibial-fibular synostosis to produce a functioning below-knee amputation. Type III deficiencies are extremely rare. They can be treated by reconstruction or foot ablation and prosthetic fitting.

Congenital Posteromedial Bowing of the Tibia

Posteromedial bowing of the tibia is a benign congenital anomaly without fracture or pseudarthrosis. It is characterized by a calcaneal valgus foot deformity, posteromedial bow of the tibia, and an eventual limb-length discrepancy of 2 to 5 cm.[15] The foot deformity usually corrects itself within the first year of life. Stretching and casting are occasionally used to improve the deformity, and, rarely, an ankle-foot orthosis is used for weight bearing. Gradual and variable correction is expected to occur over several years, until the tibia is straight or has a mild S shape (**Figure 7**). Treatment of the tibial deformity consists of observation versus cor-

rection of the limb-length discrepancy and residual bow with guided growth or osteotomy at one or two levels with or without distraction osteogenesis at one site. Contralateral epiphysiodesis may be considered in individuals with a limb-length discrepancy but no residual tibia bow.

Congenital Pseudarthrosis of the Tibia

The incidence of congenital pseudarthrosis of the tibia is 1 in 150,000 live births. Half of the patients with pseudarthrosis of the tibia, fibula, or both also are diagnosed with neurofibromatosis. Congenital pseudarthrosis of the tibia is characterized by anterolateral bowing, in contrast to the anterior bowing in fibular hemimelia and posteromedial bowing of the tibia. In congenital pseudarthrosis of the tibia, the tibia is shortened. The apical dysplasia ranges from fracture with atrophy of the fracture ends to failure of tubulation of the diaphysis, with a sclerotic or cystic appearance that eventually develops into a pseudarthrosis. Fracture develops within 4 to 5 years of diagnosis in most patients with no pseudarthrosis. To prevent fracture, a knee-ankle-foot orthosis is used in infants. When children begin to walk, an ankle-foot orthosis is used. Full-time bracing is required until skeletal maturity to prevent fracture or a recurrence of fracture after successful surgical treatment.

Different treatment options are available after pseudarthrosis occurs. Amputation, the option of last resort, is considered only after failure of consolidation using a combination of three other methods of treatment.[16-18] The first method involves extraperiosteal pseudarthrosis excision and intramedullary stabilization of the tibia and fibula. An autogenous bone graft, with or without iliac crest periosteum, is used at the resection site. In recent reports, the use of recombinant bone morphogenetic proteins produced mixed results. The success rate for intramedullary nailing and bone grafting approaches 80% to 90%, although the pseudarthrosis may recur and necessitate repeated bone grafting, with or without bone stimulation units. After surgery, children are placed in a cast for 3 to 4 months and then in an ankle-foot orthosis, with the ankle locked.

The second treatment option is external fixator application and bone transport. This method is best used in children who were not successfully treated using the first method or who are older. The pseudarthrosis is resected, and the two bone ends are impacted. A ring fixator is applied. A proximal corticotomy allows for distraction and recouping of the limb-length discrepancy, and the distal fixation allows for compression at the pseudarthrosis site. As in other techniques, autogenous bone graft and bone morphogenetic protein are used to facilitate union at the distal site. The success rate of this method is 70% to 90%. Variations include implantation of an intramedullary nail throughout the distraction process or after union has been obtained.

The third option involves the use of a vascularized fibula in patients who have been unsuccessfully treated with the first two methods or who have marked bone loss and atrophy. The bone graft is stabilized with a plate or an external fixator and immobilized for several months. The success rate of this method is 80% to 90%.

Congenital Dislocation of the Knee

Unilateral or bilateral congenital dislocation of the knee occurs in approximately 1 in 100,000 live births. Females are more commonly affected than males.[19] There is a 50% incidence of hip dysplasia, clubfoot deformity, or congenital vertical talus in these patients. Bilateral deformity is associated with other conditions, such as spina bifida, arthrogryposis, or Larsen syndrome. Congenital dislocation of the knee is classified as hyperextension, subluxation, or knee joint dislocation. Hyperextension deformities (passive flexion past 45°) occur in patients with a history of breech birth or oligohydramnios. Treatment is nonsurgical and consists of stretching, casting, and use of an orthotic device such as a Pavlik harness. Patients with knee subluxation have flexion limited to less than 45°. Anterior subluxation of the tibia onto the distal aspect of the femur can be seen on radiographs. A dislocated knee has a completely displaced tibia with a severely shortened and fibrotic quadriceps tendon and an absent suprapatellar pouch. In severe cases, the hamstrings may be anteriorly displaced to the axis of rotation of the knee, and a valgus rotatory instability of the knee may be noted. Surgical treatment is considered for patients who have a fixed knee dislocation or a knee subluxation that was not improved to more than 90° using nonsurgical methods. Two surgical approaches have been described. For children younger than 3 months, a section of the quadriceps tendon and suprapatellar retinaculum is performed, followed by early motion. For older children, a VY quadricepsplasty is performed, with release of the contracted structures of the suprapatellar pouch and the quadriceps tendon, followed by long-term physical therapy and splinting.

Congenital Patella Dislocation

Congenital dislocation of the patella is rare. It is characterized by an irreducible, usually lateral dislocation of the patella. The knee may have a genu valgum deformity and a flexion contracture secondary to the lateral displacement of the patella. The treatment is surgical and consists of quadriceps immobilization, imbrication and advancement of the vastus medialis obliquus, and medialization of the patella within the extensor retinaculum.

Pediatric Foot Conditions

Pediatric foot conditions range from benign deviations from normal, to congenital conditions requiring treatment, to acquired deformities that may be a harbinger of other conditions. It is important to accurately diagnose each condition, reassuring the family if treatment is not needed, treating the condition nonsurgically or surgically when needed, and referring patients to other specialists if the deformity was caused by a more central pathology.

Congenital Vertical Talus

Congenital vertical talus is a rare foot deformity. In approximately 50% of patients, it is associated with spina bifida, arthrogryposis, sacral agenesis, diastematomyelia, or chromosomal abnormalities. If no such association is apparent, MRI evaluation of the spine and pelvis is indicated to rule out spinal dysraphism and other anomalies of the lumbosacral plexus. The equinus and valgus position of the congenital vertical talus results from a posterolateral contracture of the Achilles and peroneal tendons. The midfoot is dorsiflexed on the hindfoot as a result of a concurrent anterior contracture of the extensor hallucis longus, the anterior tibialis, and the extensor digitorum longus. This contracture leads to a dorsally dislocated navicular and a predominant talus head on the plantar aspect of the foot. Severe cases also have a concurrent dorsal cuboid dislocation on the head of the calcaneus. Radiographic evaluation includes AP and lateral views in forced plantar flexion and dorsiflexion. The forced plantar flexion lateral view is required to confirm continued dorsal displacement of the first metatarsal axis to the longitudinal axis of the talus. In some patients, the forced plantar flexion lateral radiograph shows colinearity of the first metatarsal and the longitudinal axis of the talus, suggesting that the primary disorder is a posterior lateral contracture. Such a foot is termed an oblique talus.

A child with mild or oblique congenital vertical talus can be treated by plantar flexion stretching, followed by percutaneous Achilles tendon lengthening. Casting may have a role in treatment of patients with true congenital talus.[20] In this method, plantar flexion casting is performed to stretch the anterior structures and reduce the midfoot. The talonavicular joint is then pinned, and percutaneous Achilles tendon lengthening is performed to reduce the posterior contracture. In children 2 years of age or younger, surgical reconstruction involves lengthening the Achilles, peroneus longus, and peroneus brevis tendons and performing a posterolateral subtalar release. The navicular on the head of the talus is then released, reduced, and pinned. The tibialis anterior, extensor hallucis longus, and extensor digitorum longus tendons are lengthened. Older children with residual deformities may require a salvage procedure, such as a naviculectomy, triple arthrodesis, or subtalar fusion.

Calcaneal Valgus Foot

Calcaneal valgus foot positioning is one of the most common deformities of newborn infants. The condition arises from intrauterine positioning. No treatment is needed, because spontaneous improvement is expected. The foot position of congenital vertical talus and spinal dysraphism can be similar, although in congenital vertical talus, a proximal migration of the calcaneus in the fat pad appears because of posterior contracture. In addition, the midfoot is usually stiffer than is seen in the calcaneal valgus foot. Dorsiflexion positioning of the foot may result from paralysis of the gastrocnemius muscle and subsequent dorsal positioning of the foot, as in a patient with an unrecognized spinal dysraphism. It is important to confirm that the gastrocnemius is functioning.

Clubfoot

The incidence of idiopathic clubfoot varies among ethnic groups, but the overall incidence is approximately 1 in 1,000 live births. The ratio of males to females is 3:1, and the deformity is bilateral in 40% of patients. A strong genetic component is present; the incidence in families with an affected individual is as much as 10 times higher than that in the general population. Clubfoot can be associated with neuromuscular syndromes and chromosomal abnormalities.

At birth, the entire foot appears to be severely inverted and supinated. The forefoot is adducted and pronated relative to the midfoot and hindfoot. The hindfoot is in varus and equinus. Although the entire foot is supinated, the forefoot is pronated relative to the hindfoot, resulting in cavus. Anatomically, adductus is caused by medial displacement and inversion of a wedge-shaped navicular. The navicular articulates with the medial aspect of the head of the talus, which has a medially directed neck and is in close proximity to the medial aspect of the tibia. The cuboid is also adducted in front of the calcaneus and along with the metatarsals, thus further adducting the midfoot. Hindfoot varus is caused by the adducted and inverted position of the calcaneus under the talus. The distal end of the calcaneus lies directly underneath the head of the talus and is not in the normal lateral position. Equinus deformity is caused by shortening of the extrinsic tendons, such as the gastrocnemius-soleus complex, tibialis posterior, and long toe flexors. The talus is plantar flexed in the ankle plafond, and the posterior ankle and subtalar capsules are also tight. Several classification systems appear to have moderate reproducibility and clinical relevance. Recently, an atypical clubfoot has been identified within the idiopathic clubfoot designation. It is a shorter foot with a first ray proximally recessed from the other four toes. In addition, a deep plantar crease extends from the medial arch to the lateral border of the foot. This foot tends to be fatter and have a higher cavus than is usually seen, and it is much more difficult to treat because of the intrinsic stiffness.

The goal of treatment of idiopathic clubfoot is to produce a flexible, painless plantigrade foot. Long-term results have dismissed the concept that achieving normal-appearing radiographs is essential; no correlation has been shown between radiographic parameters and long-term function. A clubfoot is initially treated nonsurgically. In the United States, the Ponseti method has become the standard for correction of a clubfoot deformity.[21-24] The protocol consists of stretching and manipulating the foot and applying successive holding casts. To stretch the ligaments and gradually correct the deformity, the foot is manipulated for a period of 1 to 3 minutes. The correction is maintained for 5 to 7 days with a well-molded plaster cast extending from the toes to the upper third of the thigh, with the knee at 90° flexion. Clubfoot correction usually requires five or six cast changes. Most patients require a percutaneous tenotomy of the Achilles tendon and posttreatment bracing with a foot abduction orthosis to maintain correction. Some patients eventually require additional treatment with manipulation and casting. Comparable success has been achieved in some European centers using a nonsurgical method of taping, physical therapy, and continuous passive motion.

Nonsurgical treatment is somewhat successful for all patients, and surgery is needed only for patients with residual deformity. Limited posterior releases and tendon transfers have been effective in children between 2 and 3 years of age. Older children who have a residual clubfoot deformity may also benefit from tendon transfers, midfoot osteotomies for residual forefoot adductus, or both. Hindfoot calcaneal sliding osteotomy may be needed in older children with residual varus deformity.

Metatarsus Adductus

Metatarsus adductus is another foot deformity common in newborn infants. The incidence approaches 1 in 1,500 live births, and one half of patients have bilateral involvement. The exact cause of metatarsus adductus is not known, although intrauterine positioning may be a factor. It was believed that patients with metatarsus adductus had higher rates of developmental dysplasia of the hip, but studies have not confirmed this theory. On physical examination, the forefoot is deviated medially with respect to the hindfoot, which is positioned in valgus. The deformity can be classified by its magnitude, as well as the stiffness of the metatarsus adductus.

The primary treatment of flexible metatarsus adductus is observation. Most patients have a benign natural history, with good correction of the deformity by age 4 years. Mild residual deformity is rarely a problem. Patients with rigid, severe metatarsus adductus can be treated with manipulation and serial casting after the age of 6 months. Manipulation involves abduction of the forefoot against counterpressure placed over the calcaneal cuboid joint. To maintain the correction after manipulation, children are placed in a long leg plaster cast, and the cast is changed every 2 weeks for three or four sessions. After the deformity is fully corrected, the child must wear a Denis Browne bar and shoes to prevent a recurrence. Surgical intervention can be used for the rare child with severe, stiff residual deformity.

Skewfoot

Skewfoot is a rare deformity characterized by medial deviation of the forefoot with lateral translation of the

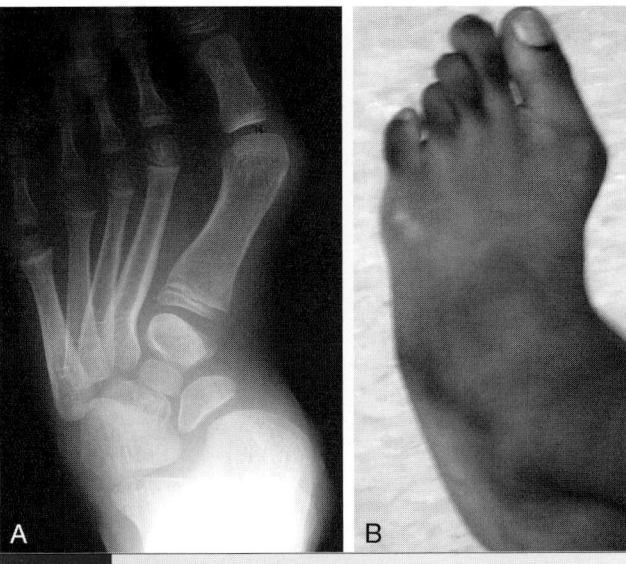

Figure 8 **A,** AP radiographic and **B,** photographic views of a skewfoot, which is characterized by forefoot abduction and lateral translation of the midfoot on a hindfoot that is in valgus.

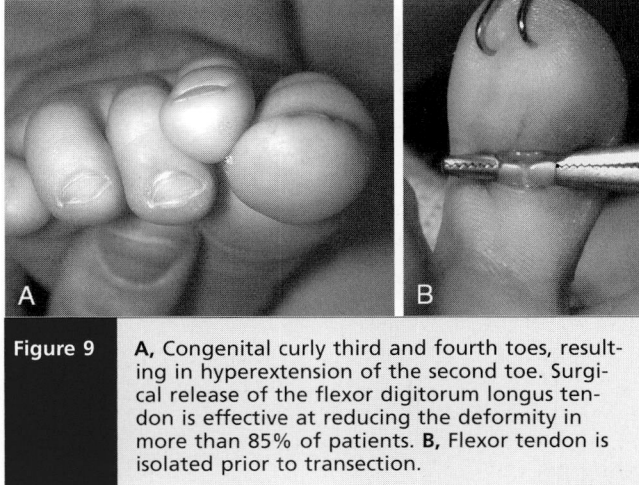

Figure 9 **A,** Congenital curly third and fourth toes, resulting in hyperextension of the second toe. Surgical release of the flexor digitorum longus tendon is effective at reducing the deformity in more than 85% of patients. **B,** Flexor tendon is isolated prior to transection.

midfoot and valgus positioning of the hindfoot (**Figure 8**). Skewfoot has also been called Z-foot or serpentine foot. The pathogenesis and natural history of this deformity are unknown. It is difficult to distinguish skewfoot from metatarsus adductus in a young child because of the unossified midfoot bones. As the child grows and the midfoot develops, radiographs show an uncovering of the talus because of lateral translation of the navicular and a lateral offset of the first metatarsal axis in line with the longitudinal axis of the talus. A valgus hindfoot is seen. Treatment with Achilles tendon stretching and a soft orthotic device with talus head support is indicated only if the child has callosities or pain with ambulation. If these conditions persist, surgery may be indicated, consisting of Achilles fascial lengthening, calcaneal lengthening osteotomies, and first cuneiform opening wedge osteotomies, with or without talonavicular joint reefing.

Congenital Lesser Toe Deformities

Although congenital curly toe deformity is common, its true incidence and natural history are unknown. The deformity frequently is bilateral, and it usually involves the third or fourth toes. In many children, it progressively corrects itself with time. Treatment with stretching and taping may be of benefit in a very mild deformity. Surgical treatment is indicated in patients who have a symptomatic deformity with pain or a nail bed deformity from abnormal positioning. Surgical release of the long toe flexor at the distal interphalangeal joint is effective in 85% to 90% of patients with congenital curly toes (**Figure 9**).

Congenital overriding fifth toe, defined as an adducted and dorsiflexed and medially deviated lesser toe,

is bilateral in 30% of patients. It is caused by subluxation or dislocation of the fifth metatarsophalangeal joint, without associated clawing of the interphalangeal joints. The treatment for mild cases is taping. One Half of patients request surgical intervention, involving capsular reconstruction and relocation, to correct painful shoe wear problems.

Flexible Flatfoot

Approximately 40% of infants are born with a flatfoot or planovalgus deformity, but the prevalence decreases to 10% in early adolescence. In most patients, this condition should be considered normal. Flatfoot deformities can be classified as rigid or flexible, depending on the mobility of the hindfoot. When the patient is standing on the toes, the valgus positioning in flexible feet repositions itself to a varus alignment. A rigid hindfoot does not have subtalar motion, either with toe standing or manipulation. Patients with a rigid hindfoot should be suspected of having a tarsal coalition or another subtalar pathology. Anatomically, both hindfoot valgus and a compensatory forefoot supination deformity are present. A tight Achilles tendon may be a component for patients with painful callosities over the head of the talus. These patients may have some intrinsic ligamentous laxity or a component of external tibial torsion that accentuates the biomechanical abnormalities of the midfoot breech. Strengthening, stretching, and a soft accommodating shoe insert may be helpful for these patients. Surgical intervention to correct a painful flatfoot is rarely necessary and generally involves a combination of osteotomies and Achilles tendon lengthening. A sliding calcaneal osteotomy can correct the hindfoot valgus, but a plantar base closing wedge osteotomy of the first cuneiform may be needed to correct the supination deformity. Alternatively, a calcaneal lengthening osteotomy can be performed, with or without a cuneiform osteotomy. In this procedure, peroneal tendon lengthening and talus-navicular reefing may also be needed.

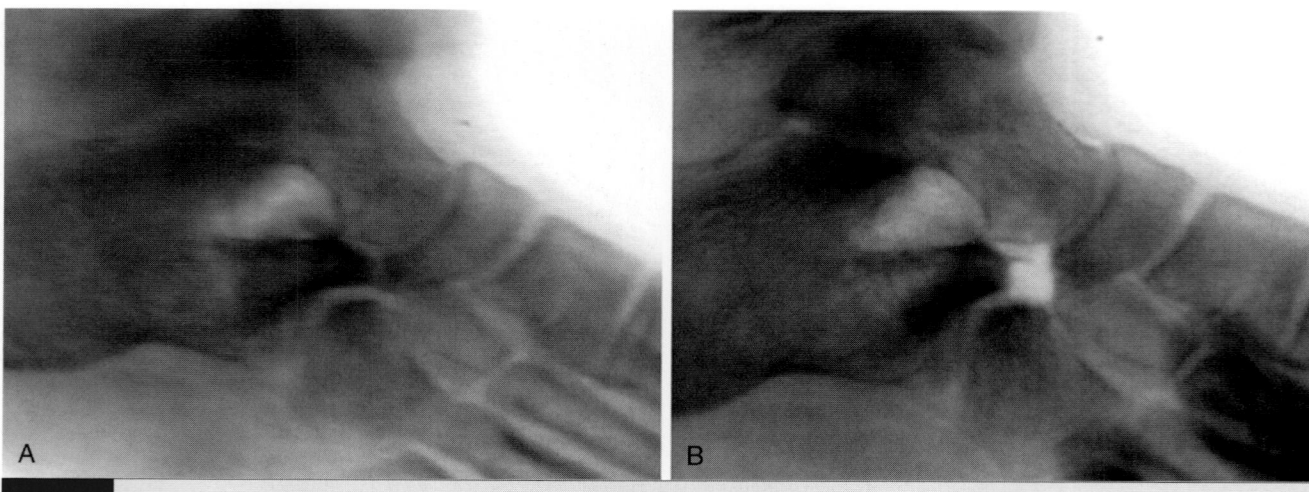

Figure 10 Preoperative **(A)** and postoperative **(B)** fluoroscopic images of a calcaneal navicular coalition. The extensor digitorum brevis muscle or fat is interposed to prevent recurrence into the resected area.

Tarsal Coalition

A tarsal coalition is an abnormal fibrous, cartilaginous, or bony connection between bones of the midfoot or hindfoot.[25] The most common is the calcaneonavicular coalition, and the second most common is the subtalar coalition. The remaining 10% arise within the calcaneocuboid or navicular–first cuneiform joint. Coalitions are bilateral in 50% to 60% of patients, and they can be inherited in an autosomal dominant pattern.

The cause and incidence of tarsal coalition is unknown, although it is occasionally seen with fibular hemimelia or clubfoot deformity. Approximately 25% of patients report activity-related pain on the dorsolateral and occasionally the posteromedial aspect of the ankle and hindfoot, and they may have spasm of the peroneal muscles. It is important to realize that inflammation of the subtalar joint from infection or inflammatory arthropathy can also produce peroneal spasm. The onset of pain usually occurs in children with a calcaneonavicular coalition between 8 and 12 years of age and in children with a subtalar coalition occurring after 12 years of age. The child may have a history of inversion ankle injuries caused by limited subtalar motion. On physical examination, hindfoot mobility is decreased. The hindfoot does not invert as it normally does during toe standing.

The calcaneonavicular coalition is best seen on oblique radiographic views. On a lateral radiograph, a long anterior process of the calcaneus, called the anteater sign, may also be noted. Subtalar coalitions can be suspected based on the presence on a lateral radiograph of a condensation underneath the medial facet of the calcaneus, called the C sign. A traction spur on the talus neck may appear, most likely as a stress reaction from increased movement of the talonavicular joint and not as a sign of arthritis. Occasionally a subtalar coalition is detected on the Harris radiographic view. CT can be used to confirm the diagnosis and rule out the presence of other coalitions. If CT is not conclusive,

MRI can be used to document the presence of abnormal fibrous tissue and inflammation in adjacent joints and bones. A bone scan and blood work may be needed to rule out inflammatory processes in patients who have significant subtalar loss of motion, pain, inflammation, and negative imaging studies. Increased bone scan uptake in the sustentaculum tali may indicate fibrous coalition.

The initial treatment of symptomatic coalition is nonsurgical and includes activity modification, anti-inflammatory drugs, an orthotic device, or a short leg walking cast. This regimen is successful in approximately one third of patients. With successful resection **(Figure 10)** and interposition of fat or extensor digitorum brevis muscle, patients with calcaneal-navicular coalitions do well. Resection of a subtalar coalition may be indicated if the total area is less than 50% of the subtalar joint. The results of subtalar resection and interposition of fat or split flexor hallucis tendon are less predictable than the results of calcaneal-navicular coalition, possibly because of the coalition size or excessive valgus deformity. Other surgical options include osteotomy to correct residual valgus positioning and arthrodesis of the subtalar joint in patients with joint arthritis or those who had unsuccessful earlier surgery.

Cavus Foot Deformity

Cavus is an acquired deformity caused by an elevated longitudinal arch as a result of plantar flexion and pronation of the first metatarsal.[26,27] Affected feet can be further described by associated hindfoot deformities, such as valgus, varus (cavovarus foot), or calcaneus (calcaneal cavus) positioning. Cavus results from muscle imbalances in both the intrinsic and extrinsic muscle groups. Weakness of the anterior tibialis with strong peroneus longus muscle tone is believed to be one of the factors causing a plantar flexed first metatarsal. Atrophy of the intrinsic muscles leads to metatarsophalangeal hyperextension deformities, which promote ca-

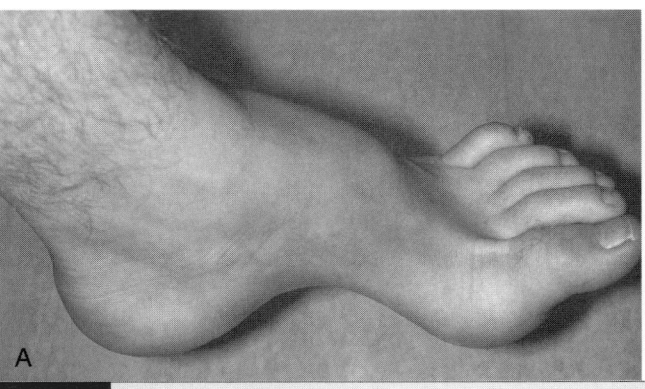
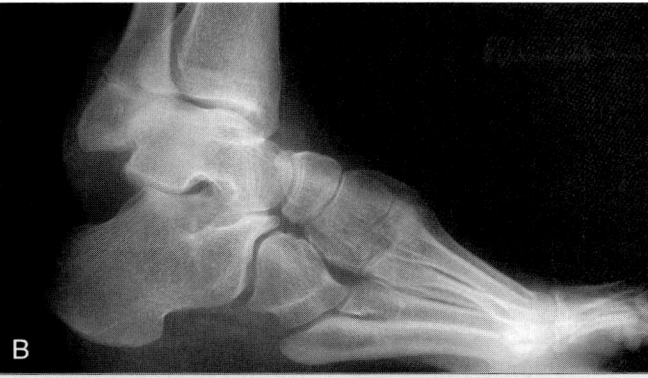

Figure 11 **A,** A cavovarus foot deformity in a 19-year-old man with Charcot-Marie-Tooth disease. **B,** Lateral radiograph shows hindfoot varus with obliquity of the subtalar joint; the cavus deformity is a result of an elevated calcaneal pitch and a dropped first metatarsal.

vus via tightening of the plantar fascia, and interphalangeal flexion deformities, which promote clawing. Varus results from tripod positioning from the dropped first ray. A strong posterior tibialis muscle and weak peroneus brevis tendon can also promote inversion or varus of the hindfoot. In many patients, bilateral deformity is associated with hereditary sensorimotor neuropathies, such as Charcot-Marie-Tooth disease, Friedreich ataxia, and many other neurologic disorders. Unilateral deformities can be associated with anatomic spinal dysraphism, such as diastematomyelia or tethering of the cord. Because of the high rate of neurologic pathology, all patients with cavus deformities require detailed physical examination with testing of reflexes, strength, and sensation. Appropriate genetic testing, electromyograms, nerve conduction velocities, and MRI, with referral to a pediatric neurologist, are usually indicated to confirm the diagnosis.

On radiographs, a patient with a cavus deformity has a plantar flexed first metatarsal with an increased talus-first metatarsal angle. In addition, the calcaneal-first metatarsal axis, which normally is 150°, is increased and representative of the cavus positioning. Obliquity of the subtalar joint and parallel orientation of the talus and calcaneus document hindfoot varus. Claw toe deformities can be seen on a lateral radiograph (**Figure 11**).

Conservative management of a cavus foot deformity includes stretching of the tight plantar fascia and Achilles tendon and strengthening of the anterior tibialis and hindfoot everters. The use of a flexible ankle-foot orthosis and arch support can relieve the plantar pressures and prevent rapid progression of the deformity. Surgical intervention is indicated for a patient with a progressive painful deformity or significant ankle instability. A range of procedures can be considered, including a combination of tendon and muscle lengthening, transfers, and osteotomies. Claw toe deformities can be treated with extensor tendon transfer to the neck of the metatarsal, in addition to flexor digitorum longus tenotomies or resection arthrodesis of the interphalangeal joints. Fusion is appropriate only for patients with a se-

verely stiff, rigid deformity or for those with ataxia, because reliable results cannot be expected from muscle transfers.

Accessory Navicular

Approximately 10% of the general population have an accessory navicular. It is often bilateral and is more common in girls than boys. A prominence is noted on the plantar medial aspect of the foot at the base of the navicular, within the substance or the insertion of the posterior tibialis tendon. Accessory navicular can be classified as type I, a small sesamoid bone in the substance of the posterior tibialis tendon itself; type II, a large wedge-shaped bone fragment that appears to be congruous with the navicular, either through a synchondrosis or synovial joint; or type III, a large horn-shaped navicular, most likely resulting from an earlier fusion of a type II deformity.

In a patient who has pain, tenderness can be found over the prominent aspect of the accessory bone. The nonsurgical options include rest, anti-inflammatory medicines, and a shoe insert with good arch support to decrease the strain of the posterior tibialis tendon and provide built-in relief by diminishing direct pressure over the bony prominence. A period of cast immobilization can be used to decrease inflammation. If pain persists, surgical intervention, with simple excision and reattachment of any disturbed posterior tibialis tendon, may be needed (**Figure 12**).

Juvenile Hallux Valgus

Juvenile bunion deformities usually occur in girls. Their true incidence is unknown. A prominence of the medial aspect of the first metatarsal head with lateral deviation of the great toe may be associated with an Achilles tendon contracture and foot flattening. Standing AP and lateral radiographs of the forefoot can help in determining the location of the deformity. Juvenile bunion deformities sometimes are associated with an increased intermetatarsal angle (greater than 10°) or an increased distal metatarsal articular angle.[28] Pain is rarely present over the medial aspect of the distal head of the first

6: Pediatrics

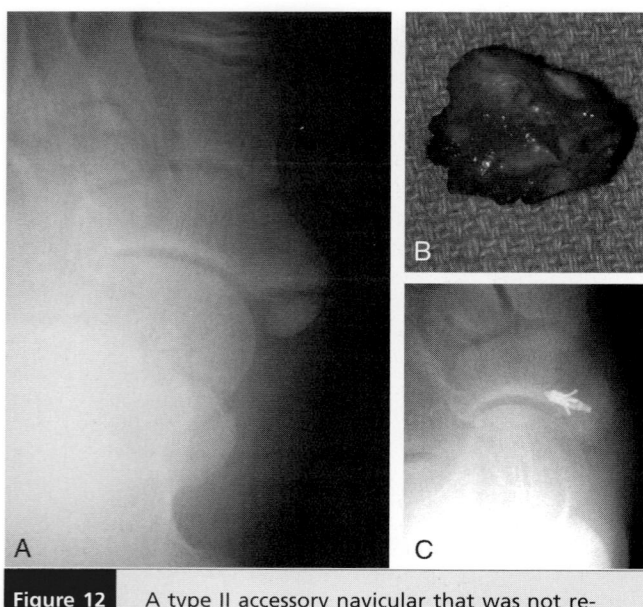

Figure 12 A type II accessory navicular that was not responsive to conservative treatment was treated with simple excision and reattachment of the posterior tibialis with a suture anchor. **A,** Preoperative AP radiograph of the foot. **B,** Intraoperative photograph of resected accessory navicular. **C,** Postoperative AP radiograph.

metatarsal.

Treatment is based solely on the presence of symptoms. Children who are asymptomatic should not undergo any form of treatment. A child with pain on the medial aspect should wear shoes with a wide toe box. Arch supports can help with the flatfoot deformity, and nighttime splinting may be of some benefit in correcting the deformity.

Surgical treatment of a symptomatic, recalcitrant juvenile bunion deformity is problematic, because the rate of recurrence is high. Families should be strongly encouraged to avoid surgery until the patient stops growing. The extremely rare surgery for juvenile bunion deformity consists of a combination of bony osteotomy and soft-tissue rebalancing.

Osteochondrosis of the Foot

Osteochondrosis of the navicular, also called Köhler's disease, affects boys more often than girls. The child has midfoot pain and an antalgic gait caused by a tendency to walk on the outside of the foot. The diagnosis is made from characteristic radiographic findings that include flattening, sclerosis, and patchy ossification of the navicular, as well as changes similar to those seen in Legg-Calvé-Perthes disease. The natural history is benign; the symptoms can be expected to resolve and the navicular to develop normally. Occasionally, the use of a short leg cast can shorten the duration of symptoms. A short leg walking cast appears to offer no benefit over a nonwalking cast.

Older children and adolescents are affected by Freiberg's infraction, which is more common in girls than in boys. Forefoot pain occurs with activity and is accompanied by swelling and tenderness at the second metatarsal head and occasionally at the first, fourth, and fifth metatarsal heads. Radiographs may show subchondral lucencies, sclerosis, and, eventually, flattening of the articular surface of the metatarsal head. The differential diagnosis includes infection, rheumatoid arthritis, and metatarsal stress fracture. In most patients, the activity-related pain and swelling will resolve, and radiographs will show remodeling of the articular surface. The nonsurgical treatment includes activity modification and the use of a shoe insert. Residual pain can be ameliorated with short-term cast immobilization. Surgical intervention, which may be needed for a patient with enduring pain, includes joint débridement, metatarsal head dorsiflexion osteotomy, or, in rare patients, resection of the metatarsal head.

Annotated References

1. Beals RK, Stanley G: Surgical correction of bowlegs in achondroplasia. *J Pediatr Orthop B* 2005;14:245-249.

    In a long-term retrospective review of 21 patients with achondroplasia who were treated with osteotomy, fibular epiphysiodesis, or the Ilizarov method, the Ilizarov method was found to be the best treatment of proximal deformity in young children. Distal osteotomy was preferable for distal deformities in older children.

2. Price CT, Izuka BH: Osteotomy planning using the anatomic method: A simple method for lower extremity deformity analysis. *Orthopedics* 2005;28:20-25.

    A method of deformity analysis using the anatomic axes is presented.

3. Novais E, Stevens PM: Hypophosphatemic rickets: The role of hemiepiphysiodesis. *J Pediatr Orthop* 2006;26: 238-244.

    A review from the literature of patients with hypophosphatemic rickets who were treated with hemiepiphyseal stapling concluded that this technique is minimally invasive and may be safely used with good success, even in young children. It can be repeated as necessary.

4. Park SS, Gordon JE, Luhmann SJ, Dobbs MB, Schoenecker PL: Outcome of hemiepiphyseal stapling for late-onset tibia vara. *J Bone Joint Surg Am* 2005;87:2259-2266.

    This large retrospective review of patients with late-onset tibia vara treated with hemiepiphyseal stapling found that the technique is safe and effective if the deformity is mild or moderate. It is particularly effective in children who are younger than 10 years. Level of evidence: Therapeutic level IV.

5. Langenskiöld A: tibia vara: A critical review. *Clin Orthop Relat Res* 1981;158:77.

6. Holsalkar HS, Jones S, Hartley J, Hill R: Three-

dimensional tomography relapsed infantile Blount's disease. *Clin Orthop Relat Res* 2005;431:176-180.

Three-dimensional CT is useful in patients with relapsed infantile Blount's disease, especially those who will be treated with hemiplateau evaluation to correct the intra-articular deformity.

7. Gordon JE, King DJ, Luhmann SJ, Dobbs MB, Schoenecker PL: Femoral deformity in tibia vara. *J Bone Joint Surg Am* 2006;88:380-386.

This retrospective evaluation of 73 patients with tibia vara documented distal femoral deformity. In patients with infantile tibia vara, the distal femur may have mild varus to mild valgus alignment. Patients with adolescent tibia vara may have more significant distal varus, which on average is 30% of the knee deformity.

8. Gordon JE, Heidenreich FP, Carpenter CJ, Kelly-Hahn J, Schoenecker PL: Comprehensive treatment of late-onset tibia vara. *J Bone Joint Surg Am* 2005;87:1561-1570.

A comprehensive treatment algorithm for patients with late-onset tibia vara is presented. Patients were treated with distal femoral osteotomy or stapling, proximal tibial osteotomy, distal tibial osteotomy, or hemiepiphyseal stapling. The comprehensive approach allowed restoration of the mechanical and anatomic axes of the lower limb in the hope of preventing later degenerative arthrosis.

9. Schoenecker P, Rich M: The lower extremity, in Morrissy RT, Weinstein SL (eds): *Lovell and Winter's Pediatric Orthopaedics*, ed 6. Philadelphia, PA, Lippincott Williams and Wilkins, 2006.

This classic text discusses concepts and procedures related to the lower extremity.

10. Greulich W, Pyle S: *Radiographic Atlas of the Skeletal Development of the Hand and Wrist.* Stanford, CA, Stanford University Press, 1959.

11. Song HR, Oh CW, Mattoo R, et al: Femoral lengthening over an intramedullary nail using the external fixator: Risk of infection and knee problems in 22 patients with a follow-up of 2 years or more. *Acta Orthop* 2005;76:245-252.

In a retrospective review of 22 patients after femoral lengthening over an intramedullary nail, deep intramedullary infection associated with a previous history of trauma or infection developed in 13%. Knee complications occurred in 18%, most of whom had lengthening of more than 20%.

12. Kocaoglu M, Eralp L, Kilicoglu O, Burc H, Cakmak M: Complications encountered during lengthening over an intramedullary nail. *J Bone Joint Surg Am* 2004;86-A:2406-2411.

In one of the most extensive reports of distraction osteogenesis over an intramedullary nail (42 segments and 35 patients), the overall complication rate was comparable to that seen in standard limb lengthening. More severe complications occurred with lengthening of more than 6 cm or 20% of the original bone length. The authors concluded that lengthening over an intramedullary nail improves patient comfort and reduces the time for external fixation.

13. Gabos PG, El Rassi G, Pahys J: Knee reconstruction in syndromes with congenital absence of the anterior cruciate ligament. *J Pediatr Orthop* 2005;25:210-214.

In four selected patients with congenital anterior cruciate ligament absence, intra-articular reconstruction restored knee stability.

14. Wada A, Fujii T, Takamura K, Yanagida H, Urano N, Yamaguchi T: Limb salvage treatment for congenital deficiency of the tibia. *J Pediatr Orthop* 2006;26:226-232.

Seven patients (nine limbs) with tibial hemimelia underwent limb salvage. Patients with type II underwent proximal synostosis and centralization of the foot on the distal fibula. Their outcomes were good. Patients who underwent Brown centralization procedures had progressive knee flexion contractures and persistent ligamentous instability.

15. De Maio F, Corsi A, Roggini M, Riminucci M, Bianco P, Ippolito E: Congenital unilateral posteromedial bowing of the tibia and fibula: Insights regarding pathogenesis from prenatal pathology. A case report. *J Bone Joint Surg Am* 2005;87:1601-1605.

In an anatomic and histologic evaluation of an aborted fetus with posterior medial bowing of the tibia, the authors hypothesize that posterior medial bowing of the tibia may result from a placental abnormality resulting in compressing events and leading to the deformed bone.

16. Dobbs MB, Rich MM, Gordon JE, Szymanski DA, Schoenecker PL: Use of an intramedullary rod for the treatment of congenital pseudarthrosis of the tibia: Surgical technique. *J Bone Joint Surg Am* 2005;87(suppl 1):33-40.

A method of intramedullary stabilization and bone grafting as the primary treatment of congenital pseudarthrosis of the tibia is elegantly illustrated.

17. Lee FY, Sinicropi SM, Lee FS, Vitale MG, Roye DP Jr, Choi IH: Treatment of congenital pseudarthrosis of the tibia with recombinant human bone morphogenetic protein-7 (rhBMP-7): A report of five cases. *J Bone Joint Surg Am* 2006;88:627-633.

Five patients were treated with BMP-7 for congenital pseudarthrosis of the tibia. On follow-up, isolated use of BMP-7 was not found to increase rates of healing, compared with historical controls.

18. Dobbs MB, Rich MM, Gordon JE, Szymanski DA, Schoenecker PL: Use of an intramedullary rod for treatment of congenital pseudarthrosis of the tibia: A long-term follow-up study. *J Bone Joint Surg Am* 2004;86-A:1186-1197.

A long-term retrospective study of 21 patients with congenital pseudarthrosis of the tibia found that 16 patients had satisfactory results at an average 14-year follow-up. Initial consolidation occurred in 18 patients, although

6: Pediatrics

multiple refractures and deformities required further surgery.

19. Manner HM, Radler C, Ganger R, Grill F: Dysplasia of the cruciate ligaments: Radiographic assessment and classification. *J Bone Joint Surg Am* 2006;88:130-137.

    Radiographic and MRI findings were correlated in patients with congenital longitudinal deformity. Notch view radiographs can suggest the absence of one or both of the cruciate ligaments.

20. Dobbs MB, Purcell DB, Nunley R, Morcuende JA: Early results of a new method of treatment for idiopathic congenital vertical talus. *J Bone Joint Surg Am* 2006;88:1192-1200.

    In two institutions, a new closed method of treating congenital vertical talus was studied. The method consisted of manipulation and reduction of the midfoot deformity, followed by talonavicular joint pinning and percutaneous Achilles tendon lengthening. The preliminary results were provocative and justify attempting this method before extensive surgical release.

21. Dobbs MB, Nunley R, Schoenecker PL: Long-term follow-up of patients with clubfeet treated with extensive soft-tissue release. *J Bone Joint Surg Am* 2006;88:986-996.

    At a mean 30-year follow up, 45 patients who underwent surgical treatment of 73 clubfeet were evaluated. Significant limitation of foot function was found, and greater disability was associated with extensive soft-tissue release or multiple procedures. The authors concluded that conservative management of clubfoot using the Ponseti approach is preferred. If residual deformity is present, an à la carte approach can avoid the long-term morbidity of extensive releases.

22. Templeton PA, Flowers MJ, Latz KH, Stephens D, Cole WG, Wright JG: Factors predicting the outcome of primary clubfoot surgery. *Can J Surg* 2006;49:123-127.

    In a retrospective analysis of 63 families of children treated with surgical management of clubfoot, 19% of children who underwent clubfoot surgery required further surgery. Outcomes were generally considered good, although results were better in children treated at approximately 1 year of age rather than during the first 6 months of life.

23. Dobbs MB, Rudzki JR, Purcell DB, Walton T, Porter KR, Gurnett CA: Factors predictive of outcome after use of the Ponseti method for the treatment of idiopathic clubfeet. *J Bone Joint Surg Am* 2004;86-A:22-27.

    In this retrospective study of 51 patients with 86 idiopathic clubfeet treated with the Ponseti method, a higher rate of recurrence was found in children of noncompliant families. Poor compliance was associated with lower educational level. The authors suggested that additional resources be devoted to families at high risk of noncompliance. Level of evidence: Prognostic level II-1.

24. Richards BS, Johnston CE, Wilson H: Nonoperative clubfoot treatment using the French physical therapy method. *J Pediatr Orthop* 2005;25:98-102.

    A follow-up of 98 patients with 142 clubfeet treated with the nonsurgical physical therapy method from France concluded that the method significantly reduced the need for surgical treatment, with 49% requiring formal open surgical releases.

25. El Rassi G, Riddle EC, Kumar SJ: Arthrofibrosis involving the middle facet of the talocalcaneal joint in children and adolescents. *J Bone Joint Surg Am* 2005;87:2227-2231.

    In 19 patients with residual anterolateral ankle pain and stiffness consistent with tarsal coalition, exploration of the sustentaculum tala and medial facet revealed synovial thickening and fibrosis, despite negative CT and MRI findings. Following resection of this stiff tissue, most patients improved. Bone scanning and uptake in the medial facet appear to be suggestive of this clinical syndrome. Level of evidence: Therapeutic level IV.

26. Wicart P, Seringe R: Plantar opening-wedge osteotomy of cuneiform bones combined with selective plantar release and Dwyer osteotomy for pes cavovarus in children. *J Pediatr Orthop* 2006;26:100-108.

    Using a treatment algorithm for cavovarus feet, 26 children with 36 affected feet received surgical correction consisting of an open-wedge osteotomy of the first cuneiform and selected plantar release with hindfoot osteotomy. The average follow-up was 7 years, and the percentage of cavus correction approached 75%. The authors concluded that treatment was satisfactory.

27. Wines AP, Chen D, Lynch B, Stephens MM: Foot deformities in children with hereditary motor and sensory neuropathy. *J Pediatr Orthop* 2005;25:241-244.

    Data are presented on 104 feet in 52 patients with hereditary motor and sensory neuropathy. A cavovarus deformity was present in 65% of feet, 22% had a planovalgus deformity, and the remainder had no significant deformity. Only 45% of patients had similar, symmetric involvement of both feet. Surgical treatment was more likely to be indicated in patients with cavovarus rather than planovalgus foot deformities. Surgery was required in slightly fewer than one half of children affected with hereditary motor and sensory neuropathy.

28. Johnson AE, Georgopoulos G, Erickson MA, Eilert R: Treatment of adolescent hallux valgus with the first metatarsal double osteotomy: The Denver experience. *J Pediatr Orthop* 2004;24:358-362.

    Nine patients (14 feet) were treated with double first-metatarsal osteotomy for adolescent bunion deformities at an average age of 15 years. A review found that 90% had good or excellent results. The authors concluded that this procedure is effective and reliable.

Chapter 62

Injuries and Conditions of the Pediatric and Adolescent Athlete

Mininder S. Kocher, MD, MPH   Jason Andersen, AB

Introduction

Sports injuries are being seen with increased frequency in pediatric and adolescent athletes as a result of increased participation in higher competitive levels at younger ages, increased recognition of injuries in this age group, and the advent of arthroscopy and MRI. The pediatric athlete differs from the adult athlete in terms of physiology, growth, psychology, and skill level. Injury patterns are age- and sport-specific. An understanding of the special considerations of the pediatric athlete and the common injury patterns is necessary for the successful management of sports injuries in these patients.

Special Considerations of the Young Athlete

Growth and Development

Childhood and adolescence are dynamic periods in terms of skeletal, sexual, and neuromuscular development. It is essential that the physician determine the young athlete's stage of growth and development because the progression of certain injury patterns is often related to growth. For example, Osgood-Schlatter disease (OSD) is frequently seen during the adolescent growth spurt. Management of specific injuries may be based on the child's stage of development. For example, anterior cruciate ligament (ACL) injuries may be treated with physeal-sparing techniques in prepubescent patients, whereas transphyseal techniques are used in adolescent patients. Anatomic changes with growth may predispose young athletes to certain injury patterns. For example, femoral anteversion, external tibial torsion, genu valgum, and pes planus may contribute to patellofemoral dysfunction.

In addition to chronologic age, skeletal age and physiologic age are important to determine. Skeletal age is typically determined using hand and wrist radiographs per the method of Greulich and Pyle. Physiologic age is determined using the Tanner stage of sexual development (**Table 1**). Flexibility changes with periods of growth should be routinely assessed by examination of hyperextension of the metacarpophalangeal joints, abduction of the thumb, and hyperextension of the el-

bow. Neuromuscular development should also be routinely assessed by examination of coordination and fine motor skills.

Training

Traditionally, strength training was discouraged in the pediatric population because of the perceived risk of growth disturbances and other injuries. Research over the past 20 years has demonstrated that not only can strength training be a safe and effective component of any comprehensive fitness program, but it can also provide clear health benefits to the pediatric age group.[1] These benefits include improved athletic performance as a result of increased coordination, muscle strength, and power, in addition to enhancement of long-term health as a result of increased cardiorespiratory fitness, reduced risk of injury, and improved bone mineral density and blood lipid profile. In the preadolescent, strength increases occur in the absence of muscle hypertrophy, likely because of neurogenic adaptation, with loss of strength benefits after 6 weeks of discontinuation of the strength training. In contrast, strength training during and after puberty is further enhanced by the hormonally induced increase in muscle growth that occurs in both males and females. Although the risk of injury associated with strength training is real, research shows that it is no greater than in any other sport when adult supervision is available to ensure that proper techniques and safety precautions are used.[1]

The increased popularity of endurance sports such as swimming, running, rowing, and cycling among children has heightened the awareness of aerobic training. The ability to enhance the aerobic capacity of children through endurance training remains a controversial topic; many of the studies to date have been methodically flawed and largely neglected children.[2]

Thermoregulation

There are several physiologic characteristics unique to the pediatric population that contribute to the thermoregulatory disadvantage they face in extreme climatic conditions, including increased surface area to body mass ratio, reduced sweating capacity, greater generation of metabolic heat per mass unit, and a

6: Pediatrics

Table 1

Tanner Staging Classification of Secondary Sexual Characteristics

Tanner Stage		Male	Female
Stage 1 (Prepubertal)	Growth	5-6 cm/y	5-6 cm/y
	Development	Testes < 4 mL or < 2.5 cm No pubic hair	No breast development No pubic hair
Stage 2	Growth	5-6 cm/y	7-8 cm/y
	Development	Testes 4 mL or 2.5-3.2 cm Minimal pubic hair at base of penis	Breast buds Minimal pubic hair on labia
Stage 3	Growth	7-8 cm/y	8 cm/y
	Development	Testes 12 mL or 3.6 cm Pubic hair over pubis Voice changes Muscle mass increases	Elevation of breast; areolae enlarge Pubic hair of mons pubis Axillary hair Acne
Stage 4	Growth	10 cm/y	7 cm/y
	Development	Testes 4.1-4.5 cm Pubic hair as adult Axillary hair Acne	Areolae enlarge Pubic hair as adult
Stage 5	Growth	No growth	No growth
	Development	Testes as adult Pubic hair as adult Facial hair as adult Mature physique	Adult breast contour Pubic hair as adult
Other		Peak height velocity: 13.5 years	Adrenarche: 6-8 years Menarche: 12.7 years Peak height velocity: 11.5 years

slower rate of heat acclimatization. A large surface area to body mass ratio is disadvantageous in hot, humid weather because it provides a larger area for heat influx, thereby raising the body's core temperature and increasing the risk of heat-induced illnesses. Despite children having a greater density of sweat glands per skin area than adults, sweating capacity is restricted because of a lower sweating rate and a higher sweating threshold. As a result, the ability to dissipate body heat by evaporation is reduced in children until the transition is made to an adult sweating pattern in late puberty. The reluctance of children to drink during prolonged exercise further exacerbates this thermoregulatory disadvantage. The American Academy of Pediatrics recommends prehydration and enforced periodic drinking during the course of prolonged exercise.[3]

Performance-Enhancing Substances

The use of performance-enhancing substances among adolescents is increasing as a result of media exposure, the availability of so-called natural supplements, the absence of formal drug testing in schools, and the increasingly competitive nature of youth sports. Pediatric athletes are at high risk of being exposed to these drugs because of increased susceptibility to societal pressures at a time when they are often dealing with complex developmental and psychosocial changes. The use of an-

drogenic steroids is widespread and has been estimated at 4% to 12% of male adolescents and 0.5% to 2% of female adolescents in the 1990s despite the banning of these substances by almost every major athletic governing body.[4]

Common Injury Patterns

Over the past 30 years there has been a significant increase in the number of children and adolescents participating in physical activity and team sports, with the largest increase among adolescent females.[5] The overall trend has seen a shift from the largely unstructured, unsupervised "free play" of the early 20th century to the evolution of organized and highly structured youth sports activities. It is estimated that up to 30 million children participate in organized sports in the United States. The Youth Risk Behavior Survey (YRBS) was a large population-based study performed throughout the 1990s, enabling accurate assessment of the emerging trends in youth sports participation. Results from the 1997 survey reported that 62% of US high school students participated in one or more sports teams, with most playing in a combination of both school and nonschool teams.[5] Although the number of women participating in sports teams has increased fivefold over the past 30 years, a disparity continues to exist between genders according to the 1997 YRBS study.

Increased youth participation in sports and physical activities has resulted in an increase in sports-related injuries secondary to trauma and overuse. The annual rate of sports injuries within the United States is approximately 3 million, with up to 70% of those resulting from youth sports activities.[5] The financial costs of managing these injuries in 1996 were well in excess of $1 billion. Pediatric sports injuries are often unique not only in terms of the underlying pathology but also the challenges in managing these injuries. Many patients participate in multiple teams during a given sports season, the rest periods between seasons are short or nonexistent, and there is increasing demand for sporting success from parents, schools, and sporting establishments. Among school athletes, football has the highest rate of injury, with wrestling a close second. Cheerleading has the highest rate of catastrophic injuries. The rate of injury in both males and females at high school and college levels is comparable, with the exception of knee injuries, which are greater in females at the college level.

Shoulder Injuries

Acromioclavicular Joint Injury

A fall onto the point of the shoulder causes acromioclavicular (AC) separations in older adolescents and lateral clavicle physeal fractures in children. The athlete reports pain and deformity around the AC joint. With either injury, displacement of the lateral clavicle occurs superiorly through a tear in the thick periosteal tube surrounding the distal clavicle. The lateral clavicular epiphysis along with the AC and coracoclavicular ligaments may remain intact to the periosteal tube. Radiographs are usually sufficient to evaluate the injury, and stress radiographs with 5 to 10 lb of traction may aid in delineating the degree of instability. The Rockwood classification identifies pediatric AC injuries based on the position of the lateral clavicle and the accompanying injury to the periosteal tube.[6] Injury types I to III involve progressive disruption of the AC ligaments and periosteal tube with increasing superior displacement of the lateral clavicle. Type IV, V, and VI demonstrate posterior, superior subcutaneous, and inferior displacement of the lateral clavicle, respectively.

Nonsurgical treatment is usually indicated for the typical physeal fracture seen in children younger than age 13 years. These injuries exhibit a great potential for healing and remodeling. Type IV, V, and VI injuries with large displacement may require surgical stabilization, usually in the form of periosteal tube repair without internal fixation. For late adolescent and adult type true AC joint separations, nonsurgical management results in good outcomes for type I and II injuries, whereas surgical management is indicated for type IV, V, and VI injuries. The management of type III injuries in the older adolescent athlete remains controversial, with initial nonsurgical management recommended most often.

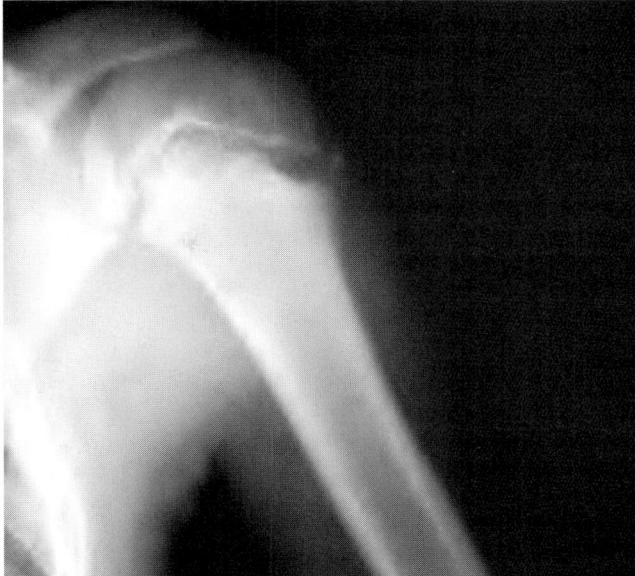

Figure 1 Little leaguer's shoulder. Widening of the proximal humeral physis associated with repetitive overuse.

Little Leaguer's Shoulder

"Little leaguer's shoulder" is a chronic stress fracture of the proximal humeral physis resulting from the repetitive large rotational torques involved in throwing.[7] This condition is most commonly seen in high-performance male pitchers age 11 to 13 years. Poor throwing mechanics and frequent pitching may predispose these children to injury. Patients report shoulder pain and there is widening of the proximal humeral physis on radiographs (**Figure 1**). Treatment involves rest from pitching, often for the remainder of the season, with a vigorous preseason conditioning program and limits on the frequency of pitching during the subsequent year (**Table 2**). Proximal humeral growth arrest is extremely rare. Proper throwing mechanics should be stressed with an emphasis on control instead of speed.

Glenohumeral Instability

Traumatic anterior dislocation is the most common type of instability seen in adolescent athletes. These injuries are usually the result of trauma, and anteroinferior capsulolabral separation (Bankart lesion) is usually present (**Figure 2**). Rates of recurrent instability in adolescents and young adults vary from 75% to 95% in several studies.[8] Nevertheless, the adolescent patient should be counseled that recurrence is likely. Controversy exists regarding optimal management of a first-time dislocation: initial surgical treatment versus initial nonsurgical treatment. Surgical treatment may result in improved outcomes.[9] Nonsurgical treatment typically consists of a period of immobilization followed by progressive motion and strengthening. Immobilization in a position of external rotation is gaining favor because there may be better approximation of the labral tear to

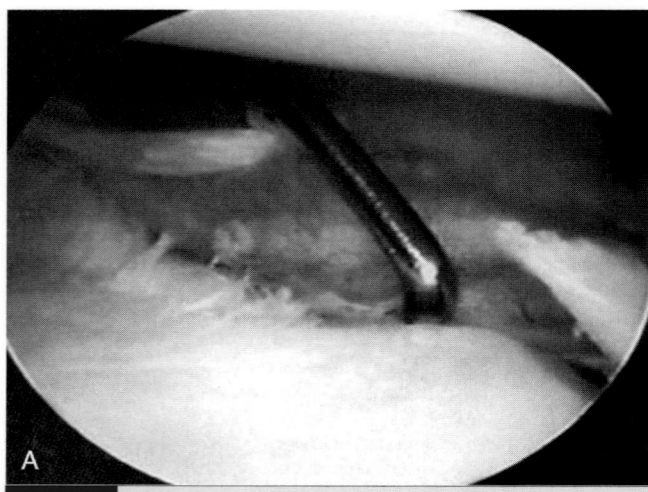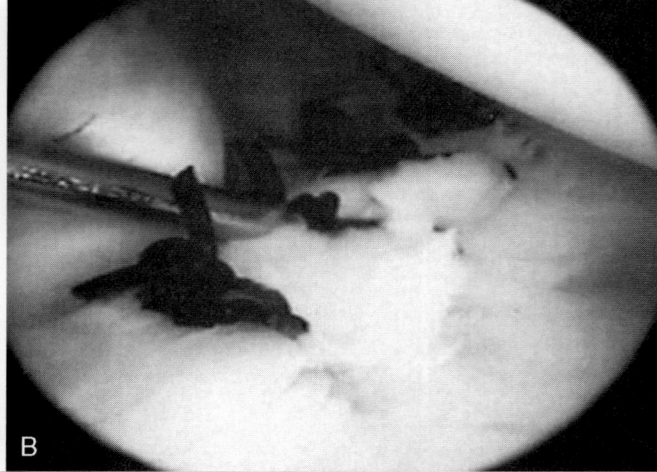

Figure 2 Anterior glenohumeral instability. Arthroscopic appearance of Bankart lesion before (**A**) and after (**B**) arthroscopic repair.

Table 2

New Throwing Guidelines From Little League Baseball

League Age (years)*+	Pitches Allowed Per Day
17-18	105
13-16	95
11-12	85
10 and younger	75

*Pitchers league ages 7 through 16 must adhere to the following rest requirements:
- If a player pitches 61 or more pitches in a day, 3 calendar days of rest must be observed.
- If a player pitches 41 to 60 pitches in a day, 2 calendar days of rest must be observed.
- If a player pitches 21 to 40 pitches in a day, 1 calendar day of rest must be observed.
- If a player pitches 1 to 20 pitches in a day, no calendar day of rest is required before pitching again.

+Pitchers league age 17 to 18 years must adhere to the following rest requirements:
- If a player pitches 76 or more pitches in a day, 3 calendar days of rest must be observed.
- If a player pitches 51 to 75 pitches in a day, 2 calendar days of rest must be observed.
- If a player pitches 26 to 50 pitches in a day, 1 calendar day of rest must be observed.
- If a player pitches 1 to 25 pitches in a day, no calendar day of rest is required before pitching again.

the glenoid for healing.[10] For recurrent instability, surgical management is indicated, consisting of a Bankart type of capsulolabral repair, performed either open or arthroscopically[11] (Figure 2).

Multidirectional instability with ligamentous laxity is more frequently seen in the adolescent female athlete without a clear history of trauma and may occur during gymnastics, throwing, hitting, swimming, or overhead serving. Initially, there are painless episodes of subluxation with spontaneous reduction. Examination reveals signs of multidirectional instability, including the sulcus sign and excessive translation with anterior and posterior drawer tests or the load and shift test. Signs of generalized ligamentous laxity are frequently present. A vigorous rehabilitation program stressing rotator cuff strengthening and scapulothoracic dynamics is successful in most patients. Surgical management of multidirectional instability is infrequently required.

Little Leaguer's Elbow
The term "little leaguer's elbow" describes a group of pathologic entities about the elbow joint in young throwers.[12] The entities include medial epicondyle fragmentation and avulsion, growth alteration of the medial epicondyle, osteochondritis dissecans (OCD) of the capitellum, deformation or OCD of the radial head, hypertrophy of the ulna, and olecranon apophysitis. OCD of the capitellum may also occur in high-performance female gymnasts. Most patients with little leaguer's elbow present with medial elbow complaints: medial pain and decreased throwing effectiveness/distance. Medial tension overload results from repetitive valgus stress and flexor forearm pull. Changes are age dependent. During childhood, irregular appearance of the secondary centers of ossification of the medial epicondyle may be seen. In adolescence, with increasing muscle strength, avulsion fracture of the medial epicondyle may occur (**Figure 3**). After fusion of the medial epicondyle in young adulthood, injuries of the ulnar collateral ligament and flexor muscle origin become more apparent. Laterally, repetitive valgus compression may lead to damage of the radiocapitellar articulation. OCD can affect both the capitellum and the radial head. Changes include chondromalacia with softening and fissuring of the articular surface, subchondral collapse, and bony eburnation. OCD of the capitellum can present with wide variations in radiographic appear-

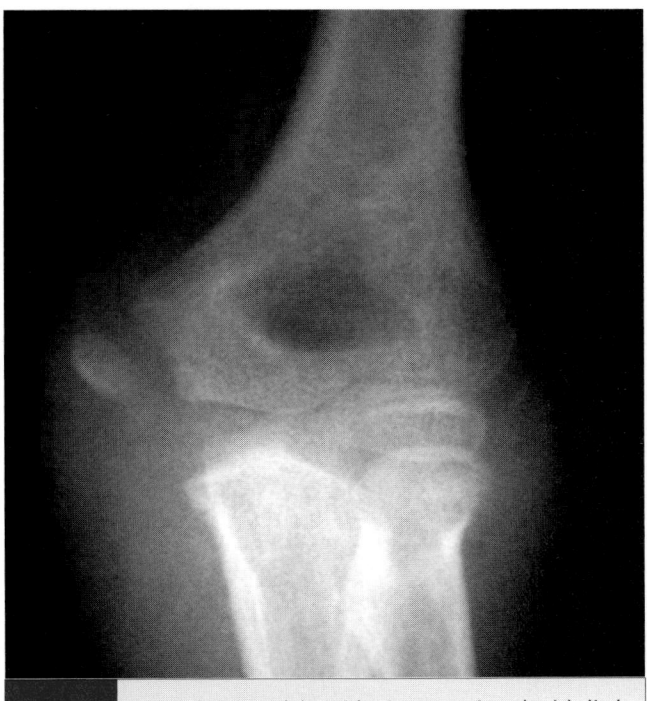

Figure 3 Medial epicondyle widening associated with little leaguer's elbow.

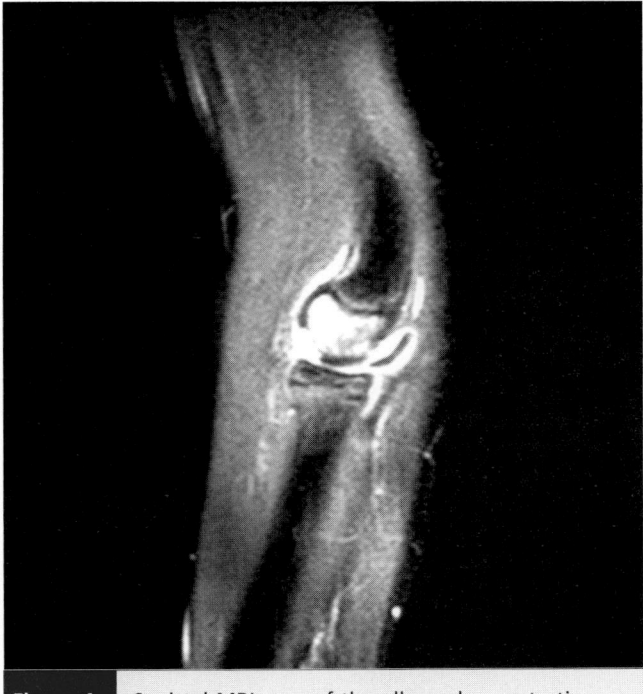

Figure 4 Sagittal MRI scan of the elbow demonstrating chondral defect of the capitellum associated with OCD.

ance depending on the extent of osteonecrosis and the presence of loose bodies (**Figure 4**). MRI has provided the opportunity for early diagnosis, before radiographic changes occur. Pain, tenderness, and contracture dominate the clinical presentation. OCD of the capitellum must be differentiated from Panner's disease, which is an osteochondrosis seen typically in boys age 5 to 12 years without a history of overuse and which usually resolves spontaneously. Additional lateral injuries seen during throwing in the skeletally immature athlete include lateral apophysis avulsion from traction during follow-through and radial physeal injury from repetitive valgus overload. Posterior elbow pain in throwers is frequently caused by the powerful contraction of the triceps in the early acceleration phase coupled with the impaction of the olecranon into its humeral fossa in the late follow-through phase of throwing. Olecranon apophysitis, avulsion fracture, posteromedial osteophytes, and loose bodies may form.

Treatment of little leaguer's elbow is directed at removing the recurrent microtrauma. Cessation of all throwing until the elbow is asymptomatic followed by reassessment of throwing mechanics and number of pitches thrown is essential.[13] Range of motion exercises and dynamic splinting may be useful for contractures. Arthroscopy is useful for assessing chondral injury, removal of loose bodies, and management of OCD through drilling or fragment fixation. Management of displaced medial epicondyle fractures is controversial in pediatric orthopaedics; however, open reduction and internal fixation of displaced medial epicondyle fractures is generally indicated in the throwing athlete be-

cause of the importance of maintaining the origin of the anterior band of the ulnar collateral ligament. When instituted early, treatment of little leaguer's elbow is generally favorable.

Wrist and Hand Injuries

In most sports, the hand and wrist are exposed and thus are vulnerable to injury. Injury patterns are sport-specific, with macrotraumatic injury or repetitive microtraumatic injury depending on the demands placed on the upper extremity. Injuries are also age-specific, related to the stage of skeletal development. In several large studies of pediatric and adolescent athletic injuries, hand and wrist injury rates vary from 15% to 65% of all injuries in pediatric and adolescent athletes depending on the sport involved.[14] Injuries to the hand are particularly common during basketball, football, boxing, softball, skateboarding, and alpine skiing. Repetitive stress injuries, particularly of the wrist, are common in gymnasts.

Wrist Injuries

Wrist pain has become common in young, highly competitive gymnasts related to chronic, repetitive upper extremity weight bearing during growth and development. Distal radial physeal stress fracture may occur with radiographs showing widened physes (**Figure 5**), cystic changes, and distal metaphyseal beaking.[15] Treatment is rest with or without casting. Distal radial physeal arrest may occur, which may result in ulnar-carpal impaction and triangular fibrocartilage complex tears.

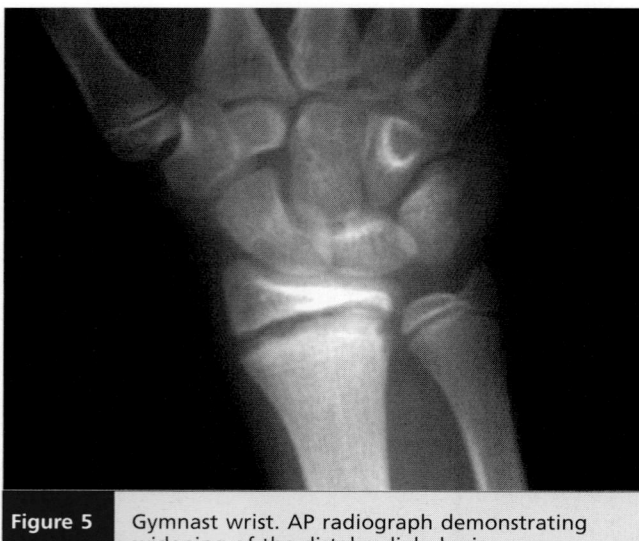

Figure 5 Gymnast wrist. AP radiograph demonstrating widening of the distal radial physis.

Stress fracture of the scaphoid waist also can be seen, particularly in competitive gymnasts. Initial radiographs are often negative, with follow-up radiographs revealing a stress fracture.

Ligamentous injuries of the wrist are unusual in children but are being seen with increased frequency in the adolescent athlete engaged in high-level sports. The volar intercarpal ligaments, particularly the radioscapholunate and radioscaphocapitate ligaments, are important stabilizers of the wrist. Patients present with wrist pain and limited motion. Radiographs may reveal widening of the scapholunate interval or alteration of the scapholunate angle (normal 30°–60°). Wrist arthrography, MRI, and arthroscopy can be used to further delineate the extent of ligamentous injury. Partial injuries are treated with immobilization. Acute complete ligamentous injuries are treated with ligament repair and Kirschner wire fixation. Chronic carpal instability is usually treated with limited carpal fusions or proximal row carpectomy, often with unpredictable results.

Hand Injuries

The thumb metacarpophalangeal joint is commonly injured, particularly during skiing. In adults and older adolescents, injury to the ulnar collateral ligament of the thumb metacarpophalangeal joint occurs ("gamekeeper's or skier's thumb"). In children and adolescents, physeal fracture at the base of the proximal phalanx is more common. The ulnar collateral ligament inserts onto the proximal phalangeal epiphysis, thus predisposing the patient to a Salter-Harris type III fracture, which may involve a large portion of the articular surface. Nondisplaced fractures and partial ulnar collateral ligament injuries are treated with 4 to 6 weeks of immobilization in a short arm-thumb spica cast. Displaced fractures are treated with open reduction and internal fixation.

The "jammed finger" is the most common joint injury in the pediatric and adolescent athlete's hand. Ax-

ial compressive forces applied to the end of the finger can result in proximal interphalangeal (PIP) joint hyperextension with subluxation or dislocation of the joint. This injury is common in sports that involve catching a ball, such as basketball or football. Reduction of the dislocated joint is accomplished by linear traction. Volar plate injury/avulsion or volar Salter-Harris type III fracture may be associated, but rarely requires fixation. Treatment involves a brief period of immobilization (using a dorsal aluminum/foam splint) followed by edema control (using an elastic bandage) and motion (buddy-taping to adjacent digit) to avoid stiffness and a fixed flexion deformity. Most athletes can return to sports (with buddy-taping) in 1 to 2 weeks; however, pain and swelling may persist for months.

Mallet finger is the most common injury occurring at the distal interphalangeal (DIP) joint, resulting from hyperflexion injury producing either extensor tendon (terminal tendon) rupture or Salter-Harris type III avulsion of the distal phalangeal epiphysis. The patient is unable to actively extend the DIP joint; however, there is full passive motion. Unless there is significant displacement of a substantial epiphyseal fragment, the DIP joint should be splinted with a dorsal splint in full extension for approximately 6 weeks. Terminal tendon repair may be necessary if an extensor lag persists after 10 weeks, considered an unusual occurrence.

Hip and Pelvis Injuries

Apophyseal avulsion injuries are common among skeletally immature athletes because of the inherent weakness of the open apophysis.[16] Avulsion fractures result from indirect trauma caused by sudden, violent, or unbalanced muscle contraction and are most commonly associated with rapid acceleration and deceleration and jumping. Although avulsion fractures can occur at any major muscle attachment, the three most common sites of avulsion injuries are the anterosuperior iliac spine (**Figure 6, A**), the anteroinferior iliac spine, and the ischial tuberosity (**Figure 6, B**), because of the violent contraction of the sartorius, rectus femoris, and hamstring muscles, respectively.[17] Avulsion fractures of the lesser trochanter can also occur (**Figure 6, C**).

Controversy exists regarding the optimal management of avulsion fractures, particularly those involving the ischial tuberosity. Typically, initial management will be conservative (rest and ice application, followed by protected weight bearing with crutches) until symptoms resolve. Thereafter, progression to light isometric stretching and full weight bearing is indicated. Patients may return to full sports participation once full strength and a pain-free range of motion is achieved. The need for surgical intervention is rare and typically is based on ongoing symptoms and the degree of bony displacement. As a general rule, large fragments displaced more than 2 cm may require surgical fixation; however, the optimal timing of surgical intervention remains unclear.

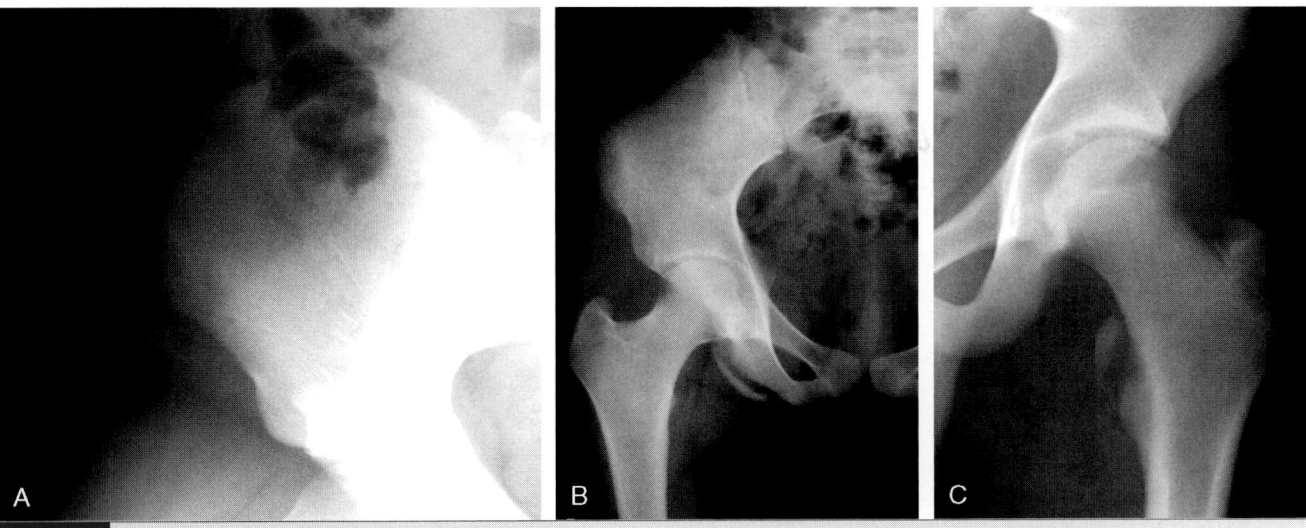

Figure 6 Apophyseal avulsion fractures of the pelvis. Anterosuperior iliac spine (**A**), ischium (**B**), and lesser trochanter (**C**).

Knee Injuries
Osgood-Schlatter Disease/Sinding-Larsen-Johansson Syndrome
OSD is the most common traction apophysitis and overuse injury to the knee in adolescent athletes. The condition develops from repetitive microtrauma to the tibial tubercle at the time of formation of the secondary ossification center.[18] Symptoms typically occur at the onset of the growth spurt in adolescent boys, usually age 13 to 14 years (range, age 10 to 15 years). The condition is activity related with higher prevalence rates in participants of jumping sports such as basketball or volleyball. As the participation of girls in sports has increased, so has their incidence of OSD, typically occurring at age 10 to 11 years. Symptoms include the insidious onset of a low-grade ache associated with activity that is localized to the area of the tibial tubercle. On examination, there is tenderness and sometimes swelling over the tubercle and adjacent patellar tendon, often with a bony or cartilaginous prominence. Radiographs may show a simple bony prominence of the tubercle with fragmentation of the ossific nucleus or a free bony fragment proximal to the tubercle in the patellar tendon. Exercises should be instituted to restore strength and flexibility to the extensor mechanism because OSD is often associated with a tight quadriceps that becomes weaker with the onset of pain. Activity should be limited, with 2 to 3 weeks of relative rest. If walking is uncomfortable, protective crutch ambulation with a knee immobilizer can be used while the patient initiates the stretching and strengthening program. If symptoms are severe, a cylinder cast for 2 to 4 weeks with crutch ambulation can be used. Symptoms may recur with resumption of sports, requiring a repeat cycle of rest, strengthening, stretching, and activity modification. However, the process is usually self-limited, stopping when growth stops and the tibial tubercle apophysis matures and fuses. Patients are more likely to have chronic symptoms after skeletal maturity if initial radiographs show fragmentation of the apophysis. Surgical excision may be necessary for patients in whom nonsurgical management has failed and who have free ossific nuclei over the tubercle or within the patellar tendon. Excision before skeletal maturity may be complicated by residual bony prominences, decreased range of motion, and recurvatum deformity.

Sinding-Larsen-Johansson syndrome is an overuse traction apophysitis at the proximal patellar tendon insertion onto the inferior patellar pole. This condition is similar to OSD, except that it occurs at the opposite end of the patellar tendon and is analogous to jumper's knee in the skeletally mature athlete. The condition is most common in adolescent boys age 9 to 13 years. On examination, there is tenderness over the distal pole of the patella and adjacent patellar tendon insertion. Frequently, the quadriceps will be tight but relatively weak. Lateral radiographs may show elongation of the distal patellar pole or fragmentation with ossicle formation. Fragmentation may also represent a patellar sleeve fracture or nonpathologic multicentric centers of ossification, found in 2% to 5% of normal adolescents. A radiograph of the opposite knee is helpful for differentiation. Treatment of this condition is similar to that of OSD, and includes relative rest, cross-training, and quadriceps strengthening and stretching. Symptoms are usually self-limited. If symptoms are severe, immobilization can be used to attain some healing before beginning muscle rehabilitation.

Patellofemoral Disorders
Patellofemoral dysfunction is common in the pediatric and adolescent athlete and includes a range of conditions including patellofemoral dysplasia, patellofemoral pain, and patellofemoral instability. Anterior knee pain and patellofemoral instability can be chronic, frustrating conditions for both the patient and the clinician;

6: Pediatrics

however, they can be treated successfully through an understanding of risk factors and patellofemoral biomechanics, a careful physical examination and accurate diagnosis, and a rational treatment plan.

The etiology of patellofemoral disorders is often multifactorial. Patellofemoral dysplasia may have genetic or developmental etiology. Joint laxity and connective tissue disorders may predispose to instability. Dysplasia of the patellofemoral joint, including hypoplasia of the trochlear groove, may also predispose to dysfunction. Rapid growth in adolescents may lead to imbalances around the patellofemoral articulation. The thicker and less compliant vastus lateralis and iliotibial band may exert a relatively unbalanced, laterally directed force. Quadriceps tightness may also lead to patella alta. Because the reaction forces across the patellofemoral joint are so high, the resultant changes in patellar tracking may contribute to the onset of anterior pain and instability. The onset of symptoms may be from repetitive overuse or from direct trauma.

Patients with patellofemoral pain typically report poorly localized anterior knee pain, which is often correlated with activity or positioning. The pain is usually of a dull, achy nature without mechanical symptoms. The pain may worsen with jumping and climbing activities or may be present with prolonged sitting. Patients with patellofemoral instability may report frank dislocation or subtle subluxation, depending on the magnitude of instability, or giving way. The history should include previous treatment, activity limitations, and the status of the contralateral knee. On examination, patellofemoral tracking, tilt, translation, crepitus, apprehension, and grind testing should be performed. In addition to physical examination of the patellofemoral joint, assessment should include gait evaluation, lower-extremity alignment, Q angle, hip examination, foot examination, knee stability, generalized ligamentous laxity, and knee range of motion. Routine four-view radiographic images of the knee (AP, lateral, tunnel, and skyline views) should be obtained in the pediatric patient with unilateral symptoms, significant initial symptoms, or symptoms unresponsive to management. Osteochondral fracture of the patella may be appreciated on radiographs; however, a substantial number of chondral or osteochondral fractures are undetected by plain radiography. A multitude of radiographic measurements of the patellofemoral relationship exist, including assessments of patellofemoral dysplasia, congruence, tilt, subluxation, and patellar height. CT may be of additional benefit in assessing patellofemoral anatomy. MRI may be helpful to detect associated chondral injuries and injury to the medial patellofemoral ligament.

The mainstay of treatment of patellofemoral pain is nonsurgical.[19] Exercises should be prescribed to stretch the iliotibial band and mobilize the patella, although the efficacy of physical therapy is unproven.[20] Medial quadriceps strengthening should be done by progressive resistive exercises. Ability to straight leg raise 12 lb for 3 sets of 10 repetitions correlates with the resolution of symptoms in most patients. Short-arc (less than 40°) exercises may benefit the tracking mechanism but should be avoided if they are painful. Children should be encouraged to refrain from activities that produce high patellofemoral compressive forces such as running, jumping, climbing, squatting, and other long-arc knee extension or hyperflexion activities. Although the scientific basis remains conjectural, neoprene elastic braces with a patella cutout may provide physical or psychological comfort. In addition, patellar taping, using the technique of McConnell, can be taught to the patient. Foot orthotics may also be of some use for minor lower-extremity malalignments. Most patients with patellofemoral pain can be successfully treated with nonsurgical treatment; however, supervised therapy for up to 6 months may sometimes be necessary. If symptoms recur, return to physical therapy usually results in resolution. In patients who are not responding to treatment, chronic regional pain syndrome should be considered. In recalcitrant cases, surgery may be considered. Lateral retinacular release has been widely used for the surgical treatment of patellofemoral pain; however, results are unpredictable. Patellofemoral realignment procedures, such as medial plication and vastus medialis advancement, may be considered if there is patellofemoral malalignment.

Management of patellofemoral instability is based on the magnitude of instability, frequency of instability, presence of associated injuries, and patellofemoral alignment.[21] Management of the acute traumatic patellofemoral dislocation is controversial. Some have advocated initial surgical management to repair the medial patellofemoral ligament to reduce the risk of recurrent instability. Others have advocated nonsurgical treatment, reserving surgical treatment for those who progress to subsequent instability.[22] Chondral or osteochondral loose bodies may occur in up to 40% of traumatic patellofemoral dislocations. In these patients, initial surgical management is indicated. Patients with atraumatic patellofemoral instability typically have subluxation episodes with underlying risk factors including ligamentous laxity and patellofemoral malalignment. Nonsurgical treatment is usually recommended in these patients. Nonsurgical treatment of patellofemoral instability consists of rehabilitation, patellofemoral bracing, and correction of malalignment such as pronation and pes planovalgus. Rehabilitation is focused on stretching of lateral structures, patellar mobilization, and strengthening of the medial quadriceps. Surgical treatment of patellofemoral instability includes proximal and distal realignment procedures. Proximally, lateral release, medial plication, vastus medialis advancement, and medial patellofemoral ligament repair or reconstruction may be performed. Distally, tibial tubercle metallization or anteromedialization osteotomy may be performed. In skeletally immature patients, tibial tubercle osteotomy is contraindicated because of the risk of growth disturbance of the apophysis with resultant recurvatum deformity. In these patients, semitendinosus transfer (Galeazzi procedure) or patellar tendon hemitransfer (Roux-Goldthwaite procedure) may be performed.

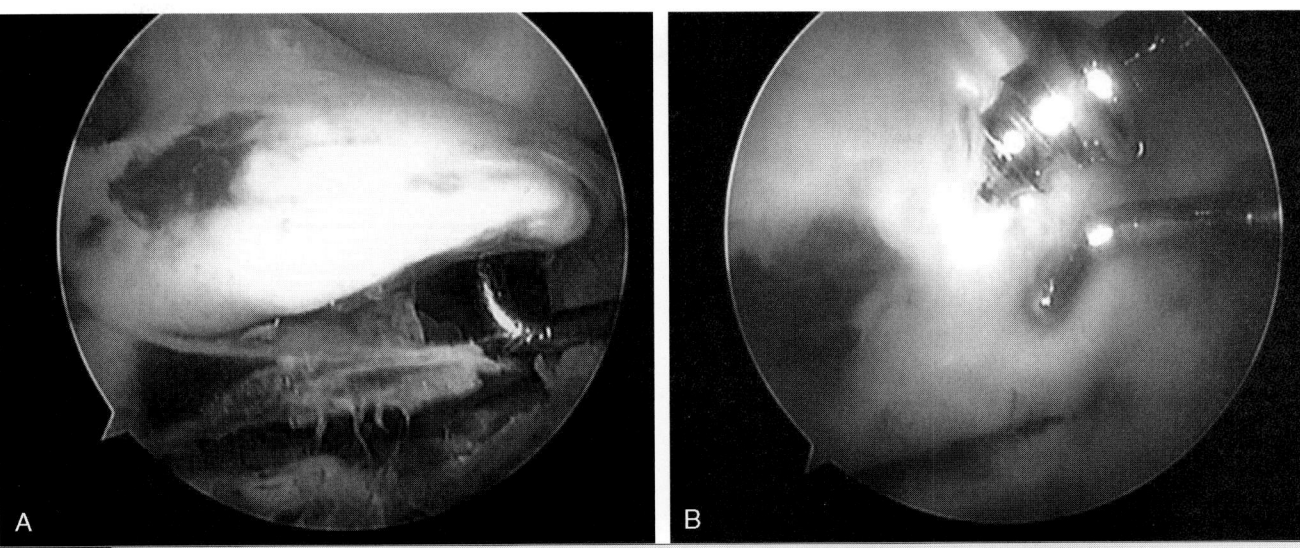

Figure 7 Epiphyseal cannulated screw fixation of a tibial spine fracture. **A,** Displaced fracture. **B,** Screw fixation.

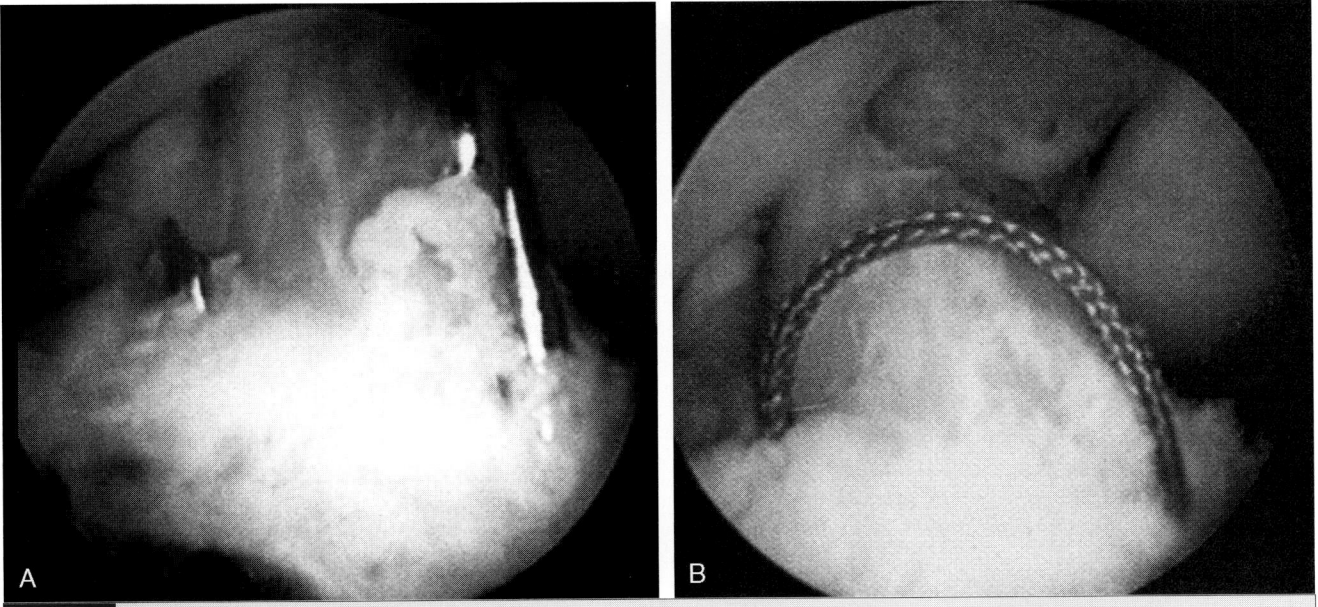

Figure 8 Suture fixation of a tibial spine fracture. **A,** Guide wires brought through the tibial spine fragment. **B,** Suture fixation.

Tibial Spine Fracture

Tibial spine fracture results from avulsion of the intercondylar tibial eminence from the tibia. Classification typically follows that described by Myers and McKeever:[23] nondisplaced (type 1), partially displaced (type 2), completely displaced (type 3). Type 1 fractures are commonly treated nonsurgically with immobilization via casting. Type 2 and 3 fractures can be treated with closed reduction in knee extension. Arthroscopic or open reduction and internal fixation is required for those fractures that do not reduce. Meniscal entrapment under the tibial spine fragment is not uncommon in type 3 fractures. Internal fixation can be performed with cannulated screws (**Figure 7**), suture (**Figure 8**), wires, or bioabsorbable fixation. Early motion is required to avoid the complication of arthrofibrosis. Even after anatomic reduction and internal fixation, persistent laxity of the knee may persist because of plastic deformation of the ACL.[24]

Meniscal Tears

The exact incidence of meniscal injuries in children and adolescents is unknown. Meniscal injuries are rare in children younger than 10 years, unless associated with

6: Pediatrics

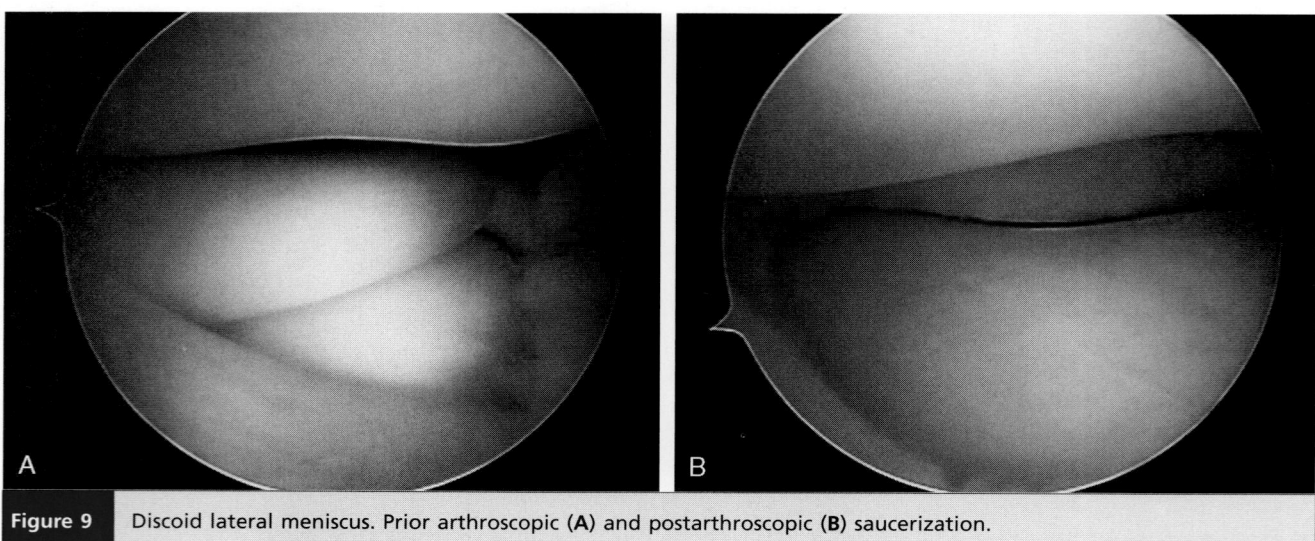

Figure 9 Discoid lateral meniscus. Prior arthroscopic (**A**) and postarthroscopic (**B**) saucerization.

a discoid meniscus. The incidence of meniscal as well as other intra-articular disorders increases with age. Meniscal injury patterns in children differ from those in adults.[25] It is estimated that longitudinal tears comprise 50% to 90% of meniscal tears in children and adolescents. Bucket-handle displaced tears are not uncommon. Also in these age groups, meniscal injuries are commonly associated with ACL injuries.

Some small, nondisplaced meniscal tears in the outer vascular region of the meniscus may heal or may become asymptomatic. Nonsurgical treatment usually consists of rehabilitation of the injured knee while avoiding pivoting and sports activity until symptoms resolve. However, most meniscal tears in pediatric patients are larger and require surgical treatment. In children and adolescents, meniscal repair should be attempted instead of partial meniscectomy for middle third tears because of greater healing potential in this age group, the long life span of these patients, the poor results of total and near-total meniscectomy, and the lack of longer-term results of partial meniscectomy.[25]

Discoid Lateral Meniscus

The true incidence of discoid lateral meniscus is unknown, as many children may remain asymptomatic. Very few actually present with a true snapping knee. Discoid morphology almost exclusively occurs within the lateral meniscus, but medial discoid menisci have also been reported. In addition, the incidence of bilateral abnormality has been reported to be as high as 20%.[26] The clinical presentation of a discoid lateral meniscus can be highly variable. Symptoms are often related to the type of discoid morphology present, peripheral stability of the meniscus, and the presence or absence of an associated meniscal tear.[27] Discoid lateral meniscus has been classified by the Watanabe classification based on morphology and stability, with type I being completely discoid, type II being partially discoid, and type III being a hypermobile variant of any morphology that lacks meniscotibial ligaments.[25]

Several treatment options exist for discoid lateral meniscus. For asymptomatic discoid lateral menisci, even if found incidentally on arthroscopy, conservative treatment is indicated. For stable, complete, or incomplete discoid menisci, partial meniscectomy or saucerization is the treatment of choice (**Figure 9**). If meniscal instability with detachment also exists, meniscal repair can also be performed. Traditionally, complete meniscectomy via open or arthroscopic means was suggested for such lesions. However, the long-term results of complete meniscectomy and near-total meniscectomy in children are poor with early degenerative changes. Although there may be a rare instance in which salvage of a discoid meniscus may seem unobtainable, better arthroscopic technology and techniques have made meniscal preservation the ideal treatment through saucerization and repair. Postoperatively, protected motion and weight bearing followed by progressive mobilization and rehabilitation is necessary. This plan of action may be challenging in younger children who are unable to ambulate effectively with crutches or comply with motion and weight-bearing restrictions.

Osteochondritis Dissecans

OCD is a relatively common cause of knee pain and dysfunction in the child and adolescent. Notch radiographs and MRI are useful in identifying and staging the OCD lesion (**Figure 10**). OCD is an acquired condition affecting subchondral bone that manifests as a pathologic spectrum of conditions, including softening of the overlying articular cartilage with an intact articular surface, early articular cartilage separation, partial detachment of an articular lesion, and osteochondral separation with loose bodies.[28] The etiology of OCD remains speculative; however, repetitive microtrauma is a common association. OCD of the knee has been classified based on anatomic location, surgical appearance, scintigraphic findings, and age. OCD of the knee is often subcategorized into a juvenile form and an adult form depending on the status of the distal femoral phy-

6: Pediatrics

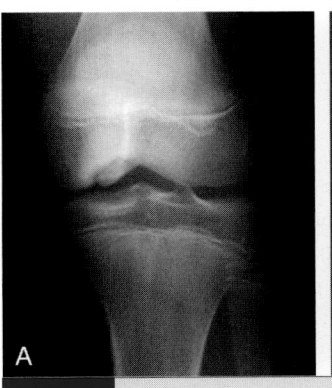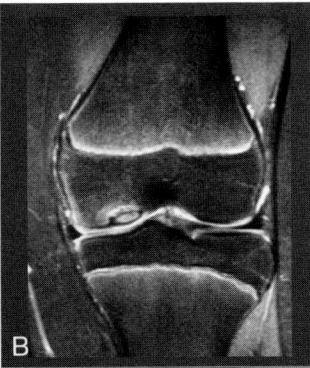

Figure 10 OCD of the knee. **A,** AP radiograph. **B,** Corresponding coronal MRI scan.

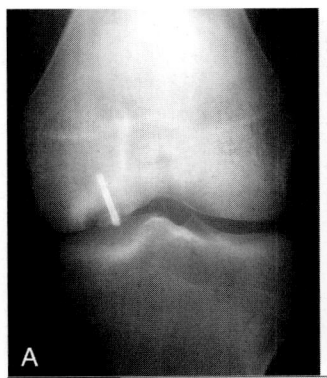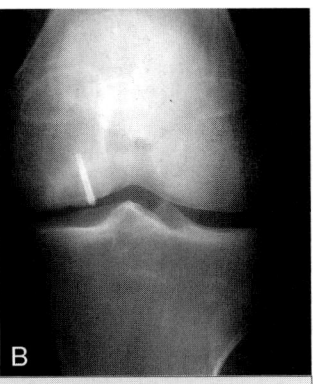

Figure 11 Fixation of unstable OCD lesion of the knee. **A,** Immediate postoperative AP radiograph, and **B,** 3-month postoperative radiograph demonstrating lesion healing.

sis. In most instances, adult OCD is believed to be the persistence of a juvenile OCD lesion that did not heal, although de novo adult OCD lesions have been described. Juvenile OCD has a much better prognosis than adult OCD, with more than 50% of patients demonstrating healing within 6 to 18 months of nonsurgical treatment. In patients with adult OCD, healing is more likely with surgical intervention. Adult OCD and juvenile OCD that does not heal have potential for later sequelae including osteoarthritis.

The treatment of OCD of the knee depends on the stage of the lesion and the physiologic stage of the patient.[28] Stable lesions in patients with open growth plates are typically treated nonsurgically, with cessation of impact activities. Healing rates are estimated at 40% to 70%. Lesions in atypical locations such as the lateral femoral condyle or patellofemoral articulation have lower healing rates. Surgical treatment is indicated for stable lesions that have undergone unsuccessful nonsurgical treatment or for unstable lesions. Surgical options include in situ drilling, fixation, fragment removal, and chondral resurfacing. Retrograde transarticular drilling and anterograde epiphyseal drilling have high healing rates for stable lesions.[29] Internal fixation for unstable lesions is relatively successful in juvenile OCD, with healing rates of 85% (**Figure 11**). Removal of large fragments typically is associated with a poor long-term prognosis. The results of chondral resurfacing techniques have not been well studied for skeletally immature patients.

ACL Injury

Intrasubstance ACL injuries in children and adolescents were once considered rare, with tibial eminence avulsion fractures considered the pediatric ACL injury equivalent. However, intrasubstance ACL injuries in children and adolescents are occurring with increased frequency and have received increased attention. ACL injury has been reported in 10% to 65% of pediatric knees with acute traumatic hemarthroses.[30]

Management of these injuries is controversial. Nonreconstructive treatment of complete tears typically results in recurrent functional instability with risk of in-

jury to meniscal and articular cartilage. Conventional adult ACL reconstruction techniques place the patient at risk for potential iatrogenic growth disturbance because of physeal violation. Growth disturbances after ACL reconstruction in skeletally immature patients have been reported.[31] Surgical techniques to address ACL insufficiency in skeletally immature patients include primary repair, extra-articular tenodesis, transphyseal reconstruction, partial transphyseal reconstruction, and physeal-sparing reconstruction. Primary ligament repair and extra-articular tenodesis alone have had poor results in children and adolescents, similar to adults. Transphyseal reconstructions with tunnels that violate both the distal femoral and proximal tibial physes have been performed with hamstring autograft, patellar tendon autograft, and allograft tissue (**Figure 12**). Partial transphyseal reconstructions violate only one physis with a tunnel through the proximal tibial physis and over-the-top positioning on the femur or a tunnel through the distal femoral physis with an epiphyseal tunnel in the tibia. A variety of physeal-sparing reconstructions have been described to avoid tunnels across either the distal femoral or proximal tibial physis[32] (**Figure 13**).

Management of ACL injuries in skeletally immature patients is based on physiologic age (**Figure 14**). In prepubescent patients, nonsurgical treatment may be considered initially to delay surgery if there is no gross instability or a repairable meniscus tear. Consideration should be given to physeal-sparing reconstruction in these young patients because of the amount of growth remaining.[32] In adolescent pubescent patients with significant growth remaining, surgical treatment is typically advocated and transphyseal techniques with a soft-tissue graft and metaphyseal fixation appear safe and effective.

Foot and Ankle Injuries

Talus OCD

OCD in the ankle typically affects the talus. The most common symptoms and findings include tenderness over

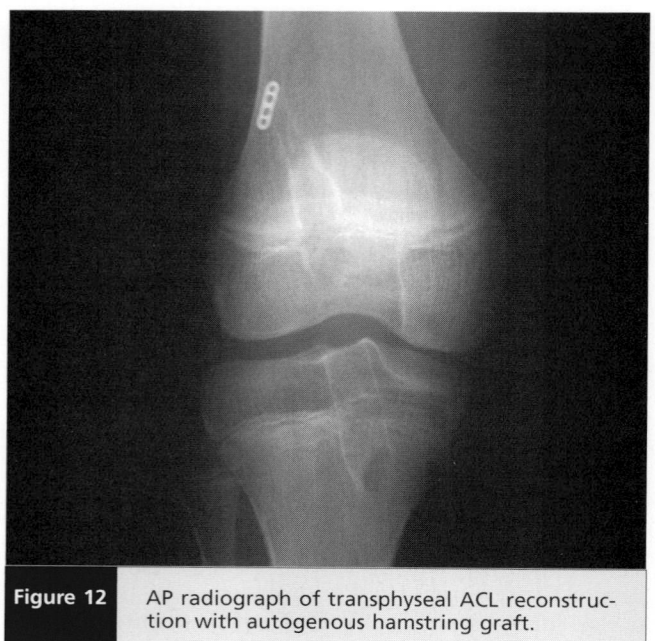

Figure 12 AP radiograph of transphyseal ACL reconstruction with autogenous hamstring graft.

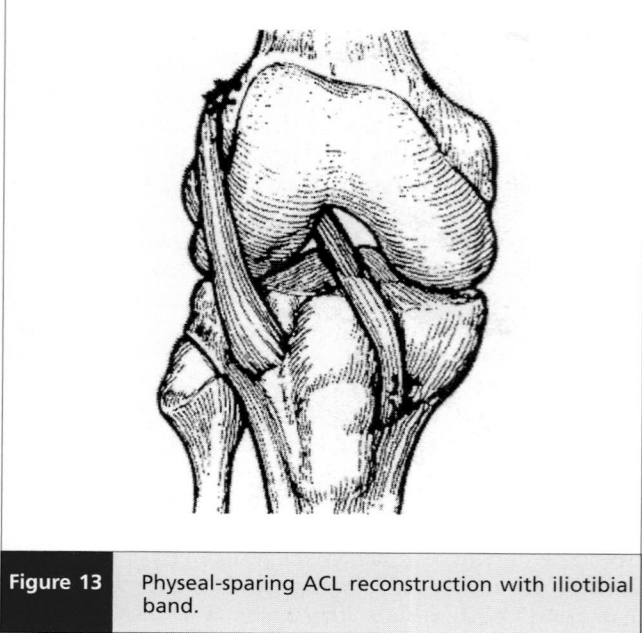

Figure 13 Physeal-sparing ACL reconstruction with iliotibial band.

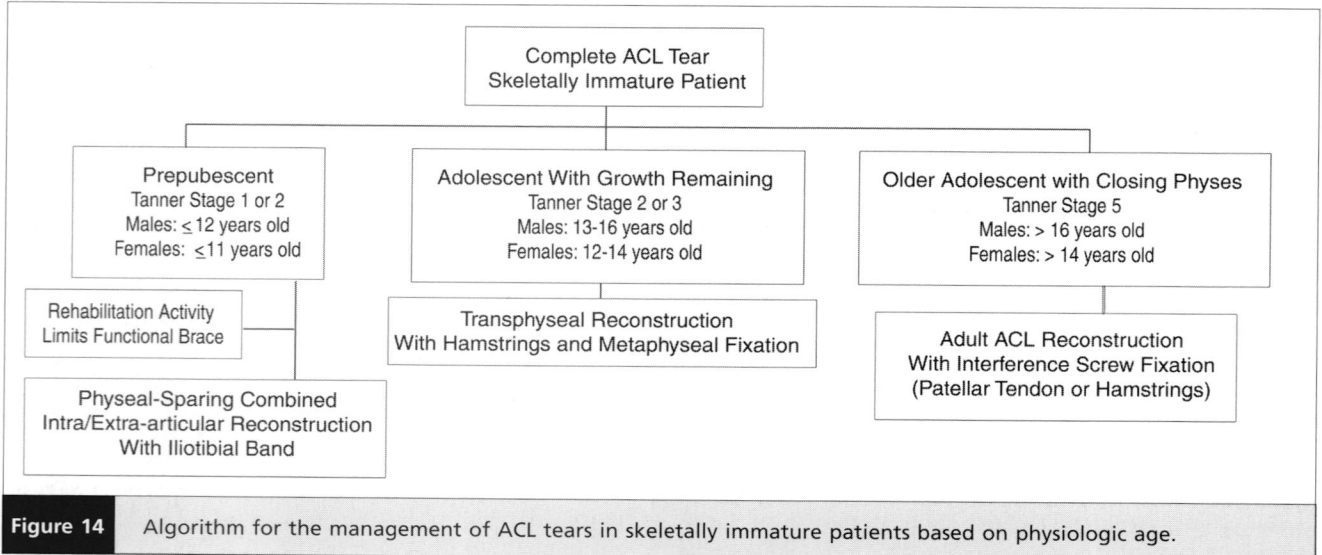

Figure 14 Algorithm for the management of ACL tears in skeletally immature patients based on physiologic age.

the talus, reduced ankle motion, and decreased range of motion.[33] Nonsurgical treatment is recommended initially, unless the lesion is unstable. Surgical treatment is indicated for stable lesions that have undergone unsuccessful nonsurgical treatment and for unstable lesions. Surgical methods include drilling, fixation, or chondral resurfacing techniques. Arthroscopic ankle surgery is usually performed. Medial malleolar osteotomy for access to posteromedial lesions may be contraindicated by open medial malleolar physes.

Sever's Disease
Apophysitis of the calcaneal tuberosity is a frequent cause of heel pain in the pediatric athlete.[33] This condi-

tion typically occurs in running and jumping athletes. Clinically there is pain with palpation of the calcaneal tuberosity. Treatment usually involves rest from impact activity, heel cord stretching, and a heel cup.

Tarsal Coalition
Tarsal coalition may present as recurrent ankle sprains in an adolescent athlete with a rigid flatfoot deformity.[33] The most common coalitions are talocalcaneal coalition and calcaneonavicular coalition. Nonsurgical treatment consists of stretching and use of orthotic devices. Surgical treatment is indicated when nonsurgical treatment has failed. Calcaneonavicular coalition is usually treated with excision. Talocalcaneal coalition

may be treated with excision or fusion depending on the extent of coalition.

Spine

Back pain and injuries to the thoracolumbar spine are common in the school-age athlete. Spine-related conditions account for almost 10% of athletes' medical conditions and approximately 75% of high-performance athletes have some sort of back pain.[34] Particular sports that require repetitive or high-velocity twisting or bending such as gymnastics, dancing, football, and rowing have a predilection for back injuries. With the increasing number of young athletes pursuing rigorous training and intense competition in some of these sports at an early age, the prevalence of back pain in the school-age athlete may be expected to increase. In the school-age athlete with back pain, a specific diagnosis such as spondylolysis, spondylolisthesis, apophysitis, tumor, or infection should be sought. Macrotrauma and microtrauma must be distinguished. The growing athlete has several unique risk factors relevant to the adolescent spine. The growth cartilage of the vertebral end plates and apophyses are more susceptible to injury.

Spondylolysis

Mechanical injury to the pars interarticularis is a common source of discomfort in young athletes involved in competitive sports. Approximately 50% of patients with spondylolysis relate the onset of symptoms to competitive sports training. In a study of 177 male high school and college athletes, approximately 21% showed radiographic evidence of spondylolysis.[34] The average age of diagnosis in the symptomatic school-age athletic population is 15 to 16 years old. Approximately 85% of spondylolysis occurs at the L5 level.

It is postulated that spondylolysis and isthmic spondylolisthesis represent acquired fatigue fractures as a result of repeated microtrauma. Shear stresses of 400 to 600 N caused by hyperextension, flexion, and torsion are concentrated across the pars interarticularis, an area calculated to be only 0.75 cm² at L5. Repetitive hyperextension loading sports such as gymnastics, blocking in football, hurdling, ballet dancing, volleyball spiking, competitive diving, tennis serving, weight lifting, rowing, and swimming turns all have been associated with spondylolysis. Pars defects occur four times more frequently in young female gymnasts than the general female population. Anatomic variations such as transitional vertebrae, spina bifida occulta, and an elongated pars may be seen.

It is essential to make the diagnosis and initiate protective treatment as early as possible. The onset of symptoms typically coincides with the adolescent growth spurt and the onset of strenuous, repetitive training. In athletes, symptoms are usually insidious, aching low back pain that does not radiate. Initially, the pain is elicited by strenuous activity; however, the pain often becomes progressively more severe and is associated with activities of daily living. Physical examination may demonstrate paraspinal tenderness, limited motion, hyperlordosis, and hamstring tightness. Typically, pain can be reproduced with hyperextension and occasionally can be localized with ipsilateral hyperextension. Initial diagnostic work-up includes radiographs of the lumbosacral spine. If spondylolysis is suspected but not demonstrated on plain films, single photon emission CT (SPECT) scanning is particularly sensitive in detecting pars defects. Alternatively, oblique linear tomography or CT scanning may show the established pars lesion.

The type of treatment is dependent on the athlete's age, type of sport activity, severity of symptoms, and risk of progression. Risk factors for slip progression include slip percentage of more than 50%, high slip angle, spina bifida, convex sacral contour, ligamentous laxity, and the adolescent age group.[34] The asymptomatic individual should be periodically followed clinically and radiographically if there are risk factors for progression. The symptomatic adolescent athlete can initially be treated with restriction of athletic activity and an abdominal/back strengthening program. Use of a rigid polypropylene lumbosacral brace constructed with 0° of lumbar flexion (antilordosis) may promote healing of the pars defect, although its use is controversial.[35] Bracing regimens typically consist of full-time brace use and activity restriction, followed by some limitations of activity and part-time brace use, followed by a gradual return to activity. Patients who fail to improve after nonsurgical treatment may require surgery; however, this is uncommon. Management of spondylolisthesis in the adolescent athlete depends on the degree of slippage and the severity of symptoms. Fortunately, it is rare to see progressive listhesis in the adolescent-onset stress fracture pars defect seen in young athletes. The asymptomatic athlete with less than 25% spondylolisthesis should be allowed to participate in all sports, including contact sports, while being followed periodically for progression. Asymptomatic athletes with 25% to 50% slippage fall into a controversial category. Observation for progression has been advocated, along with avoidance of contact sports, or surgical management if the patient wishes to return to competitive sports. A slip of more than 50% in the immature spine should be stabilized, even in an asymptomatic individual, because of the high risk of progression.

Mechanical Back Pain

Mechanical back pain secondary to acute or chronic musculoligamentous strains and sprains is rare in the prepubertal athlete and should be a diagnosis of exclusion in children with low back pain. Such back pain is believed to represent overuse or stretch injuries of the soft tissues, including the muscle-tendon unit, ligaments, joint capsules, and facets. This back pain is more commonly seen in the older age group and may be related to the adolescent growth spurt. Young athletes with mechanical back pain may be predisposed to injury because of weak abdominal musculature, tight lumbodorsal fascia, tight hamstrings, limited lumbar motion, and poor training technique. The pain is often nondescript, exac-

6: Pediatrics

erbated by activity, and relieved by rest. Red flags to suggest a more serious etiology of back pain such as tumor or infection include night pain, neurologic symptoms, or fever and chills. Physical examination in patients with mechanical back pain reveals paraspinal muscle tenderness, decreased flexibility, and limited spinal motion. Radiographs are normal. Acutely, treatment consists of rest. Massage, nonsteroidal anti-inflammatory drugs, and phonophoresis may be helpful. Once the acute phase has resolved, a rehabilitation program consisting of posture control, abdominal strengthening, and flexibility is initiated. Return to sports activity is gradually allowed with resolution of pain and return of strength and flexibility. Proper technique, conditioning, and stretching are emphasized.

Annotated References

1. Faigenbaum AD: Strength training for children and adolescents. *Clin Sports Med* 2000;19:593-619.

2. Baquet G, van Praagh E, Berthoin S: Endurance training and aerobic fitness in young people. *Sports Med* 2003;33:1127-1143.

3. Climatic heat stress and the exercising child and adolescent. American Academy of Pediatrics. Committee on Sports Medicine and Fitness. *Pediatrics* 2000;106:158-159.

4. Pate RR, Trost SG, Levin S, Dowda M: Sports participation and health-related behaviors among US youth. *Arch Pediatr Adolesc Med* 2000;154:904-911.

5. Washington RL, Bernhardt DT, Gomez J, et al: Organized sports for children and preadolescents. *Pediatrics* 2001;107:1459-1462.

6. Rockwood C: Fractures of outer clavicle in children and adults. *J Bone Joint Surg Br* 1982;64:642-649.

7. Cahill BR, Tullos HS, Fain RH: Little league shoulder: Lesions of the proximal humeral epiphyseal plate. *J Sports Med* 1974;2:150-152.

8. Hovelius L: Anterior dislocation of the shoulder in teenagers and young adults: Five-year prognosis. *J Bone Joint Surg Am* 1987;69:393-399.

9. Bottoni CR, Wilckens JH, DeBerardino TM, et al: A prospective, randomized evaluation of arthroscopic stabilization versus nonoperative treatment in patients with acute, traumatic, first-time shoulder dislocations. *Am J Sports Med* 2002;30:576-580.

10. Itoi E, Hatakeyama Y, Kido T, et al: A new method of immobilization after traumatic anterior dislocation of the shoulder: A preliminary study. *J Shoulder Elbow Surg* 2003;12:413-415.

11. Bottoni CR, Smith EL, Berkowitz MJ, Towle RB, Moore JH: Arthroscopic versus open shoulder stabilization for recurrent anterior instability: A prospective randomized clinical trial. *Am J Sports Med* 2006;34:1730-1737.

In a clinical trial of 64 patients with recurrent anterior shoulder instability randomized to arthroscopic versus open stabilization, the authors found no difference in recurrence rates or functional outcome. Patients who underwent open stabilization lost more motion. These results suggest similar functional outcome and recurrence rate from contemporary arthroscopic stabilization.

12. Klingele KE, Kocher MS: Little league elbow: Valgus overload injury in the pediatric elbow. *Sports Med* 2002;32:1005-1015.

13. Lyman S, Fleisig GS, Andrews JR, Osinski ED: Effect of pitch type, pitch count, and pitching mechanics on risk of elbow and shoulder pain in youth baseball pitchers. *Am J Sports Med* 2002;30:463-468.

14. Kocher MS, Waters PM, Micheli LJ: Upper extremity injuries in the paediatric athlete. *Sports Med* 2000;30:117-135.

15. Roy S, Caine D, Singer KM: Stress changes of the distal radial epiphysis in young gymnasts: A report of twenty-one cases and a review of the literature. *Am J Sports Med* 1985;13:301-308.

16. Kocher MS, Tucker R: Pediatric athlete hip disorders. *Clin Sports Med* 2006;25:241-253.

This review article provides an overview of the common hip and pelvis injuries in the pediatric athlete, including soft-tissue injuries, apophyseal injuries, slipped capital femoral epiphysis, Legg-Calvé-Perthes disease, and internal derangements such as labral tears, loose bodies, and chondral injuries.

17. Rossi F, Dragoni S: Acute avulsion fractures of the pelvis in adolescent competitive athletes: Prevalence, location and sports distribution of 203 cases collected. *Skeletal Radiol* 2001;30:127-131.

18. Gholve PA, Scher DM, Khakharia S, Widmann RF, Green DW: Osgood Schlatter syndrome. *Curr Opin Pediatr* 2007;19:44-50.

This review article discusses the etiology, risk factors, nonsurgical treatment, and surgical treatment of Osgood-Schlatter syndrome.

19. Thabit G III, Micheli LJ: Patellofemoral pain in the pediatric patient. *Orthop Clin North Am* 1992;23:567-585.

20. Heintjes E, Berger MY, Bierma-Zeinstra SM, Bernsen RM, Verhaar JA, Koes BW: Exercise therapy for patellofemoral pain syndrome. *Cochrane Database Syst Rev* 2003;4:CD003472.

21. Hinton RY, Sharma KM: Acute and recurrent patellar instability in the young athlete. *Orthop Clin North Am* 2003;34:385-396.

22. Nikku R, Nietosvaara Y, Aalto K, Kallio PE: Operative treatment of primary patellar dislocation does not improve medium-term outcome: A 7-year follow-up report and risk analysis of 127 randomized patients. *Acta Orthop* 2005;76:699-704.

    The authors report the minimum 5-year results from their randomized clinical trial of nonsurgical treatment versus proximal realignment surgery in 127 patients. They found no difference in outcome between the treatment methods. In general, there was worse functional outcome for female patients, young patients, and dislocations with loose bodies, and contralateral patellar instability. These results do not support advocates of surgical management of initial patellar dislocations.

23. Meyers MH, McKeever FM: Fracture of the intercondylar eminence of the tibia. *J Bone Joint Surg Am* 1970; 52:1677-1684.

24. Kocher MS, Foreman ES, Micheli LJ: Laxity and functional outcome after arthroscopic reduction and internal fixation of displaced tibial spine fractures in children. *Arthroscopy* 2003;19:1085-1090.

25. Kocher MS, Klingele KE, Rassman S: Meniscal disorders: Normal, discoid, and cysts. *Orthop Clin North Am* 2003;34:329-340.

26. Mintzer CM, Richmond JC, Taylor J: Meniscal repair in the young athlete. *Am J Sports Med* 1998;26:630-633.

27. Klingele KE, Kocher MS, Hresko MT, Gerbino PG, Micheli LJ: Discoid lateral meniscus: Prevalence of peripheral rim instability. *J Pediatr Orthop* 2004;24:79-82.

    In this consecutive series of 112 pediatric patients (128 knees) who underwent arthroscopic evaluation and treatment of a discoid lateral meniscus, the authors found that 62.1% (n = 54) were complete discoid lateral menisci and 37.9% (n = 33) were incomplete discoid lateral menisci. An associated meniscal tear was present in 69.5% (n = 89) of all knees studied. Overall, 28.1% (n = 36) of discoid lateral menisci had peripheral rim instability: 47.2% (n = 17) were unstable at the anterior-third peripheral attachment, 11.1% (n = 4) at the middle-third peripheral attachment, and 38.9% (n = 14) at the posterior-third peripheral attachment. Peripheral rim instability was significantly more common in complete discoid lateral menisci (38.9% versus 18.2%; P = 0.043) and in younger patients (8.2 versus 10.7 years; P = 0.002). The authors suggest that the frequency of peripheral instability mandates a thorough assessment of meniscal stability at all peripheral attachments during the arthroscopic evaluation and treatment of discoid lat-

    eral meniscus, particularly in complete variants and in younger children.

28. Kocher MS, Tucker R, Ganley T, Flynn JM: Current concepts: Management of osteochondritis dissecans of the knee. *Am J Sports Med* 2006;34:1181-1191.

    This review article discusses the etiology, classification, nonsurgical treatment, and surgical treatment of OCD of the knee.

29. Kocher MS, Micheli LJ, Yaniv M, Zurakowski D, Ames A, Adrignolo A: Functional and radiographic outcome of juvenile osteochondritis dissecans of the knee treated with transarticular drilling. *Am J Sports Med* 2001;29: 562-566.

30. Stanitski CL, Harvell JC, Fu F: Observations on acute knee hemarthrosis in children and adolescents. *J Pediatr Orthop* 1993;13:506-510.

31. Kocher MS, Hawkins RJ, Saxon HS, Hovis WD: Management and complications of anterior cruciate ligament injuries in skeletally immature patients: A survey of The Herodicus Society and The ACL Study Group. *J Pediatr Orthop* 2002;22:452-457.

32. Kocher MS, Garg S, Micheli LJ: Physeal-sparing anterior cruciate ligament reconstruction in skeletally immature prepubescent children. *J Bone Joint Surg Am* 2005; 87:2371-2379.

    The authors describe a physeal-sparing, combined intra-articular and extra-articular reconstruction technique in prepubescent skeletally immature children. In 44 prepubescent patients who were in Tanner stage 1 or 2 (with a mean chronologic age of 10.3 years), the authors found excellent results with this technique with excellent functional outcome and no cases of growth disturbance. Two patients underwent a revision reconstruction for graft failure at 4.7 and 8.3 years postoperatively. The authors suggest that this technique may be preferable to transphyseal reconstruction in these very young patients, given the amount of growth remaining.

33. Chambers HG: Ankle and foot disorders in skeletally immature athletes. *Orthop Clin North Am* 2003;34: 445-459.

34. Sassmannshausen G, Smith BG: Back pain in the young athlete. *Clin Sports Med* 2002;21:121-132.

35. Micheli LJ, Hall JE, Miller ME: Use of modified Boston brace for back injuries in athletes. *Am J Sports Med* 1980;8:351-356.

6: Pediatrics

Chapter 63

Skeletal Dysplasias, Connective Tissue Diseases, and Other Genetic Disorders

Eric D. Shirley, MD   Michael C. Ain, MD

Introduction

Genetic and molecular biology research continues to advance knowledge of skeletal dysplasias, connective tissue diseases, and other genetic diseases with orthopaedic manifestations. The ability to recognize these manifestations continues to be of great importance for an orthopaedic surgeon, who may be the first physician able to make the diagnosis.

Skeletal Dysplasias

Skeletal dysplasias are a heterogeneous group of disorders caused by abnormalities in bone growth or cartilage. Most skeletal dysplasias result in body disproportion and short stature (defined as height more than 2 standard deviations below the population mean). Skeletal dysplasias can be classified by short limb or short trunk disproportion, location of the short segment, pattern of bone involvement (including spine and epiphyseal involvement), or specific gene defect. The evaluation includes a complete history, physical examination, and skeletal survey. A genetics consultation can clarify the diagnosis and assist in addressing associated medical conditions.[1] Prenatal diagnosis can be made if ultrasonography reveals skeletal shortening.

Disease-specific and condition-specific treatment focuses on preventing future limitations and addressing deformity and pain. The presurgical considerations include assessment of cervical instability in certain dysplasias as well as the anesthesia risks associated with oropharyngeal or laryngeal malformations.

The use of growth augmentation for patients with skeletal dysplasias remains controversial, and most patients with short stature do not believe augmentation is necessary. The possible indications include marked stature deficit, reduced function of the upper or lower limbs, the patient's subjective negative judgment of his or her own stature, and the negative impact of short stature on the patient's personality, behavior, and social relations. Lower extremity limb lengthening can be per-

formed on the femur, tibia, or both. Humeral lengthening is also required if lower extremity lengthening or spinal fusion to the sacrum would worsen the disproportion or impede activities of daily living and personal hygiene.[2] Alternatively, a limited amount of growth augmentation can be achieved through growth hormone therapy.[3]

Achondroplasia and Related Disorders

Mutations in the fibroblast growth factor receptor-3 (*FGFR-3*) gene can result in several skeletal dysplasias of different severity, including achondroplasia, hypochondroplasia, and thanatophoric dysplasia.

Achondroplasia

Achondroplasia, the most common skeletal dysplasia, has an incidence of 1 in 30,000 persons. It is characterized by rhizomelic shortening. The inheritance pattern is autosomal dominant, although the condition results from sporadic mutations in more than 90% of patients. A single amino acid substitution results in stabilization of the FGFR protein, with accumulation on the cell surface and uncontrolled activation on the receptor. This sustained FGFR activity results in growth retardation in the proliferative zone of the physis. The risk of having a child with achondroplasia is associated with increased paternal age.

Achondroplasia is characterized by normal trunk length, frontal bossing, and trident hands. The condition is diagnosed via prenatal ultrasonography or at birth. Foramen magnum and upper cervical stenosis can occur during the first 2 years of life. Stenosis may result in cervicomedullary cord compression, which is manifested by hypotonia, delayed development, weakness, and apnea; the diagnosis is confirmed through a sleep study and MRI (**Figure 1**). Surgical decompression alleviates the stenosis to decompress the brain stem and spinal cord.

Other spinal manifestations include thoracolumbar kyphosis and spinal stenosis. Thoracolumbar kyphosis can occur when the child begins to sit, and the risk of kyphosis can be decreased by not forcing or encouraging

6: Pediatrics

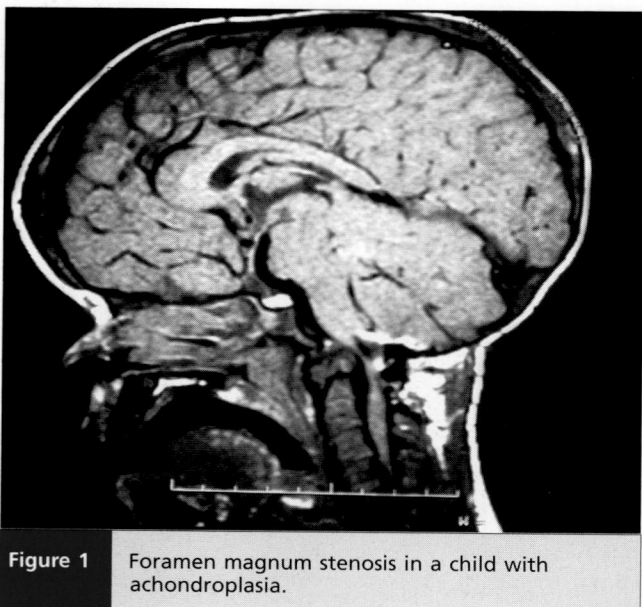

Figure 1 Foramen magnum stenosis in a child with achondroplasia.

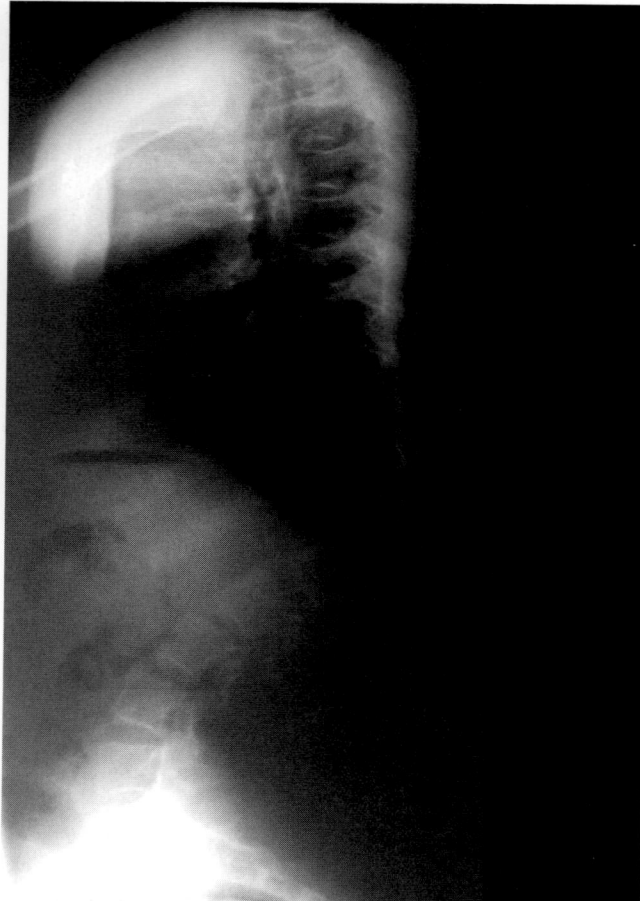

Figure 2 Lateral radiograph showing thoracolumbar kyphosis in a child with achondroplasia.

the child to sit upright until he or she is ready to do so. The kyphosis typically resolves when the child begins to walk, at 18 to 24 months of age. Bracing is indicated for progressive kyphosis with apical wedging (**Figure 2**). Spinal fusion is indicated if severe kyphosis persists despite bracing, but the specific indications, including the child's age and the degree of kyphosis, remain unclear.[4]

The achondroplastic spine is characterized by cranial-to-caudal narrowing of the lumbar interpedicular distance and shortened pedicles.[5] Lumbar spinal stenosis usually occurs in the adult patient, but it can begin as early as the second decade of life. Symptomatic stenosis requires wide decompression to avoid an early recurrence. Because wide decompression in the skeletally immature patient with achondroplasia has been associated with early postlaminectomy kyphosis, concurrent spinal fusion is recommended.[6]

Lower extremity malalignment typically is characterized by genu varum.[7] The cause of genu varum in patients with achondroplasia is a controversial topic.[8] Surgical treatment is indicated for symptoms, including pain or fibular thrust, or progressive deformities. Osteotomies are performed at the site of the deformity. Associated tibial torsion should be corrected concurrently.

Other orthopaedic clinical characteristics of achondroplasia include flexion contractures of the elbows, subluxation of the radial heads, and ligamentous laxity. The nonorthopaedic manifestations include recurrent otitis media, obstructive sleep apnea, decreased respiratory drive, decreased pulmonary function, hydrocephalus, and lifetime difficulty with weight control.

Hypochondroplasia and Thanatophoric Dysplasia
Hypochondroplasia and thanatophoric dysplasia are secondary to a *FGFR-3* mutation. The inheritance pattern of hypochondroplasia is autosomal dominant, and

its clinical characteristics are similar to, but milder than, those of achondroplasia. More phenotypic heterogeneity is seen in hypochondroplasia, probably because of mutations arising in different portions of the *FGFR-3* gene. The manifestations include short stature, lumbar spinal stenosis, and genu varum. The characteristics of thanatophoric dysplasia include rhizomelic shortening, platyspondyly, a protuberant abdomen, and a small thoracic cavity. Thanatophoric dysplasia is severe and almost always fatal before the patient reaches 2 years of age.

Disorders Related to Type II Collagen Abnormalities
These disorders include spondyloepiphyseal dysplasia (SED) congenita, SED tarda, and Kniest dysplasia.

SED Congenita and SED Tarda
SED congenita is caused by mutations in the collagen type II α-1 chain (*COL2A1*), which encodes type II collagen. The inheritance pattern is autosomal dominant, but most patients acquire the disease through new mutations. This extremely rare dysplasia is characterized by short stature, short trunk, short limbs, and abnor-

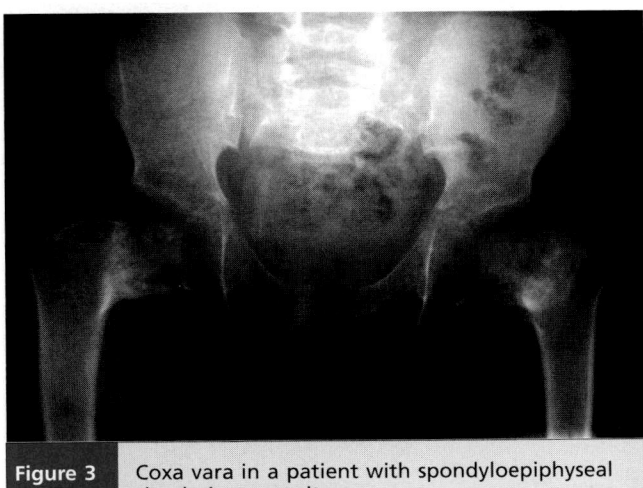

Figure 3 Coxa vara in a patient with spondyloepiphyseal dysplasia congenita.

mal formation of the long bone epiphyses, with variable metaphyseal involvement.

Odontoid hypoplasia or ligamentous laxity can result in atlantoaxial instability, which can progress to cervical myelopathy.[5] Instability should be evaluated during infancy and continuously monitored. Symptomatic or excessive instability requires fusion with decompression if stenosis is present.

Lower extremity malalignment can be caused by coxa vara, genu valgum, or distal tibia valgus (Figure 3). The evaluation of coxa vara is complicated by delayed ossification of the femoral capital epiphysis. Abnormal epiphyseal development typically results in early degenerative joint disease, which may require total joint arthroplasty during young adulthood. Other manifestations include retinal detachment, severe myopia, and sensorineural hearing loss.

SED tarda is milder than SED congenita and may not be diagnosed until school age, unlike SED congenital, which may be diagnosed at birth. SED tarda can result from a mutation in type II collagen, but the mechanism has not been shown. Several patterns of transmission have been reported, of which X-linked transmission is the most common. The manifestations include odontoid hypoplasia, scoliosis, and osteoarthritis.

Kniest Dysplasia
Kniest dysplasia, an autosomal dominant disorder caused by mutations in the *COL2A1* gene, is characterized by a trunk that is disproportionately shorter than the limbs and dumbbell-shaped long bones with broad metaphyses and irregular dysplastic epiphyses (Figure 4). The other manifestations include odontoid hypoplasia, kyphosis, mild scoliosis, joint contractures, and limb malalignment.[5] Degenerative arthritis can develop as early as the second decade of life. Other characteristics include midface hypoplasia, myopia, retinal detachment, and deafness.

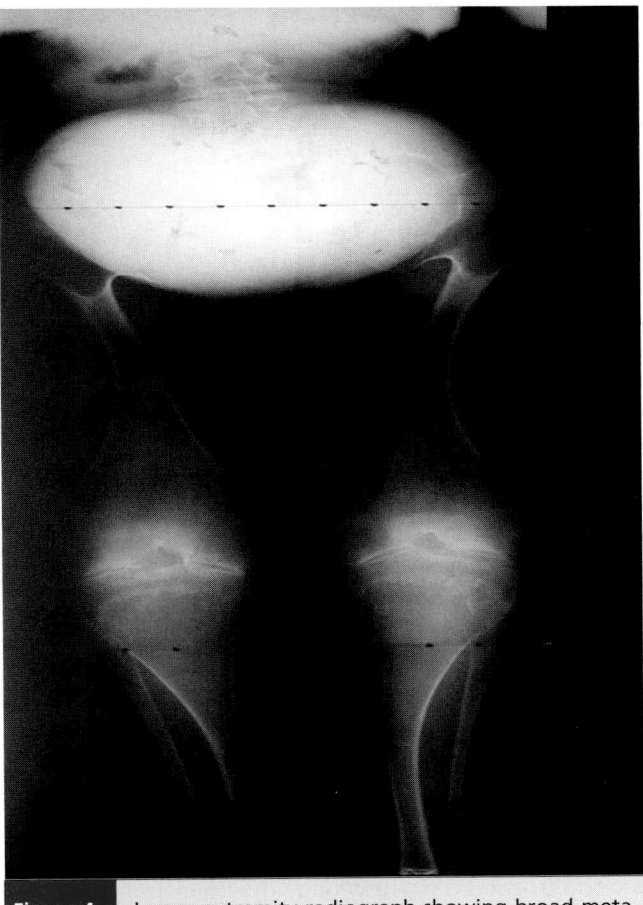

Figure 4 Lower extremity radiograph showing broad metaphyses in a patient with Kniest dysplasia.

Disorders Caused by Abnormalities in Genes Important in Normal Skeletal Development
This spectrum of disorders includes cleidocranial dysostosis and nail-patella syndrome.

Cleidocranial Dysostosis
Cleidocranial dysostosis is caused by a mutation of the core-binding factor α-1 (*CBFA1*) gene, a transcription factor that activates osteoblast differentiation. The inheritance pattern is autosomal dominant. Cleidocranial dysostosis is characterized by clavicle hypoplasia with an increased ability to appose the shoulders, widening of the symphysis pubis, and coxa vara. Clavicle hypoplasia does not require treatment. Valgus osteotomy is indicated for coxa vara with a neck shaft angle less than 100° and an associated Trendelenburg gait. Other manifestations include delayed closure of the anterior fontanel sutures, mild short stature, genu valgum, scoliosis, pes planus, and shortened middle phalanges of the third, fourth, and fifth fingers.

Nail-Patella Syndrome
Nail-patella syndrome is caused by mutations of the Lim homeobox transcription factor 1-β gene, which is involved in determining dorsoventral patterning of the

6: Pediatrics

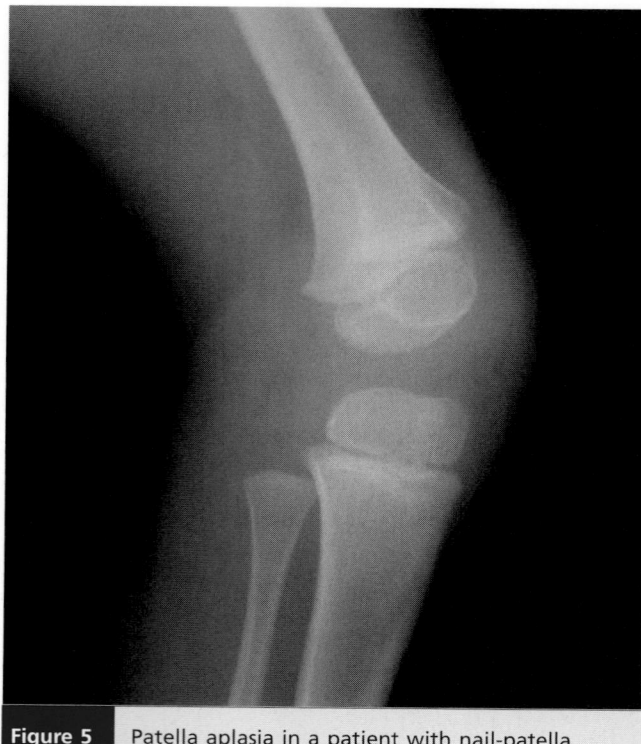

Figure 5 Patella aplasia in a patient with nail-patella syndrome.

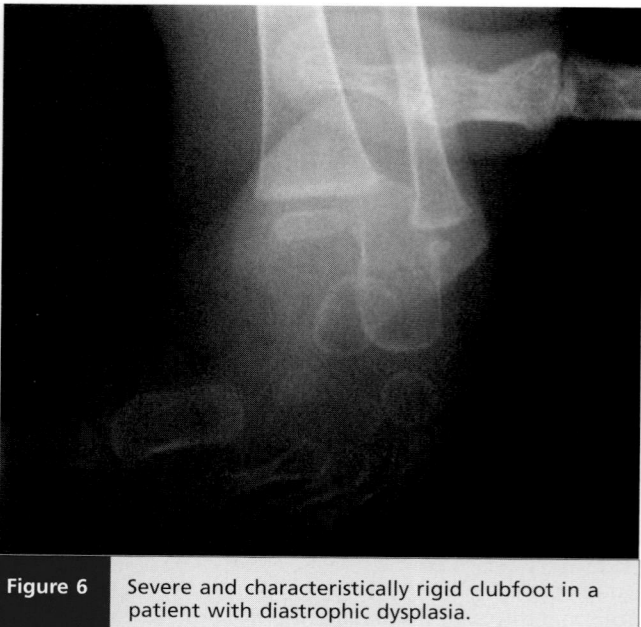

Figure 6 Severe and characteristically rigid clubfoot in a patient with diastrophic dysplasia.

limb bud. The inheritance pattern is autosomal dominant. The manifestations of nail-patella syndrome include aplasia or hypoplasia of the patella, condylar dysplasia, an intra-articular spectrum in the knee, dysplastic or aplastic nails, iliac horns, and posterior dislocation of the radial head[9] (**Figure 5**). Knee deformity and patellar realignment may require soft-tissue releases and osteotomies, and symptomatic radial head dislocation may also require surgical treatment. The medical complications include renal failure and glaucoma.

Disorders Caused by Abnormalities in Genes That Play a Role in the Processing of Proteins

This group of disorders includes diastrophic dysplasia and the mucopolysaccharidoses.

Diastrophic Dysplasia

Diastrophic dysplasia is caused by mutations in the sulfate transporter gene. It primarily affects cartilage, because of the presence of negatively charged sulfate groups in proteoglycan molecules. This dysplasia is extremely rare, except that in Finland 1% to 2% of the population are carriers. The inheritance pattern is autosomal recessive. The manifestations include cauliflower ear, marked short stature with rhizomelic shortening, cervical kyphosis, kyphoscoliosis, hitchhiker thumbs, severe clubfeet, skew foot, joint contractures, and severe osteoarthritis. Most cervical kyphoses are resolved with time and growth, but surgery is required if mye-

lopathy or progressive kyphosis or kyphoscoliosis occurs. If the kyphosis exceeds 60° and/or the apex vertebra is round or triangular and totally displaced posteriorly, then progression is likely.[10] The clubfoot in diastrophic dysplasia is typically rigid and often recurs after complete release[11] (**Figure 6**). Hip and knee flexion contractures may require releases with or without osteotomies. End-stage osteoarthritis can be treated with total joint arthroplasty.

Mucopolysaccharidoses

The mucopolysaccharidoses, a group of lysosomal storage diseases, are subdivided by enzymatic deficiency. The most common are type I (Hurler syndrome) and type IV (Morquio syndrome). The inheritance pattern is autosomal recessive, with the exception of type II (Hunter syndrome), which is X-linked. The manifestations vary by type. In general, these dysplasias are characterized by short stature, stiff joints, oval vertebral bodies, and capacious acetabuli.

Mucopolysaccharidoses type IV (Morquio syndrome) has three forms, which are distinguished by severity. The manifestations include short trunk dwarfism, genu valgum, ligamentous laxity, early hip and knee arthritis, platyspondyly, and odontoid hypoplasia. Surgery may be required for limb malalignment and C1-C2 instability. Other characteristics of Morquio syndrome include corneal opacity and cardiorespiratory disease.

Advances in medical therapy have increased the life expectancy of patients with mucopolysaccharidoses. Bone marrow transplantation has been used to treat patients with Hurler syndrome and other mucopolysaccharidoses. As life expectancy has increased, the number of musculoskeletal conditions, including end-stage arthritis, has also increased.

Other Skeletal Dysplasias

Metaphyseal Chondrodysplasia

The metaphyseal chondrodysplasias are a group of disorders characterized by metaphyseal involvement with epiphyseal preservation, short stature, and genu varum.

The Schmid type, which is most common, is caused by an α-1 chain of type X collagen (*COL110A1*) mutation. The inheritance pattern is autosomal dominant. The manifestations are mild, including moderate short stature, waddling gait, and genu varum. The Jansen type is caused by a mutation in the parathyroid receptor gene that regulates the differentiation of growth plate chondrocytes, and inheritance is also autosomal dominant. It is characterized by short stature with extremity malalignment. The McKusick type, also known as cartilage-hair hypoplasia, is caused by a mutation of the *RMRP* gene (ribosomal nucleic acid component of mitochondrial ribosomal nucleic acid processing endoribonuclease). The manifestations include atlantoaxial instability, ligamentous laxity, genu varum, pectus abnormalities, fine hair, and increased risk of viral infection and malignancy.

Pseudoachondroplasia

Pseudoachondroplasia is caused by a mutation in the cartilage oligomeric matrix protein (*COMP*) gene. COMP is an extracellular matrix glycoprotein found in the territorial matrix surrounding chondrocytes. The inheritance pattern is autosomal dominant.

Pseudoachondroplasia is characterized by involvement of the spine, metaphyses, and epiphyses; facial features may be normal or delicate. The manifestations include a short trunk and rhizomelic or mesomelic shortness, ligamentous laxity, odontoid hypoplasia, scoliosis, platyspondyly, hip subluxation, and lower extremity malalignment. Surgery may be required for atlantoaxial instability. Bracing is indicated for scoliosis between 25° and 45°, and spinal fusion is indicated for larger curves. Femoral and iliac osteotomies often are needed for hip subluxation. Lower extremity malalignment, characteristically manifested by windswept knees (**Figure 7**), can be corrected with femoral and tibial osteotomies. The deformity should not be overcorrected; otherwise, windswept knees in the other direction will occur.

Multiple Epiphyseal Dysplasia

Multiple epiphyseal dysplasia includes a spectrum of disorders resulting from different mutations. Mutations have been identified in the *COMP* gene (as in pseudoachondroplasia), *COL9A2* (collagen, type IX, α-2), and *COL9A3* (collagen, type IX, α-3). The inheritance pattern usually is autosomal dominant.

Multiple epiphyseal dysplasia is characterized by short stature with epiphyseal dysplasia and delayed ossification. The features include genu valgum, early osteoarthritis, and hip osteonecrosis. Treatment modalities for the hip are similar to the containment methods used for Legg-Calvé-Perthes disease, and realignment osteotomies may be required for genu val-

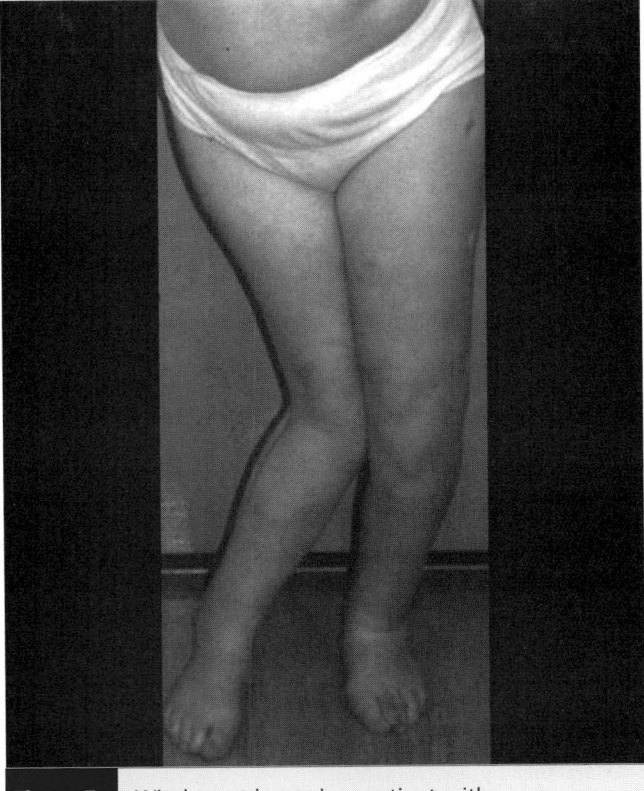

Figure 7 Windswept knees in a patient with pseudoachondroplasia.

gum. Progressive hip or shoulder arthritis can require arthroplasty.

Chondroectodermal Dysplasia

Chondroectodermal dysplasia, also known as Ellis-van Creveld syndrome, is a generalized defect of maturation of endochondral ossification. It is caused by mutation in the Ellis-van Creveld gene, the function of which is unknown. The inheritance pattern is autosomal recessive. The manifestations include short stature with meso-acromelic shortening, medial spikes from the iliac bones, genu valgum, hypoplasia of the lateral femoral epiphysis, and postaxial hand polydactyly. Osteotomies or hemiepiphysiodesis can be required to correct genu valgum. Other key features include congenital heart disease, dysplastic nails and teeth, and sparse, thin hair (**Figure 8**).

Connective Tissue Diseases

Connective tissue disorders can arise from inherited collagen or fibrillin abnormalities. The resultant abnormal extracellular matrix leads to pathology in the bone, vascular system, and viscera.

Ehlers-Danlos Syndrome

Ehlers-Danlos syndrome, the most common heritable disorder of connective tissue, is characterized by abnor-

6: Pediatrics

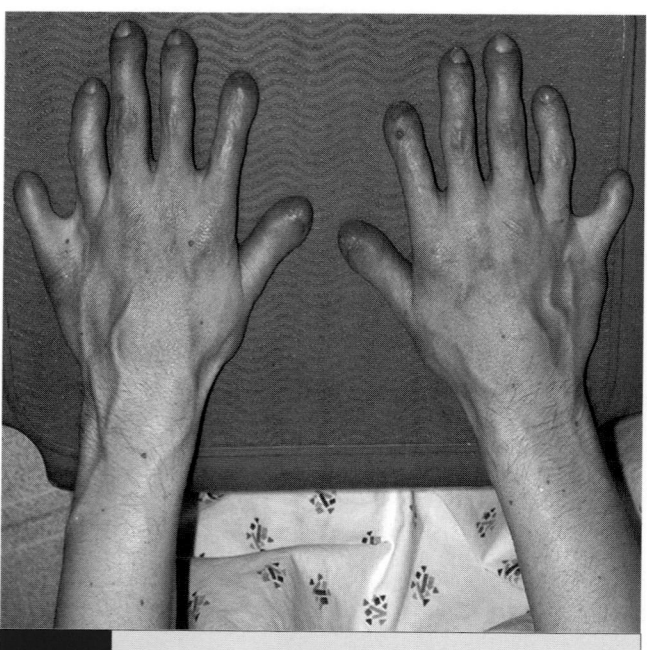

mal collagen synthesis and cross-linking. The major clinical characteristics are hyperextensibility of the skin, joint hypermobility, and generalized connective tissue fragility.[12] Manifestations are heterogeneous; hypermobility is the most characteristic symptom. According to the Villefranche system (Table 1), Ehlers-Danlos syndrome has six subtypes, of which the hypermobility and vascular subtypes are the most common. Other forms of Ehlers-Danlos syndrome also exist, including the periodontal friability and the poor clotting/fibronectin-deficient subtypes. Treatment is symptom based. For joint instability caused by hypermobility, nonsurgical treatment options should be exhausted before surgical intervention.

Marfan Syndrome

Marfan syndrome, a heritable disorder of connective tissue, involves the skeletal, ocular, and cardiovascular systems. Its prevalence is 2 to 3 individuals per 10,000. Marfan syndrome is caused by mutations of the fibrillin-1 (*FBN1*) gene, located on chromosome 15. *FBN1* is the main component of the 10- to 20-mm extracellular microfibrils involved in elastogenesis, elasticity, and homeostasis of elastic fibers. More than 500 *FBN1* mutations have been identified. The inheritance

Table 1

Villefranche Classification of Ehlers-Danlos Syndrome

Type	Biochemical Defect	Inheritance	Major Criteria	Other Characteristics
Classic	Type V collagen (*COL5A1, COL5A2*) in 50% of patients	Autosomal dominant	Soft, hyperextensible skin; easy bruising; atrophic scars; joint hypermobility; varicose veins	Scoliosis, high vertebral height, chronic musculoskeletal pain, velvety skin, hypotonia, aortic root dilatations
Hypermobility	Unknown	Autosomal dominant	Soft skin, large and small joint hypermobility and instability, chronic pain, scoliosis	Recurrent dislocation of shoulder, patellofemoral joint, ankle; musculoskeletal pain; aortic root dilatations
Vascular	*COL3A1* mutations	Autosomal dominant; rarely, autosomal recessive	Arterial, intestinal, and uterine fragility (with risk of spontaneous rupture); thin, translucent skin; easy bruising	Hypermobility of small joints, clubfoot, aortic root dilatations
Kyphoscoliosis	Lysyl hydroxylase deficiency	Autosomal recessive	Soft skin, severe hypotonia at birth, scoliosis, joint laxity, scleral fragility, and globe rupture	Easy bruising, tissue fragility, arterial rupture, osteopenia, phenotype similar to that of Marfan syndrome
Arthrochalasis	*COL1A1* and *COL1A2* mutations	Autosomal dominant	Bilateral hip dislocations, severe joint hypermobility, soft skin	Skin hyperextensibility, hypotonia, osteopenia, kyphoscoliosis
Dermatosparaxis	Type I collagen N mutations	Autosomal recessive	Severe redundant skin	Easy bruising, large hernias, premature rupture of fetal membranes

Table 2

Ghent Diagnostic Criteria for Marfan Syndrome*

System	Major Criteria	Minor Criteria	Minimum Criteria Required for Diagnosis
Musculoskeletal	Pectus carinatum; pectus excavatum requiring surgery; reduced upper to lower segment ratio or arm span: height >1.05; wrist and thumb signs; scoliosis > 20° or spondylolisthesis; reduced elbow extension; pes planus; protrusio acetabuli	Moderately severe pectus excavatum; joint hypermobility; highly arched palate with crowding of the teeth; facies (dolichocephaly, malar hypoplasia, enophthalmos, retrognathia, down-slanting palpebral fissures)	Two or more major criteria or one major plus two minor criteria
Ocular	Ectopia lentis	Abnormally flat cornea; increased axial length of globe; hypoplastic iris or hypoplastic ciliary muscle causing decreased miosis	Two minor criteria
Cardiovascular	Dilatation of ascending aorta +/– aortic regurgitation and involving sinuses of Valsalva; dissection of ascending aorta	Mitral valve prolapse +/– regurgitation, dilated main pulmonary artery in patients younger than 40 years; calcified mitral anulus in patients younger than 40 years; dilated or dissection of descending aorta in patients younger than age 40 years	One major or one minor criterion
Family or genetic history	Parent, child, or sibling meeting diagnostic criteria; mutation in *FBN1* known to cause Marfan syndrome; inherited haplotype around *FBN1* associated with Marfan syndrome in family	None	One major criterion
Skin and integument	None	Stretch marks not associated with pregnancy, weight gain, or repetitive stress; recurrent incisional hernias	One minor criterion
Dura	Lumbosacral dural ectasia by CT or MRI	None	The major criterion
Pulmonary	None	Spontaneous pneumothorax or apical blebs	One minor criterion

*Requirements for the diagnosis of Marfan syndrome for the index case: If family history is not contributory, then major criteria in at least two different organ systems and involvement of a third organ system. If a mutation known to cause Marfan syndrome is present, then one major criterion in one organ system and involvement of a second organ system. Requirements for a relative on an index case: Presence of a major criterion in the family history and one major criterion in an organ system and involvement of a second organ system.
(Adapted with permission from DePaepe A, Devereux RB, Dietz HC, Hennekam RC, Pyeritz RE: Revised diagnostic criteria for the Marfan Syndrome. Am J Med Genet 1996;62:417-426.)

pattern is autosomal dominant, although approximately 25% of patients have new mutations and linkage to *FBN1* has been excluded in some patients. In 2004, mutations of transforming growth factor-β-receptor-2 (*TGFßR2*) on chromosome 3 were identified as the Marfan syndrome type II gene.[13] *FBN1* and transforming growth factor-β (TGF-β) signaling are functionally related in the extracellular matrix.

Marfan syndrome is characterized by greater than normal height, disproportionately long arms, arachnodactyly, pectus excavatum and carinatum, ligamentous laxity, and cardiopulmonary and ocular abnormalities. The orthopaedic characteristics include scoliosis, protrusio acetabuli, and planovalgus feet.[14] The current diagnostic criteria for Marfan syndrome, called the Ghent criteria, are based on clinical findings and family history (Table 2). The role of genetic testing in establishing the diagnosis is limited, because testing for *FBN1*

6: Pediatrics

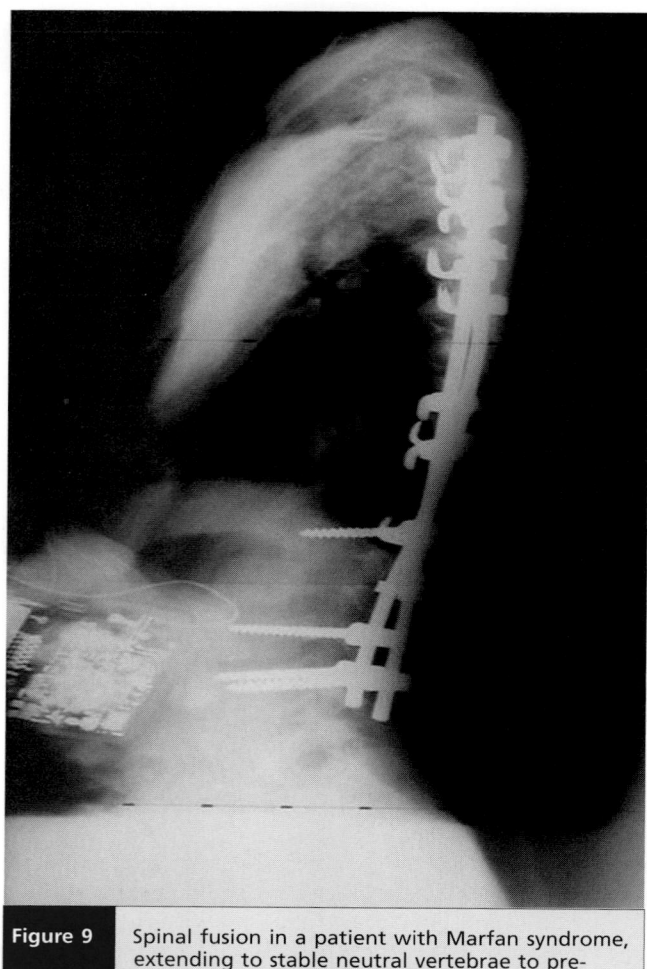

Figure 9 | Spinal fusion in a patient with Marfan syndrome, extending to stable neutral vertebrae to prevent postoperative curve decompensation.

mutations is neither sensitive nor specific for Marfan syndrome. By making the diagnosis and arranging for cardiovascular evaluation, the orthopaedic surgeon can help prevent sudden death in these patients.

Scoliosis occurs in approximately 60% of patients with Marfan syndrome and has characteristics that differ from those of idiopathic scoliosis. Bracing is less effective in these patients than it is for those with idiopathic scoliosis. Curves greater than 25° in patients with Marfan syndrome and a Risser sign of less than 2 are likely to progress and require spinal fusion.[15] Preoperative spinal MRI is necessary, because as many as 60% of patients have dural ectasias. Preoperative cardiopulmonary evaluation is also mandatory. The risk of blood loss, infection, dural tear, instrumentation failure, pseudarthrosis, and curve decompensation is increased in patients with Marfan syndrome.[16] Strong consideration should be given to extending the fusion to neutral and stable vertebrae in both planes to prevent curve decompensation and instrumentation failure[16] (**Figure 9**).

Protrusio acetabuli typically remains asymptomatic until degenerative changes occur. The indications for surgery are not well established for patients with an open triradiate cartilage and progressing protrusio acetabuli. Closure of the triradiate physis to interrupt progression is one option. In older patients with protrusio acetabuli, the treatment options include total hip replacement and valgus intertrochanteric osteotomy (for a patient with minimal arthritis).[17]

The most life-threatening complication of Marfan syndrome is thoracic aortic aneurysm, leading to aortic dissection, rupture, or both. Other cardiopulmonary manifestations include mitral valve abnormalities, dilatation of the aortic root, aortic regurgitation, and spontaneous pneumothorax. Because of the use of β-blockers and other modern cardiovascular treatment regimens, the average life span of a patient with Marfan syndrome is 70 years.

Osteogenesis Imperfecta

Osteogenesis imperfecta (OI) is a hereditary disorder characterized by osteopenia, frequent fractures, progressive deformity, and chronic bone pain. Most patients with a clinical diagnosis of OI are positive for a mutation in one of the two genes (*COL1A* and *COL2A*) that encode α chains of type I collagen, localizing to chromosomes 17 and 7, respectively.[18] In other patients, the cause of the condition is unclear. The clinical characteristics of OI include bone fragility with frequent fractures, joint laxity, protrusio acetabuli, kyphoscoliosis, basilar invagination, gray-blue sclerae, dentogenesis imperfecta, and premature deafness.

The frequency of fractures can be reduced by implanting telescoping, single nonelongating, or dual nonelongating intramedullary rods into the long bones. Osteotomy performed before rod insertion can also realign the mechanical axes. For a child with severe OI, the rods are inserted before the child begins to walk.[19] The period of postoperative immobilization should be as short as possible to prevent disuse osteopenia. As the child grows, the bones outgrow the rods, and placement of new implants is required to avoid fracture in unsupported segments.

Spinal fusion may be required to prevent scoliosis progression.[18] Bracing is an ineffective treatment for OI. For severe forms, surgery typically is indicated when the scoliosis reaches 35°; for mild forms, surgery is indicated at 45°. The symptoms of basilar invagination typically appear during the third or fourth decade of life but may begin earlier. They include apnea, altered consciousness, lower cranial nerve deficits, myelopathy, and ataxia. The treatment is transoral decompression, followed by posterior fusion and fixation.

Bisphosphonates can be used to increase the bone mass of patients with OI. Intravenous pamidronate can increase bone mineral density, decrease the incidence of fractures, improve ambulatory ability, decrease levels of urinary biochemical markers of bone turnover, and increase cortical thickness on radiographs. Treatment with bisphosphonates has not been shown to affect growth or fracture healing, but delayed healing has been reported after osteotomies for extremity realignment.[20] The use of oral bisphosphonates does not require repeated hospital admission or intravenous administration. A 2-year partially randomized prospective trial comparing the use of oral alendronate with intravenous pamidronate in children with OI showed equivalent efficacy in decreasing fracture occurrence and increasing total-body bone mineral density, spine bone mineral density, and linear growth. None of the children in the oral alendronate group had gastrointestinal problems.[21] The optimum route and duration, the result if therapy is discontinued, and the long-term consequences of therapy have not been established.

Disorders Caused by Chromosome Abnormalities

Trisomy 21 (Down Syndrome)

Trisomy 21 or Down syndrome is the most common chromosomal abnormality. The risk increases with maternal age; it is 1 in 1,500 for mothers 15 to 29 years of age and 1 in 50 for mothers older than 45 years of age. Amniocentesis can be used for prenatal diagnosis if screening laboratory tests are positive. Diagnosis at birth is made on recognition of characteristic facial features and a single transverse flexion crease in the palm, called the simian crease. Achievement of developmental milestones is delayed, and most children do not walk until they are 2 to 3 years of age. Short stature is characteristic, as is a broad-based, toed-out, waddling gait.

C1-C2 instability occurs in approximately 10% of patients. In the presence of myelopathy, fusion is indicated for an atlanto-dens interval greater than 10 mm, although a high complication rate should be anticipated.[22] In general, patients with an atlanto-dens interval of 4.5 mm to 10 mm and no neurologic findings are advised to avoid high-risk sports such as football and diving. Occipitoaxial instability and scoliosis can also occur; the latter is more common in institutionalized patients.

Patients may have hip instability, characterized by subluxation secondary to the degree of ligamentous laxity. Acetabular dysplasia may develop in late childhood and progress into maturity.[23] The treatment is controversial. Some authors recommend bracing for 6 to 8 months if the patient is younger than 6 years. Surgery has been associated with a high failure rate, although some authors reported good results.[23] Slipped capital femoral epiphysis also occurs in patients with trisomy 21; it is associated with an increased risk of osteonecrosis. Patellofemoral instability can occur as a result of ligamentous laxity. Lower extremity alignment often is characterized by genu valgum. Polyarticular arthropathy occurs in approximately 10% of patients. Other manifestations of trisomy 21 syndrome include pes planovalgus and hallux varus, mental retardation, duodenal atresia, hypothyroidism, leukemia, and congenital heart disease, which affects 50% of patients, typically as a septal defect.

Turner Syndrome

Turner syndrome can be defined as a combination of characteristic physical features and complete or partial absence of one of the X chromosomes, frequently accompanied by cell mosaicism. The effects of the single X chromosome depend on whether it was derived from the father or mother and probably are caused by imprinting. The incidence is 1 in 3,000 live births. The manifestations include short stature, webbed neck, low hairline, cubitus valgus, genu valgum, and scoliosis. There is a high incidence of fractures secondary to underlying osteoporosis.

Treatment with exogenous estrogen allows affected females to pass through puberty and develop secondary sexual characteristics. Growth hormone treatment can increase height. The treatment of scoliosis in Turner syndrome is similar to that of idiopathic scoliosis, although delayed skeletal maturation allows for a long period of scoliosis curve progression.

Disorders Caused by Abnormalities in Tumor-Related Genes

Disorders that are caused by mutations of tumor-related genes and have orthopaedic manifestations include neurofibromatosis (NF) and hereditary multiple exostosis.

Neurofibromatosis

NF is divided into three types: NF1 (von Recklinghausen disease), NF2 (associated with bilateral vestibular schwannomas), and segmental NF (with the features of NF1 but involving a single body segment). NF1, the most common single gene disorder, occurs in 1 in 3,000 live births and results from a gene-encoding neurofibromin.[24] Neurofibromin helps regulate cell growth through the RAS signaling pathway. The inheritance pattern is autosomal dominant.

Diagnostic criteria for a conclusive diagnosis of NF1 were established by the National Institutes of Health Consensus Development Conference[24] (Table 3). The risk of malignancy is increased in a patient with NF1 and includes a 10% lifetime risk of a malignant peripheral nerve sheath tumor,[1] which typically arises within a plexiform neurofibroma. Pheochromocytoma, astrocytoma, and brainstem glioma also occur.

Patients with NF1 may develop cystic lesions in long bones and congenital tibia dysplasia. Congenital tibial dysplasia includes a spectrum from anterolateral tibial bowing to pseudarthrosis (Figure 10). To prevent fracture, prophylactic application of a total-contact ankle-foot orthosis is indicated before a child reaches walking age. After the child begins walking, a knee-ankle-foot orthosis is needed. Treatment of established pseudarthrosis is initiated when the symptoms are not being controlled by the orthosis. The treatment consists of pseudarthrosis excision, bone grafting, intramedullary fixation, or Ilizarov fixation. Vascularized bone grafting, typically from the contralateral fibula, is an alternative.[24]

6: Pediatrics

Table 3

National Institutes of Health Criteria for Diagnosis of NF1

Criterion*	Minimum Number (If Applicable)
Café-au-lait spots	6
Neurofibromas, plexiform neurofibromas	2
Axillary freckling	
Optic glioma	
Lisch nodules (iris hamartomas)	2
Distinctive osseus lesion	1
First-degree relative with NF1	1

*The presence of two or more criteria is required for diagnosis.
NF1=neurofibromatosis-1
(*Adapted with permission from Crawford AH, Schorry EK: Neurofibromatosis update.* J Pediatr Orthop *2006;26:413-423.*)

Scoliosis occurs in approximately 20% of patients with NF1. The curves are classified as dystrophic or nondystrophic. Nondystrophic curves have radiographic features similar to those of idiopathic scoliosis and are treated similarly. Nondystrophic curves can modulate into dystrophic curves,[25] which are short (fewer than six segments) and sharp and have enlarged neural foramina. Dystrophic curves typically occur in patients who are younger than 6 years and are associated with scalloped endplates and rib penciling. They progress rapidly, are resistant to bracing, and may have an associated sagittal plane deformity. Surgical treatment may be required, using growing-rod instrumentation in younger children or combined anterior and posterior fusion in older children. Preoperative CT and MRI are helpful to identify defective pedicles and dural ectasias. The risk of pseudoarthrosis after spine surgery is higher in NF than idiopathic scoliosis, and thus circumferential fusion is often preferred.

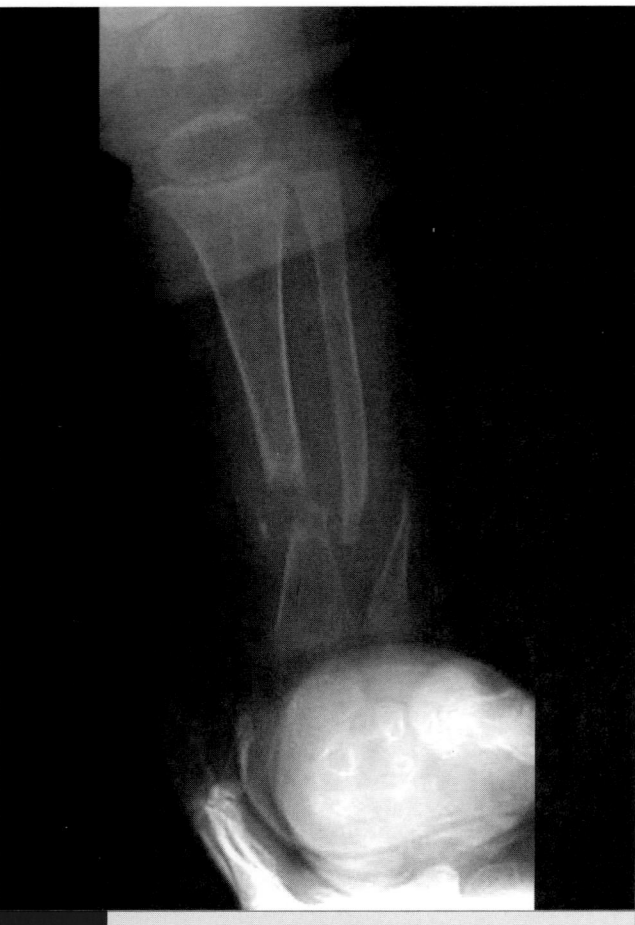

Figure 10 Congenital pseudarthrosis of the tibia and fibula in a patient with neurofibromatosis.

Annotated References

1. Unger S: A genetic approach to the diagnosis of skeletal dysplasia. *Clin Orthop Relat Res* 2002;401:32-38.

2. Aldegheri R, Dall'Oca C: Limb lengthening in short stature patients. *J Pediatr Orthop B* 2001;10:238-247.

3. Kanazawa H, Tanaka H, Inoue M, Yamanaka Y, Namba N, Seino Y: Efficacy of growth hormone therapy for patients with skeletal dysplasia. *J Bone Miner Metab* 2003;21:307-310.

4. Ain MC, Shirley ED: Spinal fusion for kyphosis in achondroplasia. *J Pediatr Orthop* 2004;24:541-545.

   The treatment of persistent thoracolumbar kyphosis with combined anterior and posterior fusion is described. Level of evidence: IV.

5. Bethem D, Winter RB, Lutter L, et al: Spinal disorders of dwarfism: Review of the literature and report of eighty cases. *J Bone Joint Surg Am* 1981;63:1412-1425.

6. Ain MC, Shirley ED, Pirouzmanesh A, Hariri A, Carson BS: Postlaminectomy kyphosis in the skeletally immature achondroplast. *Spine* 2006;31:197-201.

   A review of 10 consecutive skeletally immature patients with achondroplasia who developed early postlaminectomy thoracolumbar kyphosis after surgical decompression for spinal stenosis found that all patients required subsequent spinal fusion. The authors recommend fusion at the time of decompression in the skeletally immature patient with achondroplasia. Level of evidence: IV.

7. Bailey JA II : Orthopaedic aspects of achondroplasia. *J Bone Joint Surg Am* 1970;52:1285-1301.

8. Ain MC, Shirley ED, Pirouzmanesh A, Skolasky RL, Leet AI: Genu varum in achondroplasia. *J Pediatr Orthop* 2006;26:375-379.

   The authors evaluated the long leg radiographs of 48 children with achondroplasia. They found that the degree of fibular overgrowth was not associated with the alignment of the lower extremity. Level of evidence: IV.

9. Beguiristain JL, de Rada PD, Barriga A: Nail-patella syndrome: Long term evolution. *J Pediatr Orthop B* 2003;12:13-16.

10. Remes V, Marttinen E, Poussa M, Kaitila I, Peltonen J: Cervical kyphosis in diastrophic dysplasia. *Spine* 1999; 24:1990-1995.

11. Ryoppy S, Poussa M, Merikanto J, Marttinen E, Kaitila I: Foot deformities in diastrophic dysplasia: An analysis of 102 patients. *J Bone Joint Surg Br* 1992;74:441-444.

12. Stanitski DF, Nadjarian R, Stanitski CL, Bawle E, Tsipouras P: Orthopaedic manifestations of Ehlers-Danlos syndrome. *Clin Orthop Relat Res* 2000;376:213-221.

13. Mizuguchi T, Collod-Beroud G, Akiyama T, et al: Heterozygous TGFBR2 mutations in Marfan syndrome. *Nat Genet* 2004;36:855-860.

    The genetic heterogeneity of Marfan syndrome and a direct link between a connective tissue disorder and TGF-β signaling in humans is shown.

14. Joseph KN, Kane HA, Milner RS, Steg NL, Williamson MB Jr, Bowen JR: Orthopedic aspects of the Marfan phenotype. *Clin Orthop Relat Res* 1992;277:251-261.

15. Sponseller PD, Bhimani M, Solacoff D, Dormans JP: Results of brace treatment of scoliosis in Marfan syndrome. *Spine* 2000;25:2350-2354.

16. Jones KB, Erkula G, Sponseller PD, Dormans JP: Spine deformity correction in Marfan syndrome. *Spine* 2002; 27:2003-2012.

17. Van de Velde S, Fillman R, Yandow S: Protrusio acetabuli in Marfan syndrome: History, diagnosis, and treatment. *J Bone Joint Surg Am* 2006;88:639-646.

    This current concepts review summarizes the characteristics and treatment of protrusio acetabuli in patients with Marfan syndrome. The authors promote closure of the triradiate cartilage when it is still open and the protrusio is progressing. Level of evidence: V.

18. Zeitlin L, Fassier F, Glorieux FH: Modern approach to children with osteogenesis imperfecta. *J Pediatr Orthop B* 2003;12:77-87.

19. Joseph B, Rebello G, B CK: The choice of intramedullary devices for the femur and the tibia in osteogenesis imperfecta. *J Pediatr Orthop B* 2005;14:311-319.

In this review of the results of intramedullary rodding in patients with OI, dual Rush rods and Sheffield telescoping rods were found to be superior to a single Rush rod in the femur. In the tibia, a single Rush rod was as effective as a Sheffield rod. Level of evidence: IV.

20. Munns CFJ, Rauch F, Zeitlin L, Fassier F, Glorieux FH: Delayed osteotomy but not fracture healing in pediatric osteogenesis imperfecta patients receiving pamidronate. *J Bone Miner Res* 2004;19:1779-1786.

    This study evaluated bone healing on radiography after lower limb fractures and intramedullary rodding procedures. Pamidronate was associated with delayed healing after osteotomy, but not after fracture. Level of evidence: IV

21. DiMeglio LA, Peacock M: Two-year clinical trial of oral alendronate versus intravenous pamidronate in children with osteogenesis imperfecta. *J Bone Miner Res* 2006; 21:132-140.

    The authors partially randomized children to receive intravenous pamidronate or oral alendronate. At 2-year follow-up, oral and intravenous therapies were found to be equally effective in increasing total-body bone mineral density, spine bone mineral density, and linear growth and in decreasing bone turnover and fracture incidence. Level of evidence: II.

22. Doyle JS, Lauerman WC, Wood KB, Krause DR: Complications and long-term outcome of upper cervical spine arthrodesis in patients with Down syndrome. *Spine* 1996;21:1223-1231.

23. Katz DA, Kim YJ, Millis MB: Periacetabular osteotomy in patients with Down's syndrome. *J Bone Joint Surg Br* 2005;87:544-547.

    The authors reviewed the results of eight dysplastic acetabuli in skeletally mature patients treated with modified Bernese periacetabular osteotomy. All eight hips remained clinically stable at follow-up. Level of evidence: IV.

24. Crawford AH, Schorry EK: Neurofibromatosis update. *J Pediatr Orthop* 2006;26:413-423.

    The authors reviewed the manifestations and treatment options for NF. In addition, the current developments in molecular genetics are discussed. Level of evidence: V.

25. Durrani AA, Crawford AH, Chouhdry SN, Saifuddin A, Morley TR: Modulation of spinal deformities in patients with neurofibromatosis type 1. *Spine* 2000;25:69-75.

6: Pediatrics

Chapter 64

Neuromuscular Disorders in Children

James J. McCarthy, MD   James T. Guille, MD   David A. Spiegel, MD

Cerebral Palsy

Cerebral palsy (CP), the most common neuromuscular disorder in children, affects more than 1 in 500 children in the United States. It has been defined as "a group of disorders of the development of movement and posture, causing activity limitation, attributed to nonprogressive disturbances that occurred in the developing fetal or infant brain."[1] The severity and distribution of CP varies greatly from patient to patient, depending on the extent of the underlying central nervous system injury.

The belief that CP is the result of poor obstetric care is a misconception. In fact, improvements in obstetric care have led to increased survival of very small preterm infants, who have a high incidence of CP.[2] In addition, current fertility treatments have led to an increase in births of twins and higher order multiples, in whom the rate of CP is as much as four times that of children born singly.[1]

Assessment

The history of a child with CP should include birth history, developmental milestones, prior treatments, therapy routine, and other medical issues such as speech, swallowing, hearing, and seizure disorders. A diagnosis other than CP should be considered in the absence of corroborative perinatal history, family history of neurologic disorders, or neurologic progression.

Careful physical examination of a child with CP is important, although often difficult and time consuming. A child who uses a wheelchair should be examined while sitting in the wheelchair and, if applicable, walking with assistive devices. To properly assess tone and range of motion, especially of the lower extremities, the child should be examined on an examination table, or in the parent's lap, if age-appropriate. The assessment should include muscle tone, strength, and range of motion, as well as the fit and function of orthotic devices. It is important to differentiate increased spasticity from true joint contractures. The diarthrodial muscles, which are muscles that cross two joints, appear to be more significantly affected in children with CP; they are assessed by specific examination maneuvers (Table 1). The Adams forward-bend test or a simple examination of the spine in the nonambulatory child can yield evidence of scoliosis and should be performed at each clinic visit; if there is any concern, spine radiographs should be obtained. Hip abduction should be measured and documented; if hip abduction is limited, radiographs should be obtained to assess for hip subluxation.

Table 1

Physical Examination Maneuvers for Assessment of a Child With Cerebral Palsy

Test	Purpose	Procedure
Thomas	Isolate a true hip flexion contracture by stabilizing the pelvis	With patient in supine position, contralateral hip is flexed to stabilize the pelvis (with the lumbar spine in neutral alignment). The index hip is allowed to extend. The angle between the femur and the horizontal is the hip flexion contracture.
Ely-Duncan	Determine rectus femoris tightness	The patient is in the prone position and the knee is flexed. The test is positive if the pelvis lifts off the table (hip flexion) as the knee is flexed. The degree of knee flexion at which hip flexion occurs can be recorded.
Popliteal angle	Determine hamstring tightness	The patient is in the supine position, the hip is flexed to 90°, and the knee is extended. The angle of knee flexion in this position is the popliteal angle.
Silfverskiöld	Isolate soleus muscle tightness with gastrocnemius relaxed	The patient is in the supine position. To isolate soleus tightness, the knee is flexed to 90°, and the ankle is dorsiflexed with the foot in a neutral position. To measure gastrocnemius-soleus complex tightness, the measurement is compared with the same measurement with the knee extended.

6: Pediatrics

Table 2

Impairments Associated With Cerebral Palsy in Children

Impairment	Prevalence (%)
Speech	80
Visual	75
Gastrointestinal or feeding	50
Cognitive (IQ < 50)	50
Malnutrition or excessive weight	50
Chronic pain	70
Seizure disorder*	20-40
Hearing	15

*Most common in hemiplegic and quadriplegic patients

Motion analysis is used to acquire data for assessment of temporal spatial parameters (velocity, cadence, step length), kinematics (position), and kinetics (moments and force), as well as electromyographic data. The uses of motion analysis extend beyond preoperative evaluation to postoperative assessment, objective measurement of surgical outcomes, monitoring of ambulatory function over time, assessment of the usefulness of bracing or other assistive devices, and research.[3]

CP can be classified according to neuropathic type, anatomic location of involvement, ambulatory status, and functional status. The Gross Motor Function Classification System is reliable, repeatable over time,[4] and closely correlated with other measures of function. The 1:2:4:8 rule is useful in predicting the patient's future ambulation ability: a patient who has more than two primitive reflexes at the age of 1 year, cannot sit independently by the age of 4 years, or cannot walk by the age of 8 is unlikely ever to be able to walk independently. Children with CP often have other impairments that directly affect their care and that the orthopaedic surgeon should take into account (Table 2). Goals such as improving communication, ability to perform activities of daily living, and general mobility are often more important to the patient than improving ambulatory ability.

Chronic pain is currently recognized as a concern in adults and children with CP. One recent study found that more than half of the children with CP reported recurrent chronic pain of at least moderate intensity that often interfered with activities of daily living and sleep.[5] Their bone density is often significantly lower than that of age-matched children. Pamidronate has been shown to significantly improve bone mineral density, although the degree of improvement varied greatly and had largely disappeared 2 years after treatment.[6]

Nonsurgical Treatment

Tone Management

Muscle hypertonicity associated with CP can interfere with positioning, standing, or sitting, and it can lead to contractures or loss of range of motion. The most commonly administered oral medication is baclofen, which inhibits the release of excitatory neurotransmitters in the spinal cord. When baclofen is administered orally, the dosage required to achieve the desired reduction in spasticity may result in sedation. Baclofen can also be administered through an implanted intrathecal pump, which delivers the medication directly to the spinal cord and is titrated to effect. Although baclofen is effective in reducing muscle tone and pain in selected patients, as many as 20% of patients experience complications, including catheter failure, infection, skin breakdown, and may be associated with the development of scoliosis. If necessary, the dosage must be gradually tapered off; sudden discontinuation, even of the oral form, can cause a severe withdrawal reaction, with seizures, increased tone, hallucinations, and rarely, death.

The use of botulinum toxin has been shown to elicit short-term improvement in motion and function.[7] Botulinum toxin causes paralysis by blocking acetylcholine release at the neuromuscular junction. It is reconstituted with preservative-free sterile saline and injected into the motor end point of the muscle; electrical stimulation is commonly used to identify the best injection site.[8] Muscles with increased spasticity are usually targeted for injection; the most common are the gastrocnemius, hamstrings, hip adductors, and tibialis posterior. Weakness begins approximately 3 days after the injection, reaches the maximum effect at 3 weeks, and disappears by 4 to 6 months because of resprouting of terminals from the axon.

Selective dorsal rhizotomy divides selected dorsal nerve rootlets from L1 to S2. It has been shown to reduce spasticity and improve function in carefully selected patients with diplegic CP.[9] Care must be taken to exclude patients who either are too weak or rely on their hypertonicity to function. Extensive postoperative physical therapy is needed, and orthopaedic surgery is often performed after selective dorsal rhizotomy. Complications are uncommon; they include bowel and bladder incontinence, weakness, change or loss of sensation, spinal deformity, and hip subluxation.

Therapy

Patients with CP commonly receive ongoing occupational, physical, and speech therapy to maintain function. The intensity of therapy is often increased after surgical or other interventions. The current emphasis is on strengthening the muscles of children with CP through innovative treatment options such as treadmill training and functional electrical stimulation.[10]

Orthotic Devices

Children with CP often use orthotic devices. The most common is the ankle-foot orthosis (AFO). Solid AFOs are used to improve overall stability and prevent plantar flexion contracture. If the patient hyperextends the knee during stance, a slight degree of dorsiflexion should be incorporated into the orthotic device. If the patient has a crouched gait, a floor-reaction orthotic device should be used. For a child who has sufficient ankle range of motion, a hinged AFO permits greater movement for higher level activities such as stair climbing. Lower braces, such as supramalleolar or in-shoe orthotic devices, cannot affect ankle motion and are used for isolated flexible pronation or supination deformities.

Orthotic devices can also be used in an attempt to maintain range of motion and prevent deformity. Despite the widespread use of orthotic devices, their effectiveness has not been proven.

Surgical Treatment

Surgical treatment options for children with CP are numerous, but the recommendations of experienced surgeons vary. It is important to minimize the number of surgical treatments, maintain reasonable expectations, and communicate clearly with the patient and caregivers. In general, surgery should be avoided within the first 4 to 6 years of age to allow an assessment of improvement with growth and development and avoid recurrence or overcorrection, unless the child's hip is at risk of subluxation. In ambulatory children, multilevel surgery at age 6 to 8 years can be considered for improvement of ambulatory function. For nonambulatory children, surgery is performed primarily to treat hip subluxation, progressive scoliosis, or foot deformity, or to lengthen soft tissue to improve positioning for standing, transferring, sitting, or shoe wear.

Rotational deformities can develop in children with CP. Unlike anteversion in the typically developing child, these deformities may become more noticeable over time. Careful preoperative assessment is needed to determine the source of the rotation (femoral anteversion, tibial torsion, or foot deformity) and the best means of correcting it.

Spine

Scoliosis is common in children with CP. The overall incidence is approximately 20%, but in nonambulatory children with spastic quadriplegic CP, the incidence can be as high as 65%. Scoliosis in children with neuromuscular disorders differs from idiopathic scoliosis in that the curve is more likely to progress, even after skeletal maturity; the curve begins at an earlier age; and bracing is less effective in preventing progression, although a soft orthosis may improve sitting balance. Unlike the curve pattern of idiopathic scoliosis, the typical curve in CP is long, C-shaped, kyphoscoliotic, and it may result in pelvic obliquity. Larger curves are associated with an increase in hip and pelvic deformity; the association between functional decline and scoliosis is less clear.[11] Small curves can typically be addressed with modification of the seating system, such as changing the position of the lateral supports on a wheelchair.

Patients with curves that have progressed beyond 40° to 50° are candidates for spinal fusion. The primary surgical goal is a corrected, well-balanced spine over a level pelvis that will result in a solid fusion. Al-

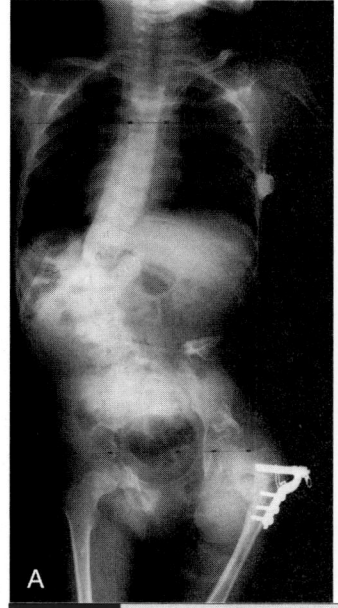
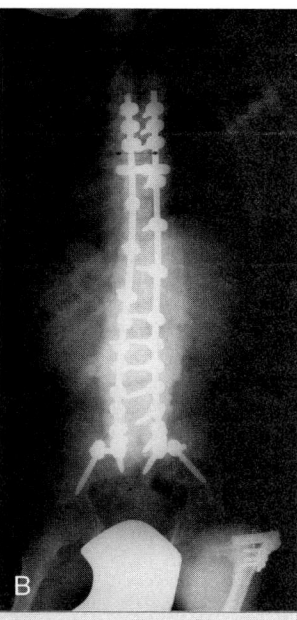

Figure 1   **A,** AP radiograph of a 10-year-old boy with quadriplegic CP showing a 50° left lumbar curve and 20° pelvic obliquity. **B,** Postoperative AP radiograph taken after posterior spinal fusion with pedicle screw fixation and sacral and iliac screw fixation to the pelvis.

though there is little evidence that posterior spinal fusion results in significant functional gains, most studies have found that sitting balance, appearance, and caregivers' assessment improved after spinal fusion.[12]

Multisegmental fixation is commonly performed using sublaminar wires in combination with Luque rods or a unit rod with pelvic fixation. Newer options such as pedicle screws also are being used[13] (**Figure 1**). Fixation should extend proximally to the upper thoracic spine (T1-T2) to prevent progressive upper thoracic kyphosis or junctional problems. Fixation should extend distally to L3-L4 if pelvic obliquity is less than 10° and the patient is ambulatory; otherwise, fixation should extend to the pelvis. Complications are common; they include hardware failure, gastrointestinal and/or pulmonary complications, neurologic complications, and death.

Sagittal plane spinal deformities include lumbar hyperlordosis (related to hip flexion contractures) and thoracic hyperkyphosis (related to poor trunk control). Cervical spondylotic myelopathy also has been reported, most commonly in adults with athetoid CP. The condition is commonly overlooked because of the patient's underlying CP and gradual functional decline.[14]

Hip

Approximately one third of children with CP develop hip subluxation. The incidence of hip subluxation increases with increased motor involvement.[15] The children at most risk are those with severe spasticity, adduction contractures, and pelvic obliquity on the higher

6: Pediatrics

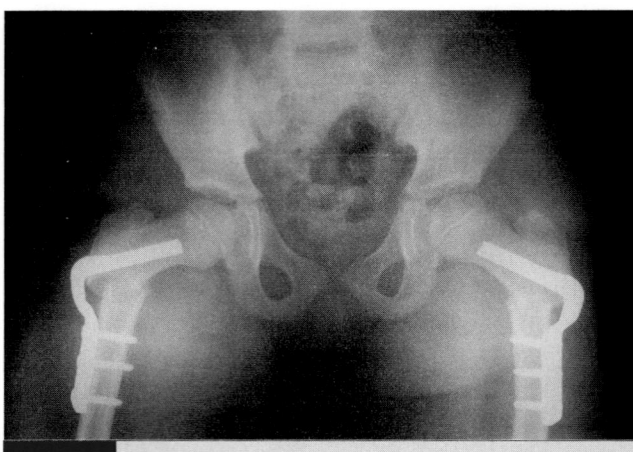

Figure 2 AP radiograph of the pelvis taken after bilateral varus derotational osteotomies with blade plates.

side. Their hip range of motion should be routinely monitored, especially for adequate abduction and extension, and AP radiographs of the hips should be taken.

Hip subluxation is one of the few indications for orthopaedic surgery in the younger child. For these children, early adductor release and hip flexor lengthening may prevent the need for more extensive bony surgery, even if radiographs show little or no subluxation. If the subluxation is more severe, especially in the setting of bony changes, varus derotational osteotomy with internal fixation is performed (**Figure 2**). If acetabular dysplasia is present, a pelvic osteotomy may be indicated. The complications include resubluxation, osteonecrosis, and heterotopic ossification. For a painful dislocated hip with secondary radiographic changes, a salvage procedure such as a femoral head resection or valgus osteotomy should be considered. Although most researchers recommend surgery to maintain hip reduction, the long-term consequences of hip dislocation in an adult with CP are not clear.[16]

Knee
Tight hamstrings and knee flexion contractures often develop in children with CP. In ambulatory children, these can result in a crouched gait pattern and increased effort to walk, as well as increased stress and eventually pain across the patellar femoral joint. The treatment includes hamstring lengthening and, if necessary, extension casting for the flexion contractures.[17] The use of other techniques, such as distal hamstring transfers and extension osteotomies combined with advancement of the patellar tendon, has recently been reported.[18] If rectus femoris spasticity inhibits knee flexion in swing, a rectus femoris transfer can be performed.

Ankle and Foot
Equinus contracture is the most common deformity in children with CP. Because the recurrence rate after lengthening is high in young children, treatment of the young child is typically nonsurgical and consists of therapy, bracing, botulinum toxin injections, and serial casting. If these treatments are ineffective, surgical lengthening is indicated. Selective recession of the gastrocnemius is generally preferred to Achilles tendon lengthening to prevent loss of push-off strength or overlengthening and crouched gait in children with diplegic CP. Prior to gastrocnemius or Achilles tendon lengthening, the hamstrings should be assessed and, if necessary, lengthened.[19]

Equinus contracture generally progresses in children with diplegic CP to an equinovalgus foot deformity, which results in a break in the midfoot and often a flatfoot deformity. Conservative treatment can be aimed at stretching the heel cord and positioning the hindfoot in a relatively neutral position. Surgery is indicated for a painful foot that cannot be adequately braced. Surgery includes gastrocnemius lengthening and a lateral stabilization technique such as a lateral opening-wedge calcaneal osteotomy or, for severe deformities, an arthrodesis.

Equinovarus foot deformity is more common in children with hemiplegic CP. Treatment involves lengthening of the gastrocnemius-soleus complex and either a split transfer of the tibialis posterior or lengthening of the tibialis posterior and split transfer of the tibialis anterior, depending on the muscle that appears to be the primary deforming force.[20] Fine-wire electromyography performed during motion analysis and the confusion test, in which a seated patient is asked to flex the hip against the examiner's hand resulting in obligatory cocontraction of either the tibialis anterior or posterior, can help to identify the muscle firing out of phase.

Myelomeningocele

Myelomeningocele is a congenital malformation of the spinal column and neural elements, in which absence of the posterior elements is associated with a cystic expansion of the meninges, which contain the spinal cord and nerve roots. The incidence is approximately 1 in 1,000. The risk can be significantly reduced during pregnancy, by maternal folic acid supplementation.[21] Myelomeningocele can be detected though prenatal ultrasound screening and maternal serum α-fetoprotein level testing. Closure is performed within 24 to 48 hours after the infant is born. Many patients require shunting for hydrocephalus. More than 80% of patients live at least 16 years, but survival into the fourth decade is less likely for patients who require shunting.[22] Latex allergy is almost universal in children with myelomeningocele; exposure to latex can be life threatening, and avoidance of latex is critical.

Myelomeningocele is a disorder of the central nervous system. Coexisting conditions within the neural axis can include hydrocephalus, Arnold-Chiari malformation, syringomyelia, intraspinal anomalies of various types, and tethering of the spinal cord. The differential diagnosis of neurologic deterioration includes shunt malfunction, hydrocephalus, tethered cord, and brainstem compression (Arnold-Chiari malformation). Clinical manifestations of neurologic deterioration include progressive scoliosis, back or leg pain, increasing spasticity, development or progression of a foot deformity, and changes in bowel or bladder function. Sleep apnea appears in 20% of patients and is a common cause of death.[23] A standardized clinical assessment that includes manual muscle testing should be performed at intervals of 6 to 12 months to identify such changes.

The early results of an ongoing, multicenter study of fetal closure of myelomeningocele found a decrease in the incidence of Arnold-Chiari malformation and a reduced need for cerebrospinal fluid shunting, but fetal closure has not been shown to improve neurologic function.[24]

Orthopaedic Treatment

The orthopaedic treatment of myelomeningocele is designed to improve function. The surgical goals are dependent on the patient's ambulatory status, which relates to the neurosegmental level of the myelomeningocele. For nonambulatory patients, the goal is a stable seating posture with a straight spine, level pelvis, and adequate lower extremity motion. For ambulatory patients, treatment focuses on maximizing ambulatory ability by maintaining or restoring range of motion, correcting malalignment, and providing the most appropriate orthotic device. Patients with thoracic and upper lumbar myelomeningocele often achieve a standing posture or limited ambulation with orthotic support during childhood, but ultimately in adolescence and adulthood they must rely on a wheelchair for mobility. Patients with midlumbar involvement who have functional quadriceps usually are community or household ambulators, possibly with the use of an assistive device. Patients with lower lumbar- and sacral-level myelomeningocele are community ambulators.

Hip
Hip flexion contracture is common, regardless of ability to walk. In ambulatory patients, it results from unopposed action of the hip flexors, and in nonambulatory patients, it results from the postural effects of muscle imbalance. The consequence of hip flexion contracture in an ambulatory patient is an increase in anterior pelvic tilt during gait, which predisposes the patient to crouch and may interfere with bracing. Surgical treatment is indicated for symptomatic contractures greater than 20°. It involves soft-tissue release of nonfunctional muscle or lengthening of functional muscle. In nonambulators, hip flexion deformity may be associated with abduction and external rotation, which can impair positioning. When symptomatic, a flexion-abduction contracture is treated with the Ober-Yount soft-tissue release procedure.

The treatment recommendations for hip subluxation or dislocation have evolved in response to observation that preserving the patient's motion is more important than hip reduction, and that reconstructive surgery

complications, especially stiffness, are common and may worsen the prognosis. A patient with a mobile dislocated hip fares better than a patient with a stiff relocated hip. Surgical reduction is considered for ambulatory patients with lower lumbar and sacral involvement, especially those with unilateral disease. These patients are community ambulators.

Knee and Lower Leg
The knee problems associated with myelomeningocele include flexion and extension contractures, torsional deformities, and valgus during the stance phase of gait. Flexion contracture results in a crouched gait with quadriceps overload and decreased endurance. The degree of knee flexion during ambulation is often greater than is measured during physical examination. Surgical treatment is indicated if the deformity is greater than 20° and interferes with ambulation. Hamstring lengthening alone may not be sufficient. Children with myelomeningocele often have a fixed flexion deformity that must be treated using a posterior capsular release or gradual distraction. Extension contractures are less common, and motion may be improved by lengthening the extensor mechanism. Casting should be avoided because of the high risk of skin breakdown in children with decreased sensation.

Foot
Foot deformities are common in both ambulatory and nonambulatory patients. The goal of treatment is a mobile, braceable foot. Arthrodesis should be avoided in patients with diminished sensation. Clubfoot is treated by circumferential soft-tissue release using tenotomy or tendon excision;[25] recurrent deformities may require talectomy or a lateral column shortening. Congenital vertical talus is treated by soft-tissue release with or without transfer of the tibialis anterior to the talar neck. Calcaneus deformity results from weakness or absence of gastrocnemius-soleus complex function; simple release of the tibialis anterior is preferable to posterior transfer.

Valgus deformity can originate in the ankle or hindfoot; standing radiographs of both the foot and ankle may be required to clarify the location of the deformity. Ankle valgus can be treated either by screw epiphysiodesis (medial malleolus) or supramalleolar osteotomy. Hindfoot valgus can be treated by tenotomy of the peroneal muscles (with or without peroneus tertius and lesser toe extensors), and a calcaneal-lengthening osteotomy.

Spine
Scoliosis occurs in as many as 90% of patients with an affected neurosegmental level of L1 or higher, compared with 5% to 25% of patients affected at the lower lumbar or sacral level. The scoliosis is most commonly paralytic, with a long, C-shaped thoracolumbar or lumbar curve, although congenital scoliosis also can occur. Paralytic curves greater than 40° progress at an approximate rate of 5° per year. A severe curve may impair sitting bal-

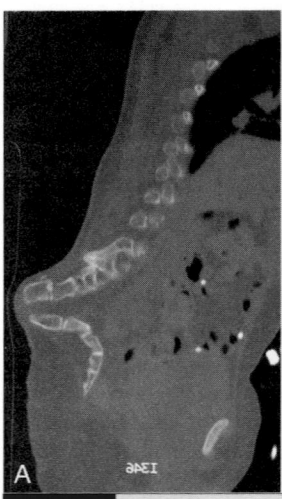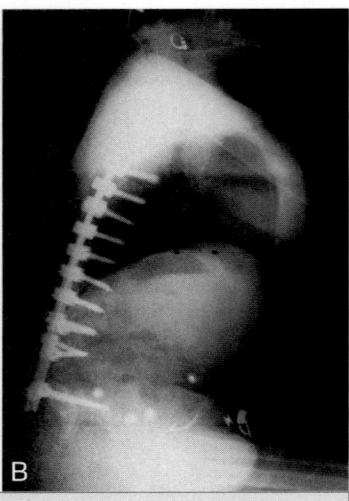

Figure 3 **A,** Preoperative CT scan of a 14-year-old girl with myelomeningocele, showing a lateral kyphotic deformity. **B,** Postoperative lateral radiograph taken after kyphectomy and instrumentation.

ance, and the patient may need to use an upper extremity to maintain upright positioning. Rapid progression of curvature can indicate spinal cord tethering and should prompt a neurosurgical evaluation. Tethered cord release can stabilize smaller curves (less than 40°). Although bracing does not arrest progression, an orthosis can improve sitting balance and slow progression of the deformity. Delaying surgical treatment allows time for the child's trunk height to increase, but this advantage must be weighed against the difficulty of treating a larger, stiffer curve. Spinal fusion is indicated for patients with a progressive curvature greater than 50° and poor sitting balance. An anteroposterior spinal fusion offers the best chance of achieving a solid arthrodesis. Coronal balance is most related to sitting balance. Most patients require fixation to the pelvis, although more limited arthrodesis may be successful in patients with less than 10° of pelvic obliquity. Complications are frequent; they include wound infection, implant failure with or without pseudarthrosis, and a host of medical complications.[26] Self-catheterization may be more difficult after fusion, and the loss of trunk mobility can make transfers more challenging.

Kyphosis, which most commonly occurs in the lumbar spine, is often congenital and is identified in 8% to 15% of patients. Patients must sit with the trunk flexed, and this positioning can compress the abdominal contents and reduce pulmonary function. Bracing is technically difficult and does not arrest progression. Although indications for surgery are debated, the most common indication is recurrent skin breakdown, which often leads to sepsis. Surgical treatment involves correction of the deformity and spinal arthrodesis. The most common approach is a kyphectomy, in which resection of the apical vertebral segment and often a part of the proximal lordotic segment is combined with a long posterior fusion extending to the sacrum (**Figure 3**).

Decancellation of multiple apical vertebral bodies is a successful alternative procedure that may reduce the risk of pseudarthrosis and implant failure. Because the spinal cord does not need to be resected, the potential for acute intraoperative hydrocephalus should be decreased or eliminated. Techniques for lumbopelvic fixation include the Galveston technique, which involves intrailiac extension of the spinal rods; the S-rod technique, in which precontoured rods are placed anterior to the sacral ala; and the Warner and Fackler technique, in which precontoured rods are placed through the first sacral foramina.[27] Complications are frequent, and revision surgery is often required.

Muscular Dystrophy

Duchenne muscular dystrophy, the most common form of muscular dystrophy, occurs in 1 of every 3,300 males and can occur in females who have Turner's syndrome. An X-linked recessive defect in chromosome Xp21 leads to an absence of the dystrophin gene, which is critical for the stability of cell membranes. Duchenne muscular dystrophy is typically diagnosed in children 3 to 5 years of age who have delayed motor milestones, a waddling gait or toe walking, a positive Gower's sign, and pseudohypertrophy of the calves. Upper extremity weakness develops a few years later. Most children stop ambulating by late childhood and die from respiratory failure before they are 30 years old. Aggressive pulmonary care can prolong their life span. The orthopaedic manifestations of Duchenne muscular dystrophy include scoliosis, foot deformities, and increased fracture risk.

Most patients with muscular dystrophy develop a progressive scoliosis, especially after they begin full-time wheelchair use. The scoliosis is a typical neuromuscular, long C-shaped thoracolumbar curve with pelvic obliquity. Wheelchair modifications and a soft thoracolumbosacral orthosis can improve the sitting posture of a child with a small, flexible curve but do not prevent curve progression. It is important to perform posterior spinal fusion early, before pulmonary function declines. Recent research has found that administration of steroids can slow the progression of scoliosis and delay the need for surgery,[28] although steroid use is associated with complications including obesity, osteopenia leading to fracture, and cataracts.

Preoperative electrocardiography and echocardiography should be performed to evaluate cardiac myopathy. Pulmonary function studies should be used to evaluate forced vital capacity, which should be at least 35%. Some patients require a prophylactic tracheostomy. Because of the risk of malignant hyperthermia and large intraoperative blood loss, an anesthesiologist should be consulted.

The standard treatment of scoliosis is with segmental instrumentation from T2 to the pelvis, using either a unit rod and sublaminar wires or pedicle screws and iliac bolts. The fusion can be stopped at L5 for smaller curves with no pelvic obliquity.

6: Pediatrics

Table 3

Genetic Characteristics of Neuromuscular Diseases

Disease	Chromosome	Gene	Mode of Inheritance	Diagnostic Sample
Duchenne muscular dystrophy	Xp21	Dystrophin	X-linked recessive	DNA analysis Creatine kinase (elevated) Muscle biopsy
Facioscapulohumeral dystrophy	4q35	Undetermined (low D_4Z_4 repeats)	Autosomal dominant	DNA analysis
Spinal muscular atrophy	5q	Survival motor neuron	Autosomal recessive	DNA analysis Muscle biopsy
Charcot-Marie-Tooth disease (type 1A)	17	Peripheral myelin protein 22	Autosomal dominant	DNA analysis Electrodiagnostics
Friedreich's ataxia	9	Frataxin	Autosomal recessive	DNA analysis

Table 4

Spinal Muscular Atrophy Classification

Type	Name	Age of Diagnosis	Age of Death	Ambulatory Status
I (severe)	Werdnig-Hoffman	< 6 months	< 2 years	Unable to walk
II (moderate)	Intermediate form (Dubowitz)	6-24 months	< 4th decade	Unable to walk but able to sit
III (mild)	Kugelberg-Welander	> 24 months	> 4th decade	Able to walk

Equinovarus foot deformity develops in most boys with Duchenne muscular dystrophy. Although foot surgery probably prolongs the ability to ambulate, the role of surgery for children who are full-time wheelchair users is controversial.

Facioscapulohumeral muscular dystrophy is characterized by weakness of the shoulder and proximal arm, scapular winging, facial weakness, and decreased flexion and abduction of the shoulder. It is an autosomal dominant condition resulting from deletions of a tandem repeat in the terminal region of chromosome 4; 95% of patients show penetrance by age 20 years. Involvement is asymmetric; the facial muscles and the muscles in the lower extremities may be affected. An infantile form of the condition appears during the first years of life and is associated with bilateral facial weakness, scapular winging, shoulder weakness, lumbar lordosis and hip flexion contracture, foot drop, sensorineural hearing loss, and retinal vasculopathy.

Both scapulothoracic fusion and scapulopexy (fixation without fusion) have been shown to improve shoulder abduction and flexion, improve cosmesis, and decrease pain.[29] Stabilization of the scapula to the posterior chest wall permits abduction and flexion of the deltoid muscle (until it is affected by the disease).

Becker muscular dystrophy is also X-linked recessive, and its incidence is 1 in 30,000 males. It is clinically similar to Duchenne muscular dystrophy but less severe. Becker muscular dystrophy becomes evident in late childhood, and patients are able to walk until young adulthood. These patients have a longer life span than patients with Duchenne muscular dystrophy. Ge-

netic characteristics of common neuromuscular diseases are outlined in **Table 3**.

Spinal Muscular Atrophy

Spinal muscular atrophy is an inherited autosomal recessive neuromuscular disorder that occurs in 1 of 6,000 to 10,000 children. A mutation of the survival motor neuron gene on chromosome 5q is present in almost all patients. The disorder is characterized by a progressive, symmetric loss of muscle function caused by the loss of anterior horn cells in the spinal cord. Diagnosis is made through muscle biopsy or DNA analysis. Type I, acute infantile spinal muscular atrophy, also called Werdnig-Hoffman disease, is a fatal condition that appears in children who are age 6 months or younger. Global weakness in the extremities, loss of deep tendon reflexes, and characteristic tongue fasciculations are followed by death from respiratory complications within the first 2 years of life. Type II, chronic infantile spinal muscular atrophy, appears between the ages of 6 months and 2 years as global muscle weakness in the extremities, especially the legs. These children may learn to sit, but they will never walk. Type III spinal muscular atrophy, or Kugelberg-Welander syndrome, is diagnosed after the age of 2 years, when proximal weakness becomes apparent. Most of these children can ambulate, although in adulthood they must use a wheelchair (**Table 4**).

Almost all patients with types II and III spinal muscular atrophy develop a progressive scoliosis with curve

6: Pediatrics

patterns similar to those seen in idiopathic scoliosis.[30] Bracing is contraindicated because of the compromised respiratory system. The timing of surgery is variable, but progressive increases in curve magnitude and stiffness are indications for spinal fusion. An anterior approach should be avoided because of the accompanying insult to the chest wall and respiratory system. Posterior spinal fusion with segmental spinal instrumentation from T1 to the pelvis has achieved good results.[31] Hip dysplasia occurs in more than half of these patients, but it is usually not symptomatic, and surgical treatment is recommended primarily for ambulatory patients.

Charcot-Marie-Tooth Disease

The hereditary motor sensory neuropathies are a group of progressive peripheral neuropathies. Charcot-Marie-Tooth (CMT) disease is the most common inherited neurologic disorder, with an incidence of 1 per 10,000 children. CMT is characterized by slowly progressing sensory loss accompanied by muscle atrophy, weakness, and diminished deep tendon reflexes. CMT disease most commonly is diagnosed during the second decade of life, when the patient develops an abnormal gait, weakness, previously unrecognized hip dysplasia, or bilateral cavovarus feet.

Type I CMT disease, the demyelinating form, affects 60% to 80% of patients with CMT. Type II, the axonal form, affects most of the remaining patients; other forms are rare. CMT disease is usually inherited in an autosomal dominant pattern, although autosomal recessive, X-linked, and sporadic incidence has been reported. Many genes can contribute to the various forms of CMT disease; the most common mutation involves the peripheral myelin protein 22 gene on chromosome 17, which results in autosomal dominant CMT disease type IA.

Hip dysplasia develops in approximately 10% of patients with CMT disease. It usually appears in the second or third decade of life as an asymptomatic condition. When pain and gait abnormalities develop, surgical treatment may be indicated. The reported likelihood of nerve injury in the operated extremity has led some to recommend intraoperative monitoring with somatosensory- or motor-evoked potentials.[32] Scoliosis (usually an idiopathic type) develops in approximately 10% of patients with CMT disease; the treatment techniques and levels of fusion are the same as those used for idiopathic scoliosis. The difficulty of neurophysiologic monitoring before and during spine surgery may necessitate the use of a wake-up test for spinal cord monitoring.

Progressive bilateral cavovarus is the most common foot deformity in patients with a hereditary motor sensory neuropathy.[33] Of all patients with bilateral cavovarus feet, 78% are diagnosed with CMT; if the patient also has a family history of CMT, the likelihood of a CMT diagnosis is 91%.[34] The classic cavovarus foot has a high arch, dropped first metatarsal, hindfoot

varus, and forefoot cavus. The lesser toes may have some degree of clawing. These problems are caused by a cascade of foot muscle weakness and, over time, joint rigidity. Patients may experience foot pain, and wearing shoes may be difficult. Treatment includes the use of orthotic devices for symptomatic treatment and an AFO for a drop foot. Plantar fascia release and tendon transfer are performed for passively correctable deformities, and osteotomy is performed for fixed bony deformities. A lateral radiograph of the foot during the Coleman block test helps in distinguishing flexible and rigid deformities of the foot. A calcaneal osteotomy should be performed for a fixed hindfoot deformity. A triple arthrodesis should be avoided, if possible.

Friedreich's Ataxia

Friedreich's ataxia, the most common cause of inherited ataxia, is autosomal recessive, with an incidence of 1 in 40,000 children. It is caused by an expanded guanine-adenosine-adenosine trinucleotide repeat in both copies of the frataxin gene on chromosome 9. Patients usually have a triad of symptoms: ataxia, spasticity, and loss of deep tendon reflexes. The condition usually appears during the second decade of life, and patients die of cardiomyopathy before 30 years of age.

Patients with Friedreich's ataxia may have equinovarus or cavovarus feet that make standing or walking difficult. Surgery can improve function and provide a stable plantigrade foot, although there is a high complication rate. Other modalities, including splinting, botulinum toxin type A injection, and physical therapy can be used to prevent or delay foot deformity.[35]

Idiopathic or long thoracolumbar scoliosis develops in 80% of patients. Bracing is generally ineffective. As is true for CMT disease, standard principles of surgical treatment should be applied, and routine fusion to the pelvis does not appear to be warranted. Cardiac clearance is crucial before surgery.

Annotated References

1. Topp M, Huusom LD, Langhoff-Roos J, et al: Multiple birth and cerebral palsy in Europe: A multicenter study. *Acta Obstet Gynecol Scand* 2004;83:548-553.

   This article defines the increased risk of multiple births. The rate of CP is four times higher with multiple births.

2. Wilson-Costello D, Friedman H, Minich N, Fanaroff AA, Hack M: Improved survival rates with increased neurodevelopmental disability for extremely low birth weight infants in the 1990s. *Pediatrics* 2005;115:997-1003.

   The researchers compared mortality and morbidity rates for preterm infants (500 g to 999 g) during two successive periods (1982 to 1989 and 1990 to 1998). They found that survival rates improved from 49% to 67% but the rate of neurologic abnormalities, including CP, increased from 16% to 25%.

3. Noonan KJ, Halliday S, Browne R, O'Brien S, Kayes K, Feinberg J: Interobserver variability of gait analysis in patients with cerebral palsy. *J Pediatr Orthop* 2003;23:279-287.

4. Palisano R, Rosenbaum P, Walter S, Russell D, Wood E, Galuppi B: Development and reliability of a system to classify gross motor function in children with cerebral palsy. *Dev Med Child Neurol* 1997;39:214-223.

5. Engel JM, Petrina TJ, Dudgeon BJ, McKearnan KA: Cerebral palsy and chronic pain: A descriptive study of children and adolescents. *Phys Occup Ther Pediatr* 2005;25:73-84.

   A structured survey of 20 youths with CP revealed that 70% experienced chronic pain on a daily or weekly basis.

6. Bachrach SJ, Kecskemethy HH, Harche HT, Lark RK, Miller F, Henderson RC: Pamidronate treatment and posttreatment bone density in children with spastic quadriplegic CP. *J Clin Densitom* 2006;9:167-174.

   Among nine patients with CP who were treated with pamidronate, bone-density Z scores improved from −3.6 to −1.7. Scores approached pretreatment levels 34 months after treatment.

7. Steenbeek D, Meester-Delver A, Becher JG, Lankhorst GJ: The effect of botulinum toxin type A treatment of the lower extremity on the level of functional abilities in children with cerebral palsy: Evaluation with goal attainment scaling. *Clin Rehabil* 2005;19:274-282.

   A single-blinded randomized study found that 9 of 11 children had significant improvement in 18 of 33 goals after treatment with botulinum toxin A.

8. Chin TY, Nattrass GR, Selber P, Graham HK: Accuracy of intramuscular injection of botulinum toxin A in juvenile cerebral palsy: A comparison between manual needle placement and placement guided by electrical stimulation. *J Pediatr Orthop* 2005;25:286-291.

   An evaluation of 1,372 injections (226 children) found that the accuracy of manual needle placement compared with that of electrical stimulation was acceptable only for injections of the gastrocnemius-soleus complex. The authors recommend using electrical stimulation or another guidance technique to aid needle placement in other muscles.

9. Engsberg JR, Ross SA, Collins DR, Park TS: Effect of selective dorsal rhizotomy in the treatment of children with cerebral palsy. *J Neurosurg* 2006;105(suppl 1):8-15.

   Carefully selected children with CP gained more strength, velocity, and gross motor function through selective dorsal rhizotomy and physical therapy than through physical therapy alone.

10. Damiano DL, Abel MF: Functional outcomes of strength training in spastic cerebral palsy. *Arch Phys Med Rehabil* 1998;79:119-125.

11. Kalen V, Conklin MM, Sherman FC: Untreated scoliosis in severe cerebral palsy. *J Pediatr Orthop* 1992;12:337-340.

12. McCarthy JJ, Dandrea L, Clements D, Betz R: The evaluation and treatment of scoliosis in the child with cerebral palsy. *J Am Acad Orthop Surg* 2006;14:367-375.

    The article presents a general review of the assessment and treatment of scoliosis in children with CP.

13. Teli MG, Cinnella P, Vincitorio F, Lovi A, Grava G, Brayda-Bruno M: Spinal fusion with Cortrel-Dubousset instrumentation for neuropathic scoliosis in patients with cerebral palsy. *Spine* 2006;31:E441-E447.

    The use of segmental, third-generation instrumentation for spinal fusion resulted in lasting correction of spinal deformity, improved quality of life, and a lower pseudo-arthrosis rate (compared with reports of older techniques).

14. Durufle A, Petrilli S, Le Guiet JL, et al: Cervical spondylotic myelopathy in athetoid cerebral palsy patients: About five cases. *Joint Bone Spine* 2005;72:270-274.

    Athetoid CP developed in five patients with spondyloid cervical myelopathy. The diagnosis was often overlooked because of the underlying neurologic condition and its slow progression.

15. Soo B, Howard JJ, Boyd RN, et al: Hip displacement in cerebral palsy. *J Bone Joint Surg Am* 2006;88:121-129.

    In 323 children with CP, the overall incidence of hip dysplasia was 35%; hip dysplasia affected no Gross Motor Function Classification System level I patients, but it affected 90% of level V patients.

16. Noonan KJ, Jones J, Pierson J, Honkamp NJ, Leverson G: Hip function in adults with severe cerebral palsy. *J Bone Joint Surg Am* 2004;86-A:2607-2613.

    Neither hip subluxation-dislocation nor osteoarthrosis was associated with hip pain or decreased function in adults profoundly affected by CP. Level of evidence: Prognostic level II-1.

17. Westberry DE, Davids JR, Jacobs JM, Pugh LI, Tanner SL: Effectiveness of serial stretch casting for resistant or recurrent knee flexion contractures following hamstring lengthening in children with cerebral palsy. *J Pediatr Orthop* 2006;26:109-114.

    In this study of 46 children with CP, the mean flexion contracture decreased from 17.6° to 8.1° after 30 days of casting.

18. Ma FY, Selber P, Nattrass GR, Harvey AR, Wolfe R, Graham HK: Lengthening and transfer of hamstrings for a flexion deformity of the knee in children with bilateral cerebral palsy: Technique and preliminary results. *J Bone Joint Surg Br* 2006;88:248-254.

    The authors describe their technique for hamstring transfer and the resulting improvements in gait after the surgery.

19. Karol LA: Surgical management of the lower extremity in ambulatory children with CP. *J Am Acad Orthop Surg* 2004;12:196-203.

    This article presents a comprehensive review of surgical assessment and management of the lower extremity in children with CP.

20. Michlitsch MG, Rethlefsen SA, Kay RM: The contributions of anterior and posterior tibialis dysfunction to varus foot deformity in patients with cerebral palsy. *J Bone Joint Surg Am* 2006;88:1764-1768.

    In this study of 78 patients with CP (88 feet), the muscular contributor to varus deformity was found to be the anterior tibialis in 30 feet, the posterior tibialis in 29, both in 27, and another contributor in 2.

21. Morrow JD, Kelsey K: Folic acid for prevention of neural tube defects: Pediatric anticipatory guidance. *J Pediatr Health Care* 1998;12:55-59.

22. Davis BE, Daley CM, Shurtleff DB, et al: Long-term survival of individuals with myelomeningocele. *Pediatr Neurosurg* 2005;41:186-191.

    The probability of survival to 16 years was 85%, with no significant survival difference between patients with a shunt and those without. The probability of survival at age 34 years was less for those with a shunt (75% versus 94%).

23. Kirk VG, Morielli A, Brouillette RT: Sleep-disordered breathing in patients with myelomeningocele: The missed diagnosis. *Dev Med Child Neurol* 1999;41:40-43.

24. Tulipan N: Intrauterine closure of myelomeningocele: An update. *Neurosurg Focus* 2004;16:E2.

    This article presents a review of the benefits and risks of intrauterine closure of myelomeningocele.

25. Flynn JM, Herrera-Soto JA, Ramirez NF, Fernandez-Feliberti R, Vilella F, Guzman J: Clubfoot release in myelodysplasia. *J Pediatr Orthop B* 2004;13:259-262.

    Seventy-two clubfeet were treated by an extensive posteromedial release including tenotomy, without internal fixation. After 8 years, the results were graded as good (62.5%), fair (25%), or poor (12.5%). No relationship was found between outcome and functional motor level or age.

26. Guille JT, Sarwark JF, Sherk HH, Kumar SJ: Congenital and developmental deformities of the spine in children with myelomeningocele. *J Am Acad Orthop Surg* 2006; 14:294-302.

    This article is a comprehensive review of spinal deformity in patients with myelomeningocele.

27. Akbar M, Bremer R, Thomsen M, et al: Kyphectomy in children with myelodysplasia: Results 1994-2004. *Spine* 2006;31:1007-1013.

    Twenty-four pediatric patients were treated with the Warner and Fackler technique (mean age, 7.6 years). After 3 years, the mean improvement in kyphosis was from 124° to 48°. Sitting balance was improved, although complications were frequent.

28. Alman BA, Raza SN, Biggar WD: Steroid treatment and the development of scoliosis in males with Duchenne muscular dystrophy. *J Bone Joint Surg Am* 2004;86: 519-524.

    Thirty of 54 boys with Duchenne muscular dystrophy (7 to 10 years of age) were treated with deflazacort. Scoliosis developed in 67% of the untreated patients and 17% of the treated patients. Level of evidence: Therapeutic level II-1.

29. Diab M, Darras BT, Shapiro F: Scapulothoracic fusion for facioscapulohumeral muscular dystrophy. *J Bone Joint Surg Am* 2005;87:2267-2275.

    This study of 11 patients found that fixation of the scapula to the chest wall improved shoulder flexion and abduction, improved cosmesis, and decreased pain. Level of evidence: Therapeutic level IV.

30. Kouwenhoven JW, Van Ommeren P, Pruijs HE, Castelein RM: Spinal decompensation in neuromuscular scoliosis. *Spine* 2006;31:E188-E191.

    In a group of patients with Duchenne muscular dystrophy, CP, spinal muscular atrophy, and spina bifida, right-sided thoracic and thoracolumbar curves or left-sided lumbar curves predominated.

31. Wimmer C, Wallnofer P, Walochnik N, Krismer M, Saraph V: Comparative evaluation of Luque and Isola instrumentation for treatment of neuromuscular scoliosis. *Clin Orthop Relat Res* 2005;439:181-192.

    The Luque-Galveston and Isola instrumentation techniques yielded similar results for scoliosis, lumbar sagittal, and pelvic obliquity correction, as well as complication rate.

32. Chan G, Bowen JR, Kumar SJ: Evaluation and treatment of hip dysplasia in Charcot-Marie-Tooth disease. *Orthop Clin North Am* 2006;37:203-209.

    The authors present an excellent review of hip dysplasia in CMT disease based on 20 years of experience.

33. Wines AP, Chen D, Lynch B, Stephens MM: Foot deformities in children with hereditary motor and sensory neuropathy. *J Pediatr Orthop* 2005;25:241-244.

    A study of 104 feet of 52 patients with a hereditary motor sensory neuropathy found cavovarus in 66% of the feet, planovalgus in 22%, and no deformity in 12%. All deformities were bilateral. Level of evidence: Therapeutic level IV.

34. Nagai MK, Chan G, Guille JT, Kumar SJ, Scavina M, Mackenzie W: Prevalence of Charcot-Marie-Tooth disease in patients who have bilateral cavovarus feet. *J Pediatr Orthop* 2006;26:438-443.

    A chart review found a 78% probability that a patient with bilateral cavovarus feet would be diagnosed with CMT disease.

35. Delatycki MB, Holian A, Corben L, et al: Surgery of equinovarus deformity in Friedreich's ataxia improves mobility and independence. *Clin Orthop Relat Res* 2005;430:138-141.

Active prevention and aggressive treatment of estab-lished foot deformity resulted in improved quality of life and independence in 36 patients with Friedreich's ataxia. Level of evidence: Therapeutic level IV.

6: Pediatrics

Chapter 65

Pediatric Tumors, Infections, and Hematologic Diseases

Mark C. Gebhardt, MD   Megan E. Anderson, MD   Samantha A. Spencer, MD

Benign Bone Tumors

Most patients with benign bone tumors present with pain. In children, pain-related symptoms are not always clear and can include development of a limp or decreased use of the limb, scoliosis related to muscle spasm, fracture, or gigantism in a digit. The pain of a benign tumor is often worse with activity and weight bearing because of the bone's weakened structure and, except for osteoid osteoma, is infrequent at night or at rest. There may be no response to the usual nonsurgical treatment for traumatic injuries, such as rest and ice application. Patient age is an important factor in narrowing the differential diagnosis. Physical examination may be normal with the exception of point tenderness in the area of the lesion or deformity related to pathologic fracture. The diagnosis can often be made based on the plain radiograph alone. Benign lesions are geographic and frequently have a thin sclerotic rim. They may thin the cortex and even slowly expand it, but usually the periosteum will be intact, with no associated soft-tissue mass. Treatment ranges from observation for inactive lesions to curettage and grafting or even resection for more aggressive lesions.

Bone-Forming Tumors

Osteoid Osteoma

Although most common in adolescence, osteoid osteoma may present in children of any age. This tumor is more common in boys and, although it can be found in any bone, approximately 50% are located in the tibia and femur. The tumor incites a marked inflammatory response presumably because of the production of prostaglandins. The result is a significant amount of pain that is sharp, boring, independent of activity, and worse at night; this pain responds to aspirin and nonsteroidal anti-inflammatory drugs (NSAIDs). Plain radiographs may only show marked sclerosis with a smooth fusiform shape. CT is the optimal imaging modality for this tumor; fine cuts are likely to demonstrate a nidus of less than 1 cm (**Figure 1**). Interpretation of MRI studies may be confusing because there is usually extensive edema about the lesion. Bone scans show a

focal area of increased uptake. Observation is a reasonable option for these lesions; they will "burn out" without treatment, although that may take several years. Surgical excision may result in significant morbidity in searching for the true nidus and reconstructing the bony defect. Radiofrequency ablation has become much more widely used with success rates that are comparable to excision and very low morbidity.[1]

Osteoblastoma

Osteoblastoma is much less common than osteoid osteoma. It is a larger tumor (> 2 cm) but has histologic findings similar to osteoid osteoma. Patients are often adolescents or young adults, with more males than females affected. These tumors are most frequently found in the posterior elements of the spine, but also can be present in the metadiaphyseal regions of long bones. Presentation is similar to that of osteoid osteoma, but these tumors do not respond well to NSAIDs. Neurologic symptoms are more common, likely because of this tumor's larger size and spinal location. Imaging reveals an expansile lesion that may be radiolucent, radiodense, or mixed and around which the periosteum is intact. A significant inflammatory reaction with edema on an MRI and uptake on a bone scan is often present. These lesions can be hard to differentiate from osteosarcoma histologically. Because of that and the tendency

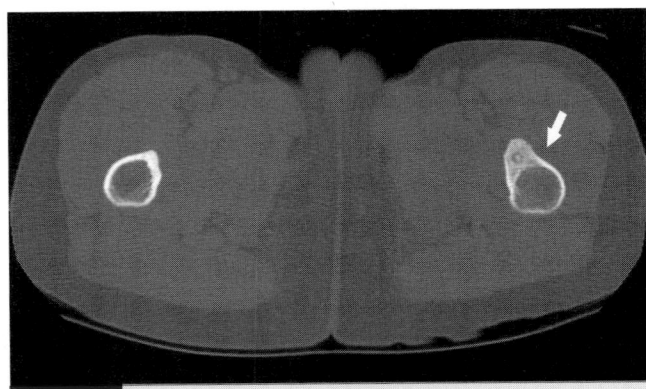

| Figure 1 | Axial CT scan of the femur of an 8-year-old child shows the radiolucent nidus and surrounding sclerosis of an osteoid osteoma. |

6: Pediatrics

for recurrence of the lesion, complete excision with aggressive curettage or resection of an involved expendable bone is recommended. Careful pathologic analysis of the entire lesion can then be performed.

Cartilage-Forming Tumors

Chondroblastoma

Most often occurring in the second decade of life, chondroblastomas are uncommon tumors that present in children around the time of physeal closure. They are most often seen in the distal femur and proximal tibia, proximal humerus, and proximal femur where they are notable for their epiphyseal location. These tumors often cause significant pain and restricted motion of the neighboring joint. Radiographs show a radiolucent lesion in the epiphysis that may have fine stippled calcification within it; the lesion can range from a subtle geographic abnormality with a sclerotic rim to an expansile lesion covered by intact periosteum only. MRI reveals a significant amount of reactive edema. CT will often show a thin rim of intact cortex or periosteum in an expanded appearance around the lesion. A bone scan will show intense uptake. These lesions are quite active, requiring extensive curettage with adjuvant therapy with agents such as phenol or liquid nitrogen. Excision and reconstruction of the defect may be challenging because of the proximity of the joint surface and the physis. Recurrence can be as high as 20% and is associated with incomplete removal of the tumor, especially in younger patients in whom curettage may not be as aggressive in an effort to avoid growth disturbance.[2] However, because so many of these patients are near skeletal maturity, the open physis is not necessarily a significant cause for concern.[3] Some of these lesions (1% or less) are very aggressive and may even develop pulmonary metastases, which occurs most frequently in patients who have had a local recurrence that indicates a more aggressive natural biology.[3] Many such patients succumb to their disease, in contrast with patients with metastatic deposits of giant cell tumor.[2,3]

Chondromyxoid Fibroma

Chondromyxoid fibroma is a very rare tumor with a high rate of local recurrence but no associated metastatic potential. Patients are usually between the ages of 10 and 30 years. Lesions are purely radiolucent and located eccentrically in the metaphyseal regions of predominantly the distal femur, proximal tibia, and distal tibia as well as the pelvis. The cortex is often thinned and the lesions can be mildly expansile with a "soap bubble" appearance. Extended curettage with the addition of adjuvant therapy and bone grafting is the most common treatment method, and is associated with a recurrence rate of 25% to 30%.[4]

Osteochondroma

Also called osteocartilaginous exostosis, this lesion is exophytic, projecting from the surface of a bone and away from the neighboring joint. These lesions are common and occur most often in children in the second decade of life. The most common locations are the metaphyses of the femur, tibia, and humerus, but pelvic and scapular locations are also common sites. These lesions share the medullary cavity with the bone from which they originate, and the normal cortex is continuous with the cortex of the lesion. A cap of mature hyaline cartilage and perichondrium is present on the outer aspect of the lesion and it appears similar to a normal growth plate on microscopic examination. This cap will grow as long as the child is still growing, and may become quite thick. Growth, new pain, or an irregular, thick (greater than 1.5 cm is often used as a parameter) cartilage cap after skeletal maturity may indicate malignant transformation; this is an extremely rare development, occurring in fewer than 1% of patients with solitary osteochondromas. Most osteochondromas can be observed unless they are painful or fracture occurs. Symptomatic lesions can be excised with predictably good results. Excision involves removing the osteochondroma at its base, flush with the normal bone, and the entire cartilage cap and perichondrium; recurrence is uncommon.

Multiple hereditary exostoses is an autosomal dominant disorder with variable penetrance. Affected patients may have just a few isolated osteochondromas and no skeletal deformities and others may have lesions from every bone, with associated skeletal deformities and short stature.[5] Mutations in the EXT1 and EXT2 genes, which encode glycoproteins involved in endochondral ossification, occur in most patients with this disorder. Beyond the skeletal deformities that may require corrective surgery, these patients also may require closer surveillance and intervention because of a higher risk of malignant transformation (approximately a 3% lifetime risk).[5]

Enchondroma/Chondroma

Enchondromas are tumors of hyaline cartilage in the intramedullary cavity of a bone and periosteal chondromas on the surface. Enchondromas are more commonly present in adulthood, and are discussed in more detail in chapter 17. In children, periosteal chondromas occur particularly in the humerus and small tubular bones of the hand. These tumors appear similar histologically, with mature hyaline cartilage arranged in a lobular configuration, except that periosteal chondromas tend to be more cellular than enchondromas.

Enchondromatosis takes the form of two genetic but not familial conditions: Ollier's disease and Maffucci's syndrome. In the former, patients have multiple enchondromas predominantly in the metaphyses of long bones, skeletal deformities, limb-length discrepancies, and are of short stature. Maffucci's syndrome has similar characteristics, but these patients also may have multiple vascular lesions. Most patients present early in life with these clinical findings. Efforts to determine the molecular defect causing these syndromes have not yet been successful, but it is presumed to be an abnormal signaling pathway in the cartilage cell. The enchondromas tend to be larger and more expansile than isolated lesions. Histologically, the cartilage is more cellular with some pleomorphism and atypia noted. Orthopaedic surgical intervention is often necessary for the deformities and these patients require lifetime follow-up for malignant transformation. The risk for malignant transformation is approximately 3% to 5% in patients with Ollier's disease. The risk of malignancy is higher in patients with Maffucci's syndrome and may involve not only chondrosarcomas, but also vascular and other malignancies.

Fibrous Tumors

Nonossifying Fibroma
Most nonossifying fibromas are discovered as incidental findings. Occasionally, they can be large enough to place the bone at risk for pathologic fracture and cause mechanical pain. The radiographic appearance (**Figure 2**) is diagnostic and demonstrates a purely radiolucent lesion that is eccentrically located in the metaphysis of a long bone. The cortex can be thinned and gently expanded, and there is a rim of dense bone around the periphery of the lesion. Most lesions can be observed without treatment because they will heal over time. It can sometimes be difficult to predict which lesions are at risk for pathologic fracture and thus warrant surgical intervention. According to a recent study, quantitative CT for biomechanical modeling has allowed greater accuracy in predicting fracture risk.[6] With these lesions, curettage and grafting has a high success rate and is associated with a low rate of recurrence.

Osteofibrous Dysplasia
Osteofibrous dysplasia, also known as Campanacci's disease, occurs commonly in the anterior cortex of the tibia in children in the first decade of life and may cause bowing, pathologic fracture, and/or pain. The lesions may be multiple along the tibia and may also involve the ipsilateral fibula. Radiographically, the cortex is focally expanded in a smooth lobular pattern with a radiolucent lesion and surrounding sclerosis beneath. The course of osteofibrous dysplasia is somewhat unpredictable: some patients have no change in their lesions over many years, some lesions spontaneously regress, and others become aggressive locally. This aggressive form is difficult to differentiate from adamantinoma and is discussed in chapter 17. Surgery or prophylactic bracing may be indicated for persistent symptoms or pathologic fracture. Surgical procedures most often require resection of part of the bone and reconstruction, as recurrence rates are quite high with curettage alone.

Fibrous Dysplasia
Fibrous dysplasia can be monostotic or polyostotic. In the latter form, it usually predominates in one half of the skeleton and may be associated with McCune-

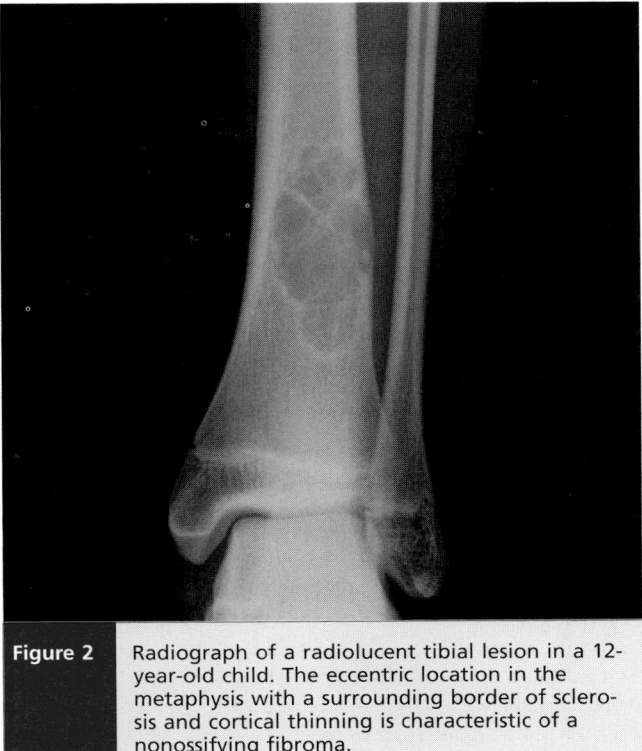

Figure 2 Radiograph of a radiolucent tibial lesion in a 12-year-old child. The eccentric location in the metaphysis with a surrounding border of sclerosis and cortical thinning is characteristic of a nonossifying fibroma.

Albright syndrome (café-au-lait spots, endocrine abnormalities). Deformity and pain are believed to be the result of multiple nondisplaced fractures and are more common in polyostotic fibrous dysplasia. Radiographically, fibrous dysplasia lesions are described as having a "ground glass" appearance, although they also may have areas of cyst formation. Endosteal scalloping and cortical expansion are usually present, and these long lesions tend to occur in the long bones. The dysplastic osteoblasts have a mutation in the α subunit of the stimulatory G protein.[7] Observation is reasonable for most small, asymptomatic lesions, but curettage and grafting with prophylactic fixation may be necessary for painful lesions with deformity or impending pathologic fracture, especially in the lower extremity. In patients with polyostotic fibrous dysplasia, bisphosphonates have been helpful to reduce fracture rates and bone pain, and increase radiographic healing.[8]

Cystic Lesions

Unicameral Bone Cyst
Unicameral bone cysts are common in skeletally immature patients who usually present for treatment of pathologic fractures. The proximal femur and proximal humerus are predominant locations for unicameral bone cysts. These fluid-filled cysts are usually asymptomatic until the patient experiences a pathologic fracture. Radiographs show a radiolucent lesion centrally located in the metaphysis (**Figure 3**). The cortex is often

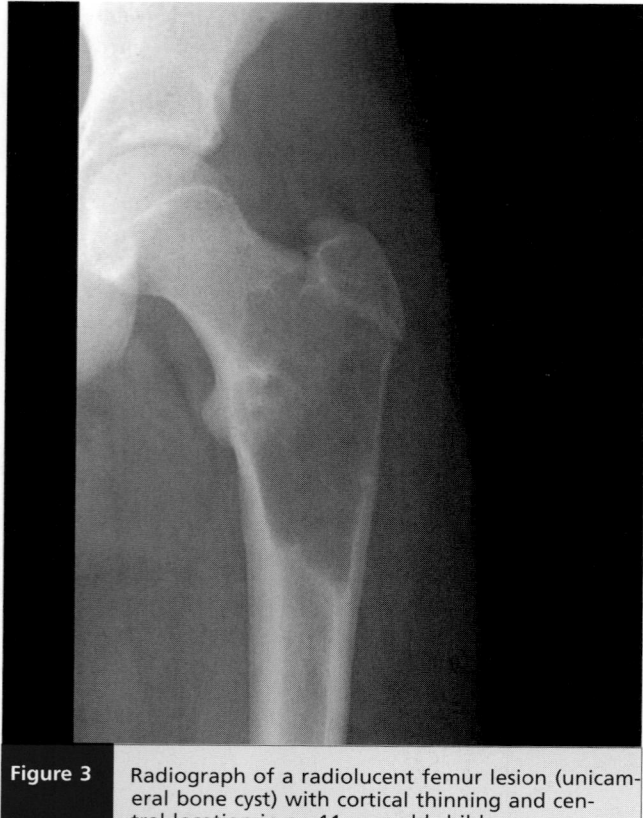

Figure 3 Radiograph of a radiolucent femur lesion (unicameral bone cyst) with cortical thinning and central location in an 11-year-old child.

though aneurysmal bone cysts were originally believed to be reactive lesions, recent research has demonstrated recurrent cytogenetic abnormalities that result in the upregulation of the ubiquitin protease *USP6* gene.[10] Most patients are younger than age 20 years and have pain from the lesion and also from mechanical symptoms related to weakening of the bone. Aneurysmal bone cysts are eccentric metaphyseal lesions that are radiolucent, often with thin, fibrous septae containing bone. The periphery of the cyst usually has a thin periosteal rim that may or may not be mineralized. These cysts expand the cortex beyond the limit of the width of the physis and can have a "blown-out" appearance because of cortical thinning. MRI and CT can be used to show intact periosteum and no true soft-tissue mass. Fluid-fluid levels are also seen on MRI scans of these blood-filled lesions, but they are not pathognomonic (telangiectatic osteosarcoma and unicameral bone cysts are examples of other lesions that can also have fluid-fluid levels). Aneurysmal bone cysts may also be secondary to other lesions such as chondroblastomas, osteoblastomas, giant cell tumors, and even osteosarcomas. Aneurysmal bone cysts are locally aggressive lesions that most often require open treatment. Aggressive curettage with adjuvant therapy and bone grafting is most commonly used, but is associated with a recurrence rate of approximately 20%. In lesions that are difficult to approach surgically, such as those in the spine and pelvis, percutaneous injection of sclerosing agents or demineralized bone matrix with bone marrow aspirate has been used with success.[11,12] Radiation has also been used for control of large unresectable or recurrent lesions but is best avoided because of the risk of secondary malignancy.[13]

extremely thin, but the lesion is usually not wider than the neighboring physis. Treatment involves first allowing the fracture to heal; however, the unicameral bone cyst will persist in most instances. Many of these cysts still also present a risk for pathologic fracture; quantitative CT can be a useful tool to assess fracture risk in questionable or incidentally discovered cysts.[6] Surgical intervention can involve open curettage and grafting, aspiration of fluid, and injection with steroid, demineralized bone matrix, bone marrow aspirate, and/or various combinations of these substances, and many other approaches including elastic intramedullary nail fixation to prompt cyst healing and bone stabilization.[9] No single approach has proved to be optimal. Several fillers have been described, including steroid, demineralized bone matrix, bone marrow aspirate, calcium sulfate, and various combinations of these materials. The lower morbidity of aspiration and injection, with healing rates that can be comparable to the open procedure, lead many surgeons to recommend this procedure as the first-line surgical treatment. However, curettage and bone grafting is usually recommended for very large lesions, lesions with displaced pathologic fractures that require open reduction, and multiple recurrent lesions.

Aneurysmal Bone Cyst
Aneurysmal bone cysts are less common than unicameral bone cysts, and tend to be more aggressive. Al-

Other Benign Bone Lesions

Langerhans Cell Histiocytosis
Langerhans cell histiocytosis, previously called eosinophilic granuloma, includes a wide spectrum of diseases. Patients may have isolated or multiple bone lesions, multiple granulomas with diabetes insipidus and exophthalmos (Hand-Schüller-Christian disease), or aggressive phagocytic syndromes such as Letterer-Siwe disease. Although Langerhans cell histiocytosis with bone involvement alone occurs in children of all ages, affected patients tend to be very young (age 1 to 5 years) and report pain or pathologic fracture. The most common location for a bone lesion is the skull, but the femur, tibia, ribs, vertebrae (often presenting as vertebra plana), scapula, and mandible are also frequently involved. Isolated bone lesions often heal after pathologic fracture and will also heal in response to an injection of steroid. Curettage alone is also often successful, but not usually required. Multifocal or multisystem disease may warrant medical treatment with systemic steroids and/or chemotherapy.

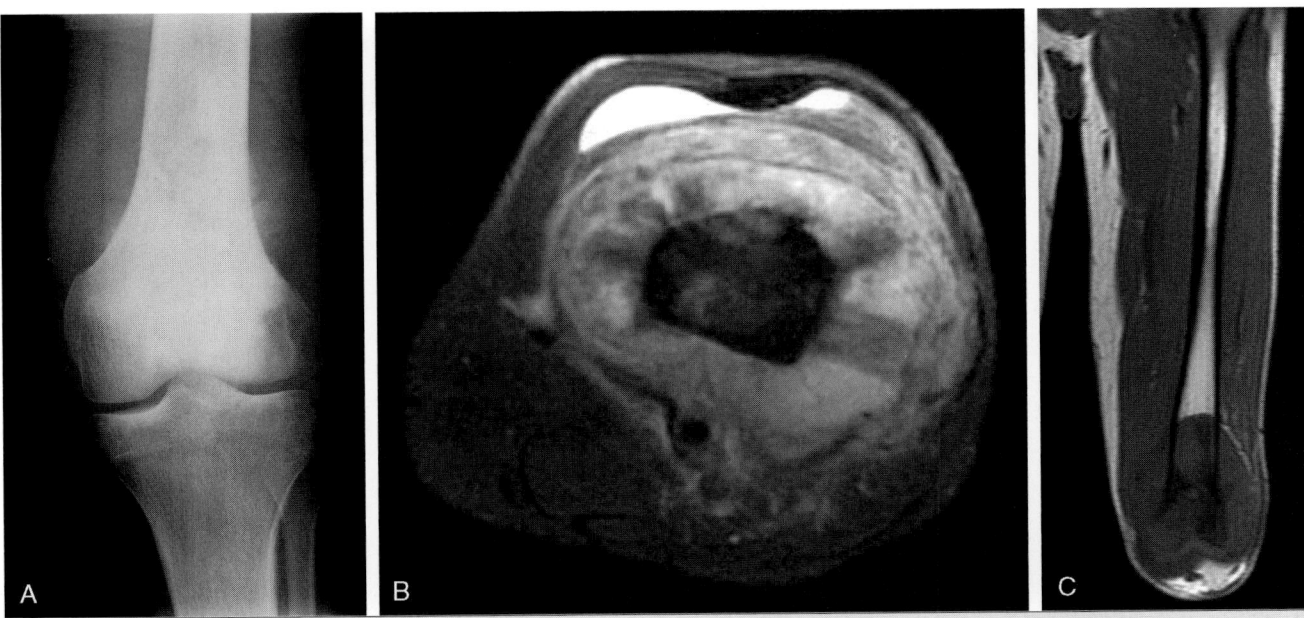

Figure 4 **A,** Radiograph of a painful lesion in the distal femur of a 17-year-old patient shows mixed radiolucent and radiodense areas and aggressive periosteal new bone formation. **B,** The T2-weighted axial MRI scan with fat saturation technique reveals the large, circumferential, associated soft-tissue mass that abuts the vessels posteriorly. **C,** The coronal T1-weighted MRI scan (**C**) includes the entire femur to allow evaluation of the extent of intramedullary disease (this is hypointense compared with the hyperintense normal marrow fat) and skip metastases.

Malignant Bone Tumors

Malignant bone tumors in children are uncommon, but primary sarcomas are more common than metastatic bone disease. The most frequent presenting symptom is pain. Worrisome characteristics include pain at rest or at night, pain independent of activity level, and pain that is gradually worsening or severe. A good principle is that extremity pain that does not resolve or worsens in a child should be evaluated to exclude the possibility of a tumor. Occasionally, the presence of a mass also prompts medical evaluation, but this is almost always in association with pain. Patients are usually otherwise healthy and do not appear ill, with the exception of some patients with Ewing's sarcoma and patients with leukemia who have a bone lesion. Laboratory studies may show elevation of alkaline phosphatase and lactate dehydrogenase levels. Imaging studies should always begin with a plain radiograph. Malignant bone lesions typically do not have sharp borders and are described as permeative. Aggressive periosteal reaction is often apparent in the form of "onion-skinning," sunburst appearance, and Codman triangles. The cortex may be destroyed in areas, and tumor may extend outside of the bone as a soft-tissue mass. MRI of the primary tumor should include the entire bone to evaluate for skip metastases, resectability, and joint involvement. The soft-tissue mass is more evident as are vital neurovascular structures, so MRI is relied on heavily for surgical planning. Staging should include a CT of the chest and a bone scan, because the lungs and other bones are the most common sites, respectively, for metastasis of pri-

mary bone sarcomas. Positron emission tomography (PET) currently is not used routinely, although the indications for its use will likely expand to staging of sarcomas; it may be preferable to a bone scan in determining sites of metastatic disease and response to preoperative chemotherapy.[14] Biopsy should be approached in a manner so that the tumor tract can be excised with definitive surgery, which requires careful planning and a multidisciplinary team.[15] Open biopsy offers the advantage of having more tissue for review, but advances in percutaneous needle biopsy techniques have resulted in greater reliability and less morbidity than an open biopsy.

Osteosarcoma

Osteosarcoma is a highly malignant spindle cell sarcoma in which the sarcoma cells directly produce osteoid or bone. It is more common in male adolescents,[16] but there is a second peak in incidence in males and females between the ages of 60 and 70 years (believed to be caused by Paget's osteosarcoma). Lesions are most commonly located in the metaphyses of long bones, particularly around the knee, and often have areas of radiodensity admixed with areas of radiolucency on radiographs (**Figure 4**). Although 10% to 20% of patients have gross evidence of metastases at presentation, all patients with osteosarcoma should be considered as having micrometastatic disease. The discovery of effective chemotherapy has had the most significant effect on survival rate, which now approaches 70%. Doxorubicin, high-dose methotrexate, and cisplatin are used most frequently, and ifosfamide is currently under fur-

6: Pediatrics

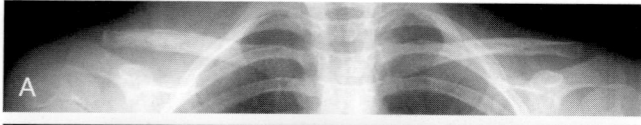

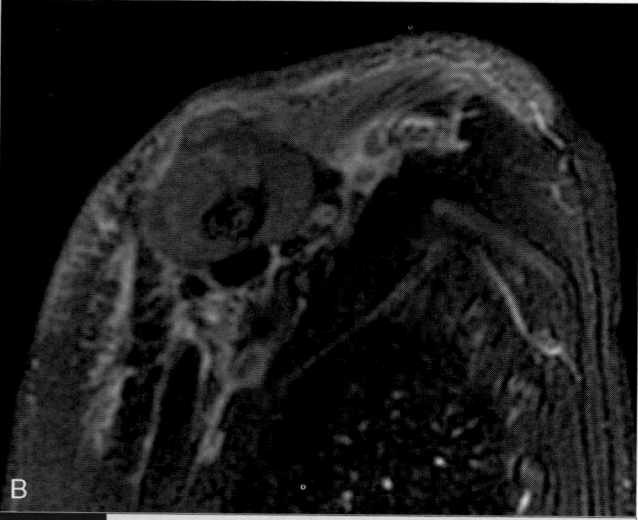

Figure 5	**A,** Radiograph of the shoulders of a 6-year-old patient with right shoulder pain shows a permeative lesion with aggressive periosteal reaction in the right clavicle, which is notably asymmetric from the left. **B,** The sagittal T2-weighted MRI scan with fat saturation shows the associated extension of the tumor as a circumferential soft-tissue mass.

common). This results in a novel gene whose protein product is a transcription factor, EWS/FLI1. Patients range in age from 5 to 30 years, are more often male and Caucasian than female and nonwhite.[16] Ewing's sarcoma is more common in the long bones, such as the pelvis, ribs, spine, scapula and clavicle, where it is most often diaphyseal (**Figure 5**). Imaging reveals a permeative lesion, usually in association with a large soft-tissue mass. The most common site of metastasis is the lung and other bones, but unlike osteosarcoma, Ewing's sarcoma may also metastasize to the bone marrow. Thus, bone marrow biopsy is part of the staging. All patients with Ewing's sarcoma also are considered to have micrometastatic disease. Before chemotherapy, the condition was almost universally fatal. Current survival rates reach approximately 60% to 80% after treatment with doxorubicin, vincristine, actinomycin D, cyclophosphamide, and ifosfamide/etoposide along with adequate local control.[18] Surgery and/or radiation are used for local control of the primary tumor. Surgery is favored if there is a good chance of obtaining negative margins because the risk of secondary malignancy and other complications associated with radiation are avoided. Chemotherapy is administered before local control (neoadjuvant chemotherapy) because it often results in a dramatic decrease in the size of the soft-tissue mass, making limb salvage or resection at other sites more feasible. Survival rates reach approximately 70% to 80% for nonmetastatic disease, and 10% to 20% with metastatic disease. Negative prognostic factors include the presence of metastatic disease (lung metastasis only is better than other sites such as bone marrow or another bone), high lactate dehydrogenase levels that do not decrease with the use of chemotherapy, residual viable tumor in the resected specimen after neoadjuvant chemotherapy, pelvis location, large tumor size, and age older than 10 years.[19] Bone marrow transplant and other drugs including targeted therapy for the EWS-FLI1 fusion product and CD99 are under investigation.

Surgery

Surgery for primary sarcomas of bone is done using either a wide resection (removing the tumor, the reactive zone, and a cuff of normal tissue) or radical resection (removing the tumor and the entire compartment(s) it involves). Both limb salvage and amputation techniques are used. If resection can be performed with a margin of normal tissue around the tumor and with sparing of the neurovascular bundle, limb salvage is usually possible. In this scenario, various methods such as autograft, allograft, metal prostheses, and combinations thereof are used to reconstruct the defect. Each of these methods has associated risks including nonunion, fracture, infection, prosthetic wear and loosening, and the need for further surgery.[20,21] In growing children, future limb-length inequality may present a unique challenge. Contralateral epiphysiodesis is reasonable in older children. In the youngest patients, amputation may be a better alternative. Rotationplasty is a reasonable option

ther investigation. Patients who do not respond to standard chemotherapy or those who relapse have a poorer prognosis than those who have a good histologic response to currently available chemotherapy agents.[17] Surgical resection of the primary tumor is most often done after two or three cycles of chemotherapy have been administered. This offers the advantage of determining response to chemotherapy by estimating the percentage of necrosis in the resected tumor and possibly then changing the postoperative drug regimen. It is also believed to increase the safety of limb-salvage surgery. Negative prognostic factors are metastatic disease (at presentation is worse than late relapse), axial location, large tumor size, presence of skip metastases, pathologic fracture, less than 90% tumor necrosis, and elevated alkaline phosphatase and lactate dehydrogenase levels. Rate of survival is approximately 60% to 80% for patients with nonmetastatic disease and 10% to 20% for patients with metastatic disease at presentation. Complete excision of all of the metastatic disease, if possible, will improve the patient's prognosis.

Ewing's Sarcoma

Ewing's sarcoma is the second most common malignant bone tumor in children. The histogenesis remains uncertain (possibly neuronal), but cytogenetic evaluation has revealed a consistent reciprocal translocation t(11;22) in most tumors (other translocations are less

for very young patients with lower extremity sarcomas; it allows a longer stump for better prosthetic limb function and some continued growth from the remaining physis.[22] The technology for expandable prostheses has now improved so that they are another option for very young children. Most of these prostheses involve mechanical lengthening through a percutaneous incision, but some can be lengthened noninvasively using electromagnetic waves.[23] Long-term studies are underway.

Soft-Tissue Tumors

Most patients with a soft-tissue tumor present simply with a lump. Benign tumors tend to be painless and may enlarge very slowly. Malignant tumors tend to enlarge with time, although some, such as synovial sarcoma, can have a very indolent presentation. Mild trauma often brings the tumor to the attention of the patient or parent and may sometimes confound the presenting symptoms. Radiographs may show the soft-tissue shadow of the mass, fat density in lipomas, phleboliths in vascular malformations, and calcification in myositis ossificans. Approximately 15% to 20% of synovial sarcomas have calcification within them. Ultrasound is helpful to demonstrate flow in vascular malformations, and solid or cystic quality of the tumor. It is also helpful to follow the size of a soft-tissue mass over time to aid in needle biopsy of a soft-tissue lesion. MRI is the gold standard for soft-tissue imaging because it allows detailed examination of the mass and of the normal anatomy around the mass. MRI is thus essential in the staging of all soft-tissue sarcomas, and can be diagnostic of particular tumors such as lipomas and pigmented villonodular synovitis. However, most soft-tissue masses are nonspecifically hypointense on T1-weighted sequences and hyperintense on T2-weighted images. The administration of gadolinium may help distinguish a more concerning enhancing mass from a nonenhancing benign mass or hematoma. The only advantage of CT over MRI is in demonstrating mineralization within a soft-tissue mass or pulmonary metastases in the staging for soft-tissue sarcomas. PET is now being used more frequently in the staging of soft-tissue sarcomas, in determining response to adjuvant treatment, and as a surveillance tool for local recurrence.[24]

Benign Soft-Tissue Tumors

Lipoma

Lipomas are the most common soft-tissue tumor overall, but are less common in children. They are benign collections of adipocytes and can be seen in the subcutaneous tissues or muscle. Lipoblastomas are also included in the differential diagnosis for fatty tumors in infants. Histologically, these tumors differ from standard lipomas in their cellular immaturity and local recurrence. Observation and marginal excision are treatment options for these tumors.

Vascular Malformation

These are the most common benign soft-tissue tumors in children. These lesions can be superficial or deep, small or very large, and consist of capillaries, arteries, veins, lymphatic vessels, or combinations of these. The superficial hemangioma tends to appear just after birth, grows rapidly, and then involutes over time, usually not requiring treatment. Larger vascular malformations are usually present from birth and do not typically regress, but do not become noticeable until they grow in proportion to the child and become more prominent. Superficial capillary lesions usually present as port-wine stains and are often treated with laser therapy. Arterial, venous, and lymphatic malformations are deeper and can become very large. They can be observed if they are asymptomatic, or excised or treated with sclerotherapy or embolization if they are large or symptomatic. Surgery may be challenging because of the difficulty in differentiating tumor from normal muscle and the potential for substantial intraoperative blood loss. A wide margin is advisable because recurrence rates are high.

Aggressive Fibromatosis

Also known as extra-abdominal desmoid tumors, these are aggressive but nonmetastatic lesions usually seen in older children and adults to approximately 40 years of age. These are usually deep masses along a fascial plane with microscopic invasion of neighboring muscle and fat tissue that can extend much beyond the palpable or visualized mass. Wide excision is indicated, but even so, is associated with a high rate of recurrence. Because of the risk of secondary malignancy, radiation in children is used only in selected patients when surgical resection is not possible or in recurrent disease. Low-dose vinblastine and methotrexate are also used in this scenario or when there are multiple areas of involvement in the same limb.

Malignant Soft-Tissue Tumors

Rhabdomyosarcoma

Rhabdomyosarcoma is the most common soft-tissue malignancy in children. There are several subtypes, but in the extremity, only alveolar and embryonal rhabdomyosarcoma are encountered. The alveolar subtype is more common in an extremity location and carries a worse prognosis overall than the embryonal subtype. Alveolar rhabdomyosarcoma has specific chromosomal translocations: t(2;13) or t(1;13) resulting in PAX3-FKHR or PAC7-FKHR fusion products, respectively. The former carries a worse prognosis than the latter.[25] Most patients are younger than 10 years; patients with the alveolar subtype are adolescents.

Much like osteosarcoma and Ewing's sarcoma, patients with rhabdomyosarcoma are considered to have micrometastatic disease at presentation. Overall survival for rhabdomyosarcoma before the advent of effective chemotherapy was approximately 25%, but is now more than 70% with multimodal therapy.[26] Approxi-

6: Pediatrics

mately 20% of patients present with gross evidence of metastatic disease and the most common sites are the lung, bone marrow, and bone. Staging involves CT of the chest, bone marrow biopsy, and a bone scan. In extremity rhabdomyosarcoma, lymphatic spread is not uncommon, making nodal sampling or sentinel biopsy necessary. Vincristine, actinomycin D, and cyclophosphamide are chemotherapeutic agents often given in the neoadjuvant setting for treatment of extremity tumors. Patients who have the alveolar subtype of rhabdomyosarcoma are treated with radiation in addition to surgical resection for tumor control. Overall survival is approximately 60% for patients with nonmetastatic alveolar rhabdomyosarcoma and 30% for patients with distant metastases. Within the alveolar subtype, negative prognostic factors include incomplete resection of disease, large tumor size, and regional lymph node involvement.[27]

Synovial Sarcoma

The second most common soft-tissue malignancy in children, synovial sarcoma also has a specific translocation: t(X;18). This results in a fusion product of the *SYT* gene with either SSX1, SSX2, or SSX 4. The SYT-SSX1 fusion protein is correlated with poor outcome.[28] Intra-articular location is extremely rare, and the actual histogenesis is uncertain. It is not uncommon for patients to have a mass for many years before the diagnosis is made. Pulmonary metastases are most common. CT of the chest is part of staging, but because nodal spread is also noted, lymph node sampling or sentinel node biopsy is also indicated. Treatment involves wide excision, with adjuvant radiation used in children mostly in the setting of positive margins. The role of chemotherapy is not completely clear, but some benefit is noted with doxorubicin and ifosfamide.[29] Like other sarcomas with known translocations, the fusion protein in synovial sarcoma is a potential target for developing specific and more effective agents.

Infantile Fibrosarcoma

Although extremely rare, infantile fibrosarcoma is unique in children. It also has a specific translocation, t(12;15) resulting in the *TEL/TRKC* fusion gene and/or trisomy of chromosome 8, 11, 17, and 20. Infantile fibrosarcoma is quite aggressive locally, but only rarely metastasizes. Complete resection is usually curative, but may not be possible for some tumors or may result in significant disfigurement and loss of function. Chemotherapy given in a neoadjuvant setting has been helpful and successful in these patients.[30]

Pediatric Musculoskeletal Infections

Serious pediatric bone and joint infections are sometimes difficult to diagnose at the onset. The patient often has history of a limp pain, and antecedent trauma. Frequently a concurrent upper respiratory infection

clouds the picture. By focusing on objective markers, grave complications such as postinfectious arthritis, growth disturbance, chronic infection, and death can be avoided.[31]

Osteomyelitis

Osteomyelitis affects 1 in 5,000 children younger than 13 years, boys more often than girls. The most common sites of osteomyelitis, in descending order, are the distal femur, pelvis, tibia, calcaneus, and humerus. Acute hematogenous infection is most common. Blood-borne bacteria deposit in the metaphysis adjacent to the physis and are able to proliferate because of relatively low blood flow and oxygen tension. The most common infecting organism is *Staphylococcus aureus* followed by group A streptococcus and *Streptococcus pneumoniae*.

Evaluation begins with a detailed history and physical examination. Joints and limbs should be examined for warmth, swelling, erythema, and range of motion. Basic laboratory workup includes a complete blood count with differential, and assessment of erythrocyte sedimentation rate (ESR), C-reactive protein (CRP), and blood cultures. Lyme serology and a tuberculosis test should be added as needed. After infection, ESR peaks at 3 to 5 days and takes 1 to 2 weeks to decline after treatment; CRP rises within 24 to 48 hours and should fall within 24 hours after treatment with antibiotics. White blood cell count (WBC) is elevated in 25% of patients with osteomyelitis, ESR in 90%, and CRP in 98%. Blood cultures are positive in one third of patients. Bone cultures, which may be obtained by needle aspiration of a superficial area or by open biopsy in the operating room, have a higher yield but may be negative in up to 50% of patients. Plain radiographs should be obtained but show little change in the first 2 weeks of infection. A bone scan is an excellent screening study[31] (Figure 6). MRI is useful to evaluate a joint once the source of infection is localized and is particularly valuable for assessment of pelvic infections (Figure 7).

Treatment with intravenous antibiotics should be instituted after cultures are obtained. Empiric coverage is usually with cefazolin unless the patient is allergic (otherwise, clindamycin or vancomycin are usually used) or if methicillin-resistant *S aureus* (MRSA) is suspected vancomycin is used (linezolid can be used if the patient is allergic to vancomycin). Surgical drainage is reserved for subperiosteal abscesses or sequestra. Hospital discharge occurs after clinical improvement and 24 hours of apyrexia. In general, intravenous antibiotics are continued at least until the patient is afebrile and clinical improvement for extremity osteomyelitis with a nonresistant bacteria is seen (courses vary from 1 to 3 weeks of intravenous antibiotics), usually followed by a course of oral antibiotics to complete a 4- to 6-week total course of treatment. Proximal femoral and pelvic osteomyelitis are treated with a longer course of intravenous antibiotics, often for 6 weeks. Patients with osteomyelitis who have been adequately treated should

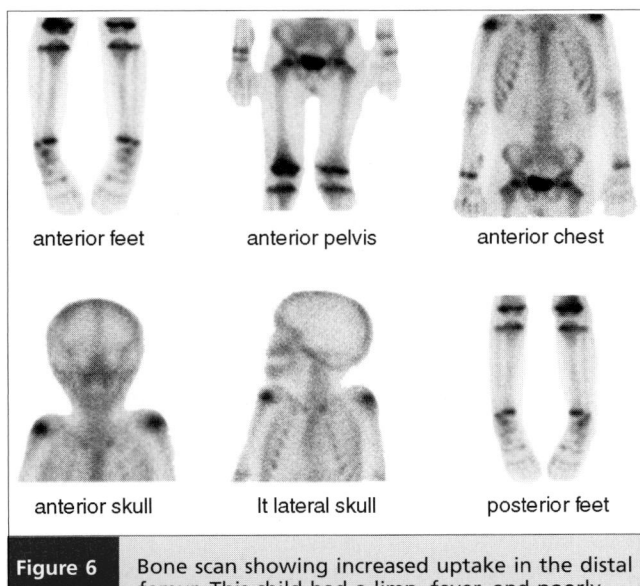

anterior feet   anterior pelvis   anterior chest

anterior skull   lt lateral skull   posterior feet

Figure 6	Bone scan showing increased uptake in the distal femur. This child had a limp, fever, and poorly localized pain. The bone scan helped pinpoint the location of infection; subsequent results from core needle biopsy showed methicillin-sensitive *S aureus*.

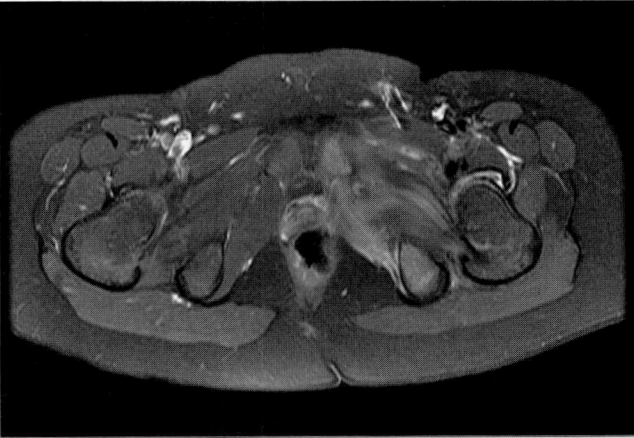

Figure 7	Postgadolinium sequence MRI scan showing enhancement in the ischium consistent with osteomyelitis. This child had a limp, fever, and elevated inflammatory markers. Hip ultrasound was negative, but the physical examination indicated a hip or pelvic source of symptoms.

experience rapid improvement. If not, the patient should be reevaluated for an abscess or adjacent joint septic arthritis. It should be remembered that Ewing's sarcoma, particularly of the pelvis, can present in the same manner as osteomyelitis, with pain, fever, and an elevated ESR.[31]

Subacute osteomyelitis has a more indolent presentation and is usually caused by a less virulent staphylococcal strain. A Brodie's abscess (radiolucent round lesion) may be seen; drainage is controversial. Treatment with antibiotics and a thorough evaluation for an underlying tumor is indicated. Chronic osteomyelitis is characterized by bone necrosis, often with a piece of necrotic bone (sequestrum) in an abscess cavity. Radiographs show extensive bone destruction and new bone formation (involucrum). Surgical débridement is often necessary, and antibiotic courses are 3 to 6 months.

Septic Arthritis
Septic arthritis may occur from hematogenous seeding, direct inoculation, or local spread from an adjacent metaphyseal osteomyelitis. The proximal femur, proximal humerus, proximal radius, and distal lateral tibia have intra-articular metaphyses that are at risk for adjacent septic arthritis. Septic arthritis is most common in the hip (35%), the knee (35%), the ankle (10%), and the shoulder/elbow/wrist (15%). Once infection occurs, the joint space fills with an inflammatory effusion mostly composed of polymorphonuclear cells. The proteolytic enzymes from the polymorphonuclear cells and the bacteria begin eroding articular cartilage in as few as 6 hours. Thus, septic arthritis is a surgical emergency.

For the limping, febrile child, the differential diagnosis is broad and includes toxic synovitis, inflammatory arthritis, a reactive effusion to an adjacent osteomyelitis, Lyme disease, a psoas abscess, a retrocecal appendicitis, cancer such as Ewing's sarcoma, osteosarcoma, or leukemia, and sacroiliac joint infection. There are some established criteria that are useful in assessing suspected septic arthritis in a child. Inability to weight bear, fever, WBC greater than 12,000/mm³, and ESR greater than 40 mm/hr were evaluated in two sequential studies at one institution for their predictive value in differentiating toxic synovitis from septic arthritis of the hip. The likelihood of septic arthritis was less than 10% with one positive predictor and greater than 93% with four positive predictors in both studies.[32,33] More recent work expanded these criteria to include CRP with the same trend.[34]

In addition to complete blood count with differential, ESR, CRP, and blood cultures, a throat culture/rapid strep test should be done, along with blood tests for antistreptolysin O and Lyme antibodies, gonococcal swabs of mucosal surfaces, and tuberculosis tests as indicated. Widening of the joint space of the hip may be present on plain radiographs. Ultrasound is an excellent method to assess effusion. If effusion is present, an aspiration for a cell count and Gram stain/culture should be performed. If the WBC is greater than 50,000/mm³, septic arthritis is likely and surgical drainage or in some cases serial aspiration is recommended. For WBC less than 50,000/mm³, more testing and a rheumatology consultation may be indicated. For a WBC of between 25,000 and 50,000/mm³, a surgical washout of the joint may still be appropriate at the discretion of the treating surgeon.

Treatment of septic arthritis is surgical drainage for a positive joint aspiration or if clinical suspicion warrants. For the hip, an anterior approach with a capsular window and drain is usually used. A core needle biopsy of the femoral neck/acetabulum to assess for osteomy-

6: Pediatrics

elitis may be appropriate. For other joints, either arthroscopic or open irrigation and débridement may be used. Intravenous antibiotics are instituted once cultures are obtained with empiric staphylococcal coverage until sensitivities are available. In more than a third of cases, positive culture data are not obtained. Alternative antibiotics to cover resistant organisms and consultation with an infectious disease specialist are helpful steps. Once the child is ambulatory and afebrile with decreasing levels of CRP and a normal peripheral WBC, many centers switch to appropriate oral antibiotics for 1 month of treatment. The child who does not rapidly improve after surgical drainage should be further evaluated. Additional imaging studies to evaluate for adjacent metaphyseal osteomyelitis with subperiosteal abscess and reaccumulation of pus in the joint may be valuable.

In the neonate, particularly in the neonatal intensive care unit, multiple joints may be seeded from intravenous and arterial lines; gram-negative bacteria are more common. Premature infants often cannot mount a febrile response, so an aggressive search for other sites of infection is warranted. Antibiotic coverage should be broad spectrum and include gram-negative rod coverage. Because these premature infants are often too unstable for transport to the operating room, bedside serial aspiration may be necessary.[30-34]

Methicillin-Resistant *S Aureus*
In a Houston pediatric hospital, methicillin resistance has been found in 74% of community-acquired *S aureus* skin infections since 2001.[35] MRSA is a virulent organism associated with higher rates of subperiosteal abscesses, multiple surgical procedures, longer hospital stays, and prolonged intravenous antibiotics. Community-acquired and hospital-acquired MRSA have different genetic profiles. Reduced affinity penicillin-binding protein is encoded by the *mecA* gene, which resides on the staphylococcal cassette chromosome mec (SCCmec). SCCmec types I-III are typically found in hospital-acquired MRSA, often carry other antibiotic-resistant genes, and rarely carry the Panton-Valentine leukocidin (*PVL*) gene. The *PVL* gene encodes cytolytic proteins that target neutrophils, macrophages, and monocytes and cause local tissue necrosis. Community-acquired MRSA with SCCmec type IV frequently carries the *PVL* gene and is believed to have led to several deaths in previously healthy children. Community-acquired MRSA with SCCmec types IV and V rarely has other antibiotic-resistant genes. Other virulent genes such as enterotoxins have also been identified. Treatment may include vancomycin, daptomycin, linezolid, and quinupristin/dalfopristin for hospital-acquired MRSA; for community-acquired MRSA, trimethoprim-sulfamethoxazole and clindamycin and in adults, tetracyclines or fluoroquinolones. A high level of vigilance is necessary as treatment protocols must be more aggressive with MRSA. Obtaining culture data from the infected part and treating empirically for MRSA in some regions is appropriate. Consultation with an infectious disease specialist is helpful.[35]

Diskitis
Back pain with point tenderness in a child should raise the possibility of diskitis. The presentation is often insidious, and the child may be afebrile. Usually the ESR is elevated. MRI is the best initial test to evaluate disk space narrowing and adjacent edema; radiographs demonstrate disk space narrowing much later in the course of the disease. Although diskitis was once considered a sterile inflammatory process, current evidence is more suggestive of true infection. Treatment consists of rest, a brace for comfort, and empiric *S aureus* coverage for 6 weeks.[36]

Chronic Recurrent Multifocal Osteomyelitis
This is a rare condition and is a diagnosis of exclusion. Two or more bony lesions that are warm, painful, and radiolucent with well-defined radiodense borders and minimal periosteal reaction are common clinical characteristics. The most common bones affected are the tibia, fibula, femur, and clavicle in the metaphyseal regions; occasional vertebra plana is seen. The disease course is one of exacerbations and remissions lasting at least 6 months and up to 2 to 4 years, with no response to antibiotics and no bacterial pathogen found on culture. The natural history is self-limiting, although this may take years. The ESR is elevated but the peripheral WBC is usually normal. Pathologic evaluation shows histology similar to chronic osteomyelitis with necrotic bone and a mixed cell infiltrate including histiocytes and plasma cells. Psoriasis-like plaques on the hands and feet with nail changes may be seen. Treatment is supportive with nonsteroidal anti-inflammatory drugs and observation as well as constant skepticism about the diagnosis. Rarely, an affected bone such as a clavicle may require resection to relieve symptoms.[31,37]

Lyme Disease
Lyme disease is caused by the spirochete *Borrelia burgdorferi* carried by tiny *Ixodes* deer ticks. The infections most commonly occur in spring and summer. According to the 2004 Centers for Disease Control and Prevention data, New York had 5,100 cases, followed by Pennsylvania, New Jersey, and other Northeastern locations. The early disease course in the first 3 to 30 days after the tick bite includes the target-like erythema migrans rash in 70% to 80% of affected patients and a flulike illness. In the untreated patient, late presentations include Bell's palsy, other neurologic symptoms, and cardiomyopathy; but the most common late presentation is a recurrent indolent arthritis of large joints in 60% of patients that will resolve and return if untreated. The most common joint affected is the knee. A large effusion is often present that is painful but tolerant of a short arc of motion. A lower WBC count than that of a septic joint is characteristic. The peripheral WBC, ESR, and CRP levels may be elevated, but high fever is less likely. MRI of a knee with Lyme arthritis

characteristically will show myositis, adenopathy, but no subcutaneous edema; MRI of a knee with septic arthritis will show subcutaneous edema and lacks myositis and adenopathy.[38] The diagnosis of Lyme disease is established by a blood test for Lyme antibody with enzyme-linked immunosorbent assay followed by a confirmatory Western blot. Treatment should be based on available information, and the treating surgeon should not wait for the Lyme test results before treating a joint suspicious for septic arthritis. Treatment at first is intravenous ceftriaxone for broad coverage until the Lyme antibody blood test results are known, followed by oral amoxicillin or doxycycline for 10 to 20 days.[39]

Pediatric Orthopaedic Hematology

Leukemia

Leukemia is the most common cancer of childhood and acute lymphoblastic leukemia represents 80% of all leukemias. Because this condition is now treatable, it is imperative to recognize leukemia early. Musculoskeletal pain is the presenting symptom in 40% to 60% of children with multiple joint involvement, with migratory symptoms that may mimic septic or inflammatory arthritis. Metaphyseal bands are characteristic on radiographs, but many types of bony lesions are seen. Constitutional symptoms (flulike illness, fatigue) are often present. Laboratory blood tests in early acute lymphoblastic leukemia often show anemia or even pancytopenia; it is important to remember that they are occasionally normal, and the orthopaedic surgeon may have the first opportunity to make the diagnosis. A bone marrow aspiration is diagnostic. Patients are treated with chemotherapy.

The orthopaedic surgeon should be aware that these children are susceptible to osteonecrosis that is often multifocal, presumably from high-dose steroids. Treatment initially includes protective weight bearing and observation, and recovery is usually slow. Core decompression or joint arthroplasty is occasionally indicated. Bone pain is also common. This may be caused by the leukemic infiltrate in the marrow and/or the chemotherapeutic agents (particularly steroids). Vincristine and vinblastine may cause peripheral neuropathy and even foot drop. Treatment with gabapentin and an ankle-foot orthosis may help until the neuropathy and tibialis anterior weakness resolve.[40]

Sickle Cell Disease

The severity of sickle cell disease correlates with the number of inherited alleles of hemoglobin-S; homozygotes are far more profoundly affected. The trait is believed to be an evolutionary adaptation to resist malaria and is seen in patients with ethnic heritages from areas where malaria is endemic, such as Africa. Osteomyelitis can mimic a sickle cell crisis in that both conditions cause fever, bone pain, and a high ESR/CRP. Osteomyelitis should be suspected if a patient fails to improve after 24 to 48 hours of hydration and pain management.

S aureus remains the most common organism, but *Salmonella* and other enteric bacteria must be considered in the antibiotic coverage. These infections are believed to occur from intestinal infarcts because of sickling red cells that release enteric bacteria into the bloodstream.[31]

Osteonecrosis commonly occurs in patients with sickle cell anemia, most frequently manifested in the hip and proximal humerus. It is bilateral in 50% of cases, and the outcome is worse in older patients. Both osteonecrosis and osteomyelitis can present in similar fashions with abnormal bone scans. Recent work suggests that a combination of both a bone marrow scan and a bone scan may help differentiate the two because the bone marrow scan will have normal uptake in osteomyelitis and abnormal but decreased uptake in acute bone infarction. MRI may also be helpful in making a diagnosis.[41]

Hemophilia

The most common types of hemophilia are caused by a deficiency of factor VIII or IX, carried in a sex-linked recessive inheritance pattern. Orthopaedic surgeons are consulted for hemarthroses and muscle hematomas. The treatment is to replace the deficient clotting factor immediately up to a level of 100% for 7 to 10 days. Conservative management is indicated unless there is a dense collection or a nerve palsy. If aspiration or drainage is considered, the clotting factor must be replaced first; more factor is likely to be needed during the postoperative period. Working together with an experienced hematologist will ensure proper treatment of the child. Affected joints should be splinted for only 1 to 2 days, then active motion should be instituted to avoid contracture. If recurrent hemarthroses occur in a joint, synovectomy (either open, arthroscopic, or chemical) may be beneficial.[42,43]

Annotated References

1. Rimondi E, Bianchi G, Malaguti MC, et al: Radiofrequency thermoablation of primary non-spinal osteoid osteoma: Optimization of the procedure. *Eur Radiol* 2005;15:1393-1399.

   Ninety-seven patients with nonspinal osteoid osteoma treated with radiofrequency ablation were reviewed, with focus on technical pearls. Pain relief was achieved in 85% of patients with one treatment and in 15% with two treatments; only two patients required excision for nonresponsive pain. There were no complications.

2. Suneja R, Grimer RJ, Belthur M, et al: Chondroblastoma of bone: Long-term results and functional outcome after intralesional curettage. *J Bone Joint Surg Br* 2005;87:974-978.

   A retrospective review of 53 patients with chondroblastoma treated with curettage alone is presented. Of seven patients (13.2%) with a local recurrence that was treated successfully, three had repeat curettage, two had endoprosthetic replacement, and one had amputation. One patient died as a result of metastatic disease and recurrence despite amputation. Mean functional scores were good.

3. Lin PP, Thenappan A, Deavers MT, Lewis VO, Yasko AW: Treatment and prognosis of chondroblastoma. *Clin Orthop Relat Res* 2005;438:103-109.

   A retrospective study of 82 patients with chondroblastoma with a focus on prognostic factors for local recurrence and metastasis is presented. Neither an open physis nor younger age affected local recurrence; however, inadequate surgery and biologic aggressiveness did. Pelvis location was associated with a worse prognosis. Level of evidence: IV.

4. Lersundi A, Mankin HJ, Mourikis A, Hornicek FJ: Chondromyxoid fibroma: A rarely encountered and puzzling tumor. *Clin Orthop Relat Res* 2005;439: 171-175.

   The characteristics of chondromyxoid fibroma based on 30 patients are reviewed. Most patients were treated with curettage with or without allograft chips or polymethylmethacrylate. Four patients underwent resection. Local recurrence occurred in seven patients (23%); there were no instances of metastatic spread. Functional outcome was good. Level of evidence: IV.

5. Stieber JR, Dormans JP: Manifestations of hereditary multiple exostoses. *J Am Acad Orthop Surg* 2005;13: 110-120.

   A thorough review of multiple hereditary exostoses is presented, with a focus on current knowledge of pathogenesis and skeletal deformities.

6. Snyder BD, Hauser-Kara DA, Hipp JA, Zurakowski D, Hecht AC, Gebhardt MC: Predicting fracture through benign skeletal lesions with quantitative computed tomography. *J Bone Joint Surg Am* 2006;88:55-70.

   Quantitative CT was compared with current radiographic guidelines for accuracy in predicting fracture in patients with a benign skeletal lesion. The quantitative CT was more accurate, resulting in a better tool for predicting fracture risk and thus determining the need for surgical intervention. Level of evidence: III.

7. Gu W, Ogose A, Matsuba A, et al: Activating Gs alpha mutation rarely occurs in musculoskeletal tumors other than fibrous dysplasia. *Anticancer Res* 2006;26: 1611-1614.

   Gs alpha mutations have been identified in almost all cases of fibrous dysplasia. Sixteen cell lines and 173 musculoskeletal tumor tissues were evaluated for this mutation and it was only identified in fibrous dysplasia. There is no correlation with this mutation and the development of a sarcoma.

8. Lala R, Matarazzo P, Andreo M, et al: Bisphosphonate treatment of bone fibrous dysplasia in McCune-Albright syndrome. *J Pediatr Endocrinol Metab* 2006;19(suppl 2):583-593.

   Fourteen patients with McCune-Albright syndrome were administered pamidronate according to alkaline phosphatase levels. Long-term therapy resulted in reduced fracture rate, decreased bone pain, and radiologic evidence of long bone lesion healing.

9. de Sanctis N, Andreacchio A: Elastic stable intramedullary nailing is the best treatment of unicameral bone cysts of the long bones in children: Prospective long-term follow-up study. *J Pediatr Orthop* 2006;26: 520-525.

   Forty-seven patients with unicameral bone cysts were treated with elastic intramedullary nailing, one of many modalities for treatment. Based on plain radiographs, 31 (66%) were completely healed and 16 (34%) were healed with residual radiolucency; thus, all of the lesions responded to the treatment.

10. Oliveira AM, Perez-Atayde AR, Inwards CY, et al: USP6 and CDH11 oncogenes identify the neoplastic cell in primary aneurysmal bone cysts and are absent in so-called secondary aneurysmal bone cysts. *Am J Pathol* 2004;165:1773-1780.

    Seventy percent of 52 primary aneurysmal bone cysts were found to have a rearrangement of *CDH11* and/or *USP6*. This abnormality was only seen in the spindle cells in the walls of the aneurysmal bone cysts, thus identifying the likely neoplastic cell. It was not observed in 17 secondary aneurysmal bone cysts, indicating that these lesions may be reactive whereas primary aneurysmal bone cysts are neoplastic.

11. Rastogi S, Varshney MK, Trikha V, Khan SA, Choudhury B, Safaya R: Treatment of aneurysmal bone cysts with percutaneous sclerotherapy using polidocanol: A review of 72 cases with long-term follow-up. *J Bone Joint Surg Br* 2006;88:1212-1216.

    Sclerotherapy with polidocanol was used to treat 72 patients with aneurysmal bone cysts. A clinical response was noted in 84.5% of patients with a mean of three injections and average length of treatment of 1 year. Two patients had a recurrence; both were treated successfully with repeat injection. The authors highlight the low morbidity of this approach, especially in surgically inaccessible sites.

12. Docquier PL, Delloye C: Treatment of aneurysmal bone cysts by introduction of demineralized bone and autogenous bone marrow. *J Bone Joint Surg Am* 2005;87: 2253-2258.

    Thirteen primary aneurysmal bone cysts were treated with demineralized bone matrix and bone marrow aspirate. All except two healed and there were no recurrences. This newer and less invasive approach to treat aneurysmal bone cysts likely merits further investigation. Level of evidence: IV.

13. Mendenhall WM, Zlotecki RA, Gibbs CP, Reith JD, Scarborough MT, Mendenhall NP: Aneurysmal bone cyst. *Am J Clin Oncol* 2006;29:311-315.

    An overall review of aneurysmal bone cysts with a focus on treatment options is presented. The authors recommend surgery as the preferred modality, noting a high cure rate, but also success in using low-dose radiation for a small subset of aneurysmal bone cysts that are not resectable, are locally aggressive, or that recur.

14. Kneisl JS, Patt JC, Johnson JC, Zuger JH: Is PET useful in detecting occult nonpulmonary metastases in pediatric bone sarcomas? *Clin Orthop Relat Res* 2006;450: 101-104.

PET was used to evaluate nonpulmonary metastatic disease in 55 patients with bone sarcomas. Four of the 12 patients in whom positive results were found had a resultant change in treatment (3 patients had Ewing's sarcoma and 1 had osteosarcoma). The authors recommend PET as a routine screening method for patients with Ewing's sarcoma, not for those with osteosarcoma. Level of evidence: II.

15. Mankin HJ, Mankin CJ, Simon MA: The hazards of biopsy revisited: Members of the Musculoskeletal Tumor Society. *J Bone Joint Surg Am* 1996;78:656-663.

16. Stiller CA, Bielack SS, Jundt G, Steliarova-Foucher E: Bone tumors in European children and adolescents, 1978-1997: Report from the Automated Childhood Cancer Information System project. *Eur J Cancer* 2006; 42:2124-2135.

This article presents a large population study of data on 5,572 patients with malignant bone tumors in which demographic information, incidence, and survival were analyzed.

17. Longhi A, Errani C, De Paolis M, Mercuri M, Bacci G: Primary bone osteosarcoma in the pediatric age: State of the art. *Cancer Treat Rev* 2006;32:423-436.

This article presents a comprehensive review of the approach to treatment for pediatric patients with osteosarcoma with a focus on past progress and the need for new drugs and methods.

18. Bernstein M, Kovar H, Paulussen M, et al: Ewing's sarcoma family of tumors: Current management. *Oncologist* 2006;11:503-519.

An overall review of Ewing's sarcoma, including presentation, prognosis, multidisciplinary management, and late effects of therapy, is presented.

19. Bacci G, Longhi A, Ferrari S, Mercuri M, Versari M, Bertoni F: Prognostic factors in non-metastatic Ewing's sarcoma tumor of bone: An analysis of 579 patients treated at a single institution with adjuvant or neoadjuvant chemotherapy between 1972 and 1998. *Acta Oncol* 2006;45:469-475.

This article presents a retrospective review of 579 patients with nonmetastatic Ewing's sarcoma treated at a single institution with a focus on prognostic factors. The authors indicate the need to stratify patients according to prognostic factors to be able to best treat them with the least morbidity and most efficacy.

20. Brigman BE, Hornicek FJ, Gebhardt MC, Mankin HJ: Allografts about the knee in young patients with high-grade sarcoma. *Clin Orthop Relat Res* 2004;421: 232-239.

One hundred three patients with bone sarcomas were treated with allograft reconstruction. Outcome was good or excellent in 49%, fair in 14%, and failure occurred in 37% over long-term follow-up. Infection oc-

curred in 16%, fracture in 27%, and nonunion in 34%. Fourteen patients eventually required amputation.

21. Biau D, Faure F, Katsahian S, Jeanrot C, Tomeno B, Anract P: Survival of total knee replacement with a megaprosthesis after bone tumor resection. *J Bone Joint Surg Am* 2006;88:1285-1293.

Ninety-one patients who underwent reconstruction after bone sarcoma resection with a GUEPAR oncologic knee prosthesis (Benoist Girard, Bagheaux, France) were evaluated. Median duration of prosthetic survival was 130 months for the distal femur and 117 months for the proximal tibia. Allograft-prosthetic composites fared worse than reconstructions using a metal or plastic sleeve. Although this is an earlier genearion prosthesis, this study demonstrates the common complications encountered with this difficult reconstruction. Level of evidence: II.

22. Fuchs B, Sim FH: Rotationplasty about the knee: Surgical technique and anatomical considerations. *Clin Anat* 2004;17:345-353.

This review article discusses the technique for rotationplasty with a focus on the unique anatomic concerns.

23. Neel MD, Wilkins RM, Rao BN, Kelly CM: Early multicenter experience with a noninvasive expandable prosthesis. *Clin Orthop Relat Res* 2003;415:72-81.

24. Schuetze SM, Rubin BP, Vernon C, et al: Use of positron emission tomography in localized extremity soft tissue sarcoma treated with neoadjuvant chemotherapy. *Cancer* 2005;103:339-348.

PET was used to follow treatment response to chemotherapy in 46 patients with high-grade soft-tissue sarcomas. Tumors with a baseline maximum standard uptake value (SUVmax) of 6 or a decrease in the SUVmax of less than 40% had a statistically significantly higher risk of disease recurrence and metastasis than those with a decrease of 40% or more. In this manner, PET can be used to stratify treatment groups and monitor response.

25. Sorensen PH, Lynch JC, Qualmon SJ, et al: PAX3-FKHR gene fusions are prognostic indicators in alveolar rhabdomyosarcoma: A report from the Children's Oncology Group. *J Clin Oncol* 2002;20:2672-2679.

26. Pastore G, Peris-Bonet R, Carli M, Martinez-Garcia C, Sanchez de Toledo J, Steliarova-Foucher E: Childhood soft tissue sarcomas incidence and survival in European children (1978-1997): Report from the Automated Childhood Cancer Information System project. *Eur J Cancer* 2006;42:2136-2149.

A population-based study of 5,802 pediatric patients with soft-tissue sarcoma is presented. Incidence, survival, and prognostic factors are reported.

27. Meza JL, Anderson J, Pappo AS, Meyer WH: Analysis of prognostic factors in patients with nonmetastatic rhabdomyosarcoma treated on Intergroup Rhabdomyosarcoma Studies III and IV: The Children's Oncology Group. *J Clin Oncol* 2006;24:3844-3851.

Prognostic factors were identified by analyzing patient

and disease characteristics as they related to outcome in two large national trials for nonmetastatic rhabdomyosarcoma. This has been crucial in stratifying patient subsets in future trials so that therapy can be adapted based on risk category.

28. Ladanyi M, Antonescu CR, Leung DH, et al: Impact of SYT-SSX fusion type on the clinical behavior of synovial sarcoma: A multi-institutional retrospective study of 243 patients. *Cancer Res* 2002;62:135-140.

29. Brecht IB, Ferrari A, Int-Veen C, et al: Grossly-resected synovial sarcoma treated by the German and Italian Pediatric Soft Tissue Sarcoma Cooperative Groups: Discussion on the role of adjuvant therapies. *Pediatr Blood Cancer* 2006;46:11-17.

    Adjuvant chemotherapy was administered to 150 patients with nonmetastatic synovial sarcoma after surgical resection, with many patients also receiving adjuvant radiotherapy. Five-year overall survival was 77% and event-free survival was 89%. Size and local invasiveness were significant factors, but surgical margin was not. Adjuvant chemotherapy was recommended for higher risk pediatric patients with synovial sarcoma.

30. Loh ML, Ahn P, Perez-Atayde AR, Gebhardt MC, Shamberger RC, Grier HE: Treatment of infantile fibrosarcoma with chemotherapy and surgery: Results from the Dana-Farber Cancer Institute and Children's Hospital Boston. *J Pediatr Hematol Oncol* 2002;24:722-726.

31. Stans AA: Osteomyelitis and septic arthritis, in Morrissy RT and Weinstein SL (eds): *Lovell and Winter's Pediatric Orthopaedics*, ed 6. Philadelphia, PA, Lippincott Williams & Wilkins, 2006, pp 439-491.

    This chapter provides a comprehensive discussion of various pediatric infections encompassing recent advances.

32. Kocher MS, Zurakowski D, Kasser JR: Differentiating between septic arthritis and transient synovitis of the hip in children: An evidence-based clinical prediction algorithm. *J Bone Joint Surg Am* 1999;81:1662-1670.

33. Kocher MS, Mandiga R, Zurakowski D, Barnewolt C, Kasser JR: Validation of a clinical prediction rule for the differentiation between septic arthritis and transient synovitis of the hip in children. *J Bone Joint Surg Am* 2004;86:1629-1635.

    The authors prospectively examined children with an irritable hip using the previously studied criteria of fever, refusal to weight bear, ESR greater than 40, WBC greater than 12,000/mm^3 and found a similar trend that more positive factors yielded an increased likelihood of true septic arthritis, although lower than from the original 1999 study. Level of evidence: I-1, diagnostic study.

34. Caird MS, Flynn JM, Leung YL, Millman JE, D'Italia JG, Dormans JP: Factors distinguishing septic arthritis from transient synovitis of the hip in children: A prospective study. *J Bone Joint Surg Am* 2006;88: 1251-1257.

    The authors prospectively followed 53 children who underwent hip aspiration for suspicion of septic arthritis and found that fever was the best predictor, followed by elevated CRP and ESR levels, refusal to weight bear, and an elevated WBC. CRP greater than 2.0 was an independent risk factor for septic arthritis. Level of evidence: I.

35. Deresinski S: Methicillin-resistant staphylococcus aureus: An evolutionary, epidemiologic, and therapeutic odyssey. *Clin Infect Dis* 2005;40:562-573.

    This article presents an excellent overview of MRSA, including differences in the genetics of hospital-acquired and community-acquired MRSA.

36. Fernandez M, Carrol CL, Baker CJ: Discitis and vertebral osteomyelitis in children: An 18-year review. *Pediatrics* 2000;105:1299-1304.

37. Schultz C, Holterhus PM, Seidel A, et al: Chronic recurrent multifocal osteomyelitis in children. *Pediatr Infect Dis J* 1999;18:1008-1013.

38. Ecklund K, Vargas S, Zurakowski D, Sundel RP: MRI features of Lyme arthritis in children. *AJR Am J Roentgenol* 2005;184:1904-1909.

    MRI appearances of Lyme disease are unique and include muscular edema and lymphadenopathy; MRI may be useful in diagnosing Lyme arthritis.

39. Centers for Disease Control and Prevention Website. Available at: http://www.cdc.gov/ncidod/dvbid/lyme/index.htm.

    An excellent overview of Lyme disease with recent demographics is presented.

40. Gallagher DJ, Phillips DJ, Heinrich SD: Orthopedic manifestations of acute pediatric leukemia. *Orthop Clin North Am* 1996;27:635-644.

41. Skaggs DL, Kim SK, Greene NW, Harris D, Miller JH: Differentiation between bone infarction and acute osteomyelitis in children with sickle-cell disease with use of sequential radionuclide bone-marrow and bone scans. *J Bone Joint Surg Am* 2001;83:1810-1813.

42. Dunn AL: Management and prevention of recurrent hemarthrosis in patients with hemophilia. *Curr Opin Hematol* 2005;12:390-394.

    Destructive arthropathy from recurrent hemarthrosis is a major complication in patients with hemophilia. Recent advances have shown that with aggressive factor replacement for bleeding episodes and arthroscopic synovectomy, outcomes may be improved.

43. Dunn AL, Busch MT, Wyly JB, Sullivan KM, Abshire TC: Arthroscopic synovectomy for hemophilic joint disease in a pediatric population. *J Pediatr Orthop* 2004; 24:414-426.

    The authors present a case series of 69 arthroscopic synovectomies in 44 hemophiliac pediatric patients with median follow-up of 79 months. Median bleeding frequency declined 84%; rehabilitation was not problematic.

Index

Page numbers with *f* indicate figures
Page numbers with *t* indicate tables

A

A delta fibers
  pain sensations and, 259
Abatacept
  description of, 224
  dosage, 222*t*
  efficacy, 222*t*
  mechanisms of action, 222*t*
  side effects, 222*t*
Abbreviated Injury Scale (AIS), 140
ABCDE acronym, 118–119
Abduction splinting, 716–717
Abductor pollicis brevis, 234*f*
Abductor pollicis longus, 347*f*
Abscesses
  epidural, 598–599
  treatment, 252*t*–253
Accessory navicular, 753, 754*f*
Acetabular components, 83, 416
Acetabular dysplasia, 717–718, 781
Acetabular fractures
  classification of, 393*f*
  cobalt-chromium alloy cup and, 81–82
  deep venous thrombosis and, 394–395
  heterotopic ossification and, 394
  pediatric
    characteristics, 705
    complications, 706
    imaging, 705
    treatment, 706
  posterior wall, 394
  treatment, 393–394
Acetabular osteotomy, 717
Acetabulum
  bone loss, 419, 420*f*, 420*t*
  defect classification, 419*f*
  normal, 412*f*
  retroversion, 413*f*
  shallow, 413*f*
Acetaminophen
  for acute preoperative pain, 264–265
  for osteoarthritis, 228
  for postoperative pain, 264
  poisoning by, 264–265
  treatment with, 25
Acetylsalicylic acid sensitivity, 124
Achilles tendon lengthening, 511, 515
Achondroplasia
  characteristics, 773–774
  foramen magnum stenosis, 774*f*
  genetic factors, 773
  incidence, 773
  thoracolumbar kyphosis in, 774*f*
Acquired immunodeficiency syndrome.
  See also Human immunodeficiency
  virus (HIV)
  preoperative assessments, 109–110
  septic arthritis and, 247

Acrocephalopolysyndactyly. *See*
  Carpenter's syndrome
Acrocephalosyndactyly. *See* Apert's
  syndrome
Acromioclavicular joints
  imaging, 277
  injuries in young athletes, 759
  pathology, 277
  reconstruction, 308*f*
Acromioclavicular separations, 307–308
Actinomyces israelii, 597
Actinomycin D, 802
Activated partial thromboplastin time,
  preoperative, 108
Activities of daily living, 383, 383*f*
Acupuncture, 268*t*, 269
Acute neuropathy, causes of, 237
Acute normovolemic hemodilution, 151
Adalimumab
  for ankylosing spondylitis, 226–227
  dosage, 222*t*
  efficacy, 222*t*
  mechanisms of action, 222*t*, 223
  perioperative, 112
  for psoriatic arthritis, 227
  side effects, 222*t*
Adamantinomas, 207, 207*f*
Adams forward-bend test, 697, 785
ADAMTS-5, 24, 25
Adduction-abduction rotation patterns,
  380
Adductor pollicis, 347*f*
Adhesion molecules, 38
Adjacent-segment degeneration, 544
Adolescent idiopathic scoliosis, 697, 699*f*
Adolescents
  as athletes, 757–771
  elbow dislocations in, 663–664
  idiopathic scoliosis, 697, 699*f*
  Osgood-Schlatter disease, 757, 763
  septic arthritis in, 248
  tibia vara, 745, 745*f*
  use of performance-enhancing
    substances, 758
Adult acquired flatfoot deformity
  extra-articular osteotomy in, 515*f*
  hindfoot dysfunction and, 513–514
  stages of, 514*t*
Adult respiratory distress syndrome
  (ARDS)
  in bilateral femoral shaft fractures, 430
  femoral reaming and, 429
  femoral shaft fractures, 431
  polytrauma patients, 140–141
Adult scoliosis, 603–614. *See also*
  Idiopathic scoliosis; Scoliosis
Advanced Cardiac Life Support (ACLS)
  recertification, 119
Advanced Trauma Life Support (ATLS)
  assessment of pelvic injuries, 389
  on femoral shaft fractures, 427
  on hip dislocations, 399
  manual, 137
  recertification in, 119

Aeromonas, 477
Age/aging. *See also* Skeletal age; Tanner
  staging
  bone mineral density and, 192
  carpal tunnel syndrome and, 357
  chondrosarcoma types and, 204
  determination of, 757
  disk biomechanics and, 535
  disk changes in, 28–29
  fracture healing and, 478
  fracture risk and, 192*t*
  hip fractures and, 401, 401*t*
  musculoskeletal tumors and, 198
  osteoporosis and, 193
  preoperative assessments, 109
  sarcopenia in, 37
  vertebral ossification, 691
  vitamin D levels and, 191
Agency for Healthcare Research and
  Quality (AHRQ), 166*t*
Aggrecans, 23, 28
Aggressive fibromatosis, 209, 803
AIDS. *See* Acquired immunodeficiency
  syndrome
Albumin, serum levels, 109
Albuterol (salbutamol), 124, 125
Alcohol abuse
  acetaminophen poisoning in, 264
  bone disorders and, 192
Alendronate, 194–195, 781
Alkaline phosphatase levels, 405
Allen's test
  in ulnar artery thrombosis, 361, 369
  in vasospastic conditions, 370
Allergic reactions, anaphylaxis in, 125
Allergic rhinitis, 124
Allgower-Donati flap stitches, 505
Allman classification of fractures, 287
Allodynia, 261
Allografts
  articular cartilage, 452
  bone, 16–17
  impaction method, 16
  infection associated with, 254
  in nonunions, 16
  osteoarticular replacement, 452
Alpha (α) angle, 715, 716*f*
α-fetoprotein, 788
Altruism, trust and, 6
Alumina ceramic
  bearings from, 81
  brittle fracture of, 81
  squeaking, 81
Alumina-zirconia composites, 81
Alveolar rhabdomyosarcomas, 803–804
Ambulatory Care Quality Alliance, 168*t*
Amenorrhea, secondary causes of, 131*t*
American Academy of Orthopaedic
  Surgeons (AAOS)
  American Board of Orthopaedic
    Surgery and, 3
  Code of Medical Ethics and
    Professionalism for Orthopaedic
    Surgeons, 6

Index

Index

Index

age-based options, 710–712, 711*f*
bone healing and, 15
femoral shaft fractures, 430
metaphyseal fractures, 672*f*
pediatric patients, 660–663
in syndesmosis injuries, 494–495
Fixed sagittal imbalance, 609*t*
Flatfoot deformity, 751
Flexible flatfoot, 751
Flexion-distraction injury, 694
Flexion-extension gap balancing, 466
Flexion-extension rotation patterns, 379–380
Flexor carpi radialis, 367*f*
Flexor digitorum profundus, 42
Flexor tendon injuries
lacerations, 353*f*
pediatric patients, 675
zones of, 353, 353*f*, 354*f*
Floating shoulder injuries, 292–293
Fluorine-18 deoxyglucose positron emission tomography (FDG-PET), 101–102, 243
Fluoroquinolone, 245
Fluoroscopic stress testing, intraoperative, 494
Focal neuropathies
in diabetes, 237
myelin disturbances and, 234
Focal scoliosis, 582
Fondaparinux, 147, 148, 420, 480
Food and Drug Administration
approval process for devices, 8
on screening of tissue donors, 16
Foot
arthroscopy of, 516
burning sensation, 237
calcaneus deformity, 789
common tumors of, 198*t*
congenital absence of rays, 746
forefoot fractures, 737
imaging, 90
injuries in athletes, 767–769
midfoot fractures, 737
in myelomeningocele, 789
pediatric conditions, 749–754
prostheses, 524
puncture wounds, 738
tarsometatarsal injuries, 737
traumatic amputations, 737–738
traumatic injuries, 735–738
valgus deformity, 789
Foramen magnum stenosis, 774*f*
Foraminal stenosis, 620*f*
Forces
definition, 67
units of, 67
Forearm fractures
classification of, 669–670
diaphyseal, 329–330
pain related to, 669
pediatric patients, 669
Forearm trauma, 319–332
Forefoot
adduction in clubfoot, 750
fractures, 737
function of, 490
Forest plots, 180*f*

Forestier's disease, 574–575
Formoterol, 124
Fractures. *See also Specific* bones
bone grafting and, 13–22
clinical risk factors for, 194*t*
external fixation, 142
greenstick, 671–673
healing cascade, 13–15, 13*f*
open
antibiotics in, 139–140
polytrauma patients, 139–140
pathologic
femoral, 407
Mirels scoring system for, 214, 214*t*
in transitional cell carcinoma, 215
plate fixation
load sharing, 75
in polytrauma patients, 142
risk of, 192*t*
stabilization of, 142
transphyseal, 663*f*
transverse, 709
triplane, 736*f*
Frankel Impairment Scale, 580
Free radicals, neutralizing of, 83, 84*t*
Freiberg's infraction, 754
Frequency-selective fat saturation imaging, 97, 98*f*
Friedreich's ataxia
cavovarus foot deformity in, 753
genetic characteristics of, 791*t*
pediatric patients, 792
Functional somatic syndrome. *See* Repetitive strain injury
Fungal infections, 247
Funnel plots, 180, 180*f*

G

Gabapentin, 267, 807
Gait. *See also* Walking
adduction-abduction rotation patterns, 380
analysis in pediatric patients, 741
anteroposterior translation patterns, 381
biomechanics of, 379–387
internal-external rotation patterns, 380–381
osteoarthritis and, 385
stance phase, 379, 380*f*
swing phase, 379
Galeazzi fractures, 673–674
Galeazzi sign, 715
Galveston technique, 790*f*
Ganglionectomy, 370
Ganglions, 370
Garden classification, 401–402, 402*f*
Gardner-Wells tongs, 139
Gartland injuries, 661
Gastroplasty, 110
Gelatinase, 28
Genu varum, malalignment, 774
Gender
ACL injuries, 449
athletes, 129–130
carpal ossification sequence, 673*t*
carpal tunnel syndrome and, 158–159

chondrosarcoma types and, 204
Ewing's sarcoma and, 204
forearm fracture rates, 669
Madelung's deformity, 684
osteoporosis and, 407–408
proximal humeral fractures and, 293
radiation-induced sarcoma and, 203
scapholunate intervals, 673*t*
Gene therapy, 37
Gentamicin, 245, 477
Genu valgum, 743*f*, 775
Genu varum, 741
Geodes, 94
Geriatric patients, preoperative assessments, 109
Ghent diagnostic criteria, 779, 779*t*
Giant cell tumor of bone, 371
description, 206–209
distal radius, 372*f*
spinal, 636*t*–637*t*, 637–639
treatment of, 212
Giant cell tumors of the tendon sheath, 370
Ginkgo, perioperative, 111
Ginseng, perioperative, 111
Glasgow Coma Scale, 119
Glatiramer acetate, 239
Glenohumeral instability
Bankart lesion, 760*f*
posterior, 306
in young athletes, 759–760, 760*f*
Glenohumeral ligament attachments, 306*f*
Glenoid
biologic resurfacing, 315
erosion, 313
glenohumeral ligaments, 306*f*
hypoplasia, 682
inverted pear, 306
normal labrum position, 304*f*
soft-tissue graft to, 315*f*
Glenoid fossa fractures
mechanisms of injury, 291
surgical treatment, 291–292
Glenoid neck fractures
mechanisms of injury, 291
presentation, 291
radiography, 292*f*
surgical treatment, 291, 292*f*
Gliosis, neurorestoration and, 54
Glomus tumors, 370–371, 371*f*
Glucocorticoids
lumbar disk herniation and, 553
in rheumatoid arthritis, 225
Glucosamine
for cartilage degeneration, 25
for osteoarthritis, 228–229
perioperative, 111
Glucose tolerance, impaired, 237
Glutamate, pain and, 259
Glycosaminoglycan (GAG) chains
in articular cartilage, 23
destruction of, 247
in intervertebral disks, 27
in ligaments, 40
in tendons, 40
GM-1 ganglioside, 53
Gonococcal swabs, 805–806
Grafton DBM, 18
Gram stains, 242–243

Index

Index

Index

Myelomas
  corticosteroids in, 635
  incidence of, 208
  pathogenesis of, 208
  spinal, 638t–639t, 643–644
Myelomeningocele
  description, 696
  kyphosis in, 790f
  overview, 788–789
  treatment, 789–790
Myelopathy, causes of, 544–547
Myelopathy, cervical. See Cervical
  myelopathy
Myo-D marker, 201
Myoblasts, 35
Myocarditis, 128
Myofibers
  contractile elements, 35
  formation of, 35
  hyperplasia, 37
  structure, 36f
  types of, 35–36, 36t
Myogenin, 201
Myositis ossificans, 97
Myotomes
  cervical, 233t
  lumbosacral, 233t
Myxoid liposarcomas, 197t, 210, 211f

N

N-telopeptides, 192
Nafcillin, 129
Nail bed disruption, 675
Nail-patella syndrome, 683, 775–776,
  776f
Naloxone, 53
Nandrolone decanoate, 131
Nandrolone phenpropionate, 131
Nasogastric tubes, 137
Natalizumab, 239
National Acute Spinal Cord Injury Study
  (NASCIS), 52–53, 139, 695
National Athletic Trainers' Association
  (NATA), 118
National Board of Medical Examiners
  (NBME), 4
National Collegiate Athletics Association,
  130
National Commission for the Protection
  of Human Subjects of Biomedical and
  Behavioral Research, 7
National Commission on State Workman's
  Compensation Laws, 157
National Football League, 130
National Guideline Clearinghouse (NGC),
  166t, 170
National Heart, Lung, and Blood Institute,
  150
National Institute for Occupational Safety
  and Health (NIOSH), 157
National Institute of Arthritis,
  Musculoskeletal, and Skin Diseases, 174
National Institutes of Health (NIH)
  corporate consulting activities within, 10
  funding for research, 173
  Glucosamine/Chondroitin Arthritis
    Intervention Trial, 25

National Osteoporosis Foundation, 408
National Quality Forum (NQF), 167t,
  168–169
National Surgical Infection Prevention
  Project, 110
Navicular
  accessory, 753, 754f
  anatomy, 488
  avulsion fracture of, 737
  osteochondrosis of, 754
Navicular fractures
  classification, 489, 489f
  incidence, 737
  injury patterns, 488–489
    body fractures, 489
    dorsal lip fractures, 488
    stress fractures, 489
    tuberosity fractures, 488
  radiographic evaluation, 488
Neck pain
  after trauma, 565
  axial, 541–542
Necrotizing fasciitis, 251t
Nedocromil, 124
Needle biopsies, 594
Neer classification, 289–290, 293
Neer trauma series, 293
Negative predictive value (NPV), 183
Neisseria gonorrhoeae, 247, 249
Neonates, septic arthritis in, 248, 249, 806
Neoplasms, appendicular skeleton, 92.
  See also Bone tumors; Cancer; Tumors;
  Specific neoplasms
Nerve compression syndromes, 357–360
Nerve conduction velocity studies
  in brachial plexus injuries, 55–56
  in carpal tunnel syndrome, 357
  in cervical radiculopathy, 543
  in compression neuropathies, 59
  neuromuscular evaluation using,
    233–236
  in pronator syndrome, 359
Nerve grafts
  conduits, 354
  sources, 57
  vascularized, 56
Nerve growth factor (NGF), 39f, 354
Nerve palsy, 431
Nerve roots
  cross-section, 532f
  pain syndromes and, 543t
  scapular pain and, 233
Nerve transfers
  in brachial plexus injury, 57
  donors, 57
Nerves
  imaging of, 100
  muscle contraction and, 35
Neuraxial blocks, 266, 267
Neurofibromas, spinal, 641
Neurofibromatosis (NF)
  description, 781–782
  diagnosis, 781, 782f
Neurofibromin, 781
Neurogenic claudication, 555t, 559,
  653–654
Neurogenic shock
  etiology of, 137

presentation of, 52
  in spinal cord injury, 52
  thoracolumbar fractures and, 579
Neuromas, 523
Neuromuscular disorders
  in children, 785–795
Neuromuscular evaluation, 233
Neuronal plasticity, 261
Neuropathies, disorders associated with,
  236–239
Neuroprotection, 53–54
Neurorestoration, 54–55
Neurotransmitters, 259
Neurotrophic growth factors, 54
Neurotrophin-3 (NT-3), 54
Neutrophils, in muscle healing, 38
New Injury Severity Score (NISS), 140
Nicotine, bone healing and, 14
Nimodipine, 53
Nitrous oxide
  in pediatric patients, 669
Nociception, mediation of, 259
Nodes of Ranvier, 59
Nonsteroidal anti-inflammatory drugs
  (NSAIDs)
  for acute preoperative pain, 264
  for ankylosing spondylitis, 226
  bone healing and, 14
  in carpal tunnel syndrome, 357
  in cartilage degeneration, 25
  impact on in ligament healing, 42
  in low back pain, 559
  in lumbar disk herniation, 553
  mechanisms of action, 110–111
  in muscle healing, 38–39
  in muscle injury, 39f
  for osteoarthritis, 227–228
  pain perception and, 259
  postoperative, 268t
  preoperative use of, 110
  for rheumatoid arthritis, 221
Nonhemorrhagic shock, 137
Nonossifying fibroma
  description, 799
  tibial, 93f
  treatment of, 212
Nonunions
  allograft use, 16
  femoral shaft fractures, 431–432
  Ilizarov treatment, 481–482
  ruling out infections, 480–481
  tibial fractures, 480f
  in tibial fractures, 479–482
Nortriptyline, 268–269
Notochordal cells, function, 536
NS-398, in muscle healing, 38–39
Nuclear imaging, 199–200
Nuclear medicine, 101–102
Nucleus pulposus
  anatomy, 27
  apoptosis, 536
  compressive loading of, 535
  degenerative processes, 536
  development of, 534–535
  function, 531
  nutritional environments, 28
Null hypothesis, 181–183
Nuremberg Code, 7

Nutritional status
 bone formation and, 14
 calcium levels, 190–191
 disk degeneration and, 536
 in female athletes, 129–130
 fracture healing and, 478
 medical history and, 192
 pediatric fractures and, 669
 postoperative infections and, 593
 preoperative assessments, 109
Nutritional supplements, 25

O

Obesity
 carpal tunnel syndrome and, 158–159
 osteoarthritis and, 228
 preoperative assessment, 107
Obesity hypoventilation syndrome, 107
Observational studies, 177, 178t
Occipital condyle fractures, 566
Occipitoatlantal dislocation, 692–693
Occipitoaxial instability, 781
Occipitocervical dislocations
 associated injuries, 566
 classification, 566
 mechanisms of injury, 566
 treatment, 566
Occupational Safety and Health Act, 157
Occupational Safety and Health
 Administration (OSHA), 157
Occupational therapy, 786
Odontoid fractures, 569–571
 in children, 692
 classification of, 570–571, 571f
 incidence, 569–570
 mechanisms of injury, 569
 treatment, 569–570
Odontoid hypoplasia, 775
O'Driscoll classification, 321, 322, 323f
Oestern and Tscherne classification, 474
Olecranon
 examination of, 279
 overhead traction, 662
Olecranon fractures, 326–328
 complications, 328
 Mayo classification, 326–328, 328f
 open reduction and fixation, 329f
 outcomes, 328, 329f
 pediatric patients, 664
 stress-type, 281
 treatment, 327–328
Olecranon osteotomy, 339
Olfactory ensheathing cells (OECs), 54
Oligomenorrhea, 130
Ollier's disease, 371, 798–799
Omega-e polyunsaturated fatty acids, 125
Omovertebral bar, 682
On-call physicians, 9
Oncology, musculoskeletal, 197–219. See
 also Specific cancers
Open-book injuries, 138
Open reduction of closed fractures with
 internal fixation
 clavicle fractures, 288
 glenoid neck fractures, 291
 Lisfranc's injuries, 487–488
 proximal humerus fractures, 294

surgical prophylaxis for, 242t
 in syndesmosis injuries, 494–495
Opioid receptors, classes of, 265
Opioids, 265, 268t
Ordinal data, description of, 180–181
Orthopaedic research, 173–187–13. See
 also Study design
 clinician-scientist in, 173
 funding for, 173–174
Orthopaedic Research and Education
 Foundation (OREF), 174
Orthopaedic Research Society, 173
Orthopaedic scientists, 173–174
Orthopaedic surgeons
 assessments of work-related injuries,
  158
 emergency department coverage by,
  8–10
Orthopaedic surgery
 blood management in, 149–152
  intraoperative, 151–152
  postoperative, 152
  preoperative, 150–151
 damage control, 141–142
 evidence-based practice guidelines, 169
 formal surgical care processes, 170t
 infections in, 241–257
 prophylaxis for, 242t
 quality in, 165–171
Orthopaedic Trauma Association (OTA),
 323–324, 325f, 402
Orthosis, selection of, 566
Ortolani maneuver, 717
Ortolani test, 715
Os odontoideum, 695
Osborne's ligament, 339
Osgood-Schlatter disease (OSD)
 in adolescents, 757, 763
 in athletes, 763
 presentation, 763
Osseous stabilization, 245
Ossification sequence, 673t
Osteoarthritis
 ankle, 512f
 antibiotic-impregnated beads, 245
 cartilage degeneration in, 24
 chondroitin sulfate in, 228–229
 description, 227
 disease-modifying drugs, 25–26
 distal interphalangeal joint, 94, 94f
 doxycycline for, 229
 elbow, 336
 erosive, 94, 94f
 exercise in, 228
 gait analysis and, 385
 genetic factors, 25
 glucosamine for, 228–229
 hand, 94f
 imaging of, 93–95
 initiation, 385
 knee, 228
 Knee Injury and Osteoarthritis Outcome
  Score, 457
 matrix metalloproteinases in, 229
 of metacarpophalangeal joints, 366
 obesity and, 228
 pain management, 227–228
 progression

gait analysis and, 385
 predictors of, 457
 prostaglandin E in, 228
 proximal interphalangeal joint, 94, 94f
 rifampin for, 245
 shoulder
  hemiarthroplasty, 315–316
  total arthroplasty, 315–316
 tetracyclines for, 229
 tobramycin for, 245
 topical products for, 229
 treatment, 25, 227–229
 trimethoprim-sulfamethoxazole for, 245
 vancomycin for, 245
 weight loss for, 228
Osteoblasts, function of, 190–191
Osteoblastogenesis, regulation of, 189t
Osteoblastomas
 description, 797–798
 imaging, 797
 presentation, 797
 spinal, 636t–637t, 642
Osteoblasts, function of, 189
Osteocalcin, in bone healing, 14
Osteocartilaginous exostosis, 798
Osteochondritis, 249
Osteochondritis dissecans (OCD)
 in athletes, 766–767
 capitellar, 281–282
 etiology, 766–767, 767f
 fixation, 767f
 talus, 767–768
Osteochondromas
 description, 798
 spinal, 636t–655.3t, 642, 642f
Osteochondromatosis, 684
Osteochondroplasty, 415–416
Osteochondrosis, 754
Osteoclasts, function, 14
Osteocytes, development of, 189
Osteofibrous dysplasia, 207, 207f, 799
Osteogenesis imperfecta (OI)
 description, 780
 fractures, 192, 780
 spinal fusion in, 780
 treatment, 780–781
Osteogenesis imperfecta tarda, 664
Osteogenic protein-1 (OP-1). See Bone
 morphogenetic proteins (BMPs), BMP-7
Osteogenic sarcomas, 638t–639t, 644
Osteoid osteomas
 description, 797
 imaging, 797, 797f
 radiofrequency coagulation, 97, 98f
 spinal, 636t–637t, 642
 treatment, 797
Osteolysis
 polyethylene components and, 83
Osteolysis, periprosthetic, 418
Osteomalacia
 causes of, 195
 drug-induced, 194t
Osteomyelitis
 adult, 243–246
 algorithm for, 244f
 chronic, 252t, 805
 chronic recurrent multifocal, 806
 classification of, 243

Index

Q

Quadriceps tendon rupture, 480
Quadrilateral space syndrome, 278
Quadriplegia, 49
Quality management, 165–171
Quasistatic tensile testing, 40, 41*f*

R

Race, work-related illnesses and, 160
Radial clubhand. *See* Radial longitudinal deficiency
Radial collateral ligament (RCL) sectioning, 333
Radial dysplasia. *See* Radial longitudinal deficiency
Radial fractures
  distal aspect
    displaced, 349*f*
    healing, 671*f*
    imaging, 347
    outcomes, 348–349
    pediatric patients, 671–673
    treatment, 348–349
  head
    classification, 319, 319*f*
    complications, 320
    imaging, 319
    treatment, 319–320, 320*f*
  metaphyseal, 672*f*
  neck, 664*f*
  proximal aspect, 665
  shaft, 670–671
Radial head
  congenital dislocation, 683
  dislocation, 683
  osteochondritis dissecans in, 760
Radial longitudinal deficiency, 683–684
Radial nerve
  compression of, 361
  iatrogenic injuries to, 345
  neuroma, 354*f*
Radiation-induced sarcomas, 203
Radicular plexopathy, 237
Radiculopathy
  C6, 575*f*
  cervical, 542–544
  lumbar disk herniation and, 553
Radiocapitellar plica, 282
Radiofrequency ablation, 797
Radiofrequency coagulation, 97
Radiography
  in adult scoliosis, 604
  in axial neck pain, 542
  axillary views, 89
  of calcaneus fractures, 503
  cervical spine injury evaluation, 565
  clavicle fractures, 287, 287*f*, 288*f*
  in diagnosis of infections, 243
  of distal tibial pilon fractures, 498*f*
  elbow imaging, 279
  in epidural abscesses, 599
  of femoral shaft fractures, 427
  of hand and wrist, 372
  of hip arthritis, 411–412
  lateral C-spine, 139
  of limb deformities, 741

  in limb-length discrepancy, 746
  in lumbar disk herniation, 552
  in lumbar spinal stenosis, 555
  of malignant bone tumors, 801
  Merchant views, 457
  musculoskeletal imaging, 89–90
  Neer trauma series, 293
  olecranon stress fracture, 281
  in osteomyelitis, 245
  of pelvis, 412*f*, 413*f*
  in polytrauma patients, 137
  in sagittal plane deformity, 611
  scapula fractures, 291
  serendipity view, 287, 290
  shoulder evaluation, 303
  of soft-tissue tumors, 803
  in spinal infections, 593, 595–596
  in spinal trauma, 691
  of spondylolisthesis, 619
  of spondylolysis, 617
  sunrise views, 457
  in thoracolumbar trauma, 580–581
  of three-dimensional motion, 379
  weight-bearing, 458*f*
Radioulnar synostosis, 683
Radius, distal aspect. *See also* Radial entries
  giant cell tumor, 372*f*
  normal alignment, 348*f*
Radotermin. *See* Growth and differentiation factor-5 (GDF-5)
Randomization, definition of, 177*t*
Raynaud's disease, phenomenon, 369
Reactive arthritis, 227
Recall biases, 175
Receptor activator of nuclear factor κB (RANKL), 190, 208
Recertification, process of, 4
RECQL4 gene mutations, 197
Rectus femoris, spasticity, 788
Reflex examination, 233
Regan-Morrey classification, 321, 322*f*
Regression models, 182
Regulatory Ethics Paradigm, 8
Rehabilitation
  gait training, 524
  for multidirectional instability, 275
  in work-related illnesses, 160
Reinfusion drains, blood, 152
Relocation test, shoulder instability, 274, 302, 302*f*
Renal failure, chronic, 107-108
Repetitive microtrauma, 274
Repetitive strain injury, 157
Repetitive trauma injury, 157
Research
  ethics, 7–8
  health outcomes research, 183–184
  study design, 175–177
Resection arthroplasty, 416
Residual limb pain, 523
Resistance training, 36–37
Resource-Based Relative Value Scale system, 9
Restriction, definition of, 177*t*
Retinoblastoma gene, 197
Revascularization
  bone grafts and, 15

  evaluation by MRI, 502
  fracture healing and, 13
Reverse Bennett's fractures, 346
Review of systems, 313
Rhabdomyosarcomas, 803–804
Rheo knee, 526
Rheumatoid arthritis (RA)
  antirheumatic drugs, 25
  cartilage degeneration in, 24
  cytokines in, 223*t*
  description, 221
  hindfoot dysfunction and, 514
  imaging of, 95
  of metacarpophalangeal joints, 366
  pathology, 221–222
  perioperative medications, 111–112
  shoulder, 95
  treatment, 221, 222*t*
Rheumatoid factor, 95*f*, 221
Ribs, common tumors of, 198*t*
Rickets
  causes of, 194*t*, 195
  fractures and, 192
Rifampin, 245
Ringer's solution, lactated, 137
Risk factors, determination of, 177
Risser stages, 697
Rituximab
  description of, 224–225
  dosage, 222*t*
  efficacy, 222*t*
  infusion reactions, 225
  mechanisms of action, 222*t*
  side effects, 222*t*
RMRP gene, 777
Rockwood classification, 307
Rofecoxib, withdrawal of, 228, 264
Rolando's fractures, 347, 347*f*
Ropivacaine, 266
Rotator cuff disease
  arthroscopic repair, 317
  pathogenesis, 276
  treatment, 276
Rotatory subluxation, 692
Rothmund-Thomson syndrome, 197
Round cell liposarcoma, 197*t*
Rowe scores, 306
Rubenstein-Taybi syndrome, 685
Ruedi and Allgower classification, 497
Russell-Taylor classification, 406

S

S-100 marker, 201
S-curve, description of, 242
SACH (solid ankle, cushion heel) prostheses, 525
Sacral nuclei, 49
Sacral slope, normal values, 621*f*, 621*t*
Sacrum, common tumors of, 198*t*
Sagittal balance, 610, 610*f*
Sagittal plane deformity
  in adult scoliosis, 608–614
    causes, 609*t*
    classification, 609
    clinical history, 610–611
    disease burden of, 610
    etiology, 609

Index

medial, 443
radiographic evaluation, 441, 441f
treatment
nonsurgical, 441–442
surgical, 442, 442f
Tibialis tendon dysfunction, 380
Tibiofemoral joint dislocations, 445
Tibiofibular ligament, imaging of, 494
Tile classification, 389, 392–393
Tillaux fractures, 734
TIMP-1 gene, 28
Tinel's sign, 359
Tissue banks, tissue from, 16
Tissue donors, screening of, 16–17
Tissue engineering, 26–27, 43
Tissue factor, coagulation cascade and, 145
Tissue inhibitors of matrix
metalloproteinases (TIMPs), 28
Tobacco use, fracture healing and, 478
Tobramycin, 245
Topical products, for osteoarthritis, 229
Torque, effects of, 75
Torsional loads, 74–75
Torticollis
painful, 692
Sprengel's deformity and, 682
Torus fractures, 671
Total ankle arthroplasty, 512–513, 513f
failed, 513
Total disk replacement, artificial, 559
Total hip arthroplasty (THA)
complications, 419–421
dislocations, 420
infections, 420
limb-length discrepancy, 420
mortality rates, 419
neurovascular injury, 419–420
displaced femoral neck fractures, 404
failure, periprosthetic osteolysis and, 418
minimally invasive, 417
primary, 416–417
acetabular components, 416–417
bearing options in, 417
femoral components, 416–417
large femoral heads, 417
total hip resurfacing, 417
revision, 417–418
thromboembolic disease after, 148
Total hip replacement (THR)
bearing materials
ceramic, 81–82
cross-linked polyethylene, 82–84
metal-on-metal, 79–80
wear-in phase, 79
Total joint arthroplasty
infection management, 467
salvage, 467
two-stage reimplantation, 467
perioperative antibiotics, 110
surgical prophylaxis for, 242t
thrombus formation and, 146
Total knee arthroplasty (TKA)
arthrodesis, 254
complications
arthrofibrosis, 465
extensor mechanism failure, 464–465

infections, 464
MCL injury, 464
periprosthetic fractures, 465
stiffness, 465
thromboembolic disease, 464
computer navigation, 464
design issues
high-flexion designs, 463
mobile-bearing devices, 463
modularity, 463
failure, wear and, 467f
infected, salvage of, 467
outcomes, disease variables, 459–460
pain management, 464
patellar resurfacing, 463–464
polyethylene liners, 463f
reference lines, 461f
revision
bone loss management, 466
component removal, 466
component retention, 466
fixation, 466
pain evaluation, 465–466
patellar management, 466–467
preoperative planning, 466
surgical technique
alignment, 461
approaches, 460
constraint, 462–463
fixation, 461
soft-tissue balancing, 461–462
thromboembolic disease after, 148
Total knee replacement
bearing materials, 84–85
bilateral, 384
Total shoulder arthroplasty
hemiarthroplasty *versus*, 315–316
Total surface-bearing (TSB) sockets, 524
Traction, overhead olecranon, 662
Tramadol hydrochloride, 265
Trampolines, forearm fractures and, 669
Tranexamic acid, 151–152
Transcutaneous electrical nerve stimulation (TENS), 268t, 269
Transforaminal lumbar interbody fusion (TLIF), 559
Transforming growth factor-β
bone healing and, 16
disk degeneration and, 28
in muscle healing, 38
in muscle injury, 39f
Transforming growth factor-β1, 40
Transforming growth factor-β-inducible early gene-1, 41
Transfusion reactions, nonhemolytic, 152
Transfusions
allergic reactions to, 108
allogenic, 152
autogenous blood donation, 108
autologous donation, 150–151
blood substitutes, 8
complications, 150–152
Creutzfeldt-Jakob disease transmission, 149
donor-directed donations, 151
indications for, 108–109, 152
preoperative evaluation, 150
Transglenoid drilling, 304

Transitional cell carcinoma of the bladder, 215
Transphyseal fractures, 663f
Transplantation, neuronal, 54
Transverse fractures, 709
Trapeziometacarpal arthritis, 249
Trauma. *See also* Polytrauma patients
axial skeleton, 90–91
cervical spine injuries, 565–578
cumulative, 157–164
responses to, 261f
risk of infection and, 241
to shoulder joints, 287–299
thoracolumbar, 579–591
Trauma centers, 9
Trauma scores, 140
Traumatic spondylolisthesis, 568–569, 568f
Trendelenburg gait, 719, 741
Trendelenburg sign, 380, 411
Treponema pallidum, 597
Triangular fibrocartilage complex (TFCC) injuries
anatomy, 350f
classification, 349–350
DRUJ stability and, 349
repair, 349–350
Tricortical bone grafting, 307
Tricyclic antidepressants (TCA)
in fibromyalgia, 229
pain management using, 268–269
Trigger digits, congenital, 686–687
Trigger points, axial neck pain and, 541
Trimalleolar fractures, 496
Trimethoprim, 146
Trimethoprim-sulfamethoxazole, 129, 245
Triplane fractures, 734, 736f
Trisomy 21, 685, 781
Tuberculin purified protein derivative (PPD) skin test, 598
Tuberculosis screening, 227, 805–806
Tuft fractures, phalangeal, 343, 675
Tumor biology, 197
Tumor necrosis factor-α
antibodies to, 553
disk degeneration and, 28
drugs targeting, 223t
secretion of, 221–222
Tumor necrosis factor-α antagonists, 222–224, 222t, 226–227
Tumors. *See also Specific* tumors
benign pediatric, 797–800
bone matrix patterns, 200f
commonly seen, 198t
growth patterns, histologic, 201t
malignant pediatric, 801–803
margins of, 198, 199f
radiographs of, 198
soft-tissue, 209–212, 803–804
spinal, 635–647
presentation, 635
staging system, 641f
translocations in, 197t
Tunnel view, knee, 90
Tunneled sural island pedicle flaps, 477
Turner's syndrome, 781, 790
"Two-hit" hypothesis, 141
Two-point discrimination test, 357